Treatment of the Postmenopausal Woman

Basic and Clinical Aspects

SECOND EDITION

Treatment of the Postmenopausal Woman

Basic and Clinical Aspects

SECOND EDITION

EDITOR

Rogerio A. Lobo, M.D.

Department of Obstetrics and Gynecology
Columbia University
College of Physicians & Surgeons
New York, New York

LIPPINCOTT WILLIAMS & WILKINS
A **Wolters Kluwer** Company
Philadelphia · Baltimore · New York · London
Buenos Aires · Hong Kong · Sydney · Tokyo

Acquisitions Editor: Lisa McAllister
Managing Editor: Susan Rhyner
Production Editor: C.J. Goldsbury
Manufacturing Manager: Dennis Teston
Cover Designer: Patricia Gast
Compositor: Lippincott Williams & Wilkins Desktop Division
Printer: Courier Westford

© 1999 by LIPPINCOTT WILLIAMS & WILKINS
227 East Washington Square
Philadelphia, PA 19106-3780 USA
LWW.com

Library of Congress Cataloging-in-Publication Data

Treatment of the postmenopausal woman : basic and clinical aspects /
    editor, Rogerio A. Lobo.—2nd ed.
       p. cm.
    Includes bibliographical references and index.
    ISBN 0-7817-1559-8
    1. Menopause— Complications.   2. Menopause—Hormone therapy.
I. Lobo, Rogerio A.
    [DNLM: 1. Climacteric—physiology.   2. Estrogen Replacement
Therapy.   3. Women's Health.   WP 580 T784 1999]
RG186.T73   1999
618.1′75—dc21
DNLM/DLC
For Library of Congress   99-34504
                                     CIP

10 9 8 7 6 5 4 3 2 1

Contents

Contributing Authors

Michael R. Adams, D.V.M.
Professor
Department of Pathology/Comparative Medicine
Wake Forest University School of Medicine
Medical Center Boulevard
Winston-Salem, NC 27157

Mary S. Anthony, M.S.
Research Associate
Department of Pathology
Wake Forest University School of Medicine
Medical Center Boulevard
Winston-Salem, NC 27157

David Archer, M.D.
Professor
Department of Obstetrics and Gynecology
Eastern Virginia Medical School
601 Colley Avenue
Norfolk, VA 23507

Cecilia A. Artacho, M.S.
Department of Obstetrics and Gynecology
Columbia University College of Physicians &
*   Surgeons*
622 West 168 Street
New York, NY 10032

Gloria A. Bachmann, M.D.
Professor & Chief
Department of Obstetrics, Gynecology, and
*   Reproductive Sciences;*
Chief of OB/GYN Service
Department of Obstetrics & Gynecology
University of Medicine & Dentistry of
*   New Jersey*
Robert Wood Johnson Medical School
Clinical Academic Building
125 Paterson St.
New Brunswick, NJ 08901

Randall B. Barnes, M.D.
Associate Professor
Department of Obstetrics and Gynecology
University of Chicago
5841 South Maryland Avenue
Chicago, IL 60637

Leslie Bernstein, Ph.D.
Professor
Department of Preventive Medicine
University of Southern California School of
*   Medicine*
1442 Eastlake Avenue, MS-44
Los Angeles, CA 90089

Mark P. Brincat, Ph.D. (Lond.), F.R.C.O.G.
Director
Department of Obstetrics and
*   Gynaecology*
St. Luke's Hospital;
Dean, Faculty of Medicine & Surgery
University of Malta Medical School
MSIDA MSD 07 Malta;

Helen M. Buckler, D.M., F.R.C.P.
Consultant Physician & Endocrinologist
Department of Endocrinology
Salford Royal NHS Trust
Salford, Manchester, M68 HD
England, United Kingdom

Irina D. Burd, B.A.
Department of Obstetrics & Gynecology
University of Medicine & Dentistry of
*   New Jersey*
Robert Wood Johnson Medical School
Clinical Academic Building
125 Paterson St.
New Brunswick, NJ 08901

Henry Burger, M.D., F.R.A.C.P.
Professor
Department of Endocrinology
Prince Henry's Institute of Medical
*   Research*
Monash Medical Center
Monash University
246 Clayton Road
Clayton, Melbourne 3168
Victoria, Australia

John Buster, M.D.
Professor
Department of Obstetrics and Gynecology;
Director, Division of Reproductive
   Endocrinology and Infertility
Baylor College of Medicine
6550 Fannin, Suite 801
Houston, TX 77030

Peter R. Casson, M.D.
Associate Professor
Department of Obstetrics and Gynecology
University of Ottawa
Civic Parkdale Clinic
737 Parkdale Ave., Suite 510
Ottawa, Ontario, Canada K1Y 1J8

Vito Cela, M.D.
Department of Reproductive Medicine and
   Child Development
Division of Obstetrics and Gynecology
University of Pisa
Via Roma 67
Pisa, Italy 56123

Judi Lee Chervenak, M.D.
Assistant Professor
Department of Obstetrics, Gynecology
   & Women's Health
Albert Einstein College of Medicine
1300 Morris Park Avenue, Room 316
The Bronx, NY 10461

Claus Christiansen, M.D.
Scientific Consultant
Center for Clinical and Basic Research
222 Ballerup Byvej
Ballerup, DK-2750
Denmark

Thomas B. Clarkson, D.V.M.
Professor
Department of Comparative Medicine
Wake Forest University School of Medicine
Medical Center Boulevard
Winston-Salem, NC 27157-1040

J. Mark Cline, D.V.M., Ph.D.
Associate Professor
Department of Pathology, Section on
   Comparative Medicine
Wake Forest University School of Medicine
Medical Center Boulevard
Winston-Salem, NC 27157-1040

John A. Collins, M.D.
Professor
Department of Obstetrics and Gynecology
McMaster University;
Active Staff
Department of Obstetrics and Gynecology
Hamilton Health Sciences Corporation
1200 Main Street West, 3N52
Hamilton, Ontario, Canada L8N 3Z5

Peter Collins, M.D., F.R.C.P.
Honorary Consultant Cardiologist
Department of Cardiac Medicine
Royal Brompton Hospital;
Reader
Department of Cardiac Medicine
National Heart & Lung Institute
Imperial College School of Medicine
Dovehouse Street
London, SW3 6LY
England, United Kingdom

Felicia Cosman, M.D.
Associate Professor of Clinical Medicine
Department of Medicine
Columbia University College of Physicians
   & Surgeons
New York, NY;
Osteoporosis Specialist /Endocrinologist
Department of Medicine
Helen Hayes Hospital
Route 9W
West Haverstraw, NY 10993

Eileen DeMarco, M.D.
Assistant Clinical Professor
Department of Obstetrics and Gynecology
Columbia-Presbyterian Medical Center;
Department of Obstetrics and Gynecology
Columbia University College of Physicians
   & Surgeons
622 West 168 Street
New York, NY 10032

M. Dören
Department of Obstetrics and Gynecology
Wesstfalische Wilhelms-Universitat
Munster, Germany

Richard Eastell, M.D., F.R.C.P.
Professor
Bone Metabolism Group
University of Sheffield
Northern General Hospsital
Sheffield, S5 7AU
England, United Kingdom

Gary A. Ebert, M.D.
Instructor
Department of Obstetrics, Gynecology, and
  Reproductive Sciences
University of Medicine & Dentistry of New Jersey
Robert Wood Johnson Medical School
125 Paterson St.
New Brunswick, NJ 08901-1977

Ian S. Fraser, M.D., F.R.A.N.Z.C.O.G.
Visiting Medical Officer
Department of Reproductive Endocrinology and
  Infertility
King George V Hospital;
Professor of Reproductive Medicine
Department of Obstetrics and Gynecology
University of Sydney
Sydney, New South Wales 2006
Australia

Adriane Fugh-Berman
Assistant Clinical Professor
Department of Health Care Sciences
George Washington University School of
  Medicine
2150 Pennsylvania Avenue, #2B417
Washington, D.C. 20037

Ray Galea, M.D., M.R.C.O.G.
Senior Registrar
Department of Obstetrics and Gynecology
St. Luke's Hospital
Gwardamangia, Malta

Harry K. Genant, M.D.
Professor of Radiology, Medicine,
  Epidemiology, and Orthopedic Surgery
Department of Radiology
University of California, San Francisco
San Francisco, CA 94143-0628

Ian Godsland, Ph.D.
Senior Lecturer
Wynn Institute for Metabolic Research
21 Wellington Road
St. John's Wood
London NW8 9SQ
England, United Kingdom

George Gorodeski, M.D., Ph.D.
Associate Professor
Departments of Reproductive
  Biology/Physiology/Biophysics
Case Western Reserve University School of
  Medicine;
Department of Obstetrics and Gynecology
University MacDonald Women's Hospital,
  University Hospitals of Clevelend
11100 Euclid Avenue
Cleveland, OH 44106

Francine Grodstein, Sc.D.
Assistant Professor
Department of Medicine
Brigham & Women's Hospital, Harvard
  Medical School
181 Longwood Avenue
Boston, MA 02115

Rosemary A. Hannon, Ph.D.
Research Associate
Bone Metabolism Group
University of Sheffield
Northern General Hospital
Sheffield, S5 7AU
England, United Kingdom

Victor W. Henderson, M.D., M.S.
Volk Professor of Neurology
Professor of Gerontology/Psychology
University of Southern California School of
  Medicine
1420 San Pablo Street (PMB-B105)
Los Angeles, CA 90089

William H. Hindle, M.D.
Professor
Department of Clinical Obstetrics and
  Gynecology
University of Southern California School
  of Medicine;
Director, Women's and Children's
  Hospital
LAC/USC Medical Center
1240 North Mission Road, Room L-1022
Los Angeles, CA 90033

Andrew R. Hoffman, M.D.
Geriatrics Research, Education, and
  Clinical Center
Medical Service, Department of Veterans
  Affairs
Palo Alto Health Care System;
Division of Endocrinology,Gerontology &
  Metabolism
Department of Medicine
Stanford University
Stanford, CA 94305

Christian Holinka, Ph.D.
President
PharmConsult
140 Seventh Avenue, Suite 7A
New York, NY 10014

Diane M. Jacobs, Ph.D.
Assistant Professional Neuropsychologist
Department of Neurology
Columbia-Presbyterian Medical Center;
Assistant Professor of Clinical Neuropsychology
Department of Neurology and the
  Gertrude H. Sergievsky Center
Columbia University College of Physicians and
  Surgeons
630 West 168 Street
New York, NY 10032

Richard Jaffe, M.D.
Associate Professor
Division of Obstetric and Gynecological
  Ultrasound
Department of Obstetrics and Gynecology
Sloane Hospital for Women
Columbia-Presbyterian Medical Center
622 West 168 Street
New York, NY 10032

C. Conrad Johnston, Jr., M.D.
Distinguished Professor
Department of Medicine/Endocrinology
Indiana University School of Medicine
545 N. Barnhill Drive, Emerson Hall 421
Indianapolis, IN 46202

Jennifer Kelsey, Ph.D.
Professor
Division of Epidemiology
Stanford University School of Medicine
Department of Health, Research & Policy
Stanford, CA 94305-5092

Ronald M. Krauss, M.D.
Senior Scientist and Head
Department of Molecular Medicine
Lawrence Berkeley National Laboratory
University of California
Donner Laboratory, Room 459
Berkeley, CA 94720

Fredi Kronenberg, Ph.D.
Associate Professor
Department of Rehabilitation Medicine
Columbia University College of Physicians
  & Surgeons
630 West 168 Street, Box 75
New York, NY 10032

Seth G. Levrant, M.D.
Partners in Reproductive Health
16345 South Harlem Ave., Suite 1W
Tinley Park, IL 60477

Robert Lindsay, M.B.Ch.B., Ph.D., F.R.C.P.
Professor of Clinical Medicine
Department of Medicine
Columbia University College of Physicians
  & Surgeons
New York, NY;
Chief of Internal Medicine
Helen Hayes Hospital
Route 9W
West Haverstraw, NY 10993

Rogerio A. Lobo, M.D.
Willard C. Rappleye Professor of OB/GYN
Chairman, Department of Obstetrics and
  Gynecology
Columbia University College of Physicians
  & Surgeons;
Director, Sloane Hospital for Women
Columbia-Presbyterian Medical Center
622 West 168 Street, 16th floor
New York, NY 10032

Jorge L. Londono, M.D.
Department of Obstetrics and Gynecology
University of South Florida
4 Columbia Drive
Tampa, FL 33606

Christopher Longcope, M.D.
Professor
Department of Obstetrics and Gynecology
University of Massachusetts Medical School;
Attending Physician
Division of Endocrinology
University of Massachusetts Memorial Health
  Care
University Campus
55 Lake Avenue North, S4-721
Worcester, MA 01655-0321

Neil J. MacLusky, Ph.D.
Professor of Reproductive Science in OB/GYN
Department of Obstetrics and Gynecology
Center for Reproductive Sciences
Columbia University College of Physicians
  & Surgeons
622 West 168 Street
New York, NY 10032

Robert Marcus, M.D.
Professor of Medicine
Stanford University School of Medicine;
Director, Aging Study Unit
Veteran Affairs Medical Center
3801 Miranda Avenue
Palo Alto, CA 94304

Lars-Åke Mattson, M.D., Ph.D.
Department of Obstetrics and Gynecology
Sahlgrens University East
S-41685 Göteburg, Sweden

Richard Mayeux, M.D., M.S.
Professor
Gertrude H. Sergievsky Center
Taub Center for Alzheimer Disease Research
Departments of Neurology and Psychiatry
Columbia-Presbyterian Medical Center
19th Floor, Room 312A
622 West 168 Street
New York, NY 10032

Frederick Naftolin, M.D., D.Phil.
Chief, Department of Obstetrics and
    Gynecology
Yale/New Haven Hospital;
Professor and Chairman
Department of Obstetrics and Gynecology
Yale University School of Medicine
333 Cedar Street, 335 FMB
New Haven, CT 06515

Morris Notelovitz, M.D., Ph.D.
Consultant
Women's Medical & Diagnostic Center
The Climacteric Clinic, Inc.
222 S.W. 36th Terrace, Suite 1C
Gainesville, FL 32607

Annlia Paganini-Hill, Ph.D.
Professor
Department of Preventive Medicine
University of Southern California School
    of Medicine
1721 Griffin Avenue, Room 205E
Los Angeles, CA 90089-9680

Jinha M. Park, B.A.
Department of Pathology
University of Southern California School
    of Medicine
Norris Comprehensive Cancer Center
1441 Eastlake Avenue
Los Angeles, CA 90089

John J. Park, B.A.
Department of Pathology
University of Southern California School
    of Medicine
Norris Comprehensive Cancer Center
1441 Eastlake Avenue
Los Angeles, CA 90089

Anna K. Parsons, M.D.
Associate Professor
Director, Image-based Gynecology Clinic
Attending Staff
Department of Obstetrics and Gynecology
Tampa General Hospital;
Department of Obstetrics and Gynecology
University of South Florida
4 Columbia Drive, Room 529
Tampa, FL 33606

Nancy A. Phillips, M.D., F.A.C.O.G.
Consultant
Department of Obstetrics and Gynecology
Wellington Hospital, Capital Coast Health Ltd.;
Senior Lecturer
Department of Obstetrics and Gynecology
University of Otago
P.O.B. 7343
Wellington, New Zealand

James H. Pickar, M.D.
Vice President
Women's Health Research
Wyeth-Ayerst Research
145 King of Prussia Rd.
Radnor PA 19087

Malcolm C. Pike, Ph.D.
Professor and Flora L. Thornton Chair
Department of Preventative Medicine
University of Southern California School of
    Medicine
Norris Comprehensive Cancer Center
1441 Eastlake Avenue
Los Angeles, CA 90089

Michael Press, M.D., Ph.D.
Professor
Department of Pathology
University of Southern California School of
    Medicine
Norris Comprehensive Cancer Center
1441 Eastlake Avenue, Room 5409
Los Angeles, CA 90089

Thomas C. Randall, M.D.
Assistant Professor
Division of Gynecologic Oncology
Department of Obstetrics and Gynecology
University of Pennsylvania Health System;
Department of Obstetrics and Gynecology
University of Pennsylvania
3400 Spruce Street
Philadelphia, PA 19104

Veronica Ravnikar, M.D.
Professor
Department of Obstetrics and Gynecology
University of Massachusetts Memorial
  Health Center
UMASS Campus
55 Lake Avenue North, S4-717
Worcester, MA 01655

Robert W. Rebar, M.D.
Chief, Department of Obstetrics and Gynecology
University Hospital;
Professor and Director
Department of Obstetrics and Gynecology
University of Cincinnati Medical Center
231 Bethesda Avenue
Cincinnati, OH 45267-0526

Catherine A. Roca, M.D.
Senior Staff Fellow
Behavioral Endocrinology Branch
National Institute of Mental Health
10 Center Drive
Bethesda, MD 20892

Raymond C. Rosen, Ph.D.
Professor
Department of Psychiatry;
Co-Director, Center for Sexual & Marital Health
University of Medicine & Dentistry of New Jersey
Robert Wood Johnson Medical School
675 Hoes Lane
Piscataway, NJ 08854

Ronald K. Ross, MD
Professor & Chairman
Department of Preventive Medicine
University of Southern California School of
  Medicine
1442 Eastlake Avenue, Room 8302B
Los Angeles, CA 90089-9181

Stephen C. Rubin, M.D.
Professor
Department of Obstetrics and Gynecology
University of Pennsylvania;
Chief, Division of Gynecologic Oncology
University of Pennsylvania Health System
3400 Spruce Street
Philadelphia, PA 19104

David Rubinow, M.D.
Clinical Director & Chief
Behavioral Endocrinology Branch
National Institute of Mental Health
10 Center Drive, MSC 1276
Bethesda, MD 20892

Göran N. Samsioe, M.D., Ph.D.
Professor
Department of Obstetrics and Gynecology
Lund University;
Senior Consultant
Department of Obstetrics and Gynecology
Lund University Hospital
SE-221 85 Lund, Sweden

Mary Sano, Ph.D.
Associate Professor
Gertrude H. Sergievsky Center
Taub Center for Alzheimer Disease Research
Department of Neurology
Columbia-Presbyterian Medical Center
19th Floor, Room 312A
622 West 168 Street
New York, NY 10032

Nanette F. Santoro, M.D.
Professor
Department of Obstetrics, Gynecology &
  Women's Health;
Director, Division of Reproductive
  Endocrinology & Infertility
Albert Einstein College of Medicine
1300 Morris Park Avenue, Room 316
The Bronx, NY 10461

Mark V. Sauer, M.D.
Professor
Department of Obstetrics and Gynecology
Columbia University College of Physicians &
  Surgeons;
Chief, Division of Reproductive Endocrinology
Columbia-Presbyterian Medical Center
622 West 168 Street, PH16-28
New York, NY 10032

Isaac Schiff, M.D.
Joe V. Meigs Professor of Gynecology
Department of Obstetrics and Gynecology
Harvard Medical School;
Chief, Vincent Memorial OB/GYN Service
Department of Obstetrics and Gynecology
Massachusetts General Hospital
55 Fruit Street, VBK 113
Boston, MA 02114

James J. Schlesselman, Ph.D.
Professor
Department of Epidemiology & Public Health
University of Miami School of Medicine;
Chief, Division of Biostatistics
Sylvester Comprehensive Cancer Center
1550 NW 10th Avenue
Miami, FL 33136

Peter J. Schmidt, M.D.
Chief, Unit on Reproductive Endocrine Studies
Behavioral Endocrinology Branch
National Institute of Mental Health/
*   National Institute of Health*
10 Center Drive
Bethesda, MD 20892-1276

Barbara B. Sherwin, Ph.D.
Co-Director, Menopause Clinic
McGill Center for Reproduction
Royal Victoria Hospital;
Professor
Departments of Psychology/Obstetrics
*   and Gynecology*
McGill University
1205 Dr. Penfield Avenue
Montreal, Quebec
Canada, H3A 1B1

Donna Shoupe, M.D.
Professor
Department of Obstetrics and Gynecology
University of Southern California School
*   of Medicine*
1240 North Mission Road, L946
Los Angeles, CA 90033

Charles W. Slemenda
Department of Medicine
Indiana University School of Medicine
545 N. Barnhill Drive
Indianpolis IN 46202

Leon Speroff, M.D.
Professor
Department of Obstetrics and Gynecology
Oregon Health Sciences University
3181 SW Sam Jackson Park Road (UHN70)
Portland, OR 97201-3098

Darcy V. Spicer, M.D.
Associate Professor
Department of Medicine
University of Southern California
*   School of Medicine*
Norris Comprehensive Cancer Center
1441 Eastlake Avenue
Los Angeles, CA 90089

Meir J. Stampfer, M.D., Dr. P.H.
Physician
Department of Medicine
Brigham and Women's Hospital;
Professor
Department of Epidemiology and Nutrition
Harvard School of Public Health
181 Longwood Avenue
Boston, MA 02115

Frank Z. Stanczyk, Ph.D.
Professor of Research
Department of Obstetrics and Gynecology
University of Southern California School
*   of Medicine;*
Director, Reproductive Endocrine Research
*   Laboratory*
Women's & Children's Hospital,
*   Room 1M2*
1240 North Mission Road
Los Angeles, CA 90033

Julie Anne Stein, M.D.
Clinical Instructor
Department of Obstetrics and Gynecology
University of Michigan
1500 East Medical Center Drive,
*   L4000 Women's*
Ann Arbor, MI 48109

Jay M. Sullivan, M.D. (Deceased)
Former Professor of Medicine
Chief, Division of Cardiovascular
*   Diseases*
Bowld Hospital
University of Tennessee, Memphis
951 Court Avenue, Room 353D
Memphis, TN 38163

Helena J. Teede, M.B.B.S.
NH & MRC Research Fellow
Staff Endocrinologist
Department of Medicine
Monash Medical Center
Monash University
Clayton, Melbourne 3168
Victoria, Australia

Anna N.A. Tosteson, Sc.D.
Associate Professor
Departments of Medicine/Community and
*   Family Medicine*
Dartmouth Medical School
One Medical Center Drive, HB 7505
Lebanon, NH 03756

Wulf H. Utian, M.B.B.Ch., Ph.D.
Director, Department of Obstetrics and
*   Gynecology*
University MacDonald Women's
*   Hospital, University Hospitals of*
*   Cleveland;*
Professor
Department of Reproductive Biology
Case Western Reserve University
11100 Euclid Avenue
Cleveland, OH 44106

Cornelis van Kuijk, M.D., Ph.D.
University of Amsterdam
Department of Radiology
Academic Medical Center
Meibergdreef 9
1105 AZ Amsterdam
The Netherlands

Michelle P. Warren, M.D.
Wyeth Professor of Women's Health
Departments of Obstetrics and
  Gynecology/Medicine
Columbia University College of Physicians
  & Surgeons;
Medical Director
Center for Menopause, Hormonal Disorders
  & Women's Health
Columbia-Presbyterian Medical
  Center
16 E 60 Street , Suite 490
New York, NY 10022

Milton C. Weinstein, Ph.D.
Henry J. Kaiser Professor of Health Policy and
  Management
Center for Risk Analysis
Harvard School of Public Health
718 Huntington Avenue
Boston, MA 02115

Scott A. Washburn, M.D,
Active Staff
Department of Obstetrics and Gynecology
Forsyth Medical Center;
Clinical Assistant Professor
Departments of Obstetrics & Gynecology,
  and Pathology
Wake Forest University Baptist Medical Center
Medical Center Boulevard
Winston-Salem, NC 27157

Janice D. Wagner, D.V.M., Ph.D.
Associate Professor
Department of Pathology/Comparative Medicine
Wake Forest University School of Medicine
Medical Center Boulevard
Winston-Salem, NC 27157

J. Koudy Williams, D.V.M.
Department of Comparative Medicine
Wake Forest University School of Medicine
Medical Center Boulevard
Winston-Salem, NC 27157

Ralf C. Zimmermann, M.D.
Assistant Professor
Departments of Obstetrics and
  Gynecology/Psychiatry
Columbia University College of Physicians
  & Surgeons
630 West 168 Street
New York, NY 10032

Acknowledgements

Once again I owe my friends greatly for contributing to this edition: for many authors of the first edition extensive revisions have been made. I am also indebted to the new contributors who were sought out because of their expertise in the field.

This project could not have been completed without the tireless help of my office and Reba Nosoff in particular. Most of all I wish to acknowledge the support and patience of my family, Jessie, Maggie, and Ross.

Preface to the First Edition

This book provides an overview of the major issues affecting perimenopausal and postmenopausal women and offers various options for treatment. For the perimenopausal or early postmenopausal woman, the book also discusses the options that women now have to bear children, if they so desire. The primary emphasis, however, will be on the nonreproductive issues affecting postmenopausal women. As menopause merely refers to the cessation of menses, I view the term menopausal to be too imprecise and therefore prefer to use the term postmenopausal, which will appear throughout this book.

One-third of a woman's life is spent in the estrogen-deficient, postmenopausal state. It has been estimated that, by the year 2000, there will be 35 million women over age 65 and 5 million over age 85, increasing by the year 2040 to approximately 65 million women over 65 and 10 million over 85! Less than 20% of women over 65 are neither receiving hormonal therapy nor any other non-hormonal modalities to prevent and/or treat osteoporosis and cardiovascular disease.

A woman at age 50 with no unusual risk factors has a life expectancy of 82.8 years. Her lifetime risk of developing cardiovascular disease is 46.1% and of dying of it is 31%. For stroke, these figures are 19.8% and 8%. For hip fracture, the risk of its occurrence is 15.3% and 1.5% for death as a sequelum. There is a 10.2% lifetime risk of developing breast cancer and a 3% probability of dying of it. For women with a uterus, there is a 2.6% lifetime risk of developing endometrial cancer and only a 0.3% chance of dying from it. These major health issues will be discussed in detail as will non-threatening issues such as hot flashes, vulvovaginal complaints, psychological well-being and life-style considerations. Hormonal therapy not only assists in the prevention of the diseases just mentioned, but also increases the quality of life and life expectancy.

The book covers the basic as well as the clinical aspects of treatment and care for the postmenopausal woman. It is intended to be useful for all students of the field. Each section begins with an overview that provides the reader with highlights and occasionally points out limitations.

I hope the reader will enjoy this book. It will provide a basis and rationale for strategies that can result in better health care for the mature woman, a growing segment of the U.S. population and the world.

Rogerio A. Lobo, M.D.

Preface to the Second Edition

This second edition of *Treatment of The Postmenopausal Woman* has been expanded. Chapters have been added as the field has broadened and at the suggestion of readers of the first edition.

As women's health issues have achieved greater prominence in our society, and as a larger segment of the population enters menopause, a firm foundation in options for the treatment of postmenopausal women seems more important than ever. The intent here is to provide concise, clear, and up to date information of a basic and clinical nature on issues facing postmenopausal women. It is my hope that this book will be helpful to practitioners from many disciplines, as well as to researchers in the field.

Each section of the book begins with an introduction which helps to summarize the key issues discussed therein, and also offers a personal perspective and update if appropriate. I hope the reader enjoys the book, and that it will be helpful in providing the best quality of care to the health of women.

Rogerio A. Lobo, M.D.

Treatment of the Postmenopausal Woman: Basic and Clinical Aspects, Second Edition, edited by Rogerio A. Lobo, Lippincott Williams & Wilkins, Philadelphia © 1999.

CHAPTER 1

The Menopause: A Signal for the Future

Leon Speroff

Throughout recorded history, multiple physical and mental conditions have been attributed to the menopause. Although medical writers often wrote colorfully in the past, they were also less than accurate, unencumbered by scientific information and data. A good example of the stereotypical, inaccurate thinking promulgated over the years is the following passage, which was written in 1887 (1).

> The ovaries, after long years of service, have not the ability of retiring in graceful old age, but become irritated, transmit their irritation to the abdominal ganglia, which in turn transmit the irritation to the brain, producing disturbances in the cerebral tissue exhibiting themselves in extreme nervousness or in an outburst of actual insanity.

The belief that behavioral disturbances are related to manifestations of the female reproductive system is an ancient one that has persisted in contemporary times. This belief regarding menopause is not totally illogical; there is reason to associate the middle years of life with negative experiences. The events that come to mind are impressive: onset of a major illness or disability (even death) in a spouse, relative, or friend; retirement from employment; financial insecurity; the need to provide care for very old parents and relatives; and separation from children. It is therefore not surprising that a middle-age event, the menopause, shares in this negative outlook.

The scientific study of all aspects of menstruation has been hampered by the overpowering influence of social and cultural beliefs and traditions. Problems arising from life events have often been erroneously attributed to the menopause. However, data, especially more reliable community-based longitudinal data, have established that the increase of most symptoms and problems in middle-aged women reflects social and personal circumstances, not the endocrine events of the menopause (2–8).

The Massachusetts Women's Health Study, a large and comprehensive prospective, longitudinal study of middle-aged women, provides a powerful argument that menopause is not and should not be viewed as a negative experience by most women (3,9). The cessation of menses was perceived by these women (as by the women in other longitudinal studies) to have almost no impact on subsequent physical and mental health. Most women expressed positive or neutral feelings about menopause. An exception was the group of women who experienced surgical menopause, but the reasons for the surgical procedure usually were more important than the cessation of menses.

Alterations in menstrual function are not symbols of some ominous "change." There are good physiologic reasons for changing menstrual function, and understanding the physiology can do much to reinforce a healthy, normal attitude. Attitude and expectations about menopause are important. Women who have been high users of health services and who expect to have difficulty do experience greater symptoms and higher levels of depression (4,9). The symptoms that women report are related to many variables within their lives, and the hormonal change at menopause cannot be held responsible for the common psychosocial and lifestyle problems we all experience. It is time to stress the normalcy of this physiologic event. Menopausal women do not suffer from a "hormone deficiency disease," and postmenopausal hormone therapy should be viewed as specific treatment for symptoms in the short term and preventive pharmacology in the long term.

It can be further argued that physicians have had a biased negative point of view because most women who are healthy and happy do not seek contact with physicians (10,11). Clinicians must be familiar with the facts about menopause and have an appropriate attitude and philosophy regarding this period of life. Medical intervention at this point of life should be regarded as an opportunity to provide and reinforce a program of preventive health care. The issues of preventive health care for women are

L. Speroff: Department of Obstetrics and Gynecology, Oregon Health Sciences University, Portland, Oregon 97201.

familiar ones. They include family planning, cessation of smoking, control of body weight and alcohol consumption, prevention of cardiovascular disease and osteoporosis, maintenance of mental well-being (including sexuality), cancer screening, and treatment of urologic problems.

AGE OF MENOPAUSE

Menstrual irregularity is the only marker used to define and establish the perimenopausal transition. The **menopause** is permanent cessation of menstruation after the loss of ovarian activity. Menopause is derived from the Greek words, *men* (month) and *pausis* (cessation). The years before menopause that encompass the change from normal ovulatory cycles to cessation of menses are known as the **perimenopausal transitional** years, marked by irregularity of menstrual cycles. **Climacteric** indicates the period when a woman passes from the reproductive stage of life through the perimenopausal transition and the menopause to the postmenopausal years. Climacteric is derived from the Greek word for ladder.

Designating the average age of menopause has been somewhat difficult. Based on cross-sectional studies, the median age was estimated to be between 50 and 52 (12). These studies relied on retrospective memories and the subjective vagaries of the individuals being interviewed. Until recently, studies with longitudinal follow-up to observe women and record their experiences as they pass through menopause were hampered by relatively small numbers. The Massachusetts Women's Health Study provided data from 2,570 women (13).

The median age for menopause in the Massachusetts Study was 51.3 years. Only current smoking could be identified as a cause of earlier menopause, with a shift of approximately 1.5 years. Factors that did not affect the age of menopause included the use of oral contraception, socioeconomic status, and marital status. A median age of menopause means that only one-half the women have reached menopause at this age. In the classic longitudinal study by Treolar, the *average* age of menopause was 50.7 years, and the range that included 95% of the women was 44 to 56 years (14). In a survey in the Netherlands, the average age of menopause was 50.2 years (15). About 1% of women experience menopause before the age of 40 (16).

Clinical impression has suggested that mothers and daughters tend to experience menopause at the same age, and two studies indicate that daughters of mothers with an early menopause (before age 46) also have an early menopause (17–19). There is sufficient evidence to believe that undernourished women and vegetarians experience an earlier menopause (17,20). Because of the contribution of body fat to estrogen production, thinner women experience a slightly earlier menopause (21). Consumption of alcohol is associated with a later menopause (18). This is consistent with the reports that women who consume alcohol have higher blood and urinary levels of estrogen and greater bone density (22–26).

There is no correlation between age of menarche and age of menopause (14,15,17). In most studies, race, parity, and height have no influence on the age of menopause; however, two cross-sectional studies found later menopause to be associated with increasing parity (13,15,17,21). Two studies have found that irregular menses among women in their forties predicts an earlier menopause (27,28). A French survey detected no influence of heavy physical work on early menopause (before age 45) (29).

An earlier menopause is associated with living at high altitudes (30). Multiple studies have consistently documented that an earlier menopause (average of 1.5 years earlier) is a consequence of smoking. There is a dose-response relationship with the number of cigarettes smoked and the duration of smoking (31,32). Even former smokers show evidence of an impact. There is reason to believe that premature ovarian failure can occur in women who have previously undergone abdominal hysterectomy, presumably because ovarian vasculature has been compromised (33).

Unlike the decline in age of menarche that occurred with an improvement in health and living conditions, most historical investigation indicates that the age of menopause has changed little since the reports from ancient Greece (34,35). A few authorities have disagreed, concluding that the age of menopause did undergo a change, starting with an average age of about 40 years in ancient times (36). If there has been a change, however, history indicates it has been minimal. Even in ancient writings, an age of 50 is usually cited as the age of menopause.

SYMPTOMS OF MENOPAUSE

During the menopausal years, some women experience severe multiple symptoms, but others have no reactions or minimal reactions that can go unnoticed. The differences in menopausal reactions in symptoms across different cultures is poorly documented, and it is difficult to do so. Individual reporting is so conditioned by sociocultural factors that it is hard to determine what is caused by biologic or cultural variability.

Women often seek medical assistance for disturbances in menstrual pattern, hot flushes, atrophic conditions, and psychologic symptoms. Disturbances in the menstrual pattern include anovulation and reduced fertility, decreased or increased flow, and irregular frequency of menses.

Vasomotor instability results in the hallmark symptom of menopause, the hot flush (Table 1.1). The vasomotor flush is viewed as the hallmark of the female climacteric, experienced to some degree by most postmenopausal

TABLE 1.1. *Characteristics of hot flushes*

Premenopausal: 15–25% of women
Postmenopausal
    Number of flushes: 15–25% of women
    Daily flushing: 15–20% of women
    Average duration: 1–2 years
    5+ years' duration: 25% of women
Other causes
    Psychosomatic
    Stress
    Thyroid disease
    Pheochromocytoma
    Carcinoid
    Leukemia
    Cancer

women. The term *hot flush* is descriptive of a sudden onset of reddening of the skin over the head, neck, and chest, accompanied by a feeling of intense body heat and concluded by sometimes profuse perspiration. The duration varies from a few seconds to several minutes or rarely for an hour. They may occur rarely or recur every few minutes. Flushes are more frequent and severe at night (when a woman is often awakened from sleep) or during times of stress. In a cool environment, hot flushes are fewer, less intense, and shorter in duration compared with a warm environment (37).

In the longitudinal follow-up of a large number of women, fully 10% of the women experienced hot flushes before menopause, but in other studies, as many as 15% to 25% of premenopausal women reported hot flushes (13,38,39). In the Massachusetts Women's Health Study, the incidence of hot flushes increased from 10% during the premenopausal period to about 50% just after cessation of menses (13). By approximately 4 years after menopause, the rate of hot flushes declined to 20%. In a community-based Australian survey, 6% of premenopausal women, 26% of perimenopausal women, and 59% of postmenopausal women reported hot flushing (40).

Although the flush can occur in the premenopause, it is a major feature of postmenopause, lasting in most women for 1 to 2 years but in as many as 25% for longer than 5 years. In cross-sectional surveys, up to 40% of premenopausal women and 85% of menopausal women report vasomotor complaints (39). In the United States, there is no difference in the prevalence of vasomotor complaints in surveys of black and white women (41,42). In a massive review of hot flushes, it was concluded that exact estimates on prevalence are hampered by inconsistencies and differences in methodologies, cultures, and definitions (43).

The physiology of the hot flush is still not understood, but it apparently originates in the hypothalamus and is brought about by a decline in estrogen. However, not all hot flushes are caused by estrogen deficiency. Flushes

and sweating can result from diseases, including pheochromocytoma, carcinoid, leukemias, pancreatic tumors, and thyroid abnormalities (44). Unfortunately, the hot flush is a relatively common psychosomatic symptom, and women often are unnecessarily treated with estrogen. When the clinical situation is not clear, estrogen deficiency as the cause of hot flushes should be documented by elevated levels of follicle-stimulating hormone (FSH).

The correlation between the onset of flushes and estrogen reduction is clinically supported by the effectiveness of estrogen therapy and the absence of flushes in hypoestrogen states, such as gonadal dysgenesis. Only after estrogen is administered and withdrawn do hypogonadal women experience the hot flush. Although the clinical impression that premenopausal surgical castrates suffer more severe vasomotor reactions is widely held, this is not borne out in objective study (45).

Although the hot flush is the most common problem of the postmenopause, it presents no inherent health hazard. The flush is accompanied by a discrete and reliable pattern of physiologic changes (46). The flush coincides with a surge of luteinizing hormone (LH), not FSH, and is preceded by a subjective prodromal awareness that a flush is beginning. This aura is followed by measurable increased heat over the entire body surface. The body surface experiences an increase in temperature, accompanied by changes in skin conductance and followed by a fall in core temperature—all of which can be objectively measured. In short, the flush is not a release of accumulated body heat but is a sudden inappropriate excitation of heat release mechanisms. Its relation to the LH surge and temperature change within the brain is not understood. The observation that flushes occur after hypophysectomy indicates that the mechanism does not depend on LH release. The same hypothalamic event that causes flushes also stimulates gonadotropin-releasing hormone (GnRH) secretion and elevates LH. This probably results in changes in neurotransmitters that increase neuronal and autonomic activity.

Premenopausal women experiencing hot flushes should be screened for thyroid disease and other illnesses. A comprehensive review of all possible causes is available (47). Clinicians should be sensitive to the possibility of an underlying emotional problem. Looking beyond the presenting symptoms into the patient's life can be an important service to the patient and her family that eventually will be appreciated. This is more difficult than prescribing estrogen, but confronting problems is the only way of reaching some resolution. Prescribing estrogen inappropriately (i.e., in the presence of normal levels of gonadotropins) only temporarily postpones by a placebo response dealing with the underlying issues.

A striking and consistent finding in most studies dealing with menopause and hormonal therapy is a marked placebo response in a variety of symptoms, including flushing. In an English randomized, placebo-controlled study of women being treated with estrogen implants and requesting repeat implants, there was no difference in outcome in terms of psychologic and physical symptoms comparing the women who received an active implant to those receiving a placebo (48).

Atrophic conditions include atrophy of the vaginal epithelium; formation of urethral caruncles; dyspareunia and pruritus from vulvar, introital, and vaginal atrophy; and urinary difficulties such as stress incontinence, urgency, and bacterial urethritis and cystitis.

Psychologic symptoms include anxiety, mood depression, irritability, insomnia, and decreased libido. The view that menopause has a deleterious effect on mental health is not supported in the psychiatric literature or in surveys of the general population (38,39,49,50). The concept of a specific psychiatric disorder (i.e., involutional melancholia) has been abandoned. Depression is less common among middle-aged women than younger women, and the menopause cannot be linked to psychologic distress (2–8,51). The longitudinal study of premenopausal women indicates that hysterectomy with or without oophorectomy is not associated with a negative psychologic impact among middle-aged women. Longitudinal data from the Massachusetts Women's Health Study document that menopause is not associated with an increased risk of depression (52). Although women are more likely to experience depression compared with men, this sex difference begins in early adolescence, not at menopause (53).

The U.S. National Health Examination Follow-up Study includes longitudinal and cross-sectional assessments of a nationally representative sample of women. This study found no evidence linking natural or surgical menopause to psychologic distress (54). The only longitudinal change was a slight decline in the prevalence of depression as women aged through the menopausal transition. Results in this study were the same for estrogen users and nonusers.

A negative view of mental health at the time of menopause is not justified; many of the problems reported at menopause are caused by the vicissitudes of life (55,56). There are problems encountered in the early postmenopause that are seen frequently, but their causal relation with estrogen is unlikely. These problems include fatigue, nervousness, headaches, insomnia, depression, irritability, joint and muscle pain, dizziness, and palpitations. Men and women at this stage of life express a multitude of complaints that do not reveal a gender difference that could be explained by a hormonal cause (57).

Attempts to study the effects of estrogen on these problems have been hampered by the subjectivity of the complaints (i.e., high placebo responses) and the "domino effect" of what reduction of hot flushes does to the frequency of the symptoms. Using a double-blind, crossover, prospective study format, Campbell and Whitehead con-

cluded many years ago that many symptomatic "improvements" ascribed to estrogen therapy result from relief of hot flushes—a domino effect (58).

A study of 2,001 women between the ages of 45 and 55 focused on the use of the health care system by women in the perimenopausal period of life (10). Health care users in this age group were frequent previous users of health care, less healthy, and had more psychosomatic symptoms and vasomotor reactions. These women were more likely to have had a significant previous adverse health history, including a history of premenstrual complaints. This study emphasized that perimenopausal women who seek health care help are different from those who do not seek help, and they often embrace hormone therapy in the hope it will solve their problems. This population is seen most often by clinicians, producing biased opinions regarding menopause among physicians. We must be careful not to generalize to the entire female population the behavior experienced by this relatively small group of women. Most importantly, perimenopausal women who present to clinicians often end up being treated with estrogen inappropriately and unnecessarily. Nevertheless, it is well established that a woman's quality of life is disrupted by vasomotor symptoms, and estrogen therapy provides impressive improvement (59,60).

Emotional stability during the perimenopausal period can be disrupted by poor sleep patterns. Hot flushing does have an adverse impact on the quality of sleep (61). Estrogen therapy improves the quality of sleep, decreasing the time to onset of sleep and increasing the rapid eye movement (REM) sleep time (59,62). Perhaps flushing may be insufficient to awaken a woman but sufficient to affect the quality of sleep, thereby diminishing the ability to handle the next day's problems and stresses.

The overall "quality of life" reported by women can be improved by better sleep and alleviation of hot flushing. However, it is still uncertain whether estrogen treatment has an additional direct pharmacologic antidepressant effect or the mood response is an indirect benefit of relief from physical symptoms and, consequently, from improved sleep. Using various assessment tools for measuring depression, improvements with estrogen treatment have been recorded in oophorectomized women (63,64). In the large, prospective cohort study of the Rancho Bernardo retirement community, no benefit could be detected in measures of depression in current users of postmenopausal estrogen compared with untreated women (65). Treated women had higher depressive symptom scores, presumably reflecting treatment selection bias; symptomatic and depressed women seek hormone therapy. Nevertheless, estrogen therapy is reported to have a more powerful impact on women's well-being beyond the relief of symptoms such as hot flushes (66). In elderly, depressed women, improvements in response to fluoxetine were enhanced by the addition of estrogen therapy (67).

SEXUALITY AND MENOPAUSE

Sexuality is a lifelong behavior with evolving changes and development. It begins with birth (perhaps before) and ends with death. The notion that it ends with aging is inherently illogical. The need for closeness, caring, and companionship is lifelong. Old people today live longer, are healthier, have more education and leisure time, and they have had their consciousness raised in regard to sexuality.

Younger people, especially younger physicians, underrate the extent of sexual interest in older people. In a random sample of women between the ages of 50 and 82 in Madison, Wisconsin, nearly one-half reported an ongoing sexual relationship (68). In the Duke longitudinal study on aging, 70% of men in the 67 to 77 age group were sexually active, and 80% reported continuing sexual interest, whereas 50% of all older women were still interested in sex (69). In the Postmenopausal Estrogen/Progestin Interventions (PEPI) trial, 60% of women 55 to 64 years old were sexually active (70).

The decline in sexual activity with aging is influenced more by culture and attitudes than by nature and physiology (or hormones). The two most important influences on older sexual interaction are the strength of a relationship and the physical condition of each partner (70). The single most significant determinant of sexual activity for older women is the unavailability of partners because of divorce and the fact that women are outliving men. Given the availability of a partner, the same general high or low rate of sexual activity can be maintained throughout life (4,71). Longitudinal studies indicate that the level of sexual activity is more stable over time than previously suggested (72–74). Individuals who are sexually active earlier in life continue to be sexually active into old age.

GROWTH OF THE OLDER POPULATION

We are experiencing a relatively new phenomenon: we can expect to become old. We are on the verge of becoming a rectangular society, one of the greatest achievements of the 20th century. This is a society in which nearly all individuals survive to advanced age and then succumb rather abruptly over a narrow age range centering on 85 years.

In 1000 BC, life expectancy was only 18 years. By 100 BC, the time of Caesar, it had reached 25 years. In 1900 in the United States, life expectancy had reached only 49 years. In 2000, the average life expectancy is 79.7 years for women and 72.9 for men (75). Today, after a man reaches 65, he can expect to reach 80.5, and a woman who reaches 54 can expect to reach the age of 84.3 years. We can anticipate that eventually about two-thirds of the population will survive to 85 years or longer, and more than 90% will live past the age of 65, producing the nearly perfect rectangular society (76,77).

Sweden and Switzerland are closest to this demographic composition.

A good general definition of elderly is 65 and older, although it is not until age 75 that a significant proportion of older people show the characteristic decline and health problems. The elderly population is the largest contributor to illness and human need in the United States (78). There are more old people (with their greater needs) than ever before (79). In 1900, there were approximately 3 million Americans 65 years or older (about 4% of the total population). By 2030, the elderly population will reach about 57 million (17% of the total population). Population aging will soon replace population growth as the most important social problem.

Two modern phenomena have influenced the rate of change. The first was the baby boom after World War II (1946 through 1964) that temporarily postponed the aging of the population but now is causing a faster aging of the general population. The second major influence has been the modern decrease in old-age mortality. Our success in postponing death has increased the upper segment of the demographic contour. By 2050, the current developed nations will be rectangular societies. By 2050, China will contain more people older than 65 years of age (270 million) than the number of people of all ages currently living in the United States.

This is a worldwide development, not limited to affluent societies (80). The population of the earth will continue to grow until the year 2100 or 2150, when it is expected to stabilize at approximately 11 billion, and 95% of this growth will occur in developing countries. The poorest countries today (in Africa and Asia) account for about one-half of the global population, and in 2000, 87% of the world's population will be living in what are now called developing countries. In most developing countries, the complications associated with pregnancy, abortion, and childbirth are the first or second most common cause of death, and almost one-half of all deaths are children younger than 5 years of age. Limiting family size to two children would cut the annual number of maternal deaths by 50% and infant and child mortality by 50% (81). It is appropriate to focus attention on population control; however, even in developing countries, this will change. In 1950, only 40% of people 60 and older lived in developing countries. By 2025, more than 70% will live in those countries (Table 1.2).

In 1900, older men in the United States outnumbered women by 102 to 100. In the 1980s, there were only 68 men for every 100 women older than 65 years. By age 85, only 45 men are alive for every 100 women. Nearly 90% of white American women can expect to live to age 70. Vital statistics data indicate that this gender difference is similar in the black and white populations in the United States (82). Approximately 55% of girls but only 35% of boys live long enough to celebrate their 85th birthday (83).

TABLE 1.2. *Projected size of the population 60 years of age and older*

Year	World (millions)	Developing countries (millions)
1950	200	80 (40%)[a]
1975	350	178 (51%)
2000	590	355 (60%)
2025	1,100	792 (72%)

[a]The percentages within parentheses compare the populations in developing countries with the world populations. From ref. 80, with permission.

TABLE 1.3. *The older U.S. female population*

Age	1990 (millions)	2000 (millions)	2010 (millions)	2020 (millions)
55–64	10.8 (8.6%)	12.1 (9.0%)	17.1 (12.1%)	19.3 (12.9%)
65–74	10.1 (8.1%)	9.8 (7.3%)	11.0 (7.8%)	15.6 (10.4%)
>75	7.8 (6.2%)	9.3 (7.0%)	9.8 (6.9%)	11.0 (7.3%)
Total	28.7	31.2	37.9	45.9

[a]The percentages within parentheses compare the group populations with world populations. From ref. 79, with permission.

Men and women reach old age with different prospects for older age, a sex differential that in part results from the sex hormone-induced differences in the cholesterol-lipoprotein profile and other cardiovascular factors, producing a greater incidence of atherosclerosis and earlier death in men (84). The use of postmenopausal estrogen therapy, with its protective effect on atherosclerosis, may exaggerate the sex differential in mortality. From a public health point of view, the greatest impact on the sex differential in mortality would be gained by concentrating on lifestyle changes designed to diminish atherosclerosis in men: low-cholesterol diet, no smoking, optimal body weight, and active exercise.

The death rate is higher for men at all ages. Coronary heart disease accounts for 40% of the mortality difference between men and women. Another one-third is from lung cancer, emphysema, cirrhosis, accidents, and suicides. In our society, the mortality difference between men and women is largely a difference in lifestyle. Smoking, drinking, coronary-prone behavior, and accidents account for most of the higher male mortality rate after age 65. It has been estimated that perhaps two-thirds of the difference has been because of cigarettes alone, but this results from a greater prevalence of smoking among men. Women whose smoking patterns are similar to those of men have a similar increased risk of morbidity and mortality.

Perhaps because more women are smoking, drinking, and working, the mortality sex difference has begun to lessen. The U.S. Census Bureau projects that the difference in life expectancy between men and women will increase until the year 2050 and then level off (79). In 2050, life expectancy will be 82 years for women and 76.7 years for men (75). There will be 33.4 million women 65 or older, compared with 22.1 million men (Table 1.3).

Unmarried women will be an increasing proportion of the elderly. By 1983, 50% of American women between the ages of 65 and 74 were unmarried (some were divorced, but most were widowed), and after age 75, 77% were unmarried (85). One-half of men 85 or older live with their wives, but only 10% of elderly women live with their husbands. Because the unmarried tend to be more disadvantaged, there will be a need for more ser-

vices for this segment of the elderly population. Older unmarried people are more vulnerable, demonstrating higher mortality rates and lower life satisfaction.

In addition to the growing numbers of elderly people, the older population itself is getting older (86). For example, in 1984, the 65 to 74 age group was more than seven times larger than in 1900, but the 75 to 84 group was 11 times larger, and the 85 and older group was 21 times larger. The most rapid increase is expected between 2010 and 2030, when the baby boom generation hits 65. In the next century, the only age groups in the United States expected to experience significant growth will be those past the age of 55. In this elderly age group, women outnumber men by 2.6 to 1. By the year 2040, there will be 8 million to 13 million people 85 years of age or older; the estimate varies according to pessimistic to optimistic projections regarding disease prevention and treatment.

THE RECTANGULARIZATION OF LIFE

The life span is the biologic limit to life, the maximal obtainable age by a member of a species. The general impression is that human life span is increasing, but the life span is fixed, and it is a biologic constant for each species (87). Differences in species' life spans argue in favor of a species-specific genetic basis for longevity. If life span were not fixed, it would mean an unlimited increase of our elderly. But a correct analysis of survival reveals that death converges at the same maximal age; what has changed is life expectancy, the number of years of life expected from birth. Life expectancy cannot exceed the life span, but it can closely approximate it. The number of old people will eventually hit a fixed limit, but the percentage of a typical life spent in the older years will increase.

Our society has almost eliminated premature death. Diseases of the heart and the circulation and cancers are the leading causes of death. The reason for this is not an increase or an epidemic; it is a result of our success in virtually eliminating infectious diseases. The major determinant is chronic disease, affected by genetics, lifestyle, the environment, and aging itself. The major achievement left to be accomplished is in cardiovascular diseases, but even if cancer, diabetes, and all circulatory diseases were totally eliminated, life expectancy would not exceed 90 years (76).

Fries describes three eras in health and disease (88). The first era existed until sometime in the early 1900s and was characterized by acute infectious diseases. The second era, highlighted by cardiovascular diseases and cancer, is beginning to fade into the third era, marked by problems of frailty (e.g., fading eyesight and hearing, impaired memory and cognitive function, decreased strength and reserve). Much of our medical approach is still based on the first era (i.e., find the disease and cure it), but we have conditions that require a combination of medical, psychologic, and social approaches. Our focus has been on age-dependent, fatal chronic diseases. The new challenge is with the nonfatal, age-dependent conditions such as Alzheimer's disease, osteoarthritis, osteoporosis, obesity, and incontinence. It can be argued that health programs in the future should be evaluated by their impact on years free of disability, rather than on mortality.

SUCCESSFUL AGING: THE ROLE OF PREVENTIVE HEALTH CARE

Chronic illnesses are incremental in nature. The best health strategy is to change the slope, the rate at which illness develops, postponing the clinical illness, and if it is postponed long enough, effectively preventing it. There has been a profound change in public consciousness toward disease. Disease is increasingly seen as something not necessarily best treated by medication or surgery but by prevention or, more accurately, by postponement.

Postponing illness is expressed by J. F. Fries as the *compression of morbidity* (87,89). We would live relatively healthy lives and compress our illnesses into a short period just before death. Is this change really possible? The mean national body weight has decreased by 5 pounds despite a slight increase in the national average height. There has been a decrease in atherosclerosis in the United States. Reasons include changes in the use of saturated fat, more effective detection and treatment of hypertension, increased exercise, and decreased smoking.

Smoking initiation has decreased markedly in men but unfortunately has remained essentially unchanged in women. Female smokers begin smoking at a younger age. More young women (including teenagers) smoke than young men. Smoking appears to have a greater adverse effect on women compared with men (90).

Physician smokers have declined from a high of 79% to a small minority (91). The greatest decrease has been among pulmonary surgeons, and the least decrease has been among proctologists. From the mid-1970s to the early 1990s, smoking among physicians declined from 18.8% to 3.3%. Unfortunately, that still amounts to approximately 18,000 physicians who smoke. The numbers are more discouraging among our professional colleagues. From the 1970s to 1991, smoking had declined from 31.7% to 18.3% among registered nurses and from 37.1% to only 27.2% among licensed practical nurses.

In the year 2000, approximately 30% of people who have not obtained a high school diploma will be smokers, but fewer than 10% of those with higher education will be smoking. Currently, approximately 28% of men and 23% of women are smokers. Cigarette smoking therefore continues to be the single most preventable cause of premature death in the United States. The use of chewing tobacco, pipe smoking, and cigars contributes significantly to morbidity and mortality.

Physicians and older patients may be skeptical that quitting smoking after decades of smoking could be beneficial. In a longitudinal study of 2,674 persons between the ages of 65 and 74, the mortality rates for ex-smokers were no higher than for nonsmokers (92). The effects are at least partly reversible within 1 to 5 years after quitting. Even older patients who already have coronary artery disease have improved survival after they quit smoking (93). No matter how old a person is, if he continues to smoke, he has an increased relative risk of death, but if he quits smoking, his risk of death decreases.

Since 1970, the death rate from coronary heart disease has declined by approximately 50% in the United States. Between 1973 and 1987 in the United States, cardiovascular mortality declined in nearly every age group. In the combined age groups up to 54 years, cardiovascular mortality decreased 42%, and for people 55 to 84 years old, it declined by 33% (90). Despite our progress, we must continue to exert preventive efforts on the risk factors associated with cardiovascular disease, especially obesity, hypertension, and lack of physical activity.

The effort to improve the quality of life has an important value to society; it will decrease the average number of years that people are disabled and a liability. Frailty and disability have become the major health and social problems of society. Most significantly, this is a major financial challenge for health care systems and social programs. With evolution toward a rectangular society, the ratio of beneficiaries to taxpayers grows rapidly, jeopardizing the financial support for health and social programs. Compression of morbidity is at least one attractive solution to this problem.

MENOPAUSE AS AN OPPORTUNITY

Clinicians who interact with women at the time of menopause have a wonderful opportunity and therefore a significant obligation. Medical intervention at this point of life offers women years of benefit from preventive health care. This represents an opportunity that should be seized.

It is logical to argue that health programs should be directed to the young. It makes sense to create good lifelong health behavior. Although not underrating the importance of good health habits among the young, it can be argued that the impact of teaching preventive care is more observable and more tangible at middle age. The prospects of limited mortality and the morbidity of chronic diseases are now viewed with belief, understanding, and appreciation during these older years. The chance of illness is higher, but the impact of changes in lifestyle is greater.

THE MENOPAUSE AS A SIGNAL FOR THE FUTURE

The menopause should remind patients and clinicians that this is a time for education. Preventive health care education is important throughout life, but at the time of menopause, a review of the major health issues can be especially rewarding. Besides the general issues of good health, attention is being focused on cardiovascular disease and osteoporosis (because of their relationship to hormone replacement therapy).

Diseases of the heart are the leading cause of death for women in the United States, followed by malignant neoplasms, cerebrovascular disease, and motor vehicle accidents. Of the 550,000 people in the United States who die each year of heart disease, 250,000 are women (94). Nearly one-third of heart disease mortality in women occurs before the age of 65.

Most cardiovascular disease results from atherosclerosis in major vessels. The risk factors are the same for men and women: high blood pressure, smoking, diabetes mellitus, and obesity. When controlling for these risk factors, men have a risk of developing coronary heart disease over 3.5 times that of women. Even taking into consideration the changing lifestyle of women (e.g., employment outside the home), women still maintain their advantage in terms of risk for coronary heart disease. However, with increasing age, this advantage is gradually lost, and cardiovascular disease becomes the leading cause of death for older women and men.

In the past 30 years, stroke mortality has declined by 60% and mortality from coronary heart disease by 50% in the United States (90). Improvements in medical and surgical care can account for some of this decline, but 60% to 70% of the improvement results from preventive measures. Excellent data from epidemiologic studies and clinical trials demonstrate a decline in stroke and heart disease morbidity and mortality from smoking cessation, blood pressure reduction, and lowering of cholesterol (95,96). There is a strong and growing scientific basis for preventive medicine and health promotion efforts in clinical practice.

Postmenopausal hormone therapy deserves consideration as a legitimate component of preventive health care for older women. It can be argued convincingly that protection against cardiovascular disease is the major benefit of postmenopausal estrogen treatment, and the magnitude of this benefit is considerable. There is a sound

rationale for this protection in the link between cardiovascular disease and the sex hormones.

Osteoporosis is a major global public health problem, and it is epidemic in the United States, affecting more than 20 million individuals (97). The increase in osteoporotic fractures in the developed world is partly caused by an increase in the elderly population. A comparison of bone densities in proximal femur bones in specimens from a period of over 200 years suggested that women lose more bone today, perhaps because of less physical activity and less parity (98). Other contributing factors include a dietary decrease in calcium and an earlier and greater loss of bone because of the impact of smoking. Our Stone Age predecessors consumed a diet high in calcium, mostly from vegetable sources (99). However, the impact of the tremendous increase in the elderly population throughout the world cannot be underrated. Because of this demographic change, the number of hip fractures occurring in the world each year will increase approximately sixfold from 1990 to 2050, and the proportion occurring in Europe and North America will fall from 50% to 25% as the numbers of old people in developing countries increase (100).

The onset of spinal bone loss begins in the twenties, but the overall change is small until menopause. Bone density in the femur peaks in the middle to late twenties and begins to decrease around age 30. In general, trabecular bone resorption and formation occur four to eight times as fast as cortical bone. Beyond age 30, trabecular resorption begins to exceed formation by about 0.7% per year. This adverse relationship accelerates after menopause, and up to 5% of trabecular bone and 1% to 1.5% of total bone mass loss per year occurs after menopause. This accelerated loss continues for 10 to 15 years, after which bone loss is considerably diminished but continues as the aging-related loss. For the first 20 years after cessation of menses, menopause-related bone loss results in a 50% reduction in trabecular bone and a 30% reduction in cortical bone (101,102).

Estrogen therapy provides a 50% to 60% decrease in fractures of the arm and hip (103–105), and when estrogen is supplemented with calcium, an 80% reduction in vertebral compression fractures occurs (106). This reduction is seen primarily in patients who have taken estrogen for more than 5 years (107,108). Protection against fractures wanes with age, and long-term estrogen use is necessary to maximally reduce the risk of fracture after age 75.

Because most osteoporotic fractures occur late in life, women and clinicians must understand that the short-term use of estrogen immediately after menopause cannot be expected to protect against fractures in the seventh and eighth decades of life. Some long-term protection is achieved with 7 to 10 years of estrogen therapy after menopause, but the impact is minimal after age 75 (109). In a prospective cohort study of women 65 years of age or older, in the women who had stopped using estrogen and in those who were older than 75 and had stopped using estrogen even if they had used estrogen for more than 10 years, there was no substantial effect on the risk for fractures (110). The effective impact of estrogen requires initiation within 5 years of menopause and use extending into the elderly years. The protective effect of estrogen rapidly dissipates after treatment is stopped, because estrogen withdrawal is followed by rapid bone loss. In the 3- to 5-year period after loss of estrogen, whether after menopause or after cessation of estrogen therapy, there is accelerated loss of bone (111–113). Maximal protection against osteoporotic fractures therefore requires lifelong therapy, and even some long-term protection requires 10 or more years of treatment.

CONCLUSION

The menopause has been overladen with negative symbolism. Many of the behavioral complaints at the time of menopause, however, can be explained by psychologic and sociocultural influences. That is not to say that important interactions between biology, psychology, and culture do not occur, but it is time to stress the normalcy of this life event. Menopausal women do not suffer from a hormone deficiency disease. Hormone replacement therapy should be viewed as specific treatment for symptoms in the short term and preventive pharmacology in the long term.

Part of the reason for our negative stereotypical views of menopause is that the initial characterization of menopause was derived from women presenting with physical and psychologic difficulties. The variability in menopausal reactions makes the cross-sectional study design particularly unsuitable. More and larger longitudinal studies are needed to document what is normal and the variations around normal.

It is important to educate women and clinicians about the normal events of this time period. Changes in menstrual function are not symbols of some ominous change. There are good physiologic reasons for changing menstrual function, and understanding the physiology can do much to reinforce a healthy, normal attitude.

The menopause serves a useful purpose. This physiologic event brings clinicians and patients together, providing the opportunity to enroll patients in a preventive health care program. Contrary to popular opinion, menopause is not a signal of impending decline, but rather a wonderful phenomenon that can signal the start of something positive, such as a good health program. Rather than being a lightning rod for social and personal problems, menopause can be a signal for the future.

REFERENCES

1. Farnham AM. Uterine disease as a factor in the production of insanity. *Alienst Neurologist* 1887;8:532.
2. Hällström T, Samuelsson S. Mental health in the climacteric: the longitudinal study of women in Gothenburg. *Acta Obstet Gynecol Scand Suppl* 1985;130: 13–18.
3. McKinlay SM, McKinlay JB. The impact of menopause and social factors on health. In: Hammond CB, Haseltine FP, Schiff I, eds. *Menopause: evaluation, treatment, and health concerns.* New York: Alan R Liss, 1989:137–161.
4. Matthews KA, Wing RR, Kuller LH, et al. Influences of natural menopause on psychological characteristics and symptoms of middle-aged healthy women. *J Consult Clin Psychol* 1990;58:345–351.
5. Koster A. Change-of-life anticipations, attitudes, and experiences among middle-aged Danish women. *Health Care Women* 1991;12:1–13.
6. Holte A. Influences of natural menopause on health complaints: a prospective study of healthy Norwegian women. *Maturitas* 1992;14:127.
7. Kaufert PA, Gilbert P, Tate R. The Manitoba Project: a re-examination of the link between menopause and depression. *Maturitas* 1992;14:143.
8. Dennerstein L, Smith AMA, Morse C, et al. Menopausal symptoms in Australian women. *Med J Aust* 1993;159:232.
9. Avis NE, McKinlay SM. A longitudinal analysis of women's attitudes toward the menopause: results from the Massachusetts Women's Health Study. *Maturitas* 1991;13:65–79.
10. Morse CA, Smith A, Dennerstein L, Green A, Hopper J, Burger H. The treatment-seeking woman at menopause. *Maturitas* 1994;18:161–173.
11. Defey D, Storch E, Cardozo S, Diaz O, Fernandez G. The menopause: women's psychology and health care. *Soc Sci Med* 1996;42:1447–1456.
12. McKinlay SM, Bigano NL, McKinlay JB. Smoking and age at menopause. *Ann Intern Med* 1985;103:350.
13. McKinlay SM, Brambilla DJ, Posner JG. The normal menopause transition. *Maturitas* 1992;14:103–115.
14. Treolar AE. Menarche, menopause and intervening fecundability. *Hum Biol* 1974;46:89.
15. van Noord PAH, Dubas JS, Dorland M, Boersma H, te Velde E. Age at natural menopause in a population-based screening cohort: the role of menarche, fecundity, and lifestyle factors. *Fertil Steril* 1997;68:95–102.
16. Coulam CB, Adamsen SC, Annegers JF. Incidence of premature ovarian failure. *Obstet Gynecol* 1986;67:604.
17. Torgerson DJ, Avenell A, Russell IT, Reid DM. Factors associated with onset of menopause in women aged 45–49. *Maturitas* 1994;19:83.
18. Torgerson DJ, Thomas RE, Campbell MK, Reid DM. Alcohol consumption and age of maternal menopause are associated with menopause onset. *Maturitas* 1997;26:21–25.
19. Cramer DW, Xu H, Harlow BL. Family history as a predictor of early menopause. *Fertil Steril* 1995;64:740–745.
20. Baird DD, Tylavsky FA, Anderson JJB. Do vegetarians have earlier menopause? *Am J Epidemiol* 1988;128:907.
21. MacMahon B, Worcester J. Age at menopause: U.S. 1960–62. *Vital Health Stat* 1966;19:1.
22. Katsouyanni K, Boyle P, Trichopoulos D. Diet and urine estrogens among postmenopausal women. *Oncology* 1991;48:490–494.
23. Gapstur SM, Potter JD, Sellers TA, Folsom AR. Increased risk of breast cancer with alcohol consumption in postmenopausal women. *Am J Epidemiol* 1992; 136:1221–1231.
24. Gavaler JS, Van Thiel DH. The association between moderate alcoholic beverage consumption and serum estradiol and testosterone levels in normal postmenopausal women: relationship to the literature. *Alcohol Clin Exp Res* 1992; 16:87–92.
25. Holbrook TC, Barrett-Connor E. A prospective study of alcohol consumption and bone mineral density. *Br Med J* 1993;306:1506–1509.
26. Ginsburg EL, Mello NK, Mendelson JH, et al. Effects of alcohol ingestion on estrogens in postmenopausal women. *JAMA* 1996;276:1747–1751.
27. Brambila DJ, McKinlay SM, Johannes CB. Defining the perimenopause for application in epidemiologic investigations. *Am J Epidemiol* 1994;140: 1091–1105.
28. Bromberger JT, Matthews KA, Kuller LH, Wing RR, Meilahn EN, Plantinga P. Prospective study of the determinants of age at menopause. *Am J Epidemiol* 1997;145:124–133.
29. Cassou B, Derriennic F, Monfort C, Dell'Accio P, Touranchet A. Risk factors of early menopause in two generations of gainfully employed French women. *Maturitas* 1997;26:165–174.
30. Gonzales GF, Villena A. Age at menopause in Central Andean Peruvian women. *Menopause* 1997;4:32–38.
31. Willett W, Stampfer MJ, Bain C, et al. Cigarette smoking, relative weight, and menopause. *Am J Epidemiol* 1983;117:651–658.
32. Midgette AS, Baron JA. Cigarette smoking and the risk of natural menopause. *Epidemiology* 1990;1:474.
33. Siddle N, Sarrel P, Whitehead M. The effect of hysterectomy on the age at ovarian failure: identification of a subgroup of women with premature loss of ovarian function and literature review. *Fertil Steril* 1987;47:94.
34. Amundsen DW, Diers CJ. The age of menopause in classical Greece and Rome. *Hum Biol* 1970;42:79.
35. Amundsen DW, Diers CJ. The age of menopause in medieval Europe. *Hum Biol* 1973;45:605.
36. Frommer DJ. Changing age at menopause. *Br Med J* 1964;2a:349.
37. Kronnenberg F, Barnard RM. Modulation of menopausal hot flashes by ambient temperature. *J Therm Biol* 1992;17:43–49.
38. Hunter M. The South-East England longitudinal study of the climacteric and postmenopause. *Maturitas* 1992;14:17–26.
39. Oldenhave A, Jaszmann LJB, Haspels AA, Everaerd WTAM. Impact of climacteric on well-being. *Am J Obstet Gynecol* 1993;168:772–780.

40. Guthrie JR, Dennerstein L, Hopper JL, Burger HG. Hot flushes, menstrual status, and hormone levels in a population-based sample of midlife women. *Obstet Gynecol* 1996;88:437–442.

41. Schwingl PJ, Hulka BS, Harlow SD. Risk factors for menopausal hot flashes. *Obstet Gynecol* 1994;84:29–34.

42. Pham KT, Grisso JA, Freeman EW. Ovarian aging and hormone replacement therapy: hormonal levels, symptoms, and attitudes of African-American and white women. *J Gen Intern Med* 1997;12:230–236.

43. Kronnenberg F. Hot flashes: epidemiology and physiology. *Ann N Y Acad Sci* 1990;592:52–86.

44. Wilkin JR. Flushing reactions: consequences and mechanisms. *Ann Intern Med* 1981;95:468–476.

45. Aksel S, Schomberg DW, Tyrey L, Hammond CB. Vasomotor symptoms, serum estrogens and gonadotropin levels in surgical menopause. *Am J Obstet Gynecol* 1976;126:165.

46. Swartzman LC, Edelberg R, Kemmann E. The menopausal hot flush: symptom reports and concomitant physiological changes. *J Behav Med* 1990;13:15.

47. Mohyi D, Tabassi K, Simon J. Differential diagnosis of hot flashes. *Maturitas* 1997;27:203–214.

48. Pearce J, Hawton K, Blake F, et al. Psychological effects of continuation versus discontinuation of hormone replacement therapy by estrogen implants: a placebo-controlled study. *J Psychosom Res* 1997;42:177–186.

49. Ballinger CB. Psychiatric aspects of the menopause. *Br J Psychiatry* 1990;156:773–787.

50. Schmidt PJ, Rubinow DR. Menopause-related affective disorders: a justification for further study. *Am J Psychiatry* 1991;148:844–854.

51. Gath D, Osborn M, Bungay G, et al. Psychiatric disorder and gynaecological symptoms in middle aged women: a community survey. *Br Med J* 1987;294:213–218.

52. Avis NE, Brambilla D, McKinlay SM, Vass K. A longitudinal analysis of the association between menopause and depression: results from the Massachusetts Women's Health Study. *Ann Epidemiol* 1994;4:214–220.

53. Kessler RC, McGonagle KA, Swartz M, Blazer DG, Nelson CB. Sex and depression in the National Comorbidity Survey I: lifetime prevalence, chronicity and recurrence. *J Affect Disord* 1993;29:85.

54. Busch CM, Zonderman AB, Costa PT Jr. Menopausal transition and psychological distress in a nationally representative sample: is menopause associated with psychological distress? *J Aging Health* 1994;6:209–228.

55. Dennerstein L, Smith AMA, Morse C. Psychological well-being, mid-life and the menopause. *Maturitas* 1994;20:1.

56. Mitchell ES, Woods NF. Symptom experiences of midlife women: observations from the Seattle midlife women's health study. *Maturitas* 1996;25:1–10.

57. Van Hall EV, Verdel M, Van Der Velden J. "Perimenopausal" complaints in women and men: a comparative study. *J Womens Health* 1994;3:45–49.

58. Campbell S, Whitehead M. Estrogen therapy and the menopausal syndrome. *Clin Obstet Gynecol* 1977;4:31–47.

59. Wiklund I, Karlberg J, Mattsson L-A. Quality of life of postmenopausal women on a regimen of transdermal estradiol therapy: a double-blind, placebo-controlled study. *Am J Obstet Gynecol* 1993;168:824–830.

60. Daly E, Gray A, Barlow D, McPherson K, Roche M, Vessey M. Measuring the impact of menopausal symptoms on quality of life. *Br Med J* 1993;307:836.

61. Woodward S, Freedman RR. The thermoregulatory effects of menopausal hot flashes on sleep. *Sleep* 1994;17:497–501.

62. Schiff I, Regestein Q, Tulchinsky D, Ryan KJ. Effects of estrogens on sleep and psychological state of hypogonadal women. *JAMA* 1979;242:2405–2407.

63. Dennerstein L, Burrows GD, Hyman GJ, Wood C. Hormone therapy and affect. *Maturitas* 1979;1:247–254.

64. Sherwin BB. Affective changes with estrogen and androgen replacement therapy in surgically menopausal women. *J Affect Disord* 1988;14:177–187.

65. Palinkas LA, Barrett-Connor E. Estrogen use and depressive symptoms in postmenopausal women. *Obstet Gynecol* 1992;80:30–36.

66. Limouzin-Lamothe M-A, Mairon N, Joyce CRB, Le Gal M. Quality of life after the menopause: influence of hormonal replacement therapy. *Am J Obstet Gynecol* 1994;170:618–624.

67. Schneider LS, Small GW, Hamilton SH, et al. Estrogen replacement and response to fluoxetine in a multicenter geriatric depression trial. *Am J Geriatr Psychiatry* 1997;5:97–106.

68. Traupman J, Eckels E, Hatfield E. Intimacy in older women's lives. *Gerontologist* 1982;2:493.

69. Pfeiffer E, Verwoerdt A, Davis GC. Sexual behavior in middle life. *Am J Psychiatry* 1972;128:1262.

70. Greendale GA, Hogan P, Shumaker S, for the Postmenopausal Estrogen/Progestin Interventions (PEPI) Trial Investigators. Sexual functioning in postmenopausal women: the Postmenopausal Estrogen/Progestin Interventions (PEPI) trial. *J Womens Health* 1996;5:445–456.

71. Martin CE. Factors affecting sexual functioning in 60–79-year-old married males. *Arch Sex Behav* 1981;10:399.

72. George LK, Weiler SJ. Sexuality in middle and late life. *Arch Gen Psychiatry* 1981;38:919.

73. White CB. Sexual interest, attitudes, knowledge, and sexual history in relation to sexual behavior in the institutionalized aged. *Arch Sex Behav* 1982;11:11.

74. Renshaw DC. Sex, intimacy, and the older woman. *Women Health* 1983;8:43–54.

75. *Annual report of the Board of Trustees of the Federal Old-Age and Survivors Insurance and Disability Insurance Trust Funds.* Washington, DC: U.S. Government Printing Office, 1995.

76. Olshansky SJ, Carnes BA, Cassel C. In search of Methuselah: estimating the upper limits to human longevity. *Science* 1990;250:634.

77. Olshansky SJ, Carnes BA, Cassel C. The aging of the human species. *Sci Am* April,1993;268:46–52.

78. Rowe JW, Grossman E, Bond E. Academic geriatrics for the year 2000: an Institute of Medicine report. *N Engl J Med* 1987;316:1425.

79. U.S. Bureau of the Census. *Current population reports: projections of the population of the United States: 1977 to 2050.* Washington, DC: U.S. Government Printing Office, 1993.

80. Diczfalusy E. Menopause, developing countries and the 21st century. *Acta Obstet Gynecol Scand Suppl* 1986;134:45.

81. Duke RC, Speidel JJ. Women's reproductive health: a chronic crisis. *JAMA* 1991;266:1846.

82. Miles TP, Bernard MA. Morbidity, disability, and health status of black American elderly: a new look at the oldest-old. *J Am Geriatr Soc* 1992;40:1047.

83. Day JC. Bureau of the Census. Current population reports. Population projections of the United States, by age, sex, race, and Hispanic origin: 1993 to 2050. Washington, DC: U.S. Government Printing Office, 1993.

84. Hazzard WR. Biological basis of the sex differential in longevity. *J Am Geriatr Soc* 1986;34:455.

85. Keith PM. The social context and resources of the unmarried in old age. *Int J Aging Hum Dev* 1986;23:81.

86. U.S. Bureau of the Census. *Current population reports, special studies:* sixty-five plus in America. Washington, DC: U.S. Government Printing Office, 1993.

87. Fries JF, Crapo LM. *Vitality and aging.* San Francisco: WH Freeman, 1981.

88. Fries JF. The sunny side of aging. *JAMA* 1990;263:2354.

89. Fries JF. Strategies for reduction of morbidity. *Am J Clin Nutr* 1992;55:1257S.

90. Davis DL, Dinse GE, Hoel DG. Decreasing cardiovascular disease and increasing cancer among whites in the United States from 1973 through 1987. *JAMA* 1994;271:431.

91. Nelson DE, Giovino GA, Emont SL, et al. Trends in cigarette smoking among US physicians and nurses. *JAMA* 1994;271:1273.

92. Jajich CL, Ostfeld AM, Freeman DH Jr. Smoking and coronary heart disease mortality in the elderly. *JAMA* 1984;252:2831.

93. Hermanson B, Omenn GS, Kronmal RA, Gersh BJ. Beneficial six-year outcome of smoking cessation in older men and women with coronary artery disease: results from the CASS registry. *N Engl J Med* 1988;319:1365.

94. Wenger NK, Speroff L, Packard B. Cardiovascular health and disease in women. *N Engl J Med* 1993;329:247.

95. Vartiainen E, Puska P, Pekkanen J, Tuomilehto J, Jousilahti P. Changes in risk factors explain changes in mortality from ischaemic heart disease in Finland. *Br Med J* 1994;309:23.

96. Vartiainen E, Sarti C, Tuomilehto J, Kuulasmaa K. Do changes in cardiovascular risk factors explain changes in mortality from stroke in Finland? *Br Med J* 1995;310:901.

97. Dempster DW, Lindsay R. Pathogenesis of osteoporosis. *Lancet* 1993;341:797.

98. Lees B, Molleson T, Arnett TR, Stevenson JC. Differences in proximal femur bone density over two centuries. *Lancet* 1993;341:673–675.

99. Eaton SB, Nelson DA. Calcium in evolutionary perspective. *Am J Clin Nutr* 1991;54:281S.

100. Cooper C, Campion G, Melton LJ III. Hip fractures in the elderly: a world-wide projection. *Osteoporos Int* 1992;2:285.

101. Ettinger B. Prevention of osteoporosis: treatment of estradiol deficiency. *Obstet Gynecol* 1988;72:125.

102. Lindsay R. Prevention and treatment of osteoporosis. *Lancet* 1993;341:801.

103. Weiss NC, Ure CL, Ballard JH, Williams AR, Daling JR. Decreased risk of fractures of the hip and lower forearm with postmenopausal use of estrogen. *N Engl J Med* 1980;303:1195.

104. Ettinger B, Genant HK, Cann CE. Long-term estrogen replacement therapy prevents bone loss and fractures. *Ann Intern Med* 1985;102:319.

105. Kiel DP, Felson DT, Anderson JJ, Wilson PWF, Moskowitz MA. Hip fracture and the use of estrogen in postmenopausal women: the Framingham Study. *N Engl J Med* 1987;317:1169.

106. Riggs BL, Seeman E, Hodgson SF, Taves DR, O'Fallon WM. Effect of the fluoride/calcium regimen on vertebral fracture occurrence in postmenopausal osteoporosis. *N Engl J Med* 1982;306:446.

107. Quigley MET, Martin PL, Burnier AM, Brooks P. Estrogen therapy arrests bone loss in elderly women. *Am J Obstet Gynecol* 1987;156:1516.

108. Lafferty FW, Fiske ME. Postmenopausal estrogen replacement: a long-term cohort study. *Am J Med* 1994;97:66.

109. Felson DT, Zhang Y, Hannan MT, Kiel DP, Wilson PWF, Anderson JJ. The effect of postmenopausal estrogen therapy on bone density in elderly women. *N Engl J Med* 1993;329:1141–1146.

110. Cauley JA, Seeley DG, Ensrud K, et al. Estrogen replacement therapy and fractures in older women. *Ann Intern Med* 1995;122:9–16.

111. Lindsay R, MacLean A, Kraszewski A, Clark AC, Garwood J. Bone response to termination of estrogen treatment. *Lancet* 1978;1:1325.

112. Horsman A, Nordin BEC, Crilly RG. Effect on bone of withdrawal of estrogen therapy. *Lancet* 1979;2:33.

113. Christiansen C, Christiansen MS, Transbol IB. Bone mass in postmenopausal women after withdrawal of oestrogen/gestagen replacement therapy. *Lancet* 1981;1:459.

SECTION I

Ovarian Senescence

Ovarian failure usually occurs over several years. This is the case whether the timing of menopause is premature or occurs during the usual age range of 40 to 58 years. Failure denotes both the cessation of endocrine function, which is predominantly that of estradiol 17β, as well as gametogenic failure which is associated with the inability to conceive. The latter occurs many years before menopause while estradiol 17β only plummets about 6 months before the permanent cessation of menses.

In this first section, three world-renowned experts will describe various aspects of ovarian failure. First, Robert Rebar will discuss the ramifications of premature ovarian failure. Next, Mark Sauer will discuss how older women, or those with premature failure, may achieve pregnancy. Finally, Christopher Longcope will set the stage for future therapeutic discussions by reviewing the endocrinology of menopause and the postmenopausal women.

As with each section of this book, this first section on ovarian senescence is meant to be able to stand on its own. In the ensuing sections, various aspects of the natural and untreated postmenopausal state will be presented. The basis for various treatment options will also be discussed.

Treatment of the Postmenopausal Woman: Basic and Clinical Aspects, Second Edition, edited by Rogerio A. Lobo, Lippincott Williams & Wilkins, Philadelphia © 1999.

CHAPTER 2

Premature Ovarian Failure

Robert W. Rebar

EARLY REPORTS OF PREMATURE OVARIAN FAILURE

Menopause, defined strictly as the last episode of menstrual bleeding, typically occurs around age 51 and is generally considered premature if it occurs before the age of 40 years. De Moraes and Jones (1) first defined premature menopause or premature ovarian failure as consisting of the triad of amenorrhea, hypergonadotropinism, and hypoestrogenism in women younger than 40 years of age. Why the cessation of reproductive life should occur prematurely has been of great interest to clinicians and remains enigmatic in most cases.

How little is known about premature menopause is less surprising in view of how little is known about normal menopause. The events that signal menopause are unclear. Depletion of oocytes is obviously an important factor, and it has been documented that follicle depletion accelerates just before menopause (2). Although a few follicles may be present at menopause, they do not respond to follicle-stimulating hormone (FSH) and luteinizing hormone (LH). In an unsuccessful effort to stimulate follicular development and estradiol secretion, the hypothalamus signals the pituitary gland to secrete still more FSH and LH. An increase in serum FSH levels is an early sign heralding the cessation of ovarian function.

Preliminary studies of strains of mice indicate that specific genes are important in controlling the number of oocytes ovulated and presumably the timing of the cessation of reproductive function (3). Although these data are difficult to extrapolate to humans, given what is known about the control of ovarian function by the X chromosome (4), it is not difficult to believe that inherited tendencies are important. Any role for ovarian inhibin and its

feedback action on pituitary FSH secretion also remains to be explored.

The hypothalamic-pituitary axis is also potentially important in the regulation of the onset of menopause. Although oocyte depletion may provide the major reason for the occurrence of menopause in humans, numerous animal studies document changes in neurotransmitter and in central nervous system feedback responses to estrogen with aging. Aging ovaries transplanted to young rodents cycle normally, whereas young ovaries transplanted to aged animals do not function well (5). Extrapolation of such data to humans is difficult.

The concept that women younger than 40 with "hypergonadotropic" amenorrhea by definition should have depletion of their oocytes and premature ovarian failure was supported by the findings of Goldenberg et al. (6). They reported in 1973 that women who had basal FSH levels of greater than 40 mIU/mL 2nd IRP-hMG without exception had no viable oocytes on ovarian biopsy.

The belief that the ovarian failure observed in such young women was permanent was first questioned by several isolated case reports documenting the initiation or resumption of cyclic menses or pregnancy in affected women. Several large series have confirmed these case reports (7). In one of those reports, we documented pubertal progression in two young girls with elevated serum FSH levels and multiple endocrine deficiencies (i.e., hypoparathyroidism and hypoadrenalism) and suggested that waxing and waning autoimmune dysfunction might account for the transient nature of the ovarian "failure" (8). O'Herlihy et al. (9) reported that up to one-fourth of younger women with elevated FSH levels in the menopausal range resume ovulation spontaneously and that a few will conceive. In 1982, we reported that 9 of 18 young women with presumptive ovarian failure had circulating levels of estradiol typical of women with functioning ovarian follicles and that four of the nine women who had ovarian biopsies had viable oocytes (10). Circulating concentrations of

R. W. Rebar: Department of Obstetrics and Gynecology, University of Cincinnati Medical Center, Cincinnati, Ohio 45267-0526.

serum progesterone typical of ovulation were observed in five women, and a spontaneous pregnancy occurred in one. Aiman and Smentek (11) reported that 18% of 157 women reported in the literature who had ovarian biopsies had specimens containing apparently viable oocytes. They also observed that 14 of the women had conceived after the ovarian failure had been diagnosed.

Several series have confirmed ovarian follicular activity in many women with ovarian failure. Hague et al. (12) reported evidence of ovarian follicular activity in 12 (17.1%) of 93 women with amenorrhea and elevated FSH levels. By pelvic ultrasound, Conway et al. (13) identified follicular activity in 65 (60%) of 109 women with idiopathic premature ovarian failure. Bone mineral density was lower in women in whom ovaries were not identified on ultrasound (n = 26) compared with those in whom follicles larger than 4 mm were identified (n = 57). Similarly, Nelson et al. (14) documented ovarian follicular activity by serum estradiol levels of greater than 50 pg/mL in nearly 50% of 65 women with karyotypically normal spontaneous premature ovarian failure and imaged an antral follicle in more than 40% (27) of the women. These observations led us to suggest that this disorder involved more than just the premature cessation of ovarian function and might more appropriately be called *hypergonadotropic amenorrhea* (13)—at least until such time as it was apparent that the premature loss of ovarian function was permanent.

CLINICAL FEATURES OF PREMATURE OVARIAN FAILURE

To define the clinical spectrum of women with hypergonadotropic amenorrhea, Rebar and Connolly (15) compiled the data from 115 affected women seen sequentially between 1978 and 1988. Initial inclusion criteria were amenorrhea of three or more months' duration, age less than 40 years at the onset of the amenorrhea, and circulating FSH levels of more than 40 mIU/mL on at least two occasions. Several interesting differences and similarities existed between those with primary and those with secondary amenorrhea and are summarized in Table 2.1.

In more than 75% of the patients, symptoms of estrogen deficiency, most commonly hot flushes and dyspareunia, were evident, but these symptoms were far more common in those with secondary amenorrhea. Failure to develop mature secondary sex characteristics and chromosomal abnormalities were far more common in those with primary amenorrhea. Chromosomal abnormalities were present in more than one-half of the women with primary amenorrhea, who tended to have deletions of all or a part of one X chromosome, whereas those with secondary amenorrhea more commonly had an additional X chromosome.

Easily detected immune disturbances occurred in approximately 20% of the patients. Thyroid abnormalities were most common, with five women having Hashimoto's thyroiditis, two developing primary hypothyroidism, one developing subacute thyroiditis, and one having Graves' disease. Three asymptomatic patients had high titers of antimicrosomal antibodies. One of the women had vitiligo and hypoparathyroidism; one had Addison's disease; and one additional woman had insulin-dependent diabetes mellitus.

A relatively small number of the women in this series, all with secondary amenorrhea, had received chemotherapy with alkylating agents and in some cases radiation therapy as well before developing hypergonadotropic amenorrhea. The effects of alkylating agents and radiation therapy on ovarian function have been recognized for several years (16). As young women with childhood malignancies, especially the various leukemias and lymphomas, are treated and cured, the incidence of such patients will no doubt increase.

Four of the patients with secondary amenorrhea and normal karyotypes had a family history of early menopause before age 40. Four others reported a temporal relationship between the onset of amenorrhea and various

TABLE 2.1. *Features of women with primary and secondary amenorrhea*

Characteristics	Primary amenorrhea[a]	Secondary amenorrhea[a]	Significant difference[b]
Number of patients	18 (15.7)	97 (84.3)	$p < 0.001$
Symptoms of estrogen deficiency	4 (22.2)	83 (85.6)	$p < 0.001$
Incomplete sexual development	16 (88.9)	8 (8.2)	$p < 0.001$
Karyotypic abnormalities	10 (55.6)	6/45 (13.3)[c]	$p < 0.01$
Immune abnormalities	4 (22.2)	16 (16.5)	NS
Spinal bone density <90% of controls	3/4 (75)[c]	13/22 (59.1)[c]	NS
Progestin-induced withdrawal bleeding	2/9 (22.2)[c]	36/70 (51.4)[c]	NS
Pregnancies before diagnosis	0	33 (34.0)	$p < 0.025$
Evidence of ovulation after diagnosis	0	23 (23.7)	$p < 0.05$
Pregnancies after diagnosis	0	8 (8.2)	NS

NS, not significant.
[a]Values in parentheses are percentages of the total number of primary and secondary cases.
[b]Results were calculated using the chi-square test.
[c]Percentages are determined for the number of cases per total number tested in each group.
Adapted from ref. 15.

infections, including chicken pox, shigellosis, malaria, and an undefined viral syndrome.

Spinal bone density, as evaluated by dual photon absorptiometry, was less than 90% (range, 62% to 105%; mean, 85.7%) of the mean value observed in age-matched controls in 16 of the 26 women who underwent such testing. Progestin-induced withdrawal bleeding, presumably an indication of endogenous estrogen levels and activity, occurred in just under 50% of the women tested. Withdrawal bleeding even occurred in two of the nine individuals with primary amenorrhea who were challenged. There was, however, no correlation between the response to exogenous progestin and subsequent ovulation.

None of the women with primary amenorrhea ever ovulated or conceived with her own oocytes. In contrast, over one-third of the women with secondary amenorrhea were pregnant at least once before developing hypergonadotropic amenorrhea, and almost one-fourth had evidence of ovulation after the diagnosis was established. However, only one-ninth (8.2%) of those with secondary amenorrhea later conceived.

Twenty-five of the patients with secondary amenorrhea were treated with clomiphene citrate to induce ovulation, but only four (16%) ovulated, as determined by serial ultrasound and serum progesterone levels. Because each of the four who ovulated had evidence of spontaneous episodic ovulation before therapy, it is unclear if the clomiphene actually induced ovulation or if ovulation occurred in association with clomiphene on the basis of chance alone. Fourteen women were suppressed for 1 to 3 months with large doses of exogenous estrogen and then administered human menopausal gonadotropins (from 50 to 100 ampules, with each ampule containing 75 IU of FSH and 75 IU of LH). We subsequently administered menotropins to five additional women suppressed previously for 1 to 3 months with a gonadotropin-releasing hormone agonist. Two of the patients suppressed with the agonist had evidence of significant follicular activity and ovulation, and one conceived. Ovulation induction is unlikely to be successful in these women.

Twelve women with secondary amenorrhea had ovarian biopsies, with apparently viable oocytes found in seven of the specimens. However, two of the eight subsequent pregnancies occurred in women with no follicles observed on biopsy. Seven of these eight pregnancies occurred while the patients were taking exogenous estrogen; the remaining pregnancy in this series occurred in response to clomiphene administration. Five of the eight pregnancies resulted in live term births, two ended in spontaneous abortion, and one was ended by elective abortion. Only three patients with primary amenorrhea underwent gonadal biopsy; the two with 46,XY karyotypes had dysgerminomas. The one additional patient had fibrous streaks.

These observations lead to the conclusion that hypergonadotropic amenorrhea is a heterogeneous disorder. No doubt many of these young women have premature ovarian failure, but others do not, as documented by subsequent ovulations and pregnancies. It would also seem logical to conclude that premature ovarian failure might be the end result of several varied disorders. Ovarian biopsy cannot be recommended in view of documented pregnancies in women who had no follicles found on biopsy. Because of the low incidence of ovulation and pregnancy among women undergoing ovulation induction, it is likewise difficult to recommend such efforts.

Moreover, these clinical observations stress the importance for subsequent management of measuring basal FSH levels in all amenorrheic women. Progestin-induced withdrawal cannot be used to identify women with chronic anovulation from those with impending ovarian failure.

PREVALENCE OF PREMATURE OVARIAN FAILURE

Estimation of the prevalence of premature ovarian failure in the general population is difficult. De Moraes-Ruehsen and Jones (1) found that 7% of 300 consecutive women presenting with amenorrhea had premature ovarian failure. Aiman and Smentek (11) combined the observations of several investigators to estimate the frequency of the disorder among American women. Based on the assumptions that 43 million American women were of reproductive age in 1985 and that the incidence of amenorrhea was 3%, they concluded that the frequency of premature ovarian failure is approximately 0.3%, with 129,000 American women being affected in that year. Alper et al. (17) estimated that 5% to 10% of women with secondary amenorrhea have this disorder. Coulam et al. (18) examined the medical records of 1,858 women living in Rochester, Minnesota, in 1950 and calculated that the risk of experiencing menopause before age 40 was 0.9%.

CAUSES OF PREMATURE OVARIAN FAILURE

De Moraes-Ruehsen and Jones (1) suggested three possible explanations for the early completion of atresia that they believed to exist in women with hypergonadotropic amenorrhea and premature ovarian failure: decreased germ cell endowment, accelerated atresia, and postnatal germ cell destruction. Because these possibilities cannot hold in individuals in whom many follicles still remain, some block to gonadotropin action in ovarian follicles must exist.

In view of data that even postmenopausal women may have a few remaining follicles (19,20) and previously cited information that follicle number decreases rapidly in the last several months before menopause (2), it is possible that a few women who are truly perimenopausal may ovulate or conceive. Among the various causes of hypergonadotropic amenorrhea that can be identified, some are present only in those who have no oocytes, whereas others may have the potential for ovulation and spontaneous pregnancy. Possible causes of hypergonadotropic amenorrhea and premature ovarian failure are listed in Table 2.2.

TABLE 2.2. *Causes of hypergonadotropic amenorrhea*

I. Genetic and cytogenetic causes
   A. "Familial" premature ovarian failure
      1. FSH receptor mutations
      2. Fragile X permutations
   B. Structural alterations or absence of an X chromosome
   C. Trisomy X with or without mosaicism
   D. Associated with myotonia dystrophica
II. Enzymatic defects
   A. 17α-Hydroxylase deficiency
   B. Galactosemia
III. Physical insults
   A. Ionizing radiation
   B. Chemotherapeutic agents
   C. Viral infection
   D. Cigarette smoking
   E. Surgical extirpation
IV. Immune disturbances
   A. Associated with other autoimmune disorders
   B. Isolated
   C. Congenital thymic aplasia
V. Defects in gonadotropin structure or actions (genetic?)
   A. Secretion of biologically inactive gonadotropin
   B. α or β subunit defects
   C. Gonadotropin receptor or postreceptor defects
   D. Circulating FSH-binding inhibitors
VI. Idiopathic

FSH, follicle-stimulating hormone.

Genetic and Cytogenetic Causes

Familial Premature Ovarian Failure

Several reports have described individual families with vertical transmission of premature ovarian failure, implying autosomal dominant, sex-linked inheritance (21–23). In such families, the cause may be one of the three reasons postulated by de Moraes-Ruehsen and Jones (1). The number of oocytes differs widely among various strains of mice (24). Moreover, individual mice (3,24) and humans (25–27) have markedly different rates of follicular atresia. It is possible that the cause of the premature ovarian failure occurring in some individuals with the neurologic disorder myotonia dystrophica also is caused by a decreased endowment in germ cell number or accelerated atresia (28).

Molecular biology has provided explanations for some familial cases of hypergonadotropic ovarian failure. Aittomäki et al. (29) showed that a mutation in exon 7 of the FSH receptor gene located on chromosome 2P, in which an Ala to Val substitution at residue 189, was present in six Finnish families with multiple affected women. The histologic appearance of the ovaries of women with this FSH receptor mutation showed hypoplasia with few primordial follicles (30). None had the appearance of complete ovarian dysgenesis with streak ovaries. That such FSH receptor abnormalities are rare causes of ovarian failure is suggested by a study in Great Britain failing to identify any such mutations in 30 women with sporadic premature ovarian failure and in 18 women with familial premature ovarian failure (31).

Women carrying one X chromosome with a fragile X permutation have an increased prevalence of premature menopause (32). Fragile X syndrome is the most common inherited form of male retardation and is caused by an expansion of a trinucleotide repeat sequence in the first exon of the *FMR1* gene (Xq27.3). The full fragile X mutation occurs when the number of trinucleotide repeats is in excess of 200 and when gene transcription fails and the FMR1 protein is not expressed (33). In normal individuals, there are fewer than 50 trinucleotide repeats at this fragile site, and a fragile X premutation is said to occur when 50 to 200 trinucleotide repeats exist. Fragile X permutations occur at least 10 times more frequently in women with premature ovarian failure than in the general population (34). However, no causal link has been shown. Because the *FMR1* gene is expressed in the brain and in the gonad, the fragile X premutation may not be as innocent as one thought (35).

Gonadal Dysgenesis

Studies of individuals with gonadal dysgenesis have documented that two intact X chromosomes are needed for normal maintenance of oocytes. The gonads of 45,X fetuses contain the normal complement of oocytes at 20 to 24 weeks of fetal age, only to have those oocytes rapidly undergo atresia so that virtually none remain at birth (36). Structural abnormalities of the X chromosome also can affect ovarian function and have been found in women with premature ovarian failure (7,11,37). Even submicroscopic deletions of a portion of the X chromosome apparently can lead to premature ovarian failure (38).

Trisomy X with or without Mosaicism

An excess of X chromosomes also may be found in some women who develop premature menopause (39). Patients have developed normal secondary sex characteristics and only later presented with secondary hypergonadotropic amenorrhea. Reports of the triple-X syndrome associated with immunoglobulin deficiency (40) and Marfan syndrome (41), together with the observation that control of T-cell function may be related to the X chromosome (42), suggest a possible association between immunologic abnormalities and triple-X females with premature ovarian failure.

Enzymatic Defects

17α-Hydroxylase Deficiency

The rare women with deficiency of the 17α-hydroxylase enzyme are identified easily because of the associated findings of primary amenorrhea, sexual infantilism, hypergonadotropinism, hypertension, hypokalemic alkalosis, and increased circulating levels of deoxycorticosterone and progesterone (43–45). Ovarian biopsies have revealed numerous large cysts and follicular cysts, with complete failure of follicular maturation (45).

Galactosemia

Women with galactosemia develop amenorrhea with elevated gonadotropin levels even when treatment with a galactose-restricted diet begins at an early age (46,47). Although the cause of the premature ovarian failure in galactosemia is unknown, it is tempting to speculate that the carbohydrate moieties on gonadotropin molecules are altered such that they are biologically inactive or their metabolism is changed. Unfortunately, this postulate does not coincide with experimental data suggesting a direct effect of galactose on the oocyte. Pregnant rats fed a 50% galactose diet delivered pups with significantly reduced numbers of oocytes, apparently because of decreased germ cell migration to the genital ridges (48).

Physical Insults

Oocytes may be destroyed by any of several environmental insults, including ionizing radiation, various chemotherapeutic agents, certain viral infections, and even cigarette smoking (49).

Ionizing Radiation

Approximately 50% of individuals who receive 4 to 5 cGy to the ovaries for more than 4 to 6 weeks, as may occur in treatment for Hodgkin's disease, develop permanent hypergonadotropic amenorrhea (16,50,51). For any given dose of radiation, the older the woman, the greater is the likelihood of her developing amenorrhea. It appears that a total of 8 cGy is sufficient to result in permanent sterility in all women (50,51).

That the amenorrhea after radiation therapy is not always permanent was reported by Jacox in 1939 (52). The transient nature of the amenorrhea in some women suggests that some follicles may be damaged but not destroyed by relatively low doses of radiation. Although it is common practice to transpose the ovaries surgically outside of the field of irradiation, it is not clear just how fertile such women ultimately are.

Chemotherapeutic Agents

As more and more young women treated for childhood malignancies, especially leukemias and lymphomas, survive for several years, it has become obvious that chemotherapeutic agents may produce temporary or permanent ovarian failure (16,53–57). The alkylating agents, particularly cyclophosphamide, are most likely to affect reproductive function. In general, the younger the woman at the time of therapy, the more likely it is that ovarian function will not be compromised by chemotherapy. The number of oocytes present at the time of therapy may

determine whether ovarian function becomes compromised; the greater the number of oocytes, the more likely it is that normal ovarian function will persist. The frequency of congenital anomalies does not appear to be increased in the children of women previously treated with chemotherapy (58). However, dactinomycin may be associated with an increased risk of congenital heart disease, and further studies in this area are needed.

Viral and Other Agents

Although several viruses are believed to have the potential to cause ovarian destruction, confirming that such is the case in humans is difficult. Morrison et al. (59) reported three presumptive cases in which "mumps oophoritis" preceded premature ovarian failure, including cases in which the mother documented mumps parotiditis and abdominal pain during pregnancy just before delivery of a daughter. Although there is no evidence that cigarette smoking leads to premature menopause, data do show that cigarette smokers experience menopause several months before nonsmokers (60).

Immune Disturbances

Any role for immune disturbances in the cause of hypergonadotropic amenorrhea remains controversial. Several autoimmune abnormalities may be associated with hypogonadotropic amenorrhea (Table 2.3). However, the incidence of autoimmune abnormalities in normal women is unknown, and it be that their incidence is not increased in cases of ovarian failure. Moreover, it is not clear whether

TABLE 2.3. *Autoimmune disorders associated with premature ovarian failure*

Alopecia
Anemia, both acquired hemolytic and pernicious
Asthma
Chronic active hepatitis
Crohn's disease
Diabetes mellitus
Glomerulonephritis
Hypoadrenalism (Addison's disease)
Hypoparathyroidism
Hypophysitis
Idiopathic thrombocytopenia purpura
Juvenile rheumatoid arthritis
Keratoconjunctivitis and Sjögren's syndrome
Malabsorption syndrome
Myasthenia gravis
Polyendocrinopathies (type I, type II, and unspecified)
Primary biliary cirrhosis
Quantitative immunoglobulin abnormalities
Rheumatoid arthritis
Systematic lupus erythematosus
Thyroid disorders, including Graves' disease and thyroiditis
Vitiligo

Adapted from refs. 7 and 61.

the autoimmune disturbances play any role in the development of hypergonadotropic amenorrhea. As is characteristic for other autoimmune disturbances, the ovarian failure in affected women may wax and wane, and pregnancies may occur early in the disease process.

In a review tabulating 380 cases of premature ovarian failure in the literature, LaBarbera et al. (61) found that 17.5% had a definite autoimmune disorder associated with their ovarian failures. Additional evidence that hypergonadotropic amenorrhea may have an autoimmune origin in at least some cases has been provided by sporadic case reports documenting return of ovarian function after immunosuppressive therapy or recovery from an autoimmune disease (62–64). In a few cases, lymphocytic infiltrates suggesting autoimmune dysfunction have been observed in ovarian biopsy specimens (65).

Still other immune abnormalities have been identified in some patients with premature ovarian failure. Enhanced release of leukocyte migration inhibition factor by peripheral lymphocytes has been observed after exposure of the lymphocytes to crude ovarian proteins (66,67). A significant association of early ovarian failure with human leukocyte antigen DR3 has been observed (68), perhaps suggesting a genetic susceptibility to autoimmunity in some individuals. Several years ago McNatty et al. (69) reported complement-dependent cytotoxic effects on cultured granulosa cells, as documented by inhibition of progesterone production and cell lysis, in sera from 9 of 23 patients with hypergonadotropic amenorrhea and Addison's disease. Cellular immune abnormalities, including abnormalities in the numbers or function of peripheral monocytes and of subsets of T cells and B cells, have also been observed in women with premature ovarian failure (70).

Indirect immunofluorescence of ovarian biopsy specimens has revealed antibodies reacting with various ovarian components in some patients (71). Circulating immunoglobulins to ovarian proteins have been detected by immunocytochemical techniques by several investigators (61). Using a solid-phase, enzyme-linked immunosorbent assay, we have detected antibodies to ovarian tissue in 22% of karyotypically normal women with premature ovarian failure (72,73). The most thorough study is that of Chiauzzi et al. (74), who documented that two patients with ovarian failure and myasthenia gravis had circulating immunoglobulin G that blocked binding of FSH to its receptor. However, it is important to reiterate that ovarian autoantibodies may not be the cause of ovarian failure. The ovarian failure instead may result from cell-mediated autoimmunity, and autoantibodies may appear only because of the resultant cell death. However, Anasti et al. (75) failed to demonstrate the presence of blocking antibodies to LH or FSH receptors in any of 38 premature ovarian failure patients studied.

There has been increasing interest in the relation between the immune system and reproductive system. Miller and Chatten (76) documented that congenitally

athymic girls dying before puberty had ovaries devoid of oocytes on autopsy. Data from our laboratory suggest that the thymus gland may be necessary early in development for normal gonadotropin function. Congenitally athymic mice, well known to develop premature ovarian failure, have lower gonadotropin concentrations prepubertally than do their normal heterozygous littermates (77). These hormonal alterations and the accelerated loss of oocytes can be prevented by thymic transplantation at birth (78). In comparing ovarian development in the rodent to that of the primate, it is essential to recognize that development occurring during the first few weeks of life in the mouse occurs *in utero* in the human female. Thymic ablation in fetal rhesus monkeys in late gestation is associated with a marked reduction in oocyte number at birth (79). One possible explanation for the association of thymic aplasia and ovarian failure may be found in our observation that peptides produced by the thymus can stimulate release of gonadotropin-releasing hormone (GnRH) and consequently LH (80).

Organ-specific autoimmunity may be directed against intracellular enzymes, particularly those involved in hormone synthesis (70,81). For example, thyroid peroxidase is a major thyroid autoantigen for autoimmune hypothyroidism and the 21-hydroxylase enzyme is the foremost autoantigen in Addison's disease. One group has identified 3β-hydroxysteroid dehydrogenase as an autoantigen in 20% of women with premature ovarian failure (82). This also may be an epiphenomenon of ovarian inflammation rather than causal for the development of ovarian failure.

From a theoretical viewpoint, identifying patients with an autoimmune origin for their hypergonadotropic amenorrhea is important because affected patients may be treated effectively early in the disease process before all viable oocytes are destroyed.

Defects in Gonadotropin Structure or Action

Abnormal structure, secretion, or metabolism of gonadotropins in some women may form the basis for early ovarian failure. The concept of secretion of altered molecular forms of FSH with reduced or absent biologic activity leading to accelerated follicular atresia, even as a rare cause for premature ovarian failure, is appealing. This is especially true given evidence that normal levels of gonadotropins are required early in development: fetal hypophysectomy in rhesus monkeys leads to the newborn having no oocytes in their ovaries (83). Moreover, cases of male pseudohermaphroditism with immunologically active but biologically inactive LH are well documented (84,85). Altered forms of immunoreactive LH and FSH have been reported in urinary extracts from women with premature ovarian failure compared with those from oophorectomized and postmenopausal women (86), suggesting that metabolism or excretion of gonadotropins is altered in some cases of this disorder. However, using two different probes for the β subunit of FSH and two probes for the FSH receptor gene, one group failed to find any mutations in a small group of patients (87). These findings do not exclude mutations in other patients and in different portions of the molecule.

Interference with FSH action at the ovarian level may lead to early ovarian failure. Theoretically, defects in FSH receptor structure [as reported in the Finnish study (29)], FSH receptor antibodies, competitive inhibitors to FSH binding, and defects in postreceptor systems that mediate hormone action are each possible. Sluss and Schneyer (88) reported identifying two individuals in a group of 27 with hypergonadotropic amenorrhea (and intermittent evidence of ovarian function) whose sera had low-molecular-weight FSH receptor-binding activity that was an antagonist of FSH action. Even when this inhibitor was removed from the serum, FSH levels were elevated in both patients. Their studies cannot eliminate the possibility that this FSH binding inhibitor is merely produced secondarily to development of ovarian insensitivity to FSH. Other possible defects in gonadotropin action remain to be identified. All of these disorders may be genetic abnormalities.

Idiopathic Causes

The diagnosis of "idiopathic" causes of premature ovarian failure is a diagnosis of exclusion, but no definitive cause is identified in most cases of hypergonadotropic amenorrhea. It is likely that additional causes of this entity will be recognized as more is learned about premature ovarian failure.

Resistant Ovary Syndrome: A Term No Longer Useful

As originally defined, the resistant ovary or Savage syndrome was found in young amenorrheic women with elevated peripheral gonadotropin levels, normal but immature follicles in the ovaries, a 46,XX karyotype, mature secondary sex characteristics, and decreased sensitivity to stimulation with exogenous gonadotropin (89). Individuals fulfilling these criteria may have any of several different causes for their hypergonadotropic amenorrhea. Moreover, regardless of the cause, these features may be common to all individuals with hypergonadotropic amenorrhea at some time during the disease process before final loss of all oocytes. As a consequence, use of the term *resistant ovary* will become less and less useful as understanding of ovarian failure increases and is already of severely restricted value.

EVALUATION OF PATIENTS WITH HYPERGONADOTROPIC AMENORRHEA

Young women with hypergonadotropic amenorrhea should be evaluated to identify specific, potentially treat-

able causes and other potentially dangerous associated disorders. A thorough history and physical examination are always warranted. A maturation index and evaluation of the cervical mucus may help determine if any endogenous estrogen is present.

Simple laboratory tests should be performed to exclude thyroid disease, hypoparathyroidism, hypoadrenalism, diabetes mellitus, and other evidence of autoimmune dysfunction. The extent of such testing is unclear, but a reasonable set of tests are listed in Table 2.4. In addition to the clinical evaluation of estrogen status, measurement of circulating LH, FSH, and estradiol concentrations on more than one occasion may help determine if any functional follicles are present. If the estradiol concentration is greater than 50 pg/mL or the LH level is greater than the FSH (in terms of mIU/mL) in any sample, a few viable oocytes must be present. Irregular uterine bleeding, indicative of continuing estrogen production, also suggests the presence of remaining functional oocytes. Identifiable follicles on transvaginal ultrasonography also can be used to identify women with remaining oocytes (90) and are present in a large percentage of affected women (12,13,90).

If available, testing of the patient's serum for antibodies to endocrine tissues, including the ovary, may be of some value. The difficulty with this recommendation is the fact that there are no readily available tests for antibodies to any specific antigens. Antibodies may develop because of cytotoxicity in the ovary and may not cause ovarian failure.

For which patients chromosomal studies should be conducted is also unclear. It would seem prudent to obtain a karyotype for women with the onset of hypergonadotropic amenorrhea before the age of 30 to identify those with various forms of gonadal dysgenesis, individuals with mosaicism, those with trisomy X, and those with a portion of a Y chromosome. If a Y chromosome is present, gonadal extirpation is warranted because of the

TABLE 2.4. *Evaluation of hypergonadotropic amenorrhea in young women*

Complete history and physical examination
Maturation index
Karyotype (may be limited to women with onset before age 30)
Complete blood cell count with differential cell count, sedimentation rate, total serum protein and albumin-globulin ratio, rheumatoid factor, antinuclear antibody
Fasting blood sugar level, serum calcium and phosphorus concentrations, evaluation of adrenal status
Thyroxine, thyroid-stimulating hormone, anti-thyroglobulin and anti-microsomal antibodies or anti-thyroid stimulating immunoglobulins (TSI)
Luteinizing hormone, follicle-stimulating hormone, and estradiol levels on at least two occasions
Evaluation of bone density

Adapted from ref. 7.

increased risk of malignancy (91–93). Chromosomal evaluation also may be warranted to exclude familial transmission in women who develop hypergonadotropic amenorrhea after the birth of daughters.

Although controversial, ovarian biopsy does not appear justified in women with hypergonadotropic amenorrhea and a normal karyotype. It is not clear how the results would alter therapy. Aiman and Smentek (15) reported one of their two patients who eventually conceived had no oocytes found on biopsy. Similarly, Rebar and Connolly (13) observed that two of eight subsequent pregnancies among 97 women with secondary hypergonadotropic amenorrhea occurred in women with no follicles present in ovarian tissue obtained by laparotomy. As observed by Aiman and Smentek (11), if five sections of an ovarian biopsy are examined and each is 6 μm thick, the presence of follicles is sought from a sample representing less than 0.15% of a 2 × 3 × 4 cm ovary. The absence of follicles on biopsy may not be representative of the remainder of the ovary. Moreover, affected individuals almost always require estrogen replacement regardless of the results of the biopsy.

Evaluation of bone density appears warranted in women with hypergonadotropic amenorrhea because of the high incidence of osteopenia (13,15,90). Periodic assessment may be warranted, regardless of therapy, to assess the rapidity of bone loss. Similarly, monitoring patients for the development of autoimmune endocrinopathies may be warranted even if all tests are normal when the patient is first evaluated; development of other disorders after diagnosis of hypergonadotropic amenorrhea does occur (15).

THERAPY

It is reasonable to treat all young women with hypergonadotropic amenorrhea with exogenous estrogen whether they are interested in childbearing or not. The accelerated bone loss and increased risk of cardiovascular disease frequently accompanying this disorder may be prevented by administration of exogenous estrogens (90,94). Although it also appears that women with premature ovarian failure are at reduced risk of breast cancer (95) and probably venous thrombosis, the hope is that administration of exogenous estrogen merely returns these relative risks to those found in normal premenopausal women.

Almost all spontaneous pregnancies in women with this disorder occur during or after estrogen administration (15,96). Even with exogenous estrogens, however, the probability of spontaneous pregnancy appears to be less than 10%. The pregnancy rate is low despite the fact that one-fourth or more of women ovulate after the diagnosis of hypergonadotropic amenorrhea is made. Because of the possibility of pregnancy, women taking exogenous estrogens in any form, even as part of oral contraceptive agents, should be advised to contact their physician if

they develop any signs or symptoms of pregnancy or do not have withdrawal bleeding. Although it may not be necessary to advise the use of barrier forms of contraception, the possibility of pregnancy must be discussed. Oral contraceptives or sequential estrogen-progestin therapy may be used, but sequential therapy is more physiologic. These young women may require twice as much estrogen as menopausal women to alleviate signs and symptoms of hypoestrogenism.

Several isolated case reports have suggested that ovarian suppression with estrogen or a GnRH agonist followed by stimulation with human menopausal gonadotropin may be efficacious in inducing ovulation and allowing conception (97–100). Most of these reports emanate from one group. Larger series suggest the possibility of successful ovulation induction and pregnancy is small and may be no greater than what concurs spontaneously in these patients (14,15,101).

In vitro fertilization involving oocyte donation clearly provides individuals with hypergonadotropic amenorrhea with the greatest likelihood of bearing children. The first successful case of oocyte donation in humans was reported in 1984. A young women with ovarian failure was given oral estradiol valerate and progesterone pessaries to prepare the endometrium for transfer of a single donated oocyte after fertilization with her husband's sperm (102). Since then, several programs using oocyte donation have been successful because of improvements in transvaginal ultrasonography allowing follicular aspiration and oocyte collection without surgery, improvements in success with embryo cryopreservation and subsequent embryo transfer to the donor at a later time, and an improved ability to synchronize artificial cycles in the recipient with the hyperstimulation cycles in the donor, generally by use of GnRH agonists (103–105). Several replacement protocols have been developed for the donor with hypergonadotropic amenorrhea, including use of oral, transvaginal, and transdermal administration of estradiol and oral, transvaginal, and intramuscular administration or progesterone. If pregnancy develops from the transferred embryo, given the absence of functional gonads in the recipient, exogenous supplementation with estradiol and progesterone must be continued until placental production of progesterone is well established. Success rates generally have exceeded those observed in standard *in vitro* fertilization programs (103–106). Oocyte donation offers the possibility of pregnancy to all women with premature ovarian failure so long as a normal uterus is present.

REFERENCES

1. De Moraes M, Jones GS. Premature ovarian failure. *Fertil Steril* 1967;18:440.
2. Richardson SJ, Senikas V, Nelson JF. Follicular depletion during the menopausal transition: evidence for accelerated loss and ultimate exhaustion. *J Clin Endocrinol Metab* 1987;65:1231–1237.
3. Spearow JL, Barkley M. Mapping genes controlling induced ovulation rate in

mice [Abstract #1462]. Abstracts of the 74th Annual Meeting of The Endocrine Society, San Antonio, TX, June 24–27, 1992:417.

4. Simpson JL, Rebar RW. Normal and abnormal sexual differentiation and development. In: Becker KL, Bilezikian JP, Bremner, et al., eds. *Principles and practice of endocrinology and metabolism,* 2nd ed. Philadelphia: JB Lippincott, 1995.

5. Parkening TA, Collins TJ, Elder FFB. Orthotopic ovarian transplantations in young and aged C57BL/6J mice. *Biol Reprod* 1985;32:989–997.

6. Goldenberg RL, Grodin JM, Rodbard D, Ross GT. Gonadotropins in women with amenorrhea. *Am J Obstet Gynecol* 1973;116:1003–1012.

7. Rebar RW, Erickson GF, Coulam CB. Premature ovarian failure. In: Gondos B, Riddick D, eds. *Pathology of infertility.* New York: Thieme Medical Publishers, 1987;123–141.

8. Lucky AW, Rebar RW, Blizzard RM, Goren EM. Pubertal progression in the presence of elevated serum gonadotropins in girls with multiple endocrine deficiencies. *J Clin Endocrinol Metab* 1977;45:673–678.

9. O'Herlihy C, Pepperell RJ, Evans JH. The significance of FSH elevation in young women with disorders of ovulation. *BMJ* 1980;281:1447.

10. Rebar RW, Erickson GF, Yen SSC. "Idiopathic premature ovarian failure": clinical and endocrine characteristics. *Fertil Steril* 1982;37:35–41.

11. Aiman J, Smentek C. Premature ovarian failure. *Obstet Gynecol* 1985;66:9–14.

12. Hague WM, Tan SL, Adams J, Jacobs HS. Hypergonadotropic amenorrhea—etiology and outcome in 93 young women. *Int J Gynaecol Obstet* 1987;25: 121–125.

13. Conway GS, Kaltsas G, Patel A, Davies MC, Jacobs HS. Characterization of idiopathic premature ovarian failure. *Fertil Steril* 1996;65:337–341.

14. Nelson LM, Kimzey LM, Merriam GR. Gonadotropin suppression for the treatment of karyotypically normal spontaneous premature ovarian failure: a controlled trial. *Fertil Steril* 1992;57:50–55.

15. Rebar RW, Connolly HV. Clinical feature of young women with hypergonadotropic amenorrhea. *Fertil Steril* 1990;53:804–810.

16. Siris ES, Leventhal BG, Vaitukaitis JL. Effects of childhood leukemia and chemotherapy on puberty and reproductive function in girls. *N Engl J Med* 1976; 294:1143–1146.

17. Alper MM, Garner PR, Cher B, Seibel MM. Premature ovarian failure. *J Reprod Med* 1986;31:699–708.

18. Coulam CB, Adamson SC, Annegers JF. Incidence of premature ovarian failure. *Obstet Gynecol* 1986;67:604–606.

19. Costoff A, Mahesh VB. Primordial follicles with normal oocytes in the ovaries of postmenopausal women. *J Am Geriatr Soc* 1975;23:193–196.

20. Hertig AT. The aging ovary—a preliminary note. *J Clin Endocrinol Metab* 1944; 4:581–582.

21. Coulam CB, Stringfellow SS, Hoefnagel D. Evidence for a genetic factor in the etiology of premature ovarian failure. *Fertil Steril* 1983;40:693–695.

22. Mattison DR, Evans MI, Schwimmer WB, et al. Familial premature ovarian failure. *Am J Hum Genet* 1984;36:1341–1348.

23. Starup J, Philip J, Sele V. Oestrogen treatment and subsequent pregnancy in two patients with severe hypergonadotropic ovarian failure. *Acta Endocrinol* 1978;89:149–157.

24. Jones EC, Krohn PL. The relationship between age, numbers of oocytes and fertility in virgin and multiparous mice. *J Endocrinol* 1961;21:469–495.

25. Baker TG. A quantitative and cytological study of germ cells in human ovaries. *R Soc Lond Proc Series B Biol Sci* 1963;158:417–433.

26. Block E. Quantitative morphological investigations of the follicular system in women: variations at different ages. *Acta Anat* 1952;14:108–123.

27. Block E. A quantitative morphological investigation of the follicular system in newborn female infants. *Acta Anat* 1953;17:201–206.

28. Harper PS, Dyken PR. Early onset dystrophia myotonia. *Lancet* 1972;2:53–55.

29. Aittomäki K, Lucena JLD, Pakarinen P, et al. Mutation in the follicle-stimulating hormone receptor gene causes hereditary hypergonadotropic ovarian failure. *Cell* 1995;82:959–968.

30. Aittomäki K, Herva U-H, Juntunen K, et al. Clinical features of primary ovarian failure caused by a point mutation in the follicle-stimulating hormone receptor gene. *J Clin Endocrinol Metab* 1996;81:3722–3726.

31. Conway E. Hoppner W, Gromoll J, Simoni M, Conway GS. Mutations of the FSH receptor gene are rare in familial and sporadic premature ovarian failure. *J Endocrinol* 1997;152[Suppl]:P257(abst).

32. Turner G, Robinson H, Wake S, Martin S. Dizygous twinning and premature menopause in fragile X syndrome [Letter]. *Lancet* 1994;344:1500.

33. Jacobs PA. Fragile X syndrome. *J Med Genet* 1991;28:809–810.

34. Conway GS, Hettiarachchi S, Murray A, Jacobs PA. Fragile X permutations in familial premature ovarian failure. *Lancet* 1995;346:309–310.

35. Hinds HL, Ashley CL, Sutcliffe JS, et al. Tissue specific expression of FMR-1 provides evidence for a functional role in fragile X syndrome. *Nat Genet* 1993;2: 197–200.

36. Singh RP, Carr DH. The anatomy and histology of XO human embryos and fetuses. *Anat Rec* 1966;155:369–381.

37. Kinch RAH, Plunkett ER, Smout MS, Carr DH. Primary ovarian failure: a clinicopathological and cytogenetic study. *Am J Obstet Gynecol* 1965;91:630–644.

38. Krauss CM, Turksoy RN, Atkins L, Laughlin C, Brown LG, Page DC. Familial premature ovarian failure due to an interstitial deletion of the long arm of the X chromosome. *N Engl J Med* 1987;317:125–131.

39. Villanueva AL, Rebar RW. The triple X syndrome and premature ovarian failure. *Obstet Gynecol* 1983;62:705–735.

40. Sills JA, Brown JK, Grace S, Wood SM, Barclay GR, Urbaniak SJ. XXX syndrome associated with immunoglobulin deficiency and epilepsy. *J Pediatr* 1978; 93:469–471.

41. Smith TF, Engel E. Marfan's syndrome with 47,XXX genotype and possible immunologic abnormality. *South Med J* 1981;74:630–632.

42. Purtillo DT, DeFlorio D Jr, Hutt LH, et al. Variable phenotypic expression of an X-linked recessive lymphoproliferative syndrome. *N Engl J Med* 1977;279: 1077–1082.

43. Bigleri EG, Herron MA, Brust N. 17-Hydroxylation deficiency in man. *J Clin Invest* 1966;45:1946–1954.

44. Goldsmith O, Solomon DH, Horton R. Hypogonadism and mineralocorticoid excess: the 17-hydroxylase deficiency syndrome. *N Engl J Med* 1967;277: 673–677.

45. Mallin SR. Congenital adrenal hyperplasia secondary to 17-hydroxylase deficiency: two sisters with amenorrhea, hypokalemia, hypertension, and cystic ovaries. *Ann Intern Med* 1969;70:69–75.

46. Hoefnagel D, Wurster-Hili D, Child EL. Ovarian failure in galactosemia. *Lancet* 1979;2:1197.

47. Kaufman FR, Kogut MD, Donnell GN, Goebelsmann U, March C, Koch R. Hypergonadotropic hypogonadism in female patients with galactosemia. *N Engl J Med* 1981;304:994–998.

48. Chen Y-T, Mattison DR, Feigenbaum L, Fukui H, Schulman JD. Reduction in oocyte number following prenatal exposure to a diet high in galactose. *Science* 1981;214:1145–1147.

49. Verp MS. Environmental causes of ovarian failure. *Semin Reprod Endocrinol* 1983;1:101–11.

50. Ash P. The influence of radiation on fertility in man. *Br J Radiol* 1980;53: 271–278.

51. Ray GR, Trueblood HW, Enright LP, Kaplan HS, Nelsen TS. Oophoropexy: a means of preserving ovarian function following pelvic megavoltage radiotherapy for Hodgkin's disease. *Radiology* 1970;96:175–180.

52. Jacox HW. Recovery following human ovarian irradiation. *Radiology* 1939;32: 538–545.

53. Damewood MD, Grochow LB. Prospects for fertility after chemotherapy or radiation for neoplastic disease. *Fertil Steril* 1986;45:443–459.

54. Horning SJ, Hoppe RT, Kaplan HS, Rosenberg SA. Female reproductive potential after treatment for Hodgkin's disease. *N Engl J Med* 1981;304:1377–1382.

55. Koyama H, Wada T, Nishizawa Y, et al. Cyclophosphamide-induced ovarian failure and its therapeutic significance in patients with breast cancer. *Cancer* 1977; 39:1403–1409.

56. Stillman RJ, Schiff I, Schinfeld J. Reproductive and gonadal function in the female after therapy for childhood malignancy. *Obstet Gynecol Surv* 1982;37: 385–393.

57. Whitehead E, Shalet SM, Blackledge G, Crowther D, Beardwell CG. The effect of combination chemotherapy on ovarian function in women treated for Hodgkin's disease. *Cancer* 1983;52:988–993.

58. Green DM, Zevon MA, Lowrie G, Seigelstein N, Hall B. Congenital anomalies in children of patients who received chemotherapy for cancer in childhood and adolescence. *N Engl J Med* 1991;325:141–146.

59. Morrison JC, Givens JR, Wiser WL, Fisk SA. Mumps oophoritis: a cause of premature menopause. *Fertil Steril* 1975;26:655–659.

60. Jick H, Porte J, Morrison AS. Relation between smoking and age of natural menopause. *Lancet* 1977;1:1354–1355.

61. LaBarbera AR, Miller MM, Ober C, Rebar RW. Autoimmune etiology in premature ovarian failure. *Am J Reprod Immunol Microbiol* 1988;16:115–122.

62. Bateman BG, Nunley WC, Kitchin JD III. Reversal of apparent premature ovarian failure in a patient with myasthenia gravis. *Fertil Steril* 1983;39:108–110.

63. Coulam CB, Kempers RD, Randall RV. Premature ovarian failure: evidence for the autoimmune mechanism. *Fertil Steril* 1981;36:238–240.

64. Lucky AW, Rebar RW, Blizzard RM, Goren EM. Pubertal progression in the presence of elevated serum gonadotropins in girls with multiple endocrine deficiencies. *J Clin Endocrinol Metab* 1977;45:673–678.

65. Rabinowe SL, Berger MJ, Welch WR, et al. Lymphocyte dysfunction in autoimmune oophoritis: resumption of menses with corticosteroids. *Am J Obstet Gynecol* 1986;81:348.

66. Edmonds M, Lamki L, Killinger DW, Volpé R. Autoimmune thyroiditis, adrenalitis, and oophoritis. *Am J Med* 1973;54:782–787.

67. Pekonen F, Siegberg R, Mäkinen T, Miettinen A, Yli-Korkala O. Immunological disturbances in patients with premature ovarian failure. *Clin Endocrinol (Oxf)* 1986;25:1–6.

68. Walfish PG, Gottesman IS, Shewchuk AB, Bain J, Hawe BS, Fared NR. Association of premature ovarian failure with HLA antigens. *Tissue Antigens* 1983;21: 168–169.

69. McNatty KP, Short RV, Barnes EW, Irvine WJ. The cytotoxic effect of serum from patients with Addison's disease and autoimmune ovarian failure on human granulosa cells in culture. *Clin Exp Immunol* 1975;22:378–384.

70. Hoek A, Shoemaker J, Drexhage HA. Premature ovarian failure and ovarian autoimmunity. *Endocr Rev* 1997;18:107–134.

71. Muechler EK, Huang K-E, Schenk E. Autoimmunity in premature ovarian failure. *Int J Fertil* 1991;36:99–103.

72. Kim JG, Anderson BE, Rebar RW, LaBarbera AR. Determination by ELISA of antiovarian antibodies in premature ovarian failure [Abstract 0-100]. Program of the 45th Annual Meeting of the American Fertility Society, San Francisco, November 13–16, 1989:542.

73. Kim MH. "Gonadotropin-resistant ovaries" syndrome in association with secondary amenorrhea. *Am J Obstet Gynecol* 1974;120:257.

74. Chiauzzi V, Cigorraga S, Escobar ME, Rivarola MA, Charreau EH. Inhibition of follicle-stimulating hormone receptor binding by circulating immunoglobulins. *J Clin Endocrinol* 1982;54:1221–1228.

75. Anasti JN, Flack MR, Froelich J, Nelson LM. The use of human recombinant gonadotropin receptors to search for immunoglobulin G-mediated premature ovarian failure. *J Clin Endocrinol Metab* 1995;80:824–828.

76. Miller ME, Chatten J. Ovarian changes in ataxia telangiectasia. *Acta Paediatr Scand* 1967;56:559–561.

77. Rebar RW, Morandini IC, Erickson GF, Petze JE. The hormonal basis of reproductive defects in athymic mice. I. Diminished gonadotropin concentrations in prepubertal females. *Endocrinology* 1981;108:120–126.

78. Rebar RW, Morandini IC, Benirschke K, Petze JE. Reduced gonadotropins in athymic mice: prevention by thymic transplantation. *Endocrinology* 1980;107:2130–2132.

79. Healy DL, Bacher J, Hodgen GD. Thymic regulation of primate fetal ovarian-adrenal differentiation. *Biol Reprod* 1985;32:1127–1133.

80. Rebar RW, Miyake A, Low TLK, Goldstein AL. Thymosin stimulates secretion of luteinizing hormone-releasing factor. *Science* 1981;214:669–671.

81. Weetman AP. Autoimmunity to steroid-producing cells and familial polyendocrine autoimmunity. *Baillieres Clin Endocrinol Metab* 1995;9:157–174.

82. Arif S, Vallian S, Farazneh F, et al. Identification of 3 beta-hydroxysteroid dehydrogenase as novel target of steroid-producing cell autoantibodies: association of autoantibodies with endocrine autoimmune disease. *J Clin Endocrinol Metab* 1996;81:4439–4445.

83. Gulyas BJ, Hodgen GD, Tullner WW, Ross GT. Effects of fetal or maternal hypophysectomy on endocrine organs and body weight in infant rhesus monkeys *(Macaca mulatta)*: with particular emphasis on oogenesis. *Biol Reprod* 1977;16:216–227.

84. Axelrod L, Neer RM, Kliman B. Hypogonadism in a male with immunologically active biologically inactive luteinizing hormone: an exception to a venerable rule. *J Clin Endocrinol Metab* 1979;48:279–287.

85. Park IJ, Burnett LS, Jones HW Jr, Migeon CJ, Blizzard RM. A case of male pseudohermaphroditism associated with elevated LH, normal FSH and low testosterone possibly due to the secretion of an abnormal LH molecule. *Acta Endocrinol* 1976;83:173–181.

86. Silva de Sa MF, Matthews MJ, Rebar RW. Altered forms of immunoreactive urinary FSH and LH in premature ovarian failure. *Infertility* 1988;11:1–11.

87. Whitney EA, Layman LC, Lanclos KD, Wall SW, McDonough PG. Polymerase chain reaction and southern analysis of the follicle-stimulating hormone receptor gene in women with 46,XX premature ovarian failure [Abstract 903]. Abstracts of the 74th Annual Meeting of The Endocrine Society, San Antonio, Texas, June 24–27, 1992:277.

88. Sluss PM, Schneyer AL. Low molecular weight follicle-stimulating hormone receptor binding inhibitor in sera from premature ovarian failure patients. *J Clin Endocrinol Metab* 1992;74:1242–1246.

89. Jones GS, de Moraes-Ruehsen M. A new syndrome of amenorrhea in association with hypergonadotropinism and apparently normal ovarian follicular apparatus. *Am J Obstet Gynecol* 1969;104:597–600.

90. Metka M, Holzer G, Heytmanek G, Huber J. Hypergonadotropic hypogonadic amenorrhea (World Health Organization III) and osteopenia. *Fertil Steril* 1992;57:37–41.

91. Manuel M, Katayama KP, Jones HW Jr. The age of occurrence of gonadal tumors in intersex patients with a Y chromosome. *Am J Obstet Gynecol* 1976;124:293–300.

92. Schellhas HF. Malignant potential of the dysgenetic gonad, part I. *Obstet Gynecol* 1974;44:298–309.

93. Schellhas HF. Malignant potential of the dysgenetic gonad, part II. *Obstet Gynecol* 1974;44:455–462.

94. van der Schouw YT, van der Graaf Y, Steyerberg EW, Eijkemans MJ, Banga JD. Age at menopause as a risk factor for cardiovascular mortality. *Lancet* 1996;347:714–718.

95. Snowden DA, Kane RL, Beeson WL, et al. Is early menopause a biological marker of health and aging? *Am J Public Health* 1989;79:709–714.

96. Alper MM, Jolly EE, Garner PB. Pregnancies after premature ovarian failure. *Obstet Gynecol* 1986;67:595–625.

97. Check JH, Chase JS. Ovulation induction in hypergonadotropic amenorrhea with estrogen and human menopausal gonadotropin therapy. *Fertil Steril* 1984;42:919–922.

98. Check JH, Chase JS, Spence M. Pregnancy in premature ovarian failure after therapy with oral contraceptives despite resistance to previous human menopausal gonadotropin therapy. *Am J Obstet Gynecol* 1989;160:114–115.

99. Check JH, Chase JS, Wu CH, et al. Ovulation induction and pregnancy with an estrogen-gonadotropin stimulation technique in a menopausal woman with marked hypoplastic ovaries. *Am J Obstet Gynecol* 1989;160:405–406.

100. Check JH, Wu CH, Check M. The effect of leuprolide acetate in aiding induction of ovulation in hypergonadotropic hypogonadism: a case report. *Fertil Steril* 1988;49:542–543.

101. Ledger WL, Thomas EJ, Browning D, Lenton EA, Cooke ID. Suppression of gonadotropin secretion does not reverse premature ovarian failure. *J Obstet Gynecol* 1989;96:196–199.

102. Lutjen P, Trounson A, Leeton J, et al. The establishment and maintenance of pregnancy using *in vitro* fertilization and embryo donation in a patient with primary ovarian failure. *Nature* 1984;307:174–175.

103. Chan CLK, Cameron IT, Findlay JK, et al. Oocyte donation and *in vitro* fertilization: clinical state of the art. *Obstet Gynecol* 1987;42:350–362.

104. Sauer MV, Paulson RJ. Oocyte donation for women who have ovarian failure. *Contemp Obstet Gynecol* 1989;Nov:125–135.

105. Lydic ML, Liu JH, Rebar RW, Thomas MA, Cedars MI. Success of donor oocyte IVF-ET in recipients with and without premature ovarian failure. *Fertil Steril* 1996;65:98–102.

106. Rebar RW, Cedars MI. Hypergonadotropic amenorrhea. In: Filicori M, Flamigni C, eds. *Ovulation induction:* basic science and clinical advances. Amsterdam: Elsevier Science, 1994:115–121.

Treatment of the Postmenopausal Woman: Basic and Clinical Aspects, Second Edition, edited by Rogerio A. Lobo, Lippincott Williams & Wilkins, Philadelphia © 1999.

CHAPTER 3

Reproductive Options for Perimenopausal and Menopausal Women

Mark V. Sauer

Since 1990, there has been a substantial increase in the number of older women interested in fertility care. This rise followed the publication of successful pregnancies in menopausal women undergoing oocyte donation, which focused international attention on the reproductive interests of women in their 40s and 50s (1). More than 3,000 cases of oocyte donation are performed in the United States, mostly for perimenopausal and menopausal patients. Similarly, more than 4,000 cases of *in vitro* fertilization are initiated annually in women older than 40 years of age, as reported by the Society for Assisted Reproductive Technology (SART) and the Centers for Disease Control (CDC) (Table 3.1 and Fig. 3.1) (2). However, despite the rising enthusiasm for fertility care, success rates in older women using their own oocytes have not significantly improved and remain low compared with rates observed in younger patients (Fig. 3.2). Poor outcomes are linked to ovarian senescence, which contributes to exaggerated infertility and pregnancy wastage in this population. Unless the aging gamete is replaced, most efforts at assisted reproduction are destined to fail once perimenopausal signs and symptoms are present.

The term *fecundity* refers to a woman's natural ability to reproduce. A fecundability rate is often used to describe the monthly conceptions among couples within a population. Fecundability rates have been calculated for many different populations and vary slightly according to cultural, religious, and sexual practices. However, a feature common to all groups is the inevitable decline in fertility that accompanies aging.

Women most often conceive and deliver a child while in their twenties. Typically, fertility rates decline during the fourth decade of life, reaching a nadir by the time women enter their early forties (Fig. 3.3) (3). The inevitable loss of fertility is readily apparent when reviewing the birth rates of "natural populations." Natural populations are composed of individuals who do not practice contraception. Within natural populations, fertility remains relatively stable until women reach approximately 30 years of age, when a significant fall occurs. By age 35, delivery rates are reduced by one-half, and by age 45, live births are diminished by 95% from values seen in the same population at age 25 (4).

Comparing figures from natural populations to delivery rates in the U.S. population at large, similar trends are apparent (5). Less than 1% of all live births occur in women older than 40 years. By age 47, this is further reduced to a mere 0.01% of deliveries (6). Although the lay press has popularized menopausal pregnancies, few women are able to successfully deliver a healthy baby beyond the age of 45 without assistance from oocyte donation.

Further complicating the decreasing fertility rate of older women is the exponential rise in the incidence of aneuploidy that occurs in their conception cycles. This leads to an elevated rate of miscarriage and an increase in the number of observed anomalies in the delivered offspring. For example, at age 25, only 10% of clinically diagnosed pregnancies end in spontaneous abortion (7). By age 45, the spontaneous abortion incidence is 40% to 50%. The association between spontaneous abortion and maternal age is further demonstrated by reviewing studies of women undergoing artificial insemination using donor sperm (8).

Pregnancy wastage is thought to result principally from spontaneous mutations within resting oocytes. Throughout life, human eggs are suspended in development at the diplotene stage of meiosis I. As time passes, gametes become particularly susceptible to environmental toxins and spontaneous mutations. The oocytes residing in the

M. V. Sauer: Department of Obstetrics and Gynecology, Columbia University College of Physicians & Surgeons, New York, New York 10032.

TABLE 3.1. *National Registry of in vitro fertilization results from the Society for Assisted Reproduction and the Centers for Disease Control: 1995 calendar year*

Data category	Patient age (years)			Total
	<35	35–39	>39	
Cycles performed	21,019	16,738	8,159	45,906
Pregnancy/initiated cycle	29.7%	23.4%	13.2%	24.4%
Births/initiated cycle	25.3%	18.2%	8.0%	19.6%
Births/embryo transfer	30.6%	23.6%	11.6%	25.1%
Canceled cycles	9.1%	14.8%	21.5%	13.6%

Adapted from ref. 2.

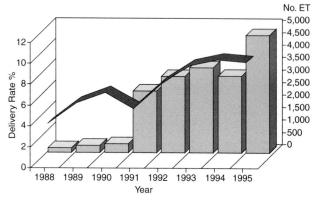

FIG. 3.2. Although the number of cases of *in vitro* fertilization in women older than 40 years has increased, success rates have remained relatively unchanged during the past 10 years.

ovaries during the perimenopause have been present since before birth. The protracted process of oocyte aging seems to exert its deleterious effects primarily on the cell nucleus, as evidenced by the positive correlation of maternal age with chromosomal aberrations. As a result, trisomy is witnessed in only 0.1% of newborns of 25-year-old mothers, rising to 2% as maternal age reaches 45 years (9). The meiotic competence of *in vitro* matured human oocytes is influenced adversely by age, with an increased frequency of errors in chromosome segregation at the first meiotic division (Table 3.2) (10). Almost 50% of ova karyotyped for women older than 35 who are undergoing *in vitro* fertilization are aneuploid (11), and 60% to 75% of biopsied normal-appearing embryos of women between the ages of 36 and 43 years are aneuploid (12,13) (Table 3.3). These findings agree with observations that a high percentage of abortuses are chromosomally abnormal (14). In a teleologic sense, preimplanta-

tion and postimplantation losses protect the species from unwanted genetic mutations while simultaneously minimizing the health risks posed by pregnancy in the older individual.

Although less well defined, adverse reproductive events also occur in men older than 55 years of age. Advanced paternal age has been associated with trisomies and the iso-X syndrome (15,16). Other reproductive hazards include an increased incidence of chronic genitourinary ailments, particularly prostatitis and epididymitis, which affect fertilization *in vivo* and *in vitro*. Chronic infections are difficult or impossible to eradicate using antibiotic therapy. Even when infections are successfully treated, lingering inflammation in the genitourinary tract may produce leukocytospermia, which is known to inhibit fertilization *in vitro* (17).

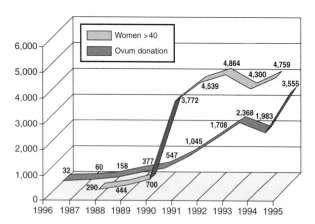

FIG. 3.1. Increasing numbers of cases of conventional *in vitro* fertilization are initiated in women of advanced reproductive age annually as reported to the Society for Assisted Reproductive Technology. Parallel increases in the number of cycles of oocyte donation probably reflect the rising interest by older recipients, many of whom have failed traditional treatments.

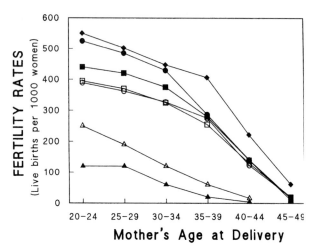

FIG. 3.3. Fertility rates in natural populations compared with those in United States populations. ♦, Hutterites, United States, 20th century; ●, Burgeoisie, Geneva, 17th century; ○, Burgeoisie, Geneva, 16th century; ■, French village, 17th century; □, Iranian village, 20th century; ▲, United States, 1955; △, United States, 1981. (From ref. 1, with permission.)

TABLE 3.2. *Aberrations in Metaphase II spindle formation and chromosomal alignment related to the age of the patient*

Patient age (years)	Oocytes with aberrations
<35	11%
≥35	71%

Adapted from ref. 10.

When pregnancy occurs in women of advanced reproductive age, the obstetric risks are increased. Delayed childbearing is associated with adverse perinatal outcomes as observed in the Swedish Medical Birth Register (18). This review focused on the obstetric experience of 173,715 nulliparous Nordic women who were 20 years or older. Mothers older than 40 years experienced an approximately 1.5- to 2.0-fold increased risk for growth retardation, preterm birth, and late fetal and early neonatal deaths compared with women younger than 25. Stillbirth rates also rise sharply after age 40 (19). As a population, women older than 35 are considered "high risk" because of their increased likelihood for developing gestational diabetes, hypertension, preterm labor, and growth retardation (9).

The prevalence of childlessness and infertility in older couples is difficult to ascertain. However, a progressive increase in the number of childless couples has been described. It is estimated that 5% of childless couples in their early 20s wish to begin a family, compared with more than 60% of couples in their 40s (20). Biologically, women may be best suited to reproduce while in their 20s. However, psychosocially, many young individuals are neither in a position to raise a child nor desirous to begin a family. Demographic data from the United States have shown that women older than 30 are giving birth to their first child in increasing numbers, up from 40,000 in 1970 to approximately 100,000 by 1980 (21). Reasons given for this delay include the pursuit of educational and vocational goals, later marriages, an increased prevalence of divorce, and the widespread availability of effective birth control. Many women are electing to begin a family

later in life as a result of second marriages. Unfortunately, many individuals are unaware of the change in fertility status that naturally occurs with advancing age and suddenly find themselves unable to conceive despite having had little or no problem in the past. Among women older than 40 interested in oocyte donation in one survey, two-thirds had never delivered a baby, and 51% were recently remarried (22).

In general, women older than 40 seeking fertility care have poor success rates (23–27) (Fig. 3.4). Registries that track and tally success rates for assisted reproduction have reported similar findings from various parts of the world (28–30). However, the pregnancy rates logged in the medical literature overestimate the likelihood of achieving pregnancy, because many women entering treatment are dropped from therapy because of poor responses to controlled ovarian hyperstimulation.

In essence, evolution has precluded many modern women from reproducing after the age of 40 and certainly by age 50, when most individuals experience complete cessation of ovulatory function. Unlike other mammals, the humans ovaries have exhausted their supply of oocytes by the time menopause occurs (31). Less than

TABLE 3.3. *Blastomere biopsies taken from human embryos generated from older in vitro fertilization patients*

Biopsy results	Patient age (years) <40	≥40
Embryos biopsied	135	110
Normal karyotype	39%	28%
Abnormal karyotype	61%	72%
Aneuploid	10%	12%
Haploid	2%	2%
Polyploid	10%	13%
Mosaic	38%	45%

Adapted from ref. 13.

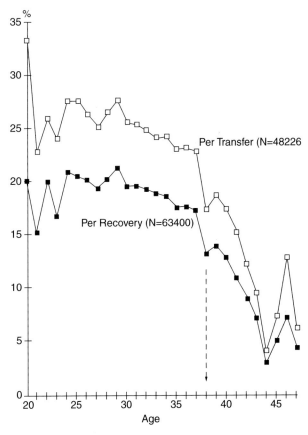

FIG. 3.4. Pregnancy rates for assisted reproduction fall to very low levels after the age of 40, as demonstrated by the French National Register on *in vitro* Fertilization (FIVNAT) data of 5,500 cycles.

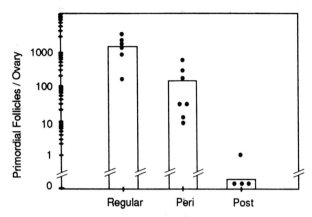

FIG. 3.5. Relation between the number of primordial follicles per ovary and menstrual status in 17 women between the ages of 45 and 55. Regular, regular menses: peri, perimenopausal erratic bleeding patterns; post, postmenopausal amenorrhea. (From ref. 26, with permission.)

0.001% of the ovary's original complement of oocytes are ever ovulated. Histologic studies reveal that, regardless of chronologic age, only a few thousand eggs remain by menopause (32). Despite the compensatory rise in stimulating pituitary gonadotropin, this cohort is unlikely to be recruited. Cadaver studies indicate a decline in follicular mass with advancing age, insinuating that accelerated rates of follicular atresia occur during the last decade of reproductive life. Ovaries removed from healthy women of various ages and analyzed for the presence of gametes demonstrate an accelerated depletion of oocytes as menopause approaches. The largest turnover of oocytes occurs before birth, with a steady decline from approximately 7 million oocytes at 20 weeks' gestation, to about 2 million at the time of delivery (33). At menarche there are about 300,000 eggs, and by menopause, few primordial follicles remain (31) (Fig. 3.5).

NATURAL FERTILITY IN THE PERIMENOPAUSE

Despite the low incidence of pregnancy in women of advanced reproductive age, spontaneous conceptions do occur even in the face of elevated gonadotropins. However, reports of healthy older women undergoing artificial insemination demonstrate reduced fecundity, with cumulative pregnancy rates approximating 40% (34,35). Spontaneous abortions are common and occur in as many as one-half of the clinical pregnancies reported for these women. A high percentage of losses result from aneuploidy. Anomalies in live births are also increased. For instance, Down syndrome occurs in 0.5 to 0.7 per thousand live births in 25-year-old mothers, but the number rises to 75.8 to 152.7 per thousand live births by age 49 (36). Of 2,404 amniocenteses performed because of advanced maternal age, 2.4% were discovered to be aneuploid, and 50% of these were trisomy (37).

As a measure of reproductive reserve, serum follicle-stimulating hormone (FSH) levels drawn on the third day of the menstrual cycle have been used as prognostic indicators before in vitro fertilization (38). Levels above 15 mIU/mL are associated with decreased success rates, and when greater than 25 mIU/mL, pregnancy rarely occurs. Elevated values are observed with increasing frequency when evaluating women older than 40 years of age and are common in most women older than 45. An increase in early follicular phase FSH coincides with the period in which diminished fecundity rates are witnessed. The follicular phase shortens during this time, and the elevated gonadotropins represent compensatory stimulation resulting from a progressively dwindling number of functioning follicles.

The identification and accurate measurement of inhibin, a glycoprotein heterodimer produced by the granulosa cells in response to FSH, has provided further insight into the effect of age on folliculogenesis. Inhibin correlates with follicular function and granulosa cell competence and is decreased with age (39,40). Inhibin measured in the follicular fluid of hyperstimulated ovaries aspirated for purposes of in vitro fertilization reflects correlations among the number of recruited follicles, oocytes retrieved, and embryos produced. Not surprisingly, inhibin was reduced in women experiencing a poor response to ovarian hyperstimulation (41). As a serum marker, it may be a more sensitive prognostic indicator of ovarian reproductive competence than levels of serum FSH. After menopause, inhibin is undetectable in serum samples. It appears that a state of "reproductive menopause" exists up to 10 years before the cessation of menses heralds the onset of the "endocrine menopause" (Fig. 3.6) (42). Traditional therapies designed to enhance fertility during this transition period are likely to fail, and live births occur in fewer than 5% of treatment cycles (43,44).

The diminished capacity to conceive and carry babies to term typically has been blamed on the ovaries and uterus. A large drop in available oocytes for recruitment and ovulation accompanies senescence in the ovary. Higher rates of chromosomally abnormal eggs exist in the remaining oocytes. However, in laboratory animals, the uterus also undergoes age-related changes responsible for diminished implantation and pregnancy rates. As a result, older animals eventually are unable to achieve pregnancy despite the transfer of embryos produced by younger donors. The number of implantations per animal and the proportion of mice found to have any implantation a week postconception declined significantly by 9 months of age (45). Similarly, older mice were in other studies observed to have fewer implantation sites and subsequently were observed to be twice as likely to resorb an early pregnancy compared with younger animals (46). Correlates using other laboratory animals also exist, including a reduction in litter size with age observed in the hamster (47). In younger animals, 31% of the losses resulted from preimplantation death, and

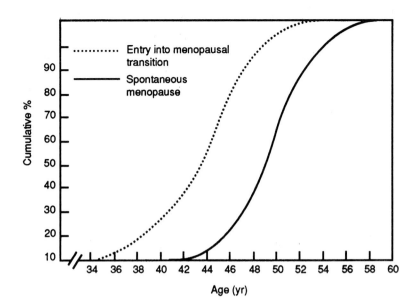

FIG. 3.6. Rising follicle-stimulating hormone values that mark the beginning of the *reproductive menopause* precedes actual cessation of bleeding or *endocrine menopause*. (From ref. 37, with permission.)

69% were from postimplantation events. However, in senescent hamsters, a reversed scenario was observed, with preimplantation death occurring in 64% and postimplantation losses seen in 36% of cases. The higher overall loss rates of older animals were thought to be a consequence of less viable ova. When senescent hamsters received ovarian grafts from younger animals, they were better able to support transferred blastocysts, implying the aging corpus luteum also plays a role in the early establishment and maintenance of pregnancy (48).

Although the number of implants is significantly reduced in mated female hamsters, the number of decidual reactions per uterine horn is the same in older animals and younger females (49). This may reflect delayed or abnormal patterns of embryonic development in the blastocysts of older individuals. Abnormal concepti may be secondary to impaired oocyte quality or perhaps be secondary to effects of the oviductal environment that alters early preimplantation development. Many possible factors influence the relationship between the conceptus and the endometrial environment. These include the rate and normal pattern of development of ova within the older female reproductive tract, delayed uterine sensitivity to blastocyst implantation secondary to a decreased capacity of older uterine tissue to take up steroids, and the less efficient uterine response to a decidualizing stimulus as seen in aging mice, rats, and hamsters (50).

Similarly, the age-related decline in human fertility may partly be caused by "uterine factors" (51). Uterine receptivity is best measured by comparing individual embryo implantation rates in humans of various ages undergoing *in vitro* fertilization and embryo transfer. Women younger than 30 years of age approach rates as favorable as 20% per embryo transferred, decreasing to 9% for women 36 years of age and older (52). After age 40, individual embryo implantation rates are less than 5%

(53). Alterations in uterine blood flow also occur with declining levels of estradiol, which may adversely affect the local endometrial environment (54). The identification of estrogen receptors in the wall of human uterine arteries supports this hypothesis (55). Fibrotic changes found in the walls of the uterine artery muscular further accent physiologic changes accounting for decreases in local blood flow (56). Approximately one-half of spontaneously aborted pregnancies are chromosomally normal, implying a local endomyometrial factor may be responsible for the loss. Whether this is a primary target organ event or secondary to the inability of the aging corpus luteum to support the pregnancy remains conjectural.

Unfortunately, it is not possible to dissociate the gamete from the influence of the local environment when studying normal postfertilization development and implantation. Oocyte and embryo donation to older women, using gametes obtained from younger individuals, provides an ideal opportunity to ascertain the contribution of each of these two variables independently from each other. When prescribed hormone replacement, the endometria of menopausal women between 40 and 60 years of age exhibit normal histologic and steroid receptor response (56). Likewise, endometria of younger women with ovarian failure are indistinguishable from older women on similar replacement regimens (Fig. 3.7). When adequate doses of exogenous estrogen and progesterone are delivered, most uteri respond appropriately and demonstrate normal endometrial morphology, regardless of the patient's age or diagnosis. The high rate of implantation and delivered pregnancies reported in women of advanced reproductive age undergoing oocyte donation is testimony to the normalcy and receptivity of a uterine environment refurbished through hormone replacement. Success rates are three to five times higher than older women using their own eggs undergoing standard *in vitro* fertilization (Table 3.4) (53).

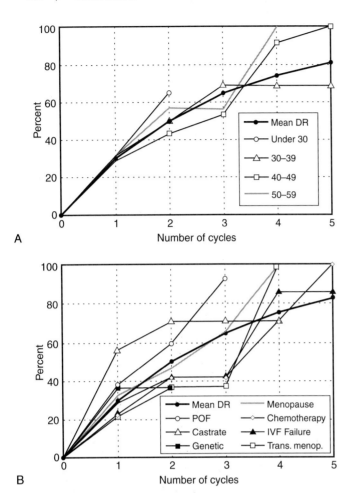

A

B

FIG. 3.7. A: Cumulative delivery rates as calculated by life-table analysis notes better than a 50% likelihood of pregnancy success by the third attempt at oocyte donation regardless of the age of the recipient. DR, delivery rate. **B:** Cumulative delivery rates are the same for patients of all ages and diagnoses undergoing oocyte donation through five cycles of therapy, with cumulative success exceeding 80%. (From ref. 72, with permission.)

DEVELOPMENT OF OOCYTE AND EMBRYO DONATION AND ITS APPLICATION IN OLDER WOMEN

The ability to transfer preimplantation embryos conceived *in vitro* or *in vivo* from one female to another has been performed in more than a dozen different mammals (57). First demonstrated in the mouse, this method was popularized by the animal husbandry business and revolutionized the cattle breeding industry (58). More than 100,000 calves are born annually as a result of refinements in this technique. Transfer of zygotes to recipient animals, synchronized to the menstrual cycle of donors, results in the establishment of pregnancy in 25% to 50% of transfer cycles.

Modification of these techniques led to the establishment of the first embryo donation pregnancy in humans in 1983 (59). Early attempts focused on the nonsurgical obtainment of embryos conceived *in vivo* from spontaneously ovulating cycles using uterine lavage. However, natural cycles produced morphologically normal embryos in only 25% of attempts, and as a result, pregnancies in recipients occurred in only 10% to 12% of initiated cycles (60). Unlike the experience in cattle, efforts to maximize the number of embryos retrieved by superovulating human donors were unsuccessful and resulted in a high rate of complications (61,62).

Controlled ovarian hyperstimulation of oocyte donors followed by *in vitro* fertilization and embryo transfer to women with premature ovarian failure was reported in 1983 and resulted in a successful pregnancy in one of seven women undergoing treatment (63). During the next 10 years, increasing numbers of studies employing a variety of transfer techniques were published with high rates of successful implantation and pregnancy (Table 3.5) (64–68).

Surprisingly, in women with hypergonadotropic hypogonadism receiving sex steroid replacement and donated

TABLE 3.4. *Results of the transfer of fertilized donor ova in women 40 years and older with ovarian failure compared with women younger than 40 years with ovarian failure and women 40 years and older undergoing standard in vitro fertilization and embryo transfer*

Variable	≥40 Years, donor IVF	<40 Years, donor IVF	≥40 Years, standard IVF
Number of recipients	65	35	57
Number of recipient cycles	93	46	79
Number of oocytes/recipients	15.2 ± 9.0	15.3 ± 6.8	6.7 ± 4.1[a]
Fertilization rate (%)	48.2	62.0[b]	39.2
Number of transfer cycles	86	43	70
Number of embryos transferred per cycle	4.4 ± 1.0	4.7 ± 0.7	2.9 ± 1.2[a]
Implantation rate per transferred embryo (%)	19.7	15.9	4.8[a]
95% Confidence limits	6.1, 24.5	11.1, 21.7	2.3, 8.7
Ratio of clinical pregnancies per ET (%)	34/86 (39.5%)	14/43 (30.2)	8/70 (11.4)
95% Confidence limits	29.2, 50.7	19.1, 48.5	5.1, 21.3
Ratio of ongoing pregnancies per transfer	29/86 (33.7)	13/43 (30.2)	6/70 (8.6)
95% Confidence limits	23.9, 44.7	17.2, 46.1	3.2, 17.7

ET, embryo transfer; IVF, *in vitro* fertilization.
[a]p <0.05, comparing women 40 years of age and older undergoing standard IVF with either group undergoing oocyte donation.
[b]p <0.05, comparing women younger than 40 years of age undergoing oocyte donation with either group of women 40 years of age and older.
Data from ref. 38, with permission.

REPRODUCTIVE OPTIONS AND MENOPAUSE / 29

TABLE 3.5. *Performance characteristics for a variety of techniques used throughout the 1980s to establish pregnancy in functionally agonadal women using donated oocytes*

Investigator	Method	Transfer attempts	Pregnancies
Rosenwaks, 1987	IVF	32	8
Formigli, 1987	Uterine lavage	17	8
Asch, 1988	GIFT	8	6
Devroey, 1988	IVF	42	10
	GIFT/ZIFT	7	3

IVF, *in vitro* fertilization; GIFT, gamete intrafallopian transfer; ZIFT, zygote intrafallopian transfer.
Data from ref. 47, with permission.

oocytes fertilized *in vitro*, clinical pregnancy rates and individual embryo implantation rates are significantly increased over values normally seen in women attempting *in vitro* fertilization using their own oocytes (43). This is attributed to the provision of large numbers of high-quality oocytes for *in vitro* fertilization produced by young, fertile donors, combined with the enhanced endometrial environment provided by the orderly deliverance of controlled doses of estrogen and progesterone. In this manner, embryo quality is maximized and endometrial receptivity simultaneously enhanced (69).

By 1990, reports of successful pregnancies in menopausal women beyond the age normally considered to be "premature" appeared (53,70). Reluctance to transfer embryos to women older than 40 was based on the general belief that a "uterine factor" precluded implantation and pregnancy in aging animals. However, preliminary trials of oocyte donation in menopausal women demonstrated similar success rates for implantation and pregnancy as younger recipients. Obstetric outcomes were favorable, and miscarriage rates were reduced below that normally seen in older mothers (43).

CHILDBEARING BY THE PERIMENOPAUSAL AND MENOPAUSAL WOMAN

Most women interested in oocyte donation appear to be perimenopausal, usually between the ages of 40 and 50 years (Table 3.6) (1,2). Older patients traditionally had

TABLE 3.6. *Oocyte donation: 1995 annual tally as reported in the National Registry of the Society for Assisted Reproductive Technology and the Centers for Disease Control*

Donation data	Recipient age (years)			Total
	<35	35–39	>39	
Embryo transfers	572	668	2,112	3,352
Birth per embryo transfer rate	30.8%	35.8%	36.7%	35.5%

Adapted from ref. 2.

the worst prognosis for fertility using natural or assisted reproductive techniques.

In many 40-year-old patients, ovarian function is still intact, because ovulatory cycles usually continue throughout the 5- to 10-year transition period that defines the perimenopause. However, using oocyte donation, women of advanced reproductive age have pregnancy rates similar to younger recipients with ovarian failure. For purposes of donor synchronization and to avoid an untimely premature ovulation in recipients, which would create a progestational endometrium, it is preferable to downregulate the pituitary of cycling women with a gonadotropin-releasing hormone (GnRH) agonist before prescribing standard hormone replacement.

Demographic differences are apparent in older recipients seeking services compared with women with premature ovarian failure (22). As a group, they are more likely to be divorced and remarried, have frequently been previously pregnant, and often have undergone an elective termination. Their incomes are generally high. They are commonly employed in a full-time vocational pursuit and in many cases are professionally educated. A large percentage of patients have undergone cosmetic surgery, usually in an attempt to maintain a youthful appearance.

Larger series reports continue to document the efficacy of oocyte donation while demonstrating the safety of the method (71). In reviewing two large series of oocyte donation, similar success in pregnancy and delivery rates were demonstrated in women with various ages and diagnoses (Table 3.7 and Fig. 3.8) (72,73). Endometrial biopsies of recipients aged 50 to 60 years suggests that the uterus maintains its ability to respond normally if given pharmacologic doses of sex steroid (56,74). Embryo implantation

TABLE 3.7. *Cumulative pregnancy success rates for oocyte donation following repeated attempts at embryo transfer*

Attempts	Pregnancies	Cumulative pregnancy rate	Deliveries	Cumulative delivery rates
1	212 (53.4%)[a]	53.4%	169 (42.6%)[b]	42.6%
2	70 (47.0%)	75.4%	52 (34.9%)	62.6%
3	26 (46.4%)	86.8%	21 (39.6%)	77.4%
≥4	28 (60.7%)	94.8%	12 (42.8%)	88.7%

[a]Parenthetic numbers are pregnancy rates for the groups indicated.
[b]Parenthetic numbers are the delivery rates for the groups indicated.
Adapted from ref. 73.

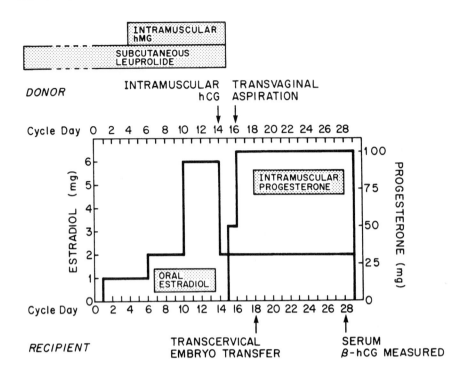

FIG. 3.8. Regimen of hormone replacement used to synchronize oocyte donors and embryo recipients.

and pregnancy rates in this very advanced reproductive age group parallel that seen in younger women (Table 3.8).

Despite the published success of the technique, few practitioners have extended oocyte donation to women older than 50 years of age (75). Concerns include the unknown risks to the elderly gravidarum, issues of longevity in the delivering parents, and the "unnatural" method inherent to the process of establishing the gestation (76,77). The recommendation to extend therapy to 50-year-old women has been made with cautious reservation by the American Society for Reproductive Medicine and with the proviso that recipients be adequately screened medically and psychologically (78). As many as 20% to 30% of potential recipients of advanced reproductive age may fail the screening process and ultimately

be precluded from treatment (43). However, after comprehensive medical screening, women found to be emotionally and physically fit have performed well in their attempts at pregnancy, and outcomes have been good.

SCREENING AND PREPARATION OF POTENTIAL RECIPIENTS

Screening potential candidates for oocyte donation has centered on testing their overall health. Although the probabilities for establishing pregnancy in recipients may be dramatically altered using oocyte donation, obstetric risks are age related and therefore significantly increased in the older population. Testing cardiovascular health is important, because the stress of pregnancy on the heart is significant. For this reason, baseline assessments of diabetes, hyperlipidemia, and exercise tolerance are also indicated. A generalized search for occult malignancies has uncovered several cancers, including breast, uterine, and cervical carcinomas and lymphoma and melanoma. Table 3.9 lists the surveillance tests most often used in screening older recipients.

Women undergoing embryo transfer have successfully used a variety of hormone replacement regimens. Most commonly, oral estradiol, micronized or as the valerate form, has been prescribed. Delivery may be accomplished in a sequential step-up fashion to mimic the normal fluctuations in serum estradiol levels (79) or delivered as a fixed continuous dose (80). Pregnancy rates are similar using either approach. When following the step-up approach, synchronization with the donor undertaking ovarian hyperstimulation requires the recipient begin medication 4 to 5 days in advance of the donor's injecting

TABLE 3.8. *Results of transfer of fertilized donor ova in women 50 and older with ovarian failure*

Variable	Result
Number of recipients	14
Number of recipient cycles	22
Number of oocytes per recipient	12.6 ± 4.4
Fertilized oocytes/oocytes retrieved	126/278
Fertilization rate (%)	45%
Number of transfer cycles	21
Number of embryos transferred per cycle (mean ± SD)	4.1 ± 1.4
Implantation rate per transferred embryo (ET) (%)	19%
Ratio of clinical pregnancies per ET (%)	8/21 (38%)
Ratio of ongoing pregnancies or deliveries per ET (%)	7/21 (33%)

From ref. 68, with permission.

TABLE 3.9. *Screening examination required of couples of advanced reproductive age requesting oocyte donation*

Medical, wife only
  Electrocardiogram (treadmill if >45 years)
  Mammogram
  Chest roentgenogram
  Fasting and 2-hour postprandial serum glucose level
  Fasting cholesterol and blood lipoproteins
  Blood chemistry panel (SMA 12/60)
  Prothrombin time/partial thromboplastin time
  Thyrotropin (sensitive thyroid-stimulating hormone)
  Antinuclear antibody, lupus anticoagulant, anticardiolipin antibody
  Complete blood count with platelets
  Papanicolaou test
Infectious disease, both spouses
  Human immunodeficiency virus test
  VDRL test
  Hepatitis screen
Reproductive
  Transvaginal ultrasound of pelvis
  Hysterosalpingogram
  Endometrial biopsy while receiving hormone replacement
  Semen analysis and semen culture

From ref. 38, with permission.

gonadotropins. Fixed-dose regimens allow greater flexibility in scheduling. Pharmacologic levels of circulating sex steroid result from prolonged use of medicinal estrogen, and despite claims of "physiologic" replacement, serum values of estrone, estrone sulfate, and estrone glucuronide are known to be grossly elevated (81). Estrogen has also been delivered transdermally with good results. Advantages of this method include maintenance of physiologic sex steroid levels and lessened hepatic effects (82). However, many patients develop rashes and irritation at the patch sites, and multiple patches must be worn simultaneously to achieve adequate levels of estradiol.

Progesterone is needed to decidualize the endometria in preparation for embryo implantation. A variety of formulations have been used successfully (83,84). Most commonly, intramuscular progesterone given twice daily has been recommended. The need to maintain replacement steroids throughout the first trimester commonly leads to local irritation and inflammation at the injection sites. Alternate regimens include suppositories and gel-based or encapsulated micronized progesterone.

Morphologic analyses of endometrial biopsies taken from women using hormone replacement therapy have uncovered certain unique characteristics. Although histologically close to normal, "mid-luteal" samples typically demonstrate a delayed pattern of glandular maturation, exhibited in up 25% of samples (56). When endometria are later resampled in the cycle (day 26 to 28), biopsies are usually normal, implying a catch-up phenomenon. Transvaginal ultrasound images denote a homogeneous echo-dense pattern, with a thickness approaching 8 to 10 mm. However, pregnancies have occurred with measures as thin as 4 mm and as thick as 23 mm (86). Sex steroid receptors for progesterone and estrogen are within normal limits for luteal endometria.

In many cases, women might not have been taking hormone replacement therapy and therefore require a priming cycle to develop a full endometrial response. This occurs in approximately 5% of new cases, regardless of the recipient's age. A mock cycle enables the discovery of such individuals and permits adjusting for a hyperplastic glandular pattern of response that occasionally occurs (2%) (87). A practice transfer using an embryo transfer catheter is performed at the time of biopsy to measure the length and contour of the cavity and to ensure that a transcervical embryo transfer can easily be accomplished.

OBSTETRIC MANAGEMENT AND DELIVERY CONSIDERATIONS

Somewhat surprisingly, most women who undergo oocyte and embryo donation experience pregnancy if they attempt multiple cycles. Because most recipients are older than 40, they are considered high-risk pregnancies by their obstetricians. Further complicating care is the common occurrence of multiple gestations, seen in 20% to 40% of live births.

Pregnancies initially are documented using serum β-human chorionic gonadotropin (β-hCG) measurements and transvaginal ultrasound. Ultrasound examinations performed early in the gestation document the number of implantation sites and delineate normal embryonic growth. Commonly, supernumerary implantations occur and often fail to develop normally. In many cases, abnormal implantation sites are absorbed without incident. Other times, their collapse results in vaginal bleeding. Ultrasound is useful for identifying patients at risk. Visualizing the early pregnancy appears to facilitate the patient's acceptance of the pregnancy, many of which initially expressed difficulty in believing the pregnancy actually occurred. Serial measures of estradiol and progesterone are neither helpful nor indicated, because pharmacologic doses of hormone are delivered daily, and serum levels do not reflect the tissue response (81,88).

Referral to specialists in maternal and fetal medicine is appropriate given the age of patients. Regardless of their prior health, pregnant women older than 40 should be considered high-risk patients. Reports describe a tendency for hypertensive complications in women after oocyte donation (89). Monitoring for diabetes and early signs of hypertension is important. Serial growth assessment provides early evidence of fetal growth retardation. Late-occurring events that complicate pregnancies in the older woman, particularly stillbirth, may best be avoided by an aggressive approach to delivery. With full knowledge of the gestational age of these mothers, attempts at inducing labor near term (38 to 39 weeks) should be considered judicious. A stillbirth was reported for one / 43-

year-old woman who was allowed to continue her pregnancy beyond term (90).

FUTURE APPLICATIONS

Interest has focused on the means for rejuvenating the oocytes of older women using cytoplasm infused from younger donor oocyte (91). Similarly, nuclear transplantation techniques may allow enucleated donor oocytes to be reconstituted with the genetic material of older recipients (92), allowing women an opportunity to perpetuate their genetic lineage. It has also been suggested that women should store or bank their oocytes, similar to men and their sperm, to avoid age-related infertility later in life (93). However, given the low rate of success in using cryopreserved oocytes (94), promoting this approach for routine clinical use remains highly controversial.

The widespread application of oocyte donation to increasing numbers of women of advanced reproductive age was inevitable. Despite attempts in several countries to limit or prohibit oocyte donation (95,96), it is unlikely that legislative bodies will enact restrictive measures to preclude the extension of this method in the United States. Increasing numbers of women in their forties seek fertility care in this country. Most of these patients fail to become pregnant, and many elect a trial of oocyte donation. For older patients, oocyte donation may actually represent the only viable option for parenting, because adoption is rarely permitted in this age group.

Vigilant surveillance is imperative in the screening of these individuals. To maximize success, a thorough health assessment is mandatory. However, oocyte donation was not intended to be used indiscriminately (97). Many abnormalities are discovered, some of which do not preclude a trial, but others may dictate exclusion. This necessitates a more primary care approach by the fertility specialist and require the development of more discriminatory criteria from that usually practiced.

Concerns have been raised regarding the potential harm to "the fabric of society" brought on by allowing older individuals the chance to become parents. However, precedent exists in that many children have been reared by grandparents, and the grandparents take on most of the parenting role in many cultures. Society has been accepting of older men and younger wives starting families. Typically, in countries where restrictions on oocyte donation exist, no laws preclude males from using donated sperm or older men from procreating with their younger wives. Precluding healthy women from availing themselves of a successful alternative for reproduction while allowing their male counterparts access to such opportunity should be considered sexist and prejudicial. As in most cases of social evolution, as increasing numbers of cases accumulate, it is likely that acceptance will follow.

REFERENCES

1. Sauer MV. Treating women of advanced reproductive age. In: Sauer MV, ed. *Principles of oocyte and embryo donation.* New York: Springer-Verlag, 1998:271–292.
2. Society for Assisted Reproductive Technology and the American Society for Reproductive Medicine. Assisted reproductive technology in the United States and Canada: 1995 results generated from the American Society for Reproductive Medicine/Society for Assisted Reproductive Technology Registry. *Fertil Steril* 1998;69:389.
3. Maroulis GB. Effect of aging on fertility and pregnancy. *Semin Reprod Endocrinol* 1991;9:165.
4. Henry L. Some data on natural fertility. *Eugenics Q Z* 1961;8:81.
5. National Center for Health Statistics. Advance report of final natality statistics, 1981. *Monthly Vital Stat Rep* 1983;32:9.
6. Hansen JP. Older maternal age and pregnancy outcome: a review of the literature. *Obstet Gynecol Surv* 1986;41:726.
7. Stein ZA. A woman's age: childbearing and childrearing. *Am J Epidemiol* 1985;121:327.
8. Virro MR, Schewchuck AB. Pregnancy outcome in 242 conceptions after artificial insemination with donor sperm and effects of maternal age on the prognosis for successful pregnancy. *Am J Obstet Gynecol* 1984;148:518.
9. Cunningham FG, Levenok J. Pregnancy after 35. In: Cunningham FG, MacDonald PC, Gant NF, eds. *Williams obstetrics,* 18th ed, suppl 2. Norwalk, CT: Appleton-Century-Crofts, 1989:1–12.
10. Volarcik K, Sheean L, Goldfarb J, Woods L, Abdul-Karim FW, Hunt P. The meiotic competence of in-vitro matured human oocytes is influenced by donor age: evidence that folliculogenesis is compromised in the reproductively aged ovary. *Hum Reprod* 1998;13:154.
11. Planchot M, DeGrouchy J, Junca AM, Mandelbaum J, Salant-Baroux J, Cohen J. Chromosomal analysis of human oocytes and embryos in an *in vitro* fertilization program. *Ann N Y Acad Sci* 1988;541:384.
12. Magli MC, Gianaroli L, Munne S, Ferraretti AP. Incidence of chromosomal abnormalities from a morphologically normal cohort of embryos in poor-prognosis patients. *J Assist Reprod Genet* 1998;15:297.
13. Munne S, Marquez C, Reing A, Garrisi J, Alikani M. Chromosome abnormalities in embryos obtained after conventional *in vitro* fertilization and intracytoplasmic sperm injection. *Fertil Steril* 1998;69:904–908.
14. Lauritsen JG. Aetiology of spontaneous abortions. A cytogenetic and epidemiologic study of 288 abortuses and their parents. *Acta Obstet Gynecol Scand* 1976;52:1.
15. Magenis RE, Chamberlain J. Paternal origin of nondysjunction. In: Cruz FF, Gerald SG, eds. *Trisomy 21 Down's syndrome.* NICHD-Mental Retardation Research Center Series. Baltimore: University Park Press, 1981.
16. Lenz W. Epidemiology of congenital malformations. *Ann N Y Acad Sci* 1965;123:228.
17. Hellstrom WJG, Neal DE. Diagnosis and therapy of male genital tract infections. *Infertil Reprod Med Clin North Am* 1992;3:399.
18. Cnattingius S, Forman MR, Berendes HW, Isotalo L. Delayed childbearing and risk of adverse perinatal outcome. *JAMA* 1992;268:886.
19. Public Health Statistics 1978–84. Wisconsin Department of Health and Human Services, Bureau of Health Statistics, Madison, WI, 1985.
20. Menken J, Larsen U. Age in fertility: how late can you wait? Presented at the Annual Meeting of the Population Association of America, Minneapolis, MN, May 1984.
21. Ventura SJ. *Trends in the first order births to older mothers, 1970–79.* Department of Health and Human Services publication (PHS) no. 82-1120 (monthly vital statistics report). Hyattsville, MD: National Center for Health Statistics; 1982:31.
22. Sauer MV, Paulson RJ. Demographic differences between younger and older recipients seeking oocyte donation. *J Assisi Reprod Genet* 1992;9:400.
23. Medical Research International. *In vitro* fertilization/embryo transfer in the United States: 1985 and 1986 results from the National IVF/ET Registry. *Fertil Steril* 1988;49:212.
24. Medical Research International and the Society of Assisted Reproductive Technology. *In vitro* fertilization/embryo transfer in the United States: 1987 results from the National IVF/ET Registry. *Fertil Steril* 1989;51:13.
25. Medical Research International and the Society for Assisted Reproductive Technology. *In vitro* fertilization-embryo transfer in the United States: 1988 results from the IVF-ET Registry. *Fertil Steril* 1990;53:13.
26. Medical Research International and the Society for Assisted Reproductive Technology. *In vitro* fertilization-embryo transfer (IVF-ET) in the United States: 1989 results from the IVF-ET Registry. *Fertil Steril* 1991;55:14.
27. Medical Research International and the Society for Assisted Reproductive Technology. *In vitro* fertilization-embryo transfer (IVF-ET) in the United States: 1990 results from the IVF-ET Registry. *Fertil Steril* 1992;57:15.
28. French National Register on *in vitro* Fertilization (FIVNAT). *In vitro* fertilization: influence of women's age on pregnancy rates. *Hum Reprod* 1990;5:56.
29. Dicker D, Goldman JA, Ashkenazi J, Feldberg D, Shelef M, Levy T. Age and pregnancy rates in *in vitro* fertilization. *J In Vitro Fertil Embryo Transfer* 1991;8:141.
30. Templeton A, Morris JK. Reducing the risk of multiple births by transfer of two embryos after *in vitro* fertilization. *N Engl J Med* 1998;339:573.
31. Richardson SJ, Senikas V, Nelson JF. Follicular-accelerated loss and ultimate exhaustion. *J Clin Endocrinol Metab* 1987;65:1231.
32. Block E. Quantitative morphological investigations of the follicular system in women: variations at different ages. *Acta Anat* 1952;14:108.

33. Baker TG. A quantitative and cytological study of germ cells of human ovaries. *Proc R Soc Lond Biol* 1963;158:417.

34. Federation CECUS, Schwartz D, Mayaux MJ. Female fecundity as a function of age. *N Engl J Med* 1982;306:404.

35. Stovall DW, Toma SK, Hammond MG, Talbert LM. The effect of age and female fecundity. *Obstet Gynecol* 1991;77:33.

36. Huck E. Rates of chromosomal abnormalities at different maternal ages. *Obstet Gynecol* 1981;58:282.

37. Golbus MS, Loughman WD, Epstein CJ, Halbasch G, Stephens JD, Hall BD. Prenatal genetic diagnosis in 3000 amniocentesis. *N Engl J Med* 1979;300:157.

38. Scott RT, Toner JP, Muasher SJ, Oehninger S, Robinson S, Rosenwaks Z. Follicle-stimulating hormone levels on cycle day 3 are predictive of *in vitro* fertilization outcome. *Fertil Steril* 1989;51:651.

39. Hughes EG, Robertson DM, Handelsman DJ, et al. Inhibin and estradiol responses to ovarian hyperstimulation: effects of age and predictive value for *in vitro* fertilization outcome. *J Clin Endocrinol Metab* 1990;70:358.

40. Danforth DR, Arbogast LK, Mroueh J, et al. Dimeric inhibin: a direct marker of ovarian aging. *Fertil Steril* 1998;70:119.

41. Jacobs SL, Metzger DA, Dobson WC, et al. Effect of age on response to human menopausal gonadotropin stimulation. *J Clin Endocrinol Metab* 1990;71:1525.

42. Natchtigall RD. Assessing fecundity after age 40. *Contemp Obstet Gynecol* 1991;36:11.

43. Sauer MV, Paulson RJ, Lobo RA. Reversing the natural decline in human fertility: an extended clinical trial of oocyte donation to women of advanced reproductive age. *JAMA* 1992;268:1275.

44. Wood C, Calderon I, Crombie A. Age and fertility: results of assisted reproductive technology in women over 40 years. *J Assist Reprod Genet* 1992;9:482.

45. Harman SM, Talbert GB. The effect of maternal age on ovulation, corpora lutea of pregnancy and implantation failure in mice. *J Reprod Fertil* 1970;23:33.

46. Holinka CF, Yueh-Chu T, Caleb EF. Reproductive aging in C57B2/6J mice; plasma progesterone, viable embryos and resorption frequency throughout pregnancy. *Biol Reprod* 1979;20:1201.

47. Thorneycroft IH, Soderwall AL. The nature of the litter size loss in senescent hamster. *Anat Rec* 1969;165:343.

48. Blaha GC. The influence of ovarian grafts upon young donors on the development of transferred ova in aged golden hamsters. *Fertil Steril* 1970;21:268.

49. Maibenco HC, Krehbiel RH. Reproductive decline in aged female rats. *J Reprod Fertil* 1973;32:121.

50. Werner MA, Barnhard J, Gordon JW. The effects of aging on sperm and oocytes. *Semin Reprod Endocrinol* 1991;9:231.

51. Levran D, Ben-Shlomo I, Dor J, Ben-Rafael Z, Nebel L, Mashiach S. Aging of endometrium and oocytes: observations on conception and abortion rates in an egg donation model. *Fertil Steril* 1991;56:1091.

52. Sauer MV, Paulson RJ. Oocyte donation to women with ovarian failure. *Contemp Obstet Gynecol* 1989;34:125.

53. Sauer MV, Paulson RJ, Lobo RA. A preliminary report on oocyte donation extending reproductive potential to women over forty. *N Engl J Med* 1990;323:1157.

54. de Ziegler D, Bessis R, Frydman R. Vascular resistance of uterine arteries: physiological effects of estradiol and progesterone. *Fertil Steril* 1991;55:755.

55. Perrot-Applanat M, Groyer-Picart MT, Garcia E, Lorenzo F, Milgram E. Immunocytochemical demonstration of estrogen and progesterone receptors in muscle cells of uterine arteries in rabbits and humans. *Endocrinology* 1988;123:1511.

56. Sauer MV, Miles RA, Dahmoush L, Paulson RJ, Press M, Moyer D. Evaluating the effect of age on endometrial responsiveness to hormone replacement therapy: a histologic, ultrasonographic, and tissue receptor analysis. *J Assist Reprod Genet* 1993;10:47.

57. Buster JE, Sauer MV. Nonsurgical donor ovum transfer: new option for infertile couples. *Contemp Obstet Gynecol* 1986;28:39.

58. Seidel GE. Superovulation and embryo transfer in cattle. *Science* 1981;211:351.

59. Bustillo M, Buster JE, Cohen S, et al. Nonsurgical ovum transfer as a treatment in infertile women. *JAMA* 1984;251:1171.

60. Sauer MV, Bustillo M, Gorrill MJ, Louw JA, Marshall JR, Buster JE. An instrument for the recovery of preimplantation uterine ova. *Obstet Gynecol* 1988;71:804.

61. Sauer MV, Anderson RE, Paulson RJ. A trial of superovulation in ovum donors undergoing uterine lavage. *Fertil Steril* 1989;51:131.

62. Carson SA, Smith AL, Scoggan JL, Buster JE. Superovulation fails to increase human blastocyst yield after uterine lavage. *Prenatal Diagn* 1991;11:513.

63. Lutjen P, Trounson A, Leeton J, Findlay J, Wood C, Renou P. The establishment and maintenance of pregnancy using *in vitro* fertilization and embryo donation in a patient with primary ovarian failure. *Nature* 1984;307:174.

64. Rosenwaks Z. Donor eggs: their application in modern reproductive technologies. *Fertil Steril* 1987;47:895.

65. Navot D, Laufer N, Kopolovic J, et al. Artificially induced endometrial cycles and establishment of pregnancies in the absence of ovaries. *N Engl J Med* 1986;314:806.

66. Asch RH, Balmaceda JP, Ord T, et al. Oocyte donation and gamete intrafallopian transfer in premature ovarian failure. *Fertil Steril* 1988;49:263.

67. Abdulla HI, Baber R, Kirkland A, Leonard T, Power M, Studd JWW. A report on 100 cycles of oocyte donation: factors affecting the outcome. *Hum Reprod* 1990;5:1018.

68. Sauer MV, Paulson RJ, Macaso TM, Francis MM, Lobo RA. Oocyte and preembryo donation to women with ovarian failure: an extended clinical trial. *Fertil Steril* 1991;55:39.

69. Paulson RJ, Sauer MV, Lobo RA. Factors affecting embryo implantation after human *in vitro* fertilization: a hypothesis. *Am J Obstet Gynecol* 1990;163:2020.

70. Serhal PF, Craft IL. Oocyte donation in 61 patients. *Lancet* 1989;1:1185.

71. Lindheim SR. Indications, success rates and outcomes. In: Sauer MV, ed. *Principles of oocyte and embryo donation.* New York: Springer-Verlag, 1998:11.

72. Paulson RJ, Hatch IE, Lobo RA, Sauer MV. Cumulative conception and live births after oocyte donation: implications regarding endometrial receptivity. *Hum Reprod* 1997;12:835.

73. Remohi J, Gartner B, Gallardo E, Yalil S, Simon C, Pellicer A. Pregnancy and birth rates after oocyte donation. *Fertil Steril* 1997;67:717.

74. Sauer MV, Paulson RJ, Lobo RA. Pregnancy after age 50: applying oocyte donation to women following natural menopause. *Lancet* 1993;341:321.

75. Sauer MV, Paulson RJ. Understanding the current status of oocyte donation in the United States: what's really going on out there? *Fertil Steril* 1992;58:16.

76. Taylor PJ, Gomel V. Abraham laughed. *Int J Fertil* 1992;37:202.

77. Seibel MM. To everything there is a season. *Contemp Obstet Gynecol* 1992;37:153.

78. The American Society for Reproductive Medicine. Guidelines for gamete and embryo donation. *Fertil Steril* 1998;70[Suppl 3]:5S.

79. Sauer MV, Stein A, Paulson RJ, Moyer D. Endometrial responses to various hormone replacement regimens in ovarian failure patients preparing for embryo donation. *Int J Gynecol Obstet* 1991;35:61.

80. Leeton J, Rogers P, Cameron I, Caro C, Healy D. Pregnancy results following embryo transfer in women receiving low-dosage variable length estrogen replacement therapy for premature ovarian failure. *J In Vitro Fertil Embryo Transfer* 1989;6:232.

81. Cassadenti DL, Miles RA, Vijod A, Press M, Paulson RJ, Sauer MV. Comparing responses to varying hormone replacement regimens prior to embryo donation: a histologic, serologic, and receptor analysis. Presented at the 38th Annual Meeting of the Society for Gynecologic Investigation, San Antonio, TX, March 1992.

82. Steingold KA, Matt DW, DeZiegler D, Sealey JE, Fratkin M, Reznikov S. Comparison of transdermal to oral estradiol administration on hormonal and hepatic parameters in women with premature ovarian failure. *J Clin Endocrinol Metab* 1991;73:275.

83. Sauer MV. Hormone replacement prior to embryo donation to women with ovarian failure. *Female Patient* 1991;16:15.

84. Sauer MV. Progesterone therapy: modern uses and treatment alternatives. *Contemp Obstet Gynecol* 1997;42[Suppl]:4.

85. Gibbons WE, Toner JP, Hamacher P, Kolm P. Experience with a novel vaginal progesterone preparation in a donor oocyte program. *Fertil Steril* 1998;69:96.

86. Remohi J, Ardiles G, Garcia-Velasco JA, Gaitan P, Simon C, Pellicer A. Endometrial thickness and serum oestradiol concentrations as predictors of outcome in oocyte donation. *Hum Reprod* 1997;12:2271.

87. Sauer MV, Paulson RJ, Moyer DL. Assessing the importance of performing an endometrial biopsy prior to oocyte donation. *J Assist Reprod Genet* 1997;14:125.

88. Miles RA, Paulson RJ, Lobo RA, Press MF, Dahmoush L, Sauer MV. Pharmacokinetics and endometrial tissue levels of progesterone after administration by intramuscular and vaginal routes: a comparative study. *Fertil Steril* 1994;62:485.

89. Abdulla HI, Billett A, Kan AK, et al. Obstetric outcome in 232 ovum donation pregnancies. *Br J Obstet Gynaecol* 1998;105:332.

90. Sauer MV, Paulson RJ. Establishment of consecutive pregnancies in a menopausal woman following oocyte donation. *Gynecol Obstet Invest* 1991;32:118.

91. Cohen J, Scott R, Schimmel T, Levron J, Willadsen S. Birth of infant after transfer of anucleate donor oocyte cytoplasm into recipient eggs. *Lancet* 1997;350:186.

92. Takeuchi T, Ergun B, Huang TH, et al. Preliminary experience of nuclear transplantation in human oocytes [Abstract O-233]. Presented at the 54th Annual Meeting of the American Society for Reproductive Medicine, San Francisco, CA, October 1998.

93. Oktay K, Newton H, Aubard Y, Salha O, Gosden R. Cryopreservation of immature human oocytes and ovarian tissue: an emerging technology? *Fertil Steril* 1998;69:1.

94. Tucker MJ, Wright G, Morton PC, Massey JB. Birth after cryopreservation of immature oocytes with subsequent *in vitro* maturation. *Fertil Steril* 1998;70:578.

95. Mori T. National regulation of and achievements in assisted reproduction in Japan. *J Assist Reprod Genet* 1992;9:293.

96. Peinado JA, Russell SE. The Spanish law governing assisted reproduction techniques: a summary. *Hum Reprod* 1990;5:634.

97. Sauer MV. Motherhood at any age? Oocyte donation was not intended for everyone. *Fertil Steril* 1998;69:187.

Treatment of the Postmenopausal Woman: Basic and Clinical Aspects, Second Edition, edited by Rogerio A. Lobo, Lippincott Williams & Wilkins, Philadelphia © 1999.

CHAPTER 4

The Endocrinology of the Menopause

Christopher Longcope

The menopause is defined as the last menstrual period in a woman's life and is usually identified as such retrospectively after 12 months of amenorrhea (1). Although some women experience regular cycles until their cessation, others experience a variable time of irregular cycles often accompanied by episodes of heavy bleeding. In any one woman, it is difficult to identify any one menses as the last, although as a woman becomes older and the length of the amenorrhea increases, there is an increasing probability that she has experienced her last menses (2). The pattern of gonadotropin, estradiol, and progesterone concentrations varies among women, especially in those whose last cycles may be irregular in length (3). The endocrinology of menopause is therefore characterized by diversity, and mean data may not necessarily apply to any one individual.

OVARY

From the standpoint of the ovary, the menopause is not a sudden event but is the cumulative result of events, some of which began in fetal life. For the normal, healthy woman, ovarian size increases until early adult life, with fluctuations caused by follicle and corpora luteal growth and pregnancy. However, by the age of 40, there is a slow but steady decrease in size until menopause (4). The rate of decrease increases in the perimenopausal period (4,5), and within 5 to 10 years of menopause, the rate of decrease in size slows (5). In the younger woman, some of this loss in size reflects the loss of follicles, but the decrease after menopause more often reflects changes in supporting tissue and stromal cells.

The ovary contains its maximum number of follicles, estimated as 2×10^6 to 6×10^6 (6), during fetal development. However, even *in utero* follicles are disappearing, so that at birth the number is less, and follicles continue to disappear at a steady rate until near menopause (6–8).

This loss primarily results from atresia, not ovulation, because in 40 years of reproductive life with monthly spontaneous ovulations, only 480 follicles ovulate.

Just before menopause, there is an increase in the rate at which follicles become atretic and disappear (6,7). This increased rate of disappearance may be a reflection of the increase in follicle-stimulating hormone (FSH) levels often seen then (3), but there are few data concerning that point. The ovarian follicles in perimenopausal women, although fewer, appear to be healthy, with a low androgen to estrogen ratio in the follicular fluid (9).

Whether the ovary is without follicles at the time of menopause remains uncertain, but probably there is individual variation. One reason for the uncertainty is technologic in that a thorough search for follicles that may be 1 to 5 mm in diameter in an ovary that is 3×5 cm in diameter is a tedious process, and the number of ovaries so examined is not large. Richardson and Nelson (6) did find a few ovaries without follicles at menopause, but others have reported that the ovaries still contain primordial follicles, even in women who are 10 years postmenopausal (10–12).

As the follicles become fewer, cycle irregularity usually becomes apparent (3,13), and the frequency of ovulatory cycles decreases. The orderly pattern of estradiol increases and decreases is lost, and as long as the cycles are anovulatory, progesterone concentrations remain low (<1.0 g/mL). Even if the cycles are ovulatory, the estradiol and progesterone concentrations through these last cycles are generally less than during the cycles of younger women (3,14,15).

With the cessation of menstruation, there is a decline in estradiol concentrations that is relatively steep for the first 12 months and then shows only a slight decline over the ensuing years (16–18) (Table 4.1 and Fig. 4.1). As seen in Fig. 4.1, there is an occasional and transient increase in estradiol concentration in some women, although these fluctuations are often not associated with episodes of vaginal bleeding (14,16). Metcalf has suggested that the sensi-

C. Longcope: Departments of Obstetrics and Gynecology and Medicine, University of Massachusetts Medical School, Worcester, Massachusetts 01655.

TABLE 4.1. *Hormonal concentrations in perimenopausal and postmenopausal women stratified by months from last menses*

Months from last menses	E2 (n)	T (pg/mL)	DHEA (ng/mL)	FSH mg/mL	FSH mIU/mL
<3	40	108 ± 19[a,b]	0.21 ± 0.02	1.32 ± 0.11	27 ± 4[c]
3–9	12	32 ± 7	0.22 ± 0.02	1.33 ± 0.14	57 ± 9[d]
9–12	18	26 ± 4[d]	0.20 ± 0.02	1.51 ± 0.19	84 ± 16[d]
12–24	6	19 ± 4	0.20 ± 0.06	1.52 ± 0.19	91 ± 18[d]
>24	12	14 ± 1[d]	0.19 ± 0.02	1.53 ± 0.24	69 ± 9[d]

E2, estradiol; T, testosterone; DHEA, dehydroepiandrosterone; FSH, follicle-stimulating hormone.
[a]Means ± SE.
[b]The difference between c and d in some columns is significant, $p<0.05$ by the Bonferroni t-test.
Data from ref. 16, with permission.

tivity of the endometrium may decline at menopause as a possible reason for the continuing amenorrhea despite transient estrogen elevations (14). The transient elevations of estradiol are sometimes a reflection of activity in a residual follicle, but such activity does not appear to be associated with ovulation. Metcalf et al. (19,20) reported no instances of progesterone increase in the postmenopausal women in whom they found a transient increase in estradiol. Other data (16) confirm these observations. In other instances, the elevations are associated with stromal hyperplasia (21), and in many cases, the exact cause is uncertain.

As with estradiol, the concentration of estrone, a weaker estrogen, also falls at and after menopause (16). The pattern of this fall is similar to that of estradiol and the concentrations of these two estrogens are highly correlated although the concentration of estrone is higher than that of estradiol in contradistinction to their relationships in normal younger women.

Estrone sulfate, as a metabolite of estrone and estradiol, is present in the circulation at higher levels than estrone or estradiol, and with menopause, its concentration falls in a pattern similar to the other estrogens (16). Although estrone sulfate has no biologic activity of its own, it becomes an active estrogen when the sulfate group is cleared as can occur in many tissues. It has been postulated as an important source of estrogenic activity in the breast (22).

In reproductive-aged normal women, the ovary is the major source of estrogens. The menopause is associated with a marked decline in the ovarian secretion of estrogens (Table 4.2) such that in only about 10% of postmenopausal women does the ovary secrete significant quantities of estradiol (23). In most postmenopausal women, the major source of circulating estradiol is from the peripheral aromatization of androgens (24,25). The menopause is also associated with a decrease in ovarian androgen secretion (Table 4.2) and with a shift in the pattern of ovarian androgen secretion toward the secretion of testosterone at the expense of androstenedione (26,27). In many postmenopausal women, the ovarian secretion of testosterone is maintained at a level approaching that of younger women, although the secretion of androstenedione falls. However, the fall in the secretion of androstenedione, a major source of testosterone, results in a decline in circulating testosterone in most postmenopausal women (16).

The fall in circulating androgens appears to precede menopause, as shown for testosterone in Table 4.1 and Fig. 4.2 (16,28), and there is little or no further decline. As shown in Fig. 4.2, the levels of testosterone for most women are well below the mean in young women (0.27 ng/mL). However, the levels for some postmenopausal are above that mean. Whether these women have different menopausal symptoms is uncertain.

The levels of androstenedione are also lower in postmenopausal women (16,17,28). Although some data indicate the fall occurs before menopause (16), this has not

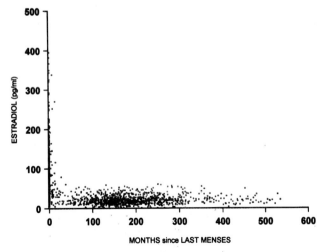

FIG. 4.1. Estradiol concentration (pg/mL) plotted against months since the last menses when the sample was obtained. Data represent 1,986 samples from 401 women.

TABLE 4.2. *Range of ovarian secretion rates of androgens and estrogens in young and postmenopausal women*

Secreted hormone	Ovary Reproductive age[a] (mg/d)	Postmenopausal (mg/d)
Estradiol	40–80	0–20
Estrone	20–50	0–10
Testosterone	50–70	40–50
Androstenedione	1–1.5	0.3–0.6

[a]Mid-follicular phase.
Data from ref. 34, with permission.

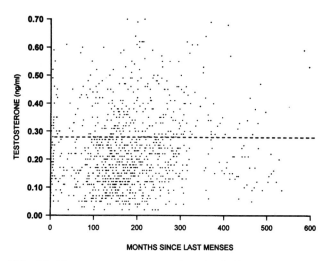

FIG. 4.2. Testosterone concentrations (ng/mL) plotted against months since the last menses when the sample was obtained. Data represent 1,921 samples from 397 women. The dashed line represents the mean value (0.28 ng/mL) for the testosterone concentration on day 5 of the cycle in 28 normal young women.

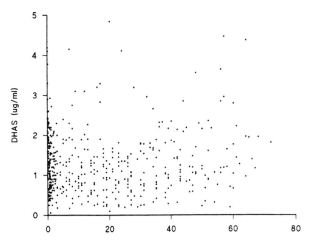

FIG. 4.3. Dehydroepiandrosterone sulfate concentrations (mg/mL) plotted against months since the last menses when the sample was obtained. Data represent 456 samples from 88 women.

been a universal finding. The levels of some circulating androgens have been reported to remain relatively stable (17) or to fall gradually after menopause (29). In any case, circulating androstenedione and testosterone levels are lower after menopause than in young women, and the decline is related to menopause.

Because there are few or no follicles in the ovary after menopause, the stromal cells are the main source of steroids. Stromal tissue from the ovaries of women up to 30 years after menopause has been shown to secrete androstenedione and estradiol *in vitro* (21). However, the ovaries of most menopausal women secrete testosterone but little androstenedione and little or no estradiol.

Luteinizing hormone (LH) receptors are present on the stromal cell in relative abundance, but FSH receptors are often not demonstrable (30). Because some stromal cells contain the aromatase complex (31), the paucity of FSH receptors may explain in part the lack of estrogen secretion from the ovary in most postmenopausal women (23,26). With the decline in follicle number, the level of circulating inhibin (32) decreases. This decrease may occur before menopause, but like changes in FSH levels, it may be variable (32). The levels of follistatin have been reported to remain relatively constant at menopause (33).

ADRENAL

Although the adrenal in young women secretes only small amounts of estrogens, it secretes a significant amount of androgen precursors such as dehydroepiandrosterone sulfate (DHEAS), dehydroepiandrosterone (DHEA), androstenedione, and the more active androgen testosterone (34). The adrenal is the only source of DHEAS (34), and if menopause caused a change in the adrenal secretion of these steroids, such a change should

be manifest by an alteration in DHEAS levels. As shown in Table 4.1 and Fig. 4.3, there is no change in the circulating levels of DHEAS related to menopause. There is a decline in the levels of DHEAS and DHEA with age (35,36), but this is independent of menopause. The circulating levels of cortisol and aldosterone also are not altered by menopause (37). The menopause is not characterized by any perturbation of adrenal steroid secretion.

HYPOTHALAMIC-PITUITARY AXIS

The hypothalamic-pituitary axis is a site in which marked changes in activity occur during and before menopause (3,18,38). The most dramatic change occurs in the secretion of FSH by the pituitary, and many women have an increase in the level of FSH even while menstrual cycles persist, albeit the cycles are often frequently irregular. In women still having cycles, the FSH concentration may be increased intermittently (32), but with the cessation of menses, FSH levels rise to a plateau within the first year (Table 4.1 and Fig. 4.4). It is probable that, with the passage of years, FSH levels will decline (39), but even in the very elderly, provided they are in good health, FSH levels remain elevated.

Although LH may be increased before menopause in some women (40), LH remains in the normal range in most of them despite the rise in FSH. At menopause, LH levels rise and plateau after about 12 months of amenorrhea (16). There may be a decline in LH levels in later years (39,41). Much of this rise is caused by the decline in ovarian estrogen secretion and the resultant loss of the negative feedback. However, the ovarian follicles are a major source of inhibin, which suppresses pituitary FSH secretion (42,43).

The increased circulating levels FSH and LH result from increased pituitary secretion of gonadotropins without a change in their metabolism (44,45). The pulses of LH and FSH are increased in amplitude but not in frequency (46), and there is an accentuated response to gonadotropin-releas-

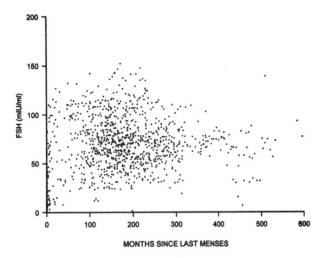

FIG. 4.4. Follicle-stimulating hormone concentrations (mIU/mL) plotted against months since the last menses when the sample was obtained. Data represent 1,972 samples from 393 women.

ing hormone (GnRH) administration in postmenopausal compared with younger women. It has been suggested that there is less inhibition by endorphins on LH pulse release to explain some of the increase in GnRH amplitude (47).

When measured by sensitive assays, the ratio of bioassayable (B) to immunoassayable (I) LH has been reported to be about two to five for women in the follicular phase of the cycle (48,49). With the menopause, the B:I ratio increases markedly to 10 to 15, depending somewhat on the standards used (45,48,49). The mechanism and importance of this rise remain uncertain.

To what degree the changes in the hypothalamic pituitary ovarian axis are caused by the ovary alone also are uncertain (50,51). There is a decrease in opioid inhibition of gonadotropin secretion in postmenopausal women, but because the opioid inhibition can be restored by estrogen replacement, it is possible that the loss of inhibition is related to the ovarian failure (47). However, it has been reported that hypothalamic pituitary events in rodents occur before ovarian failure and appear to be locally medicated (52–54). The relationship, if any, between these events and menopause in women is unsure (51,55).

HORMONE METABOLISM

Although there are marked changes in ovarian and pituitary hormone secretion, there appear to be few changes in hormone metabolism. The metabolism of LH and FSH does not appear to change at menopause (44,45). Similarly, the overall metabolism of androgens and estrogens is not altered by the relatively abrupt changes in secretion and production that occur with menopause (56). The metabolic clearance rates of testosterone and estradiol do not change across menopause (Table 4.3 and Figs. 4.5 and 4.6). Although the concen-

TABLE 4.3. *Metabolic clearance rates for estradiol and testosterone stratified by months from last menses*

Months from last menses	N	MCR^{E_2} (L/d)	MCR^T (L/d)
>3	40	1060 ± 70[a,b]	480 ± 25[b]
3–9	12	1120 ± 110	510 ± 60
9–12	18	960 ± 50	410 ± 25
12–24	6	940 ± 30	410 ± 50
>24	12	1010 ± 80	430 ± 40

E_2, estradiol; MCR, metabolic clearance rate; T, testosterone.
[a]Means ± SE.
[b]Differences between means in the same columns are not significant, $p > 0.05$ by the Bonferroni t-test.

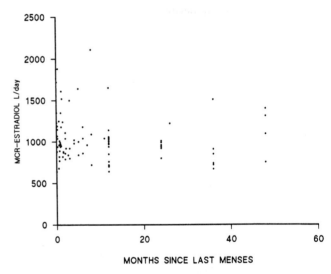

FIG. 4.5. Metabolic clearance rate (MCR) of estradiol plotted against months since the last menses when measured. Data are from 88 women.

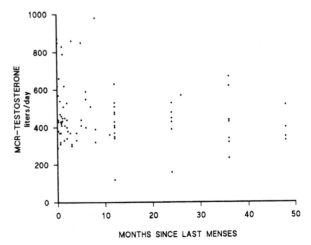

FIG. 4.6. Metabolic clearance rate (MCR) of testosterone plotted against months since the last menses when measured. Data are from 88 women.

TABLE 4.4. *Peripheral aromatization of androstenedione to estrone and of testosterone to estradiol premenopausal and postmenopausal women*

| Status | $[\rho]^{A,E1}_{BB}$ | | $[\rho]^{T,E2}_{BB}$ | |
	n	%	n	%
Premenopausal	21	1.41 ± 0.12^a	26	0.23 ± 0.02
Postmenopausal	49	2.82 ± 0.28	30	0.67 ± 0.10
	$p<0.001^b$		$p<0.001^b$	

$[\rho]^{A,E1}$, percent of androstenedione entering the blood that is converted to estrone; $[\rho]^{T,E2}$, testosterone converted to estradiol; BB, blood-blood.
^{a}Mean $\pm$ SEM.
^{b}Difference between premenopausal and postmenopausal means.

tration of testosterone does not change, that of estradiol falls, and despite this, its clearance rate is unaltered.

There is a shift in one pathway of androgen metabolism: aromatization in peripheral tissues such as adipose tissue, muscle, and probably skin. Although this change in the aromatization pathway is not great enough to be reflected in the overall metabolism of androgens, it is important to estrogen production. The peripheral aromatization of androstenedione and testosterone is significantly greater in postmenopausal women than in younger women (Table 4.4), but as shown in Fig. 4.7, the aromatization of androstenedione to estrone (percent of androstenedione entering the blood that is aromatized to estrone = $[\rho]^{A,E1}BB$) does not appear to be related to time since the last menses. The change could occur before menopause or be so gradual that little change would be observed over the course of the years shown.

With the decline in ovarian estrogen secretion, peripheral aromatization becomes the major source of estrogens in postmenopausal women (24,25). Because adipose tissue is an important site for aromatization, the increased levels of circulating estrogens in obese postmenopausal women is probably a reflection of the increased aromatization (57,58).

THYROID, PARATHYROID, AND PANCREAS

For the thyroid, parathyroid, and pancreas, changes in circulating levels of their respective hormones have been reported during aging (59–62). However, there is little or no evidence that there is a menopause-related change in the function of these glands. Leptin levels have been found to be lower in postmenopausal compared with those in premenopausal women, even when corrected for fat mass (63).

The menopause is associated with a marked decline in ovarian function manifested by a decrease in circulating estrogens and, to a somewhat lesser extent, androgens. There is an increase in pituitary gonadotropin secretion that in many women antedates a demonstrable change in ovarian cyclicity. Whether the increase in pituitary gonadotropin secretion results entirely from the change in ovarian function is somewhat uncertain. The other endocrine glands do not participate in the menopausal events or symptoms.

ACKNOWLEDGEMENTS

The author gratefully acknowledges the assistance of Dr. C. C. Johnston, Indiana University School of Medicine, in obtaining some of the data shown in this chapter. The studies were supported by grants AG-02927 and RR-750 from the National Institutes of Health.

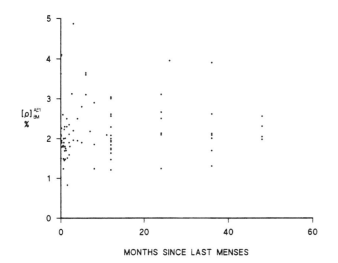

FIG. 4.7. Aromatization of androstenedione to estrone ($[\rho]^{A,E1}BB$) plotted against months since the last menses when measured. Data are from 88 women.

REFERENCES

1. Richardson SJ. The biological basis of the menopause. *Baillieres Clin Endocrinol Metab* 1993;7:1–16.
2. Cramer DW, Xu H. Predicting age at menopause. *Maturitas* 1996;23:319–326.
3. Sherman BM, West JH, Korenman SG. The menopausal transition: analysis of LH, FSH, estradiol, and progesterone concentrations during menstrual cycles of older women. *J Clin Endocrinol Metab* 1976;42:629–636.
4. Andolf E, Jörgensen C, Svalenius E, Sunden B. Ultrasound measurement of the ovarian volume. *Acta Obstet Gynecol Scand* 1987;66:387–389.
5. Goswamy RK, Campbell S, Royston JP, et al. Ovarian size in postmenopausal women. *Br J Obstet Gynaecol* 1988;95:795–801.
6. Richardson SJ, Nelson JF. Follicular depletion during the menopausal transition. *Ann N Y Acad Sci* 1990;592:13–20.

7. Gosden RG, Faddy MJ. Ovarian aging, follicular depletion, and steroidogenesis. *Exp Gerontol* 1994;29:265–274.
8. Faddy MJ, Gosden RG. A model conforming the decline in follicle numbers to the age of menopause in women. *Hum Reprod* 1996;11:1484–1486.
9. Klein NA, Battaglia DE, Miller PB, Branigan EF, Giudice LC, Soules MR. Ovarian follicular development and the follicular fluid hormones and growth factors in normal women of advanced reproductive age. *J Clin Endocrinol Metab* 1996;81:1946–1951.
10. Costoff A, Mahesh VB. Primordial follicles with normal oocytes in the ovaries of postmenopausal women. *J Am Geriatr Soc* 1975;23:193–196.
11. Gosden RG. Follicular status at the menopause. *Hum Reprod* 1987;2:617–621.
12. Thatcher SS, Naftolin F. The aging and aged ovary. *Semin Reprod Endocrinol* 1991;9:189–199.
13. Upton GV. The perimenopause: physiologic correlates and clinical management. *J Reprod Med* 1982;27:1–27.
14. Metcalf MG. The approach of menopause: a New Zealand study. *N Z Med J* 1988;101:103–106.
15. Rannevik G, Jeppsson S, Johnell O, Bjerre B, Laurell-Borulf Y, Svanberg L. A longitudinal study of the perimenopausal transition: altered profiles of steroid and pituitary hormones, SHBG and bone mineral density. *Maturitas* 1995;21:103–113.
16. Longcope C, Franz C, Morello C, Baker R, Johnston CC Jr. Steroid and gonadotropin levels in women during the peri-menopausal years. *Maturitas* 1986;8:189–196.
17. Judd HL, Fournet N. Changes of ovarian hormonal function with aging. *Exp Gerontol* 1994;29:285–298.
18. Burger HG, Dudley EC, Hopper JL, et al. The endocrinology of the menopausal transition: a cross-sectional study of a population-based sample. *J Clin Endocrinol Metab* 1995;80:3537–3545.
19. Metcalf MG, Donald RA, Livesey JH. Pituitary-ovarian function before, during and after the menopause: a longitudinal study. *Clin Endocrinol* 1982;17:489–494.
20. Metcalf MG. Incidence of ovulation from the menarche to the menopause: observations of 622 New Zealand women. *N Z Med J* 1983;96:645–648.
21. Dennefors BL, Janson PO, Knutson F, Hamberger L. Steroid production and responsiveness to gonadotropin in isolated stromal tissue of human postmenopausal ovaries. *Am J Obstet Gynecol* 1980;136:997–1002.
22. Santen RJ, Leszczynski D, Tilson-Mallet N, et al. Enzymatic control of estrogen production in human breast cancer: relative significance of aromatase versus sulfatase pathways. *Ann N Y Acad Sci* 1986;464:126–137.
23. Longcope C, Hunter R, Franz C. Steroid secretion by the postmenopausal ovary. *Am J Obstet Gynecol* 1980;138:564–568.
24. Siiteri PK, MacDonald PC. Role of extraglandular estrogen in human endocrinology. In: Greep RO, Astwood E, eds. *Handbook of physiology:* endocrinology, vol 2. Washington, DC: American Physiology Society, 1973:615–629.
25. Longcope C. The significance of steroid production by peripheral tissues. In: Scholler R, ed. *Endocrinology of the ovary.* Paris: Editions SEPE, 1978:23–35.
26. Judd HL, Judd GE, Lucas EE. Endocrine function of the postmenopausal ovary: concentration of androgens and estrogens in ovarian and peripheral vein blood. *J Clin Endocrinol Metab* 1974;39:1020.
27. Aleen FA, McIntosh TK. Menopausal syndrome: plasma levels of β-endorphin in post-menopausal women measured by a specific radioimmunoassay. *Maturitas* 1985;7:329–334.
28. Meldrum DR, Davidson BJ, Tataryn IV, Judd HL. Changes in circulating steroids with aging in postmenopausal women. *Obstet Gynecol* 1981;57:624–628.
29. Vermeulen A. Sex hormone status of the postmenopausal woman. *Maturitas* 1980;2:81–89.
30. Vihko KK. Gonadotropins and ovarian gonadotropin receptors during the perimenopausal transition period. *Maturitas* 1996;23:S19–S22.
31. Inkster SE, Brodie AMH. Expression of aromatase cytochrome P-450 in pre-menopausal and postmenopausal human ovaries: an immunocytochemical study. *J Clin Endocrinol Metab* 1991;73:717–726.
32. Burger HG. The endocrinology of the menopause. *Maturitas* 1996;23:129–132.
33. Kettel LM, DePaolo LV, Morales AJ, Apter D, Ling N, Yen SS. Circulating levels of follistatin from puberty to menopause. *Fertil Steril* 1996;65:472–476.
34. Longcope C. Adrenal and gonadal androgen secretion in normal females. *J Clin Endocrinol Metab* 1986;15:213–228.
35. Zumoff B, Rosenfeld RS, Strain GW, Levin J, Fukushima DK. Sex differences in the twenty-four-hour mean plasma concentrations of dehydroepiandrosterone (DHA) and dehydroepiandrosterone sulfate (DHAS) and the DHA:DHAS ratio in normal adults. *J Clin Endocrinol Metab* 1980;51:330–333.
36. Carlstrom K, Brody S, Lunell N, et al. Dehydroepiandrosterone sulphate and dehydroepiandrosterone in serum: differences related to age and sex. *Maturitas* 1988;10:297–306.
37. Parker L, Gral T, Perrigo V, Showsky R. Decreased adrenal androgen sensitivity to ACTH during aging. *Metabolism* 1981;30:601–604.
38. Metcalf MG, Donald RA, Livesey JH. Pituitary-ovarian function in normal women during the menopausal transition. *Clin Endocrinol* 1981;14:245–255.
39. Chakravarti S, Collins WP, Forecast JD, Newton JR, Oram D, H, Studd JWW. Hormonal profiles after the menopause. *BMJ* 1976;2:784–787.
40. Metcalf MG, Livesey JH. Gonadotropin excretion in fertile women: effect of age and the onset of the menopausal transition. *J Endocrinol* 1985;105:357–362.
41. Kwekkeboom DJ, de Jong FH, Van Hemert AM, Vandenbroucke JP, Valkenburg HA, Lamberts SWJ. Serum gonadotropins and a-subunit decline in aging normal postmenopausal women. *J Clin Endocrinol Metab* 1990;70:944–950.
42. Vale W, Rivier C, Hsueh A, et al. Chemical and biological characterization of the inhibin family of protein hormones. *Recent Prog Horm Res* 1988;44:1–34.
43. Ying S. Inhibins, activins, and follistatins: gonadal proteins modulating the secretion of follicle-stimulating hormone. *Endocr Rev* 1988;9:267–293.
44. Kohler PO, Ross GT, Odell WD. Metabolic clearance and production rates of human luteinizing hormone in pre- and post-menopausal women. *J Clin Invest* 1968;47:38–47.
45. Veldhuis JD, Urban RJ, Beitins IZ, Blizzard RM, Johnson ML, Dufau ML. Pathophysiological features of the pulsatile secretion of biologically active luteinizing hormone in man. *J Steroid Biochem* 1989;33:739–749.
46. Yen SSC, Vandenberg G, Tsai CC, Parker DC. Ultradian fluctuations of gonadotropins. In: Ferin M, Halberg F, Richart RM, Vande Wiele RL, eds. *Biorhythms and human reproduction.* New York: John Wiley & Sons, 1974:203–218.
47. Genazzani AR, Petraglia F. Opioid control of luteinizing hormone secretion on humans. *J Steroid Biochem* 1989;33:751–755.
48. Sawyer-Steffan JE, Lasley BL, Hoff JD, Yen SSC. Comparison of *in vitro* bioactivity and immunoreactivity of serum LH in normal cyclic and hypogonadal women treated with low doses of LH-RH. *J Reprod Fertil* 1982;65:45–51.
49. Chang SP, Shoupe D, Kletzky OA, Lobo RA. Differences in the ratio of bioactive to immunoreactive serum luteinizing hormone during vasomotor flushes and hormonal therapy in postmenopausal women. *J Clin Endocrinol Metab* 1984;58 925–929.
50. Wise PM, Krajnak KM, Kashon ML. Menopause: the aging of multiple pacemakers. *Science* 1996;273:67–70.
51. Knobil E, Yen SS. The advent of menopause. *Science* 1996;274:18–20.
52. Nelson JF, Felicio LS. Hormonal influences on reproductive aging in mice. *Ann N Y Acad Sci* 1990;592:8–12.
53. Wise PM, Weiland NG, Scarbrough K, Larson GH, Lloyd JM. Contribution of changing rhythmicity of hypothalamic neurotransmitter function to female reproductive aging. *Ann N Y Acad Sci* 1990;592:31–43.
54. Meites J. Aging: hypothalamic catecholamines, neuroendocrine-immune interactions, and dietary restriction. *Proc Soc Exp Biol Med* 1990;195:304–311.
55. Jones EE, Seifer DB, Naftolin F. Effects of hypothalamic-pituitary aging on reproduction. *Semin Reprod Endocrinol* 1991;9:221–230.
56. Longcope C. Hormone dynamics at the menopause. *Ann N Y Acad Sci* 1990;592:21–30.
57. MacDonald PC, Edman CD, Hemsell DL, Porter JC, Siiteri PK. Effect of obesity on conversion of plasma androstenedione to estrone in postmenopausal women with and without endometrial cancer. *Am J Obstet Gynecol* 1978;130:448–455.
58. Longcope C, Baker R, Johnston CC Jr. Androgen and estrogen metabolism in relationship to obesity. *Metabolism* 1986;35:235–237.
59. Davidson MS. The effect of aging on carbohydrate metabolism: a review of the English literature and a practical approach to the diagnosis of diabetes mellitus in the elderly. *Metabolism* 1979;28:688–705.
60. Majumdar APN, Jaszewski R, Dubick MA. Effect of aging on the gastrointestinal tract and the pancreas. *Proc Soc Exp Biol Med* 1997;215:134–144.
61. Prince RL, Dick I, Devine A, et al. The effects of menopause and age on calcitropic hormones: a cross-sectional study of 655 healthy women aged 35 to 90. *J Bone Miner Res* 1995;10:835–842.
62. Bagchi N, Brown TR, Parish RF. Thyroid dysfunction in adults over 55 years: a study in an urban US community. *Arch Intern Med* 1990;150:785–787.
63. Rosenbaum M, Nicolson M, Hirsch J, et al. Effects of gender, body composition, and menopause on plasma concentrations of leptin. *J Clin Endocrinol Metab* 1996;81:3424–3427.

SECTION **II**

The Perimenopause

Since the last edition there has been increased attention paid to the span of life called the perimenopause. This is because of increased awareness of vasomotor and other symptoms, which often begin around this time and the conflicting, yet real, needs of women during this time in terms of contraception and fertility. Little has been known about the onset and evolution of symptoms and signs of menopause as women age. Several recent longitudinal studies such as the NIH-sponsored Study of Women's Health Across the Nation (SWAN) is providing useful information and the data will increase in years to come. Recent findings from SWAN are interesting and confirmatory. A consistent decline in E_2, with rising follicle stimulating hormones (FSH) levels with age have been observed. Interestingly, Chinese women had low E_2 yet similar FSH levels when compared with Caucasians. African-American women consistently had higher adjusted bone mineral density.

There is confusion as to how the perimenopause should be defined; an introductory chapter discusses this issue. The evolution of gametogenic and endocrine failure will be discussed by Buckler and Burger & Teede respectively in the next two chapters. The perimenopause is a time when irregular menstrual bleeding is common. This will be discussed by Ian Fraser who is a world-renowned expert on dysfunctional bleeding. Chapters which follow include one on decision-making regarding treatment by Judi Lee Chervenak and Nanette Santoro, and contraceptive options in this age from David Archer. As each chapter is intended to "stand alone," the reader will note some overlap between them. Prior to menopause, vasomotor symptoms may ensue as well as other subtle mood and somatic changes. Although treatment may be challenging while menstrual cycles are still occurring, it should be considered for bothersome symptoms. Chervenak and Santoro write of "customizing" therapy, an approach I have always encouraged. Decisions regarding various treatment options and whether treatment should be initiated are complex. It is hoped that the information contained in this section will help the provider to aid women in making this decision.

Treatment of the Postmenopausal Woman: Basic and Clinical Aspects, Second Edition, edited by Rogerio A. Lobo, Lippincott Williams & Wilkins, Philadelphia © 1999.

CHAPTER 5

The Perimenopause

Rogerio A. Lobo

A large segment of the population is going through a life stage called the perimenopause. This is an important and complex period, during which many changes are occurring in unpredictable ways. This segment has been added to this edition of the book to emphasize this important passage of time. Some of these thoughts have been presented previously in other publications (1).

The term *perimenopause* has been defined several different ways. Part of the confusion results from the definition of menopause. The term *menopause* marks the cessation of menses. Women experiencing various events before and after menopause are referred to as being premenopausal or postmenopausal. Although the latter term is often used interchangeably with menopausal, this term is less precise because menopause refers only to the last menstrual period. The term *perimenopause* therefore refers to the period surrounding the last menstrual event (i.e., menopause). The term *climacteric* is another term that refers to a period from the cessation of reproductive function to an indefinite time after menopause.

Because no strict definition exists for the perimenopause, by convention, most clinicians consider women to begin the perimenopause when menses become irregular or symptoms associated with estrogen deficiency occur just before the age of menopause. Although the average age of menopause is between 51 and 52 years, some women experience menopause in their 40s, and consequently, the age span of women experiencing the perimenopause can be quite large. After menopause, occasional and unexpected ovarian activity can occur for a brief period. For many women, the postmenopausal years

begin approximately 1 year after the cessation of menses. Although a few women experience no symptoms or menstrual irregularities before an abrupt and complete cessation of menses (i.e., no perimenopause), many women may experience three or more years of changes before menopause and continue to have some episodic fluctuations of ovarian activity (with or without bleeding) for approximately 1 year after menopause.

For many women, the perimenopause is associated with confusion about their reproductive status and general health. There often are symptoms of estrogen deficiency and irregular bleeding, concerns of becoming pregnant, or concerns about not being able to conceive. These findings occur at a time when women are young (chronologically), and many women are at the peak of their careers. Physiologically, estrogen deficiency leads to an increase in the risk factors for cardiovascular disease, and bone loss begins to accelerate.

The ovary changes markedly from birth to the onset of menopause (Fig. 5.1) (2). The greatest number of pri-

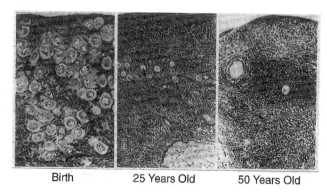

Birth   25 Years Old   50 Years Old

FIG. 5.1. Photomicrographs of the cortex of human ovaries from birth to 50 years of age. Small nongrowing primordial follicles *(arrows)* have a single layer of squamous granulosa cells. (From ref. 2, with permission.)

R. A. Lobo: Department of Obstetrics and Gynecology, Columbia University College of Physicians & Surgeons, New York, New York 10032

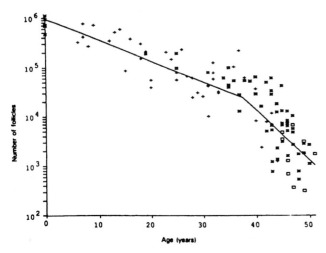

FIG. 5.2. The age-related decrease in the total number of primordial follicles (PF) within both human ovaries from birth to the menopause. As a result of recruitment (initiation of PF growth), the number of PF decreases progressively from about 1 million at birth to 25,000 at 37 years. At 37 years, the rate of recruitment increases sharply, and the number of PF declines to 1,000 at menopause (about 51 years of age). (From ref. 3, with permission.)

mordial follicles is present *in utero* at 20 weeks' gestation; they undergo a regular rate of atresia until around the age of 37. Figure 5.2 depicts the decline in primordial follicles, which becomes more rapid between age 37 and menopause; at this time, several hundred to a thousand follicles remain (3). These remaining follicles are primarily atretic in nature.

The size of the aging population is increasing worldwide. Between the years 2000 and 2025, the world population older than 60 years is expected to double, from 590 million to 1,100 million. In the United States, the number of women entering menopause will almost double in the 30 years between 1990 and 2020 (4) (Table 5.1). An increasing population of women are therefore entering the perimenopause. It is imperative that there be a greater understanding of the perimenopause, what concerns

women during this time, and what changes are expected to occur. The following chapters in this section attempt to address some of these questions.

TYPES OF OVARIAN CHANGES

Although perimenopausal changes are generally thought to be endocrine in nature, resulting in menstrual changes, a marked diminution of reproductive capacity proceeds this period by several years and may be referred to as *gametogenic ovarian failure.* The concept of a dissociation in ovarian function is appropriate. Gametogenic failure is heralded by reduced inhibin secretion, rising serum follicle-stimulating hormone (FSH) levels, and a marked reduction in fecundity. However, this occurs with normal menstrual function and no obvious endocrine deficiency and occurs as early as age 35, some 10 or more years before endocrine deficiency ensues. Although subtle changes in endocrine and menstrual function can occur for up to 3 years before menopause, it has been shown that the major reduction in ovarian estrogen production does not occur until approximately 6 months before menopause (Fig. 5.3) (5). There is also a very slow decline in androgen status (i.e., androstenedione and testosterone), which cannot be adequately detected at the time of the perimenopause. However, in comparing 24-hour levels of premenopausal and perimenopausal women, testosterone was found to decline significantly (5) (Fig. 5.4).

TABLE 5.1. *U.S. population entering the postmenopausal years, ages 55 through 64*

Year	Population
1990	10.8 million
2000	12.1 million
2010	17.1 million
2020	19.3 million

Adapted from ref. 4.

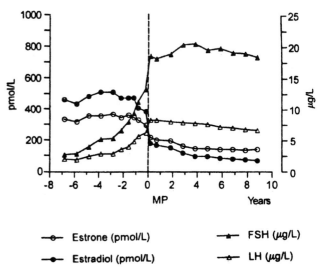

── Estrone (pmol/L)   ── FSH (µg/L)
── Estradiol (pmol/L)   ── LH (µg/L)

FIG. 5.3. Mean serum levels of follicle-stimulating hormone, luteinizing hormone, estradiol, and estrone, showing the perimenopausal transition. (From ref. 5, with permission.)

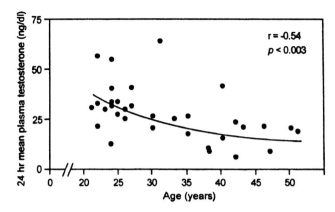

FIG. 5.4. The 24-hour mean plasma total testosterone (T) level compared with age in normal women. The regression equation was T (nmol/L) = 37.8 × age (years)$^{-1.12}$ (r = -0.54; $p < 0.003$). (From ref. 6, with permission.)

CONCLUSIONS

The perimenopause is a complex time in a woman's life, during which unpredictable and wide fluctuations in ovarian function and their physiologic consequences occur. This period usually follows a cessation in reproductive capacity (i.e., gametogenic failure) and extends into the first year after the cessation of menses (i.e., menopause). A greater understanding of this physiologic event in women is warranted, as are how women perceive of these changes and what treatments should be considered.

REFERENCES

1. Lobo RA. The perimenopause. *Clin Obstet Gynecol* 41:895–897.
2. Erickson GF. An analysis of follicle development and ovum maturation. *Semin Reprod Endocrinol* 1986;4:233–254.
3. Faddy MJ, Gosden RG, Gougeon A, Richardson SJ, Nelson JF. Accelerated disappearance of ovarian follicles in mid-life: implications for forecasting menopause. *Hum Reprod* 1992;7:1342–1346.
4. U.S. Bureau of the Census. Projections of the population of the United States: 1977 to 2050. Current Population Reports, Population Estimates and Projections, series P25, no. 704, July 1977.
5. Rannevik G, Jeppsson S, Johnell O, Bjerre B, Laurell-Borulf Y, Svanberg L. A longitudinal study of the perimenopausal transition: altered profiles of steroid and pituitary hormones—SHBG and bone mineral density. *Maturitas* 1995; 21:103–113.
6. Zumoff B, Strain GW, Miller LK, Rosner W. Twenty-four hour mean plasma testosterone concentration declines with age in normal premenopausal women. *J Clin Endocrinol Metab* 1995;80:1429–1430.

Treatment of the Postmenopausal Woman: Basic and Clinical Aspects, Second Edition, edited by Rogerio A. Lobo, Lippincott Williams & Wilkins, Philadelphia © 1999.

CHAPTER 6

The Perimenopausal State and Incipient Ovarian Failure

Helen M. Buckler

The menopause is considered to be the time that menstrual periods cease. Although menopause occurs at a specific time, the actual changes leading up to this event occur over a much longer period. As a woman approaches menopause, several biologic changes take place. The number of oocytes declines progressively from before birth but reaches critically low levels by menopause. The regular pattern of the menstrual cycle then becomes disrupted and the frequency of normal ovulatory cycles declines. There are probably changes in hypothalamic function and gonadotropin [particularly follicle-stimulating hormone (FSH)] levels increase, and those of the ovarian steroid hormones decrease. This results in changes in steroid target organs and a decline in fertility. The time from when symptoms and signs of an approaching menopause commence until 12 months after the final menstrual period is normally referred to as the *perimenopause*. The *menopausal transition* is that period from the start of the perimenopause to when menses cease.

PATHOPHYSIOLOGY OF THE MENOPAUSAL TRANSITION

Stock of Ovarian Oocytes

The ovary contains its greatest number of oocytes at around the fifth month of gestation, when about 7 million oocytes are seen. After that time, the number is continuously reduced by atresia. At birth, their number is estimated at about 1 to 2 million, and by menarche, it has fallen to 400,000. By menopause, there are only a few hundred or thousand oocytes (1–3). There appears to be a steady and approximate linear decline of follicle numbers

from menarche until around 40 years of age, but after this age, follicle numbers fall rapidly until menopause. The hormone changes occurring at the time of menopause reflect the declining ovarian follicle numbers.

Menstrual Cycle Length

For about 7 years after menarche and 8 years before menopause, there is greater variability in the intermenstrual cycle length. Between these two phases the variability is much smaller, and it is lowest between the ages of 36 and 40, just before the beginning of perimenopausal irregularity (4).

The median cycle length in the early postmenarchial years is 29 days. This drops slowly but steadily with time. At the age of 20, it is 28 days, and at age 40, it is 26 days. At the menopausal transition, the menstrual cycle length becomes highly variable but with little change in the median cycle length as long and short cycles increase in frequency. Reductions in cycle length result from a reduction in the length of the follicular phase (4).

ENDOCRINE CHANGES

Gonadotropin Levels

In women of reproductive age, before the break of regular cyclicity observed as menopause approaches, the levels of both gonadotropins have been shown to correlate positively with age (5). A progressive increase in FSH from 30 years of age onward has been reported (6). A similar correlation of FSH, but not luteinizing hormone (LH), was found when ovulatory cycles were examined in women 20 to 50 years old (7). The observed rise in FSH preceded that of LH by almost a decade. In this study, women were sampled every 5 to 7 days throughout the menstrual cycle, and a rise in LH was

H. M. Buckler: Department of Endocrinology, University of Manchester, Hope Hospital, Manchester M68HD, United Kingdom.

found only to be associated with the follicular phase, and the rise in FSH was greater over the same period. Women older than 40 have FSH levels that are significantly higher than those of younger women (5,7,8), and this hormonal status can occur in the presence of regular menstrual cycles. Lee et al. (8) investigated 94 regularly cycling women between the ages of 24 and 50 years and showed that FSH levels during the follicular phase and early postovulatory period rose significantly with increasing age despite their lack of any significant change in LH until close to the age of 50 years (8). Daily determination of gonadotropin levels in the blood of women between 46 and 51 years of age with regular cycles have also revealed an increase in FSH in the presence of normal LH levels throughout the cycle (9,10).

After a woman enters the menopausal transition, the major endocrine finding is that of significant hormonal variability. Sherman and Koreman showed that postmenopausal levels of FSH could occur in subjects during the menopausal transition and could be associated with or followed by evidence suggestive of normal ovulation and luteal function (9). Postmenopausal levels of FSH and LH have also been found accompanied by hot flushes but followed by spontaneous disappearance of the flushes and gonadotrophin levels returning to those characteristic of normal reproductive function (11). In women in the menopausal transition after establishment of irregular cycles, different patterns of gonadotropin secretion are described and may all occur sequentially in the same woman: a normal pattern similar to that in younger women, FSH and LH levels in the postmenopausal range, increase in FSH alone, and increase in LH alone. It appears that long intermenstrual intervals in this group of women are almost always associated with abnormal gonadotropin secretion, but short ones may be associated with normal gonadotropin secretion or an increase in FSH levels. Endocrine measurements may not be helpful in assessment of women during the menopausal transition because apparently ovulatory cycles may occur after the observation of FSH levels in the postmenopausal range.

Steroid Hormone Levels

Early endocrine studies of women approaching menopause suggested that this period was associated with normal urinary estrogen levels despite raised levels of gonadotropins (12,13). However, Sherman et al. (10) demonstrated lower levels of estradiol during the early follicular phase, midcycle, and the luteal phases in perimenopausal compared with young women. In a study that found that mean FSH levels in a group of normal cycling women between the ages of 45 and 49 years were twice as high as those of younger age groups; estradiol levels were also found to be lower in this age group compared with women between 30 and 39 years of age, although not when compared with even younger women (14). Two

other studies have reported normal estradiol levels in women older than 40 compared with younger women (7,8). One study suggested that the perimenopause can be associated with hyperestrogenism because overall mean estrone and conjugate estrogen excretion was greater in perimenopausal women than in younger women and that this could occur as early as 43 years of age (15). It therefore appears that in older women continuing to have regular cycles there is a selective increase in serum FSH levels as a function of increasing age, but it is not confirmed whether this is associated with significant decline in estradiol secretion.

Progesterone secretion in perimenopausal women with irregular cycles can be normal in short cycles (10,11) but can also be associated with decreased luteal phase progesterone excretion (15). These women can also go through long spells of amenorrhea in which progesterone secretion is absent. The frequency of cycles with normal ovulatory progesterone levels decreases markedly as menopause approaches (16).

From these studies, it appears as if women approaching menopause may experience a mixture of normal, short, and long cycles (17) (Fig. 6.1). Short cycles may exhibit a normal pattern or more commonly are characterized by an elevation of FSH, possibly associated with a low estradiol level or even increased estrogen secretion. Long cycles are characterized by abnormal gonadotropin and low estradiol levels for most of their length. Close to the end of such cycles, a rise in estradiol secretion is usually recorded, which may or may not be followed by indications of luteinization. Hormone changes may include normal estradiol levels associated with high gonadotropin levels (usually at the end of long cycles) and a brisk rise in gonadotropin levels after a fall in estradiol to low levels (at the end of short cycles).

Reproductive aging may also be associated with a menstrual cycle–related decrease in androgen secretion, because a decline in testosterone concentration with increasing age has been reported in premenopausal women such that levels in women in their forties are about one-third of those in their twenties (18). Moreover, diminished free testosterone and androstenedione levels were found at midcycle in older women (19). No change was found in testosterone, dyhydrotestosterone, or androstenedione levels during the 18 months after the last menstrual period in one study (20), but a small decline in testosterone and androstenedione within a 6-month period encompassing the last menstrual period was described (16). Longcope et al. (20) found that the mean concentration of testosterone in all their subjects was less than those of a group of young women. Taken together, these results indicate that a fall in circulating androgens is associated with aging and may precede menopause with a decline in levels starting during the perimenopause period. Androgens have an important role as precursors to estrogen, but they also may play a

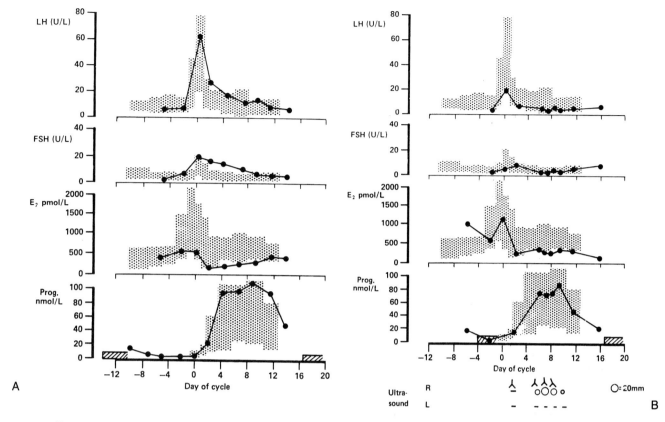

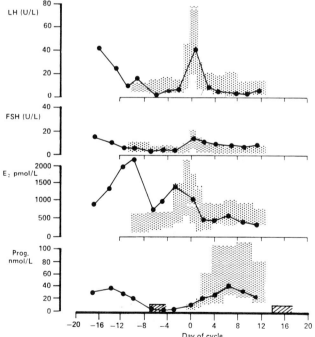

FIG. 6.1. Hormonal studies of three spontaneous cycles in a woman who went through a premature menopause 2 years later. Blood samples were obtained two to three times weekly. In the second of these three cycles, ovarian ultrasound scans were performed to monitor follicular development and ovulation. The stippled area indicates the 95% confidence limits for 30 ovulatory cycles (36). The hatched bars indicate menstruation. **A:** The first cycle studied was 30 days long. Luteinizing hormone (LH) levels were borderline high, and follicle-stimulating hormone (FSH) levels were persistently high throughout the luteal phase. Estradiol (E_2) levels rose modestly at midcycle and remained low during the luteal phase, whereas progesterone attained normal high levels. **B:** The second cycle studied was 20 days long and apparently had a short follicular phase. A modest LH peak was recorded on day 5 of the cycle. During the luteal phase, levels of both gonadotropins were borderline low, whereas a dissociation of E_2 and progesterone was seen. E_2 levels were low, and progesterone levels were normal. Ultrasound scans from day 7 of the cycle, 2 days after the LH surge, showed development of a small cystic structure during the middle of the luteal phase. **C:** The hormonal profile was assessed without ultrasound over a 30-day period, which included the luteal phase of one cycle and the whole of the following cycle. The hormone findings are bizarre and abnormal throughout. During the first of the luteal phases, LH and FSH levels were high, and E_2 levels were exceptionally so (up to 2230 pmol/L); progesterone on this occasion was within the normal range for the luteal phase, and menstruation occurred when progesterone declined in the presence of persistently high levels of circulating E_2. The following cycle was characterized by a very short follicular phase, with an LH peak recorded on day 7. LH levels were normal and FSH levels high during the luteal phase.

part in feelings of well-being and sexual function. The decreased androgen levels associated with the perimenopausal and postmenopausal states may be more important than previously thought. The strategy of androgen replacement therefore in these women merits further consideration (21).

Inhibin Levels

Inhibin refers to a family of gonadal glycoprotein hormones that consist of two dissimilar disulfide-linked subunits designated α and β. the two major inhibin species, A and B, found in humans consist of a common α subunit and one of two different β subunits, $β_a$ and $β_b$ (22). It is well established that the function of inhibin is to suppress the synthesis and secretion of FSH by direct pituitary action, and it may have local regulatory functions within the ovary (22–24).

Inhibin, like estradiol is a granulosa cell product. Unlike estradiol, ovarian follicles other than the dominant follicle significantly contribute to total circulating inhibin concentrations. Until recently, most data describing inhibin physiology have been based on an radioimmunoassay widely referred to as the Monash assay (22). However, this assay cross-reacts with nonbiologically active α-subunit precursors and with biologically active inhibin A and inhibin B. Studies using the Monash assay have shown that, in the late follicular phase of the normal menstrual cycle, inhibin and estradiol rise in parallel consistent with the finding that granulosa cells produce inhibin (25). After ovulation, inhibin rises in parallel with progesterone, and both reach a peak in the mid-luteal phase. Levels of both hormones fall before the onset of menstruation. During the luteal-follicular transition, an inverse relationship between inhibin and FSH occurs (26), with FSH secretion being maximally suppressed during the mid-luteal phase when inhibin levels are highest, suggesting inhibin has a role in regulating folliculogenesis by suppressing FSH.

Assays have been developed for measurement of inhibin A and inhibin B, and it appears as if inhibin A shows a pattern of secretion similar to inhibin as measured by the Monash assay (27). Inhibin B appears to reach peak levels in the early follicular phase and then falls throughout the remainder of the follicular phase and correlates with the early follicular phase fall in FSH (27).

Because the secretion of gonadotropins from the pituitary is under the negative feedback influence of the ovaries, removal of or damage to the ovaries results in an elevation of the peripheral concentration of LH and FSH (28). Factors responsible for the increase in FSH without a concomitant increase in LH before menopause have not been fully elucidated. Sherman and Korenman (9) postulated the existence of an ovarian regulatory hormone level capable of suppressing FSH, which could be inhibin. If inhibin levels decline in the years before menopause as a result of the decreasing follicle numbers, this could result in an increase in FSH. Inhibin is undetectable after a normal and premature menopause (29).

Data have been published for serum levels of inhibin, FSH, LH, progesterone, and estradiol in women of increasing age with regular cycles (14). A study found that the mean follicular phase levels of inhibin were lower in women between the ages of 45 and 49 years, but mean FSH levels were higher than in younger women. They concluded that these results were consistent for a role of serum immunoreactive inhibin in addition to estradiol in the regulation of FSH during the follicular phase of the menstrual cycle as a function of increasing age. The Melbourne midlife project also reported changes in inhibin in relation to the perimenopause (30). Women in this study were between 45 and 55 years of age, and blood samples were obtained between the fourth and eighth day of the menstrual cycle. Women who reported no change in menstrual frequency or flow were used as a control group. Immunoreactive inhibin levels were found to be reduced in women experiencing a change in menstrual frequency or flow compared with the control group, and inhibin levels were found to fall with increasing age.

If there is a decrease in production of estradiol by the ovary in the years approaching menopause, the negative feedback effect of estradiol on the hypothalamic pituitary axis would be removed. This may result in a gradual rise in gonadotropin levels, with FSH rising earlier and to higher levels than LH. However, after a premature menopause, physiologic estradiol supplementation cannot maintain FSH levels within the normal range (31). Although Sherman and Korenman (9) reported low estradiol concentrations during the menopausal transition, Reyes et al. (7) and Lee et al. (8) found no evidence for a decline in estradiol concentrations in women older than 40 years. Evidence that FSH is more sensitive than LH to the suppressive effects of estradiol (32) argues against an increase caused only by decreased estradiol concentration. It is possible that a decrease in estradiol may result in a greater response of FSH than LH because of differential regulation of FSH and LH secretion at the hypothalamic or pituitary level. Altered sensitivity of the aging hypothalamus and pituitary to sex steroids may manifest during the perimenopause period by differential regulation of the gonadotropins.

Fecundity decreases with increasing age in women, and to some extent, this occurs because of an increase in frequency of anovulatory cycles after the age of 40 years. Pregnancy rates also decrease with increasing age of women undergoing artificial insemination with donor sperm (33) and women undergoing *in vitro* fertilization (34). The basal FSH level strongly influences performance in an *in vitro* fertilization program (35) and is a better predictor than age for many outcome variables, including the peak estradiol level, the number of oocytes retrieved and fertilized, the number of embryos transferred, and the ongoing pregnancy rate. The elevation of early follicular phase FSH appears to represent a standard clinical marker of reduced ovarian reserve and diminished responsiveness of the ovary to ovulation induction. An elevated plasma FSH value is of strong predictive value in detecting the presence or absence of follicles in women with amenorrhea from premature ovarian failure (36). It has also been found that infertile women who have an impaired superovulation response for *in vitro* fertilization had elevated plasma FSH concentrations (37). These patients had circulating autoantibodies, and it was suggested that there might be an association with premature ovarian failure and that they might represent an early stage of this condition. There was, however, no decrease in the circulating estradiol or circulating inhibin levels. Hughes et al. (38) found an age-related reduction in inhibin, but not estradiol, during hyperstimulation. This suggests that these two hormones reflect different granulosa cell functions and that the serum inhibin response may be a sensitive and early index of declining ovarian reserve with advancing age.

Ovarian reserve describes a woman's existing reproductive potential as it relates to the process of follicular depletion and oocyte quality. The identification of markers of ovarian reserve are therefore of interest, particularly because women continue to delay childbearing. Measurement of an early follicular phase FSH level appears to be a strong predictor of a woman's ovarian reserve and of treatment success. It provides more pertinent information than chronologic age in regard to reproductive potential of an individual. However, in the later reproductive years, there is great variation among women in early follicular phase FSH levels, and the prognostic information it provides is often too late for effective intervention.

PREMATURE OVARIAN FAILURE

Premature ovarian failure is defined as the cessation of ovarian function before the age of 40 (39). It is characterized by secondary amenorrhea with elevated serum gonadotropins. Primary amenorrhea also may occur because of ovarian failure as a result of gonadal dysgenesis with a chromosome complement of 45XO (i.e., Turner's syndrome) or gonadal dysgenesis with a normal chromosomal complement. Women with gonadal dysgenesis have a decreased complement of ova from birth. Ovarian failure may be induced by exposure to external irradiation or cytotoxic chemotherapy. Ovarian function may be destroyed by viral infection or surgery. In many cases, the cause is unknown, and it is then referred to as idiopathic ovarian failure.

An association between ovarian failure and autoimmune disease has been reported (40), and these patients also produce autoantibodies to tissues other than the ovary and steroid-producing cells. The exact mechanism and importance of the autoimmune process remains unknown.

INCIPIENT OVARIAN FAILURE

It appears that normal women older than 40 years of age experience a monotropic rise in FSH as the first detectable endocrine manifestation of reproductive aging, occurring well before the cessation of menses (7–11,17). This pattern is most marked early in the follicular phase of the cycle (when estradiol levels are lowest) and is not seen in the luteal phase, in which estradiol and progesterone levels are raised. As soon as progesterone falls, FSH levels rise markedly.

It is reasonable to presume that women approaching a premature menopause would exhibit hormone changes at an earlier age that are similar to those of women approaching a normal menopausal transition. We have extensively studied a group of young infertile women with a combination of anovulation, increased FSH concentrations, and reasonably regular menses who may fall into this category (41).

An assessment of ovulation was made for women attending the infertility clinic at Hope Hospital, Manchester, United Kingdom, by combination of ultrasound and detailed hormone analysis. Experience of using this method of assessment has been presented previously (42). Scans were started from around day 7 of each cycle and then carried out on alternate weekdays. Scanning was not stopped until after the demonstration of presumptive ovulation. Serum levels of LH, FSH, estradiol, and progesterone were measured three times weekly over the whole menstrual cycle. The criteria of normal (ovulatory menstrual) cycles included a cycle length of 26 to 32 days, the presence of a well-defined midcycle peak (at least twofold rise from follicular phase levels), luteal phase length of 13 days or more, midluteal progesterone concentration greater than 25 nmol, good follicular growth, and ovulation detected ultrasonically by disappearance or collapse of the preovulatory follicle within 48 hour of the LH peak. This abnormality of a combination of anovulation, inappropriately raised FSH levels, and regular or nearly regular menstrual bleeding is thought to represent an impending premature menopause or incipient ovarian failure. These women appear to have become unable to conceive, although they maintain normal menstruation without obvious dysfunction of the reproductive axis. A group of 13 women with this abnormality underwent detailed assessment of ovulation on at least one occasion. Inhibin was measured by the Monash radioimmunoassay in these subjects (41). Details of these results are presented in Fig. 6.2. All 13 women underwent premature menopause within 5 years after completing the study.

FSH levels depend on the presence or absence of ovarian oocytes (36), and they correlate positively with age in

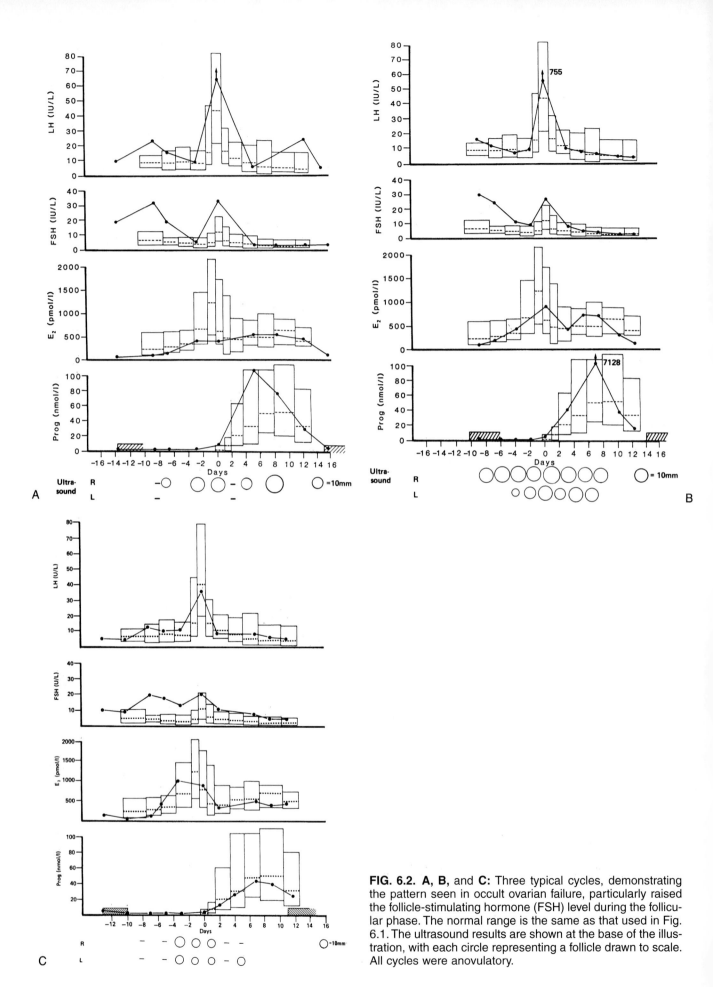

FIG. 6.2. A, B, and **C:** Three typical cycles, demonstrating the pattern seen in occult ovarian failure, particularly raised the follicle-stimulating hormone (FSH) level during the follicular phase. The normal range is the same as that used in Fig. 6.1. The ultrasound results are shown at the base of the illustration, with each circle representing a follicle drawn to scale. All cycles were anovulatory.

premenopausal women (5,7). Women older than 40 have increased FSH levels compared with those in younger women (5,8). At any age, elevation of FSH appears to be a marker of an approaching menopause (5,8). Described here is a group of patients with raised FSH levels and infertility who appear to have entered the perimenopause or menopausal transitional stage prematurely. A combination of inappropriately raised FSH levels and anovulation may be secondary to incipient ovarian failure. After a premature or normal menopause, there is reduced ovarian estradiol secretion and follicular atresia. Circulating estradiol levels were normal in the incipient ovarian failure group, suggesting normal ovarian steroid synthesis. This may be maintained by a compensatory increase in pituitary FSH secretion.

Inhibin levels are lower in women with incipient ovarian failure than in a group of normal women, and the FSH level is inversely correlated with that of inhibin (44) (Fig. 6.3). These findings are consistent with the involvement of inhibin deficiency in the elevated FSH levels and suggest that ovarian inhibin secretion declines with incipient ovarian failure. Inhibin is a granulosa cell product (22), and the decline in inhibin may be caused by a reduction in the number of follicles in the failing ovary or a reduction in the maximum ability of each granulosa cell to produce inhibin. These findings are similar to the situation in aging men, in whom immunoreactive FSH levels are higher and inhibin levels are lower than in younger men (43). In our study, estradiol levels were not found to be reduced in the incipient ovarian failure group. It does not appear that the steroidogenic activities of granulosa cells are impaired in incipient ovarian failure, although the peptide secreting abilities appear to have been reduced.

The assay of inhibin has been associated with problems. In the studies described previously, total inhibin was measured by radioimmunoassay (i.e., Monash assay). Two-site assays have been developed with specificity for inhibin A and inhibin B. These assays have been used in a study to compare circulating and follicular fluid concentrations of dimeric inhibin A and B in normal older and younger ovulatory women (44). Follicular phase inhibin B secretion was found to be decreased in older ovulatory women who demonstrated a monotropic FSH rise, whereas inhibin A secretion was found to be similar to that in younger women. They found that, although FSH concentrations were elevated and inhibin B levels reduced, estradiol concentrations were similar between the older and younger groups. The researchers speculated that decreased inhibin B secretion most likely reflects a diminished follicular pool in older women and might be an important regulator of the monotropic FSH rise. This conclusion was based on the assumption that inhibin B may be predominantly a product of the cohort of developing primary and subsequent early antral follicles, whereas inhibin A secretion is more reflective of

dominant follicle function. Decreased inhibin B levels in older women may be a result of fewer primordial to early antral follicles in the ovary, with a subsequent smaller cohort proceeding to the recruitment stage. The dominant follicle appeared to function normally in the older ovulatory women, explaining why women of advanced reproductive age demonstrate follicular phase inhibin A secretion similar to that in younger women.

During the normal menstrual cycle, levels of inhibin B rise early in the follicular phase and then progressively decrease until the midcycle LH peak, at which time another short lived surge occurs that falls for the remainder of the luteal phase (27). The timing of the early follicular rise of inhibin B suggests that it may be related to follicular maturation and raises the possibility of whether early follicular phase inhibin B measurement may be a marker of ovarian reserve. In a study to test this hypothesis, Seifer et al. (45) found that women with a low day 3 serum inhibin B concentration demonstrated a poorer response to ovulation induction and were less likely to conceive after *in vitro* fertilization treatment relative to women with a high day 3 inhibin B. It therefore appears that a low day 3 serum inhibin measurement adds further prognostic value for response to ovulation induction and as a marker of ovarian reserve to day 3 serum FSH levels.

The exact role of inhibins in the human menstrual cycle and the relative roles of inhibin B and estradiol in the regulation of pituitary FSH and the relative contribution inhibin B, estradiol and FSH play in controlling follicular maturation are not fully understood. It is unknown whether relative inhibin deficiency in patients with incipient ovarian failure is contributing to their infertility. It may be that inhibin B has a role in controlling the FSH rise that initiates each cycle. Evidence is accumulating for a paracrine role for inhibin, and inhibin B may be involved in the paracrine regulation of the follicle and may be a direct reflection of follicular and oocyte quality. Administration of exogenous LH and FSH alone to normal subjects or to patients with polycystic ovarian syndrome stimulates parallel rises in estradiol and immunoreactive inhibin, which correlate with a number of developing follicles (46,47). Inhibin may be a better marker than estradiol of follicular function and health (48). Low inhibin levels may be associated with abnormal follicular development, and in the situation of incipient ovarian failure, it may contribute to anovulation and infertility. Alternatively, the lowered inhibin concentrations may reflect altered and diminished function of the granulosa cells that may therefore contribute to oocyte viability or to the ability of fertilization to occur. The increased FSH secretion and decreased inhibin secretion and reduced frequency of ovulation may therefore be interdependent. Although most of the data suggesting that inhibin may reflect a decrease in ovarian reserve are using total inhibin measurements, it looks as if inhibin B may be more important.

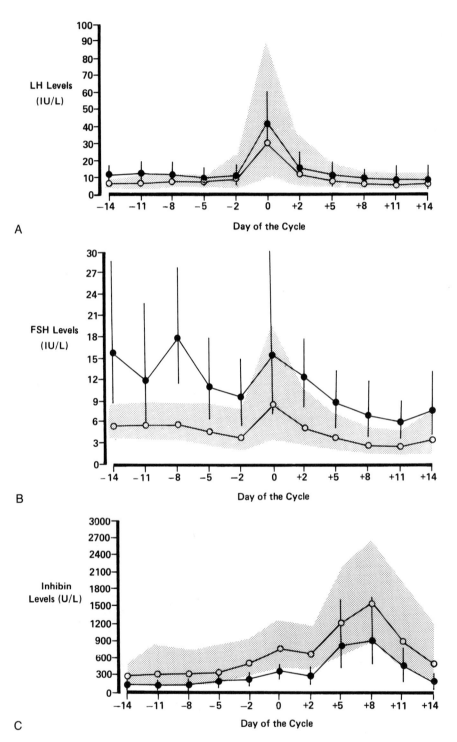

FIG. 6.3. Luteinizing hormone (LH) **(A)**, follicle-stimulating hormone (FSH) **(B)**, inhibin **(C)**, estradiol **(D)**, and progesterone **(E)** levels in all incipient ovarian failure cycles (z). The geometric mean and 67% confidence limits are shown. The geometric mean (o) and the 95% confidence limit of the normal control group are also shown in the shaded area. All data are log transformed. The baseline cycles are shown. FSH levels were raised in the ovarian failure group (p < 0.001), and this is particularly evident in the early follicular phase. Serum LH was raised on days -14 to -8 (*p* < 0.001), day -5 (*p* < 0.001), day 5 (*p* < 0.001), day 8 (*p* < 0.001), and day 11 (*p* < 0.01) relative to the LH surge. There is no difference in estradiol and progesterone levels between the study and control groups. Inhibin levels were lower in the incipient ovarian failure group throughout the cycle (*p* < 0.001). However, they showed the same pattern over a cycle as the normal group, with the highest levels in the luteal phase secreted in a pattern similar to that for progesterone secretion. There was an inverse relationship between FSH and inhibin during the follicular phase (*r* = -0.54, *p* < 0.05) and during the luteal phase (*r* = -0.52, *p* < 0.05). Inhibin was positively correlated with progesterone during the luteal phase (*r* = 0.67, *p* < 0.01). Sixty women with normal ovulatory cycles (as determined by hormone concentrations and ultrasound scanning) served as a control group for LH, FSH, estradiol, and progesterone levels. Daily venous blood samples were collected from 33 normally ovulating North American women between the ages of 21 and 35 years and were measured for inhibin by radioimmunoassay. Daily venous blood samples were also collected from 10 normal women who were judged to be ovulating normally on the basis of their menstrual calendars and luteal phase progesterone concentrations (>25 nmol/L) (22). Comparison of the inhibin data from these two groups showed no difference; the data from all the subjects were combined to give a control group of 43 subjects for comparison with inhibin levels from the incipient ovarian failure group.

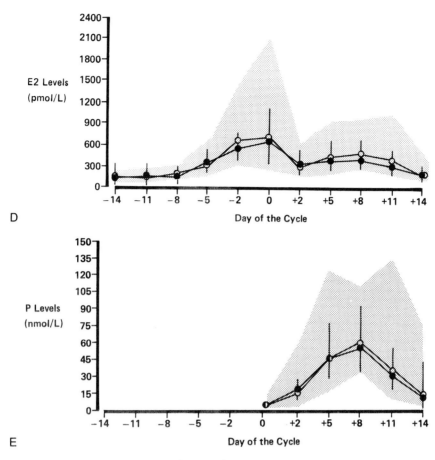

FIG. 6.3. *Continued.*

Fertility and Incipient Ovarian Failure

Ovulation is impossible if the ovary is completely devoid of follicles. However, ovulation and pregnancy have been induced in some women with premature ovarian failure with exogenous gonadotropins (49) and by estrogen and gonadotropins (50). Pregnancies have also been reported while patients were on or immediately after estrogen treatment (51–56). This may result from a reversal of the downregulation of FSH receptors because of estrogen, or the estrogen lowers the endogenous gonadotropins, and after cessation of treatment, follicular growth is triggered. However, these reports of pregnancies are usually of isolated cases and return of ovulation and pregnancy can also occur spontaneously in patients with premature ovarian failure (57–59). It may be that the association between estrogen therapy and pregnancy is only coincidental, because no controlled studies have been carried out.

In young women with regular menstrual cycles, ordered follicular growth takes place, leading to ovulation of a single dominant follicle from an initial cohort of 6 to 30 follicles, 1 to 15 mm in diameter in each ovary (60). In women during the menopausal transition, the primary change is believed to be the diminishing follicle stock (3) and a resulting reduction in suppression of gonadotropins. High FSH levels for prolonged periods are likely to result in disruptive and chaotic follicular growth. The coexistence of high LH levels may lead to erratic luteinization of follicles without ovulation. The possibility therefore exists that prolonged and effective suppression of gonadotropin levels may line up the growing follicles by allowing those that have been committed by inappropriate gonadotropin levels to regress. After a time, a new crop of healthy follicles can advance to the appropriate stage. Discontinuation of suppression can be anticipated to result in a rebound rise of gonadotropins, which could trigger normal follicular growth and ovulation for one cycle (17).

Treatment for Infertility

An attempt was made by us to suppress the raised FSH levels in the incipient ovarian failure group of patients presented earlier, using various estrogen and progestogen preparations for 4 weeks. The cycle after stopping treatment (i.e., rebound cycle) was assessed by detailed hormone and ultrasound measurements as previously described (Fig. 6.4).

We were able to induce ovulation in the rebound cycle, even when FSH levels rose to the previous inappropriately elevated levels and inhibin levels were again low in the fol-

licular phase. Unfortunately, no pregnancies occurred. These findings are consistent with the hypothesis that intraovarian inhibin has an important role in producing follicular development and oocyte maturation before ovulation. It appears as if inhibin is involved in the elevated FSH

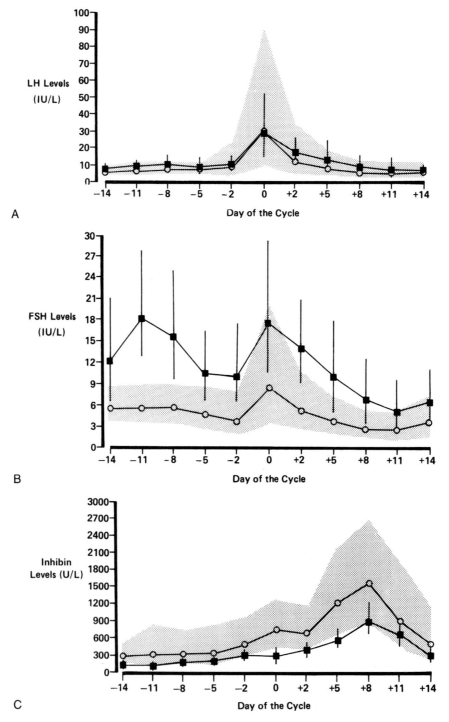

FIG. 6.4. Luteinizing hormone (LH) **(A)**, follicle-stimulating hormone (FSH) **(B)**, inhibin **(C)**, estradiol **(D)**, and progesterone **(E)** levels in ovulatory rebound cycles (n). Geometric mean and 67% confidence limits are shown. Geometric mean (○) and 95% confidence limits of the normal control group are shown in the shaded area. All data are log transformed. Twenty-two of the 39 cycles monitored resulted in ovulation of a single dominant follicle and are shown. FSH levels are still significantly raised, and inhibin levels are significantly lower than in the normal cycles. There was no difference in estradiol or progesterone concentrations.

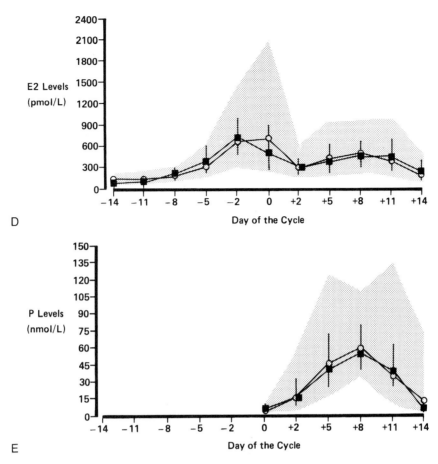

D

E

FIG. 6.4. *Continued.*

levels of incipient ovarian failure, and therefore inhibin is probably involved in the pathophysiology of the perimenopause. The normal estradiol levels in the presence of low inhibin levels suggest that in the "failing ovary" there is a disassociation between steroid and peptide secretion. Peptide secretion of the granulosa cells must be affected before the steroid-secreting capacity. Further understanding of this will help in the management of infertility seen in incipient ovarian failure and in the management of women in the perimenopausal period.

We have also tested the hypothesis that there may be a resumption of ovulatory function after suppression of the raised gonadotrophin levels in established premature ovarian failure (Fig. 6.5) (61). This study found that gonadotrophin suppression did not result in resumption of follicular activity, as was found by other researchers (62,63).

It therefore appears that there is no evidence to support a successful method for ovulation induction in women with established primary premature ovarian failure. The outlook for these women in terms of fertility is poor, and no therapy offers them any improvement in prognosis. The only chance of fertility is that offered by the development of ovum and embryo donation. Alternatively, they must be given counseling to come to terms with their infertility.

SYMPTOMS AND HEALTH ISSUES RELATED TO PERIMENOPAUSE

The perimenopause can last for years and is marked by variability and unpredictability of hormone secretion. The clinical responses to this endocrine instability include hot flushes, psychologic symptoms, and irregular endometrial bleeding. Leading up to menopause, estradiol levels may fluctuate markedly, cycle length varies, the corpus luteum may secrete less progesterone or cease secretion sooner, ovulation may not take place, and menstrual bleeding may result from estrogen withdrawal rather than progesterone withdrawal. There may be an unopposed estrogen stimulus to the endometrium, which can result in endometrial hyperplasia and abnormal uterine bleeding. Most patients with abnormal perimenopausal bleeding do not have endometrial hyperplasia, but an endometrial biopsy is often needed to confirm this. For patients with hyperplasia, cyclic progestogen therapy is used. Because of the marked fluctuations in estradiol levels in the perimenopause women can report symptoms suggestive of high estrogen levels such as bloating and breast tenderness.

About 75% of women suffer from hot flushes, which usually continue for longer than 1 year, and many women

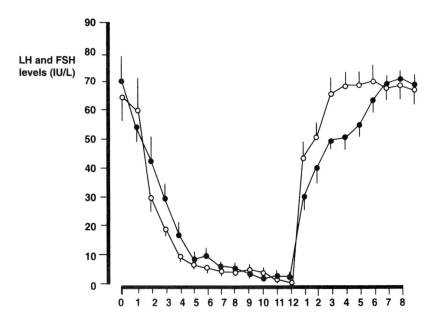

FIG. 6.5. Serum luteinizing hormone (LH, ●) and follicle-stimulating hormone (FSH, (○) basal measurement (mean and SD, n = 8) for 12 weeks of ethinyl estradiol (30 μg) and levonorgestrel (150 μg) treatment and for 8 weeks afterward. Normal early follicular phase hormone levels are 1.8 to 10.0 IU/L for LH and 1.9 to 8.5 IU/L for FSH. No follicular activity was seen on ultrasound scanning.

complain of episodes for longer than 5 years. Hot flushes usually occur for some time before menstruation completely ceases. Several studies have shown an increase in psychologic complaints at the time of menopause (64,65). Psychologic symptoms and poor sense of well-being are more common in women in the perimenopausal period compared with premenopausal or postmenopausal women (66,67).

It is unclear whether changes in female sexuality occur specifically in the perimenopause. Sexual problems are commonly found in women attending menopause clinics, but it is less clear whether sexual dysfunction occurs in the general population. Sexual desire decreases with age in both sexes, and low sexual desire is particularly common in women in their late 40s and 50s (68), but it is not known to what degree menopause specifically contributes to these changes. Vaginal dryness and dyspareunia are associated with menopause, but this may not become a significant problem until the after the menopausal transition. Negative changes in mood and poor well-being and self-esteem may also be relevant to sexual dysfunction associated with the time of menopause. Overall, there is a reduction in sexual interest and in the frequency of sexual activity and orgasm around the time of menopause, but that this may be multifactorial. Hot flushes can result in chronic sleep disturbance, which may lead to alterations of psychologic function. Whether perimenopause alters sexual function by mechanisms other than those related to hot flushes and vaginal atrophy is unknown.

Cardiovascular Risk Factors

Postmenopausal women have a higher risk of cardiovascular problems compared with premenopausal women. It is not known whether changes in cardiovascular risk fac-

tors occur during the menopausal transition. Matthews et al. (67) found no change in cardiovascular risk factors other than slight change in triglyceride levels during the perimenopause. The increase in risk of cardiovascular problems in women is partly because of an increase in age but is also related to a fall in estradiol levels during menopause. The fluctuating and eventually falling hormone levels of the perimenopause may result in subtle changes in lipids and other cardiovascular variables. It would therefore seem appropriate in women markedly at increased risk of cardiovascular disease that estrogen supplementation should be considered early in the perimenopause to minimize adverse effects on cardiovascular risk.

Changes in Bone Mineral Density

Not much is known about changes in bone density, bone loss, or bone turnover in the perimenopausal period, although there have been some reports of radial bone loss in perimenopausal women (69–71). It would therefore appear that women who are already known to be at increased risk of osteoporosis could benefit from estrogen treatment in the perimenopausal period.

The menopausal transition is associated with increased reporting of adverse symptoms. This is a time when women are more likely to see a medical practitioner. Consideration should be given at this time to the use of hormone replacement therapy to alleviate symptoms and to help reduce the risk of osteoporosis and cardiovascular disease. In women early in the menopausal transition, during which regular menses still occur and contraception may be an issue, the use of a low-dose combined oral contraceptive pill may be appropriate to suppress gonadotrophin secretion, markedly decrease the hormone fluctuations, and provide contraception. As the menopausal transition proceeds, hormone replacement therapy may then be considered for continuing treatment of hot flushes, reduced libido, and psychologic problems.

REFERENCES

1. Block E. Quantitative morphological investigations of the follicular system in women. *Acta Anat (Basel)* 1952;14:108–123.
2. Baker TG. A quantitative and cytological study of germ cells in human ovaries. *Proc R Soc Lond Biol* 1963;158:417–433.
3. Richardson SJ, Senikas V, Nelson JF. Follicular depletion during the menopausal transition: evidence for accelerated loss and ultimate exhaustion. *J Clin Endocrinol Metab* 1987;65:1231–1235.
4. Treolar AR, Bounton RE, Behn BG, Brown BW. Variation of the human menstrual cycle through reproductive life. *Int J Infertil* 1967;12:77–79.
5. Metcalf MG, Livesey JH. Gonadotrophin excretion in fertile women: effect of age and the onset of the menopausal transition. *J Endocrinol* 1985;105:357–362.
6. Ahmed Ebbiary NA, Lenton, Salt C, Ward AM, Cooke ID. The significance of elevated basal follicle stimulating hormone in regularly menstruating infertile women. *Hum Reprod* 1994;9:245–252.
7. Reyes FI, Winter JSD, Faiman C. Pituitary and ovarian relationships preceding the menopause. *Am J Obstet Gynecol* 1977;129:557–564.
8. Lee SJ, Lenton EA, Sexton L, Cooke ID. The effect on the cyclical patterns of plasma LH, FSH, oestradiol and progesterone in women with regular menstrual cycles. *Hum Reprod* 1988;3:851–855.
9. Sherman BM, Korenman SG. Hormonal characteristics of the human menstrual cycle throughout reproductive life. *J Clin Invest* 1975;55:699–706.
10. Sherman BM, West JH, Korenman SG. The menopausal transition: analysis of LH, FSH, estradiol and progesterone concentrations during menstrual cycles of older women. *J Clin Endocrinol Metab* 1976;42:629–634.
11. Metcalf MG, Donald RA, Livesey JH. Pituitary and ovarian function in normal women during the menopausal transition. *Clin Endocrinol (Oxf)* 1981;14:245–255.
12. Papanicolaou AD, Loraine JA, Dove GA, Loudon NB. Hormone excretion patterns in menopausal women. *Br J Obstet Gynaecol* 1969;76:308–316.
13. Adampoulis DA, Loraine JA, Dove GA. Endocrinological studies in women approaching the menopause. *Br J Obstet Gynaecol* 1971;76:62–79.
14. McNaughton J, Bangah M, McCloud P, Hee J, Burger H. Age-related changes in follicle-stimulating hormone, luteinizing hormone, oestradiol and immunoreactive inhibin in women of reproductive age. *Clin Endocrinol* 1992;36:339–345.
15. Santoro N, Rosenberg Brown J, Adel T, Skurnick JH. Characterisation of reproductive hormonal dynamics in the perimenopause. *J Clin Endocrinol Metab* 1996;81:1495–1501.
16. Rannevik G, Jeppsson S, Johnell O, Bjerre B, Laurell-Borulf Y, Svanberg L. A longitudinal study of the perimenopausal transition altered profiles of steroid and pituitary hormones: SHBG and bone density. *Maturitas* 1995;21:103–113.
17. Petsos P, Buckler H, Mamtora H, Anderson D. Ovulation after treatment with ethinyl-estradiol and medroxyprogesterone acetate in a woman approaching premature menopause: case report. *Br J Obstet Gynaecol* 1986;93:1155–1160.
18. Zumoff B, Stain GW, Miller LK, Rosner W. Twenty four hour mean plasma testosterone concentration declines with age in normal premenopausal women. *J Clin Endocrinol Metab* 1995;80:1429–1430.
19. Mushayandebvu T, Castracane VD, Gimpel T, Adel T, Samtoro N. Evidence for diminished mid cycle ovarian androgen production in older reproductive aged women. *Fertil Steril* 1996;65:721–723.
20. Longcope C, Franz C, Morello C, Baker K, Johnston CC Jr. Steroid and gonadotropin levels in women during the perimenopausal years 1980. *Maturitas* 1980;8:189–196.
21. Buckler HM, Robertson WR. Androgen production over the female life span. In: Wren BG, ed. *Progress in the management of the menopause.* Park Ridge, NJ: Parthenon Publishing, 1977:22.
22. Burger HG. Inhibin. *Reprod Med Rev* 1992:1–20.
23. de Jong FH. Inhibin. *Phys Rev* 1988;68:555–607.
24. Ying SY. Inhibins, activins and follistatins: gonadal proteins modulating the secretion of follicle-stimulating hormone. *Endocr Rev* 1988;9:267–293.
25. McLachlan RI, Robertson DM, Healy DL, Burger HG, de Kretser DM. Circulating immunoreactive inhibin levels during the normal human menstrual cycle. *J Clin Endocrinol Metab* 1987;65:954–961.
26. Roseff SJ, Bangah ML, Kettel LM, et al. Dynamic changes in circulating inhibin levels during the luteal-follicular transition of the human menstrual cycle. *J Clin Endocrinol Metab* 1989;69:1033–1039.
27. Groome N, Illingworth P, O'Brien M, Pair Mather J, McNeilly A. Measurement of dimeric inhibin B throughout the human menstrual cycle. *J Clin Endocrinol Metab* 1996;83:1400–1405.
28. Munro SE, Jaffe RB, Midgley AR. Regulation of human gonadotropins, changes in serum gonadotrophins in menstruating women in response to oophorectomy. *J Clin Endocrinol Metab* 1972;34:420–424.
29. McLachlan RI, Robertson DM, Healy DL, de Kretser DM, Burger HG. Plasma inhibin levels during gonadotrophin-induced ovarian hyperstimulation for IVF: a new index of follicular function. *Lancet* 1986;1:1233–1234.
30. Burger HG, Dudley I, Hopper JL, et al. The endocrinology of the menopausal transition: a cross sectional study of a population based sample. *J Clin Endocrinol Metab* 1995;80:3537–3545.
31. Lutjen PJ, Findlay JK, Trounson AO, Leeton J, Chan LK. Effect of plasma gonadotropins with cyclic steroid replacement in women with premature ovarian failure. *J Clin Endocrinol Metab* 1986;62:419–424.
32. Vaitukaitis J, Bernudez J, Cargille C, Lipsett M, Ross G. New evidence of an antioestrogenic action of clomiphene citrate in women. *J Clin Endocrinol Metab* 1971;32:503.
33. Schwartz D, Mayaux MJ. Female fecundity as a function of age results of artificial insemination in 2193 nulliparous women with azoospermic husband. *N Engl J Med* 1982;306:404–-406.
34. Hull MGR, Fleming CF, Hughes AO, McDermott A. The age related decline in female fecundity: a quantitative controlled study of implanting capacity and survival of individual embryos after *in vitro* fertilisation. *Fertil Steril* 1996;85:783–790.
35. Toner JP, Philput CB, Jones GS, Muashen SJ. Basal follicle-stimulating hormone level is a better predictor of *in vitro* fertilisation performance than age. *Fertil Steril* 1991;55:784–788.
36. Goldenberg RL, Grodin JM, Rodbard D, Ross GT. Gonadotropins in women with amenorrhea. *Am J Obstet Gynecol* 1973;116:1003–1012.
37. Cameron IT, O'Shea FC, Rolland JM, Hughes EG, de Kretser DM, Healy DL. Occult ovarian failure: a syndrome of infertility, regular menses and elevated FSH concentrations shows an impaired superovulation response for *in vitro* fertilisation (IVF). *J Clin Endocrinol Metab* 1988;67:1190–1194.
38. Hughes EG, Robertson DM, Handelsman DJ, Hayward S, Healy DM, deKretser DM. Inhibin and estradiol responses in ovarian hyperstimulation: effects of age and predictive value for *in vivo* fertilization outcome. *J Clin Endocrinol Metab* 1990;70:358–364.
39. Rebar RW, Erikson GS, Yen SSC. Idiopathic premature ovarian failure,clinical and endocrine characteristics. *Fertil Steril* 1982;37:35–41.
40. Coulam CB, Ryan RJ. Premature menopause: etiology. *Am J Obstet Gynecol* 1979;133:639–643.
41. Buckler HM, Evans CA, Mamtora H, Burger HG, Anderson DC. Gonadotrophin, steroid and inhibin levels in women with incipient ovarian failure during anovulatory and ovulatory rebound cycles. *J Clin Endocrinol Metab* 1991;72:116–124.
42. Petsos P, Chandler C, Oak M, Ratcliffe WA, Wood R, Anderson DC. The assessment of ovulation by a combination of ultrasound and detailed serial hormone profiles in 35 women with long-standing unexplained infertility. *Clin Endocrinol* 1985;22:739–751.
43. Tenover SJ, McLachlan RI, Dahl KD, Burger HG, de Kretser DM, Bremner WJ. Decreased serum inhibin levels in normal elderly men: evidence for a decline in Sertoli cell function with aging. *J Clin Endocrinol Metab* 1988;67:445–449.
44. Klein NA, Illingworth PJ, Groome MP, McNeilly AS, Battaglia DE, Soules MR. Decreased inhibin B secretion is associated with a monotropic FSH rise in older ovulatory women a study of serum and follicular fluid levels of dimeric inhibin A and B in spontaneous menstrual cycle. *J Clin Endocrinol Metab* 1996;81:2742–2745.
45. Seifer DB, Lambert-Messerlain G, Hogan JW, Gardiner AC, Frazer AS, Berk CA. Day 3 serum inhibin B is predictive of assisted reproductive technologies outcome. *Fertil Steril* 1997;67:110–114.
46. Buckler HM, Healy DL, Burger HG. Purified FSH stimulates inhibin production from the human ovary. *J Endocrinol* 1989;122:279–285.
47. Buckler HM, McLachlan RI, MacLachlan VB, Healy DL, Burger HG. Serum inhibin levels in polycystic ovary syndrome: basal levels and response to LHRH agonist and exogenous gonadotrophin administration. *J Clin Endocrinol Metab* 1988;66:798–803.
48. Buckler HM, Robertson WR, Sun JG, Morris ID. Inhibin levels may predict immunoreactive granulosa cell maturity. *Clin Endocrinol* 1992;37:552–557.
49. Amos WL. Pregnancy in a patient with gonadotrophin-resistant ovary syndrome. *Am J Obstet Gynecol* 1985;153:154–155.
50. Check JH, Chase JS. Ovulation induction in hypergonadotrophic amenorrhoea with estrogen and menopausal gonadotrophin therapy. *Fertil Steril* 1984;42:919–922.
51. Check JH, Chase JS, Spence M. Pregnancy in premature ovarian failure after therapy with oral contraceptives despite resistance to previous human menopausal gonadotrophin therapy. *Am J Obstet Gynecol* 1989;160:114–115.
52. Alper MM, Jolly E, Garner PR. Pregnancies after premature ovarian failure. *Obstet Gynecol* 1986;67:59–62s.
53. Szlachter BN, Nachtigall LE, Epstein J, Young BK, Vice G. Premature menopause: a reversible entity. *Obstet Gynecol* 1979;54:396–398.
54. Shangold MM, Turksoy RN, Bashford RA, Hammond CB. Pregnancy following the insensitive ovary syndrome. *Fertil Steril* 1977;28:1179–1181.
55. Polansky S, De Papp E. Pregnancy associated with hypergonadotrophic hypogonadism. *Obstet Gynecol* 1976;47:47–51.
56. Ylostalo P, Huhtaniemi I, Reubuka M. Induction of ovulation with low dose estrogen and progestin therapy in amenorrheic patients. *Int J Fertil* 1982;27:153–159.
57. Shapiro AG, Rubin A. Spontaneous pregnancy in association with hypergonadotrophic ovarian failure. *Fertil Steril* 1977;28:500–501.
58. Wright CSW, Jacobs HS. Spontaneous pregnancy in a patient with hypergonadotrophic ovarian failure. *Br J Obstet Gynaecol* 1979;86:389–392.
59. O'Herlihy C, Pepperell RJ, Evans JH. The significance of FSH elevation in young women with disorders of ovulation. *Br Med J* 1980;281:1447–1450.
60. McNatty GP. Ovarian follicular development from the onset of luteal regression in humans and sheep. In: Rolland R, Van Hall EY, Hillier SG, McNatty SP, Shoemaker J, eds. *Follicular maturation and ovulation.* Amsterdam: Excerpta Medica, 1982:1.
61. Buckler HM, Healy DL, Burger HG. Does gonadotrophin suppression result in

follicular development in premature ovarian failure. *Gynaecol Endocrinol* 1993;7: 123–128.

62. Menon V, Edwards RL, Lynch SS, Butt WR. Luteinizing hormone releasing hormone analogue in treatment of hypergonadotrophic amenorrhoea. *Br J Obstet Gynaecol* 1983;90:539–542.

63. Ledger WL, Thomas EJ, Browning D, Lenton EA, Cooke ID. Suppression of gonadotrophin secretion does not reverse premature ovarian failure. *Br J Obstet Gynaecol* 1989;145:360–372.

64. Ballinger CB. Psychiatric morbidity at the menopause: screening of a general population sample. *Br Med J* 1975;3:344–346.

65. Bungay GT, Vessey MP, McPherson CK. Study of symptoms in the middle life with special reference to the menopause. *Br Med J* 1980;281:181–183.

66. Hunter N, Battersby R, Whitehead M. Relationship between psychological symptoms and other complex menopausal stages. *Maturitas* 1986;8:217–228.

67. Matthew KA, Wing RR, Kuller OA, Meilahn EN, Plantiga P. Influence of the perimenopause on cardiovascular risk factors and symptoms of middle aged healthy women. *Arch Intern Med* 1994;154:2349–2355.

68. Horton K, Gath D, Dave A. Sexual function in a community sample of middle aged women with partners: effects of age, marital, socio-economic, psychiatric, gynaecological and menopause factors. *Arch Sex Behav* 1994;3: 375–395.

69. Gambacciani N, Spinetti A, Taponeco F, et al. Bone loss in perimenopausal women: a longitudinal study. *Maturitas* 1994;18:191–197.

70. Nilas L, Chistiansen C. The pathophysiology of peri- and postmenopausal bone loss. *Br J Obstet Gynaecol* 1989;96:580–587.

71. Slemenda C, Longcope C, Johnston DC, et al. Sex steroids and bone mass: a study of changes about the time of the menopause. *Br J Clin Invest* 1987;80: 1261–1269.

Treatment of the Postmenopausal Woman: Basic and Clinical Aspects, Second Edition, edited by Rogerio A. Lobo, Lippincott Williams & Wilkins, Philadelphia © 1999.

CHAPTER 7

Endocrine Changes During the Perimenopause

Henry G. Burger and Helena Teede

The estrogen deficiency state after menopause was recognized clinically more than 100 years ago. Corresponding understanding of the stable endocrine physiology in postmenopausal women is largely complete with high gonadotropin, low sex steroid, and low inhibin levels. The dynamic hormonal fluctuations that control fertile cycles during the middle reproductive years also are well understood. However, for the years of transition from the fertile, ovulatory cycles of the middle reproductive years to the stable postmenopausal estrogen deficiency state, our understanding is still evolving. Until recently, gradually declining estrogen levels accompanied by rising gonadotropins were thought to characterize the period known as the perimenopause, but conventional thinking has been challenged as the endocrine physiology of the perimenopause received increasing attention. Wide variations in hormonal profiles exist between and within individuals, and declining levels of the inhibins appear to play a pivotal role in maintaining estrogen levels until just before menopause by permitting increased levels of gonadotropins.

The perimenopause is the phase extending from the onset of symptoms of the ensuing menopause to 1 year after the final menstrual period, with a median age of onset of 45.5 to 47.5 years and an average duration of 5 years established in longitudinal studies (1,2). Perimenopausal women with a high incidence of clinical symptoms (1) seek medical consultation more frequently than premenopausal or postmenopausal women. Dysfunctional uterine bleeding is most common during perimenopause, culminating in peak rates of hysterectomy. Changes in the skeletal and cardiovascular systems have been observed even during early perimenopause. With aging of the substantial generation of "baby boomers," increasing numbers of women are becoming perimenopausal. An accurate understanding of the endocrine changes occurring during this phase of the reproductive life cycle is vital, with therapeutic and diagnostic implications.

ENDOCRINE DYNAMICS: THE NORMAL REPRODUCTIVE CYCLE

The normal hormonal dynamics of the hypothalamic-pituitary-ovarian axis control reproductive physiology during the middle reproductive years. An understanding of this control provides a background for subsequent observations throughout the perimenopause.

The pituitary is regulated by pulsatile secretion of gonadotropin-releasing hormone (GnRH) from the hypothalamus. Luteinizing hormone (LH) and follicle-stimulating hormone (FSH), produced by the pituitary in response to GnRH, regulate ovarian function. These gonadotropins are subject to predominantly negative feedback by the sex steroids estradiol and progesterone. With FSH, a dimeric glycoprotein, regulation is more complex, because it has a constitutive secretory component, in contrast to LH, which is entirely GnRH dependent. Research has demonstrated that FSH is subject to negative feedback control that is mediated by the inhibins and sex steroids. Ovarian follicular activity is reflected by production of sex steroids and peptide hormones (i.e., inhibin and activin). The sex steroids include estradiol produced by the follicle, progesterone produced by the corpus luteum after the maturation of the dominant ovarian follicle, and androgens, primarily testosterone and androstenedione, secreted by the ovarian stroma. Appreciation of the pivotal role played by the ovarian glycoproteins inhibin and activin is a recent development. The function of the inhibins includes paracrine regulation of the gonads and pituitary and closed long-loop negative feedback on FSH at the level of the pituitary (3).

Inhibin is a dimeric glycoprotein produced in the granulosa cells of the ovary (3). It has been documented to increase in puberty, fluctuate across the menstrual cycle

H. G. Burger: Department of Endocrinology, Prince Henry's Institute of Medical Research, Clayton, Victoria 3168, Australia

H. Teede: Department of Medicine, Prince Henry's Institute of Medical Research, Clayton, Victoria 3168, Australia

and become undetectable after menopause. Two major and distinct inhibin subtypes, inhibins A and B, are composed of a common α subunit and one of two β subunits, β_a and β_b. The physiologic roles of the two inhibins are distinct by virtue of their β subunits. The two subtypes display functional, structural, and molecular differences (4). Most studies of the physiology of inhibin have employed a heterologous radioimmunoassay, the Monash assay, developed in Melbourne. It is nonselective, detecting inhibins A, B, and inactive free α subunits (5). Subsequent work demonstrated that the Monash assay largely parallels the patterns seen with inhibin A. Specific, two-site assays have been developed for the measurement of inhibins A and B, and their physiology in the menstrual cycle has been documented (4,6) (Fig. 7.1).

Only inhibin B is found in male plasma, but inhibin A and inhibin B occur in women. In women, inhibin B is produced mainly by the granulosa cells of the cohort of developing follicles, and inhibin A is a product of the dominant follicle. Using the Monash assay, immunoreactive inhibin levels have been demonstrated to be the same in both ovarian veins, regardless of the side of the dominant follicle (7). This pattern contrasts with that of estradiol, which is produced primarily by the granulosa cells of the dominant follicle. No data are available for dimeric inhibin levels in the ovarian veins. Peripheral plasma levels of inhibin A increase progressively in the later part of the follicular phase, rising to a midcycle peak corresponding to the LH and FSH peak (Fig. 7.1). They then fall, only to rise again to their peak levels in the luteal phase, parallel to the patterns of estradiol and progesterone. Inhibin B peaks in the early follicular phase, then declines before a midcycle peak, and falls to low levels in the luteal phase (4,6). Data suggest that inhibin B may be less biologically active than inhibin A, although this area is still being researched (8).

At a functional level, the major role of inhibin is the negative feedback regulation of pituitary FSH secretion (3). FSH administration stimulates inhibin production (9), and inhibin levels are inversely correlated with FSH concentrations (10). Inhibin B is thought to be the predominant peptide feedback factor for FSH in the follicular phase, along with estradiol, and inhibin A may be more important in the luteal phase (4). Inhibins are also involved in paracrine regulation of the gonads. Activins, discovered during the purification of inhibin, are formed from the dimerization of two inhibin β subunits. Activins primarily act in paracrine regulatory functions in the ovary and in the pituitary, where activin B is responsible for the autonomous component of FSH secretion (11).

ENDOCRINE DYNAMICS: THE PERIMENOPAUSE

The hormonal features of the menopausal transition are still being clarified. Current understanding encompasses the exponential decline of oocyte numbers as menopause approaches, with fluctuating ovarian hormone production and altered feedback regulation on the pituitary as a result of approaching ovarian failure. The role of declining inhibin levels is significant, with reduced negative feedback on the pituitary resulting in increased FSH production. Knowledge about the endocrine changes occurring during the perimenopause is based on evidence from several different study designs, and interpreting the results of these studies has also been difficult because of the variety of definitions used for this phase of reproductive life. Many studies have related observed changes to age rather than cycle pattern or symptoms. Few longitudinal studies encompassing serum sex steroid, gonadotropin, and inhibin profiles exist, with most data being cross-sectional.

Traditional concepts about the endocrine changes characterizing the perimenopause included gradually declining estrogen levels and rising gonadotropins. However, increasing evidence suggested estrogen and FSH levels rise during the perimenopause. Reyes studied ovulating women between 20 and 50 years old. FSH levels increased with age, but estradiol did not decline before menopause (12). Lee had a similar finding, with a rising FSH concentration but no decline in levels of estradiol in a study of 94 regularly cycling women 24 to 50 years of

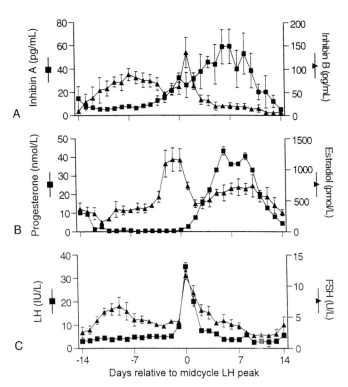

FIG. 7.1. Plasma concentrations of inhibin A **(A)**; inhibin, estradiol, and progesterone **(B)**; and luteinizing hormone (LH) and follicle-stimulating hormone (FSH) **(C)** during the menstrual cycle. Data displayed with respect to the day of the midcycle LH peak. (From ref. 4, with permission.)

age (13). FSH rose as a function of increasing age (especially in the early follicular phase and at midcycle), with a minimal rise in LH and no change in estradiol or progesterone levels. Fitzgerald observed perimenopausal women had the most variability in ovarian steroid profiles but found the mean serum estrogens were no different from those of younger women (14). The maintenance of estrogen levels for as long as possible can reduce undesirable health outcomes.

Limited longitudinal data are primarily based on urine steroid profiles. Several of these studies have documented elevated estrogen production in the setting of multiple developing follicles in perimenopausal women. Brown analyzed urinary steroid profiles in 85 "climacteric" women and demonstrated that estrogen levels fluctuated, producing periods of hyperestrogenism (15). Unfortunately, little recognition was given to these findings because they were thought to be incompatible with the conventional thinking of a slowly progressive decline in estrogen. Metcalf documented elevated FSH with high estrogen levels on 32 separate occasions in 14 perimenopausal women (16). Santoro studied daily urine profiles of perimenopausal women between the ages of 47 and 50 years who showed greater estrone conjugate excretion than did women in their middle reproductive years (17). Variability was evidenced by episodes of marked hyperestrogenism, and elevated FSH was documented in many of the women studied. These findings are consistent with erratic follicular development and occasions of multiple follicles developing at any one time (18).

These fluctuating hormone profiles can explain the variable symptoms, including those consistent with transient estrogen excess and the high incidence of dysfunctional uterine bleeding. An increase in the rate of follicle development with elevated FSH and estrogen levels has also been found (19) in adolescents with anovulatory dysfunctional uterine bleeding.

In one study (20), daily serum samples were obtained for one full cycle in cycling women early (19 to 34 years) and later (42 to 49 years) in reproductive life. Insulin-like growth factor-1 (IGF-1) and growth hormone levels in these two groups were studied. The rationale was based on observations that estradiol influences both levels and that growth hormone and IGF-1 levels decrease with age and are low after menopause. However, IGF-1 levels were not lower in older reproductive aged women in this study, perhaps consistent with maintained estrogen levels over these years, because it was again demonstrated that the older group of women had elevated FSH and elevated estradiol concentrations (Fig. 7.2). Blake et al. (20) stated, "It is important to highlight the estrogen increase because it may represent a harbinger of impending perimenopause, with therapeutic and diagnostic relevance." Given the accumulating evidence, it became increasingly obvious that the proposed declining estrogen stimulus for rising gonadotropins appeared unsustainable.

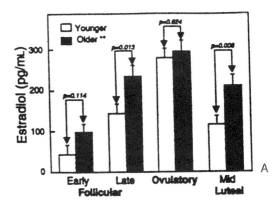

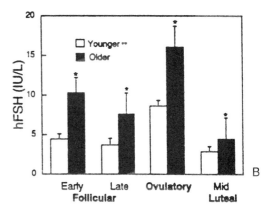

FIG. 7.2. Estradiol **(A)** and follicle-stimulating hormone (FSH) **(B)** by age group and cycle stage in younger women (19 to 34 years) and older women (42 to 47 years). (From ref. 20, with permission.)

It was necessary to postulate that other factors were responsible for the observed rise in FSH. This dilemma was touched on in the 1970s, when the observations about estrogen and FSH were first made. Sherman and Korenman observed shorter cycle length in older cycling women because of a shortened follicular phase (21). They observed elevated FSH levels and proposed that reductions in an "inhibin-like substance," similar to that found in men, could be the primary stimulus for FSH elevation. Although longitudinal studies had not been completed, further evidence to support this theory of declining inhibin before menopause was sought. Most of these studies used the nonspecific Monash assay. *In vitro* evidence for a reduced inhibin reserve with age (22) was supported by studies of *in vivo* inhibin production in women undergoing *in vitro* fertilization. Hughes (23) demonstrated that inhibin responses to gonadotropin hyperstimulation were significantly lower in women older than 35 years compared with those of younger women, whereas the estradiol responses were similar in all groups. Cross-sectional studies demonstrated declining inhibin concentrations with increasing age and elevated FSH levels (10,24,25).

The Melbourne Midlife Project, for example, is based on a cross-sectional survey of a randomly selected, community-based sample of 2,001 Melbourne women between the ages of 45 and 55 at the time of their initial interview (May 1991) (24). A longitudinal study of 437 of these women is examining many aspects of the menopausal transition. The first-year data have been analyzed cross sectionally in terms of menstrual cycle history and therefore menopausal status. Twenty-seven percent of subjects had reported no change in menstrual frequency or flow, and 23% reported a change in flow only. Nine percent reported a change in frequency without a change in flow, and 28% reported a change in frequency and flow. By the time the first-year blood sample was obtained, 13% reported at least 3 months of amenorrhea. Only those who had experienced 3 months of amenorrhea showed a statistically significant fall in estradiol, for which the geometric mean concentration was 42% of the group with no change in cycle. There was a broad spread of estradiol levels, with some greater than 1,500 pmol/L, suggesting granulosa cell hyperstimulation by elevated FSH levels. Immunoreactive inhibin was significantly lower in those who had experienced a change in frequency and flow and was the case for 38% of those in the reference group in women with 3 months of amenorrhea. Overall, the data suggested a fall in inhibin levels earlier than the fall in estradiol, consistent with the hypothesis that a declining inhibin concentration provides a mechanism that allows FSH to rise and thereby maintain intact early follicular phase estradiol concentrations.

The situation has been further clarified by comparison of early follicular-phase hormone levels in normal ovulating women between the ages of 40 and 45 with those in women between the ages of 20 and 25 years (26). A fall in the level of inhibin B in the follicular phase of the cycle appeared to account for the age-associated rise in FSH, with estradiol levels slightly higher in the older women. For inhibin decline to be a primary stimulus for FSH elevation and maintenance of estrogen levels, as we hypothesized, it is necessary to postulate that the secretion of estrogen and inhibin may reflect different aspects of granulosa cell function (27). This idea is supported by the differential response of estradiol and inhibin to ovarian hyperstimulation in older women. There is a marked follicular phase decrease in inhibin B levels in early perimenopause, defined on the basis of a reported change in menstrual cycle frequency (28), when FSH levels start to rise, but inhibin A and estradiol concentrations remain unchanged (Fig. 7.3). Only in late perimenopause (i.e., after more than 3 months of amenorrhea) do estradiol and inhibin A levels also fall, with a marked rise in FSH. This pattern would be supported by studies demonstrating different estrogen and inhibin responses to ovarian hyperstimulation.

The overall fall in inhibin levels correlates with physiologic changes occurring in the ovary as the number of fol-

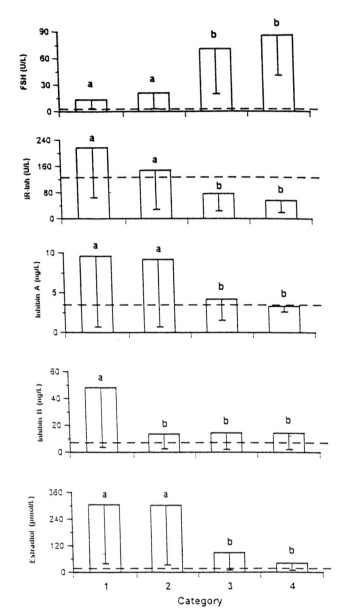

FIG. 7.3. Geometric mean levels (with lower 95% confidence intervals) of follicle-stimulating hormone (FSH), immunoreactive inhibin (IR-INH), inhibin A, inhibin B, and estradiol as a function of menopausal status in a group of 110 women from the Melbourne Mid-Life Project. Stage 1, premenopausal: no change in cycle frequency; stage 2, early perimenopausal: change in cycle frequency; stage 3, late perimenopausal: 3 to 11 months of amenorrhea; stage 4, postmenopausal: more than 12 months of amenorrhea. Values with the same superscript (a or b) are not statistically different; values with differing superscripts, $p < 0.05$. (From ref. 28, with permission)

licles, the source of inhibin production, declines dramatically. Early autopsy studies (29) counted follicle numbers in ovaries of women 7 to 44 years old. Gougeon (30) obtained ovaries after oophorectomy combined with hysterectomy from women 19 to 52 years old. Subsequent studies completed by Richardson et al. on oophorectomy specimens estimated follicle numbers in women 44 to 55 years old (31). Combining these studies and applying mathematical analysis, Richardson demonstrated a steady decline in follicle numbers from the early years until 40 years of age. After 40, there was an exponential acceleration of follicle loss. Faddy and Gosden developed a mathematical model based on histologic analysis of ovaries of 52 cycling women (32). The model predicted a decline in the number of oocytes developing to a stage at which two layers of granulosa cells surround the oocyte, from 51 per day at 24 to 25 years to 1 per day at 49 to 50 years. They hypothesized that the accelerated rate of follicular depletion was attributable to an increase in the rate of atresia of primordial follicles. This idea was consistent with the observed increasing percentages of cycles that are anovulatory as women approach menopause (33,34). The primary event that stimulates accelerated follicular depletion is not understood and remains a topic of ongoing research. Fewer FSH receptors are found on ovarian follicles in the years preceding menopause, possibly suggesting that there is a disturbance of follicular maturation and function before exhaustion of follicles (35).

Altered hypothalamic-pituitary sensitivity to hormonal factors may also contribute to perimenopausal endocrine physiology. Several observations support this theory. Estrogen suppression of the hypothalamic-pituitary axis is less complete in the perimenopausal woman, with hormone replacement therapy rarely suppressing gonadotropin production substantially. A longitudinal study compared perimenopausal women with dysfunctional uterine bleeding (DUB) to regularly menstruating control subjects (36). Basal and stimulated serial steroid and gonadotropin levels were analyzed. In contrast to controls, exogenous estradiol did not have a consistent suppressive effect on gonadotropins in women with DUB. This finding and the documentation of elevated estrogens in the presence of elevated gonadotropins indicate that feedback may be altered.

In light of the erratic and unreliable basal FSH levels during the perimenopause, other stimulatory procedures have been employed, primarily to predict fertility in women of older reproductive age. The clomiphene citrate challenge (CCC) was used to determine fertility potential in older reproductive women. In a study by Gindoff (37), responses of FSH to CCC were assessed according to menstrual cycle pattern. Younger cycling women, older cycling women, irregularly cycling women older than 35, and menopausal women were compared. The perimenopausal and postmenopausal women showed baseline elevated FSH levels. Sustained FSH elevation after CCC was obvious in the perimenopausal women. Basal estrogen levels were higher, but stimulated estrogen responses were lower in perimenopausal women (Fig. 7.4). The responses to stimulation with GnRH did not differ in any of the groups of cycling women (38).

With fluctuating but generally rising FSH, variable estradiol and falling inhibin levels, what are the patterns

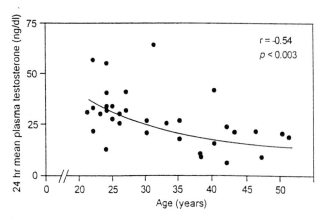

FIG. 7.4. The 24-hour mean plasma total testosterone (T) level is compared with age in normal women. The regression equation was T (nmol/L) = $37.8 \times$ age (years)$^{-1.12}$; $r = -0.54$; $p < 0.003$). (From ref. 41, with permission.)

of progesterone and androgens? Progesterone is produced primarily in the corpus luteum after ovulation. Anovulatory cycles occur with increasing frequency as menopause approaches, with 3% to 7% of cycles anovulatory in women 26 to 40 years old, but 12% to 15% were anovulatory in those between the ages of 41 and 50 (33). Anovulation may occur because of increased rates of follicle atresia. Ultimately, the level of progesterone declines as menopause approaches (17). Urinary pregnanediol levels were found to decline in perimenopausal women in studies completed in the 1970s (15). This reduction in ovulatory cycles observed in the setting of complex endocrine changes results in reduced fertility.

Androgens are primarily produced by ovarian interstitial cells and the adrenal glands. Data on androgen changes across the perimenopause and postmenopause remain controversial. A cross-sectional study of women between the ages of 40 and 60 years concluded that androgen profiles were inherently complex, with only lifestyle factors, including smoking and nutrition, showing significant influence. No clear patterns related to menopause emerged in multivariate analysis (39). In a comparison of younger cycling women, perimenopausal women, and postmenopausal women, testosterone levels were not significantly different, and the dehydroepiandrosterone sulfate concentration was lower in postmenopausal women only. We demonstrated in the longitudinal Melbourne Midlife Project that a decline in testosterone of 1.7% per year occurs in perimenopausal women, but after correction for age and body mass index, levels were found to be higher in women as they approached menopause (24). Another study found that the postmenopausal ovary maintains testosterone secretion but that less androstenedione is produced (40). There appear to be no specific changes related to the perimenopausal period, although androgen levels may fall for many years before the menopausal transition (41) (Fig. 7.4). Much of the confusion regarding androgen levels in relation to menopause may be the result of studies that compared testosterone levels in older postmenopausal women with levels in women in their 20s. It appears that the major fall in testosterone levels occurs between 20 and 40.

Based on the forgoing evidence, it is hypothesized that a fall in inhibin levels (perhaps mainly inhibin B) occurs with reproductive aging because of declining follicle number, allowing a rise in FSH, which leads to accelerated follicle development and increased estrogen secretion in perimenopausal women. Progesterone levels fall as more cycles become anovulatory, and androgens show little or no change. These endocrine changes appear to vary between and within individuals, and substantial changes have been observed from one cycle to the next. We previously concluded that for, estrogen and FSH profiles, the "most noteworthy characteristic is significant hormonal variability" (27). The only conclusion that can be made with confidence concerning hypothalamic-pituitary-ovarian function in individual perimenopausal women is that it is unsafe to generalize.

CLINICAL SEQUELAE OF ENDOCRINE CHANGES IN THE PERIMENOPAUSE

The clinical features and management of the perimenopausal woman are covered elsewhere in this book, but it is appropriate to highlight the clinical observations with direct reference to the observed endocrine changes. Women in the perimenopausal years are more likely to seek medical consultation than their premenopausal or postmenopausal counterparts (1). Vasomotor symptoms, including hot flushes, night sweats, disturbances of sexuality, and psychologic symptoms, are markedly increased in the perimenopause (42,43). Vasomotor symptoms demonstrate the most instability, probably reflecting fluctuating hormone profiles. In one review (44), the increased frequency of migraines in the perimenopause was also attributed to fluctuating hormone profiles.

Negative psychologic symptoms are most common and a sense of well-being is least available during the perimenopausal period (45). Symptoms of estrogen excess and deficiency often occur in the same individual over time. Breast tenderness, menorrhagia, migraine, nausea, shorter cycle length, and a shorter follicular phase (15,17,36), all features of estrogen excess, have been documented in the perimenopause.

Along with significant symptoms related to hormonal fluctuations, women also contend with irregular and heavy-flow menstrual cycles. Fitzgerald (14) described age-related changes in the reproductive cycle. Initially, cycles are shorter, with a shorter follicular phase progressing to increased cycle length and then to irregularity. DUB, occurring with persistent elevation of unopposed estrogens (46), occurs most frequently in perimenopausal women, who have the greatest maximal thickness of endometrium

(14) and have the highest incidence of hysterectomy. Menorrhagia occurs in 20% of perimenopausal women, compared with 9% of women in other phases of reproductive life, and differences in uterine vessel structure have been documented in perimenopausal women (47). Ironically, in 1974, on the basis of his studies of ovarian estrogen secretion in women with DUB, Fraser (46) suggested hyperestrogenism resulted from multiple follicles developing because of abnormal gonadotropin release, which was consistent with today's thinking.

HORMONE-INDUCED CHANGES IN THE PERIMENOPAUSE

Estrogen deficiency induces a rapid phase of bone turnover in the early postmenopausal period that contributes to osteoporosis in later life. The changes in bone turnover in the perimenopause evoke controversy about whether significant alterations precede the decline in estrogen levels. In a prospective study of bone loss in perimenopausal women (part of the Melbourne Midlife Project), Guthrie et al. (48) showed that maximal rates of bone loss occurred in women who became postmenopausal during the period of observation. The researchers found a statistically significant increased rate of loss in late but not early perimenopausal women. Estradiol levels are preserved in early but not late perimenopausal women. Nilas and Christiansen (49) reported radial bone loss in women during perimenopause associated with increased FSH but not with reduced estrogen levels. In a study by Steinberg (50), cross-sectional changes in bone mass density (BMD) in the perimenopause correlated inversely with FSH levels, but estrogen and testosterone levels correlated directly with lower BMD. Slemenda (51) undertook a longitudinal study over 3 years and demonstrated that women in the later phase of the menopausal transition with elevated FSH levels had reduced radial BMD but that those in the early transitional phase with irregular cycles and normal FSH levels did not have reduced BMD.

The opportunity to improve peak bone mass has passed in women reaching the menopausal transition, and further bone loss should be prevented to avoid later osteoporotic fractures. Given the emerging evidence that bone turnover increases and BMD falls preceding menopause, it may be timely to consider osteoporosis and skeletal health earlier than conventionally thought. Alterations have also been demonstrated in lipid profiles during the perimenopause, with progressive decreases in high-density lipoproteins and increases in total cholesterol preceding menopause by several years (52).

ENDOCRINE PROFILE ASSESSMENT OF THE PERIMENOPAUSAL WOMAN

In the setting of variable hormone profiles and symptoms, how should a physician approach the assessment of a perimenopausal woman? The studies of perimenopausal women have found the variations in FSH, inhibin, and estrogen levels to be transient and therefore unreliable in diagnosing approaching menopause or in predicting the stage of menopausal transition for any woman (53). Caution in interpreting hormone profile results is recommended, but if FSH assays are to be used, early follicular phase samples are the most reliable (53). A more rational alternative to hormone profile testing would be acquisition of individual longitudinal symptom data on women who present with perimenopausal complaints. The importance of daily menstrual pattern documentation was emphasized by Treloar (2). The Women's Midlife Project has demonstrated that hormone profiles correlate well with symptoms and cycle features (24). Daily symptom diaries in our hands have proven more useful than isolated steroid profiles, and they can be helpful in self-education for women and provide an assessment tool for clinicians.

CONCLUSIONS

Although the hormonal changes in perimenopausal women are still being clarified, existing data show an exponential decline in oocyte number, with consequent declining inhibin levels, fluctuating and often elevated estradiol, and generally increasing FSH levels. This hormonal milieu may be accompanied by significant symptoms and menstrual disturbances, increased bone turnover, and lipid profile changes. Improved understanding of the endocrine changes characterizing the perimenopause can assist the clinician in accurate assessment and management of patients. The ideal endocrine assessment is likely to be individual, longitudinal, and symptom based and is best achieved by the use of a perimenopause diary rather than isolated endocrine profiles.

REFERENCES

1. McKinlay SM, Brambilla DJ, Posner JG. The normal menopause transition. *Maturitas* 1992;14:103–115.
2. Treloar AE. Menstrual cyclicity and the premenopause. *Maturitas* 1981;3: 249–264.
3. Burger HG. Inhibin. *Reprod Med Rev* 1992;1:1–20.
4. Groome NP, Illingworth PJ, O'Brien M, et al. Measurement of dimeric inhibin B throughout the human menstrual cycle. *J Clin Endocrinol Metab* 1996;81:4: 1401–1405.
5. Burger HG. Clinical utility of inhibin measurements. *J Clin Endocrinol Metab* 1993;76:1391–1396.
6. Groome NP, Illingworth PJ, O'Brien M, et al. Detection of dimeric inhibin A throughout the human menstrual cycle by two-site enzyme immunoassay. *Clin Endocrinol* 1994;40:717–723.
7. Illingworth PJ, Reddi K, Smith, KB, Baird DT. The source of inhibin secretion during the human menstrual cycle. *J Clin Endocrinol Metab* 1991;73:667–673.
8. Robertson DM, Cahir N, Findlay JK, Burger HG, Groome NP. The biological and immunological characterisation of inhibin A and B forms in human follicular fluid and plasma. *J Clin Endocrinol Metab* 1997;82:889–896.
9. Hee J, MacNaughton J, Bangah M, et al. FSG induces dose-dependent stimulation of immunoreactive inhibin secretion during the follicular phase of the human menstrual cycle. *J Clin Endocrinol Metab* 1993;76:5 1340–1343.
10. MacNaughton J, Bangah M, McCloud P, Hee J, Burger HG. Age related changes in follicle stimulating hormone, luteinizing hormone, estradiol and immunoreactive inhibin in women of reproductive age. *Clin Endocrinol* 1992;36:339–345.
11. Corrigan AZ, Bilezikjian LM, Carroll RS, et al. Evidence for an autonomous role of activin B within rat anterior pituitary cultures. *Endocrinology* 1991;128: 1682–1684.
12. Reyes FI, Winter JS, Faiman C. Pituitary ovarian relationships preceding the menopause. A cross-sectional study of serum follicle-stimulating hormone, luteinizing hormone, prolactin, estradiol and progesterone levels. *Am J Obstet Gynecol* 1977; 129:557–564.
13. Lee SJ, Lenton EA, Sexton L, Cooke ID. The effect of age on the cyclical patterns of plasma LH, FSH, estradiol and progesterone in women with regular menstrual cycles. *Hum Reprod* 1988;3:851–855.
14. Fitzgerald CT, Self MW, Killick SR, Bennett DA. Age related changes in the female reproductive cycle. *Br J Obstet Gynaecol* 1994;101:229–233.
15. Brown JB, Harrisson P, Smith MA, Burger HG. Correlations between the mucus symptoms and the hormonal markers of fertility throughout reproductive life. Melbourne: Ovulation Method Research Centre of Australia, Advocate Press, 1981.
16. Metcalf MG, Donald RA, Livesey JH. Pituitary-ovarian function in normal women during the menopausal transition. *Clin Endocrinol* 1981;14:245–255.
17. Santoro N, Brown JR, Adel T, Skurnick JH. Characterization of reproductive hormonal dynamics in the perimenopause. *J Clin Endocrinol Metab* 1996;81: 1495–1501.
18. Metcalf MG, Donald RA. Fluctuating ovarian function in a perimenopausal woman. *N Z Med J* 1979;89:45–47.
19. Baird DT. Anovulatory dysfunctional uterine bleeding in adolescence. In: Flamigni C, Venturoli S and Givens JR, eds. Adolescence in females. Chicago: Year Book Medical Publishers, 1985:273–285.
20. Blake EJ, Adel T, Santoro N. Relationships between insulin-like growth hormone factor-1 and estradiol in reproductive aging. *Fertil Steril* 1997;67:697–701.
21. Sherman BM, Korenman SG. Hormonal characteristics of the human menstrual cycle throughout reproductive life. *J Clin Invest* 1975;55:699–706.
22. Pellicer A, Mari M, de los Santos MJ, Tarin JJ, et al. Effects of aging on the human ovary: the secretion of immunoreactive α-inhibin and progesterone. *Fertil Steril* 1994;61:663–668.
23. Hughes EG, Robertson DM, Handelsman DJ, Hayward S, Healy DL, DeKretser DM. Inhibin and estradiol responses to ovarian hyperstimulation: effects of age and predictive value for *in vitro* fertilization outcome. *J Clin Endocrinol Metab* 1990;70:358–364.
24. Burger HG, Dudley EC, Hopper JL, et al. The endocrinology of the menopausal transition: a cross-sectional study of a population-based sample. *J Clin Endocrinol Metab* 1995;80:3537–3545.
25. Lenton EA, Kretser DM, Woodward AJ, Robertson DM. Inhibin concentrations throughout the menstrual cycles of normal, infertile and older women compared with those during spontaneous conception cycles. *J Clin Endocrinol Metab* 1991; 73:1180–1190.
26. Klein NA, Illingworth PJ, Groome NP, McNeilly AS, Battaglia DE, Soules MR. Decreased inhibin B secretion is associated with the monotrophic FSH rise in older, ovulatory women: a study of serum and follicular fluid levels of dimeric inhibin A and B in spontaneous menstrual cycles. *J Clin Endocrinol Metab* 1996;81:2742–45.
27. Burger HG. Inhibin and steroid changes in the perimenopause. In: Lobo R, ed. *The perimenopause.* New York: Springer Verlag, 1998.
28. Burger HG, Cahir N, Robertson DM, et al. Serum inhibins A and B fall differentially as FSH rises in perimenopausal women. *Clin Endocrinol* 1998;48:809–813.
29. Block E. Quantitative morphological investigations of the follicular system in women: variations in different ages. *Acta Anat* 1952;14:108–123.
30. Gougeon A, Caractère qualitative and quantatif de la population folliculaire dans líavaire humain adulte. *Contracep Fertil Sex* 1984;12:527–535
31. Richardson SJ, Senikas V, Nelson JF. Follicular depletion during the menopausal transition: evidence for accelerated loss and ultimate exhaustion. *J Clin Endocrinol Metab* 1987;65:1231.
32. Faddy MJ, Gosden RG, Gougeon A, Richardson SJ, Nelson JF. Accelerated disappearance of ovarian follicles in mid-life: implications for forecasting menopause. *Hum Reprod* 1992;7:1342–1346.
33. Doring GK. The incidence of anovulatory cycles in women. *J Reprod Fertil* 1969; [Suppl 6]:77–81.
34. Metcalf MG. Incidence of ovulatory cycles in women approaching the menopause. *J Biosoc Sci* 1979;11:39–48.
35. Vihko KK. Gonadotropins and ovarian gonadotropin receptors during the perimenopausal transition period. *Maturitas* 1996;23[Suppl]:S19–S22.
36. Van Look PF, Lothian H, Hunter WM, Michie EA, Baird DT. Hypothalamic-pituitary-ovarian function in perimenopausal women. *Clin Endocrinol* 1977;7:13–31.
37. Gindoff PR, Schmidt PJ, Rubinow DR. Responses to clomiphene citrate challenge test in normal women through perimenopause. *Gynecol Obstet Invest* 1997;43: 186–191.
38. Schmidt PJ, Gindoff PR, Baron DA, Rubinow DR. Basal and stimulated gonadotropin levels in the perimenopause. *Am J Obstet Gynecol* 1996;175:643–650.
39. Bancroft J, Caewood EH. Androgens and the menopause: a study of 40–60-year-old women. *Clin Endocrinol* 1996;45:577–587.
40. Judd HL. Hormonal dynamics associated with the menopause. *Clin Obstet Gynecol* 1976;19:775–788.
41. Zumoff B, Strain GW, Miller LK, Rosner W. Twenty-four hour mean plasma testosterone concentration declines with age in normal premenopausal women. *J Clin Endocrinol Metab* 1995;80:1429–1430.
42. Dennerstein L, Smith AM, Morse CA, Green A, Burger H, Hopper JL. Menopausal symptomatology: the experience of Australian women. *Med J Aust* 1993;159: 232–236.
43. Mitchell ES, Woods NF. Symptom experiences of mid-life women: observations from the Seattle Midlife Womeńs Health Study. *Maturitas* 1996;25:1–10.

44. MacGregor EA. Menstruation, sex hormones and migraine. *Neurol Clin* 1997; 15:125–141.
45. Hunter M, Battersby R, Whitehead M. Relationships between psychological symptoms, somatic complaints and menopausal status. *Maturitas* 1986;8:217–228.
46. Fraser IS, Baird DT. Blood production and ovarian secretion rates of estradiol 17b and estrone in women with dysfunctional uterine bleeding. *J Clin Endocrinol Metab* 1974;39:564–569.
47. Abberton KM, Taylor NH, Healy DL, Rogers PA. Vascular smooth muscle alpha actin distribution around endometrial arterioles during the menstrual cycle: increased expression during the perimenopause and lack of correlation with menorrhagia. *Hum Reprod* 1996;11:204–211.
48. Guthrie JR, Ebeling PR, Hopper LJ, et al. A prospective study of bone loss in menopausal Australian-borne women. *Osteoporos Int* 1998;19:165–173.
49. Nilas L, Christiansen C. Bone mass and its relationship to age and the menopause. *J Clin Endocrinol Metab* 1987;65:697–702.
50. Steinberg RK, Freni-Titulaer W, Depuey EG, Miller DT, et al. Sex steroids and bone density in premenopausal and perimenopausal women. *J Clin Endocrinol Metab* 1989;69:533–539.
51. Slemenda C, Hui SL, Longcope C, Johnston CC. Sex steroids and bone mass: a study of changes about the time of menopause. *J Clin Invest* 1987;80:1261–1269.
52. Shargil AA. Hormone replacement therapy in perimenopausal women with a triphasic contraceptive compound: a three-year prospective study. *Int J Fertil* 1985;30:15–28.
53. Burger HG. Diagnostic role of follicle-stimulating hormone (FSH) measurements during the menopausal transitionóan analysis of FSH, oestradiol and inhibin. *Eur J Endocrinol* 1994;130:38–42.

Treatment of the Postmenopausal Woman: Basic and Clinical Aspects, Second Edition, edited by Rogerio A. Lobo, Lippincott Williams & Wilkins, Philadelphia © 1999.

CHAPTER 8

Changes in the Menstrual Pattern During the Perimenopause

Ian S. Fraser

The menopause is strictly defined as the last menstrual period of a woman and is therefore determined only in retrospect. Most authorities agree that menopause can be deemed to have occurred when no menstrual bleeding has occurred for 1 year in a woman of the appropriate age, especially if supported by the presence of vasomotor or other symptoms. This permanent cessation of menses is preceded by a light phase, generally lasting 2 to 5 years, usually called the *perimenopause* or *climacteric*. This phase of progressive gearing down of the ovaries continues 2 to 3 years beyond the menopause.

The perimenopause is characterized by increasing irregularity and unpredictability of the menstrual cycle. There is an increase in the incidence of short and long follicular phases, defective ovulation, anovulation, and highly erratic cycles. This pattern of increasing irregularity should be distinguished from a pattern of continuing regular menstrual cycles with superimposed episodes of intermenstrual bleeding. Different patterns of intermenstrual bleeding can be confusing when they occur in the older woman. Intermenstrual bleeding is frequently associated also with postcoital bleeding. Intermenstrual and postcoital bleeding are frequently associated with important genital tract pathology, and the physician should remain alert to ensure that such pathology is not overlooked in this age group (1). There is also increasing variability in the volume of menstrual blood loss. In this age group, menorrhagia is much more common than it is in the middle reproductive years, and it may be associated with ovulatory and anovulatory dysfunctional uterine bleeding or with pelvic pathology. Considerable sensitivity is required to distinguish "normal" perimenstrual patterns from those that may indicate pelvic pathology.

During the gearing-down phase of the perimenopause with variable and unpredictable menstrual patterns, other symptoms of menopause such as hot flashes and night sweats may also develop months or years before menopause occurs. The menstrual changes predominantly result from changes in ovarian steroid secretion as a consequence of oocyte and follicle depletion (2), but they are also influenced by age-related and pathology-related changes in the uterus.

PERIMENOPAUSAL MENSTRUAL PATTERNS

We are indebted to the huge database of prospectively collected, long-term menstrual charts, established by Alan Treloar through the Tremin Trust at the University of Minnesota, for our present understanding of the changes in menstrual patterns preceding menopause. The initial volunteers for this study were recruited in the 1930s, and numbers were progressively added over the next 40 to 50 years. Volunteers were asked to record the onset of every menstrual period from recruitment until menopause, with noted pauses for pregnancy. This unique database is supervised by the College of Nursing, University of Utah. The Treloar program initially reported on the menstrual patterns of 2,702 women followed for many years (25,825 total woman-years of menstrual experience) of whom 120 had reached menopause at the time of publication (3). Subsequent longer-term and more detailed reviews of the same cohort provided data on 324 women reaching menopause (4,5). The mean age of menopause in this group was 49.5 years, and the women had been menstruating for an average of 35.9 years. The findings of this study were supported by the large independent menstrual database collected by Vollman (6). The studies of Treloar and Vollman demonstrate an increasing irregularity of cycles as menopause approaches. This is specifically seen as a sharp increase

I. S. Fraser: Department of Obstetrics and Gynaecology, Sydney Centre for Reproductive Health Research, University of Sydney, NSW 2006, Australia.

in cycle variability in 10% to 15% of women 6 years before menopause, which includes increased numbers of short and long cycles. There was a sharp increase in variability in another 30% of women between 3 and 2 years before menopause, although most women demonstrated little change in most cycles until the last 1 to 2 years. Similar increases in variability precede menopause in Indian women (7) and probably occur in a similar manner in all ethnic groups, although the ages at which change occurs may vary slightly.

The mean and centile variations in cycle length during the years leading up to menopause are illustrated in Fig. 8.1. These data demonstrate that the mean cycle length increases from 26 days at 4 years before menopause to 27 days at 2 years before and to 28 days at 1 year before the final menstrual period (3). During the same timeframe, the 10th percentile of women experience a shortening of cycle length from 21 days through 17 days to 16 days. In contrast, women on the 80th percentile experience an increase from 29 days through 40 days up to 57 days. This figure gives a clear impression of the rapidly increasing intermenstrual intervals in some women as menopause approaches and of the contrasting shortening of intervals in others.

Figure 8.1 does not illustrate the fact that some women experience highly erratic and unpredictable variations in cycle length during this phase of life (Fig. 8.2). One of the women illustrated in Fig. 8.2 has experienced hugely varying intermenstrual intervals over 9 years, with extreme variations between 26 and 191 days in the 2 years before menopause. The other woman in Fig. 8.2 exhibited minimal variation except in the last 2 years, when the maximal variations were between 19 and 81 days, with only one cycle longer than 38 days.

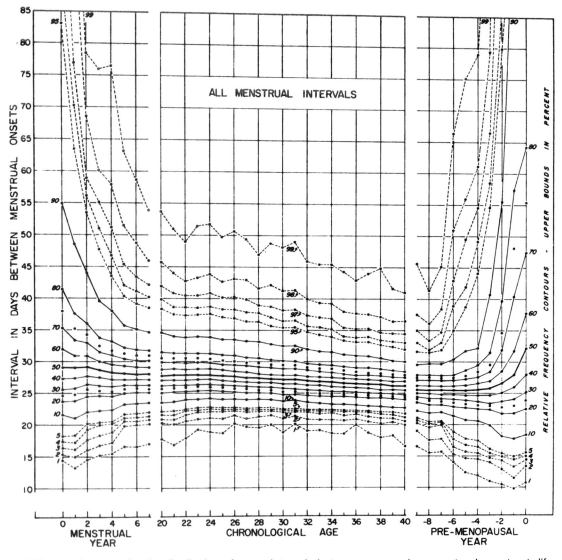

FIG. 8.1. Contours for the distribution of mean intervals between successive menstrual onsets at different ages. The right end of the graph shows menstrual intervals in the 9 years preceding the onset of menopause. (From ref. 3, with permission.)

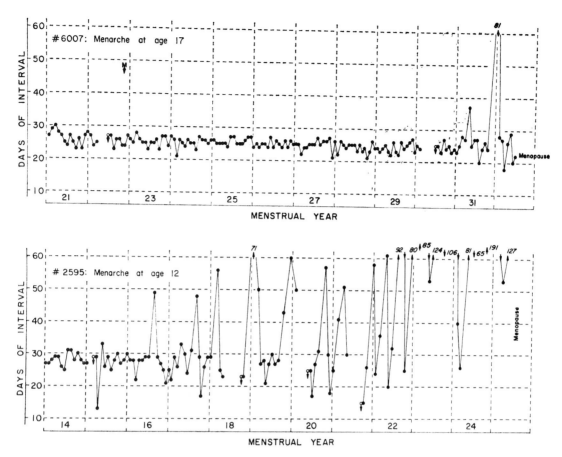

FIG. 8.2. Menstrual intervals in two women during the 11 years leading up to menopause, demonstrating extreme differences in menstrual experience during the menopausal transition. (From ref. 3, with permission.)

The data from individual women can be used to calculate the percentage probability of menopause having already occurred according to the duration of amenorrhea at different ages (8) (Table 8.1). For example, a woman who has a first episode of amenorrhea that is greater than 180 days between the ages of 45 and 49 years had a 45.5% chance of having already reached menopause. However, she also has a 54.5% chance of having one or more additional menses before menopause supervenes. Others have found that 70% of women experienced significant oligomenorrhea before menopause, while 18% experienced menorrhagia or metrorrhagia and only 12% had fairly regular cycles up to the onset of postmenopausal amenorrhea (9). The important message is that the actual occurrence of menopause is difficult to predict ahead of this event in individual women.

The increasingly erratic nature of the menstrual cycle as menopause approaches is associated with an increasing incidence of shortened follicular phases, lengthened follicular phases, defective luteal function, and anovulation (6,10,11). Data from a large cross-sectional basal body temperature chart study demonstrated that the incidence of defective luteal function increases from 8% of cycles at 31 to 35 years to 36% at 40 to 50 years of age (9). This study also demonstrated that anovulation increases from 8% at 31 to 35 years up to 16% of cycles at 45 to 50 years. This information is mirrored by the demonstration of a marked increase in the incidence of anovulation associated with cystic glandular hyperplasia of the endometrium in older women, peaking at the age of around 50 years (12,13). This condition could be

TABLE 8.1. *Probability of menopause having already occurred according to age and to duration of first episode of amenorrhea*

Duration of first amenorrheic episode (days)	Age (years)		
	45–49	50–52	>53
90–119	1	2.8	30.4
47.4			
180–209	45.5	65.2	71.9
270–299	74.1	86.3	88.6
360+	89.5	93.6	95.5

Adapted from ref. 8.

regarded as one end of the spectrum of anovulatory dysfunctional uterine bleeding, and until recently. It was graced with the name of *metropathia hemorrhagica*.

A dramatic decline in fertility precedes menopause by about 10 years, but this does not correlate directly with any changes in the menstrual pattern. Individuals may still be fertile during periods of considerable irregularity, and spontaneous pregnancies, albeit rare, can occur after the age of 50. The longstanding substantiated record of the oldest mother to give birth after a spontaneous conception is Ruth Ellis Kistler at 57 years and 129 days, but the oldest reported mother is Rossanna Dalla Corta from Italy who gave birth in 1994 at the age of 63. It is likely that further births to women in their late 50s and 60s will occur because of the application of assisted reproductive technologies (14). The incidence of such births varies widely from culture to culture, with the highest known rate in the mid-1970s being in Albania (55 per 10,000 births).

With assisted reproductive technologies, most women in their 50s and 60s who are giving birth are using donated oocytes from younger women. Nevertheless, fresh corpora lutea have been found at laparotomy even up to 3 years after the age of apparent spontaneous menopause (15). Wallace et al. (8) found menses can occur after prolonged periods of perimenopausal amenorrhea and that these cycles occasionally are ovulatory (11).

POSTMENOPAUSAL BLEEDING EPISODES

The Treloar data demonstrate that, even among women older than 52 with 1 year of amenorrhea, 4.5% have at least one more episode of menstruation (8). Vaginal bleeding occurring more than 1 year after menopause is conventionally defined as postmenopausal bleeding and must be investigated because of an incidence of 10% to 20% of underlying genital tract malignancy. Nevertheless, most such episodes of bleeding occur in the absence of pathology and are probably associated with growth and atresia of an evanescent ovarian follicle and rarely even ovulation.

MENSTRUAL BLOOD LOSS

The volume of menstrual blood loss is awkward to measure in clinical practice, and there are no longitudinal studies of menstrual blood loss through the perimenopause. Cross-sectional data are fragmentary but suggest an overall tendency toward an increase in the volume of blood loss as menopause approaches. These cross-sectional studies have demonstrated a trend toward increasing volumes of objectively measured blood loss as women grow older (16,17). In the Swedish study, the mean monthly volume rose from 28.4 mL at 15 years of age to 62.4 mL at 50 years (16). Although this mean rise could have been accounted for by substantial increases in a small proportion of the total group, Rybo et al. demonstrated a highly significant and progressive rise in menstrual blood loss, from 36 to 68 mL, in 33 women at intervals over 12 years between the ages of 38 and 50 years (18) (Fig. 8.3). Perception and tolerance play a major role in the reporting of "heaviness" of menstrual bleeding (16,19). A major proportion (more than 50%) of the volume of the menstrual flow is made up of an endometrial transudate rather than whole blood (20). This proportion does not appear to change with age and probably greatly influences women's perception of the absolute volume of her flow.

An increasing proportion of women develop menorrhagia as they move into the late reproductive years (12,16). The incidence of ovulatory and anovulatory dysfunctional uterine bleeding increases during this phase, and menorrhagia due to pelvic pathology is also more common. Few women with menorrhagia caused by dysfunctional uterine bleeding in this age group are consistently anovulatory as implied by American definitions (21), and most have ovulatory cycles from time to time (22). Some women experience true menorrhagia with measured menstrual blood loss in excess of 80 mL per month when they are placed on treatment with standard regimens of hormone replacement therapy after menopause (23,24) (Table 8.2).

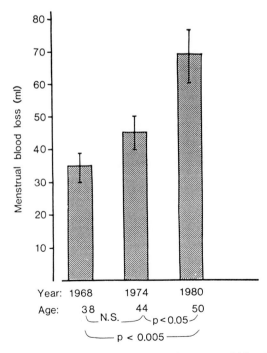

FIG. 8.3. Objective measurements of menstrual blood loss from 33 Swedish women between the ages of 38 and 50 years who were studied on three occasions during the 12-year period. (Adapted from ref. 18.)

TABLE 8.2. *Causes of perimenopausal changes in the menstrual pattern*

Oligomenorrhea and amenorrhea; short cycles; hypomenorrhea
 Natural changes in pattern and volume of menstruation with declining ovarian function
 Other pathologic causes
Intermenstrual bleeding (with or without postcoital bleeding)
 Endometrial disease: polyps, leiomyomas, endometritis, carcinoma
 Adenomyosis or endometriosis
 Cervical disease: polyps, cervicitis, ectropion, carcinoma
Menorrhagia
 Pelvic disease: leiomyomas, adenomyosis, endometriosis, endometrial polyps, endometrial adenocarcinoma, myometrial hypertrophy, arteriovenous malformations, and rare disorders
 Systemic disease: coagulation disorders, hypothyroidism, systemic lupus erythematosus, rare disorders
 Dysfunctional uterine bleeding: anovulatory, ovulatory (acute or chronic)
Acyclic bleeding
 Hypothalamic-pituitary anovulatory disturbances
 Endometrial or cervical carcinoma

Adapted from ref. 25.

CAUSES OF PERIMENOPAUSAL MENSTRUAL CHANGES

The main pathophysiologic explanation for changes in the regularity of perimenopausal cycles is failure of development of ovarian follicles as the total follicle pool is greatly depleted (2). Failure of follicle growth and lack of estradiol secretion lead to the negative feedback stimulation of FSH (and LH) secretion that eventually stimulates growth of the next follicle to enter the stage in which it becomes sensitive to FSH. This process continues erratically until no further follicles are left in the ovaries. There is also a possibility that some women develop independent disturbances of hypothalamic-pituitary function. Various genital tract pathologies are common in this age group, and

the likelihood of finding particular pathology depends on the nature of the bleeding disturbance (Table 8.3).

Pelvic pathology is a common cause of abnormal bleeding in the perimenopausal phase. In one study of 500 perimenopausal women attending a single clinic, 20% gave a history of menorrhagia, metrorrhagia, or intermenstrual bleeding; 9% of these had a genital tract malignancy, and 14% had endometrial hyperplasia (9). Quinn et al. reported that 38% of women found to have a premenopausal endometrial carcinoma presented with regular menorrhagia, and 29% presented with irregular bleeding and 33% with irregular and very heavy bleeding (25). Benign pelvic causes of these menstrual symptoms are also common, with uterine myomas, adenomyosis, endometriosis, and endometrial polyps accounting for at least 50% of cases of menorrhagia. The remainder are caused by ovulatory and anovulatory dysfunctional uterine bleeding. The need for precision in diagnosis and evaluation has become increasingly important with the development of a widening range of options for medical and surgical management (26,27).

CONCLUSIONS

Intervals generally tend to increase, but many cycles show shortened follicular phases or anovulation. The most striking feature of the menstrual cycle in perimenopausal women is its unpredictability, with erratic and major variations in menstrual intervals, volume, and pattern of flow. Increasing volume of flow is common as women grow older, and this may be perceived as being abnormal by the woman. This symptom commonly causes social distress and concern about cancer and is relatively infrequently associated with progressive development of iron deficiency and anemia. It is a critically important clinical skill to know when to investigate perimenopausal women with menstrual changes for possible serious underlying pathology, and the physician must remain alert to ensure early detection of the 40% to 50% of endometrial cancers that manifest before menopause is reached.

TABLE 8.3. *Measured menstrual blood loss during programmed withdrawal bleeds in postmenopausal women treated with three regimens of combined sequential hormone replacement therapy*

Study	Number of women	Median MBL (mL)			Range of MBL (mL)			MBL >80 mL
		3 mo	6 mo	12 mo	3 mo	6 mo	12 mo	
Rees[23a]	50	26	23	17	1–313	2–256	1–106	13%
Sporrong[24b]	23	22	—	—	0–582	—	—	13%
Sporrong[24c]	23	16	—	—	0–346	—	—	13%

MBL, menstrual blood loss.
[a]Rees used estradiol valerate 2 mg and levonorgestrel (75 μg).
[b]Sporrong's first regimen was estradiol valerate (2 mg) and levonorgestrel (250 μg).
[c]Sporrong's second regimen was estradiol valerate (2 mg) and medroxyprogesterone (10 mg).
Data from refs. 23 and 24, with permission.

REFERENCES

1. Fraser IS, Petrucco OM. The management of intermenstrual and postcoital bleeding and an appreciation of the issues arising out of the recent medico-legal case of O'Shea v Sullivan and Macquarie pathology. *Aust N Z J Obstet Gynaecol* 1996;36:67–73.

2. Richardson SJ, Senikas V, Nelson JF. Follicular depletion during the menopausal transition: evidence for accelerated loss and ultimate exhaustion. *J Clin Endocrinol Metab* 1987;65:1231–1237.

3. Treloar AE, Boynton RE, Behn BG, Brown BW. Variation of the human menstrual cycle through reproductive life. *Int J Fertil* 1967;12:77–126.

4. Treloar AE. Menarche, menopause and intervening fecundity. *Hum Biol* 1974;46:89–107.

5. Treloar AE. Menstrual cyclicity and the premenopause. *Maturitas* 1981;3:49–64.

6. Vollman RF. *The menstrual cycle.* Philadelphia: WB Saunders, 1977.

7. Jeyaseelan L, Antonisamy B, Rao PS. Pattern of menstrual cycle length in South Indian women: a prospective study. *Soc Biol* 1992;39:306–309.

8. Wallace RB, Sherman BM, Beau JA, Treloar AE, Schlabaugh L. Probability of menopause with increasing duration of amenorrhoea in middle-aged women. *Am J Obstet Gynecol* 1979;135:1021–1024.

9. Seltzer VL, Benjamin F, Deutsch S. Perimenopausal bleeding patterns and pathologic findings. *J Am Womens Assoc* 1990;45:132–134.

10. Doring GK. The incidence of anovular cycles in women. *J Reprod Fertil* 1969; [Suppl 6]:77–81.

11. Sherman BM, Korenman SG. Hormonal characteristics of the menstrual cycle throughout reproductive life. *J Clin Invest* 1975;55:699–706.

12. Schröder R. Endometrial hyperplasia in relation to genital function. *Am J Obstet Gynecol* 1954;68:294–309.

13. Fraser IS, Baird DT. Endometrial cystic glandular hyperplasia in adolescent girls. *J Obstet Gynaecol Br Commonw* 1972;79:1009–1015.

14. Matthews P, ed. *The Guinness book of records.* Dublin: Guinness Publishing, 1996:57.

15. Novak ER. Ovulation after fifty. *Obstet Gynecol* 1970;36:903–910.

16. Hallberg L, Hogdahl AM, Nilsson L, Rybo G. Menstrual blood loss—a population study. *Acta Obstet Gynecol Scand* 1966;45:320–351.

17. Cole SK, Billewicz WZ, Thomson AM. Sources of variation in menstrual blood loss. *J Obstet Gynaecol Br Commonw* 1971;78:933–939.

18. Rybo G, Leman J, Tibblin E. Epidemiology of menstrual blood loss. In: Baird DT, Michie EA, eds. *Mechanism of menstrual bleeding.* New York: Raven Press, 1983: 181–193.

19. Fraser IS, McCarron G, Markham R. A preliminary study of factors influencing perception of menstrual blood loss volume. *Am J Obstet Gynecol* 1984;149: 788–793.

20. Fraser IS, McCarron G, Markham R, Resta T. Blood and total fluid content of menstrual discharge. *Obstet Gynecol* 1985;65:194–198.

21. Cowan BD. Dysfunctional uterine bleeding: clues to efficacious approaches. In: Alexander NJ, d'Arcangues C, eds. Steroid hormones and uterine bleeding. Washington: AAAS Press, 1992:9–15.

22. Fraser IS, Baird DT. Blood production and ovarian secretion rates of oestradiol-17β and estrone in women with dysfunctional uterine bleeding. *J Clin Endocrinol Metab* 1974;39:564–570.

23. Rees MCP, Barlow DH. Quantitation of hormone replacement-induced withdrawal bleeds. *Br J Obstet Gynaecol* 1991;98:106–107.

24. Sporrong T, Rybo G, Vilbergson G, Crona N, Mattson LA. An objective and subjective assessment of uterine blood loss in postmenopausal women on hormone replacement therapy. *Br J Obstet Gynaecol* 1992;99:399–401.

25. Quinn M, Neale BJ, Fortune DW. Endometrial carcinoma in premenopausal women: a clinico-pathological study. *Gynaecol Oncol* 1985;20:298–306.

26. Hickey M, Fraser IS. Mechanisms and management of dysfunctional uterine bleeding. In: Fraser IS, Jansen RPS, Lobo R, Whitehead MI, eds. *Estrogens and progestogens in clinical practice.* London: Churchill Livingstone, 1998.

27. Cameron IT, Fraser IS, Smith SK, eds. *Clinical disorders of the endometrium and menstruation.* Oxford: Oxford University Press 1998.

Treatment of the Postmenopausal Woman: Basic and Clinical Aspects, Second Edition, edited by Rogerio A. Lobo, Lippincott Williams & Wilkins, Philadelphia © 1999.

CHAPTER 9

Decisions Regarding Treatment in the Perimenopause

Judi Lee Chervenak and Nanette Santoro

The United States population is increasing in age. Not only is the number of elderly people increasing, but this older population itself is getting older (1). As the post World War II baby boom generation reaches age 65, which will occur between the years 2010 and 2030, the most rapid increase in the elderly population is expected. As life expectancy increases, women will spend more of their lives in the postmenopausal period. Because the population is aging, it is important to identify and correct risk factors that could adversely affect health and quality of life. The perimenopause is a stage in a woman's life during which she has an opportunity to reduce her risk factors in order to maximize the quality of the rest of her life.

Natural menopause is traditionally defined as the time period that occurs after 12 consecutive months of amenorrhea. The perimenopause or climacteric refers to the time period before the onset of menopause, when changes in a woman's hormonal milieu are associated with irregular menstrual cycles and increased episodes of amenorrhea. One current clinical definition of the perimenopause is as follows: (a) a self-report of 3 to 11 months of amenorrhea or (b) increased menstrual irregularity in women who are not experiencing amenorrhea (2). This transition lasts about 4 years and usually occurs between ages 45 and 55 (2,3).

Smoking is the greatest independent risk factor for earlier menstrual irregularity and earlier menopause. Smoking causes an earlier perimenopause and menopause by about 1 to 2 years (4,5). Another strong indicator for an earlier age at menopause is a maternal history of early menopause (6).

Once a woman older than 45 has had 1 year of amenorrhea, she has less than a 10% likelihood of ever menstruating again (7). However, there is no clear-cut transition period from the pre- to the postmenopausal state. Cessation of menstrual cyclicity occurs spontaneously at some point during this transition.

Regarding the hormonal milieu of women traversing the menopause, Metcalf et al. (8) could not identify any hormonal differences between the irregular cycles of the perimenopausal woman and the immediately postmenopausal woman, except that no detectable progesterone was ever produced after a woman's final menstrual period (FMP). The preponderance of evidence now suggests that significant changes are occurring in a woman's hormonal environment during the perimenopause.

During the perimenopause, there is thought to be an increase in the number of anovulatory cycles. However, the mechanisms responsible for perimenopausal anovulation remain unclear. The anovulatory cycles occurring during the perimenopause appear similar to those occurring in adolescence and may reflect an inability to produce a luteinizing hormone (LH) surge after exposure to estrogen (9). There may be central changes in the hypothalamic-pituitary axis that affect gonadotropin secretion. This has been suggested by the lack of response to an estradiol challenge with a luteinizing hormone surge in perimenopausal women with dysfunctional uterine bleeding (9–11). However, abnormalities in ovarian steroid or peptide secretion may also play a role.

During the perimenopause, ovarian function appears to be highly variable. Length of menses varies, and anovulatory cycles become more common. Hormone levels may fluctuate widely during this time, and as estrogen levels decrease, the inherent protective effects of estrogen may

J.L. Chervenak and N. Santoro: Department of Obstetrics, Gynecology & Women's Health, Albert Einstein College of Medicine, The Bronx, New York 10461.

also decrease. Thus, the hormonal changes associated with aging may have detrimental effects that must be recognized, addressed, and ameliorated whenever possible.

CHANGES ASSOCIATED WITH AGING

Many of the physiologic changes associated with menopause occur or begin before the last menstrual period (12) and may be associated with somatic aging. Somatic aging is reflected by decreases in somatotropic axis function, adrenal androgen production, and continuous loss of bone mineral density after peak bone mass has been attained. Several hormonal systems have age-related changes that may be associated with reproductive aging (9).

The most important factor regulating the pace of the menopausal transition is ovarian function. Ovarian follicular depletion is the ultimate causative factor for perimenopause and menopause. However, the commencement of perimenopause may also result from aging-associated changes in other systems, such as the hypothalamus, pituitary, and uterus. Because none of these systems has been fully examined in the human, their contribution to the perimenopause and menopause remains unclear.

CHANGES IN THE HORMONAL ENVIRONMENT

Estrogenic Changes

Midcycle estrogen concentrations in the perimenopause have been shown to be normal or increased (13–16), while androgens have been observed to be normal or decreased, independent of major changes in sex hormone-binding globulin (17,18).

Hyperestrogenemia may be a feature of the early perimenopause, but the immediately premenopausal cycles may have decreased levels of estrogen (9,13). During the perimenopause, estradiol levels do not gradually decrease but instead fluctuate greatly around the normal range until menopause, when no more responsive follicles are available (19). Thus, as a woman ages, there is not a downward spiral in the estrogenic milieu but, instead, a "roller coaster" in estrogen production (9). This important feature of the perimenopause is clinically frustrating, as patients may complain of changing symptoms for which therapy must be customized. It is important to consider seriously a patient's complaints of irregular bleeding because the fluctuations in estrogen levels, associated with periods of hyperestrogenemia, may predispose a woman to irregular bleeding and endometrial hyperplasia with its potential sequelae. Ultrasound monitoring and biopsy may be necessary in these patients.

The etiology of the perimenopausal fluctuations in estradiol may be a decrease in the aging ovary's ability to regulate follicle-stimulating hormone (FSH) secretion. It has been suggested that day 3 serum FSH is an indirect bioassay of dimeric inhibin production at the level of the granu-

losa cell (60). Inhibin A and B both appear to be decreased in perimenopausal women. Inhibin A is believed to be a product of the dominant follicle and corpus luteum. Inhibin B is a product of smaller, preovulatory follicles and is the dominant inhibin in the follicular phase of the cycle. Different patterns of circulating inhibins A and B observed during the human menstrual cycle suggest that they may have different physiologic roles. Decreased production of both of these peptides has been reported in perimenopausal women, leading to decreased "restraint" of FSH secretion (61). Furthermore, activin A, an FSH-releasing peptide, is elevated in the follicular phase of perimenopausal women, causing further stimulation of FSH secretion (Reame, personal communication, 1997). Women with low day 3 serum concentrations of inhibin B have been shown to demonstrate a poorer response to ovulation induction than women with high day 3 inhibin B (61). It also appears that greater circulating amounts of FSH are needed to initiate folliculogenesis in reproductively aged women with "decreased follicular reserve." When all these mechanisms are active, enhanced FSH secretion may cause an "overshoot" of estradiol that results in hyperestrogenemia (9,13). In support of this concept, it appears that women in their 40s are more likely to have naturally occurring twin pregnancies than are younger women, implying that multiple folliculogenesis may be more common in this age group. Thus, although reproductive efficiency is markedly decreased in the perimenopausal woman, hormonal secretion patterns may be exuberant. The early perimenopause is therefore conceptualized as an endocrine state of compensated failure.

Although progesterone is no longer produced after a woman's final menstrual period, there exists a brief time when small amounts of estrogen may still be produced. Metcalf et al. (8) observed that although elevations in FSH and LH were common before the final menstrual cycle, episodes of significant estrogen production were not uncommon in the first year after the final menstruation.

Progestagenic Changes

Both normal (14,20–22) and decreased (13,15) corpus luteum production of progesterone have been observed in the perimenopause. It would be clinically very helpful to have further clarification regarding progesterone levels in the perimenopause because, if decreased progesterone levels are associated with increased estradiol, then this may predispose women to dysfunctional uterine bleeding and endometrial hyperplasia.

Growth Hormone Changes

Growth hormone (GH), under hypothalamic regulation by growth hormone-releasing hormone (GHRH), is a pulsatile hormone released from the anterior pituitary. Somatostatin, on the other hand, inhibits GH secretion. With aging, there is a decrease in GH secretion. It remains to be elucidated whether the decrease in GH results from increased release of somatostatin, decreased levels of GHRH, decreased sensitivity to GHRH, or a combination of these factors (9).

Significant gender differences exist in GH secretion. In women, estrogen appears to play an important role in GH secretion. There is a positive association between estrogen status and GH concentrations. Thus, in a decreased estrogenic environment, such as that found in menopause, there is decreased GH secretion (23).

Age itself may be a more important factor affecting concentrations of GH than estrogen alone. Recent studies have shown that decreased somatotropic axis activity is detectable before any changes occur in menstrual cyclicity or evidence of ovarian failure is present. Older, regularly cycling women (age 42 to 46) secrete less GH in the daytime than do younger, regularly cycling controls (aged 19 to 34). This was found to occur in the older women despite higher estradiol levels on the day of sampling (when compared with their younger controls). Older reproductive-aged women had twice the early follicular phase concentration of estradiol as did their younger controls (24).

Insulin-Like Growth Factor 1 Changes

Lower levels of insulin-like growth factor 1 (IGF-1) have been observed to be associated with elevated estradiol and decreased GH levels in older reproductive-age women (24). The mechanism by which changes in IGF-1 and GH affect perimenopausal physiology is not fully understood. Whether or not functional changes in the somatotropic axis and hormonal environment affect sensitivity to insulin remains to be shown. During the perimenopause, insulin sensitivity decreases, especially when there is a weight gain (25–27). As a woman ages, she gains weight. A prospective study of 485 middle-aged women (42 to 50 years) showed that after 3 years, the average weight gain was 2.25 to 4.19 kg. However, there were no significant differences between the amount of weight gain in premenopausal versus postmenopausal women (2.07 vs. 1.35 kg) (26). Change in weight is not entirely dependent on menopausal status.

A direct association between perimenopausal weight gain and insulin resistance was noted by Wing et al. (26). Thus, aging has been associated with decreased GH and IGF-1 levels, decreased insulin sensitivity, increased insulin resistance (28), and weight gain (29). It is important for women, especially during the perimenopausal and postmenopausal period, to control their weight to minimize their already age-associated increased risk for diseases such as cardiovascular disease.

Androgenic Changes

The three major sources for circulating androgens during the reproductive period are the ovary, the adrenal cortex, and peripheral conversion of circulating androstenedione and dehydroepiandrosterone (DHEA) to testosterone. The premenopausal ovary produces 25% of circulating testosterone, 60% of circulating androstendione, and about 20% of circulating DHEA. The adrenal cortex produces 40% of circulating androstenedione, 25% of testosterone, and almost all DHEA and DHEA sulfate (DHEAS). In the postmenopausal period, 50% of circulating testosterone levels result from peripheral conversion of androstenedione (33). Approximately 50% of postmenopausal women have androgens still produced by their ovaries, although in minimal quantity. Their physiologic significance, if any, is unknown (34).

Both adrenal and ovarian androgen levels decline commencing after age 20. By age 40, serum androgen levels are approximately half those found at age 20 (35). Most of the marked decrease in circulating C_{19} steroids and the resulting androgen metabolites occurs between ages 20 to 30 and 50 to 60 years. Smaller changes are seen after age 60 years (62). However, changes in the androgenic environment can be affected by other factors associated with aging. For example, insulin and IGF-1 can both act as stimulants of androgens by the ovarian stroma and theca tissues.

In normally menstruating women, there is a preovulatory increase in intrafollicular and peripheral androgens. At midcycle, peripheral androstenedione and testosterone increase by 15% to 20% (36). Several speculations exist regarding the role of the midcycle rise in androgens. It may help accelerate follicular atresia so that at ovulation, there is a single dominant follicle (37). Alternatively, it may be involved in the stimulation of libido: it has been shown that female-initiated sexual activity occurs most often at midcycle (38). If androgens are important in the production of a single dominant follicle and in stimulating libido, then the age-related decrease in androgens may be associated with the increased incidence of multiple pregnancy and decreased libido that has been reported in older reproductive-aged women. If this association holds true, then androgen replacement may be useful for restoring libido in symptomatic older women.

Among the adrenal androgens, DHEAS is most abundant hormone in the body. However, DHEAS is not biologically active unless it is converted to testosterone or estradiol. In the early 20s, DHEA production is maximal. With increasing age, its secretion is greatly decreased. The decrease is accelerated after menopause (19). In the elderly, concentrations of DHEAS are only about 10% those in younger persons (39). The age-associated decrease in DHEAS is independent of cortisol (40). Decreased DHEAS also appears to be independent of reproductive aging but instead represents a somatic aging event. Studies to support this belief still need to be performed (9).

Because the adrenal cortex androgens, DHEA and DHEAS, have such low intrinsic biologic activity unless converted to more active androgens, they have only recently been considered to be potentially important in immunocompetence and general well-being (29). Their role in the perimenopause has yet to be fully established. Relationships between DHEAS levels and cardiovascular morbidity and mortality that have been reported for men are not true for women. In women, although higher levels of DHEAS were associated with several major cardiovascular disease risk factors, they were not related to risk of fatal cardiovascular disease (63,64). Therefore, the role of DHEAS supplementation in the perimenopause remains to be elucidated.

Gonadotropin Level Changes

During the menopause transition, there is an increase in FSH that has been attributed to a loss of ovarian inhibin. This relationship appears to supported by available immunoassay data (14,21,41).

Although there is a progressive increase in serum levels of FSH with increasing age, there exists much overlap regarding the level and its association with the timing of menopause. Therefore, although measuring FSH may be useful in an infertility setting, it is a poor predictor of the timing of menopause (17,18). Longitudinal studies have shown that the increase in FSH occurs as early as the early 40s in normal women (42). Along with the elevation in FSH, there is a lesser, but still significant, rise in perimenstrual levels of luteinizing hormone (LH) (42). Because the age at which the rise in FSH first appears may not necessarily correlate with onset of perimenopause or menopause, monitoring of serum FSH or LH for menopause status has limited usefulness.

Gonadotropin receptor level changes have also been noted to occur during the perimenopause. A Finnish study (43) investigated FSH, LH, and 17β-estradiol levels in perimenopausal women before elective abdominal hysterectomy and salpingo-oophorectomy and measured ovarian FSH and LH receptor content. Higher serum gonadotropin levels were found in women with fewer gonadotropin receptors. Postmenopausal women had no detectable FSH or LH receptor levels. High serum gonadotropin levels in perimenopausal women suggest the presence of low or undetectable ovarian gonadotropin receptors. The authors proposed that measurement of gonadotropin receptors may be a useful indicator of ovarian status during the perimenopause.

No absolute predictors of ovarian function exist to date. The marked variations during a typical ovulatory cycle in excreted FSH and LH indicate that there is no simple measure of the effect of age on ovarian function. Thus, it is difficult to recognize early ovarian failure in the clinical setting (42).

Cycle Length Changes

As age increases, there is a significant decrease in length of the follicular phase. Although average follicular phase length in women aged 18 to 24 is 15 ± 2 days, the average in women 40 to 44 years is 10 ± 4 days (44). This follicular phase shortening appears to result from accelerated folliculogenesis during the perimenopause. This subsequently causes a 3-day decrease in the intermenstrual interval in most women (13). However, this change in length of the follicular phase is not necessarily continuous. Before the perimenopause, with increasing age there is a decrease in mean menstrual cycle length. During the perimenopause, mean cycle length becomes highly variable (45). Perimenopausal menstrual cycles are unpredictably irregular or "irregularly irregular," and there is no apparent orderly progression between the extremes of short and long cycles (45,46). The average follicular phase decrease by 3 to 4 days is clinically useful because it precedes obvious, clinically detectable endocrine changes (20). Patients with very frequent cycles or very heavy bleeding often present as a diagnostic and therapeutic challenge. For many such women, hormonal therapy with low-dose oral contraceptives may be useful.

Common Complaints Associated with the Perimenopause

Hot Flushes

The incidence of hot flushes is about 10% before the perimenopause. However, during the perimenopause, the incidence greatly increases, reaching a peak at menopause of about 50%. By about 4 years postmenopause, the incidence decreases to about 20% (3). A population-based study of subjective hot flush reporting in pre-, peri, and postmenopausal women revealed that 13% of premenopausal, 37% of perimenopausal, and 62% of postmenopausal women (as well as 15% of women on hormone replacement therapy) complained of at least one hot flush in the 2 weeks prior to the study. Although FSH levels were higher in the women with at least one hot flush per day, estradiol levels were higher in women with one or no hot flushes per week. These investigators concluded that hot flush frequency was associated with increasing FSH and decreasing estradiol levels (47).

Patients often present with a primary complaint of vasomotor symptoms. For these patients, hormonal replacement therapy may ameliorate their symptoms. Choice of hormone replacement therapy should be customized for each patient. Low-dose oral contraceptives in nonsmoking candidates or standard or low-dose estrogen replacement therapy (pill or patch) are potential choices.

Cardiovascular Changes

As a perimenopausal woman ages, her risk for cardiovascular disease increases. In fact, the leading cause of death for women in the United States, beginning at age 40, is cardiovascular disease. After age 50, women have the same rate of cardiovascular disease as 40-year-old men and eventually the same or higher rates as men in older age. After age 50, women have greater rates of hypertension than do men (31,32). The possible sequelae of these changes in weight and IGF-1 levels may have great clinical impact because they are predictive of cardiovascular disease (26,27). The perimenopause presents an opportunity for a woman to mitigate her risk factors for cardiovascular disease (weight control, diet, and exercise).

After menopause, the incidence of coronary heart disease increases, probably secondary to multiple mechanisms. Risk factors for cardiovascular disease include high cholesterol and other alterations in the lipid profile, abnormal glucose tolerance, hypertension, insulin resistance, smoking, and obesity. After the menopause, higher cholesterol, triglycerides, total/high-density lipoprotein cholesterol, insulin levels, and body weight are present (48–51).

Risk factors for cardiovascular disease can be affected by hormonal fluctuations. Estrogen may have cardioprotective effects independent of its effects on lipids, including improved pulsatility index, vasdilation, improved blood flow, and inhibition of atheromatous plaque formation (52–55).

Life-style changes can vastly ameliorate cardiovascular risk factors. These changes include exercise, weight loss, careful diet, blood-pressure monitoring, stress reduction, and cessation of smoking. The perimenopause presents an ideal time for modification of risk factors so that a woman will maximize not only her perimenopausal years but also her menopausal years.

Bone Mineral Density Changes

In the perimenopause, decreased ovarian function is associated with altered calcium metabolism and decreased trabecular bone mass (56). Peri- and postmenopausal women have significant bone loss in all skeletal sites, especially trabecular bone. Although premenopausal bone loss has been significantly associated with decreased concentrations of androgens, peri- and postmenopausal bone loss has been associated with lower levels of both androgens and estrogens. Sex steroids appear to play an important role in maintaining integrity of the skeleton throughout a woman's life (57).

Bone mass measurements, such as those used to predict postmenopausal fracture risk, may also be predictive of perimenopausal traumatic fractures. Perimenopausal fractures can be weakly but significantly predicted by bone mass quantification (especially of the lumbar spine) using dual-energy x-ray absorptiometry (DEXA) of the spine and hip. One study involving 1,000 perimenopausal women who had screening DEXA noted a 2% incidence of stress fractures in women in the 2 years before screening (58).

Although the use of urinary bone markers such as urine N-telopeptides is appealing because of its ease of use and noninvasiveness, further studies are necessary to establish the role of urinary bone markers in the clinical diagnosis of osteopenia and in care of the perimenopausal woman.

Prevention of bone loss should be encouraged early in all women. Weight-bearing exercise, calcium and vitamin D supplementation, and hormone replacement therapy should be discussed with all peri- and postmenopausal patients. If a patient has not already considered ways to reduce her risk for bone loss, the perimenopause can serve as an "alarm" so that she can take action to maximize her bone density.

HORMONE REPLACEMENT IN THE PERIMENOPAUSE

During the perimenopause, hormone replacement therapy (HRT) may reduce symptoms such as hot flushes and difficulty sleeping. One study of 32 perimenopausal women, ages 42 to 47 years, with irregular anovulatory cycles and symptoms associated with menopause, involved administration of a 6-month course of transdermal estradiol patches (0.05 mg/day for 21 days) and oral progestogens (10 mg/day for 10 days) (59). Menopausal symptoms were relieved during therapy; there were decreases in serum levels of FSH and LH and an increase in serum estradiol. FSH and LH concentrations were significantly lower than before HRT after 6 months of therapy.

If a patient complains of hot flushes, difficulty sleeping, or other complaints associated with the perimenopause, HRT is a viable option. Not only will it alleviate her symptoms such as hot flushes and thus immediately improve her quality of life, it will also reduce her risk factors for osteoporosis and cardiovascular disease, two major causes of morbidity and mortality in the older woman.

On the other hand, it is important to advise the patient that standard HRT regimens are not adequate for contraception. If a sexually active woman has less than 1 year of amenorrhea before beginning HRT, she is at a low but real risk for a possibly unwanted pregnancy. She should be advised and encouraged to consider using other forms of contraception such as barrier methods. Alternatively, very low-dose (20 µg) ethinyl estradiol-containing oral contraceptives are often appealing and well tolerated with an excellent safety profile in a nonsmoking older reproductive-aged woman. All low-dose oral contraceptives may be safely continued up to menopause.

When to switch a patient from oral contraceptives to hormone replacement therapy presents a clinical dilemma. At present, there does not exist a simple biochemical test that definitively predicts the onset of menopause. Without conclusive clinical data, it is our policy to prospectively establish a date at which oral contraceptive use will be stopped and HRT use begun. For most women, age 51— the average age at natural menopause—is a comfortable age at which to make this transition. This transition should be done in partnership with the perimenopausal patient and must take into account the fact that hormone replacement therapy is not an adequate contraceptive.

SUMMARY

The perimenopause is a poorly defined but real period in a woman's life when changes in her hormonal environment may be the cause of many clinical signs and symptoms. A woman may present with "irregularly irregular" menses, hot flushes, dysfunctional uterine bleeding, difficulty sleeping, mood changes, and osteoporosis/osteopenia. These and other complaints may result from periods of hyperestrogenemia, normal or hypoestrogenemia, decreased androgen levels, and decreased levels of GH and IGF-1 seen in the perimenopause. The treatment of the perimenopausal woman may present a clinical challenge secondary to the lack of a neatly organized transition period and to the variation that exists between women and within each woman. Therefore, it is important that we become familiar with the perimenopausal woman and her needs. The perimenopause presents an ideal time for reduction of risk factors that may affect quality of life, not just during the perimenopause but also for her postmenopausal years.

REFERENCES

1. Manton KG, Soldo BJ. Dynamics of health changes in the oldest old: New perspectives and evidence. *Milbank Q* 1985;63:206–285.
2. Brambilla D, McKinlay S, Johannes C. Defining the perimenopause for application in epidemiologic investigations. *Am J Epidemiol* 1994;140:1091.
3. McKinlay SM, Brambilla DJ, Posner JG. The normal menopause transition. *Am J Hum Biol* 1992;4:37.
4. Brambilla D, McKinlay S. A prospective study of factors affecting age at menopause. *J Clin Epidemiol* 1989;42:1031.
5. McKinlay S, Bifano N, McKinlay J. Smoking and age at menopause in women. *Ann Intern Med* 1985;103:350.
6. Cramer DW, Xu H, Harlow BL. Family history as a predictor of early menopause. *Fertil Steril* 1995;64:740.
7. Wallace R, Sherman, Bean J, et al. Probability of menopause with increasing duration of amenorrhea in middle-aged women. *Am J Obstet Gynecol* 1979;135:1021.
8. Metcalf MG, Donald RA, Livesey JH. Pituitary-ovarian function before, during and after menopause: A longitudinal study. *Clin Endocrinol* 1982;17:489.
9. Santoro N. Hormonal changes in the perimenopause. *Clin Consult Obstet Gynecol* 1996;8:2.
10. Fraser IS, Baird DT. Blood production and ovarian secretion rates of estradiol 17-beta and estrone in women with dysfunctional uterine bleeding. *J Clin Endocrinol Metab* 1974;39:564.
11. Van Look P, Lothian H, Hunter WM, et al. Hypothalamic-pituitary ovarian function in perimenopausal women. *Clin Endocrinol* 1977;7:13–31.
12. McKinlay SM. The normal menopause transition: An overview. *Maturitas* 1996;23:137.
13. Santoro N, Brown JR, Adel T, et al. Characterization of reproductive hormonal dynamics in the perimenopause. *J Clin Endocrinol Metab* 1996;81:1495.
14. Sherman BM, West JH, Korenman SG. The menopausal transition: Analysis of LH, FSH, estradiol and progesterone concentrations during menstrual cycles of older women. *J Clin Endocrinol Metab* 1976;42:629.
15. Reyes FI, Winters JS, Faiman C. Pituitary–ovarian relationship preceding the menopause: A cross-sectional study of serum FSH, LH, prolactin, estradiol and progesterone levels. *Am J Obstet Gynecol* 1977;129:557.
16. Shideler S, DeVane G, Kaira P, et al. Ovarian–pituitary hormone interactions during the perimenopause. *Maturitas* 1989;11:331.
17. Longcope C, Baker S. Androgen and estrogen dynamics: Relationships with age, weight and menopausal status. *J Clin Endocrinol Metab* 1993;76:601.
18. Longcope C, Franz C, Morello C, et al. Steroid and gonadotropin levels in women during the perimenopausal years. *Maturitas* 1986;8:189.
19. Speroff L, Glass R, Kase N, eds. *Clinical gynecologic endocrinology and infertility, 5th ed.* Baltimore: Williams & Wilkins, 1994.
20. Lenton EA, Landgren B, Sexton L, et al. Normal variation in the length of the follicular phase of the menstrual cycle: Effect of chronological age. *Br J Obstet Gynecol* 1984;91:681.
21. Sherman BM, Korenman SG. Hormonal characteristics of the human menstrual cycle throughout reproductive life. *J Clin Invest* 1975;55:669.
22. Lenton EA, Sexton L, Lee S, et al. Progressive changes in LH and FSH and LH: FSH ratios in women throughout reproductive life. *Maturitas* 1988;100:35.
23. Ho KY, Evans WS, Blizzard RM, et al. Effects of sex and age on the 24 hour profile of growth hormone secretion in man: Importance of endogenous estradiol concentration. *J Clin Endocrinol Metab* 1987;64:51.
24. Wilshire G, Loughlin J, Brown J, et al. Diminished function of the somatotropic axis in older reproductive—aged women. *J Clin Endocrinol Metab* 1995;80:608.
25. Wind RR, Matthews KA, Kuller LH, et al. Environmental and familial contributions to insulin levels in middle-aged women. *JAMA* 1992;268:1890.
26. Wing RR, Matthew KA, Kuller LH, et al. Weight gain at the time of menopause. *Arch Intern Med* 1991;151:97.
27. Wing RR, Kuller LH, Bunker C, et al. Obesity, obesity-related behaviors and coronary heart disease risk factors in black and white premenopausal women. *Int J Obesity* 1994;13:511.
28. Proudler AJ, Felton CV, Stevenson JC. Aging and the response of plasma insulin, glucose and C-peptide concentrations to intravenous glucose in psotmenopausal women. *Clin J Sci* 1992;83:489.
29. Buster JE, Casson PR, Straughn AB, et al. Postmenopausal steroid replacement with micronized dehydroepiandrosterone: Preliminary oral bioavailability and dose proportionality studies. *Am J Obstet Gynecol* 1992;166:1163.
30. Wenger NK. Coronary disease in women. *Annu Rev Med* 1994;62:20.
31. Castelli WP. Menopause and cardiovascular disease. In: Eskin BA, ed. *The menopause—comprehensive management,* ed. New York: McGraw-Hill, 1994:117–136.
32. Kannel WB. Metabolic risk factors for coronary heart disease in women: Perspective from the Framingham Study. *Am Heart J* 1987;114:413–419.
33. Longcope C. Adrenal and gonadal steroid secretion in normal females. *J Clin Endocrinol Metab* 1986;15:213.
34. Adashi EY. The climacteric ovary as a functional gonadotropin-driven androgen-producing gland. *Fertil Steril* 1994;62:20.
35. Zumoff B, Strain GW, Miller LK, et al. 24-hour mean plasma testosterone concentration declines with age in normal premenopausal women. *J Clin Endocrinol Metab* 1995;80:1429.
36. Judd LH, Yen S. Serum androstenedione and testosterone levels during the menstrual cycle. *J Clin Endocrinol Metab* 1973;36:475.
37. Mushayandebvu T, Castracane D, Santoro N, et al. Evidence for diminished mid-cycle ovarian androgen production in older reproductive aged women. *Fertil Steril* 1996;65:721.
38. Adams DB, Gold AR, Burt AD. Rise in female-initiated sexual activity at ovulation and its suppression by oral contraceptives. *N Engl J Med* 1978;299:1145.
39. Orentrelch N, Brind JL, Rizer RL, et al. Age changes and sex difference in serum dehydroepiandrosterone sulfate concentrations throughout adulthood. *J Clin Endocrinol Metab* 1984;59:551.
40. Parker LN, Odell WD. Decline of adrenal androgen production measured by radioimmunoassay of urinary unconjugated dehydroepiandrosterone. *J Clin Endocrinol Metab* 1978;47:600.
41. Buckler HM, Evans CA, Mantora H, et al. Gonadotropin, steroid and inhibin levels in women with incipient ovarian failure during anovulatory and ovulatory rebound cycles. *J Clin Endocrinol Metab* 1991;72:116.
42. Metcalf MG, Livesey JH. Gonadotropin excretin in fertile women: Effect of age and the nset of the menopausal transition. *J Endocrinol* 1985;105:357.
43. Vihko KK, Kujansuu E, Morsky P, et al. Gonadotropins and gonadotropin receptors during the perimenopause. *Eur J Endocrinol* 1996;134:357.
44. Lenton EA, Landgren BM, Sexton L. Normal variation in the length of the luteal phase of the menstrual cycle: Identification of the short luteal phase. *Br J Endocrinol Metab* 1984;91:685.
45. Treloar A, Bounton A, Benn R, et al. Variation of the human menstrual cycle through reproductive life. *Int J Fertil* 1967;12:77.
46. Metcalf MG. The approach of menopause: A New Zealand study. *NZ Med J* 1988;101:103.
47. Guthrie JR, Dennerstein L, Hopper JL, et al. Hot flushes, menstrual status and hormone levels in a population-based sample of midlife women. *Obstet Gynecol* 1996;88:437.
48. Wing RR, Matthews KA, Kuller LH, et al. Weight gain at the time of menopause. *Arch Intern Med* 1991;151:97.
49. Wing RR, Kuller LH, Bunker C, et al. Obesity, obesity-related behaviors and coronary heart disease risk factors in black and white premenopausal women. *Int J Obesity* 1994;13:511.
50. Razay G, Heaton KW, Bolton CH. Coronary heart disease risk factors in relation to the menopause. *NZ J Med* 1992;85:889.
51. Matthews K, Meilahn E, Kuller LH, et al. Menopause and risk factors for coronary heart disease. *N Engl J Med* 1989;321:641.
52. Steinleitner A, Stanczyk FZ, Levin JN. Decreased *in vitro* production of 6 keto-prostaglandin F₁ by uterine arteries from postmenopausal women. *Am J Obstet Gynecol* 1989;161:1677.
53. Wren BG. Hypertension and thrombosis with postmenopausal estrogen therapy.

In: Studd JWW, Whitehead MI, eds. *The menopause.* Oxford: Blackwell Scientific, 1989:181–189.

54. Hussman F. Long-term metabolic effects of estrogen therapy. In: Greenblatt RB, Heithecker R, eds. *A modern approach to the perimenopausal years: new developments in bioscience.* New York: W de Gruyter, 1986:163–175.

55. Adams MR, Clarkson TB, Koritnik DR, et al. Contraceptive steroids and coronary artery atherosclerosis in cynomolgus macaques. *Fertil Steril* 1987;144:41.

56. Garton M, Martin J, New S, et al. Bone mass and metabolism in women aaged 45–55. *Clin Endocrinol* 1996;44:536.

57. Slemenda C, Longcope C, Peacock M, et al. Sex steroids, body mass, and bone loss. A prospective study of pre, peri and postmenopausal women. *J Clin Invest* 1996;97:14.

58. Stewart A, Torgeson DJ, Reid DM. Prediction of fractures in perimenopausal women: A comparison of DEXA and broadband ultrasound attenuation. *Ann Rheum Dis* 1996;55:140.

59. DeLeo V, Lanzetta D, D'Antona D, et al. Transdermal estrogen replacement therapy in normal perimenopausal women: Effects on pituitary ovarian function. *Contraception* 1996;10:49.

60. Seifer DB, Gardiner AC, Lambert-Messserlian G, et al. Differential secretion of dimeric inhibin in cultured luteinized granulosa cells as a function of ovarian reserve. *J Clin Endocrinol Metab* 1996;81(2):736–739.

61. Seifer DB, Lambert-Messerlian G, Hogan JW, et al. Day 3 serum inhibin B is predictive of assisted reproductive technologies outcome. *Fertil Steril* 1997;67(1):110–114.

62. Labrie FF, Belanger A, Cusan L, et al. Marked decline in serum concentrations of adrenal C_{19} sex steroid precursors and conjugated androgen metabolites during aging. *J Clin Endocrinol Metab* 1997;82(8):2396–2402.

63. Barrett-Connor E, Goodman-Gruen D. DHEAS does not predict cardiovascular death in postmenopausal women. The Rancho Bernardo Study. *Circulation* 1995;91(6):1757–1760.

64. Barrett-Connor E, Goodman-Gruen D. The epidemiology of DHEAS and cardiovascular disease. *Ann NY Acad Sci* 1995;774:259–270.

Treatment of the Postmenopausal Woman: Basic and Clinical Aspects, Second Edition, edited by Rogerio A. Lobo, Lippincott Williams & Wilkins, Philadelphia © 1999.

CHAPTER 10

Use of Contraceptives for Older Women

David Archer

Contraception for women over the age of 35 has been contentious because of the reported increase in cardiovascular disease in women who smoke cigarettes and use oral contraceptives.

Despite a reduction in fecundity, sexually active women who are perimenopausal require contraception. Older women can utilize a variety of contraceptive options based on their life style and individual preferences. The final decision on which contraceptive method to recommend should be based on a knowledge of the patient's history and physical findings, current frequency of coital activity, and prior contraceptive experiences. The information obtained by the physician or health care provider concerning these three parameters will allow for a frank discussion of the risks and benefits of the contraceptive options available and open a dialogue with the patient in order to reach a decision on the best method for her use. Currently available contraceptive options are listed in Table 10.1.

This review discusses each of these methods with the intent that they be used for healthy women over the age of 35 years. Healthy women are those individuals who have no known risk factor for cardiovascular disease and are not taking any chronic medication other than thyroid replacement therapy on a regular basis. Use of other chronic medications for concurrent medical problems requires evaluation and knowledge of the interaction between the medication and oral or implantable steroidal contraceptives. The risk factors for cardiovascular disease are listed in Table 10.2.

ORAL CONTRACEPTIVES

Combination oral contraceptives (COCs) are one of the best options because of their ease of administration and known benefits for reduction in the incidence of functional ovarian cysts, pelvic inflammatory disease, ovarian cancer, and endometrial cancer. The reluctance to use them in older women has in part been because of the perception that they increase the risk of cardiovascular events in older women. As described below, this is not the case, making COCs a first choice for these women.

The COCs have been available since 1960. They consist of an orally active estrogen, generally ethinyl estradiol, and a synthetic progestin. All of the formulations on the United States market have undergone clinical trials that have shown them to be safe and effective in preventing pregnancy. There has been a steady reduction in the amount of estrogen and progestin in COCs since their introduction. This has been driven by the concern that some of the adverse side effects are related to the dose of the estrogen and by the pervasive philosophy of using the

TABLE 10.1. *Available contraceptive options for older women*

Combination oral contraceptives
Progestin-only methods
   Subcutaneous levonorgestrel implants
   Depo-medroxyprogesterone acetate
   Oral miniprogestin pills
Intrauterine devices
   Copper-containing
   Progesterone-releasing
Barrier devices
   Condoms: male and female
   Spermicides
   Diaphragms
   Cervical caps
Symptothermal or rhythm methods

D. Archer: Department of Obstetrics and Gynecology, Eastern Virginia Medical School, Norfolk, Virginia 23507.

TABLE 10.2. *Risk factors for cardiovascular disease*

Hypertension
Smoking cigarettes
Diabetes mellitus
Pregnancy induced hypertension
Dyslipidemias
Family history of early age onset of cardiovascular disease
Obesity
Androgen excess states

TABLE 10.3. *Combination oral contraceptives containing 20 mg of ethinyl estradiol*

Name	Progestin	Progestin concentration (mg)
Loestrin	Norethindrone acetate	1.000
Mircette	Desogestrel	0.150
Alesse	Levonorgestrel	0.100

least amount of a medication that can be proven to be effective.

At the present time there are three COC formulations on the United States market that contain 20 μg of ethinyl estradiol (see Table 10.3). All of these formulations have pregnancy rates (Pearl indices) of less than one pregnancy per 100 women per year.

Associated with the reduction in the estrogen dose has been the development of new progestational compounds. The first progestins marketed in the United States were 19-norsteroids derived from testosterone. Although ethyndiol diacetate was first marketed, it is converted to norethindrone, the biologically active form (1). Norethindrone has been further modified to create what are called gonane progestins. Norgestrel or its active isomer levonorgestrel is the principal compound.

The last 15 years have seen further modification in the steroidal configuration of levonorgestrel to yield three progestins known as norgestimate, desogestrel, and gestodene.

EFFICACY

Oral contraceptives are designed to prevent pregnancy. The measure used for assessment of efficacy is the occurrence of pregnancy in a group using the Pearl index. The Pearl index is the number of pregnancies that occur in a known number of women during 1 year of use of a contraceptive agent, divided by 100 (79). For example, one pregnancy in 100 women using COCs for 1 year is a Pearl index of 1.0. All COCs on the U.S. market have a Pearl index of ≤1.25. The contraceptive effectiveness of COCs can also be calculated with life table analysis (79).

Women over the age of 35 have been found to have a reduction in their fecundity (2). It is obvious that this reduction does not reach zero, and these women are still at

risk for pregnancy. In fact, unintended pregnancies are a major problem in older women, where the use of therapeutic abortion is as high as that found in teen-age women.

BENEFITS OF ORAL CONTRACEPTIVES IN WOMEN OVER 35 YEARS OF AGE

1. Contraception. The principal benefit of COCs is their ability to allow a couple to determine when they want a pregnancy. The utilization of oral contraceptives has been limited in older women because of the concern of cardiovascular events (see below). Current evidence indicates that for women with no cardiovascular risk, COCs are a highly effective and safe method. A low-dose estrogen-containing (35, 30, or 20 μg) COC should be the principal form used. Contraception is accomplished in several ways. The principal mechanism is the inhibition of ovulation; second is alteration in the receptivity of the cervical mucus for sperm penetration, and third is a change in the endometrium that may alter or inhibit implantation (3–6).

2. Reduced incidence of ectopic pregnancy. Associated with the reduction in the occurrence of pregnancy is a concomitant reduction in ectopic pregnancy (7). This is obvious because inhibition of ovulation is one of the major mechanisms of action of COCs. Thus, the reduction in intrauterine pregnancies should be mirrored with a similar decline in ectopic pregnancies. The COCs have been shown to reduce the incidence of functional ovarian cysts (3,8,9). In fact, COCs are indicated for the treatment of functional ovarian cysts, although it may require one to two cycles before the ovarian cyst regresses.

3. Pelvic inflammatory disease. Use of COCs has been reported to decrease the incidence of pelvic inflammatory disease (PID). The occurrence and incidence of cervical colonization with *N. gonorrheae* and *C. trachomatis* is not reduced, but the findings of clinical PID have been found to be decreased in women using COCs (8).

4. Endometrial and ovarian neoplasia. The COCs have been found to reduce the incidence of endometrial cancer by at least 40% (80–83). This protective effect is apparent after 1 year of use, and the incidence remains reduced for 15 years, which is the length of the follow-up studies reported to date. The mechanism of action is thought to be progestin altering the endometrium. In support of this hypothesis is the finding of an enhanced reduction of adenocarcinoma incidence in women who have used a low dose estrogen with a potent progestin. The COCs reduce the incidence of ovarian neoplasia by 40% (8,84). The duration of this effect is also 15 years following 1 year or more of use of COCs. Recent data indicate that reduction in the incidence of ovarian cancer is

also applicable to women who have a strong history of inheritable breast and ovarian cancer (87). These women often have *BrCa1* or *BrCa2* present on genotyping. The inhibition of ovulation is felt to be the principal mechanism whereby ovarian neoplasia is interdicted by COCs.

5. Irregular or excessive uterine bleeding. The COCs have been used for the treatment of irregular or heavy uterine bleeding associated with anovulation, uterine fibroids, and women presenting with dysfunctional uterine bleeding (90). Clinical evidence of the COCs efficacy for each of these clinical conditions is sparse. They have been shown to reduce the amount of bleeding in normal women, but no published data are available for women with menorrhagia.

6. Bone mineral density. The COCs have been reported to enhance bone mineral density in older women (10–12). This attribute would make them a logical choice for perimenopausal women, who would need to have a bone bank of increased bone mineral density before menopause.

ADVERSE EVENTS ASSOCIATED WITH ORAL CONTRACEPTIVES

Myocardial Infarction

Myocardial infarction has been reported to be increased in women over the age of 35 who use COCs and who smoke (13,14). Recent epidemiologic studies have indicated that in healthy women who do not smoke, there is no increased risk of myocardial infarction (14–16). The Transnational Study at one time felt that desogestrel containing COCs would actually reduce the incidence of myocardial infarction in women compared to other progestins (17,18). In women over the age of 35 who do not have any cardiovascular risk, COCs are indicated as an effective means of contraception (see Table 10.2). I recommend that the 20-µg preparations be used if a woman is started on COCs at this age.

Cerebral Vascular Disease

Cerebral vascular disease, or stroke, has been implicated as being increased in women who use COCs (19). This increase in the incidence has been linked to the dose of estrogen, with a reduction in the incidence of stroke associated with a decrease in estrogen dose. The overall incidence of stroke is rare in women under the age of 45 (20,21). A significant increase in stroke is associated with advancing age. Smoking is a risk factor for stroke in both pre- and postmenopausal women. Recent data have found an increased incidence of both thrombotic and hemorrhagic stroke in women who smoke (21). In women without risk factors, the current or past use of COCs was not associated with an increase in the incidence of either thrombotic or hemorrhagic stroke (19,21). Women under treatment for diabetes mellitus or hypertension were found to have a significant increase in the relative risk for stroke (21). These data indicate that other disease states contribute significantly to the cause of stroke in women and not the hormones in COCs.

Venous Thromboembolism

Use of COCs has been linked with the occurrence of deep vein thrombosis (DVT) and pulmonary embolism (PE) (22,23). The occurrence of DVT has been linked to the dosage of ethinyl estradiol (EE$_2$) in the COCs. Reductions in the ethinyl estradiol dose from over 50 µg to the current formulations containing 20 to 35 µg have reduced the incidence and relative risk from venous thromboembolism (VTE). The reports from three recent studies indicate that the relative risk for DVT is approximately 2.0 for COCs with less than 35 µg of ethinyl estradiol (22–24). These results translate into an actual incidence of two to four cases of DVT per 10,000 women at risk per year. Controversy has arisen from these papers in regard to an increased incidence of VTE in women using third-generation COCs such as norgestimate, desogestrel and gestodene. Compared to second-generation COCs such as levonorgestrel, the epidemiologic studies have found a relative risk of 1.5 or 2.0 for VTE in young women using third-generation COCs compared to second-generation COCs (levonorgestrel). Recent publications have discussed the potential biases in each of these studies in order to explain the increased relative risk with the newer progestational COCs (23,25–27). One of the biases identified is the healthy user effect (28,29). Physicians will not or do not change COC formulations in women without problems. A second bias is the attrition of susceptibles. This hypothesis states that there is a pool of women who are more likely to develop VTE when placed on COCs. This group of women could develop a DVT and/or PE after having a VTE diagnosed. The patient who develops a DVT on COCs is no longer a candidate for COCs.

New starters on COCs can include a pool of susceptible women within the larger cohort of women who are not susceptible to VTE. Therefore, use of newer formulations of COCs can have a larger at-risk group of women than the older formulations because of their inclusion as new starters. These findings could result in the apparent increased incidence of DVT in current users of desogestrel- or gestodene-containing products.

These points have been extensively debated in the literature. At present, the most important point that has been made is that there is no biologic plausibility for the results of an increase in VTE incidence in women on third-generation progestational agents. Estrogens have always been implicated in the etiology of VTE. The low-dose 20 μg ethinyl estradiol products available should have an even lowered incidence of VTE.

Weight Gain

One of the principal reasons for discontinuation of COCs is real or perceived weight gain. Clinical trials that are performed for the introduction or licensing of COCs have failed to show any significant weight gain in participants during the clinical trial (30,31). Despite this, there remains a strong feeling that COCs will cause weight gain. The most common reasons for weight gain are lack of exercise and overeating. Counseling is required for weight gain, but its effectiveness in modifying behavior is limited.

Headaches

Headache is a ubiquitous symptom and is reported in about 10% of women participating in clinical trials of COCs (32). This figure always seems high, but this is because of the lack of an appropriate control group. Menstrual-related headaches are those that are associated with the onset of menstruation and are cyclic and repetitive in nature. The management of these headaches can be a problem. Recently, the extended use of COCs for 42 days or longer in a continuous fashion has been described (33). This may be used for the management of menstrual migraines, but the physician should be aware that continuous use of COCs could result in the onset of breakthrough bleeding in these women. When breakthrough bleeding occurs, the COCs should be stopped for 3 to 5 days. After this, you can reinitiate the COCs in a continuous fashion.

A second option is to use a transdermal delivery system of estradiol-17β (E_2) as a bridge during the placebo or pill free days of the COC cycle. This will theoretically prevent the fall in serum E_2 levels, which are thought to be the stimulus for the headache. The recent introduction of COCs with a reduced pill free interval (Mircette, *Organon, Inc,West Orange, NJ*) may be useful in this instance, but there are no data indicating efficacy for menstrual migraine.

Migraine headache is also associated with the withdrawal of the estrogen in the COC preparation. The migraine literature indicates that there is an increased incidence of migraine headache in COC users. The COC literature is sparse in this regard, but a recent review indicates that migraine headache sufferers do not have an increased incidence of occurrence of headaches while using COCs (34). A trial of COCs is indicated in women with a history of migraine headaches. This can be viewed as a therapeutic trial. In women with no increase in frequency or intensity of their migraine headaches, continued use of COCs is indicated. The use of progestin only contraceptives, either oral, injection, or implantation, may be indicated in women who continue to have frequent or severe migraine headaches.

INTRAUTERINE DEVICES

Intrauterine devices offer a significant alternative for older women. They are a highly effective means of contraception and have few systemic side effects. Intrauterine devices (IUDs) have been linked to an increased incidence of pelvic inflammatory disease (PID) (35–37). Early articles from the Centers for Disease Control implied that there was an increased risk of PID in users of IUDs (35). A more recent review of the CDC data does not support an increase in the incidence of PID in monogamous couples (91). The increased incidence is found in divorced or unmarried women and is strongly linked to the number of sexual partners. A large multicenter, multinational trial reported by the World Health Organization also indicated that there is no increase in the incidence of PID in women using IUDs. There is evidence for an increase in what appears to be PID in the first 3 to 4 weeks following insertion of the IUD (38). These data have led to published reports indicating that prophylactic antibiotics could or should be used at the time of insertion of the IUDs. There is no consensus on the use of antibiotics at the time of IUD insertion. At the present time in the United States there is no compelling evidence that concurrent antibiotics with insertion of the IUD prevent the occurrence of infection immediately following the insertion of the IUDs.

Intrauterine devices do not have a systemic contraceptive action. They appear to exert their effects locally, either by altering gamete function or changing the endometrial receptivity. The bulk of the data support an effect on gametes with either no or few sperm cells detected in the fallopian tubes of women using IUDs (39,40). This finding is also reflected in the lack of fertilized oocytes or embryos present in the fallopian tubes of women using an IUD.

At one time it was hypothesized that one of the mechanisms of action of the IUD was to inhibit implantation or to be an abortifacient. There is no evidence that there is any abortifacient activity associated with IUDs. Published reports have failed to find any evidence for an increased occurrence of early clinical miscarriages or evidence of human chorionic gonadotropin (hCG) in serum or urine as an indicator of pregnancy (39).

Recently we have shown that the administration of pentoxifylline (Trental, *Hoescht-Roussel, Somerville, NJ*) to rats bearing an IUD can reverse the contraceptive effect of the IUDs (41). We believe that this effect results from the action of pentoxifylline on altering the function of the endometrial leukocytes that are present in the intrauterine lumen and the endometrial stroma of women and animals bearing an IUD. Our current hypothesis is that intrauterine cytokines are involved as part of the mechanism of IUD action.

There are two different IUDs on the United States market—the copper-containing IUD known as Paraguard (*Ortho Pharmaceutical, Raritan, NJ*) and the medicated device containing progesterone, Progestasert (*ALZA Corporation, Palo Alto, CA*).

Copper-Containing IUDs

The Cu IUD is a highly effective contraceptive with a Pearl index between 1.0 and 2.5 pregnancies per 100 women per year of use. The variability of the Pearl index is related to the population under investigation. The mechanism of action of the Cu IUDs is both a foreign body reaction of the IUD frame (silicone) and the release of elemental copper, which is a known spermicide. The load or amount of copper on the devices has been variable, but the Paraguard has 380 mm^2 of surface area of copper wound on the arms and the stem of the IUD. This system has an effective duration of action of 10 years (42–45).

Side effects are uterine cramping and, in some instances, expulsion of the device. A second side effect is an increase in the amount and duration of menstrual flow. Nonsteroidal antiinflammatory agents have been shown to be effective in decreasing the amount of bleeding associated with IUDs (46). The studied doses are ibuprofen, 800 mg three times a day, and naproxen, 500 mg three to four times a day.

Progesterone-Releasing IUDs

The release of progesterone from the stem of this IUD is designed to enhance its contraceptive efficacy and to reduce expulsion. Progesterone changes the endometrial histology to one of progestational dominance, and this could be part of the mechanism of contraceptive action.

Clinical trials have found that there is a decrease in the amount of menstrual blood loss in women using a Progestasert system (46). Menstrual cramps are also decreased with this system.

The major drawback to the Progestasert is the short duration of efficacy. The Progestasert is approved for only 1 year of contraceptive use in the United States, and then it must be replaced. This results in the necessity of removal and reinsertion, which is uncomfortable and expensive for the consumer. Despite this drawback, there is little systemic effect of the released progesterone. The reduction in amount of menstrual bleeding by the Progestasert has a definite place in the management of older women who are experiencing an increase in menstrual flow.

INJECTABLE CONTRACEPTION

Injectable preparations of a progestin have been available for 30 years. The prototype is Depo-Provera, a crystalline suspension of medroxyprogesterone acetate.

A long-acting form of norethindrone enanthate (Noristerate, *Schering, Kenilworth, NJ*) is marketed outside the United States. Noristerate is administered on an every-2-month basis. Depo medroxyprogesterone acetate (DMPA) is administered at 11- to 12-week intervals. The advantage of DMPA is the fact that it contains only a progestational steroid and has no estrogen component. The contraceptive efficacy is high, on the order of less than 1.0 pregnancy per 100 women per year of use (Pearl index) (47). The advantages for older women are the lack of estrogenic side effects. Progestin-only methods may be used in women at risk for cardiovascular problems. Women who have liver dysfunction may be candidates for DMPA, but this decision should be individualized. Limited data suggest that progestin-only contraception should or could be used in women with migraine headaches. Conclusive medical evidence in this regard is lacking.

One significant drawback is the pharmacokinetic profile of DMPA. In some women, medroxyprogesterone acetate has been found to remain in the circulation for over 18 months (46). This extended duration of action has resulted in a delay in the return of ovulation and, of course, fertility. This potential problem should be discussed with women who may want to become pregnant in the future. The overall return of fertility (fecundity) is comparable to that of women stopping other forms of reversible contraception based on the cumulative pregnancy rate. There is a delay of 3 to 6 months in pregnancy rate immediately following DMPA use, but by the end of 24 months, pregnancy rates are comparable between women who used DMPA and users of other forms of reversible contraceptives.

The disadvantages for older women are the increased risk of irregular bleeding that occurs in the first year of use and the report of a decrease in bone mineral density.

Irregular bleeding is common in all progestin-only methods of contraception. The cause of the irregular bleeding is unknown. The pattern of bleeding is irregular spotting and staining without premenstrual or prodromal symptoms (89). The bleeding usually consists mainly of spotting; rarely is there an associated anemia. This irregular bleeding does not imply that there is endometrial pathology. Endometrial biopsies have demonstrated only an atrophic or progestationally suppressed endometrium. Treatment usually consists of simple reassurance and observation. In some cases, where there is concern, the use of an oral estrogen has been reported. There appears to be some efficacy in the use of ethinyl estradiol or estrone sulfate to stop the bleeding/spotting, but the improvement is minimal (48). By the end of the first year of use of DMPA, over 50% of women are not bleeding (49).

A decrease in bone mineral density (BMD) in women using DMPA has been reported (50). Peripheral serum estradiol levels were lower than those found in the early follicular phase. This study was small in terms of numbers and requires a further follow-up.

Extensive follow-up of users of DMPA has been performed by the World Health Organization (WHO) because of concerns over potential breast cancer. The report of a multinational, multicenter trial has shown only an increase in breast cancer in the first 3 months of use, and there is no increase in breast cancer with long-term (over 10 years) use of DMPA (51). There appears to be a significant reduction in the incidence of endometrial cancer in DMPA users (52). This latter fact may enhance the utility of DMPA for older women.

There is always the concern for changes in mood in older women using medroxyprogesterone acetate orally. These statements are for the most part anecdotal. The same effect on mood or depression has been sought in younger women using DMPA. No significant changes in depression scores were found in a prospective study of DMPA users (53,54).

Overall, DMPA is a reasonable alternative for contraception in older women. It has the advantage of limited motivation for the consumer. The need to return for repeat injections on a regular basis may be a significant issue for some individuals. This could result in making this a less desirable alternative for contraception in women over the age of 35 years.

IMPLANTABLE CONTRACEPTIVES

At the present time on the United States market, there is only one implantable subdermal contraceptive device. This product contains levonorgestrel (Norplant, *Wyeth-Ayerst, Philadelphia, PA*). Norplant is a six-capsule system with each capsule containing 30 mg of levonorgestrel. Norplant was developed by the Population Council beginning in 1968 to 1970. Several different progestational agents were evaluated for efficacy at that time.

Clinical trials have indicated that levonorgestrel implants have a very low contraceptive failure rate, with a Pearl index less than 0.5 pregnancies per 100 women per year (55). Levonorgestrel implants could be used in older women because they contain no estrogen, as mentioned above for DMPA. The advantages of the Norplant contraceptive devices are the fact that the consumer requires little motivation after the insertion, and the contraceptive efficacy lasts up to 5 years.

As with all progestin-only contraceptives, the side-effect profile includes irregular uterine bleeding (56). This is principally light bleeding and spotting and is similar to that described for DMPA. Thirty percent of women will experience irregular bleeding and spotting within the first 3 months after the insertion of Norplant (56,57). With continued use of Norplant, there is an increasing occurrence of no menstrual bleeding at all.

The other side effects that have been associated with the levonorgestrel system include weight gain, depression, acne, and loss of scalp hair (58–61). In terms of the latter effect, no one has reported alopecia, although a heavy loss of hair has been anecdotally reported.

The principal contraindications to Norplant utilization are active liver disease and undiagnosed uterine bleeding. Both of these conditions should be evaluated before Norplant insertion along with any other laboratory evaluation that is indicated. Overall, the Norplant system has a very positive safety profile. It has not been linked to any risk of cardiovascular disease (60,61). There is no evidence of an increased risk of venous thromboembolism with progestin-only contraceptive methods.

BARRIER CONTRACEPTIVES

There are a variety of barrier-type contraceptives available on the United States market. Physical barriers include the diaphragm, cervical cap, and male and female condoms. Listed under barriers, although not truly a physical barrier, are spermicides, usually containing nonoxynol-9, which are available in a variety of forms, including films, suppositories, and tablets.

In general, barrier contraceptives have been associated with a higher pregnancy rate than hormonal contraceptive methods. The use effectiveness rates range from 7 to 15 pregnancies per 100 women per year with a variety of barrier contraceptives (79,85). With highly motivated couples who consistently use barrier contraceptives in a reliable fashion, pregnancy rates as low as four to five pregnancies per 100 women per year have been reported. Overall, barriers offer an advantage to older women from several standpoints.

They are coitally related, and from this standpoint they require use only at the time of intercourse. In a couple with declining frequency of coital activity, this may be something that is attractive to them. Second, they do not involve hormonal medication, an intrauterine device, or an implant. From this standpoint, they are totally consumer controlled and consumer driven. Appropriate use of the barrier contraceptive is dependent on the motivation of the consumer and her partner.

Barrier contraceptives depend on the utilization of an associated spermicide to enhance their efficacy. This is true for the diaphragm, the cervical cap, and, in some instances, male and female condoms. Male and female condoms have been impregnated with nonoxynol-9 as an additional means of reducing pregnancy rates.

The spermicidal product nonoxynol-9 (N-9) is a surface-active detergent that has been shown to lyse cell membranes, resulting in sperm immobilization and/or death (86). The concentrations of N-9 in spermicide vary among preparations. Marketed preparations and their spermicidal content and concentration are shown in Table 10.4.

Barrier contraceptives, in order to be effective, should be inserted before penile penetration of the vagina. In general, for spermicides, an interval of 5 to 15 minutes

TABLE 10.4. *Firms manufacturing and/or distributing contraceptives worldwide, 1993 and 1994*

Company	Product manufactured or distributed
Aladan	Condoms
Alza	IUDs (Progestasert)
Ansell	Condoms (including one with nonoxynol-9)
Berlex	Oral contraceptives (Tri-Levlen, Levlen)
Boehringer Ingelheim	Oral contraceptives
Bristol-Myers Squibb	Oral contraceptives
Carter-Wallace	Condoms (including one spermicidally lubricated)
CCC (Canada)*	IUDs
Cervical Cap Ltd.	Cervical cap (Prentif/manufactured by Lamberts/Dalston England)
Chartex (UK)	Female condom (Femidom)
Cilar (UK)*	Oral contraceptives
Dongkuk Trading (Korea)*	Condoms
Finishing Enterprises*	IUD
Gedeon Richter (Hungary)	Emergency postcoital contraceptive (Postinor)
Gruenenthal	Oral contraceptives
Gyno Pharma[a]	IUD [CuT380A (Paragard)] (distributor)
	Oral contraceptive (Norcept)
	Diaphragms (distributor for Schmid)
Hyosung (Korea)*	Condoms
Jenapharm (Germany)	Oral contraceptives
Kinsho Mataichi (Japan)*	Spermicides
Leiras Oy Pharmaceuticals	Progestin-releasing IUD (Mirena)
	Norplant (manufacture)
Lexis	Oral contraceptives (NEE)
London Rubber	Condoms
	Diaphragms
Magnafarma	Oral contraceptives
Mayer	Condoms
Mead Johnson	Oral contraceptives (Ovcon)
Medimpex* (Hungary and United States)	Oral contraceptives/raw materials
Menarini	Oral contraceptives
Milex Products Inc.	Diaphragms (Omniflex, Wide-seal)
	Jellies and creams (Shur Seal Jel has nonoxynol-9)
National Sanitary	Condoms
Okamoto, USA	Condoms
Organon	Oral contraceptives (Marvelon, Desogen, Jenest)
Akzo (Netherlands)*	IUD (Multiload) (manufacturing subsidiary, Bangladesh)
Ortho Pharmaceutical*	Oral contraceptives (Loestrin; Ortho-Cept, Ortho-Cyclen, Other Tri-Cyclen, Ortho-Novum, Modicon)
	Diaphragms (Allflex, Ortho Diaphragm)
	Spermicides* (Gynol—octoxynol)
	IUDs
Parke-Davis (Warner-Lambert)	Oral contraceptives
Polifarma	Oral contraceptives
Reddy Health Care	Condoms
RFSU of Sweden	Condoms
Roberts	Oral contraceptives
Rugby Labs	Oral contraceptives (Genora)
Safetex	Condoms
Schering AG (Germany)*	Oral contraceptives*
	Injectables*
Schering Plough (United States)	Spermicides
Schmid	Condoms (including spermicidal condoms)
	Spermicides
	Diaphragms (distributed by GynoPharma)
Searle (Monsanto)	Oral contraceptives (Demulen)
Seohung (Korea)*	Condoms
Syntex	Oral contraceptives (Tri-Norinyll, Devcon, Norinyl, Brevicon)
Thompson Medical	Spermicides
Upjohn* (Upjohn Belgium)*	Injectable (Depo-Provera/DMPA)
Warner-Chilcott	Oral contraceptives (Nelova)
Whitehall	Sponge (Today)[b]
Wisconsin Pharmacal	Female condom (Reality)
Wyeth-Ayerst (American Home Products)	Oral contraceptives (Lo-Ovral, Nordette, Triphasil) (joint venture, Egypt, production)
	Norplant (marketing, distribution)
Wyeth-Pharma (Germany)*	Oral contraceptives
Wyeth (France)*	Oral contraceptives

Note: an asterisk indicates that the firm supplies to UNFPA procurement. Where the firm is listed with more than one product line and is a UNFPA source, the product supplied is also marked with an asterisk.

[a]GynoPharma was sold to Ortho Pharmaceuticals in summer of 1995.

[b]Whitehall decided to discontinue the Today sponge because of the costs of bringing the plant up to U.S. Food and Drug administration specifications.

Data from Frost, Sullivan. U.S. contraceptive and fertility product markets. New York: United Nations Population Fund (UNFPA), 1993 Procurement Statistics, 1993.

has been recommended between application and vaginal penetration. Clinical trials to confirm the efficacy of this time interval have not really been reported. Some spermicides on the United States market have never been tested in clinical trials. Our experience using a variety of marketed spermicidal preparations has shown that the spermicide effectively reduces the number of motile sperm seen in the postcoital test of normal couples to less than one sperm per high-powered microscopic field (62,63). There is no good correlation between the postcoital test results and the reduction in fecundity at this juncture. However, the postcoital test has been used along with *in vitro* spermicidal function as surrogates to indicate a high level of contraceptive efficacy.

Diaphragms

Diaphragms have been available for many years on the United States market and have principally been made out of latex. A coil spring is present in the outer margin as a means of holding the diaphragm in place. All diaphragms require fitting by a health care provider, and fitting changes should be performed after vaginal delivery.

The fitting is done best by using a ring-like device to measure the normal dimensions of the upper vagina. Diaphragm sizes are in millimeters, such that a #70 diaphragm is a 70 mm in transverse diameter. All marketed diaphragms, whether they be spring or arc-spring in type, rely on the application of the spermicide within the concavity and around the edges of the diaphragm to enhance their contraceptive efficacy. There are no studies that I am aware of that the diaphragm alone, without a spermicidal product, has any contraceptive efficacy. Recent clinical trials of two new barrier devices, the Lea's contraceptive and the Femcap, have been performed with and without spermicide. The postcoital test was used as the measure with the Femcap, which was tested with and without spermicide and compared to the diaphragm with spermicide (62). There was no difference in the number of sperm in the cervical mucus (average 0.1 sperm per high-power field) in each treatment area.

Similar results were found in a phase I trial of the Lea's contraceptive when it was compared with and without spermicide to a diaphragm with spermicide (64). No sperm were present in the cervical mucus of the women with a diaphragm or Lea's contraceptive with spermicide. Only two sperm were found in one woman in the group using the Lea's contraceptive alone without spermicide. The contraceptive efficacy of the Lea's contraceptive was evaluated further in a clinical trial with and without spermicide. There were more pregnancies in the nonspermicide group, but the difference was not statistically significant. The overall pregnancy rate was not different from that in historical diaphragm users (65).

Neither of these barrier devices is available on the United States market as of this time.

Condoms

Both male and female condoms are available on the United States market. Male condoms have in the past been made of latex but recently have been made of a polyurethane material that is designed to increase strength, reduce breakage, enhance heat transmission, and, therefore, increase sensation with coital activity (66–68). A variety of condom designs and colors have been used in order to enhance consumer utilization in both developing and developed countries. The addition of a spermicide to the male condom should enhance its contraceptive efficacy, but there are no identified studies that address this issue. It should be pointed out that nonoxynol-9, as well as latex, can result in allergic reactions in consumers. This reaction can take the form of a local irritation or burning, and in rare instances, an anaphylactoid reaction has been reported.

Female condoms, on the other hand, are available and are made of a polyurethane material (88). This device has a bag-like structure with an inner ring that is designed to anchor in the upper portion of the vagina and an outer ring that protrudes outside the vaginal introital area. This was designed to protect the perineum. The objective of the female condom is to allow a woman-controlled method that will prevent pregnancy and reduce the heterosexual transmission of sexually transmitted diseases such as gonorrhea, chlamydia, syphilis, and possibly HIV (69). The female condom has as its major advantage this protective effect. Its major disadvantage is its price and the fact that it is utilized only once and then is disposed of.

Spermicides

Spermicides are principally nonoxynol-9 products in the United States. They come in a variety of formulations and packaging, as shown in Table 10.4. At the present time, spermicides, like condoms, are available over the counter, but many couples are unaware of their availability, effectiveness, and utility. Use effectiveness of spermicides is on the order of condoms and diaphragms with a wide range of reported pregnancy rates (85). Many spermicides are packaged in such a manner that they can be carried in the purse or in a small wallet without contributing undue bulk. At the present time, the United States Food and Drug Administration is undertaking a review of currently marketed spermicides to document their efficacy. In general, spermicides are to be utilized before insertion of the penis. They are effective for only a one-time use, and a second episode of coital activity requires a second application of the product. Side effects associated with spermicide use have been an increased incidence of vaginitis and an increase in urethritis (70–75). Benefits have been a reduction in the transmission of sexually transmitted diseases and the fact that it is a local product without systemic effects (76–78).

SUMMARY

The contraceptive products that are available for young women are also available for women over the age of 35. However, the physician or health care provider should take into consideration the woman's medical history, physical findings, and past contraceptive utilization before recommending or prescribing any of the contraceptive options as listed in this chapter. Overall, in highly motivated individuals, even barrier contraceptives can reduce the pregnancy rate down to below five to six pregnancies per 100 women per year. The health care provider should be aware of the fact that women who are older still have a pregnancy potential and require contraception.

REFERENCES

1. Thorneycroft IH. Cycle control with oral contraceptives: A review of the literature. *Am J Obstet Gynecol* 1999;180:280–287.
2. Schwartz D, Mayaux MJ. Female fecundity as a function of age: results of artificial insemination in 2193 nulliparous women with azoospermic husbands. Federation CECOS. *N Engl J Med* 1982;306:404–406.
3. Grimes DA, Godwin AJ, Rubin A, Smith JA, Lacarra M. Ovulation and follicular development associated with three low-dose oral contraceptives: a randomized controlled trial. *Obstet Gynecol* 1994;83:29–34.
4. Killick SR, Fitzgerald C, Davis A. Ovarian activity in women taking an oral contraceptive containing 20 µg ethinyl estradiol and 150 µg desogestrel: effects of low estrogen doses during the hormone-free interval. *Am J Obstet Gynecol* 1998;179:S18–S24.
5. Lete I, Morales P. Inhibition of follicular growth by two different oral contraceptives (monophasic and triphasic) containing ethinylestradiol and gestodene. *Eur J Contracept Reprod Health Care* 1997;2:187–191.
6. Teichmann A, Martens H, Bordasch C, Petersen G, Lorkowski G. The effects of a new low-dose combined oral contraceptive containing levonorgestrel on ovarian activity. *Eur J Contracept Reprod Health Care* 1996;1:245–256.
7. Drife J. Benefits and risks of oral contraceptives. *Adv Contracept* 1990;6(Suppl):15–25.
8. Mishell DR Jr. Noncontraceptive benefits of oral contraceptives. *J Reprod Med* 1993;38:1021–1029.
9. Burkman RT. Noncontraceptive clinical benefits of oral contraceptives. *Int J Fertil* 1989;34:50–55.
10. Gambacciani M, Spinetti A, Cappagli B, et al. Hormone replacement therapy in perimenopausal women with a low dose oral contraceptive preparation: effects on bone mineral density and metabolism. *Maturitas* 1994;19:125–131.
11. Kleerekoper M, Brienza RS, Schultz LR, Johnson CC. Oral contraceptive use may protect against low bone mass. Henry Ford Hospital Osteoporosis Cooperative Research Group. *Arch Intern Med* 1991;151:1971–1976.
12. Tuppurainen M, Kroger H, Saarikoski S, Honkanen R, Alhava E. The effect of previous oral contraceptive use on bone mineral density in perimenopausal women. *Osteoporos Int* 1994;4:93–98.
13. Petitti DB, Sidney S, Quesenberry CP. Oral contraceptive use and myocardial infarction. *Contraception* 1998;57:143–155.
14. Farley TM, Collins J, Schlesselman JJ. Hormonal contraception and risk of cardiovascular disease. An international perspective. *Contraception* 1998;57:211–230.
15. Rosenberg L, Palmer JR, Sands MI, et al. Modern oral contraceptives and cardiovascular disease. *Am J Obstet Gynecol* 1997;177:707–715.
16. Sidney S, Petitti DB, Quesenberry CP Jr, Klatsky AL, Ziel HK, Wolf S. Myocardial infarction in users of low-dose oral contraceptives. *Obstet Gynecol* 1996;88:939–944.
17. Lewis MA, Spitzer WO, Heinemann LA, MacRae KD, Bruppacher R, Thorogood M. Third generation oral contraceptives and risk of myocardial infarction: an international case-control study. Transnational Research Group on Oral Contraceptives and the Health of Young Women [see comments]. *Br Med J* 1996;312:88–90.
18. Lewis MA, Heinemann LA, Spitzer WO, MacRae KD, Bruppacher R. The use of oral contraceptives and the occurrence of acute myocardial infarction in young women. Results from the Transnational Study on Oral Contraceptives and the Health of Young Women. *Contraception* 1997;56:129–140.
19. Lidegaard O, Kreiner S. Cerebral thrombosis and oral contraceptives. A case-control study. *Contraception* 1998;57:303–314.
20. Petitti DB, Sidney S, Quesenberry CP Jr, Bernstein A. Incidence of stroke and myocardial infarction in women of reproductive age. *Stroke* 1997;28:280–283.
21. Petitti DB, Sidney S, Bernstein A, Wolf S, Quesenberry C, Ziel HK. Stroke in users of low-dose oral contraceptives [see comments]. *N Engl J Med* 1996;335:8–15.
22. Venous thromboembolic disease and combined oral contraceptives: results of international multicentre case-control study. World Health Organization Collaborative Study of Cardiovascular Disease and Steroid Hormone Contraception [see comments]. *Lancet* 1995;346:1575–1582.
23. Spitzer WO, Lewis MA, Heinemann LA, Thorogood M, MacRae KD. Third generation oral contraceptives and risk of venous thromboembolic disorders: an international case-control study. Transnational Research Group on Oral Contraceptives and the Health of Young Women [see comments]. *Br Med J* 1996;312:83–88.
24. Jick H, Jick SS, Gurewich V, Myers MW, Vasilakis C. Risk of idiopathic cardiovascular death and nonfatal venous thromboembolism in women using oral contraceptives with differing progestagen components [see comments]. *Lancet* 1995 346:1589–1593.
25. Lewis MA, Heinemann LA, MacRae KD, Bruppacher R, Spitzer WO. The increased risk of venous thromboembolism and the use of third generation progestagens: role of bias in observational research. The Transnational Research Group on Oral Contraceptives and the Health of Young Women [see comments]. *Contraception* 1996;54:5–13. [Published erratum appears in *Contraception* 1996;54(2):121].
26. Lewis MA. The epidemiology of oral contraceptive use: a critical review of the studies on oral contraceptives and the health of young women. *Am J Obstet Gynecol* 1998;179:1086–1097.
27. Suissa S, Blais L, Spitzer WO, Cusson J, Lewis M, Heinemann L. First-time use of newer oral contraceptives and the risk of venous thromboembolism [see comments]. *Contraception* 1997;56:141–146.
28. Spitzer WO. The 1995 pill scare revisited: anatomy of a non-epidemic [see comments]. *Hum Reprod* 1997;12:2347–2357.
29. Spitzer WO. Bias versus causality: interpreting recent evidence of oral contraceptive studies. *Am J Obstet Gynecol* 1998;179:S43–S50.
30. Rosenberg M. Weight change with oral contraceptive use and during the menstrual cycle. Results of daily measurements [in process citation]. *Contraception* 1998;58:345–349.
31. Reubinoff BE, Grubstein A, Meirow D, Berry E, Schenker JG, Brzezinski A. Effects of low-dose estrogen oral contraceptives on weight, body composition, and fat distribution in young women. *Fertil Steril* 1995;63:516–521.
32. Archer DF, Maheux R, DelConte A, O'Brien FB. A new low-dose monophasic combination oral contraceptive (Alesse) with levonorgestrel 100 micrograms and ethinyl estradiol 20 micrograms. North American Levonorgestrel Study Group (NALSG). *Contraception* 1997;55:139–144.
33. Sulak PJ, Cressman BE, Waldrop E, Holleman S, Kuehl TJ. Extending the duration of active oral contraceptive pills to manage hormone withdrawal symptoms. *Obstet Gynecol* 1997;89:179–183.
34. Mattson RH, Rebar RW. Contraceptive methods for women with neurologic disorders. *Am J Obstet Gynecol* 1993;168:2027–2032.
35. Lee NC, Rubin GL, Borucki R. The intrauterine device and pelvic inflammatory disease revisited: new results from the Women's Health Study. *Obstet Gynecol* 1988;72:1–6.
36. Kronmal RA, Whitney CW, Mumford SD. The intrauterine device and pelvic inflammatory disease: the Women's Health Study reanalyzed [see comments]. *J Clin Epidemiol* 1991;44:109–122.
37. Grodstein F, Rothman KJ. Epidemiology of pelvic inflammatory disease. *Epidemiology* 1994;5:234–242.
38. Farley TM, Rosenberg MJ, Rowe PJ, Chen JH, Meirik O. Intrauterine devices and pelvic inflammatory disease: an international perspective [see comments]. *Lancet* 1992;339:785–788.
39. Ortiz ME, Croxatto HB, Bardin CW. Mechanisms of action of intrauterine devices. *Obstet Gynecol Surv* 1996;51:S42–S51.
40. Spinnato JA 2nd. Mechanism of action of intrauterine contraceptive devices and its relation to informed consent [see comments]. *Am J Obstet Gynecol* 1997;176:503–506.
41. Ramey JW, Starke ME, Gibbons WE, Archer DF. The influence of pentoxifylline (Trental) on the antifertility effect of intrauterine devices in rats. *Fertil Steril* 1994;62:181–185.
42. Chi IC. The multiload IUD: U.S. researcher's evaluation of a European device. *Contraception* 1992;46:407–425.
43. Kimmerle R, Weiss R, Berger M, Kurz KH. Effectiveness, safety, and acceptability of a copper intrauterine device (CU Safe 300) in type I diabetic women. *Diabetes Care* 1993;16:1227–1230.
44. Rosenberg MJ, Foldesy R, Mishell DR Jr, Speroff L, Waugh MS, Burkman R. Performance of the TCu380A and Cu-Fix IUDs in an international randomized trail. *Contraception* 1996;53:197–203.
45. Sivin I, Shaaban M, Odlind V, et al. A randomized trial of the Gyne T 380 and Gyne T 380 Slimline Intrauterine Copper devices. *Contraception* 1990;42:379–389.
46. Archer DF. Reversible contraception for the woman over 35 years of age. *Curr Opin Obstet Gynecol* 1992;4:891–896.
47. Kaunitz AM. Long-acting contraceptive options. *Int J Fertil Menopausal Stud* 1996;41:69–76.
48. Said S, Sadek W, Rocca M, et al. Clinical evaluation of the therapeutic effectiveness of ethinyl oestradiol and oestrone sulphate on prolonged bleeding in women using depot medroxyprogesterone acetate for contraception. World Health Organization, Special Programme of Research, Development and Research Training in Human Reproduction, Task Force on Long-acting Systemic Agents for Fertility Regulation. *Hum Reprod* 1996;11(Suppl 2):1–13.
49. Fraser IS. A survey of different approaches to management of menstrual distur-

bances in women using injectable contraceptives. *Contraception* 1983;28:385–397.

50. Cromer BA, Blair JM, Mahan JD, Zibners L, Naumovski Z. A prospective comparison of bone density in adolescent girls receiving depot medroxyprogesterone acetate (Depo-Provera), levonorgestrel (Norplant), or oral contraceptives. *J Pediatr* 1996;129:671–676.

51. Skegg DC, Noonan EA, Paul C, Spears GF, Meirik O, Thomas DB. Depot medroxyprogesterone acetate and breast cancer. A pooled analysis of the World Health Organization and New Zealand studies. *JAMA* 1995;273:799–804.

52. Depo-medroxyprogesterone acetate (DMPA) and risk of endometrial cancer. The WHO Collaborative Study of Neoplasia and Steroid Contraceptives. *Int J Cancer* 1991;49:186–190.

53. Westhoff C, Wieland D, Tiezzi L. Depression in users of depo-medroxyprogesterone acetate. *Contraception* 1995;51:351–354.

54. Westhoff C, Truman C, Kalmuss D, et al. Depressive symptoms and Depo-Provera. *Contraception* 1998;57:237–240.

55. Sivin I, Viegas O, Campodonico I, et al. Clinical performance of a new two-rod levonorgestrel contraceptive implant: a three-year randomized study with Norplant implants as controls. *Contraception* 1997;55:73–80.

56. Archer DF, Philput CA, Weber ME. Management of irregular uterine bleeding and spotting associated with Norplant. *Hum Reprod* 1996;11(Suppl 2):24–30.

57. Diaz J, Faundes A, Olmos P, Diaz M. Bleeding complaints during the first year of norplant implants use and their impact on removal rate. *Contraception* 1996;53:91–95.

58. Dugoff L, Jones OW 3rd, Allen-Davis J, Hurst BS, Schlaff WD. Assessing the acceptability of Norplant contraceptive in four patient populations. *Contraception* 1995;52:45–49.

59. Tang GW, Lo SS. Levonorgestrel intrauterine device in the treatment of menorrhagia in Chinese women: efficacy versus acceptability. *Contraception* 1995;51:231–235.

60. Sivin I, Alvarez F, Mishell DR Jr, et al. Contraception with two levonorgestrel rod implants. A 5-year study in the United States and Dominican Republic. *Contraception* 1998;58:275–282.

61. Sivin I, Mishell DR Jr, Darney P, Wan L, Christ M. Levonorgestrel capsule implants in the United States: a 5-year study. *Obstet Gynecol* 1998;92:337–344.

62. Mauck CK, Baker JM, Barr SP, Johanson W, Archer DF. A phase I study of Femcap used with and without spermicide. Postcoital testing. *Contraception* 1997;56:111–115.

63. Mauck CK, Baker JM, Barr SP, Johanson WM, Archer DF. A phase I comparative study of three contraceptive vaginal films containing nonoxynol-9. Postcoital testing and colposcopy. *Contraception* 1997;56:97–102.

64. Archer DF, Mauck CK, Viniegra-Sibal A, Anderson FD. Lea's shield: a phase I postcoital study of a new contraceptive barrier device. *Contraception* 1995;52:167–173.

65. Mauck C, Glover LH, Miller E, et al. Leaís shield: a study of the safety and efficacy of a new vaginal barrier contraceptive used with and without spermicide. *Contraception* 1996;53:329–335.

66. Farr G, Katz V, Spivey SK, Amatya R, Warren M, Oliver R. Safety, functionality and acceptability of a prototype polyurethane condom. *Adv Contracept* 1997;13:439–451.

67. Frezieres RG, Walsh TL, Nelson AL, Clark VA, Coulson AH. Breakage and acceptability of a polyurethane condom: a randomized, controlled study. *Fam Plann Perspect* 1998;30:73–78.

68. Rosenberg MJ, Waugh MS, Solomon HM, Lyszkowski AD. The male polyurethane condom: a review of current knowledge. *Contraception* 1996;53:141–146.

69. Elias CJ, Coggins C. Female-controlled methods to prevent sexual transmission of HIV. *AIDS* 1996;10(Suppl 3):S43–S51.

70. Berer M. Adverse effects of nonoxynol-9 [letter; comment]. *Lancet* 1992;340:615–616.

71. Feldblum PJ. Self-reported discomfort associated with use of different nonoxynol-9 spermicides [letter]. *Genitourin Med* 1996;72:451–452.

72. McGroarty JA, Reid G, Bruce AW. The influence of nonoxynol-9-containing spermicides on urogenital infection. *J Urol* 1994;152:831–833.

73. Roddy RE, Cordero M, Cordero C, Fortney JA. A dosing study of nonoxynol-9 and genital irritation. *Int J Stud AIDS* 1993;4:165–170.

74. Stafford MK, Ward H, Flanagan A, et al. Safety study of nonoxynol-9 as a vaginal microbicide: evidence of adverse effects. *J Acquir Immune Defic Syndr Hum Retrovirol* 1998;17:327–331.

75. Steiner MJ, Cates W Jr. Condoms and urinary tract infections: is nonoxynol-9 the problem or the solution? [editorial; comment] [see comments]. *Epidemiology* 1997;8:612–614.

76. Howett MK, Neely EB, Christensen ND, et al. A broad-spectrum microbicide with virucidal activity against sexually transmitted viruses. *Antimicrob Agents Chemother* 1999;43:314–321.

77. Roddy RE, Zekeng L, Ryan KA, Tamoufe U, Weir SS, Wong EL. A controlled trial of nonoxynol 9 film to reduce male-to-female transmission of sexually transmitted diseases. *N Engl J Med* 1998;339:504–510.

78. Cook RL, Rosenberg MJ. Do spermicides containing nonoxynol-9 prevent sexually transmitted infections? A meta-analysis. *Sex Transm Dis* 1998;25:144–150.

79. Hatcher RATJ, Stewart F, Stewart GK, et al. *Contraceptive technology, 16th rev ed.* Manchester, NH: Irvington Publishers, 1994:730.

80. La Vecchia C, Tavani A, Franceschi S, Parazzini F. Oral contraceptives and cancer. A review of the evidence. *Drug Safety* 1996;14(4):260–272.

81. Schlesselman JJ. Risk of endometrial cancer in relation to use of combined oral contraceptives. A practitioneris guide to meta-analysis. *Hum Reprod* 1997;12(9):1851–1863.

82. Vessey MP, Painter R. Endometrial and ovarian cancer and oral contraceptives findings in a large cohort study. *Br J Cancer* 1995;71(6):1340–1342.

83. Jick SS, Walker AM, Jick H. Oral contraceptives and endometrial cancer. *Obstet Gynecol* 1993;82(6):931–935.

84. Grimes DA, Economy KE. Primary prevention of gynecologic cancers. *Am J Obstet Gynecol* 1995;172(1 Pt 1):227–235.

85. Trussell J. Efficacy of barrier contraceptives. In: Mauck CK, Gabelnick HL, Spieler JM, Rivera R, eds. *Barrier contraceptives, current status and future prospects.* New York: Wiley-Liss, 1994.

86. Doncel GF. Chemical vaginal contraceptives: preclinical evaluation. In: Mauck CK, Gabelnick HL, Spieler JM, Rivera R, eds. *Barrier contraceptives, current status and future prospects.* New York: Wiley-Liss, 1994:147–162.

87. Narod SA, Risch H, Moslehi R, et al. Oral contraceptives and the risk of hereditary ovarian cancer. Hereditary Ovarian Cancer Clinical Study Group [see comments]. *N Engl J Med* 1998;339(7):424–428.

88. Farr G, Gabelnick H, Sturgen K, Dorflinger L. Contraceptive efficacy and acceptability of the female condom. *Am J Public Health* 1994;84(12):1960–1964.

89. Fraser IS. A survey of different approaches to management of menstrual disturbances in women using injectable contraceptives. *Contraception* 1983;28(4):385–397.

90. Shaw RW. Assessment of medical treatments for menorrhagia. *Br J Obstet Gynaecol* 1994;101(Suppl 11):15–18.

91. Archer DF. Reversible contraception for the woman over 35 years of age. *Curr Opin Obstet Gynecol* 1992;4(6):891–896.

SECTION III

Pharmacology of Hormone Replacement

In this section the chapters are designed to provide the basis for decision-making regarding hormonal therapy in postmenopausal women. Basic information regarding the physiology of estrogen replacement is provided by Randall B. Barnes and Seth G. Levrant. The choice and use of any one of these products is an individual decision and strategies for this decision-making process will appear throughout the book. The detailed pharmacology and relative potency of the various classes of progestational components is reviewed by Frank Z. Stanczyk. This information is vital in being able to prescribe appropriately. It also provides the underpinning for the understanding of individual problems that may emerge with a given prescription. These concepts will be reexplored in later chapters.

Androgen replacement therapy remains controversial but is gaining in popularity. Many women will have complaints that may warrant the consideration of androgen replacement. There are those (both physicians and patients) who feel that only the prescription of androgen and estrogen can reestablish the sense of well-being experienced prior to the menopause, particularly for those women who have experienced bilateral oophorectomy. This subject will be reviewed by John Buster and Peter Casson who have considered this issue carefully as they have designed their studies on DHEA therapy which will be reviewed specifically in Chapter 56. Most recently data has emerged for the first time that physiologic testosterone replacement in older postmenopausal women results in an increased sexual response (1).

How estrogens and progestogens may be administered is explored in a chapter on routes of administration. While a specific prescription recommendation is not offered, this chapter should provide a basis for a rationale choice of therapy, considering several options.

A discussion of the pharmacology of alternative hormonal preparations is an area of need. However, to date there is imprecise information and in certain cases, therapeutic efficacy has not been established. Nevertheless there is data, including our own, for some benefit of phytoestrogens on vasomotor symptoms. A review will be presented in Chapter 42.

REFERENCE

1. Braunstein G, Shifren J, Casson P, et al. Evaluation of transdermal testosterone replacement therapy for treatment of sexual dysfunction in surgically menopausal women–a multi-center, placebo-controlled crossover study (Abstract S56-3). Presented at the 81st Annual Meeting of the Endocrine Society, San Diego, CA, June, 1999.

Treatment of the Postmenopausal Woman: Basic and Clinical Aspects, Second Edition, edited by Rogerio A. Lobo, Lippincott Williams & Wilkins, Philadelphia © 1999.

CHAPTER 11

Pharmacology of Estrogens

Randall B. Barnes and Seth G. Levrant

ESTROGEN PRODUCTION AND ACTION

During the reproductive years, the main source of estrogen in women is the dominant follicle and the corpus luteum it subsequently forms after ovulation. The principal estrogen produced is estradiol (1). Normal ovulatory cycles result in serum estradiol levels ranging from 40 pg/mL in the early follicular phase to 250 pg/mL at midcycle and 100 pg/mL during the midluteal phase (2). Ovarian production of estradiol ranges from 60 to 600 mg/day during the menstrual cycle (3). The dominant follicle and corpus luteum account for more than 95% of the circulatory estradiol in the premenopausal women (1,4). Peripheral conversion of estrone to estradiol accounts for most of the remaining circulating estradiol (1).

Estrone, the second major human estrogen, is derived principally from the metabolism of estradiol and from the aromatization of androstenedione in adipose tissue (1). A small quantity is secreted directly by the ovary and adrenal. Serum levels during the menstrual cycle vary from 40 to 170 pg/mL, paralleling estradiol levels. The estradiol-to-estrone ratio is greater than 1.0 in premenopausal women (1).

In ovulatory perimenopausal women, the most consistent findings are a shortened follicular phase and elevated FSH throughout the cycle compared to younger ovulatory women (5–7). Perimenopausal women have been found to have increased follicular- and luteal-phase urinary estrogen excretion (7) and increased follicular-phase serum estradiol (8); however, decreased serum estradiol has also been reported throughout the menstrual cycle (5,6). Luteal phase progesterone has been found to be both normal (5,6) and decreased (8), whereas urinary pregnanediol has been found to be decreased (7). The contradictory estrogen and progesterone findings in these studies may be caused by

small sample sizes together with greater cycle variability in perimenopausal women or by differences in sampling technique. Later in the perimenopause, estrogen levels rise and fall without evidence of ovulation, and cycles become irregular (5–7). Both follicle-stimulating hormone (FSH) and luteinizing hormone (LH) levels increase, and eventually anovulation and amenorrhea occur. The ovary fails to respond to gonadotropin stimulation and estrogen deficiency results. Postmenopausal women have serum estradiol levels below 15 pg/mL and mean estrone levels of about 30 pg/mL (9–11).

In postmenopausal women, the predominant estrogen is estrone, with a reversal in the estradiol-to-estrone ratio to less than 1. The primary source of estrone is from peripheral aromatization of androstenedione. Ninety-five percent of postmenopausal androstenedione production occurs in the adrenal gland, and 5% in the ovaries. The conversion rate of androstenedione to estrone is 1% to 2% in normal premenopausal women (12–14). Increased conversion of androstenedione to estrone occurs with increasing weight (as high as 12% to 15% in women who weigh 135 to 181 kg), resulting in increased estrogen levels (11,14,15). The conversion of androstenedione to estrone increases with age (16). However, there have been conflicting reports of the changes in serum androstenedione and estrone levels that occur with aging in postmenopausal women (11,15,16).

The enzyme cytochrome P450 aromatase responsible for transforming androstenedione into estrone is present in nonendocrine tissues, including adipose tissue and stroma (14,17,18). The level of aromatase activity in stromal cells is greater than that in adipocytes (14). Aromatase activity in stromal cells can be increased up to 50-fold by glucocorticoid steroids (19). Weight loss may not decrease the aromatase activity in obese individuals, suggesting that the level of aromatase activity in stromal cells may be independent of the total mass of adipose tissue (14).

Peripheral aromatization of testosterone to estradiol and estrone contributes minimally to estradiol and estrone

R. B. Barnes: Department of Obstetrics and Gynecology, University of Chicago, Chicago, Illinois 60637.

S. G. Levrant: Partners in Reproductive Health, Tinley Park, IL 60477.

production postmenopausally (20). The primary source of estradiol in the postmenopausal women is from the peripheral conversion of estrone. The conversion between estradiol and estrone is catalyzed by 17β-hydroxysteroid dehydrogenase (17β-HSD) in the liver and other tissues (21). At least four 17β-HSD isoenzymes have been identified (22). The type 1 enzyme found in the ovary and placenta favor reduction, whereas the type 2 enzyme found in the liver and endometrium and the ubiquitous type 4 enzyme favor oxidation. Thus, the peripheral conversion between estradiol and estrone favors the formation of estrone. Fifteen percent of estradiol is converted to estrone, whereas only 5% of estrone is converted to estradiol (Fig. 11.1). The amount of estrone derived from estradiol (approximately 3 pg/mL) is extremely low because of the low concentrations of estradiol in postmenopausal women.

Another source of estrone is from the reversible metabolism of estrone-3-sulfate (estrone sulfate), which is the principal circulating estrogen in the body (23,24). Estrone sulfate is 90% bound to albumin and has a metabolic clearance rate (MCR) of 127 ± 33 L/day/m^2 (range 102 to 180) (25). Levels of estrone sulfate follow the same general patterns as estrone and estradiol, ranging from 1,000 pg/mL in the follicular phase to 1,800 pg/mL in the luteal phase (26–28). In postmenopausal women, estrone sulfate levels reach 320 pg/mL, severalfold higher than levels of serum estrone (30 pg/mL) and estradiol (13 pg/mL) (29). Sixty-five percent of estradiol and 54% of estrone are converted to estrone sulfate, while 21% of estrone sulfate is converted to estrone and only 1.5% is converted to estradiol (24).

Within tissues, particularly at the intracellular level, estradiol is the predominant estrogen, even in postmenopausal women in whom estrone is the predominant estrogen in the circulation (30). Differences in microvasculature permeability, plasma protein binding, and intracellular 17β-HSD activity are major determinants of end-target estrogen activity (30,31). Hepatic extraction of all estrogens significantly exceeds that of the brain and

uterus (32). This increased extraction of estrogen is because the liver microcirculation does not have a basement membrane, and its permeability barrier consists of only the hepatocyte plasma membrane. The extraction of estrogens by the liver, brain, endometrium, and myometrium exceed the free (dialyzable) fractions of the compounds, indicating that part of the protein-bound estrogens are available for tissue extraction (31,32). Influx of estrone sulfate and estrone into the endometrium exceeds that of the myometrium (31). Secretory endometrium, under the influence of progesterone, deactivates intracellular estradiol through type 2 17β-HSD conversion to estrone (29).

Estradiol and other unconjugated estrogens diffuse freely into cells, but estrogenic activity within a cell is dependent on the presence of the estrogen receptor (ER). The ER is a member of the nuclear receptor superfamily. The steroid hormone receptor members of the superfamily are hormone-activated regulators of transcription. When unbound, the ER is associated with a multiprotein complex that includes heat shock proteins. These proteins maintain the receptor in a conformation that allows it to bind easily to the estrogen ligand and may also prevent constitutive activity of the receptor (33). Binding of estrogen to its receptor results in receptor dimerization and binding to the palindromic estrogen receptor response element of the promoter region of estrogen-responsive genes. The receptor then interacts with the transcription initiation complex to regulate transcription (33,34). The binding affinity of the physiologic estrogens for the ER parallel their *in vivo* activity, with estradiol > estrone > estriol > catecholestrogens. The stilbene estrogens such as diethylstilbestrol have a three- to fourfold higher affinity than estradiol, whereas the triphenylethylene estrogen agonist/antagonist varies, with 4-hydroxytamoxifen having almost twice the affinity of estradiol and clomiphene and tamoxifen having 25% or less affinity for the estrogen receptor than does estradiol (35).

Recently a second estrogen receptor, ERβ, was cloned in the rat and human (36,37). The human ERβ has 47% homology with the originally cloned estrogen receptor (38,39), now ERα, with 96% homology in the DNA-binding domain and 58% in the ligand-binding domain (40). In the presence of estradiol, both receptors bind to the same DNA estrogen response element with similar affinity (41). The affinity of ERβ for natural and synthetic ligands is similar to that of ERα, except that the ERβ has a higher affinity for phytoestrogens (35). In the human, ERβ mRNA is expressed in classic estrogen-sensitive tissues such as the uterus, breast, and bone (40, 42,43). It is also expressed in human granulosa cells and spermatids, tissues devoid of ERα (40).

The discovery of ERβ has added another alternative to the discussion of how estrogen agonists, antagonists, and agonist/antagonists (selective estrogen receptor modula-

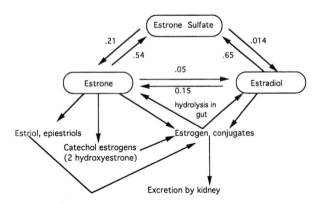

FIG. 11.1. Estrogen metabolism and conversion ratios among estradiol, estrone, and estrone sulfate.

tors) produce their varied effects by binding to the same receptor (44). The responses produced by ligand-bound receptors may be the result of a number of factors. In addition to the ligand, the ER may bind various coactivators and corepressors that affect its ability to activate transcription. The binding of these factors depends on their presence in a given cell and on the conformation of the ER, which is influenced by the specific ligand bound to it. Antagonist-specific binding sites have been described in the estrogen receptor that recognize antagonists such as 4-hydroxytamoxifen but not estrogens. Specific promoter elements may exist that bind the estrogen receptor in addition to the estrogen response element. Recently a raloxifene response element has been described that produced higher transcription activity when the ER was bound to the selective estrogen receptor modulator, raloxifene, than when it was bound to estradiol (45). Finally, different target cells may respond differently to the same hormonal stimulus because of varying ratios of ERα, ERβ, and their heterodimer.

ESTROGEN METABOLISM

Irreversible metabolism of estrogen proceeds primarily in the liver by oxidation of estrone via two different pathways (21). Hydroxylation at the 16 position on the D ring results in the formation of estriol, a biologically weak estrogen, and its isomers, epiestriols. Obesity, hypothyroidism, and cirrhosis favor the metabolism of estrone to estriol. Hydroxylation at the 2 or 4 positions on the A ring results in the formation of catechol estrogens (Fig. 11.1).

Catechol estrogens are also produced in the hypothalamus, where they may have important central nervous systems effects. Catechol estrogens competitively inhibit the enzymes tyrosine hydroxylase and catechol-O-methyl transferase. Catechol estrogens can modulate synthesis and degradation of catecholamines, dopamine and norepinephrine, neurotransmitters important in the control of gonadotropin-releasing hormone release (46). Catechol estrogen formation by A ring metabolism is favored in states of weight loss, such as in anorexia nervosa and hyperthyroidism.

Estrogen metabolism proceeds in the liver and kidney by conjugation of estriol, epiestriols, and catechol estrogens to glucuronides and sulfates, which are highly water soluble and are rapidly excreted by the kidney. The principal urinary estrogens are the conjugates of estriol and 2-hydroxyestrone (47). In addition to urinary excretion, there is a significant enterohepatic circulation of estrogen metabolites. After labeled estrone or estradiol is injected, approximately one-half is present in the urine excreted during the first 24 hours while the remainder is found in bile (48). The conjugated biliary estrogens undergo hydrolysis in the gut, and approximately 80% are reabsorbed. They are returned to the liver, where they may escape reconjugation and enter the systemic circulation, or they may be reconjugated and excreted in the urine or bile. Only about 10% of an injected estrogen will ultimately be lost in the feces. The enterohepatic circulation of estrogen metabolites may be an important factor in the prolonged effect of orally administered estrogens.

All estrogens, conjugated and unconjugated, circulate in the blood either protein bound or unbound (physiologically free). Estrogens are specifically bound with high affinity to sex hormone-binding globulin (SHBG) or loosely (nonspecifically) bound to serum albumin. Serum binding affects the availability of estrogen to diffuse across cell membranes and express biologic activity. Thirty-eight percent of estradiol is bound to SHBG, 60% is loosely bound to albumin, and approximately 2% to 3% is free to diffuse across cell membranes (49). Estrone, estriol, and estrone sulfate all bind poorly to SHBG but have a greater affinity for albumin than does estradiol. Estrone sulfate has the highest affinity for albumin, with more than 90% of circulating estrone sulfate bound to albumin (50). Alterations in SHBG levels change the concentration of unbound estradiol, altering bioavailability. Estrogen therapy, pregnancy, and hyperthyroidism increase SHBG, and hypothyroidism, androgen excess, hyperinsulinemia, and obesity lower SHBG levels (14,51,52). Obese women who are >50 lb (23 kg) above ideal body weight have serum SHBG binding capacity reduced by 20% to 30% compared to normal-weight postmenopausal women, which results in a two- to threefold increase in the free and albumin-bound fractions of estradiol (14).

The liver plays an integral role in the metabolism and excretion of estrogens and is, as importantly, influenced by estrogen status. The liver is affected by estrogens absorbed from the gastrointestinal tract (first-pass effect) and by reabsorption of estrogens secreted in the bile (enterohepatic circulation). The liver is a principal site of metabolic interconversion of estrogens as well as conjugation of estrogens in preparation for excretion into bile and by the kidney. Bioavailability of estrogens is affected by sex hormone-binding globulin and albumin, products of the liver. Estrogens, in turn, influence liver carbohydrate metabolism, lipid metabolism, bile production, and protein production (binding proteins, clotting factors, and renin substrate).

PHARMACOLOGY OF ESTROGEN PREPARATIONS

Estrogens for hormone replacement therapy may be separated by chemical composition (natural or synthetic) or by route of administration (oral or parenteral) (Tables 11.1 and 11.2). Natural estrogens include estradiol, estrone, estriol, and their conjugates, as well as conjugated equine estrogens. Synthetic estrogens include

TABLE 11.1. *Estrogen replacement therapies available in the United States*

Oral		
Conjugated equine estrogens	Premarin	0.3, 0.625, 0.9, 1.25, 2.5 mg
Esterified estrogens (75–85% estrone sulfate, 6–15% equilin sulfate derived from plant sterols)	Estratab	0.3, 0.625, 1.25, 2.5 mg
Estropipate (Piperazine estrone sulfate)	Ogen Ortho-Est	0.625, 1.25, 2.5 mg
Micronized estradiol	Estrace	0.5, 1.0, 2.0 mg
Raloxifene (selective estrogen receptor modulator)	Evista	60 mg
Oral combined		
Conjugated equine estrogens and medroxyprogesterone acetate	Prempro	0.625 mg conjugated equine estrogens and 2.5–5 mg medroxyprogesterone acetate
Esterified estrogens and methyltestosterone	Estratest	1.25 mg esterified estrogen and 2.5 mg methyltestosterone
	Estratest HS	0.625 mg esterified estrogen and 1.25 mg methyltestosterone
Transdermal		
Estradiol	Alora (twice weekly) Climara (weekly) Estraderm (twice weekly) FemPatch (weekly) Vivelle (twice weekly)	0.025, 0.0375, 0.05, 0.075, 0.1 mg of estradiol released daily (dose options for various products)
Vaginal		
Conjugated equine estrogens	Premarin vaginal cream	0.625 mg/g
Dienestrol	Ortho dienestrol cream	0.1 mg/g
Estradiol	Estring	7.5 µg
Estropipate	Ogen vaginal cream	1.5 mg/g
Micronized estradiol	Estrace vaginal cream	1.0 mg/g

ethinyl estradiol, mestranol, quinesterol, diethystilbesterol, and raloxifene. Parenteral routes of administration include injection, transvaginal (creams, tablets, and silastic rings), transdermal patch, subcutaneous pellets, intranasal, and percutaneous gel administration. Irrespective of the type of estrogen or the route of administration, there are large intraindividual and interindividual variations of serum concentrations (53,54).

Synthetic Estrogens

Synthetic estrogens that have been used for menopause estrogen replacement include ethinylestradiol; its C-3-methylated derivative, mestranol; its cyclophenyl ether, quinesterol; and the stilbene derivative diethylstilbestrol. Ethinyl estradiol, the estrogen used in most oral contraceptives, is rapidly absorbed in the gastrointestinal tract

TABLE 11.2. *Approximate serum estradiol and estrone levels after administration of various estrogen preparations*

Preparation	Daily dose (mg)	Estradiol (pg/mL)	Estrone (pg/mL)
Oral			
Conjugated equine estrogen	0.625	30–50	150
	1.25	40–60	120–200
Estropipate	0.625	35	125
	1.25	30–50	150–300
	2.5	125	360
Micronized estradiol	1	30–50	150–300
	2	50–180	300–850
Estradiol valerate	1	50	160
	2	60–70	185–300
Vaginal			
Conjugated equine estrogen	1.25	25–40	65–80
Micronized estradiol	0.5	250	130
Parenteral			
Transdermal estradiol	0.05	30–65	40–45
	0.1	50–90	30–65
Percutaneous estradiol gel	1.5	40–100	90
	3.0	60–140	45–155

after oral administration. Compared to an intravenous dose of ethinyl estradiol, the bioavailability of oral ethinyl estradiol is $59.0 \pm 13\%$ (55). An oral dose of 50 mg of ethinyl estradiol results in a blood level of 400 pg/mL. The ethinyl group at position 17α on ethinyl estradiol prevents oxidation by 17β-HSD. With D-ring metabolism impeded, the principal inactivation pathway is ring A 2-hydroxylation to catechol estrogens. Liver cytochrome P450 enzymes, the chief site of oxidative transformation of ethinyl estradiol, can become irreversibly inactivated by the intermediate compounds of ethinyl estradiol metabolism (56). The strong potency and pronounced effects on hepatic metabolism of ethinyl estradiol compared to natural estrogens are consequences of the relatively slow transformation into inactive metabolites in the hepatocytes and resultant high local concentrations during the first liver passage. Ethinyl estradiol is approximately 75 to 1,000 times more potent on a per-weight basis than conjugated equine estrogens, piperazine estrone sulfate, or micronized estradiol in terms of increasing the production of hepatic proteins (sex hormone-binding globulin, renin substrate, corticosteroid-binding globulin, and thyroid-binding globulin) (57). The minimum dosage required for a therapeutic effect, such as normalization of the calcium/creatinine ratio (10 mg), is greater than the minimum dosage that produces marked elevation in hepatic protein production (5 mg) (58).

As with natural estrogens, the major circulatory form of ethinyl estradiol is its 3-sulfate (56). Ethinyl estradiol is excreted in the urine and feces as glucuronides and sulfates and undergoes enterohepatic circulation. Ethinyl estradiol is almost exclusively bound to albumin. Vaginal administration of 50 mg ethinyl estradiol results in circulating ethinyl estradiol levels equivalent to those achieved after oral ingestion of 10 mg of ethinyl estradiol. Equivalent serum levels of ethinyl estradiol achieved after oral or vaginal administration result in similar effects on hepatic proteins (59). This suggests that the hepatic effects of ethinyl estradiol are related more to the chemical properties of ethinyl estradiol than just to the first liver pass after oral ingestion.

Mestranol is a prodrug that must be converted to ethinyl estradiol before becoming active. Quinestrol is an ester of ethinyl estradiol that has an extremely long half-life. The pharmacokinetics of mestranol and quinestrol correspond to those of ethinyl estradiol.

Raloxifene, a nonsteroidal benzothiophene derivative initially developed as a therapy for breast cancer, has been recently approved in the United States for the prevention of osteoporosis in postmenopausal women. Raloxifene is a selective estrogen receptor modulator that acts as an estrogen agonist in bone and liver but as an estrogen antagonist in the uterus and breast (60,61). It binds to recombinant human ER with an affinity similar to that of estradiol (62). Raloxifene treatment maintained bone mineral content in postmenopausal women over a period of 2 years (63) and decreased total and LDL-cholesterol. Although raloxifene had no overall effect on HDL-cholesterol, it increased HDL_2-cholesterol, but not to the same extent as did conjugated equine estrogens (64). After oral administration, raloxifene undergoes extensive first-pass metabolism to its glucuronide conjugates, which are its primary circulating forms in plasma. It is excreted mainly in the feces, with less than 6% of the dose eliminated in urine as glucuronide conjugates (Evista package insert).

Conjugated Equine Estrogens

One of the most commonly prescribed estrogen preparations for postmenopausal hormone replacement is conjugated equine estrogens (CEE). This preparation is extracted from the urine of pregnant mares and contains classical estrogens (estrone, estradiol, and estrone sulfate) and ring B unsaturated estrogens, which are not native to humans. The CEE preparation contains approximately 45% estrone sulfate, 25% equilin sulfate, 15% 17α-dihydroequilenin sulfate, and lesser amounts of the sulfate esters of equilenin, 17β-dihydroequilin, 17β-dihydroequilenin, 17β-dihydroequilenin, estradiol, 17α-estradiol, and delta-8-estrone (65,66). The pharmacokinetics of CEE is complex because of the various estrogenic components that constitute the preparation. The conversion of equilin and equilenin to 17β-dihydroequilin and 17β-dihydroequilenin by reduction of the 17-ketosteroid correspond to the conversion between estrone and estradiol. As with estrone, the major ring B unsaturated estrogens circulate in the blood as sulfate esters.

Ingestion of 10 mg of CEE, containing 4.5 mg estrone sulfate and 2.5 mg equilin sulfate, results in peak levels of 560 pg/mL equilin and 1,400 pg/mL estrone within 3 and 5 hours, respectively. After 24 hours hormone levels decrease to 125 pg/mL equilin and 280 pg/mL estrone (67). Intravenous administration results in peak levels of equilin and estrone by 20 minutes because equilin sulfate and estrone sulfate are rapidly hydrolyzed to the unconjugated steroids (68). Oral ingestion of 1.25 mg of CEE results in peak levels of 120 to 180 pg/mL of estrone and 40 pg/mL estradiol within 6 to 10 hours. Plasma estrone and estradiol values return to baseline within 48 hours (69). A significant portion of equilin sulfate and estrone sulfate are hydrolyzed to the unconjugated steroids before absorption from the gut (68). After absorption, the unconjugated estrogens undergo reconjugation in the liver to their sulfates, the main circulatory form of these hormones. The sulfated estrogens are also excreted in the bile and undergo enterohepatic recirculation (68,70). Equilin sulfate binds to albumin (74% of total) in a similar fashion to estrone sulfate (up to 88% of total) and does not bind to SHBG. Equilin sulfate is metabolized to its 17β-metabolites. 17β-Dihydroequilin, like 17β-estradiol, is more potent than its parent compound equilin and has a binding affinity to SHBG that is similar to that of 17β-estradiol (68). Equilin sulfate has a MCR of 176 ± 44 L/day/m^2 (range 93 to 342) and a half-life of 3.2 hours compared to a MCR of 94.1 ± 22 L/day/m^2 (range 39 to 141) and a half-life of 5.3 to 9 hours for estrone sulfate (68). 17β-Dihydroequilin and 17β-dihydroequilin sulfate have MCRs of $1,252 \pm 103$ L/day/m^2 and 376 ± 93 L/day/m^2, respectively, and half-lives (slow component) of 45 ± 9 minutes and 135 ± 17 minutes, respectively (71). The binding affinities for human estrogen receptor for various components of CEE follows the following order: 17β-dihydroequilin > 17β-estradiol > 17β-dihydroequilenin > estrone = equilin > 17α-dihydroequilin > 17α-estradiol > 17α-dihydroequilenin > equilenin (66,68). The pharmacokinetics of equilin sulfate is similar to that of estrone sulfate, with equilin and 17β-dihydroequilin being analogous to estrone and 17β-estradiol. About 25% of equilin sulfate is converted to equilin, which is similar to the 15% to 20% conversion rate of estrone to estrone sulfate. However, 15% of equilin sulfate is converted to 17β-dihydroequilin, which is much higher than the 1% to 3% conversion rate of estrone to 17β-estradiol (66). Metabolites of equilin sulfate are excreted in the urine mainly conjugated to glucuronic acid (70). The biologic effects of CEE are therefore a combination of primarily estrone sulfate and equilin sulfate and their respective metabolites.

Use of CEE vaginal cream results in serum levels approximately one-half to one-fourth of those obtained with comparable oral dosages (Fig. 11.2) (72–74). Each gram of vaginal cream contains 0.625 mg of CEE. Intravaginal application of 1.25 mg CEE results in peak estradiol level of 33 ± 6.6 pg/mL in 6 hours and peak estrone level of 73 ± 9.2 pg/mL in 8 hours (72). Twenty-four hours after vaginal CEE, estradiol levels did not differ significantly from baseline, and estrone levels were 50 ± 8.7 pg/mL, twice baseline level (72). Vaginal CEE, 0.3 mg, is equivalent to the effect of 1.25 mg oral CEE on vaginal cytology. However, vaginal CEE, 0.3 mg, results in minimal increases in estrone and estradiol levels that are lower than those found in the early follicular phase (74). Vaginal CEE 2.5 mg is comparable to oral CEE 0.15 to 0.625 mg in its action on hepatic markers (SHBG, TBG, and renin substrate) and calcium-to-creatinine ratios (74). Comparable serum levels of estrone and estradiol, but diminished hepatic effects, have been reported for vaginal CEE 2.5 mg compared with oral CEE 0.625 mg (29). Vaginal absorption of estrogen is erratic, and in one report four of five women had higher estradiol and estrone levels after 1.25 mg of vaginal than after 1.25 mg of oral CEE (69).

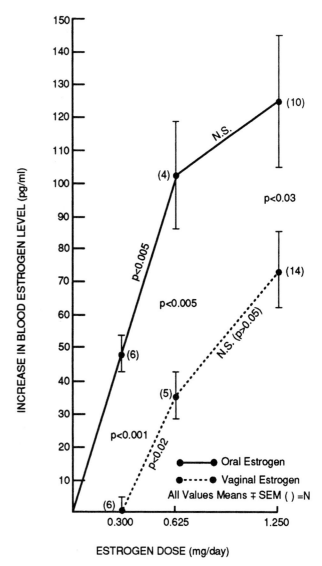

FIG. 11.2. Total plasma estrogen levels after 1 week of oral or vaginal conjugated equine estrogens. (From ref. 73, with permission.)

Estradiol and Estrone

Oral estrone and estradiol preparations include estropipate (piperazine estrone sulfate), estradiol valerate, and micronized estradiol. All oral estrogens result in higher serum estrone levels than estradiol levels because estradiol is oxidized by intestinal mucosa and liver 17β–HSD during the first hepatic passage. Estradiol and estrone are better absorbed in their conjugated or micronized forms. Oral ingestion of 1.2 mg estropipate, 1 mg of micronized estradiol, and 0.625 mg CEE result in similar maximum serum levels of estradiol and estrone of 30 to 50 pg/mL and 150 to 300 pg/mL, respectively, after 4 to 6 hours (Table 11.2) (75,76). Doses of 1.5 mg of oral estropipate and 2 mg estradiol valerate result in nearly superimposable levels of estradiol and estrone sulfate and slightly higher estrone values for estradiol valerate (Fig. 11.3) (77). Maximum levels of 300 pg/mL for estrone and 65 pg/mL for estradiol are achieved after 2 mg oral micronized estradiol (76,78). Pharmacokinetic studies of estropipate and estradiol valerate suggest similar half-life characteristics (79). Long-term use of 2 mg oral micronized estradiol results in estradiol levels of 114 ± 65 pg/mL and 575 ± 280 pg/mL for estrone (76,78). Estradiol and estrone levels after 4 weeks of 2.5 mg of estropipate daily were 126 pg/mL and 356 pg/mL, respectively (76,80). Serum levels achieved after chronic exposure to oral estrogens are slightly higher than those seen after acute dosing. This may be a result of increased levels of sex hormone-binding globulin as well as sequestration of estrogens in adipose tissue.

Most estrogens are readily absorbed across vaginal epithelium. Vaginal administration of estrogen can be via a cream, saline suspension, tablet, or vaginal ring. Micronized estradiol suspended in saline results in a more rapid absorption than micronized estradiol in cream, with peak levels occurring at 2 and 4 hours, respectively (72,81). Vaginal administration of 2 mg micronized estradiol in cream and 0.5 mg micronized estradiol saline result in comparable estradiol and estrone serum levels. Vaginal administration of estradiol bypasses the intestinal-hepatic first-pass metabolism, resulting in higher serum estradiol values than estrone values. With use of vaginal micronized estradiol in saline,

serum estradiol levels reach 29 times baseline (860 pg/mL) for 3 hours and then drop to eight times baseline level (250 pg/mL) after 6 hours, with modest increases in estrone of four times (210 pg/mL) and 2.4 times (130 pg/mL) baseline values after 3 and 6 hours, respectively (82). Vaginal administration of 0.5 mg estrone in saline resulted in serum estrone levels 14 times baseline (435 pg/mL) and estradiol serum level 3.7 times baseline (125 pg/mL) after 6 hours (82). Micronized estradiol in tablet form is also well absorbed from the vagina.

Vaginal rings consisting of crystalline estradiol mixed with a liquid polymer, polydimethysiloxane, produce sustained and fairly constant levels of estradiol for 3 months after an initial burst effect (83,84). The 100-mg, 200-mg, and 400-mg estradiol vaginal rings produce serum levels of estradiol in the range of 40 to 50 pg/mL, 70 to 80 pg/mL, and 140 pg/mL, respectively (83). Serum estrone levels increase twofold to a peak value of 55 pg/mL with the 400-mg estradiol vaginal ring (85). An intravaginal silastic ring (Estring) has recently been approved for treatment of urogenital atrophy in the United States. After an initial burst of estradiol release, the ring releases about 8 μg of estradiol daily for 3 months. Plasma levels of estradiol and estrone increase by about one-third but remain within the normal postmenopausal range (86,87). The ring increases the vaginal maturation index and relieves urogenital atrophy but has no effect on FSH, SHBG, or endometrial thickness (86,88).

Intranasal administration of estrogen suspended in saline results in rapid dissipation and low estrogen levels (81). Estradiol suspended in dimethyl-β-cyclodextrin results in peak levels within 30 minutes with a half-life of 120 to 145 minutes (89). Nasal administration of 0.34 mg estradiol results in serum levels of approximately 408 pg/mL and 136 pg/mL after 2 and 5 hours, respectively. An open nonrandomized trial found decreased FSH and LH levels and symptomatic relief in eight of nine patients over a 6-month trial (89).

Percutaneous administration of estradiol in an alcohol-based gel has been used for estrogen replacement therapy in Europe. The gel is applied to the arms, shoulders, and abdomen, dries in 2 to 5 minutes, and leaves no sticky sensation or odor. The skin, particularly the stratum corneum, acts as a reservoir for continuous release of estradiol. Five grams of gel contains 3 mg of estradiol. Generally, 1.5 mg or 3 mg of estradiol is administered. Five grams of percutaneous estradiol gel results in estradiol levels of about 100 pg/mL within 4 to 6 hours and reaches a steady state after 3 to 5 days (53,90). Administration of 3 mg and 1.5 mg of estradiol daily by percutaneous gel for 14 days results in mean estradiol serum levels of 103 ± 40 pg/mL and 68 ± 27 pg/mL, respectively, compared with 114 ± 65 pg/mL and 41 ± 14 pg/mL after 2 mg oral micronized estradiol and 50 mg/day transdermal estradiol (78). Mean serum estrone levels for percu-

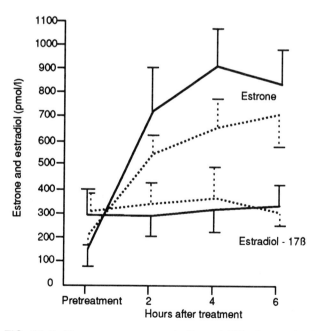

FIG. 11.3. Mean serum concentrations (±SE of mean) of estrone and estradiol before and at 2-hour intervals after oral piperazine estrone sulfate, 1.5 mg (dotted line), and estradiol valerate, 2 mg (solid line), in postmenopausal women. (From ref. 77, with permission.)

taneous estradiol 1.5 mg and 3.0 mg are 90 pg/mL and 120 pg/mL, respectively, compared with 575 pg/mL and 43 pg/mL for 2 mg oral micronized estradiol and 50 mg/day transdermal estradiol (78). Estrogen levels may be extremely variable because absorption is proportional to the surface area of application, intensity of rubbing in, and extent of removal by clothing (91).

Pellets containing crystalline estradiol, implanted underneath the skin in the subcutaneous tissue, deliver steady levels of estradiol for 6 months (92–94). Estradiol levels are highest 24 hours after insertion, reach a steady state after 1 week, and remain relatively constant for 24 weeks (93). Pellets containing 25 mg and 50 mg of estradiol result in serum estradiol levels of 50 to 70 pg/mL and 100 to 120 pg/mL, respectively (92,93). The estradiol/estrone ratio at 6 months is 1.45 and 1.59 after insertion of 25 mg and 50 mg estradiol pellets, respectively (94).

Several transdermal delivery systems of estradiol are available in the United States (Table 11.1). Estradiol is released from an alcohol gel reservoir (Estraderm) or directly from an acrylic (Alora, Climara, Vivelle) or silicon (FemPatch) adhesive matrix. The patches are designed to release 0.025 to 0.10 mg of estradiol daily for 3.5 or 7 days. With transdermal delivery, the estrogen reservoir is in the patch itself and not in the skin, as it is with the percutaneous estradiol gel. The transdermal patch is applied to the abdomen or buttock once or twice a week. The half-life of estradiol delivered from a transdermal patch is 161 ± 14 minutes in nonobese, fasting postmenopausal women (95). Maximum serum levels of estradiol are achieved within 2 to 8 hours (3,93,96,97). The 50 mg/day alcohol gel patch results in peak levels of 92 pg/mg of estradiol and 48 to 62 pg/mL of estrone within 2 to 8 hours after application (96). Long-term use results in mean serum estradiol and estrone levels of 33 to 62 pg/mL and 38 to 45 pg/mL, respectively (78,98,99). The 100 mg/day alcohol gel patch results in peak estradiol levels of 152 ± 33 pg/mL and estradiol and estrone levels of 46 to 89 pg/mL and 32 to 64 pg/mL, respectively, with long-term use (93). The 7-day adhesive matrix patch produces similar mean estradiol levels as the 3.5-day patch at both the 0.05-mg and 0.10-mg doses, but with less variation in estradiol levels (97). The mean 7-day estradiol levels were approximately 50 and 100 pg/mL for the 0.05-mg and 0.10-mg patches, respectively.

CLINICAL ASPECTS OF ESTROGEN THERAPY

Estrogen replacement is beneficial for symptomatic relief of hot flashes and genitourinary symptoms and for prevention of osteoporosis. All of the estrogen preparations previously described in appropriate doses will improve vasomotor symptoms and genitourinary symptoms. The lowest dosage that relieves symptoms and is effective in preventing osteoporosis should be used. Effective dosages for prevention of bone loss are presented in Table 11.3 (63,94,100,105). As discussed in

TABLE 11.3. *Effective daily dose for prevention of bone loss*

Conjugated equine estrogen	0.625 mg[a]
Estropipate	0.625 mg (spine)
	1.25 mg (hip)
Micronized estradiol	1.0 mg[a]
Raloxifene	60 mg
Transdermal estradiol	0.05 mg[a]
Percutaneous estradiol gel	3.0 mg

[a]Recently FDA-approved minimal effective doses include 0.3 mg of esterified estrogen, 0.5 mg of micronized estradiol, and 0.037 mg transdermal estradiol.

other chapters, estrogen replacement is probably effective in the prevention of cardiovascular disease and may help prevent other conditions such as colon cancer and Alzheimer's disease. Because the evidence for estrogen preventing these conditions is epidemiologic, the effective daily dosages for various estrogen compounds and routes of administration are unknown. However, the percentage increase in HDL- and decrease in LDL-cholesterol found with 0.625 mg conjugated equine estrogen, 2 mg micronized estradiol, and 2.5 mg estropipate are approximately the same (80,106). Likewise, the effects of various estrogens and routes of administration on the possibly harmful outcomes of estrogen replacement such as breast cancer and thromboembolic disease are unknown.

There is limited information on the interaction of diseases and drugs with estrogen in postmenopausal women receiving replacement therapy. Sex hormone binding capacity is increased in moderate smokers compared with nonsmokers (107). After ingestion of oral micronized estradiol, the change in serum estrone sulfate and estrone glucuronide is greater in postmenopausal smokers, suggesting a greater hepatic metabolism of estradiol than in nonsmokers (107). Thus, moderate smoking results in less biologically available estradiol in women taking estrogens. Postmenopausal smokers not taking estrogen replacement therapy have estrogen levels similar to those in nonsmokers (11,108). Acute alcohol ingestion resulted in a 20% increase in serum estradiol in women given estradiol transdermal patches (109), and the half-life of estradiol was increase by about 50% (110). Likewise, in women taking oral estradiol, the serum estradiol level was tripled by acute alcohol ingestion (111), but there was no effect of alcohol on estradiol levels in women not taking estrogen. Interestingly alcohol had no effect on estrone levels with transdermal or oral estradiol administration. In a case report phenytoin was found to increase estrogen clearance and reduce estrogen levels (112). Postmenopausal women with end-stage renal disease had a higher baseline serum estradiol and a greater serum estradiol response to oral estradiol administration than did normal postmenopausal controls (113).

REFERENCES

1. Baird DT, Fraser IS. Blood production and ovarian secretion rates of estradiol-17β and estrone in women throughout the menstrual cycle. *J Clin Endocrinol Metab* 1974;38:1009–1017.
2. Kletzky OA, Nakamura RM, Thorneycroft IH, Mishell DR Jr. Log normal distribution of gonadotropins and ovarian steroid values in the normal menstrual cycle. *Am J Obstet Gynecol* 1975;121:688–694.
3. Powers MS, Schenekel L, Darley PE, Good WR, Balestra JC, Place VA. Pharmacokinetics and pharmacodynamics of transdermal dosage forms of 17β-estradiol: comparison with conventional oral estrogens used for hormone replacement. *Am J Obstet Gynecol* 1985;152:1099–1106.
4. Lloyd CW, Lobotsky J, Baird DT, et al. Concentration of conjugated estrogens, androgens and gestagens in ovarian and peripheral venous plasma in women: the normal menstrual cycle. *J Clin Endocrinol Metab* 1971;32:155–166.
5. Sherman BM, Korenman SG. Hormonal characteristics of the human menstrual cycle throughout reproductive life. *J Clin Invest* 1975;55:699–706.
6. Sherman BM, West JH, Korenman SG. The menopausal transition: Analysis of LH, FSH, estradiol, and progesterone concentrations during menstrual cycles of older women. *J Clin Endocrinol Metab* 1976;42:629–636.
7. Santoro N, Brown JR, Adel T, Skurnick JH. Characterization of reproductive hormonal dynamics in the perimenopause. *J Clin Endocrinol Metab* 1996;81:1495–1501.
8. Reyes FI, Winter JSD, Faiman C. Pituitary-ovarian relationships preceding the menopause. *Am J Obstet Gynecol* 1977;129:557–564.
9. Judd HL. Hormonal dynamics associated with the menopause. *Clin Obstet Gynecol* 1976;19:775–788.
10. Laufer LR, DeFazio JL, Lu JKH, et al. Estrogen replacement therapy by transdermal estradiol administration. *Am J Obstet Gynecol* 1983; 146:533-38.
11. Cauley JA, Gutai JP, Kuller LH, LeDonne D, Powell JG. The epidemiology of serum sex hormones in postmenopausal women. *Am J Epidemiol* 1989;129:1120–1131.
12. Siiteri PK, MacDonald PC. Role of extraglandular estrogen in human endocrinology. In: Greep RO, Astwood EB, eds. *Handbook of Physiology: Endocrinology, vol 2, part 1.* Washington, DC: American Physiology Society, 1973:45.
13. Longcope C. Metabolic clearance and blood production rates of estrogens in postmenopausal women. *Am J Obstet Gynecol* 1971;111:778ó-781.
14. Siiteri PK. Adipose tissue as a source of hormones. *Am J Clin Nutr* 1987;45:277–282.
15. Meldrum DR, Davidson BJ, Tataryn IV, Judd HL. Changes in circulating steroids with aging in postmenopausal women. *Obstet Gynecol* 1981;57:624–628.
16. Hemsell DL, Grodin JM, Brenner PF, Siiteri PK, MacDonald PC. Plasma precursors of estrogen II. Correlation of the extent of the conversion of plasma androstenedione to estrone with age. *J Clin Endocrinol Metab* 1974;38:476–479.
17. Ackerman GE, Smith ME, Mendelson CR, MacDonald PC, Simpson ER. Aromatization of androstenedione by human adipose tissue stromal cells in monolayer culture. *J Clin Endocrinol Metab* 1981;53:412–417.
18. Simpson ER, Mahendroo MS, Means GD, et al. Aromatase cytochrome P450, the enzyme reponsible for estrogen biosynthesis. *Endocr Rev* 1994;15:342–355.
19. Simpson ER, Ackerman GE, Smith ME, Mendelson CR. Estrogen formation in stromal cells of adipose tissue of women: induction by glucocorticosteroids. *Proc Natl Acad Sci USA* 1981;78:5690–5694.
20. Judd HL, Shamonki IM, Frumar AM, Lagasse LD. Origin of serum estradiol in postmenopausal women. *Obstet Gynecol* 1982;59:680–686.
21. Fishman J, Bradlow HL, Gallagher TF. Oxidative metabolism of estradiol. *J Biol Chem* 1960;235:3104–3107.
22. Penning TM. Molecular endocrinology of hydroxysteroid dehydrogenases. *Endocr Rev* 1997;18:281–305.
23. Pack BA, Tovar R, Booth E, Brooks SC. The cyclic relationship of estrogen sulfurylation to the nuclear receptor level in human endometrial curettings. *J Clin Endocrinol Metab* 1979;48:420–424.
24. Ruder HJ, Loriaux L, Lipsett MB. Estrone sulfate: production rate and metabolism in man. *J Clin Invest* 1972;51:1020–1033.
25. Jasonni M, Bulletti C, Franceschetti F, et al. Metabolic clearance rate of oestrone sulphate in post-menopausal women. *Maturitas* 1984;5:251.
26. Loriaux DL, Ruder HJ, Lipsett MB. The measurement of estrone sulfate in plasma. *Steroids* 1971;18:463.
27. Wright K, Collins DC, Musey PI, Preedy JRK. A specific radioimmunoassay for estrone sulfate in plasma and urine without hydrolysis. *J Clin Endocrinol Metab* 1978;47:1092–1098.
28. Hawkins RA, Oakey RE. Estimation of oestrone sulfate, oestradiol-17b and oestrone in peripheral plasma: concentrations during the menstrual cycle and in men. *J Endocrinol* 1974;60:3–17.
29. Lobo RA. Absorption and metabolic effects of different types of estrogens and progestogens. *Obstet Gynecol Clin North Am* 1987;14:143–167.
30. King RJB, Dyer G, Collins WP, Whitehead MI. Intracellular estradiol, estrone and estrogen receptor levels in endometria from postmenopausal women receiving estrogens and progestins. *J Steroid Biochem* 1980;13:377–382.
31. Bulletti C, Jasonni VM, Ciotti PM, Tabanelli S, Naldi S, Flamigni C. Extraction of estrogens by human perfused uterus. *Am J Obstet Gynecol* 1988;159:509–515.
32. Steingold KA, Cefalu W, Pardridge W, Judd HL, Chaudhuri G. Enhanced hepatic extraction of estrogens used for replacement therapy. *J Clin Endocrinol Metab* 1986;62:761–766.
33. Beato M, Herrlich P, Schutz G. Steroid hormone receptors: Many actors in search of a plot. *Cell* 1995;83:851–857.
34. Tsai MJ, O'Malley BW. Molecular mechanisms of action of steroid/thyroid receptor superfamily members. *Annu Rev Biochem* 1994;63:451–486.
35. Kuiper GGJM, Carlsson B, Grandien K, et al. Comparison of the ligand binding specificity and transcript tissue distribution of estrogen receptors α and β. *Endocrinology* 1997;138:863–870.
36. Kuiper GGJM, Enmark E, Pelto-Huikko M, et al. Cloning of a novel estrogen receptor expressed in rat prostate and ovary. *Proc Natl Acad Sci USA* 1996;93:5925–5930.
37. Mosselman S, Polman J, Dijkema R. ERβ: Identification and characterization of a novel human estrogen receptor. *FEBS Lett* 1996;392:49–53.
38. Green S, Walter P, Kumar V, et al. Human oestrogen receptor cDNA: Sequence, expression and homology to v-*erb*-A. *Nature* 1986;320:134–139.
39. Greene GL, Gilna P, Waterfield M, et al. Sequence and expression of human estrogen receptor complementary DNA. *Science* 1986;231:1150–1154.
40. Enmark E, Pelto-Huikko P, Grandien K, et al. Human estrogen receptor β-gene structure, chromosomal localization and expression pattern. *J Clin Endocrinol Metab* 1997;82:4258–4265.
41. Pace P, Taylor J, Suntharalingam S. Human estrogen receptor β binds DNA in a manner similar to and dimerizes to estrogen receptor α. *Am Soc Biochem Mol Biol* 1997;272:25832–25838.
42. Dotzlaw H, Leygue E, Watson PH, et al. Expression of estrogen receptor-beta in human breast tumors. *J Clin Endocrinol Metab* 1996;82:2371–2734.
43. Arts J, Kuiper GGJM, Janssen JMMF, et al. Differential expression of estrogen receptors α and β mRNA during differentiation of human osteoblast SV-HFO cells. *Endocrinology* 1997;138:5067–5070.
44. Kuiper GGJM, Gustafsson JA. The novel estrogen receptor-β subtype: Potential role in the cell- and promoter-specific actions of estrogens and anti-estrogens. *FEBS Lett* 1997;410:87ó-90.
45. Yang NN, Venugopalan M, Hardikar S. Identification of an estrogen response element activated by metabolites of 17β-estradiol and raloxifene. *Science* 1996;273:1222–1224.
46. Fishman J, Norton B. Brain catecholestrogens: formation and possible functions. *Adv Biosci* 1975;15:123.
47. Fishman J. Role of 2-hydroxyestrone in estrogen metabolism. *J Clin Endocrinol Metab* 1963;23:207–210.
48. Sandberg A, Slaunwhite WR. Studies on phenolic steroids in human subjects. II. The metabolic fate and hepato-biliary-enteric circulation of C^{14} estrone and C^{14} estradiol in women. *J Clin Invest* 1957;36:1266–1278.
49. Chung-Hsiu W, Motohashi T, Abdel-Rahman HA, Flickinger GL, Mikhail G. Free and protein bound plasma estradiol 17β during the menstrual cycle. *J Clin Endocrinol Metab* 1976;43:436–445.
50. Rosenthal HE, Pietrzak E, Slaunwhite WR Jr, Sandberg AA. Binding of estrone sulfate in human plasma. *J Clin Endocrinol Metab* 1972;34:805–813.
51. Anderson DC. Sex-hormone binding globulin. *Clin Endocrinol* 1974;3:69.
52. Nestler JE. Sex hormone-binding globulin: A marker for hyperinsulinemia and/or insulin resistance? *J Clin Endocrinol Metab* 1993;76:273–274.
53. Kuhl H. Pharmacokinetics of oestrogens and progestogens. *Maturitas* 1990;12:171–197.
54. Fotherby K. Intrasubject variability in the pharmacokinetics of ethynyloestradiol. *J Steroid Biochem Mol Biol* 1991;38:733ó-736.
55. Orme M, Back DJ, Ward S, Green S. The pharmacokinetics of ethynylestradiol in the presence and absence of gestodene and desogestrel. *Contraception* 1991;43:305–316.
56. Guengerich FP. Metabolism of 17α-ethynylestradiol in humans. *Life Sci* 1990;47:1981–1988.
57. Mashchak CA, Lobo RA, Dozono-Takano R, et al. Comparison of phkarmacodynamic properties of various estrogen formulations. *Am J Obstet Gynecol* 1982;144:511–518.
58. Mandel FP, Geola Fl, Lu JKH, et al. Biologic effects of various doses of ethinyl estradiol in postmenopausal women. *Obstet Gynecol* 1982;59:673–679.
59. Goebelsmann U, Mashchak CA, Mishell DR Jr. Comparison of hepatic impact of oral and vaginal administration of ethinyl estradiol. *Am J Obstet Gynecol* 1985;151:868–877.
60. Sadovsky Y, Adler S. Selective modulation of estrogen receptor action. *J Clin Endocrinol Metab* 1998;83:3–5.
61. Mitlak BH, Cohen FJ. In search of optimal long-term female hormone replacement: The potential of selective estrogen receptor modulators. *Horm Res* 1997;48:155–163.
62. Glasebrook AL, Phillips DL, Sluka JP. Multiple binding sites for the anti-estrogen raloxifene. *J Bone Mineral Res* 1993;8:S268.
63. Delmas PD, Bjarnason NH, Mitlak BH, et al. Effects of raloxifene on bone mineral density, serum cholesterol concentrations, and uterine endometrium in postmenopausal women. *N Engl J Med* 1997;337:1641–1687.
64. Walsh BW, Kuller LH, Wild RA. Effects of raloxifene on serum lipids and coagulation factors in healthy postmenopausal women. *JAMA* 1998;279:1445–1451.
65. Bhavnani BR, Woolever CA, Henoit H, et al. Pharmacokinetics of equilin and equilin sulfate in normal postmenopausal women and men. *J Clin Endocrinol Metab* 1983;56:1048–1056.
66. Bhavnani BR. Pharmacokinetics and pharmacodynamics of conjugated equine estrogens: Chemistry and metabolism. *Proc Soc Exp Biol Med* 1998;217:6ó-16.
67. Bhavnani BR, Sarda IR, Woolever CA. Radioimmunoassay of plasma equilin

and estrone in postmenopausal women after the administration of premarin. *J Clin Endocrinol Metab* 1981;52:741–747.

68. Bhavnani BR. The saga of the ring B unsaturated equine estrogens. *Endocrine Reviews* 1988;9:396–416.
69. Englund DE, Johansson EDB. Plasma levels of oestrone oestradiol and gonadotrophins in postmenopausal women after oral and vaginal administration of conjugated equine oestrogens (Premarin). *Br J Obstet Gynaecol* 1978;85:957–964.
70. Bhavnani BR, Woolever CA, Wallace D, Pan CC. Metabolism of [³H]equilin-[³⁵S]sulfate and [³H]equilin sulfate after oral and intravenous administration in normal postmenopausal women and men. *J Clin Endocrinol Metab* 1989;68:757–765.
71. Bhavnani BR, Cecutti A. Pharmacokinetics of 17b-dihydroequilin sulfate and 17b-dihydroequilin in normal postmenopausal women. *J Clin Endocrinol Metab* 1994;78:197–204.
72. Rigg LA, Hermann H, Yen SSC. Absorption of estrogens from vaginal creams. *N Engl J Med* 1978;298:195–197.
73. Deutsch S, Ossowski R, Benjamin I. Comparison between degree of systemic absorption of vaginally and orally administered estrogens at different dose levels in postmenopausal women. *Am J Obstet Gynecol* 1981;139:967–968.
74. Mandel FP, Geola FL, Meldrum DR, et al. Biological effects of various doses of vaginally administered conjugated equine estrogens in postmenopausal women. *J Clin Endocrinol Metab* 1983;57:133–139.
75. Lobo RA, Brenner P, Mishell DR Jr. Metabolic parameters and steroid levels in postmenopausal women receiving lower doses of natural estrogen replacement. *Obstet Gynecol* 1983;62:94–98.
76. Lobo RA, Cassidenti DL. Pharmacokinetics of oral 17b-estradiol. *J Reprod Med* 1992;37:77–84.
77. Anderson ABM, Sklovsky E, Sayers L, Steele PA, Turnbull AC. Comparison of serum oestrogen concentrations in post-menopausal women taking oestrone sulphate and oestradiol. *Br Med J* 1978;1:140–142.
78. Scott RT Jr, Ross B, Anderson C, Archer DF. Pharmacokinetics of percutaneous estradiol: a crossover study using a gel and a transdermal system in comparison with oral micronized estradiol. *Obstet Gynecol* 1991;77:758–764.
79. Aedo A-R, Landgren B-M, Diczfalusy E. Pharmacokinetic properties of oral oestrone sulphate piperazine and oestradiol valerate in postmenopausal women. *Maturitas* 1984;6:79.
80. Colvin PL Jr, Auerbach BJ, Koritnik DR, Hazzard WR, Applebaum-Bowden D. Differential effects of oral estrone versus 17β-estradiol on lipoproteins in postmenopausal women. *J Clin Endocrinol Metab* 1990;70:1568–1573.
81. Rigg A, Milanes B, Villanueva B, Yen SSC. Efficacy of intravaginal and intranasal administration of micronized estradiol-17β. *J Clin Endocrinol Metab* 1975;45:1261–1264.
82. Schiff I, Tulchinsky D, Ryan KJ. Vaginal absorption of estrone and 17β-estradiol. *Fertil Steril* 1977;28:1063–1066.
83. Stumpf PG. Selecting constant serum estradiol levels achieved by vaginal rings. *Obstet Gynecol* 1986;67:91–94.
84. Stumpf PG, Maruca J, Santen RJ, Demers LM. Development of a vaginal ring for achieving physiologic levels of 17β-estradiol in hypoestrogenic women. *J Clin Endocrinol Metab* 1982;54:208–210.
85. Veldhuis JD, Samojlik E, Evans WS, et al. Endocrine impact of pure estradiol replacement in postmenopausal women: alterations in anterior pituitary hormone release and circulating sex steroid hormone concentrations. *Am J Obstet Gynecol* 1986;155:334–339.
86. Smith P, Heimer G, Lindskog M, et al. Oestradiol-releasing vaginal ring for treatment of postmenopausal urogenital atrophy. *Maturitas* 1993;16:145–154.
87. Johnston A. Estrogens pharmacokinetics and pharmacodynamics with special reference to vaginal administration and the new estradiol formulation Estring. *Acta Obstet Gynecol Scand* 1996;75:16ó-25.
88. Holmgren PA, Lindskog M, von Schoultz B. Vaginal rings for continuous low-dose release of oestradiol in the treatment of urogenital atrophy. *Maturitas* 1989;11:55–63.
89. Hermens WAJJ, Belder CWJ, Merkus JMWM, Hooymans PM, Verhoef J, Merkus FWHM. Intranasal estradiol administration to oophorectomized women. *Eur J Obstet Gynecol Reprod Biol* 1991;40:35ó-41.
90. Whitehead MI, Townsend PT, Kitchin Y, et al. Plasma steroid and protein hormone profiles in postmenopausal women following topical administration of oestradiol 17β. In: Mauvais-Jarvis P, Vickers CFH, Wepierre J, eds. *Percutaneous absorption of steroids*. New York: Academic Press, 1980:231.
91. Jewelewicz R. New developments in topical estrogen therapy. *Fertil Steril* 1997;67:1–12.
92. Lobo RA, March CM, Goebelsmann U, Krauss RM, Mishell D Jr. Subdermal estradiol pellets following hysterectomy and oophorectomy. *Am J Obstet Gynecol* 1980;138:714ó-719.
93. Stanczyk FZ, Shoupe D, Nunez V, Macias-Gonzales P, Vijod MA, Lobo RA. A randomized comparison of nonoral estradiol delivery in postmenopausal women. *Am J Obstet Gynecol* 1988;159:1540ó-1546.
94. Notelovitz M, Johnston M, Smith S, Kitchens C. Metabolic and hormonal effects of 25-mg and 50-mg 17β-estradiol implants in surgically menopausal women. *Obstet Gynecol* 1987;70:749–754.
95. Ginsburg ES, Gao X, Shea BF, et al. Half-life of estradiol in postmenopausal women. *Gynecol Obstet Invest* 1998;45:45–48.
96. Haas S, Walsh B, Evans S, Krache M, Ravnikar V, Schiff I. The effect of transdermal estradiol on hormone and metabolic dynamics over a six-week period. *Obstet Gynecol* 1988;71:671–676.
97. Gordon SF. Clinical experience with a seven-day estradiol transdermal system for estrogen replacement therapy. *Am J Obstet Gynecol* 1995;173:998–1004.
98. Steingold KA, Laufer L, Chetkowski RJ, et al. Treatment of hot flashes with transdermal estradiol administration. *J Clin Endocrinol Metab* 1985;61:627–631.
99. Ribot C, Tremollieres F, Pouilles JM, Louvet JP, Peyron R. Preventive effects of transdermal administration of 17b-estradiol on postmenopausal bone loss: a 2-year prospective study. *Gynecol Endocr* 1989;3:259–267.
100. Lindsay R, Hart DM, Clark DM. The minimum effective dose of estrogen for prevention of postmenopausal bone loss. *Obstet Gynecol* 1984;63:759–763.
101. Quigley MET, Martin PL, Burnier AM, Brooks P. Estrogen therapy arrests bone loss in elderly women. *Am J Obstet Gynecol* 1987;156:1516–1523.
102. Stevenson JC, Cust MP, Gangar KF, Hillard TC, Lees B, Whitehead MI. Effects of transdermal versus oral hormone replacement therapy on bone density in spine and proximal femur in postmenopausal women. *Lancet* 1990;335:265–269.
103. Gallagher JC, Baylink D. Effect of estrone sulfate on bone mineral density of the femoral neck and spine. *J Bone Mineral Res* 1990;5(Suppl 2):275.
104. Chetkowski RJ, Meldrum DR, Steingold KA, et al. Biologic effects of transdermal estradiol. *N Engl J Med* 1986;314:1615–1620.
105. Riis B, Thomsen K, Christiansen C. Does calcium supplementation prevent postmenopausal bone loss? *N Engl J Med* 1987;316:173–177.
106. Walsh BW, Schiff I, Rosner B, Greenberg L, Ravnikar V, Sacks FM. Effects of postmenopausal estrogen replacement on the concentrations and metabolism of plasma lipoproteins. *N Engl J Med* 1991;325:1196–1204.
107. Cassidenti DL, Vijod AG, Vijod MA, Stanczyk FZ, Lobo RA. Short-term effects of smoking on the pharmacokinetic profiles of micronized estradiol in postmenopausal women. *Am J Obstet Gynecol* 1990;163:1953–1960.
108. Cassidenti DL, Pike MC, Vijod AG, Stanczyk FZ, Lobo RA. A reevaluation of estrogen status in postmenopausal women who smoke. *Am J Obstet Gynecol* 1992:166:1444–1448.
109. Ginsburg ES, Walsh, BW, Gao X, et al. The effect of acute ethanol ingestion on estrogen levels in postmenopausal women using transdermal estradiol. *J Soc Gynecol Invest* 1995;2:26–29.
110. Ginsburg ES, Walsh BW, Shea BF, et al. The effects of ethanol on the clearance of estradiol in postmenopausal women. *Fertil Steril* 1995;63:1227–1230.
111. Ginsburg ES, Mello NK, Mendelson JH. Effects of alcohol ingestion on estrogens in postmenopausal women. *JAMA* 1996;276:1747–1751.
112. Notelovitz M, Tjapkes J, Ware M. Interaction between estrogen and Dilantin in a menopausal women. *N Engl J Med* 1981;304:788–789.
113. Ginsburg ES, Owen WF, Greenberg LM. Estrogen absorption and metabolism in postmenopausal women with end-stage renal disease. *J Clin Endocrinol Metab* 1996;81:4414–4417.

Treatment of the Postmenopausal Woman: Basic and Clinical Aspects, Second Edition, edited by Rogerio A. Lobo, Lippincott Williams & Wilkins, Philadelphia © 1999.

CHAPTER 12

Structure–Function Relationships, Potency, and Pharmacokinetics of Progestogens

Frank Z. Stanczyk

A variety of progestogens are available for treatment of women. A progesten is a substance that binds to the progesterone receptor and has progestational activity. The most widely recognized progestational activity is transformation of proliferative to secretory endometrium in estrogen-primed uteri. Progestogens are also frequently referred to as progestins and less frequently as gestagens.

Progestogens can be divided into two types: natural and synthetic (Table 12.1) (1–4). There is only one natural progestogen, and that is progesterone. Synthetic progestogens can be subdivided into those structurally related to progesterone and those structurally related to testosterone. The progestogens structurally related to progesterone can be subdivided further into pregnane and norpregnane derivatives. The pregnane derivatives consist of acetylated and nonacetylated compounds. Similarly, progestogens structurally related to testosterone can be subdivided further into compounds with and without ethinyl groups. The ethinylated derivatives can be subdivided further into estrane and gonane derivatives.

The term progestin is often used to refer to a synthetic progestogen and exclude the natural progestogen. There is, however, no rule of nomenclature that restricts the use of that term specifically for a synthetic progestogen. Thus, the terms progestogen, progestin, and gestagen can be used interchangeably to refer to either a natural or synthetic progestogen.

NATURAL PROGESTOGENS

From the practical point of view, progesterone is the only natural progesterone with significant progestational activity. The progesterone molecule contains 21 carbons

and has ketone groups at carbons 3 and 20 as well as a double bond between carbons 4 and 5 (Fig. 12.1).

SYNTHETIC PROGESTOGENS STRUCTURALLY RELATED TO PROGESTERONE

Chemical manipulation of the progesterone molecule has led to the development of potent progestogens (Fig. 12.1). Addition of a hydroxyl group at C-17 of progesterone results in a loss of progestational activity. Acetylation of the 17-hydroxyl group gives rise to 17-hydroxyprogesterone acetate, which has some progestational activity. This compound offers an important starting point in the development of a number of synthetic progestogens. Elongation of the carboxyl side-chain carbon-17 (C-17) of 17-hydroxyprogesterone acetate gives rise to long-acting progestogens, when used parenterally; examples include 17-hydroxyprogesterone caproate.

TABLE 12.1. *Classification of progestogens*

Natural: progesterone
Synthetic
  Structurally related to progesterone
    Pregnane derivatives
      Acetylated: medroxyprogesterone acetate, megestrol acetate, cyproterone, acetate, chlormadinone acetate, medrogestone
      Nonacetylated: dydrogesterone
    Norpregnane derivatives: demegestone, promegestone, nomegestrol acetate
  Structurally related to testosterome
    Ethinylated
      Estrane derivatives: norethindrone, norethynodrel, lynestrenol, norethindrone acetate, ethynodiol diacetate.
      Gonane derivatives: levonorgestrel, desogestrel, gestodene, norgestimate
    Nonethinylated: dienogest

F. Z. Stanczyk: Department of Obstetrics and Gynecology, University of Southern California School of Medicine, Los Angeles, California 90033.

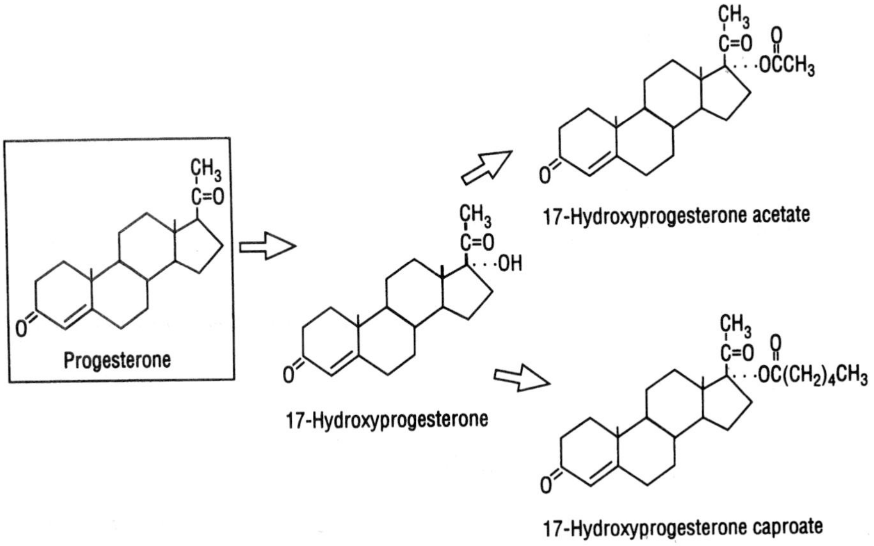

FIG. 12.1. Chemical structures of progestogens related to progesterone. (From ref. 2, with permission.)

Manipulation of the 17-hydroxyprogesterone acetate molecule, primarily at C-6, has produced potent oral as well as parenteral progestogens (Fig. 12.2). Addition of a methyl group at C-6 of 17-hydroxyprogesterone acetate gives rise to medroxyprogesterone acetate. Formation of a double bond between C-6 and C-7 of the latter compound yields megestrol acetate. Manipulation of the latter molecule by substitution of the methyl group at C-6 with a chloral group and attachment of a methylene group so that is shared jointly by C-1 and C-2 gives rise to cyproterone acetate.

SYNTHETIC PROGESTOGENS STRUCTURALLY RELATED TO TESTOSTERONE

Alteration of the testosterone molecule by addition of an ethinyl group at C-17 causes the steroid to lose androgenicity substantially and to acquire both progestational properties and oral activity. 17α–Ethinyltestosterone (also known as ethisterone) became the first orally active progestogen structurally related to testosterone (Fig. 12.3). Removal of the methyl group at C-10 of 17α-ethinyltestosterone fur-

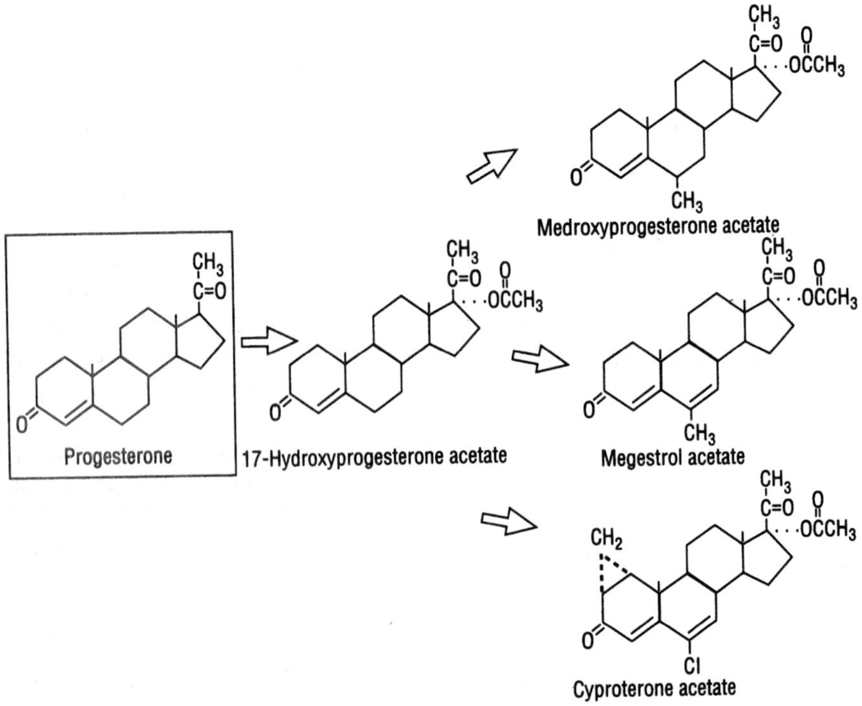

FIG. 12.2. Chemical structures of progestogens related to 17-hydroxyprogesterone acetate. (From ref. 2, with permission.)

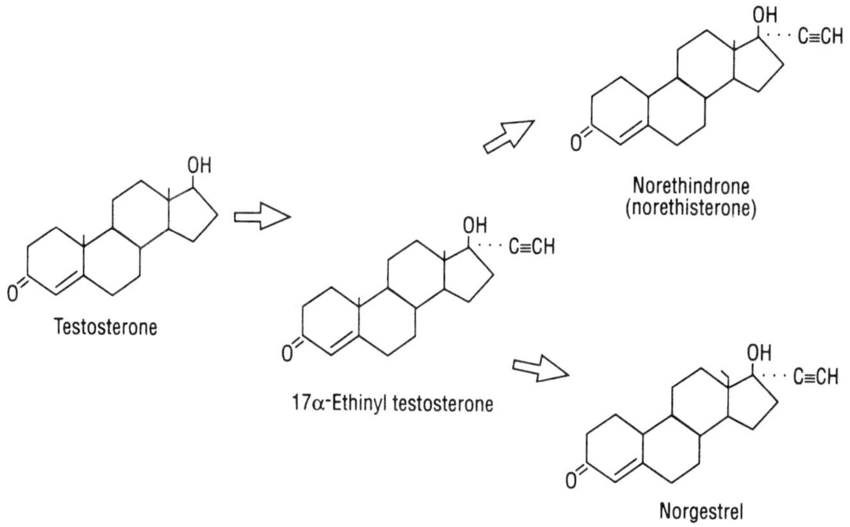

FIG. 12.3. Chemical structures of progestogens related to testosterone. (From ref. 2, with permission.)

ther increases the progestogenic activity of the molecule and virtually eliminates its androgenicity. The resulting product is norethindrone (also called norethisterone). Substitution of an ethyl group for the methyl group on C-13 of norethindrone gives rise to norgestrel, which consists of a racemic mixture of D-(-)-norgestrel (levonorgestrel) and L-(+)-norgestrel (dextronorgestrel) when synthesized. Levonorgestrel is the biologically active form of norgestrel and is one of the most potent orally active progestogens. A number of other 19-nortestosterone derivatives have been synthesized from norethindrone and levonorgestrel.

Compounds Derived from Norethindrone

Five derivatives of norethindrone are widely recognized: norethynodrel, lynestrenol, norethindrone acetate, ethynodiol diacetate, and norethindrone enanthate (Fig. 12.4). Norethynodrel differs from norethindrone by having a double bond between C-5 and C-10 instead of C-4 and C-5. Loss of the oxygenated function at C-3 gives rise to

lynestrenol. Acetylation of the 17-hydroxyl group of norethindrone yields norethindrone acetate, and subsequent reduction of the ketone group at C-3 followed by acetylation of the resulting hydroxyl group produces ethynodiol diacetate. Norethynodrel, lynestrenol, norethindone acetate, and ethinyldiol diacetate are orally active progestogens. In contrast, norethindrone enanthate is formed by esterification of norethindrone with heptanoic acid.

Compounds Derived from Levonorgestrel

Compared to the norethindrone derivatives, the compounds derived from levonorgestrel are relatively new and are sometimes referred to as the new generation of orally active progestogens. They include desogestrel, norgestimate, and gestodene (Fig. 12.5). Desogestrel is formed by removal of the oxygenated function at C-3 and addition of a methylene group at C-11. Formation of an oxime group at C-3 and an acetate group at C-17 of lev-

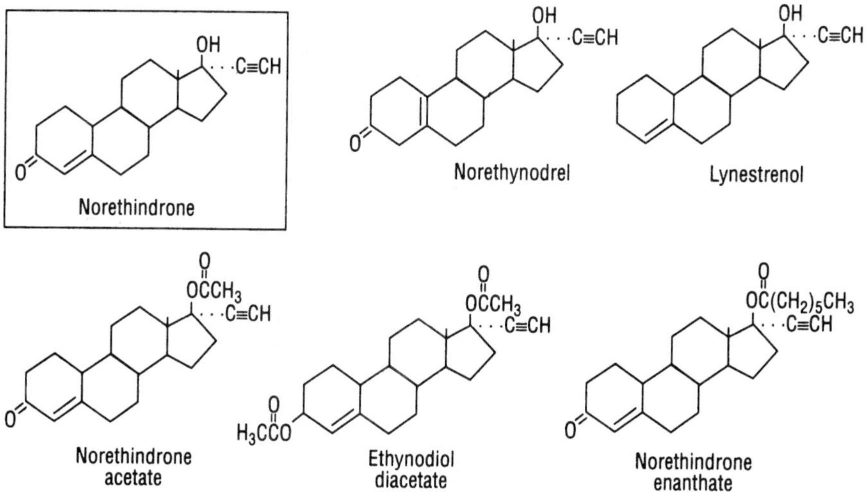

FIG. 12.4. Chemical structures of progestogens related to norethindrone. (From ref. 2, with permission.)

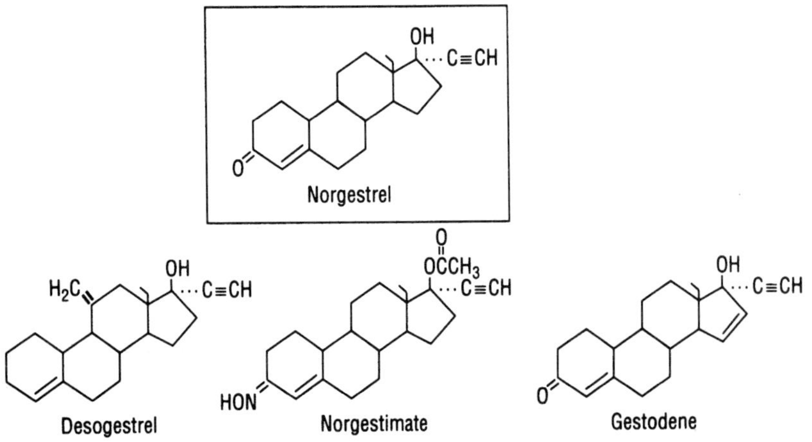

FIG. 12.5. Chemical structures of progestogens related to norgestrel. (From ref. 2, with permission.)

onorgestrel yields norgestimate. Gestodene differs structurally from levonorgestrel only in the double bond that it possesses between C-15 and C-16.

POTENCY OF PROGESTOGENS

The potency of a drug can be defined as an estimate of a specific biologic effect of the drug. From the technical point of view, a drug's potency is always related to that of a standard drug and is quantified by measuring the difference of the parallel dose-response curves produced by the standard drug and the test drug.

Problems encountered in estimating potencies of progestogens are well recognized (5–8). A variety of qualitative and quantitative tests utilizing either human or animal species to establish potencies of progestogens have been performed. The tests can be divided into the following three types: (a) in vitro receptor-binding assays, (b) bioassays, and (c) clinical tests. Unfortunately, there are difficulties in obtaining precise quantification of potencies with these tests. A major source of the difficulties can be found in the variables associated with each test. In general, the variables include (a) type of animal species, (b) type of tissue or target organ, (c) the specific response of the tissue or target organ, (d) temporal considerations (e.g., time of test following dosing), and (e) the route of, and vehicle for, drug administration. Difficulties also arise from the fact that potency estimates from animal tests cannot be extrapolated to humans. Although these difficulties exist, there is a substantial amount of information pertaining to potencies of progestogens. An overview of some of the more relevant data pertaining to progestogenic, androgenic, and estrogenic potencies of these compounds is now presented.

Progestational Potency

Receptor Binding Tests

It is well established that a steroid hormone must bind to a receptor before a hormonal action is produced. Thus, a compound should bind to the progestogen receptor before it can be considered a progestational agent. Uteri

from various animal species, including humans, in various conditions of age and pretreatment have been utilized as a source of progesterone receptors for binding studies. In practice, the binding affinity of a test steroid for the progesterone receptor is determined by the concentration of the steroid that corresponds to 50% inhibition of the total binding (IC_{50}) of a radiolabeled progestational marker (e.g., tritiated R5020) to the receptor.

Because progesterone is the natural progestational agent of all mammals, it may be considered the prototype for comparison. Progesterone intially served as the reference steroid and was utilized in conjunction with [^{3}H]progesterone in competitive binding studies with progesterone receptors. However, because most synthetic progestogens have considerably greater progestational activity than progesterone, a highly potent synthetic progestin, referred to as R5020 (17,21-dimethyl-19-nor-pregna-4,9-diene-3,20-dione), has replaced progesterone as the reference compound.

Comparison of the binding affinity of a test steroid for a specific receptor relative to that of a steroid standard is expressed by the relative binding affinity (RBA). Thus, the RBA of a test steroid for uterine progesterone receptors can be calculated from the IC_{50} of progesterone divided by the corresponding IC_{50} of the test steroid. The ratio is multiplied by 100 and expressed in percent.

Most receptor binding tests utilize an incubation procedure, usually overnight, to allow the radioligand and test substance to compete for binding to the progesterone receptors. The binding of various test substances to progesterone receptors in cytosols (105,000-g fractions) of human uterine tissues has been determined after overnight incubation at 4°C, using different progestogens (R5020, 3-ketodesogestrel, gestodene, and levonorgestrel) as reference steroids (9). Table 12.2 shows that when R5020 was employed as the reference steroid, 3-ketodesogestrel, levonorgestrel, medroxyprogesterone acetate, cyproterone acetate, and gestodene were all bound with high affinity to the progesterone receptors. The RBA values of these compounds ranged from 85% to 130% and were 2.1- to 3.2-fold higher than the RBA of progesterone (40%). No mea-

TABLE 12.2. *Relative binding affinities (%) of different progestogens for binding to human uterine progesterone receptor*

Compound	R5020	Ketodesogestrel	Gestodene	Levonorgestrel
Progesterone	40	15	2	18
Gestodene	85	110	100	150
Levonorgestrel	90	75	100	120
R5020	100	20	20	22
Org2058	350	N.D.	35	N.D.
Desogestrel	1	0.3	<0.1	0.3
3-Ketodesogestrel	130	100	55	110
Norgestimate	<0.1	<0.1	<0.1	<0.1
Cyproterone acetate	90	N.D.	N.D.	N.D.
Medroxyprogesterone acetate	115	N.D.	N.D.	N.D.

N.D., not determined.
From ref. 9, with permission.

surable binding affinity to the progesterone receptors was demonstrated for desogestrel or norgestimate.

A different pattern in hierarchy of RBA values was obtained with the test substances when 3-ketodesogestrel, gestodene, or levonorgestrel were utilized as reference steroids (Table 12.2). R5020 was only a weak competitor with respect to these reference steroids. Levonorgestrel was able to displace gestodene from the binding sites of the progesterone receptors only to a relatively moderate extent, but considerably more than 3-ketoderogestrel. The RBAs of levonorgestrel and 3-ketodesogestral were 75% and 55%, respectively. On the other hand, gestodene was a high-affinity competitor (RBAs are 110% and 150%, respectively), when either 3-ketodesogestrel or levonorgestrel was the reference steroid. The results also show that 3-ketodesogestrel had a slightly higher affinity for the uterine progesterone receptors than levonorgestrel, when either progestogen was used as the test substance. Thus, on the basis of the data shown in Table 12.2, it appears that gestodene binds to the progesterone receptors with higher affinity than either 3-ketodesogestrel or levonorgestrel, and 3-ketoderogestrel has a slightly higher affinity than levonorgestrel.

The lack of significant binding of norgestimate and desogestrel to progesterone receptors (Table 12.2) supports the view that these compounds are prodrugs and must be transformed to a biologically active form for progestogenic action. A recent study (10) analyzed the binding of not only norgestimate but also its potential metabolites to progesterone receptors. The possible metabolites included levonorgestrel-17-acetate (deoximated norgestimate), levonorgestrel-3-oxime (deacetylated norgestimate), and levonorgestrel (deoximated and deacetylated norgestimate). A cytosolic preparation from human myometrium was used in conjunction with R5020 as reference steroid, and an overnight incubation was carried out at 4°C with the test compounds. The results confirmed the lack of significant binding of norgestimate (RBA, 0.8%) to the progesterone receptors. Also, it was shown that these receptors bind to levonorgestrel-17-acetate with affinity (RBA, 110%) and levonorgestrel-3-oxime to only a small extent (RBA, 8%). The highest binding was obtained with levonorgestrel (RBA, 250%). Progesterone had an RBA of

30%. These data differ significantly from those obtained in another study (11), in which it was shown that norgestimate and levonorgestrel-3-oxime displaced [^{3}H]R5020 from estrogen-primed rabbit uterine progesterone receptors with affinities similar to that of progesterone. The findings in the two studies (10,11) just discussed not only point out the importance of choosing appropriate animal species to carry out competitive binding studies but also support the view that the progestational action of norgestimate is mediated through one or more of its metabolites.

Bioassays

The most common bioassays used to evaluate progestational potency determine the effect of the test compound on either uterine glandular proliferation, inhibition of ovulation, pregnancy maintenance, or delay of parturition in rabbits or rats. Examples of different types of bioassays are now discussed.

Uterine Glandular Proliferation

Clauberg Test. The most widely used bioassay for progestational agents has been the Clauberg test. This test is based on initial observations made by Clauberg in the 1920s. In 1934, McPhail organized these observations into specific protocols (12). In general, the test procedure involves priming immature female rabbits with estrogen, followed by either oral or parenteral treatment with the test substance. Progestogens induce the development of complicated glandular structures in the estrogenic endometrium with simple glands. A standardized scale for grading glandular proliferation of the rabbit endometrium was provided by McPhail. This scale ranges from 0, which corresponds to no glandular development, to a value of +4, corresponding to maximal glandular development. Active progestational compounds are compared at a dose level that produces a +2 on the McPhail scale.

Estimates of progestational potency for a variety of compounds by the Clauberg test are shown in Table 12.3 (8,13). This table shows that medroxyprogesterone acetate and megestrol acetate are the most potent compounds, levonorgestrel is less potent, norgestrel is half as potent as

TABLE 12.3. *Comparative activities of various progestogens in a series of assay procedures*

| | Assay | | | | | | |
| | Human | | | Laboratory Animal | | | |
Compound	Binding (%)	Delay of menses[a]	Minimum bleeding dose[b]	Clauberg	McGinty[c]	Pregnancy maintenance[c]	Delay of parturition
Progesterone	100	—	—	100	A	A	100
Levonorgestrel	95	—	—	1,800	—	A	—
Norethindrone	85	4(?)	2	8	I	I	100
Medroxyprogesterone acetate	78	22.5	—	3,500	A	A	300
Megestrol acetate	70	1.8	4–5	2,500	A	A	—
Norgestrel	49	0.125	0.5	900	A	A	1,000
Norethynodrel	5	5.3	5	?	I	I	A
Ethynodiol diacetate	5	1.5	1	240	—	—	—

[a]With 100 µg mestranol; figures are ED$_{50}$ values in milligrams.
[b]With 50 µg of ethinyl estradiol of 100 µg of mestranol; oral contraceptive values are given in milligrams.
[c]A, active; I, inactive.
From ref. 8, with permission.

its biologically active enantiomer, and ethynodiol diacetate is appreciably less potent. Both norethindrone and norethynodrel are weak progestogens in the particular conditions of the Clauberg test used to obtain the data in Table 12.3. Norethynodrel was so weak that it failed to produce a +2 McPhail value at any dose.

In a study (14) in which the Clauberg test was used to compare progestational activity among gestodene, desogestrel, 3-ketodesogestrel, and levonorgestrel, the data showed that gestodene had the highest progestogenic activity (Table 12.4). However, the data for 3-ketodesogestrel were incomplete.

Although the Clauberg test is the most widely used bioassay for progestational agents, it is subject to considerable divergence in estimates of potency (8). The variablility appears to result from differences in protocol and to

TABLE 12.4. *Comparison of progestational activity*

| Progestogen | Dose (mg/animal/day) | Inhibition of ovulation in rats[a] (%) SC | Maintenance of pregnancy in ovariectomized rats[b] (♀ day 8–autopsy day 21) (%) SC | Clauberg test in rabbits—endometrial transformation McPhail index[c] | |
				SC	PO
Gestodene	0.1	—[d]	—	—	3.5 (10)
	0.03	100 (6)	100 (6)	3.1 (9)	2.6 (10)
	0.01	100 (6)	92 (6)	1.8 (10)	1.5 (10)
	0.003	50 (6)	33 (6)	1.0 (9)	1.0 (10)
	0.001	0 (6)	0 (6)	—	—
Levonorgestrel	0.1	—	100 (5)	3.2 (11)	2.3 (10)
	0.03	100 (6)	88 (5)	2.3 (10)	1.1 (8)
	0.01	33 (6)	0 (5)	1.1 (10)	1.0 (11)
	0.003	17 (6)	—	—	—
	0.001	0 (6)	—	—	—
3-Ketodesogestrel[e]	0.1	—	88 (6)	—	—
	0.03	100 (6)	58 (6)	—	3.3 (6)
	0.01	100 (6)	57 (6)	—	2.3 (5)
	0.003	33 (6)	0 (6)	—	1.2 (5)
Desogestrel	3.0	—	100 (6)	—	—
	1.0	100 (6)	60 (5)	—	—
	0.3	33 (6)	0 (6)	—	—
	0.1	17 (6)	0 (6)	2.4 (8)	3.3 (5)
	0.03	17 (6)	0 (6)	1.2 (8)	2.8 (6)
	0.01	—	—	1.0 (7)	1.4 (8)

[a]Number in parentheses indicates number of treated animals/group.
[b]Progestogen was administered together with 1.0 µg estrone SC.
[c]Transformation: none (0) to maximal (4).
[d]Dash indicates *not tested*.
[e]Active metabolite of desogestrel.
From ref. 14, with permission.

certain peculiar observations that emerge from examination of the test results. An example of the latter situation has been described for the Clauberg test data shown in Table 12.3. The dose-response curves for most of the compounds were steep and were parallel to that of progesterone. The compounds with steep slopes had McPhail values ranging from +3 to +3.5. In contrast, the slope for norethindrone was shallow, and that for norethynodrel was virtually nonexistent. The corresponding McPhail values for these slopes were only +2 and +1.3, respectively. In addition, there were differences in the characteristic shape of the uterine glandular cells. Following treatment with medroxyprogesterone acetate, megestrol acetate, norgestrel, and progesterone, the uterine glandular cells had a low columnar shape. In contrast, the glandular cells were tall columnar, without subnuclear vacuoles after treatment with norethindrone and ethynodiol diacetate, and with subnuclear vacuoles after norethynodrel treatment. It has been pointed out that for meaningful comparisons of potencies among progestogens, it is essential that the corresponding histologic characteristics of the glandular cells be similar and that parallelism exists among the dose-response curves of the test compounds. These criteria are most often not met, resulting in erroneous conclusions about differences in the potency of progestogens.

McGinty Test. A variation of the Clauberg test was established by McGinty et al. (15). In the McGinty assay, the test compound is infused directly into a tied-off segment of the uterine lumen of estrogen-primed spayed rabbits. The vehicle-treated contralateral uterine horn may be used as a control. The McGinty test is not used routinely because it is laborious. Apparently, most of the compounds shown in Table 12.3 are active in the McGinty test, with the exception of norethindrone and norethynodrel (8,13).

Inhibition of Ovulation

Inhibition of ovulation is an important property of progestogens used for oral contraception. Bioassays in which test compounds are administered subcutaneously to rats and rabbits to determine whether or not they prevent ovulation have been used to compare progestational potencies. For example, it has been shown that doses of 3 μg of gestodene per day, administered subcutaneously, are sufficient to inhibit ovulation in the rat (14). Under the same conditions, the potency of gestodene is similar to that of 3-ketodesogestrel and is at least three times greater than that of levonorgestrel (Table 12.4).

Pregnancy Maintenance

The basis of the pregnancy maintenance test is that progesterone administration reverses abortion or resorption of the conceptus if pregnant animals of certain species are spayed after implantation. Rats are the most commonly used animals for this test. The test protocol involves ovariectomy on day 7 or 8 of pregnancy, followed by administration of different doses of the test sub-stance. The time of autopsy varies considerably from one laboratory to another. Although the results may be quantified, it is usually sufficient to express the data qualitatively. With this test, it has been shown that medroxyprogesterone acetate, megestrol acetate, norgestrel, and levonorgestrel are active, whereas norethindrone and norethynodrel are inactive (Table 12.4) (8,13). Another study showed that gestodene has the capacity to maintain pregnancy in spayed gravid rats at a dose of 3 to 10 μg/day (14). In comparison, the progestational potency of 3-ketodesogestrel is similar to that of gestodene, whereas the potency of levonorgestrel is about one-third less than that of the former compounds (Table 12.4).

Delay of Parturition

The delay-of-parturition test is based on the fact that in certain mammalian species there is a delay in delivery of the fetus at term following the administration of progesterone to the mother. This finding has been adapted to an assay protocol in which pregnant rats near term receive a progestogen before the expected delivery date, and the delay in the onset of parturition is measured. With this test, results from a study (16) shown in Table 12.3 indicate that norgestrel had a tenfold greater potency than either progesterone or norethindrone and a 3.3-fold higher potency than medroxyprogesterone acetate.

Clinical Tests

A variety of clinical tests have been used to assess the relative potency of progestogens in women. These include tests based on induction of secretory changes in the endometrium, inhibition of ovulation, and changes in vaginal cytology and cervical mucus. Because endometrial effects of progestogens are relatively simple to assess clinically, the earliest efforts to compare the potency of progestogens relied on the delay-of-menses test, which was first described by Greenblatt et al. (17). The test is based on the fact that uterine bleeding is induced by withdrawal of hormonal support of the endometrium at the end of the menstrual cycle. In general, the assay protocol involves administration of the test substance beginning on the sixth or seventh day after ovulation and continuation of treatment for 3 weeks or more. An effective progestogen will delay menstrual bleeding until 2 to 3 days after treatment is discontinued. The delay-of-menses test was subsequently standardized by Swyer and utilized for comparative potency evaluations of progestogens; this test is sometimes referred to as the Swyer-Greenblatt test.

Table 12.5 shows a variety of progestogens that were assayed for progestational potency using the Swyer-Greenblatt test (5,18). The potencies of the progestogens vary considerably, and there is a change in progestational potency when the compounds are combined with estrogen. Norethindrone has a potency similar to that of ethynodiol diacetate but approximately twofold greater than that of norethindrone acetate, medroxyprogesterone

TABLE 12.5. *Postponent of menstruation assays: various progestogens*

Drug	Number of observations	Approximate ED_{50} (mg)
Norethisterone	89	4.25
Norethisterone acetate	51	10.5
Norethynodrel	16	20
Norethynodrel + mestranol (Enovid)	28	5.3
Provera	4	>10
Provera + mestranol	21	22.5
Megestrol acetate	30	>10
Megestrol acetate + mestranol	51	1.8
Ethynodiol diacetate	9	>4
Ethynodiol diacetate + mestranol	32	1.5
Didrogesterone	9	>20
Didrogesterone + mestranol	4	>10

Modified from ref. 5, with permission.

acetate, or megestrol acetate and about fivefold higher than that of norethynodrel. The data also show that there is an increase in progestational activity following the addition of 0.1 mg of mestranol to some of the compounds; the extent of the increase varies. This observation is also evident in Table 12.6, which shows the results of testing the progestational potency of norgestrel with and without mestranol, employing the same delay-of-menses assay as that used to obtain the data in Table 12.5. The potency of norgestrel, which was similar to that of norethindrone (Table 12.5), increased by about 30-fold when 0.1 mg of mestranol was added to it. In contrast, the potency of norethynodrel increased by only fourfold when the same dose of mestranol was added (Table 12.5).

Although the Swyer-Greenblatt test is an important pharmacologic method for comparing the potency of progestogens on human endometrium, there are reservations about

the test. It has been pointed out that the data obtained in Tables 12.5 and 12.6 are not consistent with expected findings based on doses of progestogens employed in minipills, which contain no estrogen (5). On that basis, it is generally accepted that the progestational potency of norgestrel is about 10 times that of norethindrone. In contrast, the data just presented show that the progestational potencies of those two compounds are essentially the same.

Potency of orally administered progestins in women has also been studied by analyzing the biochemical and morphologic features of endometria from estrogen-primed postmenopausal women (19,20). Postmenopausal women were treated with 0.65 or 1.25 mg of conjugated equine estrogen daily each month for at least 3 months, and the effects of at least three doses of each several orally administered progestogens (norgestrel, norethindrone, medroxyprogesterone acetate, and progesterone) were assessed. The progestogens were administered on the last 6 to 12 days of monthly treatment. Curettage was performed after 6 days of progestogen treatment, when endometrial responses are maximal. The endometria were homogenized and analyzed for soluble and nuclear estradiol receptors, isocitric and estradiol dehydrogenases, protein, and DNA. Progestogen effects on epithelial morphologic features were calculated by summing up the appearances of secretory histologic features, subnuclear glycogen, giant mitochondria, and the nuclear channel system. The results show that when the progestogen effects are related to a standardized value for norethindrone, levonorgestrel is about eight times more potent than norethindrone, whereas medroxyprogesterone acetate and progesterone exhibit 9% and 0.2% of the activity of norethindrone, respectively.

In 1985, the potencies of progestogens were compared on the basis of available human data in the literature obtained from studies in which the effect of progestogens on the delay of menses, subnuclear vacuolization, and glycogen deposition, as well as on lipids and lipoproteins,

TABLE 12.6. *Postponement of menstruation assay on norgestrel*

Dose (mg)	Number of subjects	Response Positive	Response Negative	% positive
8	1	1	0	100
4	11	5	6	45
2	13	4	9	31
1	3	1	2	33
		ED_{50} 4 mg (number of observations 28)		
2 + 0.1 mestranol	10	10	0	100
1 + 0.1 mestranol	14	14	0	100
0.5 + 0.1 mestranol	13	11	2	85
0.25 + 0.1 mestranol	17	13	4	76.5
0.2 + 0.1 mestranol	2	2	0	—
0.125 + 0.1 mestranol	11	6	5	55
0.1 + 0.1 mestranol	3	0	3	0
		ED_{50} 0.125 mg (number of observations 70)		

From ref. 5, with permission.

was assessed (21). In the review of those data, the objective was to examine the scientific evidence, which generally supported the view that the potency of the progestogens used in oral contraceptive formulations marketed in the United States were similar. The conclusion of the review was that norethindrone, norenthindrone acetate, and ethynodiol diacetate are approximately equivalent in potency, whereas norgestrel and its biologically active enantiomer, levonorgestrel, are about five to ten and ten to 20 times as potent as norethindrone, respectively.

Androgenic Potency of Progestogens

The androgenic potency of a variety of progestogens has been estimated by use of tests analogous to those described for progestational activity. Examples of some these tests follow.

Androgen Receptor Binding Tests

The cytosol of rat prostate cells has a receptor that binds to androgens and has been incubated with different progestational agents to determine their ability to displace tritiated R1881 (17β-hydroxy-17-methylestra-4,9, 11-trien-3-one, methyltrienolone) from the androgen receptor. In one study (22) it was shown that, after a 15- to 17-hours incubation at 0°C, levonorgestrel, norethindrone, and medroxyprogesterone acetate had 43%, 23%, and 23% of the displacing ability of testosterone, respectively, and that this inhibition was roughly parallel to the inhibitory effect of these progestogens on luteinizing hormone (LH) release. In contrast, the displacing ability of megestrol acetate and cyproterone actate was 5% to 7.5% relative to testosterone activity, whereas norethynodrel and ethynodiol diacetate had insignificant inhibitory effect. In another study (9), various test substances were allowed to compete with [3H]R1881 for binding to androgen receptors in cytosols of prostates from castrated rats (4-hour incubation at 4°C); unlabeled R1881 was used as the reference steroid. Gestodene had the highest RBA (100%), followed by levonorgestrel (45%) and 3-ketodesogestrel (22%). Medroxyprogesterone acetate and cyproterone acetate had considerably lower RBAs (5% and 6%, respectively), whereas norgestimate had an insignificant affinity for the androgen receptor.

Bioassays

The growth response of the ventral prostate of young castrated rats to treatment with different test compounds has been utilized in bioassays to assess androgenicity. Comparison of prostatic growth effects of various progestogens relative to testosterone showed that the adrogenic potency of levonorgestrel was twice that of norgestrel and approximately tenfold and 15-fold greater than that of norethindrone and ethynodiol diacetate, respectively (Table 12.7) (8). Norethynodrel, nedroxy-

TABLE 12.7. Prostalic growth effects of various progestagens

Compound	Prostalic growth, relative potency
Testosterone	100
Levonorgestrel	15.0
Norgestrel	7.5
Norethindrone	1.6
Ethynodiol diacetate	1.0
Norethynodrel	I
Medroxyprogestrone acetate	I
Chlormadinone acetate	I
Megestrol acetate	I
Progestrone	

I, inactive.
From ref. 8, with permission.

progesterone acetate, chlormadinone acetate, megestrol acetate, and progesterone showed no androgenic activity.

Clinical Tests

Progestogens that are closely related to testosterone structurally have the potential of exhibiting androgenic side effects. However, several problems are encountered when attempts are made to evaluate the androgenic effect of 19-nortestosterone derivatives clinically (23). First, there is evidence that in addition to having potential androgenic properties, these progestogens may also have antiandrogenic, estrogenic, and antiestrogenic effects. Second, when combined oral contraceptive formulations are tested, the counterbalancing effect of the synthetic estrogen, ethinylestradiol (EE2) or mestranol, has to be considered. Furthermore, the balance between androgenic and estrogenic side effects is subject to individual variablility. Therefore, clinical effects of progestogens structurally related to testosterone are influenced by individual patient variability in sex steroid metabolism as well as sensitivity of skin to androgenic and/or skin stimuli. Because of individual variation in sensitivity, assessment of androgenic skin changes (e.g., hirsutism, sebum production, acne) has to be carried out in carefully randomized, controlled double-blind studies.

It has been suggested that the best way to assess overall clinical androgenicity may be to measure changes in a parameter that can be altered by both androgen and estrogen (23). One of the best markers of this effect in blood is the measurement of sex hormone-binding globulin (SHBG). The SHBG level is raised by estrogen and lowered by androgen.

The utility of SHBG as a marker of androgen/estrogen balance is further illustrated in Tables 12.8 and 12.9. On the basis of differences in androgenic potency observed between norgestrel and norethindrone relative to their effects on prostatic growth in rats (Table 12.7), one would predict that doses of 75 µg of norgestrel and 350 µg of

TABLE 12.8. *SHBG as a marker of androgen/estrogen balance (concentrations)*

Oral contraceptive[a]	Concentration (nmol)	
	Pretreatment	Posttreatment
NET-A 1 mg + EE 20 μg	36 ± 15	62 ± 22[b]
NET-A 1 mg + EE 50 μg	39 ± 15	81 ± 36[b]
NET 350 μg	38 ± 20	27 ± 11
DL-NG 75 μg	44 ± 20	24 ± 11[b]
NET 0.4 mg + EE 35 μg	34 ± 8	126 ± 20[c]
DL-NG 0.3 mg + EE 30 μg	51 ± 8	63 ± 8[d]

[a]SHBG, sex hormone-binding globulin; NET-A, norethindrone acetate; EE, ethinyl estradiol; NET, norethindrone; DL-NG norgestrel.
[b]$p < 0.001$.
[c]$p < 0.004$.
[d]NS, not significant.
From ref. 23, with permission.

norethindrone have approximately equal androgenic potencies. Table 12.8 shows that their effects on decreasing circulating of SHGB are similar, resulting in reduced SHGB levels of 24 ± 11 nM and 27 ± 11 nM, respectively. Increasing the EE$_2$ dose from 20 to 50 μg in combination with a constant dose (1 mg) of norethindrone acetate increases SHBG levels, demonstrating the estrogenic influence on SHBG. Additionally, using similar doses of EE$_2$ (30 μg and 35 μg) in combination with similar doses of norgestrel (0.3 μg) and norethindrone (0.4 mg) results in no significant changes in SHGB levels with the norgestrel formulation (27% increase) but a dramatic 270% increase with the norethindrone formulation (Table 12.9). This finding illustrates the profound androgenic potency difference between norgestrel and norethindrone.

Because SHBG binds with high affinity to testosterone, one important consequence of the lower circulating SHBG levels attained by levonorgestrel compared to norethindrone is that the bioavailable (non-SHBG-bound) fraction of circulating testosterone becomes larger. This fraction is considered to be readily available for either metabolism or biologic action in target tissues. Although levonorgestrel gives rise to a larger

TABLE 12.9. *SHBG as a marker of androgen/estrogen balance*

Oral contraceptive[a]	Change (%)
NET 350 μg	30 ↓
DL NG 75 mg	45 ↓
NET-A 1 mg + EE 20 μg	72 ↓
NET-A 1 mg + EE 50 μg	108 ↓
NET 0.4 mg + EE 35 μg	270 ↓
DL NG 0.3 mg + EE 30 μg	23 ↓

[a]SHBG, sex hormone-binding globulin; NET, norethindrone; DL-NG, norgestrol; NET-A, norethindrone acetate; EE, ethinyl estradiol.
From ref. 23, with permission.

bioavailable testosterone fraction than norethindrone, our findings show a suppressive effect of levonorgestrel on ovarian androgen production greater than that of norethindrone (24).

The greater suppressive effect of levonorgestrel on ovarian androgen production results in lower circulating testosterone levels and consequently a lower bioavailable testosterone concentration, which approximates that obtained with norethindrone. This is evident in data from our study (24), in which a total of 41 healthy cycling women were randomized to receive orally either 1,000 μg of norethindrone acetate combined with 20 μg of ethinylestradiol, or 100 μg of levonorgestrel in combination with 20 μg of ethinylestradiol. After 3 months of treatment, the group receiving norethindrone acetate/ethinylestradiol ($n = 20$) showed a 234% increase from baseline in serum SHBG levels as compared to 100% in the levonorgestrel/ethinylestradiol group ($n = 21$). In contrast, total testosterone levels were reduced (-21%) only by the latter group. Despite these differences, bioavailable testosterone was similarly and significantly reduced by both groups. Thus, with norethindrone acetate, the nonsignificant reduction of the ovarian androgen marker, total testosterone, required a greater increase in SHBG to achieve similar significant reduction in bioavailable testosterone as with levonorgestrel.

In the study just described, the adrenal androgen marker DHEAS and the peripheral androgen markers dihydrotestosterone and 3α–androstanediol glucuronide were each similarly and significantly reduced from baseline in both groups. On average, DHEAS and dihydrotestosterone were reduced by 20%, whereas 3α-androstanediol glucuronide, which has been shown to be an excellent marker of 5α-reductase activity and peripheral androgen action, was reduced by as much as 37%. These data demonstrate that both levonorgestrel and norethindrone in combination with ethinylestradiol have profound antiandrogenic effects with respect to androgen production when administered orally.

An important antiandrogenic effect of combined oral contraceptives is observed clinically in women who show improvement in hirsutism and acne. Studies show that within the cells of pilosebaceous units in skin, circulating androstenedione and testosterone are converted, via the enzyme 5α-reductase, to dihydrotestosterone, which is a markedly more potent androgen than testosterone. In patients with hirsutism and acne, there is increased conversion of testosterone to dihydrotestosterone, compared with nonhirsute women. However, studies show that contraceptive progestogens inhibit 5α-reductase activity. Our *in vitro* study demonstrated 50% to 60% inhibition of dihydrotestosterone formation from testosterone in genital skin by either levonorgestrel or norethindrone. These findings not only suggest a mechanism by which combination oral contraceptives may achieve their observed improvements in hair growth and acne but also demonstrate their profound antiandrogenic effects.

Estrogenic Potency of Progestogens

It is known that some progestogens exhibit estrogenic effects (5,8). The binding affinity of a variety of progestogens for the uterine estrogen receptors has been investigated using incubation procedures similar to those described for the progesterone receptor and androgen receptor assays. Weak displacement of tritiated estradiol from rabbit uterine cytosol receptors has been demonstrated by norethindrone, norethynodrel, and ethynodiol diacetate but not by levonorgestrel, medroxyprogesterone acetate, and megestrol acetate (Table 12.10) (8). In a similar study (24), relative binding affinities of a number of different progestogens were determined for binding to human estrogen receptors. The results showed no affinity of the estrogen receptor for gestodene, levonorgestrel, medroxyprogesterone acetate, or cyproterone acetate (RBAs < 0.1%).

The estrogenicity of norethindrone, norethynodrel, and ethynodiol diacetate has also been demonstrated in bioassays (Table 12.10) (8). Both norethynodrel and ethynodiol diacetate have demonstrated estrogenic effects in short-term assays for vaginal cornification in rats (Allen-Doisy vaginal smear test). In contrast, norethindrone causes vaginal changes in the rat only when long-term protocols involving the oral route of administration are used (25). It is not effective by parenteral routes of administration.

Clinical evaluation of estrogenicity, as measured by actions on the cervix and changes in vaginal cytology, shows that the estrogenic effects of norethynodrel and ethynodiol diacetate in humans parallel those in the rat (Table 12.10) (8). However, there is no clear-cut evidence that norethindrone exhibits an estrogenic effect clinically.

PHARMACOKINETICS OF PROGESTOGENS

Progesterone

When progesterone is administered orally in a crystalline form, it is poorly absorbed. However, when the particle size of crystalline progesterone is decreased by the process of micronization, the oral absorption of progesterone is increased. Micronization gives rise to a greater surface area of the compound, allowing it to be dissolved in the aqueous medium of the intestine.

In one study, circulating levels of progesterone were measured in five postmenopausal women following oral ingestion of 100 mg of the micronized steroid in the morning and 200 mg in the evening for five consecutive days (26). There was wide intersubject variation in C_{max} and t_{max} after administration of the morning and evening doses. The peak progesterone levels after the morning dose ranged from approximately 4 to 12 ng/mL and were achieved from 1 to 4 hours. After the evening dose, the levels ranged from approximately 8 to 20 ng/mL and were attained from 2 to 8 hours after dosing.

Progesterone circulates primarily in a bound form (27) and is extensively metabolized (28). Approximately 20% of the circulating progesterone is bound to corticosteroid-binding globulin (CBG), but the majority is bound to albumin. Progesterone is metabolized primarily to a variety of reduced metabolites, which include 5α-pregnanedione, 5α-pregnanedione, four different pregnanolone isomers, and eight different pregnanediol isomers. The pregnanolones and pregnanediols undergo conjugation, forming pregnanolone and pregnanediol sulfates and glucuronides, of which 5α-pregnane-3α,20α-diol-3-glucuronide is quantitatively the most important. Levels of this metabolite found in large amounts in urine during the lateral phase of the menstrual cycle and in pregnancy and correlates highly with circulating progesterone concentrations.

Progesterone also undergoes some hydroxylation. It has been shown recently that after progesterone is adminis-

TABLE 12.10. *Estrogenic effects of progestrones*

Compound	Binding constant for estrogen receptor[a]	Allen-Doisy vaginal smear (rat)[a,b]	Long-term vaginal changes (rat)[a,c]	Human effects[a]
Progestrone	I	I	I	I
Megestrol acetate	I	I	I	I
Medroxyprogesterone acetate	I	I	I	
D-Norgestrel (Levonorgestrel)	I	I	I	I
Norethindrone	6×10^{-7}	I	0.3%	I
Norethynodrel	2.8×10^{-9}	7%	2.1%	A
Ethynodiol diacetate	9.9×10^{-8}	4%	0.4%	A

[a]A, active; I, inactive.
[b]Figures express potency relative to estrone.
[c]Figures represent potency relative to ethinyl estradiol, 100%; all by oral route.
From ref. 8, with permission.

tered orally, it is hydroxylated at carbon-21 to a significant extent, forming deoxycorticosterone (DOC) (29). When equal doses of progesterone are given both orally and intramuscularly, the ratio of DOC to progesterone is much higher by the oral route despite a threefold increase in serum levels of progesterone by the intramuscular route.

Medroxyprogesterone Acetate

There is little information about the pharmacokinetics of low doses of medroxyprogesterone acetate. In one of our studies (30), 10 mg of this compound was administered orally to three women daily for five continuous days. A considerable amount of variation in serum medroxyprogesterone acetate levels was observed among the subjects (Fig. 12.6). The mean peak levels ranged

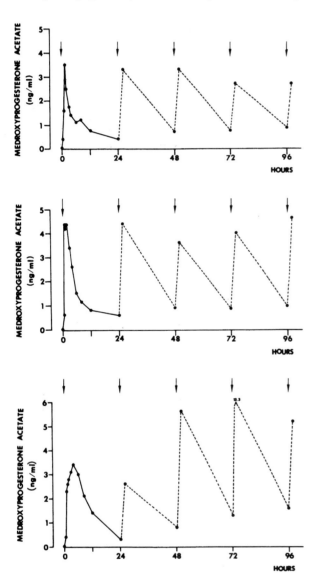

FIG. 12.6. Serum concentrations of medroxyprogesterone acetate (MPA) before and 0.5, 1, 1.5, 2, 3, 4, 6, 8, 12, and 24 hours after an initial oral dose of 10 mg of MPA, and before and 2 hours following four subsequent oral doses (10 mg) of MPA (indicated by arrows) taken by three healthy women for five consecutive days. (From ref. 31, with permission.)

from 3 to 5 ng/mL and were attained between 1 and 4 hours. The levels then fell and were approximately 0.5 ng/mL at 24 hours after dosing. In the circulation, over 90% of medroxyprogesterone acetate is bound nonspecifically to albumin (31). Its metabolic clearance rate is approximately 21 L/day/kg (32), its volume of distribution is 20 L, and the half-life of an oral dose (10 mg) of the compound is 24 hours (33). The compound undergoes ring-A reduction, hydroxylation (primarily at carbon-6 and 20), and conjugation (primarily glucuronidation) (31). The acetate group apparently remains intact.

Norethindrone

Plasma norethindrone level versus time profiles for doses of 1,000, 500, and 300 μg of norethindrone administered orally to normal cycling women are shown in Fig. 12.7 (34,35). The highest dose of norethindrone was administered in combination with 120 μg of ethinylestradiol, whereas the other two doses were given without estrogen. A dose response was obtained with all three formulations. Mean peak norethindrone levels of approximately 16, 6, and 4 ng/mL were attained with the 1,000-, 500-, and 300-μg doses of norethindrone, respectively, within 1 to 2 hours following the dosing. Thereafter, all three levels fell precipitously at first and then declined gradually until 24 hours. At that a time, the mean levels were approximately 0.5 ng/mL or less. The areas under the plasma norethindrone level-time curves (AUCs) were calculated and shown to be proportional to the administered dose.

Most of the information about the pharmacokinetics of norethindrone is based on a study (36) in which norethindrone acetate in combination with 50 μg of ethinylestradiol was administered as a single dose orally and intravenously to a group of six women. The results show that the absolute bioavailability ranged from 47% to 73% (mean ± standard deviation, 64 ± 10%). In the same study it was also shown that after the intravenous dose the mean (± standard deviation) clearance, apparent volume of distribution, and half-life of elimination were, respectively, 355 ± 68 mL/hr/kg (range 260 to 422 mL/hr/kg), 3.6 ± 2.0 L/kg (range 2.09 to 6.90 L/kg), and 8.0 ± 3.3 hours (range 5.2 to 12.8 hours). The values for these parameters were not significantly different from the corresponding values obtained after the oral dosing.

It has been shown that following the administration of norethindrone to women ($n = 10$), more than 95% of circulating norethindrone is bound to SHBG and albumin (37). The following distribution of norethindrone in serum (mean ± standard deviation) was found: SHBG-bound, 35.5 ± 13.6%; albumin-bound, 60.8 ± 12.9%; unbound, 3.7 ± 0.9%.

The metabolism of norethindrone occurs primarily by ring-A reduction, followed by conjugation with sulfuric and glucuronic acids (38). A number of investigators have attempted to demonstrate the presence of ethinylestradiol

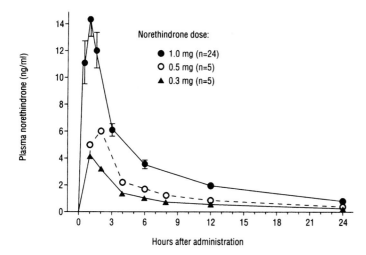

FIG. 12.7. Plasma norethindrone level-time curves for different doses of norethindrone administered orally to women. (From ref. 2, with permission.)

in the circulation following administration of commonly prescribed doses of norethindrone (1 mg or less) (38). However, there is no rigorous evidence to support such a finding. One study utilized a double-isotope technique to measure the conversion of norethindrone to ethinylestradiol in two perimenopausal women with breast cancer *in vivo* (39). The transfer constants for this conversion were 2.26% and 2.34% when calculated for blood and 2.27% and 0.38% when calculated for urine. Although the investigators of this study concluded that a small but significant proportion of norethindrone is converted to ethinylestradiol *in vivo,* it should be noted that the same conclusion may not apply to normal women.

More recently, the *in vivo* conversion of norethindrone and norethindrone acetate to ethinylestradiol was studied in postmenopausal women (40). The results show that the mean (± standard deviation) conversion ratio of norethindrone acetate to ethinylestradiol was 0.7 ± 0.2% and 1.0 ± 0.4% at doses of 5 and 10 mg, respectively. This corresponded to an oral dose equivalent of about 6 μg ethinylestradiol per milligram of norethindrone acetate. Similarly, for norethindrone, a conversion ratio of 0.4 ± 0.4% was found at a dose of 5 mg, which corresponded to an oral dose equivalent of about 4 μg ethinlyestradiol per milligram of norethindrone. On the basis of these data, it was estimated that lower doses (0.5 to 2.5 mg) of norethindrone commonly prescribed in combined oral contraceptives would add between 2 and 10 μg of ethinylestradiol to the existing ethinylestradiol dose. Similarly, the calculation for norethindrone acetate revealed that the metabolic conversion of this progestogen would increase the total dose of ethinylestradiol from 50 to 56 μg per pill. However, it should be realized that the estimations for the lower doses of norethindrone and norethindrone acetate were extrapolated from high doses of these progestogens, which were not combined with ethinylestradiol and which were administered to postmenopausal women.

On the basis of the studies carried out to date, it appears that insignificant amounts of ethinylestradiol are found in the circulation or in urine following oral administration of norethindrone or norethindrone acetate (1 mg or less) to normal women. However, whether this conversion exists at a local level in specific tissues or whether there is accumulation of these progestogens in tissues remains to be established.

Derivatives of Norethindrone

Very little is known about the pharmacokinetics of the progestogens structurally related to norethindrone. Most of the norethindrone derivatives are converted to the parent compound. Thus, norethindrone acetate and ethynodiol diacetate undergo rapid hydrolysis and are transformed to norethindrone and its metabolites. There is some evidence that lynestrenol may undergo hydroxylation at carbon-3 with subsequent oxidation of the hydroxyl group, thereby forming the parent compound. Although there is no convincing evidence for the *in vivo* transformation of norethynodrel to norethindrone, data from receptor binding tests and bioassays suggest that norethynodrel is also a prodrug.

Levonorgestrel

There has been a great deal of confusion about the nomenclature of norgestrel (38). Norgestrel is synthesized chemically, and the final product consists of a racemic mixture that can be resolved into its optically active dextrorotatory and levorotatory enantiomers. The dextrorotatory and levorotatory isomers are assigned the prefixes (+) or (D) and (−) or (L), respectively. It has been shown that (−)-norgestrel has the same stereochemistry as D-glyceraldehyde and belongs to the D-steroid group. Similarly, (+)-norgestrel belongs to the L-steroid group (41,42). It has been shown that naturally occurring steroids generally belong to the D-series and are dextrorotatory, on the basis of their absolute stereochemical configuration rotation, respectively. Although some synthetic progestogens belong to the same category as the naturally occurring ones, others such as the biologically active form of norgestrel belong to the D-series but are levorotatory. For this reason, the World Health Organization selected the name levnorgestrel for the biologically active enantiomer of norgestrel [D-(−)-norgestrel]. The name norgestrel for the racemic mixture of the compound [DL-(±)-norgestrel] remained the same. Although no name was given to the inactive dextrorotatory enantiomer [L-(−)-norgestrel], this compound is often referred to as dextronorgestrel.

As depicted in Fig. 12.8, dose-response curves are obtained when doses of 250, 150, and 75 μg of levonorgestrel are administered orally to normal cycling women (43–45). The 250-μg dose was administered in the form of the racemic mixture of norgestrel, that is, DL-(±)-norgestrel (500 μg). Also, all three levonorgestrel doses were given in combination with 30 to 50 μg of ethinylestradiol. Mean peak levels of approximately 6.0, 3.5, and 2.5 ng/mL were attained at 1 to 3 hours with the 250-, 150-, and 75-μg doses, respectively. At 24 hours, the mean levonorgestrel level was 1 to 2 ng/mL with the highest dose and less than 0.5 ng/mL with the other two doses.

Pharmacokinetic data have been obtained for the 150- and 75-μg doses of levonorgestrel (44,45) but are sparse for the 250-μg dose. The mean absolute bioavailability of levonorgestrel has been generally accepted to be virtually 100%. However, it must be realized that this conclusion is based on only two studies. In one of the studies (46), absolute bioavailabilities were determined for the 250- and 150-μg doses of levonorgestrel, each of which was administered in combination with ethinylestradiol to only five women. The absolute bioavailability for the 250-μg dose of levonorgestrel ranged from 72% to 125% (mean ± standard deviation, 99 ± 20%), and for the 150-μg dose the range was 65% to 108% (mean ± standard deviation, 89 ± 13%). Sixty percent of the subjects who received the

250-μg dose of levonorgestrel had absolute bioavailabilities substantially greater than 100%. It is not clear why the areas under the curves (AUCs) in those subjects were greater by the oral route compared to the parenteral route, unless there were methodologic problems in the study. Nevertheless, it is in correct to determine a mean absolute bioavailability using those values. In a second study (47), the absolute bioavailability of levonorgestrel was investigated using a 30-μg dose of the drug in three women; values of 80%, 83%, and 97% were obtained.

On the basis of the very limited data on the bioavailability of levonorgestrel, it appears that, in general, this drug is not subject to an appreciable first-pass effect. However, as many as 20% of women receiving the 150- or 250-μg dose of levonorgestrel may undergo a substantial first-pass effect (absolute bioavailability less than 75%).

Other pharmacokinetic parameters of levonorgestrel have been calculated following either intravenous or oral dosing. In the same study (46) in which the absolute bioavailabilities of levonorgestrel were determined for the 150- and 250-μg doses, the mean (± standard deviation) clearance, apparent volume of distribution, and half-life of elimination were found to be 105 ± 36 and 113 ± 31 mL/hr/kg, 1.9 ± 0.7 and 1.6 ± 0.7 L/kg, and 13.2 ± 6.0 and 9.9 ± 0.7 hours, for these doses, respectively, when administered intravenously. The half-life of elimination following oral dosing was similar to the values obtained after intravenous dosing.

The following distribution of levonorgestrel in serum (mean ± standard deviation) has been reported: SHBG-bound, 47.5 ± 11.7%; albumin-bound, 50.0 ± 11.0%; unbound, 2.5 ± 0.7% (37).

Norgestimate

There has been considerable controversy about whether or not norgestimate is a prodrug. Support for the view that norgestimate is a prodrug is based on the identification of levonorgestrel and four of its metabolites in urine following oral administration of radiolabeled norgestimate to four women (48). Other metabolites were isolated but were not characterized. Although these metabolites were not identified, some investigators speculate that they may be closely related in structure to norgestimate.

Evidence has been presented to support the view that norgestimate is not a prodrug. Dramatic pharmacologic differences between norgestimate and levonorgestrel were reported with respect to their effects on lipid metabolism and their binding to SHBG in women (49). However, these findings were obtained in a study in which the progestogens were administered in combination with ethinylestradiol and, in addition, slightly different doses of the estrogen were used.

Another argument presented against the concept that norgestimate is a prodrug comes from progesterone receptor binding studies (11). As mentioned earlier, it was

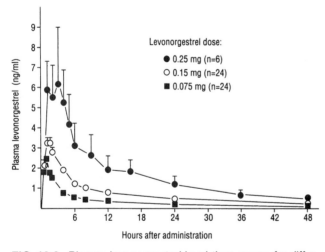

FIG. 12.8. Plasma levonorgestrel level-time curves for different doses of levonorgestrel administered orally to women. (From ref. 2, with permission.)

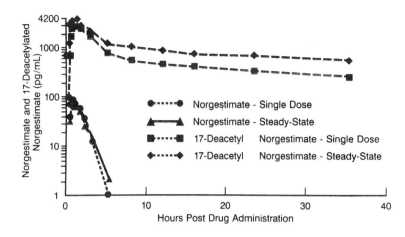

FIG. 12.9. Mean serum level of norgestimate and levonorgestrel-3-oxime after single and multiple oral dose administration of 360 μg of norgestimate in combination with 70 μg of ethinylestradiol to ten women. (From ref. 45, with permission.)

shown that the relative binding affinities (RBAs) of norgestimate and levonorgestrel-3-oxime (deacetylated norgestimate) for estrogen-primed rabbit uterine progesterone are similar to the RBA of progesterone for the same receptors. However, when human (instead of rabbit) myometrial tissue was used to study binding affinities of different progestogens to the progesterone receptors, the results showed that norgestimate binds insignificantly to the receptors (RBA, 0.8%), whereas levonorgestrel-17-acetate (deoximated norgestimate) binds substantially to the same receptors (RBA, 110%; RBA for levonorgestrel, 250%) (10). Although levonorgestrel-17-acetate shows substantial binding to the human uterine receptors *in vitro,* the levels of this metabolite in the circulation are barely detectable.

Because norgestimate is a prodrug that is metabolized to at least three major metabolites, its pharmacokinetics is difficult to study. One study (50) showed that mean peak serum levels of norgestimate were only about 100 pg/mL, following either single-dose or multiple-dose (daily for 1 week) administration of 360 μg of this progestogen in combination with 70 μg of ethinylestradiol to a group of 10 women (Fig. 12.9). It was also shown that serum levels of the deacetylated metabolite of norgestimate, levonorgestrel-3-oxime, were very high. Mean peak values of the metabolite were greater than 4 ng/mL after about 1 hour and remained elevated as long as 36 hours after treatment. Levonorgestrel levels were not measured in this study.

Desogestrel

It is well established that desogestrel is a prodrug and that its progestational action is mediated through one of its metabolites, namely, 3-ketodesogestrel. Initial evidence for this finding came from a study in which a single 2.5-mg dose of desogestrel was administered to one woman and a peak circulating level of 3-ketodesogestrel, 12.7 ng/mL, was attained within 1.5 hours after treatment (52). In contrast, the peak level of desogestrel was only

about 0.7 ng/mL. This finding was supported by data showing that [³H]3-ketodesogestrel was a major metabolite resulting from incubation of human liver homogenates with [³H]desogestrel (53). Further evidence that desogestrel acts via 3-ketodesogestrel came from a study in which 10 women received 150 μg of desogestrel in combination with 30 μg of ethinylestradiol, and another 10 women received 150 μg of 3-ketodesogestrel combined with 30 μg of ethinylestradiol (54,55). Each combination was ingested as a single dose. Large intersubject variability in serum levels of 3-ketodesogestrel was found in both groups of women (Fig. 12.10). However, no statistical difference was observed between the two groups with respect to the areas under the serum level-time curves of serum 3-ketodesogestrel.

The bioavailability of desogestrel was determined in a crossover study in which nine women received an oral dose of 150 μg of desogestrel in combination with 30 μg of ethinylestradiol, and an intravenous dose of 150 μg 3-ketodesogestrel combined with 30 μg of ethinylestradiol (56). Mean plasma levels of 3-ketodesogestrel were

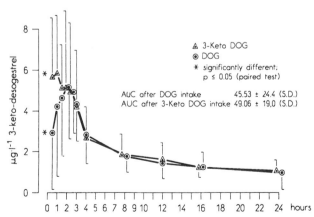

FIG. 12.10. Mean serum levels (± standard deviation) of 3-ketodesogestrel following oral administration of 150 μg of desogestrel or 150 μg of 3-ketodesogestrel in combination with 30 μg of ethinyl estradiol (EE₂) to ten women. (From ref. 51, with permission.)

higher following the intravenous dose, and large inter-subject variability was observed with both routes of administration.

The mean (± standard deviation) absolute bioavailability of 3-ketodesogestrel was 76 ± 22%. In a subsequent study (57), the mean (± standard deviation) absolute bioavailability of the same progestogen was reported to be 62 ± 7%. In the former study (56), the mean (± standard deviation) clearance of 3-ketodesogestrel following administration of 3-ketodesogestrel following administration of 3-ketodesogestrel intravenously and of desogestrel orally was 8.7 ± 2.9 and 12.1 ± 4.7 L/hr, respectively. Although the apparent volume of distribution of 3-ketodesogestrel was not reported in that study, the data were utilized by others to calculate this parameter; a value of 3.0 ± 1.3 L/kg has been reported (58).

More recently, the pharmacokinetics of 150 µg of desogestrel administered orally in combination with 30 µg of ethinylestradiol were investigated in 25 women (59). A mean C_{max} of 3.69 ± 0.97 ng/mL and a t_{max} of 1.6 ± 0.97 ng/mL were reported. In the same study, a reliable estimate of the elimination half-life of 3-ketodesogestrel was obtained by following its serum levels for up to 72 hours; the mean elimination half-life was 23.8 ± 5.3 hours. This value is approximately twice as high as that reported previously in a study in which blood samples were collected only up to 24 hours after oral or intravenous dosing (56). In most pharmacokinetic studies, blood sampling is carried out only for 24 hours.

Serum levels of 3-ketodesogestrel have also been quantified following multiple dosing with desogestrel (60). A dose of 150 µg of desogestrel in combination with 30 µg of ethinylestradiol was administered to 11 women during 12 continuous treatment cycles. Blood sampling was carried out at frequent intervals on days 1, 10, and 21 cycles 1, 3, 6, and 12. This experimental design was part of a study (61) designed to compare circulating levels of ethinylestradiol following administration of ethinylestradiol with either desogestrel or gestodene. Multiple dosing with desogestrel resulted in large intersubject variability in serum levels of 3-ketodesogestrel. Comparison of the mean serum 3-ketodesogestrel levels measured in the samples on days 1, 10, and 21 showed that the levels were relatively low on day 1 of treatment but rose progressively and were higher on day 21 of treatment in all study cycles except cycle 12.

Increases in 3-ketodesogestrel levels have been attributed to elevated serum levels of SHBG induced by the estrogenic component of the pill. In the study described above (60), the mean serum SHBG levels rose dramatically (131%) between days 1 and 10 of the first cycle but increased by only 10% between days 10 and 21 of the same cycle. On day 1 of subsequent cycles, mean SHBG levels were 84% to 115% higher than the SHBG level on day 1 of the first cycle. Also, in the subsequent cycles, the rise in mean SHBG levels between days 1 and 10 (25% to

54%) was considerably lower than the rise observed in the first cycle, and the rise in mean SHBG levels between days 10 and 21 did not exceed 20%. Mean SHBG levels on day 21 of subsequent cycles were 2.5- to 3.3-fold greater than the level on day 1 of the first cycle.

The following distribution of 3-ketodesogestrel in serum has been reported (mean ± standard deviation): SHBG-bound, 31.6 ± 12.0%; albumin-bound, 65.9 ± 11.9%, unbound, 2.5 ± 0.2% (62).

Gestodene

It has been shown that after oral administration of C-labeled gestodene to three women, the substrate was converted to reduced and hydroxylated metabolites, but a substantial number of the metabolites were not identified (63). Gestodene was not excreted in urine to any significant extent in an unchanged form, and it was not converted to levonorgestrel. It is generally accepted that gestodene is not a prodrug.

Single-dose pharmacokinetics of gestodene after intravenous and oral administration was investigated in six women who received four different treatments: 75 µg of gestodene given intravenously and 50, 75, or 125 µg of gestodene administered orally, each in combination with 30 µg of ethinylestradiol (58). After oral administration of the 50-, 75-, and 125-µg doses, maximum plasma levels of 1.0, 3.6, and 7.0 ng/mL, respectively, were attained between 1.4 and 1.9 hours posttreatment (Fig. 12.11). After the maximum levels were reached, the subsequent levels of gestodene showed two disposition phases with half-lives of approximately 1 hour and 12 to 14 hours for each of the three doses. The mean (± standard deviation) absolute bioavailability was 99 ± 11% (range 86% to 11%) for the 75-µg oral dose of gestodene. A subsequent study (57) showed that the mean (± standard deviation) absolute bioavailability of gestodene was 87 ± 19% (range 64% to 126%), when 75 µg of this drug in combination with 30 µg of ethinylestradiol was administered orally and intravenously to a group of 10 women. Thus, the data from these studies show that gestodene is highly bioavailable.

Both the clearance and volume of distribution of gestodene were calculated from data obtained in the last two studies (57,58). Values (mean ± SD) of 3.4 ± 1.5 L/hr and 0.80 ± 0.53 mL/min/kg were reported for the clearance, and 47.3 ± 24 L and 0.66 ± 0.43 L/kg for the volume of distribution, respectively. The values for the clearance and volume of distribution obtained from the former study (57) can also be expressed on the basis of an estimated average weight of 60 kg per subject; they are 0.94 ± 0.42 mL/min/kg and 0.79 ± 0.40 L/kg, respectively (4).

As mentioned earlier, a multiple-dosing study measured levels of gestodene in serum. The gestodene levels were quantified in samples obtained from 11 women at frequent intervals on days 1, 10, and 21 of several cycles

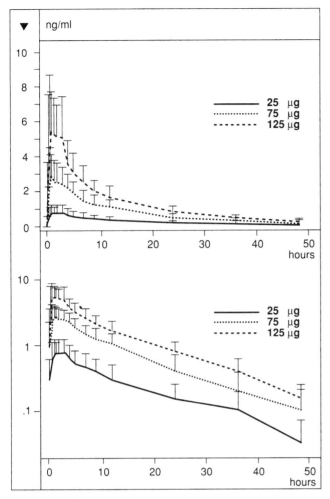

FIG. 12.11. Mean plasma levels (± standard deviation) of gestodene following oral administration of 25, 75, or 125 µg of gestodene in combination with 30 µg of ethinylestradiol to six women. (From ref. 54, with permission.)

during 12 continuous cycles of treatment with 75 µg of gestodene in combination with 30 µg of ethinylestradiol (64). The results showed large intersubject variability in the gestodene levels, a dramatic rise in the mean gestodene levels between day 1 and day 10, and a further rise between day 10 and day 21 in all study cycles. These findings are similar to those obtained when multiple dosing was performed with desogestrel.

The multiple-dosing study with gestodene/ethinylestradiol (64) also showed that the increases in mean SHBG levels during the first cycle and in subsequent cycles of treatment were very similar to the increases observed during long-term treatment with desogestrel/ethinylestradiol. There was a 2.7- to 3.0-fold increase in mean serum SHBG levels on day 21 of each cycle relative to the mean SHBG level on day 1 of the first cycle.

In a recent review, it was pointed out that after administration of 75 µg of gestodene in combination with 30 µg of ethinylestradiol to women, circulating levels of gestodene

are high relative to levels of other progestogens measured after treatment with combined steroid oral contraceptives (65). These elevated levels occur after both single and multiple doses of gestodene/ethinylestradiol. The finding is surprising because the 75-µg dose of gestodene is the lowest of any progestogen in a combination pill.

Two factors may contribute to high circulating levels of gestodene: elevated circulating SHBG levels and a high affinity of SHBG for gestodene. Elevated SHBG results from the estrogenic component of combination pills, which has been shown to increase SHBG as much as threefold from pretreatment levels (64). However, a similar increase in serum SHBG levels is found after treatment with desogestrel/ethinylestradiol, although serum 3-ketodesogestrel levels remain relatively low. It has been reported that, in serum, gestodene is distributed as follows (mean ± standard deviation): SHBG-bound, 75.3 ± 9.1%; albumin-bound, 24.1 ± 9.1%; unbound, 0.6 ± 0.1% (58). Thus, approximately 75% of total circulating gestodene is bound to SHBG, in contrast to 32% for 3-ketodesogestrel, 35% for norethindrone, and 47% for levonorgestrel (58). As a consequence, gestodene has a lower metabolic clearance rate and a greater concentration in the circulation. It is probably the affinity of SHBG for gestodene rather than an increase in circulating SHBG levels that is responsible for elevating the serum levels of this progestogen.

SUMMARY AND CONCLUSIONS

Chemical alteration of the progesterone and testosterone molecules has led to a number of synthetic progestogens that are used therapeutically. Some of these compounds (norethindrone, levonorgestrel, gestodene, medroxyprogesterone acetate, megestrol acetate) bind significantly to the progesterone receptors, and those that do not are prodrugs that exhibit progestational effects only after transformation to a biologically active metabolite. Thus, it is generally accepted that ethynodiol diacetate, norethindrone acetate, lynestrenol, and probably norethynodrel manifest their progestational activity through their parent molecule, namely, norethindrone. Similarly, desogestrel acts via 3-ketodesogestrel, whereas the progestational activity of norgestimate appears to be mediated via its metabolites, specifically deacetylated and deoximated norgestimate, and levonorgestrel.

A variety of qualitative and quantitative tests to establish progestational, androgenic, and estrogenic potencies have been performed. Typically, three categories of tests are utilized; these include (a) receptor binding assays, (b) bioassays, and (c) clinical tests. Problems encountered with these tests are well recognized. A major source of the difficulties is found in the variables associated with each test. Examples of this are evident in the three categories of the tests. In receptor binding tests, a variety of conditions have been used to determine the affinity of test substances for progesterone, androgen, and estrogen receptors. Some of the more obvious methodologic differences among studies pertain to the source (animal) and type of tissue, choice and purity of reference steroid, purity of test substance and radiolabeled steroid, incubation time and temperature, and technique for separating receptor-bound from unbound steroid. Major methodologic deficiencies in bioassays include a lack of standardized protocols and the inability to demonstrate parallelism of dose-response curves obtained for test substances relative to those for standard progestogens. This is complicated by the fact that there are many different measurable effects of progestogens about which a bioassay can be constructed. Depending on which specific biologic parameter is tested, the relative potency of a progestogen may vary greatly. A further complication is found when data obtained from biologic assays utilizing animals are extrapolated to clinical situations without demonstrating the validity of such an extrapolation. As for clinical tests used to compare potencies of progestogens, a major shortcoming in many studies in which a progestogen is tested in combination with an estrogen (usually ethinylestradiol) is the lack of recognition of the influence of the estrogenic component on the biologic action of the progestogen. Thus, it is quite evident from the numerous deficiencies found in tests used to assess progestational potencies that these tests must be standardized if we are to compare the potencies of different progestogens reliably.

Although there are weaknesses in many of the studies in which potencies of progestogens are compared, some reliable data exist and can be used to make some generalizations. On the basis of the relative binding affinities of different progestogens for the human uterine progesterone receptors, it appears that medroxyprogesterone acetate, megestrol acetate, norethindrone, levonorgestrel, 3-ketodesogestrel, and gestodene bind with high affinity to the progesterone receptors. Medroxyprogesterone acetate and megestrol acetate have less progestational activity than the 19-nortestosterone-related progestogens. In the latter group, gestodene has the highest progestational activity, followed by 3-ketodesogestrel and, closely behind, by levonorgestrel. Norethindrone, however, has only about one-tenth or less of the progestational activity of levonorgestrel. As for androgenic activity of progestogens, there has been a great deal of misinterpretation of data. Certain progestogens, such as levonorgestrel, have been labeled as androgenic on the basis of extrapolated data from animals, particularly the rat, to the human, as well as on their effect on lowering SHBG levels. In most instances, androgenicity of progestogens does not take into consideration their overall effects on lowering ovarian, adrenal, and peripheral androgen production or their inhibitory actions on 5α-reductase activity. On this basis, progestogens structurally related to testosterone can be considered antiandrogenic. Finally, as far as estrogenic properties are concerned, there is no evidence demonstrating that any of the progestogens just discussed have an estrogenic effect clinically.

Notwithstanding the widespread use of some porgestogen preparations for many years, our knowledge about the pharmacokinetics of these compounds is very limited and is derived primarily from studies of oral contraceptives in premenopausal women. Pharmacokinetic data are lacking for medroxyprogesterone acetate, megestrol acetate, cyproterone acetate, and norgestimate. Also, very little is known about the pharmacokinetics of progestogens structurally related to norethindrone. Because, in most instances, the derivatives appear to be rapidly converted to norethindrone, the pharmacokinetics of these progestogens is probably similar to that of the parent compound. There are, however, sufficient data pertaining to the pharmacokinetics of norethindrone, levonorgestrel, gestodene, and desogestrel to allow us to make comparisons among the corresponding values obtained for specific pharmacokinetic parameters of these compounds (Table 12.11).

TABLE 12.11. *Summary of the pharmacokinetic parameters and serum-binding distribution of norethindrone (NET), levonorgestrel (LNG), gestodene (GSD), and 3-ketodesogestrel (KDG)*

Parameter[a]	NET (1000 µg)	LNG (150 µg)	GSD (75 µG)	KDG (150 µg)
C_{max}(ng/ml)	15.7	3.4	3.8	2.0[b]
t_{max} (hr)	1.2	1.4	1.7	1.6[b]
F (%)	64[c]	89	99	76
$t_{1/2}\beta$ (hr)	8.0[c]	13.2	10.0	12.6
Cl (ml/hr/kg)	355[c]	105	48	174
V_d(L/kg)	3.6[c]	1.9	0.7	3.0
Binding (%)				
SHBG	35.5	47.5	75.3	31.6
Albumin	60.8	50.0	24.1	65.9
Unbound	3.7	2.5	0.6	2.5

[a]Values for the maximum concentration (C_{max}) and time to reach C_{max} (t_{max})were determined following oral dosing. The absolute bioavailability (F) was calculated after oral and intravenous dosing. The half-life of elimination ($t_{1/2}\beta$), clearance (Cl), and volume of distribution (V_d) were determined after intravenous dosing.
[b]The C_{max} and t_{max} of 3-ketodesogestrel were determined following desogestrel administration.
[c]The value was determined after norethindrone acetate administration.

The pharmacokinetic data presented in Table 12.11 were taken primarily from four different studies (36,46, 56,58), in which the progestogens were administered in combination with EE_2 to women orally and intravenously. Only mean values (without standard errors) are shown because the purpose here is to obtain a gross comparison among the values obtained for each pharmacokinetic parameter. Large intersubject and intrasubject variability in the pharmacokinetics of progestogens is well documented. Comparison of the values in Table 12.11 shows that the maxium plasma level (C_{max}) of norethindrone was approximately 4.3-fold higher than that of either levonorgestrel or gestodene. The C_{max} values of the latter two compounds were almost twice as high as that of 3-ketodesogestrel. The time to reach maximum levels (t_{max}), however, did not vary much among the four progestogens (1.2 to 1.7 hours). The higher C_{max} of norethindrone is consistent with the greater administered norethindrone dose (1,000 µg), which was about sevenfold higher than that (150 µg) of levonorgestrel and desogestrel. Although only 75 µg of gestodene was administered, compared to twice that of levonorgestrel and desogestrel, the C_{max} value of gestodene was higher than that of the latter two progestogens. This finding is consistent with the very high affinity of SHBG for gestodene. The data in Table 12.11 also show that gestodene and, to a lesser extent, levonorgestrel are 15% to 25% less bioavailable than either gestodene or levonogestrel, whereas norethindrone is considerably less bioavailable.

Of the four progestogens in Table 12.11, norethindrone had the lowest half-life and highest clearance and volume of distribution. The half-lives of levonorgestrel and 3-ketodesogestrel were similar and highest; the half-life of gestodene was a little lower. A higher half-life of gestodene was anticipated because it binds with such high affinity to SHBG. However, the clearance and volume of distribution of gestodene were very low.

Table 12.11 also shows the binding distribution of each progestogen in serum (37,62). After getsodene, the highest binding to SHBG was obtained with levonorgestrel, and this was followed by norethindrone and 3-ketodesogestrel, which had similar bindings. The unbound progestogen fractions ranged between 0.6% and 3.7%.

Obviously we know very little about the pharmacokinetics of progestogens. Not only are more studies required, but there is also a need for studies with better experimental designs. In addition, it is important to gain knowledge about the effect of the estrogenic component of combined oral contraceptives on progestogen pharmacokinetics. Furthermore, information is lacking on the pharmacokinetics of progestogens administered for prolonged periods of time. Much more research is required to obtain a better understanding of the bioequivalence and effectiveness of progestogens so that patients can be treated efficiently with these drugs.

REFERENCES

1. Henzl MR. Contraceptive hormones and their clinical use. In: Yen SSC, Jaffe RE, eds. *Reproductive endocrinology, physiology, pathophysiology, and clinical management.* Philadelphia: WB Saunders, 1986:643–682.
2. Stanczyk FZ. Pharmacokinetics of progestogens. *Int Proc J* 1989;1:11–20.
3. Stanczyk FZ. Introduction: Structure–function relationships, metabolism, pharmacokinetics and potency of progestins. *Drugs Today* 1996;32(Suppl H):1–14.
4. Stanczyk FZ. Pharmacokinetics of the new progestogens and influence of ge stodene and desogestrel on ethinylestradiol metabolism. *Contraception* 1997:55: 273–282.
5. Edgren RA, Sturtevant FM. Potencies of oral contraceptives. *Am J Obstet Gynecol* 1976;125;1029–1038.
6. Edgren RA. Progestational potency of oral contraceptives: a polemic. *Int J Fertil* 1978;23:162–169.
7. Edgren RA. Relative potencies of oral contraceptives. In: Moghissi KS, ed. *Controversies to contraception.* Baltimore: Williams & Wilkins, 1979:1–19.
8. Edgren RA. Progestogens. In: Givens JR, ed. *Clinical use of sex steroids.* Chicago: Year Book Medical Publishers, 1980:1–29.
9. Juchem M, Pollow K. Binding of oral contraceptive progestogens to serum proteins and cytoplasmic receptor. *Am J Obstet Gynecol* 1990;163:2171–2183.
10. Juchem M, Pollow K, Elger W, Hoffman G, Moebus V. Receptor binding of norgestimate—a new orally active synthetic progestational compound. *Contraception* 1993;47:283–294.
11. Phillips A, Demarest DW, Hahn F, Wong F, McGuire JL. Progestational and androgenic receptor binding affinities and *in vivo* activities of norgestimate and other progestins. *Contraception* 1990;41:399–410.
12. McPhail MK. The assay of progestin. *J Physiol* 1934;83:145–156.
13. Edgren RA, Jones RC, Peterson DL. A biological classification of progestational agents. *Fertil Steril* 1967;18:238–256.
14. Elger W, Steinbeck H, Schillinger E. Endocrine–pharmacological profile of gestodene. In: Elstein M, ed. *Gestodene, development of a new gestodene-containing low-dose oral contraception.* London: Parthenon Publishers, 1988:19–33.
15. McGinty DA, Anderson CP, McCullough NB. Effect of local application of progester one on the rabbit uterus. *Endocrinology* 1939;24:829–832.
16. Edgren RA, Peterson DL. Delay of parturition in rats by various progestational steroids. *Proc Soc Exp Biol Med* 1966;123:867–869.
17. Greenblatt RB, Jungck EC, Barfield WE. A new test of efficacy of progestational compounds. *Ann NY Acad Sci* 1958;71:717.
18. Swyer GIM, Little V. Clinical assessment of relative potency of progestogens. *J Reprod Fertil Suppl* 1968;5:63–68.
19. Whitehead MI, Townsend PT, Pryse-Davies J, Ryder TA, King RJB. Effects of estrogens and progestins on the biochemistry and morphology of the postmenopausal endometrium. *N Engl J Med* 1981;305:1599–1605.
20. King RJB, Whitehead MI. Assessment of the potency of orally administered progestins in women. *Fertil Steril* 1986;46:1062–1066.
21. Dorflinger LL, Relative potency of progestins used in oral contraceptives. *Contraception* 1985;31:557–579.
22. Labrie F, Ferland L, Lagace L, et al. High inhibitory activity of R5020, a pure progestin, at the hypothalamic–adenohypophyseal level on gonadotropin secretion. *Fertil Steril* 1977;28:1104–1112.
23. Lobo RA. The androgenicity of progestational agents. *Int J Fertil Suppl* 1988;33: 6–12.
24. Stanczyk FZ, Weber ME, Conti A, et al. Effect of low-dose oral contraceptives on adrenal, ovarian and preripheral androgen production (Abstract). *J Soc Gynecol Invest* (Suppl) 1999;6:65A.
25. Jones RC, Edgren RA. The effects of various steroids on the vaginal histology in the rat. *Fertil Steril* 1973;24:284.
26. Padwick ML, Endacott J, Matson C, Whitehead MI. Absorption and metabolism of oral progesterone when administered twice daily. *Fertil Steril* 1986;46: 402–407.
27. Westphal U. *Steroid–protein interactions II.* New York: Springer Verlag, 1986:259.
28. Briggs MH, Brotherton J. *Advances in steroid biochemistry and pharmacology.* London: Academic Press, 1970:52–85.
29. Ottosson UB, Carlstrom K, Damber JE, von Schoulz B. Conversion of oral progesterone into deoxycorticosterone during postmenopausal replacement therapy. *Acta Obstet Gynecol Scand* 1984;63:577–579.
30. Hiroi M, Stanczyk FZ, Goebelsmann U, Brenner PF, Lumkin ME, Mishell DR, Jr. Radioimmunoassay of serum medroxyprogesterone acetate (Provera) in women following oral and intravaginal administration. *Steroids* 1975;26:373–386.
31. Mathrubutham M, Fotherby K. Medorxyprogesterone acetate in human serum. *J Steroid Biochem* 1981;14:783–786.
32. Gupta C, Musto NA, Bullock LP, et al. *In vivo* metabolism of progestins. II. Metabolic clearance rate of medroxyprogesterone acetate in four species. In: Garattini S, Berendes HW, eds. *Pharmacology of steroid contraceptive drugs.* New York: Raven Press, 1977:131–136.
33. Victor A, Johansson ED. Pharmacokinetic observations on medroxyprogesterone acetate administered orally and intravaginally. *Contraception* 1976;14:319–329.
34. Stanczyk FZ, Mroszezak EJ, Ling T, et al. Plasma levels and pharmacokinetics of norethindrone and ethinylestradiol administered in solution and as tablets to women. *Contraception* 1983;28:241–251.
35. Odlind V, Weiner E, Victor A, Johansson EDB. Plasma levels of norethindrone after single oral dose administration of norethindrone and lynestrenol. *Clin Endocrinol* 1979;10:29–38.

36. Back DJ, Breckenridge AM, Crawford FE, et al. Kinetics of norethindrone in women. II. Single-dose kinetics. *Clin Pharmacol Ther* 1978;24:448–453.

37. Hammond GL, Lahteenmaki PL, Luukkainen T, et al. Distribution and percentages of non-protein bound contraceptive steroids in human serum. *J Steroid Biochem* 1982;17:375–380.

38. Stanczyk FZ, Roy S. Metabolism of levonogestrel, norethindrone, and structurally related contraceptive steroids. *Contraception* 1990;42:67–96.

39. Reed MJ, Ross MS, Lai LC, Ghilchik MW, James VHT. *In vivo* conversion of norethisterone to ethinylestradiol in perimenopausal women. *J Steroid Biochem Mol Biochem* 1990;37:301–303.

40. Kuhntz W, Huener A, Humpel M, Seifert W, Michaelis K. *In vivo* conversion of norethesterone and norethisterone acetate to ethinyl estradiol in post menopausal women. *Contraception* 1997;56:379–385.

41. Lardon A, Schindler O, Reichstein T. Eine weitere synthese voin *d,l*-aldosteron. *Helv Chim Acta* 1957;40:676–677.

42. Fieser LF, Fieser M. *Steroids.* New York: Reinhold, 1959:336.

43. Humpel M, Wendt H, Dogs G, Weib CHR, Rietz S, Speck U. Intraindividual comparison of pharmacokinetic parameters of *d*-norgestrel, lynestrenol and cyproterone acetate in 6 women. *Contraception* 1977;16:199–215.

44. Goebelsmann U, Hoffman D, Chiang S, Woutersz T. The relative bioavailability of levonorgestrel and ethinyl estradil administered as a low-dose combination oral contraceptive. *Contraception* 1986;34:341–351.

45. Stanczyk FZ, Lobo RA, Chiange ST, Woutersz TB. Pharmacokinetic comparison of two triphasic oral contraceptive formulations containing levonorgestrel and ethinylestradiol. *Contraception* 1990;41:39–53.

46. Back DJ, Bates M, Breckenridge AM, Hall JM, MacIver M. Levonorgestrel and ethinylestradiol in women—studies with Ovran and Ovranette. *Contraception* 1981;23:229–239.

47. Humpel M, Wendt H, Pommerenke G, Weib CHR, Speck U. Investigations of pharmacokinetics of levonorgestrel to specific consideration of a possible first pass effect in women. *Contraception* 1978;17:207–220.

48. Alton KB, Hetyel NS, Shaw C, Patrick JE. Biotransformation of norgestimate in women. *Contraception* 1984;29:19–29.

49. Chapdelaine A, Desmarais J-L, Derman RJ. Clinical evidence of the minimal androgenic activity of norgestimate. *Int J Fertil* 1989;34:347–352.

50. McGuire JL, Phillips A, Hahn DW, Tolman EL, Flor S, Kafrissen ME. Pharmacologic and pharmacokinetic characteristics of norgestimate. *Am J Obstet Gynecol* 1990;163:2127–2131.

51. Kuhnz W, Blode H, Mahler M. Systemic availability of levonorgestrol after single oral administration of a norgestimate-containing oral contraceptive to 12 women. *Contraception* 1993;47:283–294.

52. Viinikka L. Radioimmunoassay of a new progestogen, ORG 2969, and its metabolite. *J Steroid Biochem* 1978;10:353–357.

53. Viinikka L. Metabolism of a new synthetic progestogen, ORG 2969, by human liver *in vitro. J Steroid Biochem* 1979;10:353–357.

54. Hasenack HG, Bosch AMG, Kaar K. Serum levels of 3-ketodesogestrel after oral administration of desogestrel and 3-ketodesogestrel. *Contraception* 1986;33:591–596.

55. Hammerstein J. Prodrugs: advantage or disadvantage? *Am J Obstet Gynecol* 1990;163:2198–2203.

56. Back DJ, Grimmer SFM, Shenoy N, Orme MLE. Plasma concentrations of 3-ketodesogestrel after oral administration of desogestrel and intravenous administration of 3-ketodesogestrel. *Contraception* 1987;35:619–626.

57. Orme M, Back DJ, Ward S, Green S. The pharmacokinetics of ethinyl estradiol in the presence and absence of gestodene and desogestrel. *Contraception* 1991;43:305–316.

58. Tauber U, Tack JW, Matthes H. Single dose pharmacokinetics of gestodene in women after intravenous and oral administration. *Contraception* 1989;40:461–479.

59. Berginck W, Assendorp R, Koosterboer L, van Lier W, Voortman G, Qvist I. Serum pharmacokinetics of orally administered desogestrel and binding of contraceptive progestogens to sex hormone-binding globulin. *Am J Obstet Gynecol* 1990;163:2132–2137.

60. Kuhl H, Jung-Hoffman C, Heidt F. Serum levels of 3-ketodesogestrel and SHBG during 12 cycles of treatment with 30 μg desogestrel. *Contraception* 1988;38:381–390.

61. Jung-Hoffman C, Kuhl H. Interaction with the pharmacokinetics of ethinyl estradiol and progestogens contained in oral contraceptives. *Contraception* 1989;40:299–312.

62. Kuhnz W, Pfeffer M, Al-Yacoub G. Protein binding of the contraceptive steroids gestodene, 3-ketodesogestrel and ethinylestradiol in human serum. *J Steroid Biochem* 1990;35:313–318.

63. Dusterberg B, Tack J-W, Krause W, Humpel M. Pharmacokinetics and biotransformation of gestodene in man. In: Elstein M, ed. *Gestodene: development of a new gestodene-containing low-dose oral contraceptive.* London: Parthenon Publishers, 1987:35.

64. Kuhl H, Jung-Hoffman C, Heidt F. Alterations in the serum levels of gestodene and SHBG during 12 cycles of treatment with 30 mg ethinyl estradiol and 75 mg gestodene. *Contraception* 1988;38:477–486.

65. Fotherby K. Potency and pharmacokinetics of gestagens. *Contraception* 1990;41:533–550.

Treatment of the Postmenopausal Woman: Basic and Clinical Aspects, Second Edition, edited by Rogerio A. Lobo, Lippincott Williams & Wilkins, Philadelphia © 1999.

CHAPTER 13

Clinical Aspects of Hormonal Replacement

Routes of Administration

Rogerio A. Lobo

In this chapter, routes of administration for estrogens and progestogens in postmenopausal replacement therapy are discussed. The reader is also directed to Chapter 11, which discusses in greater detail the pharmacology of estrogen.

ROUTES OF ADMINISTRATION: ORAL THERAPY

There are many ways in which estradiol (E_2) can be delivered. For oral E_2 to be absorbed efficiently from the gastric mucosa, it needs to be administered in a micronized or conjugated form. The most common conjugated form of E_2 is E_2 valerate (E_2V), which, as discussed below, is extremely similar to micronized E_2. Unconjugated estrone (E_1) and E_2 are absorbed very inefficiently from the gastrointestinal tract. In contrast to these absorption characteristics, as discussed below, the vaginal mucosa absorbs E_2 and E_1 in an extremely efficient manner (1). In this regard, it has been suggested that E_2 is better absorbed vaginally than is E_1. Even whole tablets of micronized E_2 are well absorbed directly from the vaginal mucosa (2).

With oral therapy, E_1 is the predominant estrogen in the circulation after any oral preparation is administered (Fig. 13.1). That is because of enhanced hepatic metabolism or the first-passage uptake effect, which occurs with oral administration. When E_2 is ingested, the liver actively deactivates E_2 by its metabolism into E_1 and E_1 conjugates. Some estrogen does enter the systemic circulation as E_2. However, E_1 is the predominant estrogen after oral

E_2 administration, and the metabolites of E_1—E_1S and, more specifically, E_1 glucuronide (E_1G)—serve as markers of this first-passage hepatic interaction. This hepatic effect results in the production of hepatic globulins as well as lipoproteins, such as high-density lipoprotein (HDL)-cholesterol.

Estradiol administered systematically is converted to E_1 in blood, but the effects on the liver are only secondary, and therefore, the effects on hepatic globulins and HDL-cholesterol are far less pronounced (3). That E_1G is an important marker of the first-passage effect of oral administration is illustrated in Fig. 13.2. Within 3 hours there is approximately a threefold increase in serum E_1G with oral administration of E_2 valerate (E_2V). That does not occur, however, with the systemic routes of administration, where serum E_1G levels remain low (4).

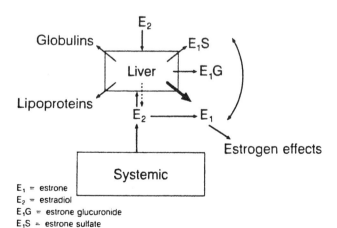

FIG. 13.1. Oral versus systemic estradiol delivery. (From Lobo RA and Cassidenti DL. *J Reprod Med* 1992;37:77.)

R. A. Lobo: Department of Obstetrics and Gynecology, Columbia University College of Physicians & Surgeons, New York, New York 10032.

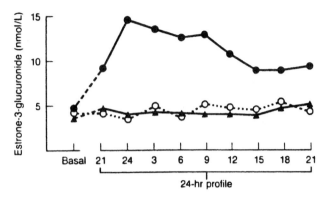

FIG. 13.2. Levels of estrone-3-glucuronide after the administration of oral estradiol valerate and percutaneous estradiol cream and implantation of subcutaneous estradiol. (From Siddle N and Whitehead M., *Contemp Obstet Gynecol* 1983;22:137.)

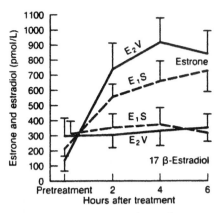

FIG. 13.3. Mean serum concentrations of estrone and 17β-estradiol before and at 2-hour intervals after the administration of 1.5 mg of oral piperazine estrone sulfate and 2 mg of estradiol valerate in postmenopausal women. (From ref. 5, with permission.)

Once in the circulation, both E_1 and E_2 will express estrogen-related effects on the brain, cardiovascular system, and bone. The end-organ response is a reflection of the levels of E_1 and E_2 achieved and is independent of whether the estrogen is derived from oral or systemic administration. However, it is well known that E_2 is more potent than E_1, and it can be estimated that the levels of E_1 in blood required to equal the biologic effects of E_2 are at least threefold greater.

COMPARISON BETWEEN THE LEVELS OF ESTROGEN ACHIEVED AFTER ORAL ESTRADIOL AND ESTRONE ADMINISTRATION

Estradiol is better absorbed in its conjugated or micronized form; the same is true of E_1. Therefore, E_1 usually is administered as the conjugate, E_1S. A study by Anderson (5) compared the levels of serum E_1 and E_2 after the administration of 1.5 mg of oral piperazine E_1S and 2 mg of E_2V. The serum levels of E_2 achieved were nearly identical (Fig. 13.3). Although the pharmacokinetics were similar, E_2V administered at a higher dose, 2 mg as compared with 1.5 mg of E_1S, resulted in levels of E_1 that were slightly higher. Serum E_1S levels after E_2V and E_1S were again almost superimposable. Peak levels of E_2, E_1, and E_1S occurred at approximately 4 hours with each preparation.

The administration of 1 and 3 mg of piperazine E_1S also suggests a linear dose-response relationship in the pharmacokinetics of E_1S administration (Fig. 13.4). Serum levels that peak at 4 hours were seen in one study (5) to be maintained for many hours. The data suggest that the half-life of E_1S is approximately 12 hours (5). Other studies that have compared the pharmacokinetics of E_2V and E_1S have also suggested similar half-life characteristics (6). The studies to date, therefore, suggest that in terms of serum E_2 and E_1 levels achieved

after oral therapy, there are no real differences between the oral administration of equal doses of the conjugated forms.

Whether there are biologic differences between the effects of E_2 and E_1 administered orally remains unclear. A study by Colvin et al. (7) suggested that with an incremental oral regimen, after the highest dose of estrogen, which was either 2.5 mg of E_1S (Ogen) or 2 mg of oral micronized E_2 (Estrace), there was a greater increase in HDL-cholesterol after E_2 was administered. Although the two doses achieved the same serum concentrations of E_1 and E_2, there also was a greater increase in HDL-cholesterol and a greater reduction in low-density lipoprotein (LDL)-cholesterol with E_2 than with piperazine E_1S (Fig. 13.5). These results suggest that with oral administration there may be some subtle biologic differences related to inherent differences in the potencies of E_2 and E_1. Clearly, more work is needed in this area.

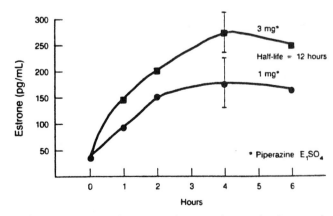

FIG. 13.4. Levels of estrone after two doses of estrone sulfate. (From ref. 5, with permission.)

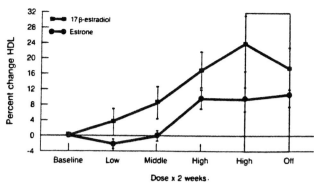

FIG. 13.5. Percentage change in high-density lipoprotein cholesterol from baseline concentrations to low, middle, and high doses of 17β-estradiol and estrone sulfate. (From ref. 7, with permission.)

PHARMACOKINETICS OF ORAL 17β-ESTRADIOL

With oral administration of 1 mg of 17β-E_2, serum levels of E_1 and E_2 increase rapidly during the first 4 to 8 hours after ingestion (8). Although interpatient variation exists, peak levels are attained by 4 hours. The levels of E_1 achieved are approximately 200 pg/mL, and the levels of E_2 are 40 to 50 pg/mL. In response to this oral dose, levels of E_1G peak within the first hour and then gradually return to normal. There is a slower, more gradual increase in E_1S, which again appears to peak at approximately 4 hours (Fig. 13.6). As has been shown in previous studies with piperazine E_1S (5), the pharmacokinetics of oral estrogen follows a linear dose-response relationship. After 2 mg of E_2, the pharmacokinetic profiles are extremely similar. The levels achieved are higher over 12 hours; the E_1 levels at 4 hours are approximately 300 pg/mL and are maintained for 12 hours. The E_2 levels reach approximately 65 pg/mL and also remain elevated for 12 hours. It has been surmised from these and other data that 12-hour levels after the acute administration of oral E_2 are representative of the 24-hour pharmacokinetic profile. That is not the case in patients receiving estrogen on a chronic basis. Once steady state occurs, within 2 to 4 weeks, the levels of E_2 and E_1 are fairly constant, and the levels seen 24 hours after dosing are generally representative of the entire 24-hour profile (7,9,10). Although serum profiles are fairly constant, there is more fluctuation with E_1 than with E_2, which remains very constant under steady-state conditions.

We have measured the levels of E_1 and E_2 after administering 2 mg daily, 2 mg twice daily (a total of 4 mg/day), and 2 mg thrice daily (6 mg/day) (Figs. 13.7 and 13.8). These doses of E_2 were taken by women with ovarian failure for the purpose of endometrial synchronization for oocyte donation and *in vitro* fertilization. This dosing, therefore, represents both chronic exposure to oral estrogen and bolus increases of 2 mg with each

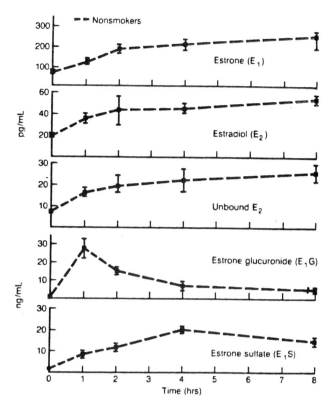

FIG. 13.6. Pharmacokinetics of 1 mg of oral 17β–estradiol over 8 hours in nonsmokers. (From Lobo RA, *J Reprod Med* 1992;37:77.)

tablet ingested to achieve total daily doses of 4 and 6 mg, respectively.

As shown, the levels of serum E_1 12 hours after administration are approximately 250 mg/mL. After 4 mg (2 mg twice daily), the 12-hour values (representative of the 24-hour profile) were approximately 560 pg/mL. After 6 mg (2 mg thrice daily), the E_1 level was 700 pg/mL 12 hours after the last 2-mg dose (Fig. 13.7). With each acute dosing of 2 mg taken to achieve the 4- or 6-mg daily dose, an acute increase of 300 to 400 pg/mL is seen in serum E_1

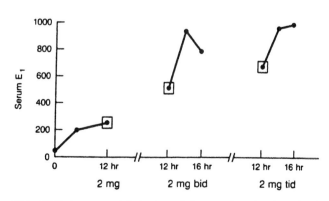

FIG. 13.7. Incremental dosing of 2 mg of oral micronized estradiol: serum estrone (E_1) levels. (From Lobo RA and Cassidenti DL. *J Reprod Med* 1992;37:77.)

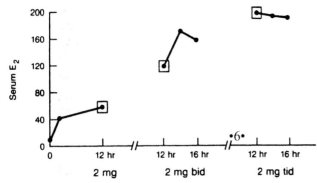

FIG. 13.8. Incremental dosing of 2 mg of oral micronized estradiol (E_2): serum E_2 levels. (From Lobo RA and Cassidenti DL. *J Reprod Med* 1992;37:77.)

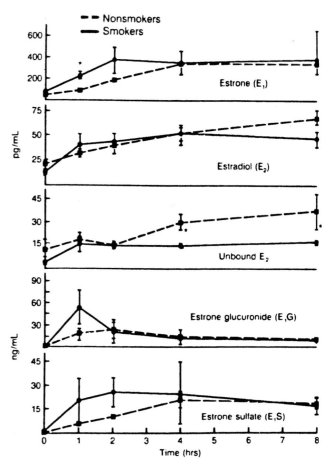

FIG. 13.9. Pharmacokinetics of 2 mg of oral 17β-estradiol over 8 hours in smokers and nonsmokers. (From Lobo RA and Cassidenti DL. *J Reprod Med* 1992;37:77.)

(Fig. 13.7). It occurs over a 4-hour period, after which serum E_1 returns to basal steady-state levels (Fig. 13.7).

A similar pharmacokinetic profile is seen for serum E_2 (Fig. 13.8). With 2 mg of oral micronized E_2, the serum levels of E_2 are 63 pg/mL. A much smaller incremental increase, of only 40 pg/mL, occurs with each dose of 2 mg. With the 4-mg dose the serum E_2 levels are approximately 121 pg/mL, and with 6 mg, approximately 200 pg/mL.

After the ingestion of various doses of conjugated equine estrogen (CEE), the levels of E_1 and E_2 are comparable, on a milligram basis, to the levels of piperazine E_1S and micronized E_2. However, CEE is more potent than E_1S and E_2. In our studies, CEE was three times more potent, on a weight basis, than either E_2S or micronized E_2 in stimulating hepatic globulin production (11). The reason is that CEE contains other estrogens that are not generally measured but that have considerable biologic potency. Specifically, equilin sulfate, which makes up approximately 25% of the dose of CEE, and its active 17β-hydroxy metabolite have been shown to be extremely potent in stimulating hepatic globulins and inducing an increase in HDL-cholesterol (12). In addition, as pointed out in Chapter 11, there are several other active metabolites in CEE. Among these the 17α-conjugate and the Δ^{5-8} estrone conjugate have known biologic activity, and the levels of these metabolites are substantial in the circulation.

EFFECTS OF SMOKING ON ESTROGEN METABOLISM

It has been suggested that smoking decreases estrogen levels in women receiving oral estrogens (13). Therefore, we reviewed the acute pharmacokinetics of E_1 and E_2 in smokers and nonsmokers in order to understand the mechanisms behind those observations. Our data suggest that although the levels of E_1 and E_2 are comparable with doses of 1 and 2 mg of oral micronized E_2, there are significantly lower levels of unbound E_2 in women who smoke. This difference is greater with the 2-mg dose than with the 1-mg dose (Fig. 13.9). The levels of the estrogen

conjugates, E_1G and E_1S, are higher after oral E_2 (10). These results suggest that with smoking there is enhanced hepatic metabolism of estrogen. This enhanced first-passage effect results in lower levels of unbound or free E_2, in large part through an increase in sex hormone-binding globulin (SHBG). Thus, smoking accelerates the hepatic metabolism of oral estrogen and also increases SHBG, resulting in lower levels of unbound E_2.

FACTORS INFLUENCING THE CHOICE OF A NONORAL ESTROGEN

Although oral estrogen may be considered a first-line approach to therapy, Table 13.1 lists some reasons for considering an alternative form of treatment.

As shown in Fig. 13.6, the pharmacodynamics of oral micronized estradiol shows abrupt increases in serum estrone, which, with its conjugates, is the predominant estrogen after oral therapy. Rarely, normal peak estrogen levels may not be achieved. This may be because of unusual hepatic enzymatic activities as well as being the

TABLE 13.1. *Reasons for considering nonoral estrogens*

Problems with absorption; concomitant medications
Smokers (>1 pack/day)
Coagulation disorders and family history of
thromboembolism
Hypertension if exacerbated by estrogen
Liver disease
Diabetes, particularly if triglycerides are increased
Nausea, GI discomfort, allergic reactions
Difficulty in control of vasomotor system
Preference/compliance

result of use of certain antiepileptic and other medications that may affect hepatic conjugation and estrogen metabolism (2-, 4-, or 16-hydroxylation). This is not frequently encountered but may be uncovered by measuring serum estrone when a patient complains of persistence of symptoms. Serum estrone should be measured instead of estradiol, and levels below 150 pg/mL 4 hours after oral dosing are suggestive of altered metabolism. This may be addressed by increasing the oral dose of estrogen or, preferably, by switching to a nonoral preparation.

As shown in Fig. 13.9 and discussed above, smoking minimally interferes with oral absorption. However, in our studies of only moderate smokers (<15 cigarettes/day), the reduction in measured estrogens from this hepatic effect were almost imperceivable and probably are not clinically relevant. This is in contrast to a Danish study (13) that suggested reduced levels with smoking. In heavy smokers (>1 pack/day), these findings may warrant increasing the oral dose or using a nonoral form of therapy that has been shown to be unaffected by smoking (14).

In contrast to the possible decreases in serum estrogen with smoking, acute alcohol ingestion raises estrogen levels over the first 4 hours. This has been shown to occur with both oral and transdermal estrogens (15,16).

Oral estrogen does not alter coagulation factors adversely, although there are minor changes observed in factors VII and X, as well as a reduction in antithrombin III. At the same time, fibrinogen decreases and plasminogen increases (17). However, after some earlier reassurance that oral estrogen does not increase the risk of thrombosis in postmenopausal women (18,19), several papers appeared simultaneously in the literature suggesting an increased risk of thromboembolism in postmenopausal women ingesting oral estrogen (20–22). Nevertheless, this increased risk is relatively low (about twofold) and results in a total of 25 cases per 100,000 women. The cases appear early in treatment with no incremental risk with time and is less than the prevalence of thromboembolism in pregnancy (approximately 60/100,000 women). On a practical basis, if a woman has other risk factors for venous thrombosis (obesity,

immobilization, etc.) or a prior history of thrombosis or a familial risk of thrombophilia, a nonoral form of estrogen should be prescribed in that there are no changes observed in any coagulation factors with "physiologic" levels of nonoral estrogen and estradiol levels in the range of 60 pg/mL (3). Note that the risk of thrombosis and thromboembolism discussed here pertains only to venous thrombosis and not to arterial thrombosis, the risk of which is not believed to be increased with oral estrogen.

Oral estrogen has been found to raise blood pressure as an "idiosyncratic reaction," and only in about 5% of cases (23). Indeed, oral estrogen has been found to lower blood pressure in both normotensive and hypertensive women (Fig. 13.10) (24). However, in those women with an unusual blood pressure response to oral estrogen, a nonoral approach should be considered.

Women with hepatocellular disease and those who have alterations in liver enzymes should not receive oral estrogen. Table 13.2 illustrates the dose-response relationship of various oral estrogens in stimulating hepatic globulin synthesis. Note that, based on these and other data, postmenopausal replacement therapy with ethinyl estradiol should be in the 5- to 7-g range (four to seven times less than the amount of ethinyl estradiol contained in oral contraceptives). Nonoral therapies, which are reviewed below, do not increase globulin production. However, with nonoral estrogen therapy, some monitoring is prudent in high-risk individuals to assure that E_2 levels remain in a physiologic range.

Estrogen increases insulin sensitivity and therefore should be of benefit for postmenopausal women who have been found to have insulin resistance, which increases further as they age (25,26). This is particularly relevant for women who have impaired glucose tolerance and in those with frank diabetes. However, oral estrogen in higher doses can also reverse sensitivity and cause worsening of insulin resistance, which does not occur with transdermal estrogen. Women who require higher doses of estrogen should benefit from a nonoral estrogen. With hyperlipidemia, and particularly for those women with diabetes who have a higher prevalence of hypertriglyceridemia, nonoral estrogen should be administered. Oral estrogen increases total triglycerides by about 25% (28). Although this is clearly the preferred approach, it is important to realize that nonoral estrogen will not increase HDL-C, unlike oral estrogen (28); low levels of HDL-C are often a characteristic of hyperlipemic and diabetic women.

Clearly there are the practical concerns of gastrointestinal irritability, nausea, and occasional allergic reactions associated with oral estrogen. The former complaints may subside with time and with the concurrent ingestion with food or at a different time during the day. Allergic reactions are linked to certain dyes used in dif-

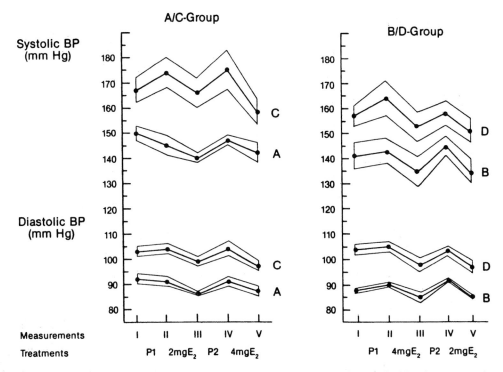

FIG. 13.10. The effect of micronized estradiol (E₂) on diastolic and systolic blood pressure in normotensive (groups A and B) and hypertensive (groups C and D) women. Shown are mean values ± SEM for blood pressure in supine position. P, placebo. (From ref. 24, with permission.)

ferent estrogen preparations and may be addressed by changing to another oral preparation.

Apart from absorption problems as noted above, some women on oral therapy do not achieve a desirable degree of relief from vasomotor symptoms. There are data to suggest that hot flushes decrease proportionately with an increase in serum E₂ (Fig. 13.11) (29). However, in women whose symptoms are difficult to control, larger doses of oral estrogen should be avoided, and a nonoral preparation should be considered. The theoretical reason for an advantage here is that nonoral estradiol therapy provides a more constant or steady-state concentration of E₂, which is also more potent than E₁. The pharmacokinetic characteristics of oral therapy show wider variations (both peak and trough values of E₁ and E₂). Abrupt reductions in serum levels of estrogen are known to precipitate symptoms.

Clearly a woman may have a preference for a nonoral preparation. Among the nonoral forms, the transdermal gel has been viewed by some women to have characteristics of a cosmetic rather than a medication. Some nonoral preparations such as the pellet and the 7-day patch provide for better compliance in that it is not necessary to remember to take a pill daily. The subcutaneous pellet, which provides E₂ for 4 to 6 months, is obviously an advantage in this regard. However, in spite of literature suggesting that the 7-day patch has such an advantage (16), this is not universally accepted.

TABLE 13.2. *Relative potency according to four parameters of estrogenicity*

	Serum FSH	Serum CBG-BC	Serum SHBG-BC	Serum angiotensinogen
Piperazine estrone sulfate	1.1	1.0	1.0	1.0
Micronized estradiol	1.3	1.9	1.0	0.7
Conjugated estrogens	1.4	2.5	3.2	3.5
Diethylstilbestrol	3.8	70	28	13
Ethinyl estradiol	80–200	1,000	614	232

CBG-BC, corticosteroid-binding globulin binding capacity; FSH, follicle stimulating hormone; SHBG-BC, sex hormone-binding globulin binding capacity.
Adapted from ref. 11.

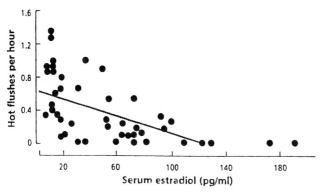

FIG. 13.11. Relationship between hot flush frequency and serum estradiol. $R = 0.6045$; $p < 0.001$. (From ref. 29, with permission.)

2. Individual women may have cutaneous sensitivities with the use of transdermal methods, and other women may feel uncomfortable with vaginal preparations. Large volumes of vaginal cream are necessary to achieve systemic levels of estrogen with vaginal therapy, although much smaller volumes and other preparations (ring, tablets) are of benefit for vulvovaginal symptomatology.

3. All nonoral preparations (apart from vaginal estrone sulfate and conjugated equine estrogen creams) increase estradiol in the circulation. Estradiol is much more potent than estrone and is thought to be more stimulatory to the breast and endometrium. However, this concern is somewhat theoretical, and there are no data to support a greater role in promoting cancer.

SELECTING A NONORAL PREPARATION

Some Drawbacks to Consider

The following are several potential drawbacks to nonoral therapy:

1. In keeping with the fact that hepatic globulins are not increased with nonoral therapy, HDL-cholesterol is also unchanged. Thus, the protective cardiovascular benefit of raising HDL-C by some 13% does not occur with nonoral therapy. Nevertheless, the absent HDL-C effect stands alone in that cholesterol and LDL-cholesterol are lowered, as is LP(a), and the oxidation of LDL-C is retarded, as it is with oral estrogen. Another potential advantage of nonoral estrogen is that there is no increase in triglycerides. All the beneficial vascular effects of E_2 (increase in nitric oxide, reduction in endothelin I, etc.) are maintained with nonoral therapy and are reviewed in Chapter 34.

Preparations Aimed at Achieving Systemic Effects

Intramuscular preparations are nonphysiologic and should be avoided. Larger fluctuations in E_2 are encountered; a supraphysiologic peak response is followed by rapid clearance and precipitation of symptoms. This requires a follow-up dose in a matter of weeks. High estrogen levels from accumulating stores in adipose have been witnessed. Perhaps because of the pharmacologic nature of intramuscular use, this form of therapy has been associated with an increased prevalence of breast cancer (31).

The E_2 patch provides predictable, near-steady-state concentrations of E_2 as shown in Fig. 13.12 (32). Data are similar for the new "matrix" patches, which are not alcohol dependent. A wide range of doses are available from several manufacturers, from 0.025 to 0.1 mg. Most symptoms require replacing a new patch at midweek, but a 7-day patch is also available (Fig. 13.13) (33). In considering

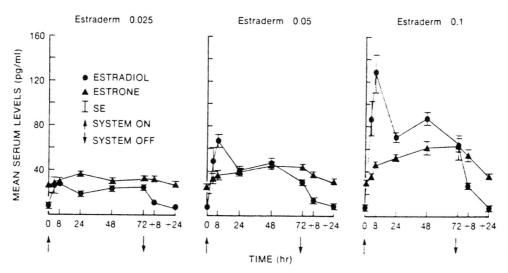

FIG. 13.12. Mean serum levels of estradiol and estrone with use of Estraderm 0.025, 0.05, and 0.1 mg per day. (From ref. 32, with permission.)

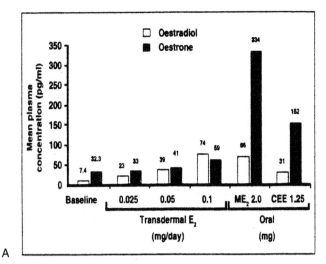
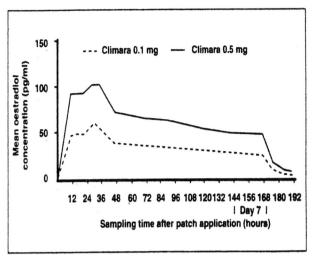

FIG. 13.13. A: Plasma estrone/estradiol levels with transdermal and oral estrogen replacement therapy. (From ref. 32, with permission.) **B:** Dose proportionality: comparison between 0.05-mg and 0.1-mg matrix patches. (From ref. 33, with permission.)

lower doses of all preparations including the low-dose patch, it is important to realize that to optimize the bone and cardiovascular benefit, an E_2 level of 60 pg/mL should be achieved. This concept has been extrapolated from several studies and has been directly assessed in the monkey model of atherosclerosis (34). However, lower levels may be effective and are preferable for some women.

The subcutaneous pellet (25 or 50 mg) provides steady-state levels for 4 to 6 months after its insertion with a trocar (35,36). This crystalline pellet is completely absorbed in about 6 months. Compared to the patch, levels are maintained with less variation for up to 6 months (Fig. 13.14) (36). Symptomatic relief and a beneficial metabolic profile have also been noted, and there is no

increase in hepatic globulin production as discussed earlier (35,36). Higher levels of E_2 achieved have been associated with small increments in HDL-cholesterol, but this is considerably less than after oral therapy.

Concerns with the pellet are the necessity for trocar insertions at 4- to 6-month intervals and the difficulty in retrieving the pellet, if needed. Another concern is the variability in the time to complete dissolution of the pellet. Symptoms typically return while E_2 levels are still above baseline. This fact and that sequestration of E_2 in adipose tissue occurs, as well as a variable release of E_2 into the circulation results in individual levels of E_2 that are not predictable. Without monitoring serum E_2, some patients have had sustained, supraphysiological levels.

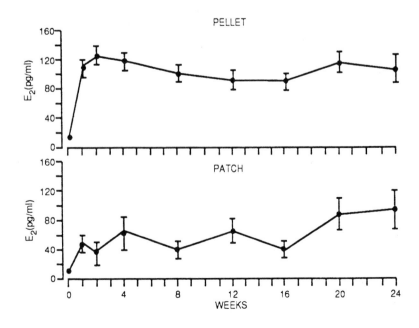

FIG. 13.14. Mean (±SE) serum estradiol (E_2) levels before and during 1 to 24 weeks of subdermal estradiol (two 25-mg pellets inserted once) and transdermal estradiol (0.1-mg/day patch applied twice weekly). (From ref. 36, with permission.)

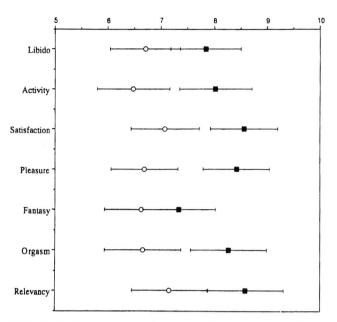

FIG. 13.15. Summary graph showing the grand mean (i.e., means of 6, 12, 18, and 24 months) for each sexuality parameter adjusted for baseline as a covariate. *Error bars* represent SEDs for each mean. If the *error bars* do not overlap for a single parameter, the difference is significant with a *p* value <0.05. (From ref. 37, with permission.)

This mode of delivery has also been used for the testosterone pellet (50 and 75 mg). Usually testosterone and E_2 are administered simultaneously. A pellet of 50 or 75 mg usually results in increments of testosterone in the 30 to 70 ng/dL range, which places serum testosterone in the normal or slightly elevated premenopausal range. Larger doses of testosterone have been used (e.g., 100 mg), which lead to levels above this range. This form of

therapy has been shown to improve symptoms without any adverse effects (Fig. 13.15) (37).

A hydroalcoholic gel, Oestrogel, available in 3 and 5 g (1.5 and 3 mg of E_2) sizes, is rubbed daily over a large surface area (e.g., thighs, arms, and abdomen). The E_2 is sequestered in the dermis and is released slowly (Fig. 13.16) (38,39). Although blood levels vary widely within a physiologic range, on an individual basis, day-to-day variation in individual women is small. Oestrogel has been found to result in good relief of symptoms, have a beneficial metabolic profile (absence of any changes in HDL-C), and to maintain bone mass. It is anticipated to be available in the U.S. market by the year 2000 and has been used in Europe and worldwide for many years.

Vaginal Preparations

As discussed in Chapter 11, small amounts of vaginal estrogen are sufficient to provide an improvement in symptoms of vulvovaginal atrophy. However, approximately four times the oral dose (e.g., 2.5 mg of conjugated equine estrogens vaginally or 4 g of cream) is necessary to achieve a systemic effect (40). This in turn is influenced by blood flow, which increases absorption as therapy continues, and the matrix (cream) of the preparation. These vary with different manufacturers, and it is the cream base that retards absorption. Absorption is greatest if estrogen is delivered in saline (1) but will vary with other preparations (41). On a practical basis, vaginal estrogen is not an efficient way to deliver estrogen if a systemic effect is desired.

As little as 0.3 mg or less of vaginal CEE cream has a significant local effect, with limited absorption. The same is the case for Estring, which is a silastic ring con-

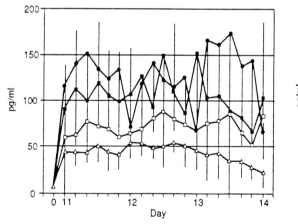

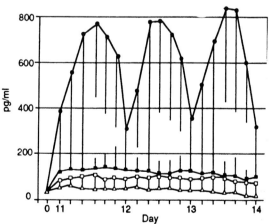

FIG. 13.16. A: Serum estradiol (E_2) levels (pg/mL; mean ± SD) in postmenopausal women treated with 0.05-mg transdermal delivery system (△), 1.5 mg of percutaneous estradiol (Oestrogel) (□), 3.0 mg of percutaneous estradiol (■), and micronized estradiol, 2.0 mg orally (●). **B:** Serum estrone (E_1) levels (pg/mL; mean ± SD) in postmenopausal women treated with 0.05-mg transdermal delivery system (△), 1.5 mg of percutaneous estradiol (Oestrogel) (□), 3.0 mg of percutaneous estradiol (■), and micronized estradiol, 2.0 mg orally (●). (From ref. 39, with permission.)

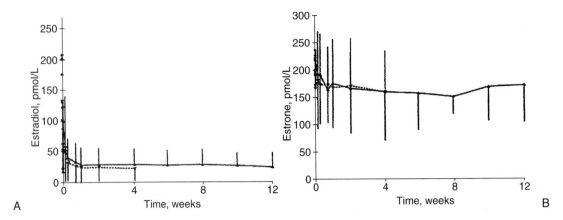

FIG. 13.17. (From Schmidt G, Anderson SB, Nordle O, et al. Release of 17-β-oestradiol from a vaginal ring in postmenopausal women: pharmacokinetic evaluation. *Gynecol Obstet Invest* 1994;38:253.

taining 2 mg of E_2 and lasts 3 months. Apart from an initial burst effect of E_2 (50 to 60 g/day), the release rate achieved is a low steady state of 7.5 mg/day for 90 days. Levels of E_2 and E_1 remain low (Fig. 13.17) (42).

Another similar product is Vagifen, which is a 6-mm-diameter tablet of 25 g E_2 placed high in the vagina with an applicator. Serum E_2 levels are not increased with a dosing regimen of once daily for 2 weeks and a maintenance regimen of twice a week. Vagifen is not yet available in the United States.

PHARMACOLOGY AND ROUTES OF ADMINISTRATION OF PROGESTOGENS

Progestogens are necessary for endometrial protection when estrogen is administered. The concerns of added progestogens are related to the type and dose of progestogens and their route of administration. Attenuation of the CV benefits of estrogen (e.g., on the rise in HDL-C and on blood flow) and mood alterations in some women have warranted the consideration of alterations in dose, type, and route of progestogen administration.

Use of Progesterone

Absorption of oral progesterone is inefficient. Rapid hepatic hydroxylation and conjugation (first-pass effects) occur, resulting in increases in pregnanediol-3-glucuronide, the major urinary metabolite. Nevertheless, oral progesterone has been used with some efficacy in postmenopausal women (43), in whom a dose of 300 mg may result in 5 to 10 ng/mL in the systemic circulation. A more efficient means of ingesting progesterone is with a micronized product. Micronized progesterone may be administered orally in 100- to 200-mg doses. When it is administered in divided doses, 100 mg at 9 AM and 200 mg at 9 PM, peak serum progesterone levels of more than 10 ng/mL are encountered (Fig. 13.18) (44). These findings were associated with significant endometrial progestational activity. It has been shown that 200 mg of micronized prog-

esterone affords sufficient endometrial protection when the equivalent of 0.625 mg of CEE is used daily (45).

Oral administration of native progesterone is nevertheless subject to first-pass effects. Characteristic of these

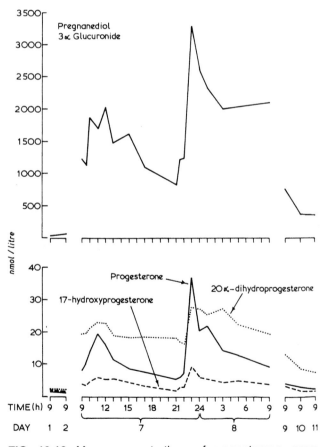

FIG. 13.18. Mean concentrations of progesterone, pregnanediol 3α-glucuronide, 17-hydroxyprogesterone, and 20α-dihydroprogesterone in the peripheral plasma of postmenopausal women before, during, and after administration of oral progesterone. Pretreatment, days 1 and 2; after 5 days of treatment with 100 mg progesterone at 9 hours and 200 mg at 21 hours, day 7; and posttreatment, days 9 to 11. (From ref. 44, with permission.)

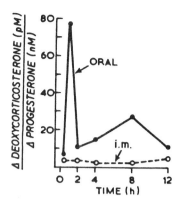

FIG. 13.19. The mean ratio between the increase in deoxycorticosterone and progesterone in plasma after oral and intramuscular administration of 100 mg of progesterone in four women in the follicular phase of the cycle. (From ref. 46, with permission.)

changes is the rapid conversion of progesterone to desoxycorticosterone, an effect that does not occur readily with the systemic route (43,44). When equal doses of progesterone are administered orally and intramuscularly, despite a threefold increase in serum levels with the intramuscular route, the ratio of desoxycorticosterone/progesterone was much higher than with the oral route (Fig. 13.19). These data, which confirm hepatic effects characteristic of first-pass phenomena, are interesting but await clinical relevance. Perhaps these and similar changes with oral progestogens would help explain unusual hypertensive and metabolic responses in some women.

Native progesterone is well absorbed vaginally and rectally (48,49) as well as nasally (50) but does not compare with the high levels achieved by the intramuscular route. These routes of administration afford much higher levels of progesterone than does the oral route, which is subject to first-pass changes. It is for the levels of progesterone that may be achieved by nonoral routes that these methods are chosen for premenopausal women (who have the need to more closely mimic the normal luteal phase). To date, no adverse effects have been documented with the use of oral native progesterone in spite of first-pass effects, and this method appears to be a good choice for postmenopausal women.

Synthetic Progestogens

Of the two classes of synthetic progestogens, the 17-acetoxy group (medroxyprogesterone acetate) has properties closest to native progesterone. Apart from the 17-acetoxy function of this class, the manipulations at C-6 (CH$_3$ for medroxyprogesterone acetate) produce increased progestational effects and oral efficacy. The 19-norprogestogens, by virtue of an ethinyl group at C-17 and the removal of the 19th carbon from C-10, have increased progestational activity, oral efficacy, and reduced androgenic activity,

even though this class is derived from testosterone. However, despite the C-17 ethinyl group, which tends to nullify androgen action, characteristics of some members of this group (particularly norethindrone and levonorgestrel) are their androgenic side effects.

Oral absorption of these synthetic progestogens is variable. For this and other reasons, it has been difficult to ascribe potency ratios for these various progestogens. The most commonly used progestogens are medroxyprogesterone acetate, norethindrone, and levonorgestrel, with medroxyprogesterone acetate constituting the majority of prescriptions for postmenopausal patients in the United States.

Absorption of medroxyprogesterone acetate after a 10-mg oral dose is fairly rapid, reaching levels of 3 to 4 ng/mL within 1 to 4 hours and declining to 0.3 to 0.6 ng/mL by 24 hours. However, these characteristics are variable, and major differences have been noted in medroxyprogesterone acetate pharmacokinetics in postmenopausal women (Fig. 13.20) (51).

Similar characteristics occur with administration of norethindrone. After ingestion of 1 mg, peak concentrations occurred within 1 hour in 16% of women, within 2 hours in 51%, and after 2 hours in 33% (52). Although these data pertain to oral contraceptive users, at least this degree of variability would be expected in postmenopausal women. In the case of 1 mg of norethindrone, peak levels of 5 ng/mL occur, which then decline to less than 1 ng/mL within 24 hours. However, these levels, although higher than those achieved with 10 mg of medroxyprogesterone acetate, are still 60% of levels achieved by parenteral administration.

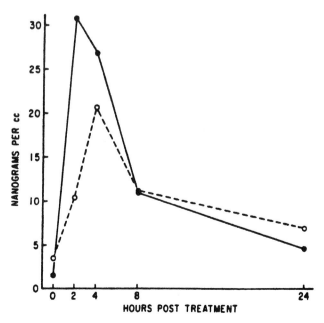

FIG. 13.20. Plasma levels of medroxyprogesterone acetate after oral administration. (From ref. 51, with permission.)

This is not the case with levonorgestrel, in which oral and parenteral administration lead to similar level (53). Thus, we see significant first-pass effects and portal-hepatic inactivation with these three progestogens. Medroxyprogesterone acetate is most affected, followed by norethindrone. Levonorgestrel is least affected. These data also correlate with the known differences in potency among these progestogens (levonorgestrel the most potent) and with the variability observed in postmenopausal endometria (medroxyprogesterone acetate, greatest variability) as reviewed elsewhere.

Clinical Effects of Administered Progestogens

As noted with the estrogens, the structure and route of administration of progestogens affect various biochemical parameters. Although first-pass effects are significant with medroxyprogesterone acetate and norethindrone, the major parameter affected is lipid metabolism. To the best of our knowledge, progestogens do not have a significant impact on binding globulins and appear to have negligible effects on clotting parameters (17,54).

Although all progestogens affect metabolism adversely to some degree, only very large doses cause elevations in LDL-cholesterol. However, a lowering of HDL-cholesterol levels, particularly the HDL_2 subfraction, is noted repeatedly (28). Although a rise from baseline is observed when CEE 0.625 mg is given with various combinations of MPA, the rise is about half that from CEE alone (Fig. 13.21) (17). The smallest attenuating effect on CEE was observed with 200 mg of micronized progesterone in the Postmenopausal Estrogen/Progestin Interventions (PEPI) Trial (Fig. 13.22) (45).

In a dose-related manner, higher doses of oral progestogens affect insulin sensitivity; and a reduction of insulin

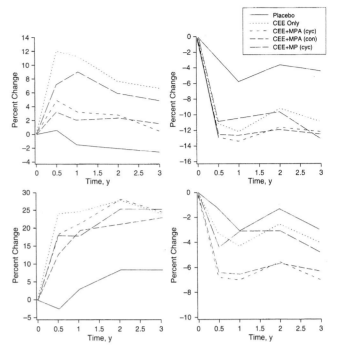

FIG. 13.22. Mean percentage change from baseline by treatment arm for high-density lipoprotein cholesterol (top left), low-density lipoprotein cholesterol (top right), triglycerides (bottom left), and total cholesterol (bottom right). (From ref. 45, with permission.)

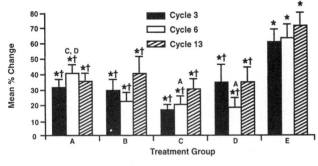

FIG. 13.21. Mean percentage change from baseline ± SE (mg/dL) in HDL_2-cholesterol at cycles 3, 6, and 13 in women treated with continuous combined regimens of conjugated estrogens and MPA (groups A and B), with sequential regimens of conjugated estrogens and MPA (groups C and D), or with conjugated estrogens alone (group E). A,C,D, significant difference between conjugated estrogens plus MPA groups. *Significant difference from baseline; †significant difference from conjugated estrogens alone. (From ref. 17, with permission.)

sensitivity occurs with 10 mg of MPA (25,26). The effects are less with 2.5 mg. However, even 0.35 mg of NET has been shown to decrease glucose tolerance slightly.

Among the negative metabolic effects, only HDL-C and insulin sensitivity stand out, and the latter is minimized by using a smaller dose of progestogen. However, some potentially disadvantageous vascular effects may also be encountered. Some women also have adverse mood effects from various progestogens. These are predominantly of the depressive type and have been considered to be similar to the premenstrual syndrome experienced by some women. Alterations from the oral route may be beneficial under these circumstances if reductions in dose and changes in the type of progestogens are not successful. As little as 2.5 mg of MPA or 0.35 mg of NET used sequentially may be sufficient to protect the endometrium.

Nonoral Progestogen Therapy

Nonoral forms of progestogens include the new transdermal preparations, vaginal preparations, and intrauterine devices. Norethindrone acetate (NET-A) (250 g) and levonogesterel (75 g) both have been combined with E_2 in matrix patches for hormonal therapy. The original concept was to develop a sequential regimen beginning with a standard matrix patch of E_2, 50 g, for 2 weeks followed by a combination patch of 50 g of E_2 with either progestogen for 2 weeks. Recently a combination matrix patch has

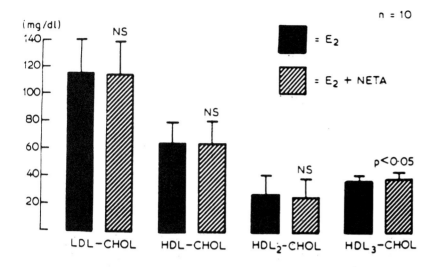

FIG. 13.23. Mean concentrations of serum lipoproteins during treatment with estradiol-TTS and estradiol and estradiol/norethisterone acetate-TTS patches. (From ref. 55, with permission.)

been approved for use in the United States. This system combines both E₂ and NET-A: 50 µg E₂ is combined with 140 or 250 µg of NET-A as a daily continuous combined regimen. Each patch has a life-span of 3½ days and needs to be changed accordingly.

Because HDL-C is not increased with transdermal E₂, there is no benefit of giving progestogens nonorally to prevent the decline in HDL-C serum with oral therapy. Indeed, the lipid and lipoprotein changes are considered neutral (Fig. 13.23) (55). Similarly, glucose and insulin data are largely unchanged from baseline levels (Fig. 13.24). Cycle control with two sequential patches with NET-A or levonogesterel have been compared, and although some small differences are appreciated between the two preparations, in general cycle control is considered to be very good (56). Thus, to date, the major advantage of the combination E₂ and progestogen patches is convenience. Although low doses of systemically administered progestogen should have metabolic advantages

over higher doses of oral therapy because of first-passage effects, to date the metabolic effects have to be considered to be neutral.

Because the only reason to administer progestogens is to achieve endometrial protection, it is attractive to consider vaginal or uterine therapy to avoid all systemic effects. We have shown that vaginal administration of micronized progesterone capsules increased uterine concentrations to levels above those measured during the luteal phase (57). Thus, serum levels may be minimized with good endometrial protection by using smaller, yet effective vaginal doses as low as 25 or 50 mg.

A progesterone gel (Crione) is a marketed product that achieves this end point. A 4% gel (45 mg) administered every other day results in adequate progestational effects to protect the endometrium while serum progesterone levels remain low (<2 ng/mL; 59) (Fig. 13.25).

Effective endometrial protection has also been accomplished with a progesterone IUD, replaced annually (60).

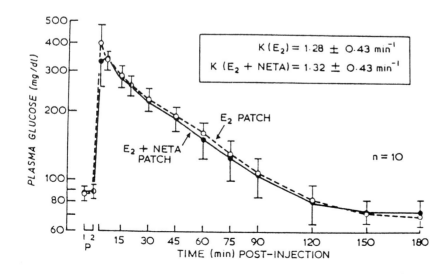

FIG. 13.24. Plasma glucose concentrations from intravenous glucose tolerance test during treatment with estradiol-TTS and estradiol/norethisterone acetate patches. (From ref. 55, with permission.)

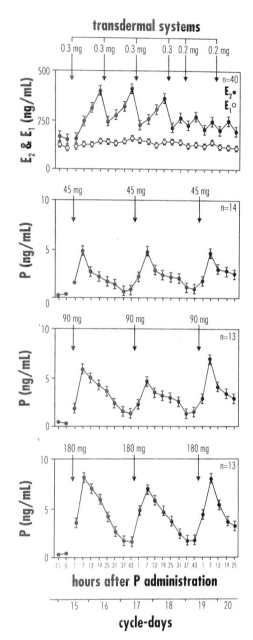

FIG. 13.25. Plasma estradiol (E₂) and estrone (E₁) (upper panel) and progesterone (P) profiles (lower panels) in groups A (45 mg), B (90 mg), and C (180 mg) from days 15 to 20. Estrogen levels fluctuated in relation to changes of transdermal systems, but the E₂-to-E₁ ratio remained greater than 1 throughout the observation interval. Overall mean progesterone levels were significantly lower in group A (2.4 ± 0.2 ng/mL) than in group B (3.6 ± 0.2 ng/mL) or C (3.4 ± 0.4 ng/mL) ($p < 0.005$). BL, baseline. (From ref. 59, with permission.)

Here a direct progestational effect on the uterus is exerted without appreciable levels of serum progesterone. A levonorgestrel IUD (20 µg/day) has been used in Europe for contraception and menorrhagia and has been found to be highly effective (61). A smaller model of this IUD, 5 to 10 µg, offers promise for use in postmenopausal women (62).

REFERENCES

1. Shiff I, Tulchinsky D, Ryan KJ. Vaginal absorption of estrone and 17-β-estradiol. *Fertil Steril* 1977;28:1063.
2. Martin PL, Yen SSC, Burmier AM, et al. Systemic absorption and sustained effects of vaginal estrogen creams. *JAMA* 1979;242:2699.
3. Chetkowski RJ, Meldrum DR, Steingold KA, et al. Biologic effects of transdermal estradiol. *N Engl J Med* 1986;314:1615.
4. Siddle N, Whitehead M; Flexible prescribing of estrogens. *Contemp Ob/Gyn* 1983;22:137.
5. Anderson ABM, Sklovsky E, Sayers L, et al. Comparison of serum oestrogen concentrations in postmenopausal women taking oestrogen concentrations in postmenopausal women taking oestrone sulphate and oestradiol. *Br Med J* 1978;1:140.
6. Aedo A-R, Landgren B-M, Diczfalusy E. Pharmacokinetic properties of oral oestrone sulphate piperazine and oestradiol valerate in post-menopausal women. *Maturitas* 1984;6:79.
7. Colvin PL Jr, Auerbach BJ, Koritnik DR, et al. Differential effects of oral estrone versus 17β-estradiol on lipoproteins in postmenopausal women. *J Clin Endocrinol Metab* 1990;70:1568.
8. Cassidenti DL, Vijod AG, Vijod MA, et al. Short-term effects of smoking on the pharmacokinetic profiles of micronized estradiol in postmenopausal women. *Am J Obstet Gynecol* 1990;163:1953.
9. Lobo RA, Brenner P, Mishell DR Jr. Metabolic parameters and steroid levels in postmenopausal women receiving lower doses of natural estrogen replacement. *Obstet Gynecol* 1983;62:94.
10. Whitehead JL, Minardi J, Kitchin Y, et al. Systemic absorption of oestrogen from Premarin vaginal cream. In: Cooke ID, ed. *The role of oestrogen/progestogen in the management of the menopause.* Lancaster, UK: MTP Press, 1978:636-71.
11. Mashchak CA, Lobo RA, Dozono-Takano R, et al. Comparison of pharmacodynamic properties of various estrogen formulations. *Am J Obstet Gynecol* 1982;144:511.
12. Lobo RA, Nguyen HN, Eggena P, et al. Biologic effects of equilin sulfate in postmenopausal women. *Fertil Steril* 1988;49:234.
13. Jensen J, Christiansen C, Rodbro R. Cigarette smoking, serum estrogens, and bone losses during hormone-replacement therapy early after menopause. *N Engl J Med* 1985;313:973.
14. Jensen JN, Christiansen C. Effects of smoking on serum lipoproteins and bone mineral content during postmenopausal hormone replacement therapy. *Am J Obstet Gynecol* 1988;159:820.
15. Ginsburg ES, Mello NK, Mendelson JH, et al. Effects of alcohol ingestion on estrogens in postmenopausal women. *JAMA* 1996;276:1747.
16. Ginsburg E, Walsh B, Gao X, Gleason R, Feltmate C, Barbieri L. The effect of acute ethanol ingestion on estrogen levels in postmenopausal women using transdermal estradiol. *J Soc Gynecol Invest* 1995;2:26.
17. Lobo RA, Pickar JH, Wild RA, Walsh B, Hirvonen E, and the Menopause Study Group. Metabolic impact of adding medroxyprogesterone acetate to conjugated estrogen therapy in postmenopausal women. *Obstet Gynecol* 1994;84:987.
18. Notelovitz M, Kitchens C, Ware M, et al. Combination of estrogen and progestogen replacement therapy does not adversely affect coagulation. *Obstet Gynecol* 1983;62:596.
19. Lobo RA. Estrogen and the risk of coagulopathy. *Am J Med* 1992;92:283.
20. Daly E, Vessey MP, Hawkins MM, Carson JL, Parimala G, Marsh S. Risk of venous thromboembolism in users of hormone replacement therapy. *Lancet* 1996;348:977.
21. Jick H, Derby LE, Myers MW, Vasilakis C, Newton KM. Risk of hospital admission for idiopathic venous thromboembolism among users of postmenopausal oestrogens. *Lancet* 1996;348:981.
22. Grodstein F, Stampfer MJ, Goldhaber SZ, et al. Prospective study of exogenous hormones and risk of pulmonary embolism in women. *Lancet* 1996;348:983.
23. Mashchak CA, Lobo RA. Estrogen replacement therapy and hypertension. *J Reprod Med* 1985;30(Suppl 10):805.
24. Luotola H. Blood pressure and hemodynamics in postmenopausal women during estradiol-17β substitution. *Ann Clin Res* 1983;15(Suppl 38):9.
25. Lindheim SR, Presser SC, Ditkoff EC, Vijod MA, Stanczyk FZ, Lobo RA. A possible bimodal effect of estrogen on insulin sensitivity in postmenopausal women and the attenuating effect of added progestin. *Fertil Steril* 1993;60:664.
26. Lindheim SR, Buchanan TA, Duffy DM, et al. Comparison of estimates of insulin sensitivity in pre- and postmenopausal women using the insulin tolerance test and the frequently sampled intravenous glucose tolerance test. *J Soc Gynecol Invest* 1994;1:150.
27. Lindheim SR, Duffy DM, Kojima T, Vijod MA, Stanczyk FZ, Lobo RA. The route of administration influences the effect of estrogen on insulin sensitivity in postmenopausal women. *Fertil Steril* 1994;62:1176.
28. Lobo RA. Effects of hormonal replacement on lipids and lipoproteins in postmenopausal women. *J Clin Endocrinol Metab* 1991;73:925.
29. Steingold KA, Laufer L, Chetkowski RJ, et al. Treatment of hot flashes with transdermal estradiol administration. *J Clin Endocrinol Metab* 1985;61:627.
30. Cano A. Compliance to hormone replacement therapy in menopausal women controlled in a third level academic centre. *Maturitas* 1995;20:91.
31. Lobo RA, Gibbons WE. The role of progestin therapy in breast disease and central nervous system function. *J Reprod Med* 1982;27:515.
32. Powers MS, Schenkel L, Darley PE, et al. Pharmacokinetics and pharmacodynamics of transdermal dosage forms of 17β-estradiol: Comparison with conventional oral estrogens used for hormone replacement. *Am J Obstet Gynecol* 1985;152:1099.

33. Gordon SF. Clinical experience with a seven-day estradiol transdermal system for estrogen replacement therapy. *Am J Obstet Gynecol* 1995;173(Part 2, Suppl):998.

34. Williams JK, Shivaly CA, Clarkson TB. Determinants of coronary artery reactivity in premenopausal female cynomolgus monkeys with diet induced atherosclerosis. *Circulation* 1994;90:983.

35. Lobo RA, March CM, Goebelsmann U, Krauss RM, Mishell DR Jr. Subdermal estradiol pellets following hysterectomy and oophorectomy. Effect upon serum estrone, estradiol, luteinizing hormone, follicle-stimulating hormone, corticosteroid binding globulin-binding capacity, testosterone-estradiol binding globulin-binding capacity, lipids and hot flushes. *Am J Obstet Gynecol* 1980;138:714.

36. Stanczyk FZ, Shoupe D, Nunez V, Macias-Gonzales P, Vijod MA, Lobo RA. A randomized comparison of nonoral estradiol delivery in postmenopausal women. *Am J Obstet Gynecol* 1988;159:1540.

37. Davis SR, McCloud P, Strauss JG, Burger H. Testosterone enhances estradiolís effects on postmenopausal bone density and sexuality. *Maturitas* 1995;21:227.

38. Whitehead MI, Townsend PT, Kitchin Y, et al. Plasma steroid and protein hormone profiles in post-menopausal women following topical administration of oestradiol 17β. In: Mauvais-Jarvis P, Vickers CFH, Wepierre J, eds. *Percutaneous absorption of steroids.* London: Academic Press, 1980.

39. Scott RT Jr, Ross B, Anderson C, Archer DF. Pharmacokinetics of percutaneous estradiol: a crossover study using a gel and a transdermal system in comparison with oral micronized estradiol. *Obstet Gynecol* 1991;77:758.

40. Mandel FP, Geola FL, Meldrum DR, et al. Biological effects of various doses of vaginally administered conjugated equine estrogens in postmenopausal women. *J Clin Endocrinol Metab* 1983;57:133.

41. Deutsch S, Ossowski R, Benjamin I. Comparison between degree of systemic absorption of vaginally and orally administered estrogens at different dose levels in postmenopausal women. *Am J Obstet Gynecol* 1981;139:967.

42. Schmidt G, Andersson SB, Nordle O, Johansson CJ, Gunnarsson PO. Release of 17-beta-oestradiol from a vaginal ring in postmenopausal women: pharmacokinetic evaluation. *Gynecol Obstet Invest* 1994;38:253.

43. Whitehead MI, Townsend PT, Gill DK, et al. Absorption and metabolism of oral progesterone. *Br Med J* 1980;280:825.

44. Padwick M, Endacott J, Matson C, et al. Absorption and metabolism of oral progesterone when administered twice daily. *Fertil Steril* 1986;46:402.

45. The Writing Group for the PEPI Trial. Effects of estrogen or estrogen/progestin regimens on heart disease risk factors in postmenopausal women. *JAMA* 1995;273:199.

46. Ottosson UB, Carlstrom K, Damber JE, et al. Serum levels of progesterone and some of its metabolites including deoxycorticosterone after oral and parenteral administration. *Br J Obstet Gynaecol* 1984;91:1111.

47. Ottosson UB, Carlstrom K, Damber JE, et al. Conversion of oral progesterone into deoxycorticosterone during postmenopausal replacement therapy. *Acta Obstet Gynecol Scand* 1984;63:577.

48. Nillus SJ, Johansson EDB. Plasma levels of progesterone after vaginal, rectal or intramuscular administration of progesterone. *Am J Obstet Gynecol* 1971;110:470.

49. Whitehead MI, Siddle NC, Townsend PT, et al. The use of progestins and progesterone in the treatment of climacteric and postmenopausal symptoms. In: Bardin CW, Milgrom E, Mauvis-Jarvis P, eds. *Progesterone and progestin.* New York: Raven Press, 1982.

50. Steege JF, Rupp SL, Stout AL, et al. Bioavailability of nasally administered progesterone. *Fertil Steril* 1986;46:727.

51. Cornette JC, Kirton KT, Duncan GW. Measurement of medroxyprogesterone acetate by radioimmunoassay. *J Clin Endocrinol Metab* 1971;33:459.

52. Fotherby K. Variability of pharmacokinetic parameters for contraceptive steroids. *J Steroid Biochem* 1983;19:817.

53. Humpel M, Wendt H, Pommerenke G, et al. Investigations of pharmacokinetics of levonorgestrel to specific consideration of a possible first-pass effect in women. *Contraception* 1978;17:207.

54. Conrad J, Cazenave B, Samama M. Antithrombin II content and antithrombin activity in estrogen-óprogestogen and progestogen-only treated women. *Thromb Res* 1980;18:675.

55. Gangar KF, Whitehead MI. Biological actions of progestins. In: Korenman SG, ed. *The menopause.* Norwell, MA: Serono Symposia, 1990.

56. Symposium ReportóFIGO, August 4. *Eur Menopause J* 1997;4:1.

57. Miles RA, Paulson RJ, Lobo RA, Press MF, Dahmoush L, Sauer MV. Pharmacokinetics and endometrial tissue levels of progesterone after administration by intramuscular and vaginal routes. A comparative study. *Fertil Steril* 1994;62:485.

58. Mezrow G, Koopersmith T, Shoupe D, Lobo RA. *Estrogen replacement therapy using micronized vaginal progesterone.* Paper presented at the 42nd annual meeting of the Society for Gynecologic Investigation, Chicago, March 15-ó18.

59. Fanchin R, DeZiegler D, Bergeron C, et al. Transvaginal administration of progesterone. *Obstet Gynecol* 1997;90:396.

60. Shoupe D, Meme D, Mezrow G, Lobo RA. Prevention of endometrial hyperplasia in postmenopausal women with intrauterine progesterone. *N Engl J Med* 1991;325:1811.

61. Suhonen SP, Allonen HO, Lahteenmaki P. Sustained-release estradiol implants and a levonorgestrel-releasing intrauterine device in hormone replacement therapy. *Am J Obstet Gynecol* 1995;172:562.

62. Wollter-Svensson L-O, Stadberg E, Andersson K, et al. Intrauterine administration of levonorgestrel 5 and 10 μg/24 h in perimenopausal hormone replacement therapy. A randomized clinical trial during one year. *Acta Obstet Gynecol Scand* 1997;76:449.

Treatment of the Postmenopausal Woman: Basic and Clinical Aspects, Second Edition, edited by Rogerio A. Lobo, Lippincott Williams & Wilkins, Philadelphia © 1999.

CHAPTER 14

Where Androgens Come From, What Controls Them, and Whether to Replace Them

John E. Buster and Peter R. Casson

Androgen production declines with advancing age (1–5). Estrogens without androgens, therefore, are probably incomplete menopause replacement. Recent studies indicate that restoration of youthful androgen levels to menopausal women may significantly retard maladies of age: cardiovascular disease, neoplasia, diabetes, immunosenescence, osteoporosis, muscular wasting, loss of libidinal interest, and depression (6–8). Despite burgeoning interest in this field, it is not clear when or how to administer androgens to menopausal women: optimal therapies and their doses are not established even though androgens alone, or in combinations with estrogens, are widely prescribed.

This chapter reviews the recent literature on where androgens come from, what controls them, and the impact of age on declining androgen production. It further examines conditions that accelerate the decline of androgens and methods and indications for replacing androgens.

WHERE ANDROGENS COME FROM AND WHAT CONTROLS THEM

The literature traditionally identifies five androgens (Table 14.1) as clinically important: dehydroepiandrosterone sulfate (DHEA-S), dehydroepiandrosterone (DHEA), androstenedione (Δ^4A), testosterone (T), and dihydrotestosterone (DHT). In women, these androgens have widely differing serum concentrations, production rates, potencies, and origins (Table 1). Although the basic 19-carbon (C_{19}) androstane nuclear structure is held in common (Fig. 14.1), effects on target tissues differ. As

examples, DHEA-S is associated with immunomodulation, enhancement of insulin effect, and osteoporosis protection, whereas libidinal drive, sex hair development, seborrhea, and acne are more associated with T (6–10). Interconversion among DHEA-S, T, and other androgens blur these distinctions (9–12).

The sources, regulation, and interconversion of these five androgens, as influenced by aging and menopausal status, are depicted (Figs. 14.2 and 14.3). They are described in detail now.

TABLE 14.1. *Androgen concentrations and relative biologic potency in reproductive-age women using testosterone as a standard of 1.0.*

Androgen	Relative bioassay potency	Representative concentration
Dihydrotestosterone	5	<5 ng/dL
Testosterone (T)	1	50 ng/dL
Androstenedione Δ^4A	0.1	100 ng/dL
DHEA	0.01	500 ng/dL
DHEA-S	0.001	200,000 ng/dL

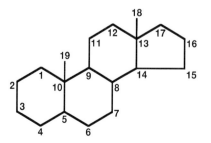

FIG. 14.1. Androstane structural nucleus (19 carbons) common to the five clinically important androgens.

J. E. Buster: Department of Obstetrics and Gynecology, Division of Reproductive Endocrinology and Infertility, Baylor College of Medicine, Houston, Texas 77030.

P. R. Casson: Department of Obstetrics and Gynecology, University of Ottawa, Ontario, Canada K1Y 1J8.

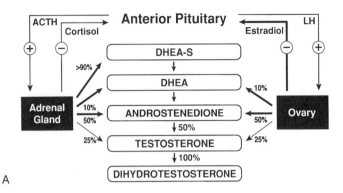

A

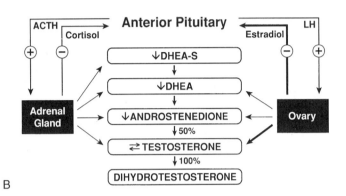

B

FIG. 14.2. Androgen dynamics in **(A)** premenopausal and **(B)** postmenopausal women. Menopausal levels of luteinizing hormone (LH) drive ovarian stroma to produce increased T, compensating in part for the age-related loss of adrenal androgens and androgen precursors.

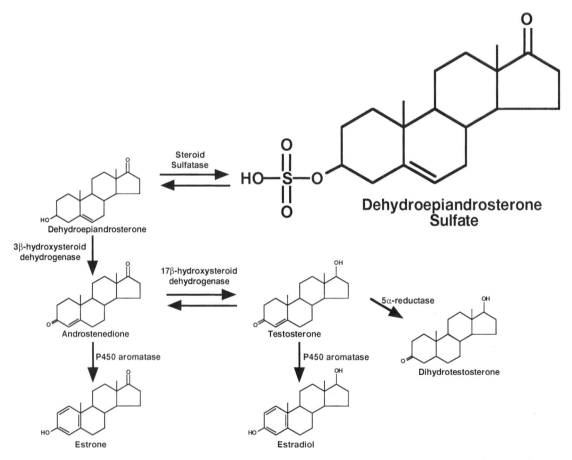

FIG. 14.3. Interconversions of five clinically important androgens from circulating dehydroepiandrosterone sulfate (DHEA-S): androstenedione (Δ^4A), testosterone (T), and dihydrotestosterone (DHT) are formed within target tissues from circulating DHEA-S. Estrone (E_1) and estradiol (E_2) are also formed within target tissues from their corresponding Δ^4 androgens, Δ^4A and T.

Dehydroepiandrosterone and Dehydroepiandrosterone Sulfate

Dehydroepiandrosterone (DHEA) and dehydroepiandrosterone sulfate (DHEA-S), collectively designated DHEA(S), are prohormones without known receptors or specific target tissue activity. DHEA-S and DHEA are secreted daily in milligram amounts by the zona reticularis (ZR) of the human adrenal cortex (11). The ZR, the sole secretory source of DHEA-S, is unique to humans and higher primates (4,13). At a rate of 8 to 16 mg/day (much less after menopause), DHEA-S production exceeds that of all other steroids (11,12). With circulating concentrations of 100- to 1,000-fold of any other androgen, DHEA-S circulates in a pool with very slow turnover. Unconjugated DHEA, also originating from the ZR, and in addition secreted by ovarian stroma (DHEA-S is not), is converted peripherally to DHEA-S. Unconjugated DHEA is a metabolic intermediate to and from DHEA-S to Δ^4A, T, and DHT (Fig. 14.3). Its production rate is 6 to 8 mg/day (less after menopause), but because it has a considerably higher metabolic clearance rate than DHEA-S, its pool turns over more quickly in circulating concentrations that are much lower than DHEA-S (11,12).

From circulating DHEA-S, bioactive androgens and estrogens are synthesized within the cells of their site of action—the target tissues (9,14–16). DHEA-S is extracted from the circulation and transferred into target cells as DHEA-S (Fig. 14.4). Once in the cell, DHEA-S is converted to DHEA by steroid sulfatase, to Δ^4A by intracellular 3β-hydroxysteroid dehydrogenase (3β-HSD), and then to T by 17β-hydroxysteroid dehydrogenase (17β-HSD) (Figs. 14.3 and 14.4). Testosterone (T) thus formed is acted on by 5α-reductase to produce DHT or, alternatively, by aromatase to produce 17β-estradiol (E$_2$)—depending on local biologic requirements and steroidogenic architecture (Figs. 14.3 and 14.4) (9,14–16). It thus appears that in both women and men (more in women), much of the biologically significant androgen production originates from cir-

culating DHEA-S with interconversion and then action occurring in target tissues. In breast, for example, approximately 75% of estrogen in premenopausal women originates from circulating DHEA-S. After menopause, virtually 100% of breast tissue estrogen comes from this source (14–16). In men, as another example, over half of prostatic T arises from circulating DHEA (Fig. 14.4) (14,17–18). Male castration, which drops circulating T precipitously, reduces prostatic DHT by only 50% to 60%. In men, therefore, DHEA-S, originating exclusively from the ZR, continues to circulate in abundance even after castration and therefore continues to exert significant androgen effect within the prostate (14,17–18). Even steroid-secreting organs themselves utilize circulating DHEA-S as a prohormone. The ovary, for example, extracts and converts circulating DHEA-S in granulosa cells of maturing follicles (19,20). Extracted DHEA-S is converted to intrafollicular T, which modulates oocyte maturation (19–20).

DHEA-S secretion, as mentioned previously, originates exclusively from the ZR (4,13). DHEA-S secretion is regulated by ACTH and several coregulatory factors that include prolactin, insulin-like growth factor (IGF-1), estrogen, and the ZR cell mass itself (21–27). The ZR is one of three adult zones of the adrenal: the outer zona glomerulosa (ZG), the middle zona fasciculata (ZF), and the inner zona reticularis (ZR) (Fig. 14.5) (4,27). The ZR

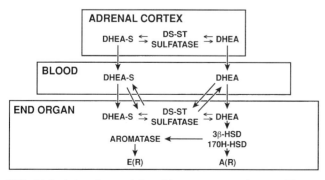

FIG. 14.4. Intracrine activity of human target tissues. These are the known biosynthetic steps involved in the formation of androgens (A) from circulating DHEA-S and estrogens (E) in human target tissue. 17OH-HSD, 17β-hydroxysteroid dehydrogenase; 3β-HSD, dehydrogenase/Δ^4–Δ^5 isomerase; R, steroid receptor. (Modified from ref. 14.)

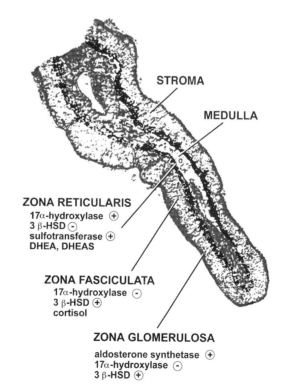

FIG. 14.5. Histologic section of the adult adrenal cortex. The adrenal cortex is divided into three zones: the outer zona glomerulosa (ZG), the middle zona fasciculata (ZF), and the innermost zona reticularis (ZR). Steroidogenic enzyme architecture unique to each zone directs the profile of steroid products secreted by each. (Adapted from ref. 28.)

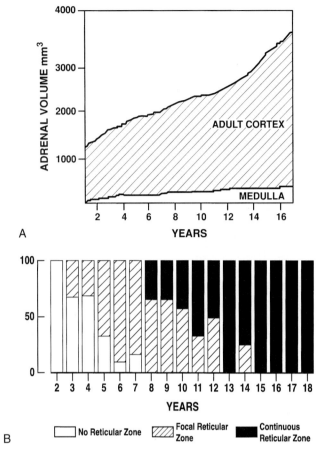

FIG. 14.6. Mass of adrenal cortex as a function of (A) age and (B) zona reticularis detected histologically as a percentage of harvested glands. Total adrenal mass increases steadily during childhood. Zona reticularis is detectable histologically as early as age 6 and is present in virtually all glands by the age of 14 years. (Adapted from ref. 29.)

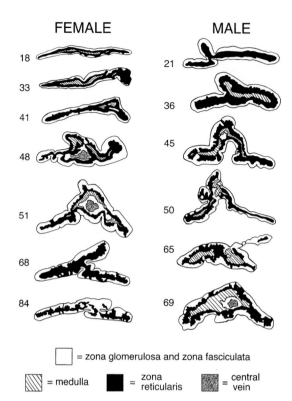

= zona glomerulosa and zona fasciculata

= medulla   = zona reticularis   = central vein

FIG. 14.8. In a process resembling apoptosis, there is a decrease in the number of functional ZR cells with age. This figure, showing 12 adrenal glands (18 to 84 years), is reproduced from one of a very small number of studies of the changes in the reticularis with aging. It shows increasing ZR irregularity rather than simple involution of the zone (32). (Adapted from ref. 33.)

becomes histologically distinct during childhood and assumes an increasing percentage of adrenal mass during the years surrounding adrenarche (Fig. 14.6) (28,29). The steroidogenic zonal architecture is determined by gene expression unique to the cells of that zone (Fig. 14.7).

Thus, ZR cells in culture have very low expression of 3β-HSD. Correspondingly, 3β-HSD is easily detected in ZF cells, which produce Δ^4 steroids in abundance: Δ^4A and cortisol, not DHEA. Thus, the ZR embodies a morphologically distinctive cell type that is genetically programmed with steroidogenic machinery devoted solely to production of Δ^5 androgens: DHEA-S and DHEA (Figs. 14.5–14.7) (4,27). DHEA, but not DHEA-S, is also

FIG. 14.7. Steroidogenic architecture of the zona reticularis. DHEA and DHEA-S are secreted by a discrete layer of cells in the adult human adrenal cortex, the zona reicularis (ZR). The key molecular feature of the ZR that results in the production of DHEA(S) is its low expression of the enzyme 3β-HSD. The zona fasciculata (ZF) has a high level of 3β-HSD, resulting in the synthesis of the glucocorticoid cortisol. Other key enzymatic differences between the zones that result in the production of different steroids by the zones are shown. (Adapted from ref. 12.)

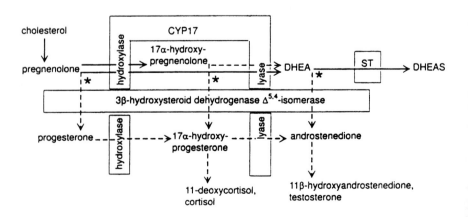

secreted by the premenopausal ovary in modest amounts (5,11,12). The postmenopausal ovarian stroma, under the influence of high undulating pituitary LH, continues to secrete DHEA in significant amounts (5,11,12,30–32).

In aging women, DHEA-S production and its circulating concentrations decline dramatically (1–4). This decline is associated with fragmentation of the ZR in a cellular process closely resembling apoptosis (33). This apoptotic process and the ZR atrophy that results are believed to represent the principal mechanism for the age-related decline in adrenal androgens (Fig. 14.8). The corpus luteum like ZR may thus be seen in nature as a temporary tissue (4)."

Androstenedione

Androstenedione (Δ^4A), the Δ^4 analog of DHEA, is also a circulating prohormone (9,11,14). It has no specific receptors or target tissue activity. In normal women, most Δ^4A found in androgen-responsive tissues has been converted to Δ^4A from circulating DHEA-S to DHEA (9,11,14). This conversion is facilitated by 3β-HSD in tar-

get tissue cells (9,14). Circulating Δ^4A is secreted by both ovarian stroma and the adrenal ZF (the zone that secretes cortisol) (4,13,27). It is not produced by adrenal ZR cells, which lack 3β-HSD activity and therefore produce DHEA (13,27). During premenopausal years, approximately 50% of secreted Δ^4A originates from the ZF, whereas the other 50% originates from ovarian stroma (11,12). Variations in circulating Δ^4A reflect its dual origins: its adrenal origin by a circadian variation and its ovarian origin by a periovulatory surge during midcycle (Fig. 14.9) (12,34).

In aging women, circulating Δ^4A decreases slightly (1,12,35). This is because even though adrenal secretion decreases, ovarian secretion continues. Presumably this represents the response of the ovarian stroma to high menopausal LH, allowing the ovary to compensate in part for a diminishing adrenal contribution (30–32,36,37).

Testosterone

Testosterone (T) is a biologically potent androgen with specific receptors and target tissues. It is secreted into the circulation by both the adrenal ZF (cortisol and Δ^4A) and the ovaries (13,27,30–32,36,37). As mentioned previously, it is also formed within target tissue from circulating DHEA-S (9). During reproductive years, approxi-

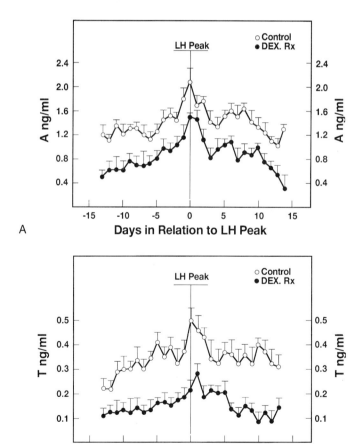

FIG. 14.9. Midcycle rise in ovarian Δ^4A (A) and T (B) in a group of women before and after 1 month of dexamethasone suppression of adrenal androgen production. Both Δ^4A and T have a midcycle increase in concentration associated with periovulatary period. (Adapted from ref. 34.)

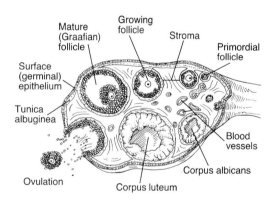
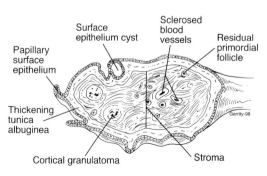

FIG. 14.10. Schematic representation of the most salient differences between the reproductive age (A) and postmenopausal (B) ovary. The stromal compartment comprises virtually all of the postmenopausal ovary. The postmenopausal ovarian stroma synthesizes and secretes considerable DHEA, Δ^4A, and T. (Adapted from ref. 39.)

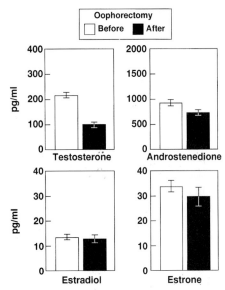

FIG. 14.11. Peripheral and ovarian vein androgen and estrogen levels in ten postmenopausal women. A dramatic stepdown gradient is demonstrated for Δ^4A and T. (Adapted from ref. 40.)

mately 25% of circulating T originates from the ovary, about 25% from the ZF, and about 50% from peripheral Δ^4A conversion (11). During reproductive years, T levels show a periovulatory rise at midcycle in association with the LH surge (Fig. 14.9) (34). Circulating T has no circadian change (11,12).

In aging women, circulating T remains stable well into the 80s (12,36,37). Although ovarian volume decreases by about 30%, ovarian stroma, driven by high undulating, menopausal LH, secretes T in increasing abundance (Figs. 14.10–14.12) (38–41). Circulating T thus decreases little after menopause even though adrenal androgen production

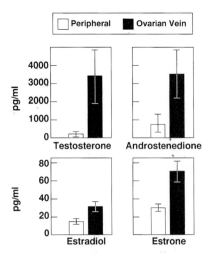

FIG. 14.12. Serum androgen and estrogen levels in 16 postmenopausal women before and after ovariectomy. Ovariectomy produces a dramatic decrease of T and some decrease of Δ^4A. (Adapted from ref. 5.)

of DHEA(S) and Δ^4A decline. A substantial ovarian contribution of T after menopause is well documented by a considerable ovarian vein–peripheral vein stepdown gradient, which is even greater in postmenopausal women (Fig. 14.9) (40,41). Removal of postmenopausal ovaries produces a 40% to 50% decrement in circulating T (Fig. 14.12) (5). Given that considerable target tissue T is transformed from circulating DHEA-S, and given that menopausal DHEA-S concentrations are very low, the impact of menopausal oophorectomy from T withdrawal at target tissues is probably clinically significant.

Dihydrotestosterone

Dihydrotestosterone (DHT), believed to be the most potent of androgens, is present primarily in target tissues. Its circulating concentrations are very low in women (34). It is secreted by the adrenal ZF (cortisol) in small amounts (4,13). DHT is produced from 5α-reduction of the 4–5 double bond in the A ring of T. In target tissues, where the receptor DHT complex has far greater affinity for genome receptor sites than does the receptor for T, DHT is a potent androgen (Figs. 14.3 and 14.4) (14). Target tissue conversion of T to DHT is believed to act as an androgen amplifier mechanism that sequesters androgens in a nonaromatizable and very potent configuration.

How Androgens Increase with Youth and Decline with Age

DHEA(S) production begins to increase at ages 7 to 8 in girls (Fig. 14.13), when the ZR first appears as a structure identifiably separate from other adrenal zones (Figs. 14.5 and 14.6) (28,29,42). This increase is associated with clinical benchmarks of adrenarche: pubic and axillary hair, emerging libidinal interest, muscle mass and strength, increased bone mass, maturation of the immune system, and increasing stature (Table 14.2; Fig. 14.14) (42). DHEA(S) concentrations reach their lifetime zenith during the decades of the 20s and 30s and then begin a gradual decline that continues into the 80s and 90s (Fig. 14.13) (2,3). Whereas circulating T, Δ^4A, and DHT fall only modestly with advancing age, it is likely that tissue production and target tissue impact fall more dramatically in concert with declining DHEA-S production because DHEA-S is the principal prohormone to these steroids (Fig. 14.3) (1). During this decline, identified clinically as postmenopausal senescence, events much the opposite of adrenarche occur: loss of pubic and axillary hair, decreased libidinal interest, loss of muscle mass and strength, loss of bone mass, immunosenescence, and decline of adult stature (Table 14.2) (43–46). Because DHEA-S is an important prohormone, it is reasonable to speculate this decline is linked to events of aging. It follows that restoration of youthful circulating DHEA-S may attenuate some aspects of aging.

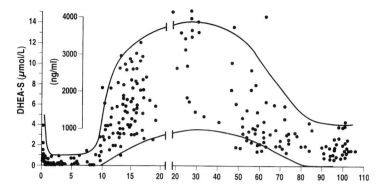

FIG. 14.13. Circulating DHEA-S in girls and women from birth to age. Graph is a composite of two studies. DHEA-S concentrations, a direct reflection of DHEA-S adrenal secretion, begins to increase in girls aged 7 to 8 **(A)**. Maximum liftetime concentrations are achieved during the decades of the 20s and 30s and begin a sustained decline through age 100 **(B)**. *Outside bands* enclose 95% of the data points. (**A**, adapted from measurements in girls from ref. 42; **B**, adapted from measurements in adult women through age 100 from ref. 2.)

TABLE 14.2. *Postmenopausal senescence as a model of reverse adrenarche analogous to events after menopause that are associated with declining DHEA-S production*

Adrenarche	Menopausal senescence
Increasing sex hair	Loss of sex hair
Increasing libido	Loss of libido
Increasing bone density	Loss of bone density
Increasing stature	Loss of stature
Increasing muscle mass	Loss of muscle mass
Immune maturation	Immunosenescence

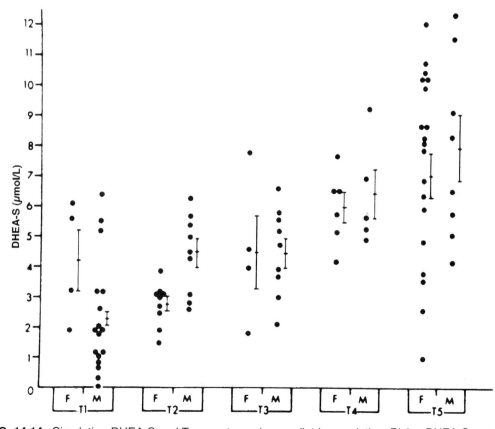

FIG. 14.14. Circulating DHEA-S and Tanner stages in a pediatric population. Rising DHEA-S concentrations are directly correlated with Tanner stage in adolescent boys and girls. (Adapted from ref. 42.)

Conditions that Accelerate Declining Androgen Production

Declining androgen production is accelerated by misadventures of advancing years.

Oophorectomy

Postmenopausal oophorectomy decreases circulating T by 40% to 50%. Perimenopausal and postmenopausal oophorectomy is associated with decreased libidinal interest, depression, and may have other long-term liabilities to include loss of bone mineral density, accelerated immunosenescence, and increased insulin resistance (5).

Pituitary/Adrenal Insufficiency

Both Sheehan's syndrome and Addison's disease are models of androgen depletion. Both are associated with muscle wasting, loss of pubic and axillary hair, decreased libidinal interest, osteoporosis, and immunosenescence.

Chronic Illness

Anorexia nervosa, advanced neoplasia, and burn trauma are all associated with low androgen concentrations and clinical manifestations of androgen depletion (46–48).

Estrogen Replacement

Estrogen replacement to menopausal women suppresses circulating DHEA-S, Δ^4A, and T; LH levels are

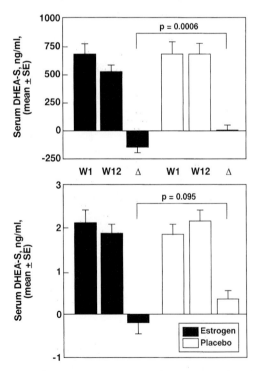

FIG. 14.15. The effect of physiologic postmenopausal estrogen replacement therapy on circulating DHEA-S and DHEA. In this randomized, prospective, blinded, placebo-controlled trial of 28 subjects, estrogen suppressed circulating DHEA-S and DHEA levels. (Adapted from ref. 49.)

also suppressed, and levels of sex hormone-binding globulin are increased (Fig. 14.15) (49).

Corticosteroid Therapy

Corticosteroids suppress ACTH and therefore ZR secretion of DHEA(S) (26). The clinical picture of Cushing's syndrome includes androgen depletion, loss of pubic and axillary hair, osteoporosis, muscle wasting, and immunosuppression. Plausibly, the serious side effects of corticosteroid suppression could be attenuated by coadministration of DHEA (50).

Clinical Expression of Androgen Deficiency

There are no agreed-on diagnostic criteria for androgen deficiency. In women, androgen deficiency is subtle in presentation and slow to evolve. Though not immediately lethal, it may accelerate aging and increase mortality. As mentioned above, events of adrenarche, a clinical model of increasing androgen effect in women (Table 14.2), are reversed with advanced age. These events have traditionally been accepted with resolve as inevitable and unpreventable ravages of aging.

New strategies to replace androgens in women are under active investigation. These are discussed now.

ANDROGEN REPLACEMENT FOR WOMEN

Available strategies involve administration of T or DHEA(S) (Table 14.3).

Testosterone Replacement

Testosterone replacement has been studied extensively in men, not women. Preparations are diverse: they can be either synthetic 17β-alkylated or 17β-esterified T substitutes or natural T. Routes of T administration can be oral, intramuscular, sublingual, subcutaneous, or transcutaneous. We examine delivery systems that have been investigated in women.

Oral Testosterone

Given orally, crystalline T is metabolized rapidly by the liver (51). Micronized oral T needs to be given in substantial amounts, and while bioavailable, the increases in serum T are erratic (52). Strategies to overcome hepatic first-pass effect on exogenous T have been devised and include various ring substitutions (Table 14.3; Fig. 14.16).

Testosterone Undecenoate

Testosterone undecenoate is a 17β-ester; this configuration renders the molecule sufficiently lipophilic to allow absorption into intestinal lymphatics, which bypass the liver, and increases bioavailability (53). To ensure absorption, T undecenoate must be administered with oleic acid and ingested 2 to 3 times a day. This formulation is not available in the United States.

TABLE 14.3. *Androgen delivery systems that are clinically available or have been investigated in women*

Route	17β-Hydroxyesters	17αAlkylated compounds	Other combinations/substitutions	Native steroid
Oral	T undecenoate	Methyl testosterone	Fluoxymesterone (Halotestine) 17 α-methyl-19-nortesterone (MENT) Danazol (Danocrine)	Miscronized T Crystalline DHEA Micronized DHEA
Intramuscular	T propionate T cypionate T enanthate T cyclohexane Carboxylate T undecenoate T buciclate	Nandrolone phenpropionate (Durabolin)		T microspheres
Sublingual				Crystalline DHEA T cyclodextrin
Subcutaneous			17 α-methyl-19-nortesterone (MENT)	T pelletsl
Transcutaneous			DHEA cream	T patch (Matrix reservoir) DHT gel 2% T gel
Vaginal				Micronized DHEA

17β-Alkylated Testosterone Derivatives

Methyl testosterone (MT) is the most widely used 17β-alkylated T derivative. For women, the various brands of MT are given, either with or without addition of oral estrogens (Estratest, Android, Testred, Virolon), mesterolone, methenolone acetate, methandrostenolone, nandrolone, phenpropionate (Durabolin), and stanozolol (Winstrol). The 17β-alkyl substitution allows escape from hepatic metabolism; these compounds circulate and exert their androgenic action as the substituted molecules (51). Because MT is not measurable by routine clinical assays, dose titration to physiologic concentrations is not possible.

In women, oral MT is commonly used at doses of 1.25 or 2.5 mg/day in combination with conjugated estrogen. Doses of MT as high as 10 mg/day have been used and are available. Androgen cotherapy (with estrogen) may have beneficial effects on bone mass, menopausal symptomatology, and libido above that seen with estrogen replacement alone (54). Significant concern exists regarding MT-induced liver toxicity and atherogenic lipid profile (55).

Historically, oral MT was used in substantial doses in men (50 to 150 mg/day) for athletic training, sex conversion, impotence, and aplastic anemia. With such doses, a high incidence of hepatic toxicity was noted, including enzyme abnormalities, peliosis hepatitis, jaundice, and some cases of hepatocellular carcinoma (55). Although many of these changes were reversible, some were not. This effect appears unique to compounds with 17β-alkylation; although rare, it has been reported with doses as low as 10 mg MT (56). Some feel that the hepatic toxicity is dose and duration related and that, in the amounts used in women, it does not constitute a significant risk. Others remain less sanguine and do not recommend MT for women (55). The longest trial of menopausal MT therapy, at 1.25 or 2.5 mg/day (with concurrent estrogen replacement), where liver function test was monitored is 1 year in length: no liver abnormalities were seen in this study (57).

Atherogenic lipid profiles are of concern. Administration of 1.25 mg of MT in conjunction with estrogen over 2 years results in a significant decline in HDL, essentially obviating any lipoprotein benefit obtained from estrogen (Fig. 14.17) (58). This effect seems

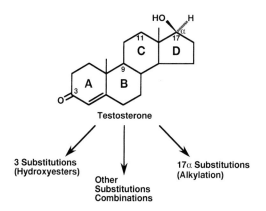

FIG. 14.16. The testosterone (T) molecule can be substituted at either the 1, 3, 9, or 17 carbon to form compounds that are orally bioavailable or lipophilic.

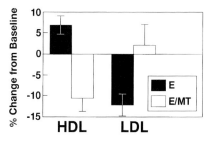

FIG. 14.17. Oral methyltestosterone (MT) given at 1.25 mg/day, in conjunction with estrogen (E), compared to the same dose of estrogen alone. This results in an arthrogenic lipoprotein profile that releases the effects of estrogen. (Adapted from ref. 58.)

unique to oral androgen administration; it is seen with oral DHEA but not with subcutaneous T pellets, despite high serum T levels (58,59). It is unknown whether this adverse lipoprotein effect actually increases cardiovascular risk.

Because of the potential hepatic toxicity, adverse lipoprotein effects, and inability to measure the hormone, oral 17β-alkylated agents in women are problematic. These problems have stimulated further research to develop alternate delivery systems.

Intramuscular Testosterone

Most of the clinical experience with intramuscular (IM) T involves 17β-ester-substituted compounds, primarily T enanthate or cypionate (Table 14.3). Experience in women is limited. Testosterone (T) and its esters have approximately the same metabolic clearance rate and plasma half-life. Slow release of the hydrophobic T ester from its oily depot accounts for its extended duration of action (53).

Unfortunately, bioavailability is erratic. Although administration of 200 to 250 mg of T enanthate or cypionate given to hypogonadal men every 2 weeks results in peak T levels in 1 to 3 days, in 10 to 14 days the levels become subphysiologic (53,55). Men often report sequential symptoms of hyper- and hypoandrogenism.

Newer parenteral T delivery systems are under development. A long-lasting subcutaneous crystalline T silastic capsule has been tested successfully in animals, but the large size needed for human use makes such a delivery system impractical (60). A mechanism to deliver T in IM-injected biodegradable microspheres is presently under development (61). In hypogonadal men, this technique provides physiologic replacement over 10 to 11 weeks. However, microsphere production technology is still developmental. Alternately, T undecenoate (1,000 mg) given IM every 6 weeks also appears to give more physiologically appropriate replacement (61). This T compound is used in China and investigational in Europe. Finally, T buciclate can be administered intramuscularly in an aqueous suspension and also provides a more physiologic T replacement pattern over 12 to 16 weeks (53).

Much of the initial research in women involving androgens, sexual function, and menopausal symptomatology was done using intramuscular T esters. Doses were pharmacologic: 150 to 200 mg of T enanthate with or without esterified estradiol given every 2 months (62,63). Although these studies demonstrated beneficial effects of T coreplacement with estrogens, serum T was extremely high (in the tumor range). Subsequent reports emerged documenting significant virilization in these women (64). Even months after stopping these agents, virilizing levels of T remained. Because of this, depot IM T esters are used infrequently.

Testosterone Implants

There is considerable clinical experience in postmenopausal women with subcutaneous crystalline T pellets (Table 14.3). These pellets are either 50 mg or 100 mg and are replaced every 3 months, usually in conjunction with an estradiol pellet (65). They deliver between 250 and 500 μg per day of T. The addition of the T pellet in several studies improved bone mass and sexual function over estrogen alone (65,66). Interestingly, serum T reaches supraphysiologic values (about 120 ng/dL), however, there appear to be no adverse changes in lipid profiles. Whether these pellets have adverse long-term effects is unknown.

Pellets are inserted with a trochar in the left or right lower quadrant of the abdominal wall. A local anesthetic is needed. The pellets must be gently placed into the subcutaneous tissue, with care taken not to crush them; the skin incision is closed with a single suture or steristrip. The insertion procedure is well tolerated, and expulsion of the pellet or infection at the site occurs infrequently. To date, these pellets represent the most physiologic method of replacing T in women (67).

Transdermal Testosterone

Transdermal T delivery for men has only recently been clinically available (53,55,68). A scrotal T matrix patch delivers 4 or 6 mg/day of T (Testoderm). These patches, 40 or 60 cm² in area, are applied to scrotal skin. Absorption is maximized by shaving this highly vascular area before patch placement. A nongenital reservoir T patch (Androderm) is also available for men. The use of two patches, applied to nonscrotal skin, will deliver 5 mg of T per day. Both of these transdermal delivery systems closely approximate the physiologic T of a eugonadal male. The scrotal patch is inconvenient, and the nongenital patches are large, bulky, and irritating.

In women, a much smaller amount of T is needed. Indeed, a transdermal matrix T patch designed specifically for women is currently under development. This patch, which delivers 150 μg of T per day, is changed every 3 to 4 days. It is now in phase II clinical trials in oophorectomized women with sexual dysfunction (N. Mazer, Theratech, Ltd., personal communication).

A 2% T or dihydrotestosterone (DHT) gel is sometimes used, usually compounded by individual pharmacies. Absorption is reported to be good after gel application (68).

Because of skin 5α-reductase activity, transcutaneously administered T, in both men and women, is converted in part to DHT. Serum DHT levels are elevated more than those of T. The degree of this conversion seems dependent on the skin area used and patch design. Whether this altered ratio of circulating T to DHT (the latter being nonaromatizable) is clinically important is not known. Improvements in transcutaneous T delivery probably represent the best future hope for physiologic T delivery to women.

Mucosal Membrane Testosterone

There are reports of intranasal and rectal administration of T (Table 14.3). Serum bioavailability is highly variable between individuals (51).

Earlier this century, sublingual T was used to treat endometriosis. More recently a sublingual T preparation for men has been developed, T cyclodextrin (53,69,70). Cyclodextrin, a carbohydrate moiety, potentiates transport across the oral mucosal membrane, allows for significant and reliable bioavailability with sublingual administration. The applicability of this technology for women remains unknown.

DHEA Replacement

As discussed earlier, there is evidence that the age-related deficiency in DHEA and DHEA-S potentiates senescent declines in immune function, bone mass, insulin sensitivity, and cognitive ability (43–46). Because, a considerable amount of biologically active T in women is derived from conversion of circulating DHEA-S, the modest age-related decline of circulating T and Δ^4A (supported by ovarian secretion) may be misleading as to the amount of androgen depletion that occurs (1,9).

Oral DHEA

Clinical experience with DHEA in older women is confused by widely varying doses, routes of administration, and formulations. It is clear that oral DHEA in small doses, 25 to 50 mg, approximates the adrenal androgen milieu of reproductive age without adverse androgenization (71,72). Unfortunately, oral DHEA results in hepatic bioconversion to downstream metabolites, such as Δ^4A and T (73). Indeed, a daily dose of 50 mg of oral DHEA not only normalizes serum DHEA and DHEA-S levels but also increases serum T to well above reproductive-age values (72). Available in the United States as a food supplement, oral DHEA represents the only readily available way of elevating serum T in a physiologically appropriate fashion using an oral route of administration while concurrently normalizing DHEA-S and DHEA values.

Nonoral DHEA

Oral DHEA has risks. We have reported one case of transient liver dysfunction after DHEA administration (73) and have also noted, along with others, adverse changes in lipoprotein profiles (decreased HDL) with very small amounts of oral DHEA (59,74). Thus, several have investigated transcutaneous or transmucosal methods of administering DHEA (75–78). There is encourag-

ing experience with transcutaneous DHEA using a topical cream (78). This area needs further investigation.

WHETHER TO REPLACE ANDROGENS

Even though androgens are commonly prescribed to women, there is little consensus on their indications. Any replacement contemplated clinically requires documentation of the deficiency by history, examination, and confirmation of subphysiologic concentrations of T and DHEA-S. Normal values for these hormones are well known, and replacement with the expectation of restoring high normal concentration seems reasonable. Testosterone (T) pellets, skin creams, and MT are the only available alternatives for replacing testosterone. A T-impregnated patch, the most attractive option, is investigational. DHEA, widely available in tablet form, is probably better replaced in percutaneous form, such as with a cream. Patch technology for DHEA is not yet available.

Androgen replacement to postmenopausal women should be considered in the following situations.

Androgen Deficiency of Aging

No criteria for intervention exists. In women with intact ovaries and normal concentrations of DHEA-S and T, androgens probably should not be given. When levels of these hormones are very low and patients manifest accelerated signs of menopausal senescence, androgen replacement, probably with estrogen, should be considered.

Women Who Have Undergone Oophorectomy

Strong arguments can be made for replacing androgens after oophorectomy. Testosterone (T) concentrations drop considerably. Testosterone (T) is the principal missing hormone, and a physiologic way of replacing T, such as MT, T implants, or a patch should be sought.

Major Endocrine Insufficiencies

Panhypopituitarism and adrenal cortical insufficiency are life-threatening medical conditions. Although regimens for replacing androgens in men are straightforward, replacement for women is more discretionary. For women afflicted with one of these conditions, androgen replacement should probably be considered with the same priority as in men. Oral DHEA is the most readily available replacement for this condition.

Chronic Wasting Diseases

Androgen administration appears beneficial to patients afflicted with chronic infectious diseases, malignancies, and following burn trauma (42). Preliminary experience with oral DHEA to HIV patients has been encouraging (79,80).

Chronic Corticosteroid Therapy

DHEA may attenuate some of the side effects of corticosteroid wasting (50). This has not been studied sufficiently to make specific recommendations. On the negative side, DHEA could also attenuate some of the therapeutic benefits of corticosteroids.

Loss of Libido

There is compelling evidence that androgens play important roles in female sexuality and that declining androgen production after menopause is a contributing factor to decreasing sexual interest expressed by many older women (81–85). Controlled studies involving estrogen replacement alone show improvement in general well-being, vasomotor symptoms, and vaginal dryness but little change in libidinal interest (86,87). The addition of injected testosterone enanthate in pharmacologic doses, however, is effective in prospective trials involving oophorectomized women (62,63). The doses utilized, however, are virilizing, and it is not likely that the doses used in these trials can be safely sustained (64). More encouraging are recent reports involving T subcutaneous implants (50 mg), which, in a 2-year randomized trial, demonstrated significant enhancement of sexual activity, satisfaction, pleasure, orgasm, and relevancy significantly better than estradiol implants alone (65–67). Furthermore, these T implants, in the doses used, did not produce hepatotoxicity, adverse effects on lipids, or virilization even though testosterone concentrations were mildly superphysiologic (65–67). The ultimate decision to replace T for loss of libido is clinical. If predisposing conditions exist (e.g., oophorectomy) that lead to low T concentrations, and indeed T concentrations are low, androgen replacement for enhancement of libido seems appropriate. Although the use of T implants or parenteral T seems the closest to physiology, some feel that oral MT preparations are also appropriate (56).

Osteopenia and Osteoporosis

The positive correlations reported between free T, DHEA, and DHEA-S and bone mineral density have provided a stimulus to investigations of androgen replacement (88–92). Human osteoblastic cells possess androgen receptors, and androgens directly stimulate human bone cell proliferation and differentation (93–94). Thus, open trials show that pharmacologic doses of androgens do increase bone mineral density and suppress biochemical markers of bone loss (96–98). This effect appears to occur in addition to the antiresorptive effects of estrogen. More recently, T implants (50 mg) replacing hormone at

a physiologic level also increased bone mineral density when used concomitantly with estradiol implants (99). The T effect significantly exceeds that of estradiol alone. Finally, DHEA applied daily in a 10% cream significantly increased bone mineral density in a group of healthy women 60 to 70 years old. The DHEA was given without estrogens (78). No specific recommendations can be made at this present time as to what androgen treatment should be used for treatment of osteoporosis and osteopenia. Future prospects for incorporating androgens into antiosteoporosis treatments are promising.

SUMMARY AND CONCLUSIONS

Increasing sophistication in the understanding of DHEA(S) kinetics readily supports the thesis that androgen production in women falls dramatically with age. This decline is exaggerated by postmenopausal oophorectomy. Estrogen replacement further exaggerates this condition. Clinical data in women using prototype T and DHEA replacement support the position that T and DHEA deficiency has adverse sequelae that can be attenuated with therapeutic androgens—probably administered as cotherapy with estrogens. Unfortunately, clinically available T and DHEA delivery systems for women need refinement. For men, androgen replacement systems are more physiologic and have been extensively exploited. As technology for nonoral physiologic T and DHEA replacement evolve for women, highly targeted and sophisticated improvements in menopausal replacement should evolve.

REFERENCES

1. Labrie F, Belanger A, Cusan L, Gomez JL, Candas B. Marked decline in serum concentrations of adrenal C_{19} sex steroid precursors and conjugated androgen metabolites during aging. *J Clin Endocrinol Metab* 1997;82:2396–2402.
2. Ravaglia G, Forti P, Maioli F, et al. The relationship of dehydroepiandrosterone sulfate (DHEAS) to endocrine-metabolic parameters and functional status in the oldest-old. Results from an Italian study on healthy free-living over-ninety-years-olds. *J Clin Endocrinol Metab* 1996;81:1173–1178.
3. Orentreich N, Brind JL, Rizer RL, Vogelman JH. Age changes and sex differences in serum dehydroepiandrosterone sulfate concentrations throughout adulthood. *J Clin Endocrinol Metab* 1984;59:551–555.
4. Hornsby PJ. Biosynthesis of DHEA-S by the human adrenal cortex and its age-related decline. *Ann NY Acad Sci* 1995;774:29–46.
5. Judd HL, Lucas WE, Yen SCS. Effect of oophorectomy on circulating testosterone and androstenedione levels in patients with endometrial cancer. *Am J Obstet Gynecol* 1974;118:793–798.
6. Casson PR, Carson SA. Androgen replacement therapy in women: myths and realities. *Int J Fertil* 1996;41:412–422.
7. Casson PR, Hornsby PJ, Ghusn HF, Buster JE. Dehydroepiandrosterone (DHEA) replacement in postmenopausal women: present status and future promise. *Menopause* 1997;4:225–231.
8. Casson PR, Buster JE. DHEA replacement after menopause: HRT 2000 or nostrum of the 90's? *Contemp Ob/Gyn* 1997;42:119–133.
9. Labrie F, Bélanger A, Simard J, Luu-The V, Labrie C. DHEA and peripheral androgen and estrogen formation: Intracrinology. *Ann NY Acad Sci* 1995;774:16–28.
10. Labrie F, Bélanger A, Cusan L, Candas B. Physiological changes in dehydroepiandrosterone are not reflected by serum levels of active androgens and estrogens but of their metabolites: intracrinology. *J Clin Endocrinol Metab* 1997;82:2403–2409.
11. Longcope C. Adrenal and gonadal androgen secretion in normal females. *Clinics in Endocrinol Metab* 1986;15:213–227.
12. Longcope C. Hormone dynamics at the menopause. *Multidiscip Perspec Menopause* 1990;592:21–30.

13. Endoh A, Kristiansen SB, Casson PR, Buster JE, Hornsby PJ. The zona reticularis is the site of biosynthesis of dehydroepiandrosterone and dehydroepiandrosterone sulfate in the adult human adrenal cortex, resulting from its low expression of 3β-hydroxysteroid dehydrogenase. *J Clin Endocrinol Metab* 1996;81:3558–3565.

14. Labrie F. Intracrinology. *Mol Cell Endocrinol* 1991;78:C113–C118.

15. Martel C, Melner MH, Gagne D, et al. Widespread tissue distribution of steroid sulfatase, 3β-hydroxysteroid dehydrogenase/Δ⁵-Δ⁴ isomerase (3β-HSD), 17β-HSD 5α-reductase and aromatase activities in the rhesus monkey. *Mol Cell Endocrinol* 1994;104:103–111.

16. Simpson ER, Zhao Y. Estrogen biosynthesis in adipose tissue. Significance in breast cancer development. *Ann NY Acad Sci* 1996;184:18–26.

17. Bélanger B, Bélanger A, Labrie F, Dupont A, Cusan L, Monfette G. Comparison of residual C-19 steroids in plasma and prostatic tissue of human, rat and guinea pig after castration: Unique importance of extratesticular androgens in men. *J Steroid Biochem* 1989;32:695–698.

18. Roy AK. Regulation of steroid hormone action in target cells by specific hormone-inactivating enzymes. *Proc Soc Exp Biol Med* 1992;199:265–272.

19. Hanings RV Jr, Flood CA, Hackett RJ, Loughlin JS, McClure NRJ. Metabolic clearance rate of dehydroepiandrosterone sulfate, its metabolism to testosterone, and its intrafollicular metabolism to dehydroepiandrosterone, androstenedione, testosterone, and dihydrotestosterone *in vivo*. *J Clin Endocrinol Metab* 1991;72:1088–1095.

20. Haning RV Jr, Hackett RJ, Flood CA, Loughlin JS, Zhao QY. Plasma dehydroepiandrosterone sulfate serves as a prehormone for 48% of follicular fluid testosterone during treatment with menotropins. *J Clin Endocrinol Metab* 1993;76:1301–1307.

21. Feher T, Szalay KS, Szilagyi G. Effect of ACTH and prolactin on dehydroepiandrosterone, its sulfate ester and cortisol reduction by normal and tumorous human adrenocortical cells. *J Steroid Biochem* 1985;23:153–157.

22. Klein NA, Andersen RN, Casson PR, Buster JE, Kramer RE. Mechanisms of insulin inhibition of ACTH-stimulated steroid secretion by cultured bovine adrenocortical cells. *J Steroid Biochem Mol Biol* 1992;41:11–20.

23. Polderman KH, Gooren LJG, van der Veen EA. Testosterone administration increases adrenal response to adrenocorticotropin. *Clin Endocrinol* 1994;40:595–601.

24. Poderman KH, Gooren LJG, van der Veen EA. Effects of gonadal androgens and estrogens on adrenal androgen levels. *Clin Endocrinol* 1995;43:415–421.

25. Parker JR, Stankovic AK, Falany CN, Grizzle WE. Effect of TGF-β on dehydroepiandrosterone sulfotransferase in cultured human fetal adrenal cells. *Ann NY Acad Sci* 1995;774:326–328.

26. Parker LN, Sack J, Fisher DA, Odell WD. The adrenarche: prolactin, gonadotropins, adrenal androgens, and cortisol. *J Clin Endocrinol Metab* 1978;46:386–401.

27. Hornsby PJ. DHEA: a biologistís perspective. *J Am Geriatr Soc* 1997;45:1395–1401.

28. Bargmann W. *Histologic and mikroskopische Anatomie des Menshen, vol 2: Organe and Systeme.* Stuttgart: Georg Thieme, 1951.

29. Dhom G. The prepuberal and puberal growth of the adrenal (adrenarche). *Beitr Pathol* 1973;150:357–377.

30. Lucisano A, Russo N, Acampora MG, et al. Ovarian and peripheral androgen and oestrogen levels in post-menopausal women: correlations with ovarian histology. *Maturitas* 1986;8:57–65.

31. Nagamani M, Hannigan EV, Dillard EA Jr, Dinh TV. Ovarian steroid secretion in postmenopausal women with and without endometrial cancer. *J Clin Endocrinol Metab* 1986;62:508–512.

32. Ushiroyama T, Sugimoto O. Endocrine function of the peri- and postmenopausal ovary. *Horm Res* 1995;44:64–68.

33. Kreiner E, Dohm G. Altersveranderungen de menschilichen Nebenniere. *Zbl Allg Pathol Anat* 1979;123:351–356.

34. Abraham GE. Ovarian and adrenal contribution to peripheral androgens during the menstrual cycle. *J Clin Endocrinol Metab* 1974;39:340.

35. Burger HG, Dudley EC, Hopper JL, et al. The endocrinology of the menopausal transition: a cross-sectional study of a population-based sample. *J Clin Endocrinol Metab* 1995;80:3537–3545.

36. Longcope C, Hunter R, Franz C. Steroid secretion by the postmenopausal ovary. *Am J Obstet Gynecol* 1980;138:564–568.

37. Vermeulen A. The hormonal activity of the postmenopausal ovary. *J Clin Endocrinol Metab* 1976;42:247–253.

38. Burger HG. The endocrinology of the menopause. *Maturitas* 1996;23:129–136.

39. Nicosia SV. Ovarian changes during the climacteric. In: *The climacteric.* New York: Plenum Press, 1986:179–199.

40. Judd HL, Judd GE, Lucas WE, Yen SCC. Endocrine function of the postmenopausal ovary: concentration of androgens and estrogens in ovarian and peripheral vein blood. *J Clin Endocrinol Metab* 1974;39:1020.

41. Chang RJ, Judd HL. The ovary after menopause. *Clin Ob/Gyn* 1981;24:181–191.

42. Babalola AA, Ellis G. Serum dehydroepiandrosterone sulfate in a normal pediatric population. *Clin Biochem* 1988;18:182–189.

43. Vermeulen A. Dehydroepiandrosterone sulfate and aging. *Ann NY Acad Sci* 1996;774:121–127.

44. Casson PR, Anderson RN, Herrod HG, et al. Oral dehydroepiandrosterone in physiologic doses modulates immune function in postmenopausal women. *Am J Obstet Gynecol* 1993;169:1536–1539.

45. Garg M, Bondada S. Reversal of age-associated decline in immune response to Pnu-imune vaccine by supplementation with the steroid hormone dehydroepiandrosterone. *Infect Immun* 1993;61:2238–2241.

46. Wild RA, Buchanan JR, Myers C, Demers LM. Declining adrenal androgens: an association with bone loss in aging women. *Proc Soc Exp Biol Med* 1987;186:355–360.

47. Parker JR, Banter CR. Divergence in adrenal steroid secretory pattern after thermal injury in adult patients. *J Trauma* 1985;25:508–510.

48. Findling JW, Buggy BP, Gilson IH, Brummitt CF, Bernstein BM, Raff H. Longitudinal evaluation of adrenocortical function in patients infected with the human immunodeficiency virus. *J Clin Endocrinol Metab* 1994;79:1091–1096.

49. Casson PR, Elkind-Hirsch KE, Buster JE, Hornsby PJ, Carson SA, Snabes MC. Effect of postmenopausal estrogen replacement on circulating androgens. *Obstet Gynecol* 1997;90:995–998.

50. Kalimi M, Shafogoj Y, Loria R, Padgett D, Regelson W. Antiglucocorticoid effects of dehydroepiandrosterone (DHEA). *Mol Cell Biochem* 1994;131:99–104.

51. Griffin JE, Wilson JD. Disorders of the tests and the male reproductive tract. In: Wilson JD, Foster DW, eds. *Williams textbook of endocrinology.* Philadelphia: WB Saunders, 1992:779–852.

52. Daggett PR, Wheeler MJ, Nabarro JDN. Oral testosterone, a reappraisal. *Horm Res* 1978;9:121–129.

53. Bhasin S, Brenner WJ. Emerging issues in androgen replacement therapy. *J Clin Endocrinol Metab* 1997;82:3–8.

54. Sands R, Studd J. Exogenous androgens in postmenopausal women. *Am J Med* 1995;98:76S–79S.

55. Wood AJJ. Drug therapy. *N Engl J Med* 1996;334:707–714.

56. Gelfand MM, Wiita B. Androgen and estrogen-androgen hormone replacement therapy: a review of the safety literature, 1941 to 1996. *Clin Ther* 1997;19:383–404.

57. Barrett-Connor E, Timmons C, Young R, Wiita B. Interim safety analysis of a two-year study comparing oral estrogen-androgen and conjugated estrogens in surgically menopausal women. *J Women Health* 1996;5:93–601.

58. Watts NB, Notelovitz M, Timmons MC, Addison WA, Wiita B, Downey LJ. Comparison of oral estrogens plus androgen on bone mineral density, menopausal symptoms, and lipid-lipoprotein profiles in surgical menopause. *Obstet Gynecol* 1995;85:529–537.

59. Casson PR, Santoro NF, Elkind-Hirsch KE, et al. Postmenopausal dehydroepiandrosterone (DHEA) administration increases free insulin-like growth factor-I (IGF-I) and decreases high density lipoprotein (HDL): a six month trial. *Fertil Steril* 1998;70:107–110.

60. Marberger H. Hormonal therapy with steroid-filled Silastic rubber implants. *Br J Urol* 1976;48:153–154.

61. Partsch CJ, Weinbauer GF, Fang R, Neischlag E. Injectable testosterone undercoate has more favorable pharmacokinetics and pharmacodynamics than testosterone enanthate. *Eur J Endocrinol* 1995;132:514–519.

62. Sherwin BB, Gelfand MM. Differential symptom response to parenternal estrogen and/or androgen administration in the surgical menopause. *Am J Obstet Gynecol* 1985;151:153–160.

63. Sherwin BB, Gelfand MM. The role of androgen in the maintenance of sexual functioning in oophorectomized women. *Psychosom Med* 1992;79:286–294.

64. Urman B, Pride SM, Yuen BH. Elevated serum testosterone, hirsutism, and virilism associated with combined androgen-estrogen hormone replacement therapy. *Obstet Gynecol* 1991;77:595–598.

65. Burger HG, Hailes J, Nelson J, Menelaus M. Effect of combined implants of oestradiol and testosterone on libido in postmenopausal women. *Br Med J* 1987;294:936–937.

66. Burger HG, Hailes J, Menelaus M, Nelson J, Hudson B, Balazs N. The management of persistent menopausal symptoms with oestradiol-testosterone implants: clinical, lipid and hormonal changes. *Maturitas* 1984;6:351–358.

67. Davis SR, Burger HG. Androgens and the postmenopausal woman. *J Clin Endocrinol Metab* 1996;81:2756–2763.

68. Wang C, Swerdloff RS. Androgen replacement therapy. *Finn Med Soc Ann Med* 1997;29:365–370.

69. Steiner B, Hull L, Callegari C, Swedloff RS. Testosterone replacement therapy improves mood in hypogonadal men—a clinical reasearch study. *J Clin Endocrinol Metab* 1996;81:3578–3583.

70. Wang C, Eyre DR, Clark R, et al. Sublingual testosterone replacement improves muscle mass and strength, decreases bone resorption, and increases bone formation markers in hypogonadal man—a clinical research center study. *J Clin Endocrinol Metab* 1996;81:3654–3662.

71. Morales AJ, Nolan JJ, Nelson JC, Yen SCC. Effects of replacement dose of dehydroepiandrosterone in men and women of advancing age. *J Clin Endocrinol Metab* 1994;78:1360–1367.

72. Casson PR, Faquin LC, Stentz FB, et al. Replacement of dehydroepiandrosterone (DHEA) enhances T-lymphocyte insulin binding in postmenopausal women. *Fertil Steril* 1995;563:1027–1031.

73. Buster JE, Casson PR, Straughn AB, et al. Postmenopausal steroid replacement with micronized dehydroepiandrosterone (DHEA): Premliminary bioavailability and dose proportionality studies. *Am J Obstet Gynecol* 1992;166:1163–1170.

74. Barnhart KT, Rader D, Freeman E, Kapoor SK, Smith P, Nestler J. *The effect of DHEA replacement on the endocrine and lipid profiles of perimneopausal women.* Paper presented at the 53rd Annual Meeting, American Society for Reproductive Medicine, Cincinnati, OH, 1997.

75. Yen SCC, Morales AJ, Khorram O. Replacement of DHEA in aging men and women: potential remedial effects. In: Bellino FL, Dayned RA, Hornsby PH, Lavrin DH, Nestler JE, eds. *Dehydroepiandrosterone (DHEA) and aging.* New York: NY Academy of Science, 1995:128–142.

76. Casson PR, Straughn AB, Milem CA, Umstot ES, Buster JE. Delivery of dehy-

droepiandrosterone (DHEA) in premenopausal women: Effects of micronization and non-oral administration. *Am J Obstet Gynecol* 1996;174:649–653.

77. Diamond P, Cusan L, Gomez JL, Belanger A, Labrie F. Metabolic effects of 12-month percutaneous dehydroepiandrosterone replacement therapy in postmenopausal women. *SO J Endocrinol* 1996;150:S43–50.

78. Labrie F, Diamond D, Cusan L, Gomez JL, Belanger A, Candas B. Effect of a 12-month dehydroepiandrosterone replacment therapy on bone, vagina, and endometrium in postmenopausal women. *J Clin Endocrinol Metab* 1997;82:3498–3505.

79. van Vollenhoven RF, Englemen EG, McGuire JL. An open study of dehydroepiandrosterone in systemic lupus erythematosus. *Arthritis Rheum* 1994;37:1305–1310.

80. Dyner TS, Lang W, Geaga J, et al. An open-label dose-escalation trial of oral dehydroepiandrosterone tolerance and pharmacokinetics in patients with HIV disease. *J Acq Immune Defic Syndr* 1993;6:459–465.

81. Nathorst-Böös J, von Schoultz B. Psychological reactions and sexual life after hysterectomy with and without oophorectomy. *Gynecol Obstet Invest* 1992;34:97–101.

82. Nathorst-Böös J, von Schoultz B, Carlström K. Elective ovarian removal and estrogen replacement therapy effects on sexual life, phsychological well-being and androgen status. *Obstet Gynaecol* 1993;14:283–293.

83. Bachmann GA, Leiblum SR, Sander B, et al. Correlates of sexual desire in postmenopausal women. *Maturitas* 1985;7:211–216.

84. Hallstrom T. Sexuality in the climacteric. *Clin Obstet Gynecol* 1977;4:227–239.

85. McCoy NL, Davidson JM. A longitudinal study of the effects of menopause on sexuality. *Maturitas* 1985;7:203–210.

86. Utian WH. The true clinical features of postmenopausal oophorectomy and their response to estrogen replacement therapy. *S Afr Med J* 1972;46:732–737.

87. Campbell S, Whitehead M. Oestrogen therapy and the menopausal syndrome. *Clin Obstet Gynecol* 1977;4:31–47.

88. Rannevik G, Jeppsson S, Johnell O, Bjerre B, Laurell-Borulf Y, Svanberg L. A longitudinal study of the perimenopausal transition: altered profiles of steroid and pituitary hormones, SHBG and bone mineral density. *Maturitas* 1995;21:103–113.

89. Nilas L, Christiansen C. Bone mass and its relationship to age and the menopause. *J Clin Endocrinol Metab* 1987;65:697–699.

90. Heiss CJ, Sanborn CF, Nichols DL. Associations of body fat distribution, circulating sex hormones and bone density in postmenopausal women. *J Clin Endocrinol Metab* 1995;80:1591–1596.

91. Davidson BJ, Ross RK, Paganini-Hill A, Hammond GD. Total and free estrogens and androgens in postmenopausal women with hip fractures. *J Clin Endocrinol* 1982;54:115–120.

92. Nordin BEC, Robertson A, Seamark RF, et al. The relation between calcium absorption, serum dihydroepiandrosterone and vertebral mineral density in postmenopausal women. *J Clin Endocrinol Metab* 1985;60:651–657.

93. Colvard DS, Eriksen EF, Keeting PE, Wilson EM, Lubahn DB. Identification of androgen receptors in normal human osteoblast-like cells. *Proc Natl Acad Sci* 1989;86:854–857.

94. Kasperk CH, Wergedal JE, Farley JR, Llinkhart TA, Turner RT, Baylink DG. Androgens directly stimulate proliferation of bone cells in vitro. *Endocrinology* 1989;124:1576–1578.

95. Ralston SH, Fogelman I, Leggate J, et al. Effect of subdermal oestrogen and oestrogen/testosterone implants on calcium and phosphorus homeostasis after oophorectomy. *Maturitas* 1984;6:341–345.

96. Henneman PH, Wallach S. The use of androgens and estrogens and their metabolic effects: A review of the prolonged use of estrogens and androgens in postmenopausal and senile osteoporosis. *Arch Intern Med* 1957;100:715–723.

97. Need AG, Horowitz M, Bridges A, Morris HA, Nordin BE. Effects of nandrolone therapy on forearm mineral content in osteoporosis. *Clin Orthop* 1987;225:273–278.

98. Chesnut CH III, Nelp WB, Baylink DJ, Denney JD. Effect of methandrostenolone on postmenopausal bone wasting as assessed by changes in total bone mineral mass. *Metabolism* 1977;26:267–277.

99. Davis SR, McCloud P, Strauss BJG, Burger HG. Testosterone enhances estradiolís effects on postmenopausal bone density and sexuality. *Maturitas* 1995;21:227–236.

SECTION IV

Symptoms and Signs
of Estrogen Deficiency

This section includes a discussion of problems associated with estrogen deficiency. Notably absent are two most important areas: that of bone loss and osteoporosis and that of cardiovascular disease. These two topics are in separate sections because of their importance and the amount of new information available.

The hallmark feature of vasomotor symptoms is the hot flash. Fredi Kronenberg provides a comprehensive review of the topic and suggests that the hot "flash" and "flush" can be used interchangeably. While this is indeed true, some purists would suggest that the hot "flush" includes the entire vasomotor episode (aura, temperature rise, and resolution phase), while the "flash" denotes the acute temperature-related phenomenon.

The effects of sex steroids on the central nervous system and mood are reviewed by Barbara B. Sherwin and David Rubinow and his colleagues. The important complaint of vulvovaginal atrophy is dealt with comprehensively by Gloria A. Bachmann, as is the significance of collagen support by Mark P. Brincat and Ray Galea. Indeed, one might consider postmenopausal osteoporosis to be a collagen-deficiency state. The final chapter in this section is a comprehensive review of the urinary tract by Eileen F. DeMarco. Urinary complaints are extremely prevalent and a major source of morbidity.

This important section includes the symptoms and signs for which hormonal and other treatments are prescribed. While most of these therapies are straightforward and logical, many gaps in our knowledge base still exist.

Treatment of the Postmenopausal Woman: Basic and Clinical Aspects, Second Edition, edited by Rogerio A. Lobo, Lippincott Williams & Wilkins, Philadelphia © 1999.

CHAPTER 15

Hot Flashes

Fredi Kronenberg

Hot flashes comprise the classic sign of menopause as well as the predominant complaint of perimenopausal and menopausal women in the United States. It was not until 1975, however, that serious scientific study of hot flashes was undertaken. In that year, a paper on the measurement of physiologic changes during hot flashes demonstrated their objective existence (1), and the phenomenon could no longer be dismissed as being "all in the head," as had often been the case.

A hot flash is a sudden, transient sensation ranging from warmth to intense heat that spreads over the body, particularly on the chest, face, and head; typically, it is accompanied by flushing and perspiration, and is often followed by a chill. In some instances, palpitations and a feeling of anxiety are present. Although these are characteristic features of a hot flash that make it an identifiable phenomenon, the magnitude and duration of any of these components can vary both within and among individuals, and not everyone experiences all of them. Some women flush, others do not; some sweat profusely, others hardly at all. Descriptions of hot flashes may also include pressure in the head or chest, a burning sensation, nausea, feelings of suffocation, and an inability to concentrate. Thus, just as the 28-day menstrual cycle is seen more in textbooks than in women, women's experiences of hot flashes are more variable than most textbook definitions.

Whether referred to as hot flashes, hot flushes, night sweats, or vasomotor symptoms (terms that are often used interchangeably), these episodic events can disrupt a woman's sense of well-being and create problems for professional and social life.

EPIDEMIOLOGY

Hot flashes primarily affect women who are in the transition to menopause or have become menopausal, whether naturally or because of medical intervention such as ovariectomy, chemotherapy, radiation, or medications that cause estrogen levels to fall. At other stages of the female reproductive life cycle, however, some women describe symptoms similar to the hot flashes of menopause. A small percentage of premenopausal women report having hot flashes, as do women during pregnancy or in the early postpartum period.

Hot flashes can also be experienced by men on abrupt loss of testicular function such as occurs following orchiectomy for prostatic or testicular cancer, following certain surgical procedures that compromise testicular function (2–5), or on administration of gonadotropin-releasing hormone (GnRH) agonists, which result in a fall in testosterone levels (6,7). Men who are hypogonadal for other reasons also can experience hot flashes (4).

Until relatively recently, most epidemiologic studies of menopause had been conducted in North America and Europe (8–13). These studies found that most women had at least some hot flashes. The incidence of hot flashes is highest in the first two postmenopausal years, ranging from 58% to 93% in these studies, and lessens over time. Reports of hot flash incidence in perimenopausal women range from 28% to 65%, and in premenopausal women, from 6% to 63%. Women with surgically induced menopause, at least for the first year postovariectomy, tend to have a relatively high prevalence of hot flashes, comparable with that of women in the first two years of natural menopause (see Tables 1 and 2 of ref. 14 for details of specific studies).

Hot flashes, although frequently occurring with menopause, are not universally experienced. Studies of menopause are now underway in countries around the world, and the data available thus far suggest that the high prevalence of hot flashes in Western societies is not matched

F. Kronenberg: Department of Rehabilitation Medicine, Columbia University College of Physicians & Surgeons, New York, New York 10032.

elsewhere. Hot flashes have been reported in many cultures, including Indian, African, Native American, Japanese, Indonesian, Mexican American, Mayan, Thai, Filipino, and Chinese (15–24). But the prevalence of hot flashes within these cultures varies widely. Thus far, the most extensively studied non-Western group has been Japanese women, who report very few hot flashes (18,25). Mayan women in Yucatan, Mexico, do not report any symptoms at menopause other than menstrual cycle irregularity (21). These studies raise interesting questions. Are the physiologic changes that are so characteristic of hot flashes in American women truly absent in other groups? Are they present but perceived differently? Are they, perhaps, not attributed to menopause? If absent or experienced by only a small percentage of the population, could this be due to diet, exercise patterns, or other cultural differences? Current research efforts may soon provide answers to some of these questions, and the results may generate leads to new methods of treatment. Increasingly, the patients in a medical practice come from a wide variety of cultural and religious backgrounds. It is necessary, therefore, to be aware of the menopausal symptoms that may be seen among women of other cultures, as well as to be sensitive to various cultural and medical traditions that might preclude a particular approach to treatment of hot flashes or include treatments not used by physicians in Western societies.

NATURAL HISTORY OF HOT FLASHES

The initial form of hot flashes and their pattern over time differ among women, but the physiologic basis for these differences in hot flash patterns and presentations has yet to be definitively explained. For some women, hot flashes begin as menstrual cycles are becoming irregular: they tend to occur when menstrual cycles are absent and disappear when menstrual cycles resume. For others, hot flashes begin when menstrual cycles are still regular, which may be well before menopause. There are also instances in which hot flashes first begin several years after menopause (14). Few investigators have asked about the age and menstrual cycle status at which hot flashes begin, but those who have asked report that for most women hot flashes begin prior to menopause (12,14,26).

The frequency, intensity, and duration of individual hot flash episodes vary both within and among individuals. Hot flashes can occur once a month or as often as every half hour. Most women with hot flashes have them infrequently, but about 10% to 15% of women have frequent, severe hot flashes (14). Women with frequent hot flashes often have relatively consistent patterns of hot flashes, at least in the short term. Over months or years, however, an individual's hot flash pattern can change. In many cases hot flashes first occur at night and eventually occur during the day as well. Generally, hot flashes tend to become less frequent over time; however, for some women, they

continue at frequent intervals until well into old age (14,27). Hot flash intensity can range from mild to very intense; it can vary in intensity over the course of one day, from day to day, or in different seasons. An individual hot flash episode typically lasts 3 to 6 minutes; it can be of briefer and it can last for more than 30 minutes.

The period of time over which hot flashes are most often experienced is 6 months to 2 years; however, women can have hot flashes for 10, 20, or even 40 years (14,26,28). Adequate data on the natural course of hot flashes are lacking because most investigators have not asked women across the life cycle whether they are having hot flashes. Most often excluded are women in their seventies and eighties; it had been assumed, incorrectly, that at this age they would no longer be experiencing hot flashes.

Although hot flashes often occur spontaneously with no observable trigger (particularly during sleep), some women report specific precipitating factors for their hot flashes. Psychologic stress is often cited, as are hot weather (particularly hot, humid weather), a confining space, caffeine, alcohol, and spicy foods (14,29,30).

Few studies have examined factors that might predispose women to hot flashes. No significant association has been found between the occurrence of hot flashes and sociodemographic variables such as employment status, social class, age, or marital status (13). Women with hot flashes are not distinguishable from those without hot flashes by age at menarche, number of pregnancies, or previous medical problems (31). One factor that has been shown to relate to the occurrence of hot flashes in menopausal women is mean body weight and percent ideal body weight. Asymptomatic women had significantly higher mean body weight, percent ideal body weight, and total circulating estrogen levels, than women with hot flashes (32). Recent data from a prospective study of the natural menopausal transition indicate that women with longer perimenopausal periods were more likely to report hot flashes than were those with a short perimenopausal period (51% vs. 39%) (33). Further research will determine whether factors such as genetics, diet, and exercise will be found to influence hot flashes.

PHYSIOLOGY OF HOT FLASHES

Thermoregulatory and cardiovascular changes that accompany a hot flash are now well documented. Characteristic patterns exist amid a range of individual variability (Fig. 15.1, Table 15.1). Knowledge of the time sequence of physiologic changes during a hot flash has grown incrementally as researchers have measured additional parameters. It is now frequently reported that many women have a premonition of an impending hot flash (an aura), which they distinguish from the hot flash itself. This prodromal feeling is often described as one of disease, anxiety, a tingling sensation, or pressure in the head (14). During this period immediately prior to the onset of

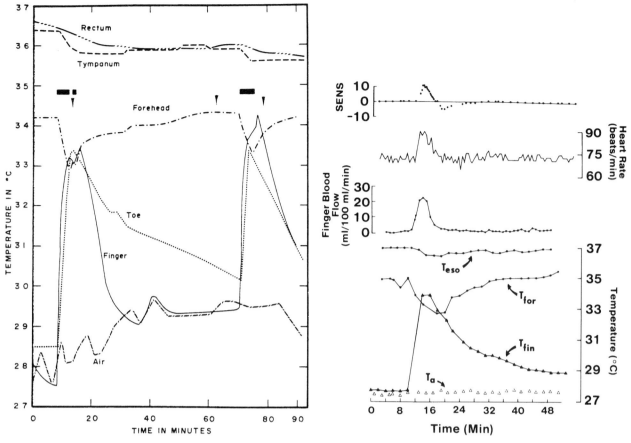

FIG. 15.1. A: Temperature responses to two spontaneous flashes (n) and evoked flash (n). ↓, Finger stab for blood sample. Nude. (From Molnar GW. Body temperatures during menopausal hot flashes. *J Appl Physiol* 1975;38:499–503.) B: Thermoregulatory and cardiovascular changes during a typical hot flash at an ambient temperature of 28°C. Subjective sensation, blood flow (finger), heart rate (30-s averages), skin resistance (chest), internal body temperature (vagina), and skin temperatures (forehead, finger) are depicted. (From Kronenberg F. Hot flashes: epidemiology and physiology. *Ann NY Acad Sci* 1990;592:52–86.)

a hot flash (approximately 5 to 60 seconds), heart rate and cutaneous blood flow begin to increase (34,35).

At the start of a hot flash typically a sudden onset of sweating occurs, primarily on the upper body but measurable throughout the body, as indicated by a rapid drop in skin resistance (increase in skin conductance) (35,36). The main sensation is one of intense heat, although internal body temperature never rises above normal. As cutaneous blood flow increases (34,35) and heart rate continues to accelerate (4 to 35 beats/minute) (34,35,37), skin temperature rises, particularly that of the fingers and toes (1° to 7°C) (1,35,38,39), and sweating continues. Evaporative cooling may cause the temperature of the wet skin to drop, particularly on the chest and forehead, where sweating

TABLE 15.1. *Clinical picture of a hot flash*

Symptom	Description
Sensation	Sudden feeling of heat and sometimes anxiety
Heart rate	Increases (5–35 bpm), sometimes felt as palpitations
Cutaneous blood flow	Increases; observed as flushing
Finger skin temperature	Rises rapidly (1–7°C) and slowly declines after hot flash ends
Sweating	Often profuse, with rapid onset; rate of evaporation depends on ambient humidity and temperature
Core temperature	Decreases (0.1–0.9°C) several minutes after hot flash starts; sometimes felt as a chill at end of hot flash
Sleeping problems	Increase in nighttime awakenings associated with hot flashes (night sweats)

bpm, beats per minute

tends to be profuse (35). Heart rate and skin blood flow peak within approximately 3 minutes of hot flash onset (34,35). To relieve the discomfort, women initiate a variety of behavioral measures to dissipate heat. The vasodilation, sweating, and behavioral responses result in heat loss and a drop in internal temperature (0.1° to 0.9°C), which reaches a nadir approximately 5 to 9 minutes after the onset of the hot flash (35,36). If significant heat loss has occurred and core temperature has dropped, the woman may experience a the sensation of a chill or even some shivering as the hot flash resolves. Factors that facilitate the return of body temperature to normal include vasoconstriction, behavior to promote warming, and, at times, an increase in metabolic rate because of shivering. Skin temperature gradually declines to its level before the hot flash. This can take 30 minutes or longer, depending on skin and ambient temperatures. No change in blood pressure has been found in association with a hot flash (34,37,40). Although sweating and the perception of heat are most intense on the upper body, the temperature of the toes increases concomitantly with finger temperature and sweating can occur over the lower body as well (1,35), demonstrating that a hot flash is a generalized physiologic phenomenon.

Subjective perception of hot flash intensity derives from to a combination of factors, including the associated sweating and increased heart rate, and probably involves other ill-defined sensations. The sensation of hot flash intensity is not a direct function of absolute skin temperature or change in skin temperature during a hot flash, because the degree to which finger skin temperature increases during a hot flash is inversely proportional to the baseline skin temperature before the hot flash (Fig. 15.2) (35,36,41). The more distal the site, the lower skin temperature is likely to be initially; therefore, the greater is the potential for an appreciable rise in skin temperature during a hot flash. As a result, in many studies finger temperature is used as an

objective indication of a hot flash. Although this is a good objective measurement in cool ambient temperature, it is less so in warm ambient temperatures when baseline skin temperature already may be high.

ENDOCRINOLOGY OF HOT FLASHES

Estrogen

Given the long-known association of hot flashes with the onset of menopause and that of menopause with a drop in circulating levels of estrogen, investigators have sought to determine whether a relationship might exist between estrogen and hot flashes. In early studies, no correlation was found between estrogen levels in the blood and the presence or absence of hot flashes in postmenopausal women (42–45), nor were any acute changes in estradiol or estrone associated with individual hot flashes (46). In other studies, postmenopausal women with severe hot flashes were found to have lower levels of circulating estrone and estradiol than did asymptomatic women (Fig. 15.3) (32, 47,48). More specifically, Erlik et al. (32) found the fraction of estradiol not bound to sex hormone-binding globulin (SHBG) to be significantly greater in asymptomatic women than in women experiencing hot flashes. Although estrogen does not appear to trigger individual hot flashes, levels of plasma estrogens do play some, as yet undetermined, role in the cause of hot flashes.

Hot flashes involve more than just the presence of low plasma estrogen levels. Throughout the postmenopausal period, estrogen levels remain low, yet some women never have hot flashes; for others, however, hot flashes occur only sporadically or soon cease. In other situations in which estrogen levels are low, such as in prepubertal girls or women with anorexia nervosa, hot flashes are not reported. Furthermore, hot flashlike episodes are reported

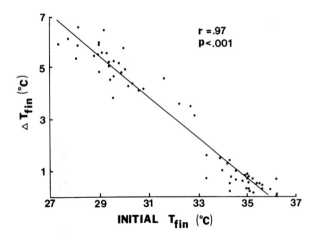

FIG. 15.2. Relationship between the maximal increase in finger temperature (T_{fin}) during a hot flash and the finger temperature immediately before the hot flash (INITIAL Tfin). (From Kronenberg F, Downey JA. Thermoregulatory physiology of menopausal hot flashes: a review. *Can J Physiol Pharmacol* 1987;65:1312-1324.)

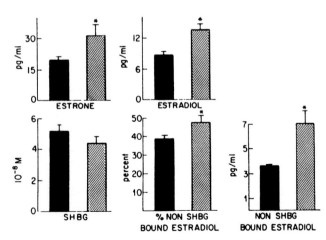

FIG. 15.3. Mean ± SE levels of estrone, estradiol, sex hormone-binding globulin (SHBG), percent non–SHBG-bound estradiol in 24 women with hot flashes (solid bars) compared with 24 asyptomatic subjects (striped bars). Asterisk (*) indicates significantly different from asymptomatic subjects. (Erlik Y, Meldrum DR, Judd HL. Estrogen levels in postmenopausal women with hot flashes. *Obestet Gynecol* 1982;59:403–407.)

during pregnancy, particularly the last trimester, when plasma estrogen level becomes particularly high (F. Kronenberg, unpublished data). Hot flashes also occur in premenopausal women during pituitary suppression with a GnRH agonist, when serum estradiol concentration is maintained at premenopausal levels (49).

What seems to be more important than levels of estrogen per se is a drop in estrogen concentration. For example, the abrupt onset of hot flashes following ovariectomy (42,50) or the administration of GnRH analogues, which cause plasma estrogen to fall (51,52), support this contention. So does the observation that postmenopausal women with gonadal dysgenesis (Turner syndrome) who have never had normal adult estrogen levels do not experience hot flashes unless they are first prescribed and then withdrawn from estrogen (38,53). Estrogen therapy generally ameliorates hot flashes; however, on discontinuation of estrogen treatment, they often return. No reports indicate whether women with hot flashes have a more precipitous natural decline in estrogen than do those who never have hot flashes.

Hot flashes have also been reported by men on acute withdrawal of testosterone, such as after total orchiectomy (2,3). The decline in testosterone as men age is far more gradual than the decline in estrogen that occurs in women, which may be the reason that hot flashes are not frequently reported in men. A sudden decrease in sex steroids in either women or men can, thus, precipitate hot flashes.

The specific role of estrogen in the cause of hot flashes remains to be fully understood. In addition to its effect on reproductive tissues, estrogen influences thermoregulatory, neural, and vascular functioning. The firing rate of thermosensitive neurons in the preoptic area of the hypothalamus in response to thermal stimuli can be modulated by estrogen (54). Estrogen also influences internal body temperature, although the direction of the effect differs between studies (55,56). The responsiveness of vascular smooth muscle to vasoactive substances such as epinephrine and norepinephrine is affected by estrogen (57), and it has been shown to be greater in women with hot flashes than in those without hot flashes (58). Thus, estrogen may have peripheral as well as central effects that are important to hot flash physiology.

Luteinizing Hormone

In addition to the study of estrogen's relationship to hot flashes, the role of gonadotropins has also been examined because gonadotropin levels become elevated at menopause. However, high gonadotropin levels are not the direct cause of hot flashes, because (a) luteinizing hormone (LH) level remains high postmenopausally, whereas hot flashes tend to lessen; (b) no differences in absolute levels of LH have been found between women with and without hot flashes (59); and (c) hot flashes can be diminished by estrogen doses insufficient to reduce LH levels in the blood (60). Furthermore, when antigonadotropins such as danazol or GnRH analogues are given to women with endometriosis, hot flashes often occur despite a decline in LH level (60).

Absolute LH level has provided little insight into the cause of hot flashes. When serial blood samples were drawn, however, LH in the peripheral circulation was found to exhibit a temporal correlation with hot flashes (Fig. 15.4); most hot flashes are accompanied by an increase in LH (38,39). The correspondence of LH pulses with hot flashes led to speculation that LH might be responsible for the initiation of hot flashes. But it was soon evident that a pulse of LH was not a necessary concomitant of hot flashes. Hot flashes can occur in women who have no episodic LH release such as (a) those having had hypophysectomy) (Fig. 15.5) (61,62); (b) premeno-

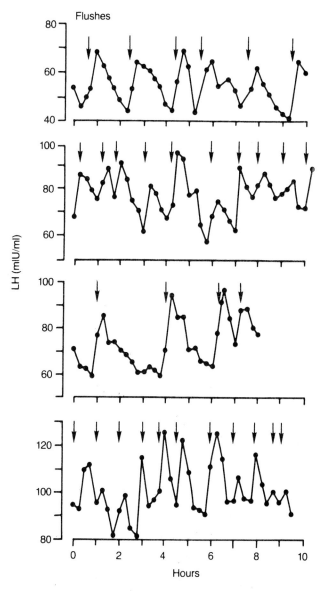

FIG. 15.4. Pattern of pulsatile luteinizing hormone (LH) release and associated menopausal flush episodes. Arrows indicate flush onset. Each part illustrates a separate 8 to 10 hour study in which blood samples were obtained at 15-minute intervals. Note that each flush is synchronized with an LH pulse. (Casper RJ, Yen SSC, Wilkes MM. Menopausal flushes: a neuroendocrine link with pulsatile luteinizing hormone secretion. *Science* 1979;205:823–825.)

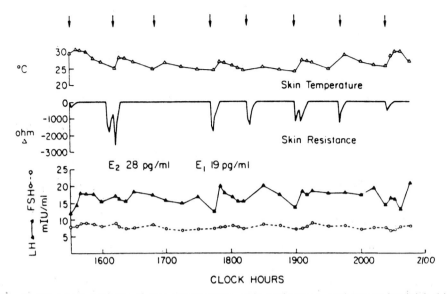

FIG. 15.5. Serial measurements of skin temperature, skin resistance, and serum luteinizing hormone (LH) and follicle-stimulating hormone (FSH) levels in a woman after hypophysectomy (patient 1). Skin resistance changes are depicted at 1-minute intervals as the change in ohms from the baseline immediately preceding the episode. Arrows mark the onsets of subjective hot flushes. E_2, estradiol; E_1, estrone. (Meldrum DR, Erlik Y, Lu JKH, Judd HL. Objectively recorded hot flushes in patients with pituitary insufficiency. *J Clin Endocrinol Metab* 1981;52:684—-687.)

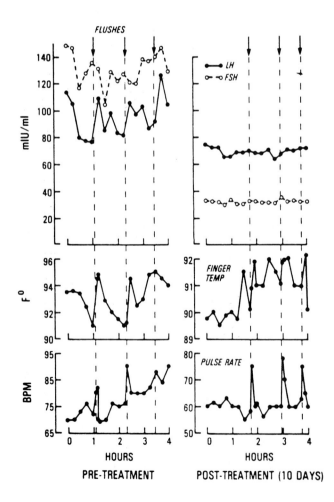

FIG. 15.6. Changes in finger temperature (°F) and pulse rate (beats/min) in association with flush episodes (arrows) and serum concentrations of luteinizing hormone (LH) (●–●) and follicle-stimulating hormone (FSH) (○–○) in a representative study of one hypogonadal subject before and after 10 days of daily luteinizing hormone releasing factor (LRF)-Ag administration (50 μg subcutaneous). (Casper RF, Yen SSC. Menopausal flushes: effect of pituitary gonadotropin desensitization by a potent luteinizing hormone releasing factor agonist. *J Clin Endocrinol Metab* 1981;53:1056–1058.)

pausal or postmenopausal women in whom pulsatile LH release has been suppressed by treatment with a GnRH agonist (Fig. 15.6) (51,63,64); and (c) women with pituitary insufficiency and hypoestrogenism (62). Ravnikar et al. (65) found a similar number of LH pulses present in women with or without hot flashes. Thus, LH secretion per se is not the immediate trigger of hot flashes.

Gonadotropin-Releasing Hormone

Because LH pulses were not found to be directly responsible for initiating hot flashes but were associated with hot flashes, it was thought that perhaps hot flashes might be initiated at the hypothalamic level and involve the releasing factor for LH. Immunoreactive GnRH measured in the peripheral circulation of women with and without hot flashes was discovered to be elevated prior to the LH pulses observed with hot flashes. Women with hot flashes also had higher mean plasma immunoreactive GnRH levels than did asymptomatic women (65). Yet women with defects in GnRH synthesis or release (isolated gonadotropin deficiency) who received estrogen treatment had hot flashes when estrogen was withdrawn

(66). When GnRH receptors were blocked with a long-acting GnRH antagonist in women who never had hot flashes, they experienced hot flashes for the first time, although LH pulses were abolished (51). Thus, episodic GnRH release is not necessary for hot flashes to occur.

Other Endocrine Studies

Several investigators have measured circulating epinephrine and norepinephrine during hot flashes with conflicting results. Casper et al. (38) found no change in epinephrine or norepinephrine in association with individual hot flashes. Given the 2 to 3 minute half-life of epinephrine and norepinephrine (67), Kronenberg et al. (35) sampled at more frequent intervals and found a significant increase in plasma epinephrine and a decrease in norepinephrine during hot flashes (Fig. 15.7). Mashchak et al. (68) found an increase in epinephrine but no change in norepinephrine levels.

Other substances that have been measured in the peripheral circulation during hot flashes are listed in Table 15.2. Circulating β-endorphin, β-lipotropin, and adrenocorticotropic hormone (ACTH) increase in association with hot flashes (Fig. 15.8) (69,70), as do cortisol,

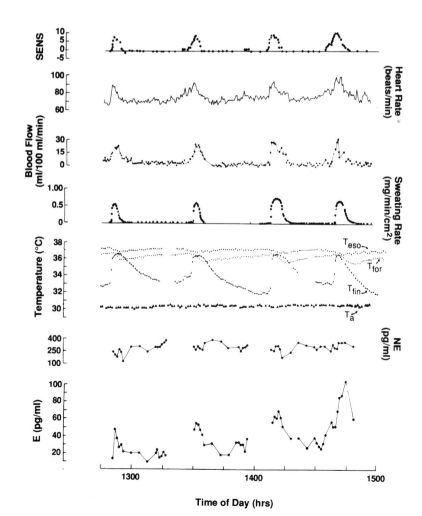

FIG. 15.7. Pattern of cardiovascular, thermoregulatory, and endocrine changes for four consecutive hot flashes over a 2-hour period. Changes in sensation (SENS), heart rate, blood flow (finger), sweating rate, temperatures (esophageal, forehead, finger, and ambient), norepinephrine (NE), and epinephrine (E) are depicted. (Kronenberg F, Downey JA. Thermoregulatory physiology of menopausal hot flashes: a review. *Can J Physiol Pharmacol* 1987;65:1312—1324.)

TABLE 15.2. *Hormone changes during hot flashes*

Substance	Response	Reference
Luteinizing hormone	Increase	35,38,39,46,68,69,153,154
Follicle-stimulating hormone	No change	39,46,68,153
	Increase	38,69
Gonadotropin-releasing hormone	Increase	65
Estradiol	No change	46
Estrone	No change	46
Dehydroepiandrosterone	Increase	46
Androstenedione	Increase	46
Progesterone	Slight increase	46
Epinephrine	Increase	35,68
	No change	38,154
Norepinephrine	No change	38,68,153
	Decrease	35
	Increase	154
Dopamine	No change	38,154
Prolactin	No change	38,46,153
Cortisol	Increase	46,69,154
	No change	155
Corticotropin	Increase	46,69
β-Endorphin	Increase	46,69
β-Lipotropin	Increase	69
Neurotensin	Increase	156
Growth hormone	Increase	46
TSH	No change	46
Glucose	No change	154
Glucagon	No change	154
Insulin	No change	154

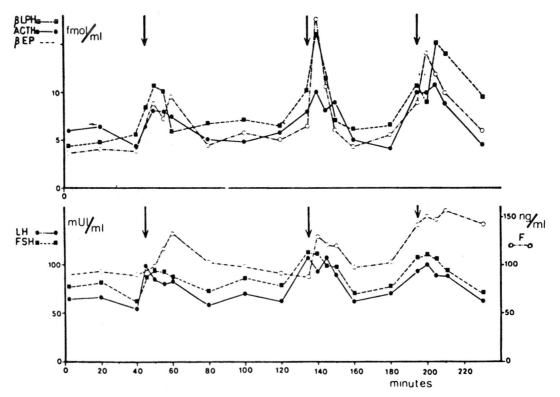

FIG. 15.8. Plasma levels of adrenocorticotropin (ACTH), β-lipoprotein (β-LPH), β-endorphin (β-EP) (top) and luteinizing hormone (LH), follicle-stimulating hormone (FSH), and cortisol (F) (bottom) in subject M.M. during observation period. Arrows indicate onset of hot flashes. (Genazzani AR, Petraglia F, Facchinetti F, Facchini V, Vope A, Alessandrini G. Increase of proopiomelancortin-related peptides during subjective menopausal flushes. *Am J Obstet Gynecol* 1984;149:775–779.)

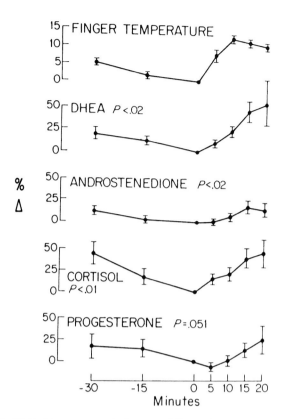

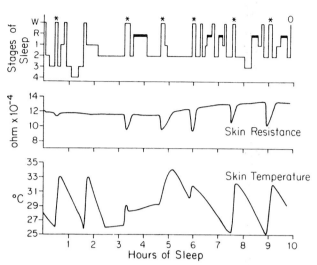

FIG. 15.10. Sleepgram and recordings of skin resistance and temperature in postmenopausal subject with severe hot flushes. Each asterisk marks occurrence of objectively measured hot flush. Open circle indicates arousal of patient by investigator at end of the study. (Erlik Y, Tataryn IV, Meldrum DR, Lomax P, Bajorek JG, Judd HL. Association of waking episodes with menopausal hot flushes. *JAMA* 1981;245: 1741–1744.)

FIG. 15.9. Mean percent change of finger temperature and serum dehydroepiandrosterone (DHEA), Δ, F, and P levels before and after objective flashes. (Meldrum DR, Tatryn IV, Frumar AM, Erlik Y, Lu KH, Judd HL. Gonadotropins, estrogens, and adrenal steroids during the menopausal hot flash. *J Clin Endocrinol Metab* 1980;50:685–689.)

dehydroepiandrosterone (DHEA), and androstenedione (Fig. 15.9) (46,69,70). Most of these substances reach peak levels after the subjective hot flash has ended. Prolactin level did not change during hot flashes. No causal relationships have been found.

HOT FLASHES AND SLEEP

One of the primary complaints of women with hot flashes is sleep disruption. They may awaken several times during the night, drenched in sweat, necessitating a change of bedding and clothes. Erlik et al. (71) used electroencephalography (EEG) to demonstrate that nocturnal awakenings in postmenopausal women with hot flashes were correlated with the occurrence of the hot flashes (Fig. 15.10). Sleep efficiency is lower and latency to rapid eye movement (REM) sleep is longer in women with hot flashes compared with those with no hot flashes (72). This disturbed sleep often leads to fatigue and irritability during the day. The frequency of awakenings and of hot flashes are reduced with estrogen treatment (Fig. 15.11) (71,73,74). Sometimes, a woman may not consciously awaken from sleep, although the EEG recording indicates

momentary arousal, yet objective physiologic measurement has documented the continuation of hot flashes throughout the night (Fig. 15.12). This sleep disturbance caused by hot flashes is a primary motivator for women to seek medical advice and pharmacologic solutions. As is discussed below, a nonpharmacologic approach may also provide nighttime relief for some women.

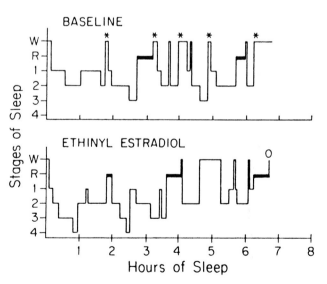

FIG. 15.11. Sleepgrams measured in symptomatic patient before and after 30 days' administration of ethinyl estradiol, 50 μg four times daily. (Erlik Y, Tataryn IV, Meldrum DR, Lomax P, Bajorek JG, Judd HL. Association of waking episodes with menopausal hot flushes. *JAMA* 1981;245: 1741–1744.)

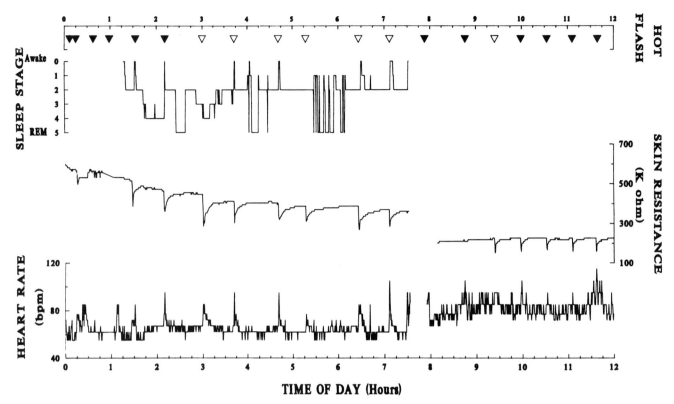

FIG. 15.12. Pattern of sleep stages, skin resistance, and heart rate for a 12-hour period (subject A-10). The solid triangles (▼) indicate reported hot flashes; open triangles (▽) indicate unreported hot flashes. Sleep stages 1 through 4, non REM sleep; stage 5, REM (rapid eye movement); absolute clock time on the abscissa. The sudden drop in skin resistance at about 7:00 AM is due to a change of skin resistance electrodes. This subject went to bed shortly after 1:00 AM and awoke at about 7:30 AM (Kronenberg F. Hot flashes: epidemiology and physiology. *Ann NY Acad Sci* 1990;592:52–86.)

AMBIENT TEMPERATURE AND HOT FLASHES

Many women find that their hot flashes worsen in warm weather. To relieve the discomfort of hot flashes, women may stand in front of an air conditioner or refrigerator, wear loose, light, nonsynthetic clothing, or open windows on cool nights. However, scant research exists on the effect of ambient temperature on hot flashes. Hot flash frequency has been found by some investigators to correlate positively with outdoor temperature (75–77), whereas others found no relationship to exist (29,30). What has long been reported anecdotally and in some uncontrolled thermal environments has now been demonstrated under controlled temperature conditions. That is, ambient temperature does significantly influence both the frequency and intensity of hot flashes. In a cool environment (19°C) women had significantly fewer and less intense hot flashes than in a warm (31°C) environment (Fig. 15.13) (77). Cooling room temperature may therefore be one way in which women can reduce their hot flashes, particularly during sleep.

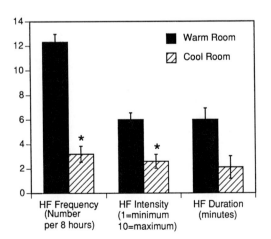

FIG. 15.13. Mean frequency, intensity, and duration of hot flashes at warm (31°C) versus cool (19°C) ambient temperatures± 1 SEM. *P < 0.05. The units of the y-axis vary with parameter, as indicated. (Kronenberg F, Barnard RM. Modulation of menopausal hot flashes by ambient temperature. *J Therm Biol* 1992;17:43—-49.)

ETIOLOGY

Several hypotheses have been presented to explain the mechanism underlying hot flashes (66,78–82). These hypotheses are based on data obtained primarily from studies of women with hot flashes in which substances measured in the peripheral circulation have been found to change in association with the hot flashes or on observations on the success of various drugs in treating hot flashes. The hypotheses discussed most widely involve adrenergic mechanisms, endogenous opioid peptide, and GnRH. Although a number of detailed reviews and critiques of the proposed models and theories to explain hot flashes exist (78,79,82), a definitive explanation still eludes us.

The hormonal milieu is obviously relevant to the occurrence of hot flashes. Although an association is found between hot flashes and low peripheral estrogen levels, hot flash episodes also occur when the estrogen level is high (e.g., late in pregnancy) and in women administered estrogen for hot flashes that occurred during pituitary desensitization with GnRH analogue (49). Their hot flashes stopped after pituitary function returned to normal, despite a relatively rapid drop in serum estradiol level. Early studies searching for a correlation between circulating estradiol levels and the occurrence of hot flashes found no association between them. More recently, studies have demonstrated that circulating estrone and estradiol levels were lower in women with than those without hot flashes (44,47,48,86). Explanations involving the acute withdrawal of sex steroids have also been offered, as hot flashes occur in most women after ovariectomy (14). However, the above-cited situation of hot flashes in the face of a rapid decrease in estrogen, point up the need for further investigation. The relationship between peripheral estrogen levels and hot flashes is undoubtedly complex, with numerous interrelated factors whose relationships have not yet been appreciated or understood.

Measurement of endocrine concomitants of hot flashes, either in terms of mean hormone levels or episodic changes, has not as yet uncovered the initiating factor or set of circumstances responsible either for triggering an individual hot flash or for providing the environment in which hot flashes will occur.

The pattern of hot flashes in menopausal women in some cultures is reported to be one of fewer hot flashes than is experienced by women in Western cultures. Neither the epidemiology of such reports or an explanatory model has been well examined. Differences in genetics, diet, or societal status of menopausal women have all been discussed in this context (18,21,87).

Descriptions of the sequence of events that characterizes a hot flash have led to proposals that hot flashes are the result of a perturbation of the brain's thermoregulatory center located in the hypothalamus. This perturbation activates mechanisms of heat loss (vasodilation, sweating, and behavioral adjustments) at hot flash onset and heat conservation (vasoconstriction, behavioral changes, and shivering) at its termination. The combination and sequence of physiologic and behavioral responses during a hot flash suggest that the phenomenon involves the coordinated action of the thermoregulatory system. The body responds as it would to dissipate excess heat in situations of overheating or fever breaking. Some studies of hot flashes did not observe an elevation of internal temperature associated with a hot flash, and described the responses as consistent with the hypothesis that a hot flash involves a transient downward resetting of the body's thermoregulatory set-point (36,88). That is, a sudden drop in set-point temperature occurs at the start of a hot flash. Because the body would then be warmer than this new set-point, the thermoregulatory system acts appropriately to cool the body. As a result, internal temperature falls. The set-point then returns to normal, and heat conservation mechanisms act to return body temperature to normal. This entire process is analogous to what happens during a fever, but the change in set-point is in the opposite direction than during fever (36,88). Pyrogenic substances can raise the set-point temperature and initiate the thermoregulatory responses that result in a fever (89). What might cause the hypothalamic resetting during a hot flash is not known.

More recent studies by Freedman et al. explored the involvement of α_2-adrenergic mechanisms in both the triggering and reduction of hot flashes. They demonstrated that yohimbine, an α_2-adrenergic antagonist, triggered hot flashes, whereas clonidine and α_2-adrenergic agonist reduced the number of hot flashes (90). These data support their hypothesis that central α_2-adrenergic receptors play a role in the initiation and inhibition of hot flashes.

Reproductive hormones modulate the functioning of the thermoregulatory system (88), as do opioid peptides (91–93), which also modulate and are influenced by reproductive hormones (94–96). Further delineation of the relationship between sex steroids, opioid peptides, and thermoregulatory function is necessary.

A coherent hypothesis should be able to accommodate the hot flash-associated thermoregulatory and neuroendocrine responses and also to explain, among other things (a) why different individuals experience hot flashes at different frequencies and for varying lengths of time; (b) why some women never get hot flashes; (c) why hot flashes begin in some women just hours after ovariectomy; (d) why some women sweat and others do not; (e) why priming with estrogen is necessary before hot flashes can occur (no hot flashes are seen in prepubertal girls, or women with gonadal dysgenesis before treatment with estrogen); (f) the similar phenomenon of hot flashes in women and men following a reduction in estrogen in women or testosterone in men; (g) why drugs such as clonidine can eliminate the sensation of hot flashes, while pulses of finger temperature and LH remain. Are there invariant components of a hot flash that are always measurable, independent of environmental conditions, age, or sex? A resolution of these questions awaits additional research, and perhaps an animal model that more closely resembles the human female in terms of both endocrine and thermoregulatory functioning.

WHY ARE HOT FLASHES A PROBLEM?

If hot flashes occur only sporadically, they are not likely to be disruptive or even more than a nuisance. But for those women with many hot flashes throughout the day, every day, hot flashes can be periodically disabling, physically draining, and they can impact negatively on work, family, and social relationships. When hot flashes disturb sleep every night, the consequences can be debilitating. Some women choose to avoid touching, hugging, or sexual activity because the skin-to-skin contact may bring on a hot flash.

Profuse sweating during a hot flash is one of the most bothersome complaints; it can be an embarrassment, particularly at work or in social situations. It can even require a change of clothing, which is not always possible or convenient. Women with severe hot flashes describe their lives as a constant struggle to achieve thermal comfort. They must adjust their behavior (such as wearing layers of clothes for easy removal, shunning synthetics for natural fibers, or carrying a fan). Some attempt to alter their immediate environment by turning on the air conditioner, opening windows, going outside if the weather is cool, or staying inside on hot humid days.

DIAGNOSIS

Most women who present with hot flashes will be perimenopausal or recently postmenopausal. Therefore, age and menstrual history (menstrual cycle irregularity, oligomenorrhea or amenorrhea) are strong indications that these are menopausally related hot flashes, as do other complaints suggestive of low estrogen (e.g., vaginal dryness and its sequelae). During the perimenopausal period, hot flashes can come and go. Menstrual cycle irregularity may correspond with these fluctuating episodes. If women are still menstruating regularly when hot flashes first occur, they may not recognize that the such episodes of feeling hot and sweating are actually hot flashes. Thus, many years of hot flashes may pass prior to menopause. Hot flashes can continue long into the postmenopausal years—sometimes throughout a woman's lifetime.

In the few cases where diagnosis of hot flashes is unclear, measurement of plasma follicle-stimulating hormone (FSH) and LH may be of value, because they are both elevated in menopausal women. Levels of these hormones can fluctuate, particularly during the perimenopause period, so multiple measurements are necessary. FSH level is a better diagnostic indicator of hot flashes than is LH because the increase in circulating LH tends to lag behind the rise in FSH. Estradiol is not a particularly good indicator on which to base diagnosis in women of premenopausal and perimenopausal ages.

Several conditions share some clinical features with hot flashes, particularly the flushing and sweating. These include hyperthyroidism, panic attacks, carcinoid syndrome, pheochromocytoma, and niacin flush.

MANAGEMENT

With adequate information and support, many women can make adjustments necessary to cope with their hot flashes. A wide range of sensations can be experienced during hot flashes, which can be upsetting if a woman is unaware of what to expect. Many of the worries related to hot flashes can be allayed if a woman is informed of what is and is not known about them. For example, it is impossible to predict exactly how long hot flashes will last; therefore, treatment duration cannot be defined. It is also important to convey that hot flashes can recur when treatment is ended.

The initial stages of management should include determining the impact level the hot flashes have on the patient and assessing how she has been coping with them. Precipitating factors (e.g., hot drinks, alcohol, caffeine, or hot environments) should be identified and the patient advised to avoid them. The patient should be made aware that stresses at home or in the workplace can make hot flashes more difficult to cope with.

Many women try to control their hot flashes by modifying their environment or behavior before consulting a physician. They change room temperature, wear light, layered clothing, and try vitamins or dietary changes that have been suggested to them. For some, these attempts may be effective and the hot flashes may become less intense or less frequent. Whereas for others, nothing they do has any impact on their relentless hot flashes. When knowledge, proscription, and behavioral changes prove insufficient, women may ask about hormone therapy.

Pharmacologic Preparations

Available therapies do not "cure" hot flashes; rather, they provide symptomatic relief by making the hot flashes less frequent or less intense; sometimes symptoms are eliminated, at least for the duration of the treatment. If hot flashes return when treatment is stopped, it is not known whether the treatment just postponed the hot flashes or whether the individual would have had hot flashes for that duration regardless of whether she had been treated. To minimize the recurrence of hot flashes, it is advisable to taper drug treatment over several weeks rather than suddenly stop it. We do not know the mechanism by which hot flashes are reduced for any of the treatments discussed below.

When various hot flash therapies are compared with a placebo, the placebo often demonstrates considerable effectiveness. Therefore, to best assess the efficacy of a treatment, it is necessary to conduct randomized, double-blind, placebo-controlled crossover studies. And, as it may take several weeks to control hot flashes effectively, studies must be sufficiently long to adequately determine how well a particular treatment works.

Estrogen

Estrogen administration is currently the most effective treatment for hot flashes. It has been used, albeit initially in the form of crude extracts, for almost 100 years. Rationale for its use is based on the association of hot flashes with the decline in ovarian function at menopause rather than on knowing what causes hot flashes.

The effect of estrogen treatment on hot flashes is not usually immediate. The full benefit may not be realized until after several months' of therapy. When treatment is discontinued, the effect on hot flashes may persist for some time, depending on the type of estrogen or route of its administration. For example, conjugated equine estrogen can remain active for several weeks after treatment has ended because of its storage in adipose tissue (97). Many patients on a cyclic estrogen regimen may find, for each cycle, that it takes several days before hot flashes diminish; however, by the end of the week in which no estrogen is taken, hot flashes will have returned. For this and other reasons, the current trend is toward continuous daily estrogen intake.

The most commonly used regimen for treating hot flashes in the United States is 0.625 to 1.25 mg of oral conjugated equine estrogen (Premarin). Many other oral preparations are available in equivalent doses (see Chapter 6). Transdermal estradiol (Estraderm 0.05 to 0.10 mg/day) has been gaining popularity. Estrogen is also available as subcutaneous implants, injectables, and vaginal creams; most are effective in treating hot flashes.

Oral estrogen has been in use for many years and has been the most extensively studied of the treatments for hot flashes. In a double-blind, placebo-controlled crossover study of conjugated equine estrogen (1.25 mg), Coope et al. (98) reported that after the first 3 months, hot flashes were reduced (approximately 90% in women on estrogen and approximately 62% in women on placebo) (Fig. 15.14). In another placebo-controlled trial, Campbell and Whitehead (99) sought to assess the efficacy of conjugated estrogen (1.25 mg) in relieving hot flashes and other symptoms of menopause such as vaginal dryness, insomnia, anxiety, irritability, and memory loss. Estrogen was significantly better than placebo in improving all these symptoms. Hot flashes were improved by 40% to 50% with estrogen and by approximately 10% with placebo (as

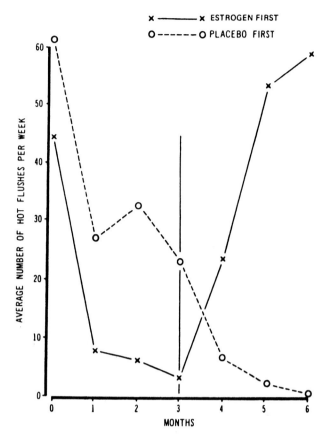

FIG. 15.14. Hot flush count during the 6-month trial. (Coope J, Thomson JM, Poller L. Effects of "natural oestrogen" replacement therapy on menopausal symptoms and blood clotting. *Br Med J* 1975;4:139—-143.)

assessed by graphic rating scores). In this study, one group of subjects had symptoms such as insomnia, but they did not have hot flashes. Treatment with estrogen improved some of their symptoms, but not their insomnia. This is in contrast to the alleviation of the insomnia for those women who also complained of hot flashes. The investigators concluded that much of the insomnia of women with hot flashes is the result of nocturnal hot flashes.

Transdermal patches that provide a continuous diffusion of estradiol are effective in reducing hot flashes. A dose–response relationship between dose of transdermal estradiol (25, 50, 100, and 200 µg/day) and hot flash frequency, using subjective and objective criteria, was demonstrated in a double-blind study by Steingold (Fig. 15.15) (100). Hot flashes were significantly reduced at all doses of estradiol, with a progressive decline in hot flashes as estradiol increased; hot flashes were not appreciably reduced by placebo. The highest dose (200 µg/day) resulted in a 91% reduction in the number of hot flashes.

Haas et al. (101) compared the effects of 6 weeks of transdermal estradiol 50 µg/day) with that of placebo, on subjectively and objectively measured hot flashes in a double-blind, placebo-controlled study. Although changes in plasma estradiol and LH levels were measurable within 8

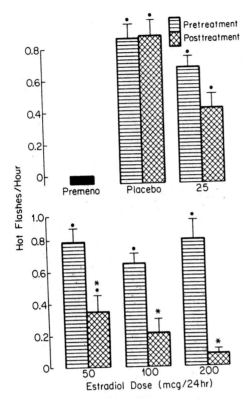

FIG. 15.15. Mean ± SE rate of occurrence of hot flashes in the study groups and premenopausal women (Premeno) before and during transdermal E₂ administration. (Steingold KA. Treatment of hot flashes with transdermal estradiol administration. *J Clin Endocrinol Metab* 1985;61:627–632.)

hours of the application of the patch, a decline in hot flashes occurred gradually over the next 4 weeks. At that point, findings were a 74% decrease in subjectively reported hot flashes and an 85% decrease in objectively monitored hot flashes (Fig. 15.16). Women on placebo

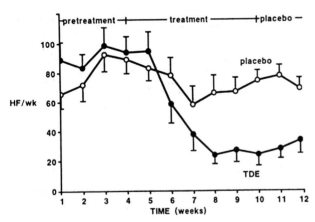

FIG. 15.16. Total subjective hot flashes (HF) recorded by patients on transdermal estradiol (TDE) patch (N = 10) and placebo (N = 8, first 7 weeks; N = 7, last 5 weeks) for each study week. (Haas S, Walsh B, Evans S, Krache M, Ravnikar V, Schiff I. The effect of transdermal estradiol on hormone and metabolic dynamics over a six-week period. *Obstet Gynecol* 1988;71:671–676.)

reported a 27% reduction in hot flashes (not statistically significant) during the first 3 weeks of the study.

Stanczyk (102) compared transdermal estradiol with subdermal estradiol. Hot flashes were eliminated in all patients, regardless of the mode of estrogen delivery.

In addition to ameliorating hot flashes, other complains that may be improved by estrogen include insomnia (74,99); vaginal dryness, memory, concentration, and lower urinary tract problems (99); and mood (99,103).

Nonestrogenic Treatments

Although most women find that estrogen relieves their hot flashes, some are found for whom estrogen is contraindicated or who find the side effects unacceptable, some whose hot flashes are not responsive to estrogen, even at elevated doses, and others who prefer not to remain on estrogen for a prolonged period of time.

Progestins

Medroxyprogesterone acetate (MPA) is a nonestrogenic steroid. Several double-blind, placebo-controlled studies have shown that MPA decreases the number of hot flashes. Injected intramuscularly, a dose of 150 mg/month MPA resulted in a 90% reduction in hot flashes, compared with a 25% reduction in the placebo group (104). The major side effect was abnormal uterine bleeding (43%). Morrison et al. (105) conducted a study of intramuscular MPA (50, 100, and 150 mg) in which a dose–response relationship was shown, with an approximate 75% improvement for those on 50 mg, and 90% to 100% relief for those on 150 mg by week 4 of treatment. Most women in the placebo group dropped out of the study. For those who remained, the placebo was ineffective. In this study, only two patients on MPA (of 36 women) had abnormal bleeding.

Taken orally, MPA has fewer side effects. In a double-blind, placebo-controlled trial, MPA (20 mg/day) resulted in an approximately 74% decline in the number of reported hot flashes by the third month of treatment; placebo caused a reduction in hot flashes of about 26% (Fig. 15.17) (106). Albrecht et al. (107) measured hot flashes both subjectively and objectively in response to 20 mg/day, oral MPA. Reported hot flashes decreased by 90% in women on MPA and by 25% in those on placebo. Finger skin temperature elevations and associated LH pulses, the objective indicators of hot flashes, were also reduced.

Another progestin, megestrol acetate (MA), has been tested and found to be effective in treating hot flashes. Oral MA significantly reduced hot flashes (no placebo control) whether measured subjectively or objectively, in a dose–response fashion with increasing doses of MA (20, 40, 80 mg/day) (Fig. 15.18). Few side effects and no abnormal bleeding or depression were reported (108).

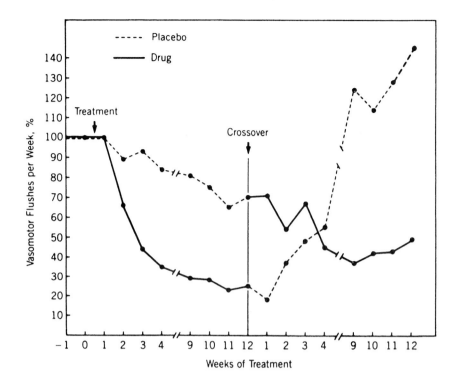

FIG. 15.17. Effect of oral medroxyprogesterone acetate on frequency of hot flashes. Mean number of vasomotor flushes as a percent change from pretreatment (week -1 to 0). (Schiff I, Tulchinsky D, Cramer D, Ryan KJ. Oral medroxyprogesterone in the treatment of postmenopausal symptoms. *JAMA* 1980; 244:1443—1445.)

Sherwin and Gelfand (109) compared women on conjugated equine estradiol alone, with those on estradiol MPA. Both regimens resulted in a reduction in hot flashes. Estradiol was administered on days 1 to 25, and MPA on days 15 to 25, leaving days 26 to 30 hormone-free. For 3 weeks of each cycle hot flashes were diminished. During the fourth week, which was hormone-free, hot flash frequency increased.

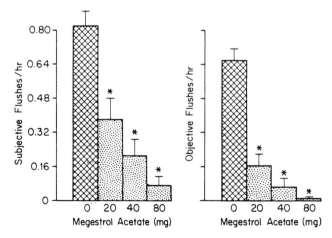

FIG. 15.18. The mean (± SE) subjective and objective flushes per hour before and following the oral administration of the various doses of megestrol acetate. *Significantly different (*P* <0.01) from baseline. (Erlik Y, Meldrum DR, Lagasse LD, Judd HL. Effect of magestrol acetate on flushing and bone metabolism in postmenopausal women. *Maturitas* 1981;3:167–172.)

Clonidine

Clonidine, an α-adrenergic receptor agonist that influences vascular responsiveness, has been used in the treatment of hot flashes. Clayden et al. (110) reported a double-blind, placebo-controlled crossover study of 86 women with hot flashes, and they demonstrated that clonidine (0.05 to 0.15 mg/day) reduced the number and intensity of hot flashes. However, as in the studies of estrogen, women on placebo also reported a reduction in hot flashes almost equal to that of women on clonidine (Fig. 15.19). Dry mouth was the primary complaint of those on clonidine. Other side effects, including insomnia, headache, depression, and nausea, were reported by both those on clonidine and those on placebo. In another study, Laufer et al. (111) demonstrated a dose–response relationship between clonidine (0.1, 0.2, 0.4 mg/day) and objectively recorded hot flashes in six women. At the highest dose, reduction in hot flashes was 46%; with placebo, reduction was small and not statistically significant. Of the initial 10 subjects, four withdrew because of side effects, which included nausea, fatigue, headaches, dizziness, and dry mouth.

When clonidine was administered intravenously to menopausal women with hot flashes, Tulandi et al. (112) obtained somewhat different results. Subjects who received clonidine (0.075 mg in 10 mL physiologic saline) reported significantly fewer hot flashes; however, objective recordings indicated a continuation of the pattern of episodic increases in finger skin temperature and the associated pulses of LH characteristic of hot flashes.

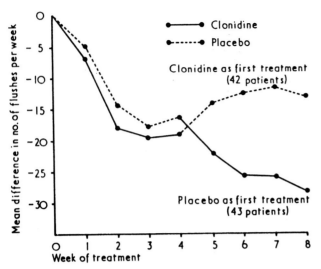

FIG. 15.19. Mean change in number of flushes from initial values. (Clayden JR, Bell JW, Pollard P. Menopausal flushing: double-blind trial of a non-hormonal medication. *Br Med J* 1974;1:409–412.)

Ginsburg et al. (113) examined vascular responsiveness in menopausal women before and after oral clonidine treatment. They measured peripheral vasodilatory responses to infusion of the vasoactive substances norepinephrine, epinephrine, and angiotensin. Forearm and hand blood flow responses in the infusions were diminished after clonidine treatment. The investigators suggest that clonidine might reduce the peripheral vasodilation that accompanies a hot flash, and that given the reduced response to angiotensin, clonidine might be acting in some way other than through peripheral adrenergic mechanisms.

Also demonstrating effectiveness in reducing hot flashes are lofexidine, another α-agonist, and α-methyldopa, whose primary metabolite, methylnorepinephrine, is a receptor agonist (114,115).

Propranolol

Propranolol, a peripherally and centrally acting β-receptor blocking agent, has been studied with mixed results. Erkkola et al. (116) reported that 60 mg/day of propranolol slightly reduced hot flashes. The reduction was from approximately 9.4 hot flashes per day to 7.8 hot flashes per day; however this study had no placebo control group. Coope et al. (75), in a randomized, double-blind, placebo-controlled trial, found 40 mg of propranolol daily to be no more effective than placebo in reducing hot flashes. The slight reduction in hot flashes was similar to that reported by Erkkola. No side effects were seen among the women on propranolol. A statistically significant reduction in hot flash frequency was reported by Alcoff et al. (117) in 70% of their subjects. However, as the extent of the reduction was not reported, it is difficult to assess whether this had clinical significance. Side effects (including lightheaded-

ness, nausea, and fatigue) occurred in 24% of those on propranolol (80 mg/day).

Bellergal

Bellergal is a combination of belladonna alkaloids, ergotamine tartrate, and phenobarbital. In a double-blind, placebo-controlled study, Lebherz and French (118) found this drug (Bellergal) to be significantly more effective than placebo in reducing subjectively reported hot flashes (60% vs. 22% decrease in hot flashes, respectively). The specific mechanism of action on hot flashes is unknown. Bellergal has sedative effects and is not a treatment of choice. One must also consider the varied actions of the three components and be aware of possible interactions with other drugs.

NONPHARMACOLOGIC APPROACHES

Hormone therapy (estrogen, with or without progesterone) is extremely efficacious in treating hot flashes, ameliorating and, in many cases, eliminating them. But some women need or desire other options, because they have medical conditions or risk factors for which estrogen is contraindicated, experience some adverse reaction to hormone therapy, or choose not to take hormones. In increasing numbers, women have been trying modes of therapy, other than conventional hormone therapy, for relief from their hot flashes.

These nonpharmacologic approaches cover a broad range of modalities, including vitamins, (in particular vitamin E), behavioral therapies (such as yoga, relaxation, and biofeedback), lifestyle changes (exercise, alcohol use, dietary changes), herbal remedies (black cohosh, ginseng, dong quai), traditional systems of medicine (such as traditional Chinese medicine or Ayurveda), homeopathy, and acupuncture. The efficacy of many of these approaches has not been rigorously evaluated. However, given the rapidly growing popularity of alternative medicine, a number of studies of alternative therapies for menopausal problems, particularly hot flashes, are being initiated or are underway.

Medicinal Herbs

Herbs have long been used by women of many cultures to reduce the discomfort of hot flashes, including herbal therapy in Western countries. However, for most herbal remedies, few clinical studies are available that provide treatment recommendations.

Black cohosh (*Cimicifugae racemosa*) is receiving increasing notice in the US marketplace, even though it its use is not new. Native American women traditionally used black cohosh to treat amenorrhea (119). It has been used in German medicine for more than 50 years, and is approved by the German Commission E (somewhat comparable to the US Food and Drug Administration [FDA]) for use in premenstrual discomfort, dysmenorrhea, and menopausal symptoms (120). Although black cohosh was reported to bind to estrogen receptors in uterus and pituitary *in vitro* (121,122), more recent reports indicate that the proliferation of estrogen receptor positive breast cancer cell lines was not promoted by an extract of black cohosh (123). Clinical studies conducted in Germany in the 1980s indicate that black cohosh reduces hot flashes in women (124–126). Determining the mechanism of action and whether it is safe for women for whom estrogen is contraindicated requires further study.

Dong quai (*Angelica sinensis*) is another herb being sold in the United States as an alternative medicine for women's health concerns. Some menopausal women who take it report that it helps relieve hot flashes (127). In a recent randomized, placebo-controlled clinical trial of dong quai for the treatment of menopausal symptoms (in 71 postmenopausal women), investigators found no statistically significant difference in the number of hot flashes, vaginal maturation index, or Kupperman index (a combined index of 11 menopausal complaints) (128). They concluded that dong quai, used alone, is not helpful in relieving menopausal symptoms. In traditional Chinese medicine, dong quai is used to maintain normal reproductive functioning and to "tonify" the reproductive system and functions of the nonreproductive system functions (129). It is typically used as one of several components of herbal formulas; it is generally not used alone. Additional studies are needed to clarify the role of dong quai, either singly or in herbal mixtures for the treatment of menopausal complaints.

Women report anecdotally that ginseng helps relieve hot flashes. Ginseng has been associated with vaginal bleeding in humans (130,131). In a recent placebo-controlled trial, ginseng (Ginsana G115) provided some symptomatic relief, particularly for depressed mood in menopausal women, and it improved general health and well-being as self-reported. It was less satisfactory in treating hot flashes (132). Ginseng boasts a broad range of pharmacologic effects, particularly on the endocrine system (133). It is still premature to assess either ginseng's effectiveness for hot flashes or its possible mechanisms of action.

Evening primrose oil is another dietary supplement readily available to women. It is discussed in some herbal literature as being beneficial for women's health problems such as mastalgia and hot flashes. It is high in the essential fatty acids linolenic acid and γ-linolenic (GLA). The literature on its value for treating premenstrual syndrome (PMS) is controversial. Although no compelling reason is found to believe that evening primrose oil would be beneficial to women with hot flashes, a randomized, double-blind, placebo controlled pilot study was undertaken to evaluate this prospect (134). No benefit over placebo was observed.

Dietary Phytoestrogens

Although some women report that particular foods (e.g., coffee, spicy foods) trigger individual hot flashes, little information is available on how long-term consumption of specific food or emphasis on certain foods in the diet might influence hormone levels and thereby effect hot flash occurrence. Many food plants contain compounds that have estrogenic activity, either directly or on being metabolized. A major classes of "phytoestrogens" is the phenolic phytoestrogens, which include isoflavones, lignans, and coumestans. Isoflavones are found in legumes such as soybeans, clover, and alfalfa. Lignan precursors are found in whole grains, and seeds, especially flaxseed (linseed), and also in rye, millet, legumes, fruits, and vegetables (135). They are broken down by bacteria in the gut to enterolactone and enterodiol, also called "mammalian lignans." Bacteria also remove a glycoside from isoflavone precursors to create the active isoflavones genistein, daidzein, and equol. Coumestans, which are found largely in legumes, tend to be more estrogenic than the isoflavones (136).

It is now well established that ingestion of plants containing phytoestrogens can cause reproductive disorders in mammals (137). A diet with substantial intake of these plants can produce estrogenlike effects in women as well. For example, ingestion of flaxseed (linseed) and clover sprouts by postmenopausal women produced changes in vaginal maturation values in an Australian study (138). In a study of a dietary soy intervention in postmenopausal American women, a slight, but not statistically significant estrogenic effect was seen on vaginal epithelium (139). It is not surprising that results differ among these studies because the food plants involved contain different classes of estrogenic compounds (lignans in the grasses and oilseeds and isoflavones in soy), with differing degrees of estrogenicity.

Although phytoestrogens tend to be only weakly estrogenic, they can be found in high levels in the body. In a study comparing American and Finnish women on three diets (omnivores, lactovegetarians, macrobiotics), excretion of the most abundant phytoestrogen was found to be highest in the macrobiotics and lowest in the omnivores (140). Postmenopausal women in Japan eating a traditional low-fat diet were found to have 100 to 1,000 times higher levels of several urinary phytoestrogens than levels of the endogenous estrogens in the urine of American or Finnish women eating an omnivorous diet (141). Traditional Asian diets are associated with a high intake of soy products. The high levels of dietary phytoestrogens have been given as an explanation for the low level of hot flashes reported by many Japanese women. Clinical studies have explored and continue to explore this link directly.

In a study designed to examine the effect of soy on hot flashes, Murkies et al. (142) compared the effect of soy flour with wheat flour supplementation in a randomized, double-blind trial. Hot flashes decreased significantly in the soy group by week 6 and in both groups by week 12. No change in vaginal maturation index was noted in either group. Excretion of urinary daidzein, an estrogenic isoflavone from soy, had increased significantly at 12 weeks in the soy group, with no significant increase in excretion of urinary phytoestrogens in the wheat group. Interpretation of these results is not clear. Wheat flour also contains phytoestrogens, but with less estrogenic potency than soy phytoestrogens. Milling supposedly removes most of the phytoestrogens from wheat (thus the choice for placebo). Sufficient critical studies on soy have yet to be done for definitive conclusions.

Brzezinski et al. (143), in a randomized, placebo-controlled study, examined the effects of a dietary supplementation with phytoestrogens on menopausal symptoms, serum estradiol, FSH, LH, SHBG, and phytoestrogens. After 12 weeks, in those with increased phytoestrogen intake (as compared with normal diet controls), SHBG level increased in and hot flashes and vaginal dryness scores were significantly reduced. These results are in contrast to those of Baird et al. (139), who did not find any changes in hot flashes after a short (4 week) intake of dietary soy (165 mg isoflavones per day).

These studies suggest that diet may play a role in modulating endocrine actions in the body. As data accumulate to elucidate the physiologic effects of the phytoestrogenic constituents of foods, we may begin to understand how diet could influence an individual's hot flash pattern, or affect whether hot flashes occur at all. How great a role diet may play and whether biologic (genetic) differences among populations result in observed differences in hot flash prevalence remain to be determined.

Vitamin E

The effectiveness of vitamin E in treating hot flashes is reported anecdotally, with little objective data available. A few clinical trials were conducted in the 1940s and 1950s. Some found vitamin E to be helpful in treating hot flashes; but, for the most part, the studies were not double-blind and placebo-controlled nor of adequate duration, given that a considerable placebo effect is found in most drug studies of hot flash therapies. In a much-cited study by Blatt et al. (144), a double-blind design (no crossover) compared the effect of vitamin E, estrogen, and a placebo on a combined group of 11 symptoms (not on hot flashes specifically) (144). Vitamin E was no more effective than placebo in treating this symptom complex. This study is cited as demonstrating a lack of effectiveness of vitamin E for treating hot flashes, a conclusion not justified from these data involving a number of combined symptoms.

In a postal survey (self-selected subjects) that included 438 women with hot flashes, 57% of these women reported having tried vitamin E specifically for their hot flashes. Of these women, 27% reported that it helped alleviate their hot flashes. But dose and duration of treatment is unknown (145).

Acupuncture

Wyon et al. (146) administered 8 weeks of acupuncture one to two times per week for 30 minutes to 24 naturally menopausal women with hot flashes. They compared two forms of acupuncture and found that both significantly reduced the daily number of hot flashes. Although controversy is found in the acupuncture field about the appropriateness of the controls used, this study is an important first step in the scientific examination of acupuncture for the treatment of hot flashes.

Osteopathy

Although some women report that chiropractic manipulation is helpful in alleviating their hot flashes (127), only one small study has been done of chiropractic or any other manual therapy. One small placebo controlled study of osteopathy demonstrated that the Fox low-force osteopathic technique reduced menopausal hot flashes (147). Given the interest (meaning visits to practitioners) many women have in chiropractic and other manual therapies for treating menopausal symptoms, further research in this area is warranted.

Behavioral Therapies

Behavioral methods for moderating hot flashes have received limited study. Freedman and Woodward (148) compared paced respiration with muscle relaxation and α-EEG biofeedback and found that paced respiration training reduced the frequency of hot flashes by approximately 40% as compared with women who received progressive muscle relaxation training or controls (11 women in each group). They obtained similar results in a more recent study with a somewhat larger subject population (N = 24) (149). Elicitation of the relaxation response for 7 weeks in a randomized, controlled study resulted in significant reductions in hot flash intensity but not in hot flash frequency (150). Results of these studies suggest the need for additional research in this area.

Exercise

Several groups have presented preliminary data suggesting that exercise moderates at least the severity, if not the frequency, of hot flashes. Because exercise has demonstrated effects on sex steroids, it is not unreasonable to think that it might influence hot flashes as well. In a study of the relationship between menopausal symptoms and aerobic fitness in healthy volunteers, Wilbur et al. (151) found that of their 375 subjects (mean age 47 year), 27% reported via a symptom check-list that they were having hot flashes or night sweats. Joint pains and backaches were the most frequently reported symptoms. A bicycle ergometer test of aerobic fitness level indicated that 54% of the sample had above-average or average fitness, 27% had average fitness, and 19% had low fitness. Hot flashes or night sweats were most prevalent in peri-menopausal women. Aerobic fitness was negatively related to hot flashes (although not statistically significant). Hammar et al. (152) reported that women who belonged to a gymnastic club had fewer hot flashes than women who did not belong, but whose physical activity was not reported. These data, although not particularly compelling, are suggestive of the positive effects of exercise and larger studies are warranted. A study comparing hormone replacement therapy and exercise would be of great interest.

CONCLUSION

We have gained considerable knowledge about hot flashes over the past two decades, although many questions remain unanswered and the specific genesis of hot flashes remains unknown. Even the role of estrogen in the cause of hot flashes or the mechanism by which estrogen relieves hot flashes are still not understood.

Although the patterns of hot flashes may be varied, they share commonalities among their physiology and subjective manifestations. The significance of hot flashes to quality of life varies greatly among women. In the United States there are currently approximately 40 million women of menopausal age. Most women will at some time experience hot flashes; for most of these women, hot flashes will last 1 to 3 years and will not be particularly frequent or disruptive. However, 3 to 5 million women will have severe and frequent hot flashes that can be physically and psychologically debilitating. These are the women who most likely will seek medical assistance.

During a hot flash, elements of the thermoregulatory, cardiovascular, and endocrine systems act in concert. These elements simultaneously serve other nonthermal functions, such as keeping blood flow and blood pressure regulated. Given human physiologic complexity, it is an immense challenge to the researcher to provide an explanation of hot flashes that integrates these various interacting physiologic factors, as well as behavioral, psychophysiological, and psychosocial components. Understanding the cause of hot flashes would provide insights into normal and abnormal changes at menopause. A more complete knowledge of the thermoregulatory, cardiovascular, and psychophysiologic factors of women with hot flashes as compared with those without hot flashes may enable us to predict who is most likely to be affected and to identify additional approaches to the management and treatment of hot flashes.

With increasing information about the factors that are predictive of hot flashes and knowledge of other heath problems that can influence treatment choice, an individualized approach to alleviating hot flashes is increasingly indicated. One dose, regimen, or approach does not fit all women, which makes it all the more urgent to understand the underlying physiology, so we can broaden the treatment options available to them.

REFERENCES

1. Molnar GW. Body temperatures during menopausal hot flashes. *J Appl Physiol* 1975;38:499–503.
2. Feldman JM, Postlethwaite RW, Glenn JF. Hot flashes and sweats in men with testicular insufficiency. *Arch Intern Med* 1976;136:606–608.
3. Steinfeld AD, Reinhardt C. Male climacteric after orchiectomy in patient with prostatic cancer. *Urology* 1980;16:620–622.
4. DeFazio J, Meldrum DR, Winer JH, Judd HL. Direct action of androgen on hot flushes in the human male. *Maturitas* 1984;6:3–8.
5. Frodin T, Alund G, Varenhorst E. Measurement of skin blood-flow and water evaporation as a means of objectively assessing hot flushes after orchidectomy in patients with prostatic cancer. *Prostate* 1985;7:203–208.
6. Linde R, Doelle GC, Alexander N, et al. Reversible inhibition of testicular steroidogenesis and spermatogenesis by a potent gonadotropin-releasing hormone agonist in normal men. *N Engl J Med* 1981;305:663–667.
7. Garnick MB, Glode LM, Smith JA Jr, Max DT. Leuprolide: a review of its effects in comparison with diethylstilboestrol in the treatment of advanced cancer of the prostate. *Br J Clin Pract* 1985;39:73–76.
8. Newton M, Odom PL. The menopause and its symptoms. *South Med J* 1964;57:1309–1313.
9. Neugarten BL, Kraines RJ. "Menopausal symptoms" in women of various ages. *Psychosom Med* 1965;27:266–273.
10. Jaszmann L, Van Lith ND, Zaat JCA. The age at menopause in the Netherlands: the statistical analysis of a survey. *Int J Fertil* 1969;14:106–117.
11. Rybo G, Westerberg H. Symptoms in the post-menopause—a population study. A preliminary report. *Acta Obstet Gynecol Scand* 1971;[Suppl 9]:25.
12. Thompson B, Hart SA, Durno D. Menopausal age and symptomatology in a general practice. *J Biosoc Sci* 1973;5:71–82.
13. McKinlay SM, Jefferys M. The menopausal syndrome. *Br J Prev Soc Med* 1974;28:108–115.
14. Kronenberg F. Hot flashes: epidemiology and physiology. *Ann NY Acad Sci* 1990;592:52–86.
15. Sharma VK, Saxena MSL. Climacteric symptoms: a study in the Indian context. *Maturitas* 1981;3:11–20.
16. Moore B. Climacteric symptoms in an African community. *Maturitas* 1981;3:25–29.
17. Wright AL. On the calculation of climacteric symptoms. *Maturitas* 1981;3:55–63.
18. Lock M, Kaufert P, Gilbert P. Cultural construction of the menopausal syndrome: the Japanese case. *Maturitas* 1988;10:317–332.
19. Agoestina T, van Keep PA. The climacteric in Bandung, West Java province, Indonesia: a survey of 1025 women between 40 and 55 years of age. *Maturitas* 1984;6:327–333.
20. Kay M, Voda AM, Olivas G, Rios F, Imle M. Ethnography of the menopause-related hot flash. *Maturitas* 1982;4:217–227.
21. Beyene Y. Cultural significance and physiological manifestations of menopause a biocultural analysis. *Cult Med Psychiatry* 1986;10:47–71.
22. Sukwatana P, Meekhangvan J, Tamrongterakul T, Tanapat Y, Asavarait S, Boonjitrpimon P. Menopausal symptoms among Thai women in Bangkok. *Maturitas* 1991;13:217–228.
23. Jalbuena JR. Menopause among Filipino women [Abstract]. *Int Meno Congr* 1990:2.
24. Liu CH. Medical care-seeking behaviour among climacteric women in Taiwan [Abstract]. *Int Meno Congr* 1980:18.
25. Lock M. Ambiguities of aging: Japanese experience and perceptions of menopause. *Cult Med Psychiatry* 1986;10:23–46.
26. Feldman BM, Voda AM, Gronseth E. The prevalence of hot flash and associated variables among perimenopausal women. *Res Nurs Health* 1985;8:261–268.
27. Voda AM, Feldman BM, Gronseth E. Description of the hot flash: sensations, meaning and change in frequency across time. In: Notelovitz M, van Keep P, eds. *The climacteric in perspective.* Lancaster, England: MTP Press, 1986:259–269.
28. Berg G, Gottqall T, Hammar M, Lindgren R. Climacteric symptoms among women aged 60 and 62 in Linkoping, Sweden, in 1986. *Maturitas* 1988;10:193–199.
29. Voda AM. Climacteric hot flash. *Maturitas* 1981;3:73–90.
30. Gannon L, Hansel S, Goldwin J. Correlates of menopausal hot flashes. *J Behav Med* 1987;10:277–285.
31. Sherman BM, Wallace RB, Bean JA, Chang Y, Schlabaugh L. The relationship

of menopausal hot flushes to medical and reproductive experience. *J Gerontol* 1981;36:306–309.

32. Erlik Y, Meldrum DR, Judd HL. Estrogen levels in postmenopausal women with hot flashes. *Obstet Gynecol* 1982;59:403–407.

33. McKinlay SM, Brambilla DJ, Posner JG. The normal menopause transition. *Am J Hum Biol* 1992;4:37–46.

34. Ginsburg J, Swinhoe J, O'Reilly B. Cardiovascular responses during the menopausal hot flush. *Br J Obstet Gynaecol* 1981;88:925–930.

35. Kronenberg F, Cote LJ, Linkie DM, Dyrenfurth I, Downey JA. Menopausal hot flashes: thermoregulatory, cardiovascular, and circulating catecholamine and LH changes. *Maturitas* 1984;6:31–43.

36. Tataryn IV, Lomax P, Bajorek JG, Chesarek W, Meldrum DR, Judd HL. Postmenopausal hot flushes: a disorder of thermoregulation. *Maturitas* 1980;2:101–107.

37. Sturdee DW, Wilson KA, Pipili E, Crocker AD. Physiological aspects of menopausal hot flash. *Br Med J* 1978;2:79–80.

38. Casper RJ, Yen SSC, Wilkes MM. Menopausal flushes: a neuroendocrine link with pulsatile luteinizing hormone secretion. *Science* 1979;205:823–825.

39. Tataryn IV, Meldrum DR, Lu KH, Frumar AM, Judd HL. LH, FSH and skin temperature during menopausal hot flush. *J Clin Endocrinol Metab* 1979;49:152–154.

40. Casper RF, Yen SSC. Neuroendocrine changes during menopausal flushes. In: Norman RL, ed. *Neuroendocrine aspects of reproduction*. New York: Academic Press, 1983:359–378.

41. Molnar GW. Investigation of hot flashes by ambulatory monitoring. *Am J Physiol* 1979;6:R306–R310.

42. Aksel S, Schomberg DW, Iyrey L, Hammond CB. Vasomotor symptoms, serum estrogens and gonadotropin levels in surgical menopause. *Am J Obstet Gynecol* 1976;12:165–169.

43. Hutton JD, Murray MAF, Jacobs HS, James VHT. Relation between plasma oestrone and oestradiol and climacteric symptoms. *Lancet* 1978;April:678–681.

44. Badawy SZA, Elliott LJ, Elbadawi A, Marshall LD. Plasma levels of oestrone and oestradiol-17B in postmenopausal women. *Br J Obstet Gynaecol* 1979;86:56–63.

45. Stone SC, Mickal A, Rye PH. Postmenopausal symptomatology, maturation index, and plasma estrogen levels. *Obstet Gynecol* 1975;45:625–627.

46. Meldrum DR, Tataryn IV, Frumar AM, Erlik Y, Lu KH, Judd HL. Gonadotropins, estrogens, and adrenal steroids during the menopausal hot flash. *J Clin Endocrinol Metab* 1980;50:685–689.

47. Hagen C, Christiansen C, Christensen MS, Transbol I. Climacteric symptoms, fat mass, and plasma concentrations of LH, FSH, Prl, oestradiol-17B and androstenedione in the early post-menopausal period. *Acta Endocrinology (Copenh)* 1982;101:87–92.

48. Mango D, Scirpa P, Battaglia F, Bini E. Plasma androstenedione and oestrone levels in the climacteric syndrome. *Maturitas* 1984;5:245–250.

49. Bider D, Ben-Rafael Z, Mashiach S, Serr DM, Blankstein J. Hot flushes during Gn-RH analogue administration despite normal serum oestradiol levels. *Maturitas* 1989;11:223–228.

50. Utian WH. The true clinical features of postmenopause and oophorectomy, and their response to oestrogen therapy. *S Afr Med J* 1972;46:732–737.

51. DeFazio J, Meldrum DR, Laufer L, et al. Induction of hot flashes in premenopausal women treated with a long-acting GnRH agonist. *J Clin Endocrinol Metab* 1983;56:445–448.

52. Lemay A, Maheux R, Faure N, Jean C, Fazekas ATA. Reversible hyperestrogenism induced by repetitive LHRH agonist administration in the treatment of endometriosis. *17th Int Congr Endocrinol* 1984:1012.

53. Yen SSC. The biology of menopause. *J Reprod Med* 1977;18:287–296.

54. Silva NL, Boulant JA. Effects of testosterone, estradiol, and temperature on neurons in preoptic tissue slices. *Am J Physiol* 1986;250:R625–R632.

55. Israel SL, Schneller O. The thermogenic property of progesterone. *Fertil Steril* 1950;1:53–64.

56. Marrone BL, Gentry RT, Wade GN. Gonadal hormones and body temperature in rats: effects of estrous cycles, castration and steroid replacement. *Physiol Behav* 1976;17:419–425.

57. Altura BM. Sex as a factor influencing the responsiveness of arterioles to catecholamines. *Eur J Pharmacol* 1972;20:261–265.

58. Ginsburg J, Hardiman P, O'Reilly B. Peripheral blood flow in menopausal women who have hot flushes and in those who do not. *Br Med J* 1989;298:1488–1490.

59. Campbell S. Double-blind psychometric studies on the effects of natural estrogens on post menopausal women. In: Campbell S, ed. *The management of the menopause and post menopausal years*. Baltimore: University Park Press, 1976:149–158.

60. Bohler CS-S, Greenblatt RB. The pathophysiology of the hot flash. In: Greenblatt RB, Mahesh VB, McDonough PG, eds. *The menopausal syndrome*. New York: Medcom Press, 1974:29–37.

61. Mulley G, Mitchell JRA, Tattersall RB. Hot flushes after hypophysectomy. *Br Med J* 1977;2:1062.

62. Meldrum DR, Erlik Y, Lu JKH, Judd HL. Objectively recorded hot flushes in patients with pituitary insufficiency. *J Clin Endocrinol Metab* 1981;52:684–687.

63. Casper RF, Yen SSC. Menopausal flushes: effect of pituitary gonadotropin desensitization by a potent luteinizing hormone releasing factor agonist. *J Clin Endocrinol Metab* 1981;53:1056–1058.

64. Lightman SL, Jacobs SJ, Maguire AK. Down regulation of gonadotropin secretion in postmenopausal women by superactive LHRH analogue: lack of effect on menopausal flushing. *Br J Obstet Gynaecol* 1982;89:977–980.

65. Ravnikar V, Elkind-Hirsch K, Schiff I, Ryan KJ, Tulchinsky D. Vasomotor flushes and the release of peripheral immunoreactive luteinizing hormone-releasing hormone in postmenopausal women. *Fertil Steril* 1984;41:881–887.

66. Gambone J, Meldrum DR, Laufer L, Chang RJ, Lu JKH, Judd HL. Further delineation of hypothalamic dysfunction responsible for menopausal hot flashes. *J Clin Endocrinol Metab* 1984;59:1097–1102.

67. Whitby G, Axelrod J, Weil-Malherbe H. The fate of H_3 (tritiated) norepinephrine in animals. *J Pharmacol Exp Ther* 1961;132:192–201.

68. Mashchak CA, Kletzky OA, Artal R, Mishell DR Jr. The relation of physiological changes to subjective symptoms in postmenopausal women with and without hot flushes. *Maturitas* 1984;6:301–308.

69. Genazzani AR, Petraglia F, Facchinetti F, Facchini V, Volpe A, Alessandrini G. Increase of proopiomelanocortin-related peptides during subjective menopausal flushes. *Am J Obstet Gynecol* 1984;149:775–779.

70. Meldrum DR, DeFazio JD, Erlik Y, et al. Pituitary hormones during the menopausal hot flash. *Obstet Gynecol* 1984;64:752–756.

71. Erlik Y, Tataryn IV, Meldrum DR, Lomax P, Bajorek JG, Judd HL. Association of waking episodes with menopausal hot flushes. *JAMA* 1981;245:1741–1744.

72. Shaver J, Giblin E, Lentz M, Lee K. Sleep patterns and stability in perimenopausal women. *Sleep* 1988;11:556–561.

73. Thomson J, Oswald I. Effect of oestrogen on the sleep, mood, and anxiety of menopausal women. *Br Med J* 1977;2:1317–1319.

74. Schiff I, Regestein Q, Tulchinsky D, Ryan KJ. Effects of estrogens on sleep and psychological state of hypogonadal women. *JAMA* 1979;242:2405–2407.

75. Coope J, Williams S, Patterson JS. A study of the effectiveness of propranolol in menopausal hot flushes. *Br J Obstet Gynaecol* 1978;85:472–475.

76. Molnar GW. Menopausal hot flashes: their cycles and relation to air temperature. *Obstet Gynecol* 1980;57:52S–55S.

77. Kronenberg F, Barnard RM. Modulation of menopausal hot flashes by ambient temperature. *J Therm Biol* 1992;17:43–49.

78. Casper RF, Yen SSC. Neuroendocrinology of menopausal flushes: an hypothesis of fluid mechanism. *Clin Endocrinol* 1985;22:293–312.

79. Rebar RW, Spitzer IB. The physiology and measurement of hot flushes. *Am J Obstet Gynecol* 1987;156:1284–1288.

80. Zichella L, Tesseri E, Falaschi P, et al. Psychoneuroendocrinology of postmenopausal hot flashes. In: Pancheri P, Zichella L, eds. *Biorhythms and stress in the pathophysiology of reproduction*. New York: Hemisphere Publishing, 1988:549–565.

81. Freedman RR, Woodward S. Behavioral treatment of menopausal hot flushes: evaluation by ambulatory monitoring. *Am J Obstet Gynecol* 1992;167:436–439.

82. Freedman RR. Biochemical, metabolic, and vascular mechanisms in menopausal hot flashes. *Fertil Steril* 1998;70:332–337.

83. Judd HL. Pathophysiology of menopausal hot flushes. In: Meites J, ed. *Neuroendocrinology of aging*. New York: Plenum Press, 1983:173–202.

84. Tulandi T, Lal S. Menopausal hot flush. *Obstet Gynecol Surv* 1985;40:553–563.

85. Ginsburg J, Hardiman P. What do we know about the pathogenesis of the menopausal hot flush? In: Sitruk-ware R, Utian WH, eds. The menopause: a hormonal replacement therapy. New York: Marcel Dekker, 1991:15–46.

86. Rannevik G, Jeppson S, Johnell O, Bjerre B, Laurell-Borulf Y, Svanberg L. A longitudinal study of the perimenopausal transition: altered profiles of steroid and pituitary hormones, SHBG, and bone mineral density. *Maturitas* 1995;21:103–113.

87. Kaufert PA, Gilbert P, Hassard T. Researching the symptoms of menopause: an exercise in methodology. *Maturitas* 1988;10:117–131.

88. Kronenberg F, Downey JA. Thermoregulatory physiology of menopausal hot flashes: a review. *Can J Physiol Pharmacol* 1987;65:1312–1324.

89. Kluger MJ. Fever: role of pyrogens and cryogens. *Physiol Rev* 1991;71:93–127.

90. Freedman RR, Woodward S, Sabharwal SC. α-adrenergic mechanism in menopausal hot flushes. *Obstet Gynecol* 1990;76:5736-578.

91. Lipton JM, Glyn JR. Central administration of peptides alters thermoregulation in the rabbit. *Peptides* 1980;1:15–18.

92. Lipton JM, Glyn JR, Zimmer JA. ACTH and alpha-melanotropin in central temperature control. *Fed Proc* 1981;40:2760–2764.

93. Murphy MT, Lipton JM. β-Endorphin: effect on thermoregulation in aged monkeys. *Neurobiol Aging* 1983;4:187–190.

94. Reid RL, Hoff JD, Yen SSC, Li CH. Effect of exogenous β-endorphin on pituitary hormone secretion and its disappearance rate in normal human subjects. *J Clin Endocrinol Metab* 1981;52:1179–1183.

95. Ferin M, Wehrenberg WB, Lam NY, Alston EF, Vande Wiele RL. Effect and site of action of morphine on gonadotropin secretion in the female rhesus monkey. *Endocrinology* 1982;111:1652–1656.

96. Wehrenberg WB, Wardlaw SL, Frantz AG, Ferin M. β-Endorphin in hypophyseal portal blood: variations throughout the menstrual cycle. *Endocrinology* 1982;111:879–881.

97. Barnes RB, Lobo RA. Pharmacology of estrogens. In: Mishell DR, ed. *Menopause: physiology and pharmacology*. Chicago: Year Book Medical Publishers, 1987:301–315.

98. Coope J, Thomson JM, Poller L. Effects of ʻnatural oestrogenʼ replacement therapy on menopausal symptoms and blood clotting. *Br Med J* 1975;4:139–143.

99. Campbell S, Whitehead M. Oestrogen therapy and the menopausal syndrome. *Clin Obstet Gynaecol* 1977;4:31–47.

100. Steingold KA. Treatment of hot flashes with transdermal estradiol administration. *J Clin Endocrinol Metab* 1985;61:627–632.
101. Haas S, Walsh B, Evans S, Krache M, Ravnikar V, Schiff I. The effect of transdermal estradiol on hormone and metabolic dynamics over a six-week period. *Obstet Gynecol* 1988;71:671–676.
102. Stanczyk FZ. A randomized comparison of nonoral estradiol delivery in postmenopausal women. *Am J Obstet Gynecol* 1988;159:1540–1546.
103. Ditkoff EC, Crary WG, Cristo M, Lobo R. Estrogen improves psychological function in asymptomatic postmenopausal women. *Obstet Gynecol* 1991;78: 991–995.
104. Bullock JL, Massey FM, Gambrell RD Jr. Use of medroxyprogesterone acetate to prevent menopausal symptoms. *Obstet Gynecol* 1975;46:165–168.
105. Morrison JC, Martin DC, Blair RA, et al. The use of medroxyprogesterone acetate for relief of climacteric symptoms. *Am J Obstet Gynecol* 1980;138: 99–104.
106. Schiff I, Tulchinsky D, Cramer D, Ryan KJ. Oral medroxyprogesterone in the treatment of postmenopausal symptoms. *JAMA* 1980;244:1443–1445.
107. Albrecht BH, Schiff I, Tulchinsky D, Ryan KJ. Objective evidence that placebo and oral medroxyprogesterone acetate therapy diminish menopausal vasomotor flushes. *Am J Obstet Gynecol* 1981;139:631–635.
108. Erlik Y, Meldrum DR, Lagasse LD, Judd HL. Effect of magestrol acetate on flushing and bone metabolism in post-menopausal women. *Maturitas* 1981;3:167–172.
109. Sherwin BB, Gelfand MM. A prospective one-year study of estrogen and progestin in postmenopausal women: effects on clinical symptoms and lipoprotein lipids. *Obstet Gynecol* 1989;73:759–766.
110. Clayden JR, Bell JW, Pollard P. Menopausal flushing: double-blind trial of a non-hormonal medication. *Br Med J* 1974;1:409–412.
111. Laufer LR, Erlik Y, Meldrum DR, Judd HL. Effect of clonidine on hot flashes in postmenopausal women. *Obstet Gynecol* 1982;6055:583–586.
112. Tulandi T, Lal S, Kinch RA. Effect of intravenous clonidine on menopausal flushing and luteinizing hormone secretion. *Br J Obstet Gynaecol* 1983;90:854–857.
113. Ginsburg J, OíReilly B, Swinhoe J. Effect of oral clonidine on human cardiovascular responsiveness: a possible explanation of the therapeutic action of the drug in menopausal flushing and migraine. *Br J Obstet Gynaecol* 1985;92:1169–1175.
114. Jones KP, Ravnikar V, Schiff I. A preliminary evaluation of the effect of lofexidine on vasomotor flushes in post-menopausal women. *Maturitas* 1985;7: 135–139.
115. Nesheim B-I, Saetre T. Reduction of menopausal hot flushes by methyldopa: a double blind crossover trial. *Eur J Clin Pharmacol* 1981;20:413–416.
116. Erkkola R, Iisalo E, Punnonen R. The effect of propranolol and oxazepam on some vegetative menopausal symptoms. *Ann Clin Res* 1973;5:208–213.
117. Alcoff JM, Campbell D, Tribble D, Oldfield B, Cruess D. Double-blind, placebo-controlled, crossover trial of propranolol as treatment for menopausal vasomotor symptoms. *Clin Ther* 1981;3:356–364.
118. Lebherz TB, French L. Nonhormonal treatment of the menopausal syndrome. *Obstet Gynecol* 1969;33:795–799.
119. Felter HW. And Lloyd JU. *Kingís American Dispensatory.* Cincinnati: The Ohio Valley Co, 1898.
120. Blumenthal M, Senior Ed. The Complete German Commission E Monographs. *Therapeutic guide to herbal medicines. Cimicifugae racemosae, Rhiizoma.* Austin: American Botanical Council and Boston: Integrative Medicine Communications, 1998:90
121. Jarry H, Harnischfeger G, Duker EM. Untersuchungen zur endokrinen wirksamkeit von inhaltsstoffen aus *Cimicifuga racemosa*: in vitro bindung von inhaltsstoffen an einen oestrogenrezeptoren. [Studies on the endocrine efficacy of the constituents of *Cimicifuga racemosa*: in vitro binding of compounds to estrogen receptors]. *Planta Med* 1985;4:291–356.
122. Duker EM, Kopanski L, Jarry H, Wuttke W. Effects of extracts from *Cimicifuga racemosa* on gonadotropin release in menopausal women and ovariectomized rats. *Planta Med* 1991;57:399-510.
123. Nesselhut T, Schellhase C, Dietrich R, Kuhn W. Untersuchungen zur proliferativen potenz von phytopharmaka mit ostrogenahnlicher wirkung bei mammakarzinomzellen. [Studies on mammary carcinoma cells regarding thr proliferative potential of herbal medications with estrogen-like effects.] *Archives Gynecol Obstet* 1993;254:817–818.
124. Stoll W. Phytopharmacon influences atrophic vaginal epithelium. Double-blind studyóvs. estrogenic substances. *Therapeutikon* 1987;1:23–31.
125. Daiber W. Klimakterische Beschwerden: ohne Hormone zum Erflog. [Climacteric complaints: success without using hormones.] *Arztl Praxis* 1983;35:1946–1947.
126. Stolze H. Der andere Weg. Klimakterische Beschwerden zu behandeln. [An alternative to treat menopausal complaints.] *Gyne* 1982;1:14–16.
127. Kronenberg F, OíLeary Cobb J, McMahon D. Alternative medicine for menopausal problems: results of a survey. *Menopause* 1994;1:171–172.
128. Hirata JD, Swiersz LM, Zell B, Small R, Ettinger B. Does dong quai have estrogenic effects in postmenopausal women? A double-blind, placebo-controlled trial. *Fertil Steril* 1997;68:981–986.
129. Noe JE. *Angelica sinensis*: a monograph. *J Natur opathic Medicine* 1997:66–72.
130. Hopkins MP, Androff L, Benninghoff AS: Ginseng face cream and unexplained vaginal bleeding. *Am J Obstet Gynecol* 1988;159(5):1121–1122.
131. Punnonen R, Lukola A. Oestrogen-like effect of ginseng. *Br Med J* 1980;281:1110.
132. Lindgren R, et al. Effects of ginseng on quality of life in postmenopausal women. *Menopause* 1997;4:4.
133. Hikino H. Traditional remedies and modern assessment: the case of ginseng. In: Wijesedera ROB, ed. *The medicinal plant industry.* Boca Raton, FL: CRC Press, 1991:149–166.
134. Chenoy R, Hussain S, Tayob Y, OíBrien PMS, Moss MY, Morse PF. Effect of oral gamolenic acid from evening primrose oil on menopausal flushing. *Br Med J* 1994;308:501–503.
135. Thompson LU, Robb P, Serraino M, Cheung F. Mammalian lignan production from various foods. *Nutr Cancer* 1991;16:43–52.
136. Miksicek RJ. Estrogenic flavonoids: structural requirements for biological activity. *Proc Soc Exp Biol Med* 1985;208:44–50.
137. Setchell KD, Gosselin SJ, Welsh MB, et al. Dietary estrogens–a probable cause of infertility and liver disease in captive cheetahs. *Gastroenterology* 1987;93: 225–233.
138. Wilcox G, Wahlqvist ML, Burger HG, Medley G. Oestrogenic effects of plant foods in postmenopausal women. *BMJ* 1990;301:905–906.
139. Baird DD, Umbach DM, Landsdell L, et al. Dietary intervention study to assess estrogenicity of dietary soy among postmenopausal women. *J Clin Endocrinol Metab* 1995;80:1685–1690.
140. Adlercreutz H, Fostis T, Bannwart C, et al. Determination of urinary lignans and phytoestrogen metabolites, potential antiestrogens and anticarcinogens, in urine of women on various habitual diets. *J Steroid Biochem* 1986;25:791–797.
141. Adlercreutz H, Hamslainen E, Gorbach S, Goldin B. Dietary phyto-oestrogens and the menopause in Japan. *Lancet* 1992;339:1233.
142. Murkies AL, Lombard C, Strauss BJG, Wilcox G, Burger HG, Morton MS. Dietary flour supplementation decreases post-menopausal hot flushes: effect of soy and wheat. *Maturitas* 1995;21:189–195.
143. Brzezinski A, Adlercreutz H, Shaoul R, Shmueli A, Tanos V, Schenker JG. Short-term effect of phytoestrogen-rich diet on postmenopausal women. *Menopause* 1997;4:89–94.
144. Blatt MHG, Wiesbader H, Kupperman HS. Vitamin E and climacteric syndrome. *Arch Intern Med* 1953;91:792–796.
145. Kronenberg F. Hot flashes: epidemiology and physiology. *Ann NY Acad Sci* 1990;592:52–86.
146. Wyon Y, Lindgrin R, Lundeberg T, Hammar M. Effects of acupuncture on climacteric vasomotor symptoms, quality of life, and urinary excretion of neuropeptides among postmenopausal women. *Menopause* 1995;2:3–12.
147. Cleary C, Fox JP. Menopausal symptoms: an osteopathic investigation. *Complementary Therapies in Medicine* 1994;2:181–186.
148. Freedman RR, Woodward S. Behavioral treatment of menopausal hot flushes: evaluation by ambulatory monitoring. *Am J Obstet Gynecol* 1992;167(2):436–439.
149. Freedman RR, Woodward S, Brown B, Javaid J, Pandey G. Biochemical and thermoregulatory effects of behavioral treatment for menopausal hot flashes. *Menopause* 1995;2:211–218.
150. Irvin JH, Domar AD, Clark C, Zuttermeister PC, Friedman R. The effects of relaxation response training on menopausal symptoms. *J Psychosom Obstet Gynedol* 1996;17:202–207.
151. Wilbur J, Dan A, Hedricks C, Holm K. The relationship among menopausal status, menopausal symptoms, and physical activity in midlife women. *Family and Community Health* 1990:67–78.
152. Hammar M, Berg G, Lindgren R. Does physical exercise influence the frequency of postmenopausal hot flushes? *Acta Obstet Gynecol Scand* 1990;69:409–412.
153. Lightman SL, Jacobs HS, Maguire AK, McGarrick G, Jeffcoate SL. Climacteric flushing: clinical and endocrine response to infusion of naloxone. *Br J Obstet Gynaecol* 1981;88:919–924.
154. Cignarelli M, Cicinelli E, Corso M, et al. Biophysical and endocrine metabolic changes during menopausal hot flashes: increase in plasma-free fatty acid and norepinephrine levels. *Gynecol Obstet Invest* 1989;27:34–37.
155. Tulandi T, Murphy BEP, Lal S. Plasma cortisol concentrations in women with menopausal flushes. *Maturitas* 1985;7:367–372.
156. Kronenberg F, Carraway RE. Changes in neurotensin-like immunoreactivity during menopausal hot flashes. *J Clin Endocrinol Metab* 1985;60:1081–1086.

Treatment of the Postmenopausal Woman: Basic and Clinical Aspects, Second Edition, edited by Rogerio A. Lobo, Lippincott Williams & Wilkins, Philadelphia © 1999.

CHAPTER 16

Impact of the Changing Hormonal Milieu on Psychologic Functioning

Barbara B. Sherwin

The steady increase in female life expectancy over the past century means that women now live one-third of their lives beyond cessation of ovarian functioning. Quality of life issues related to aging in women, therefore, have assumed increasing importance in the minds of health professionals and of women themselves.

Prominent among the complaints of perimenopausal and postmenopausal women are changes in behavior. More specifically, changes in mood, memory, and sexual functioning are frequently reported around the time of menopause. Although it must be acknowledged that sociocultural, individual, and environmental factors likely converge to influence the experience of the menopause for each woman, accumulating evidence also suggests that changes in the hormonal milieu may underlie some of the psychologic symptoms reported at this time. Moreover, to the extent that specific sex hormones can enhance specific aspects of psychologic functioning, it follows that their replacement after the menopause may serve to maintain these functions, thereby preserving the quality of life in aging women. This chapter reviews the mechanisms of action of the sex steroids on the central nervous system and the clinical literature that bears on the relationship between sex hormones and behavior with the goal of providing a clearer understanding of the role of hormones in psychologic functioning in menopausal women.

EPIDEMIOLOGY OF PSYCHOLOGIC SYMPTOMS

Before attempting to explain the manner in which changes in the endocrine milieu may precipitate psycho-

logic symptoms at menopause, it would be important to establish that these symptoms do indeed occur in a considerable number of women. Several epidemiologic studies undertaken on random samples of the population in the United States (1,2) as well as in Sweden (3) and England (4) have failed to document an increase in depressive symptoms around the time of menopause compared with other times during the lifespan. Inconsistent with these reports are the results of other studies of nonclinical populations that have found increased incidences of depressive symptoms in both perimenopausal and postmenopausal women (5–8). Interestingly, in a longitudinal survey of 2,500 middle-aged women in Massachusetts, those who had undergone a surgical menopause had high and clinically significant depression scores, whereas the naturally menopausal women did not (9).

Evidence from studies undertaken in menopause clinics tell yet a different story. Of 100 menopausal women who sought medical care in one clinic, 79% had physical symptoms such as hot flushes (also referred to as "flashes") and 65% had varying degrees of depression (10). Similarly, in a study in England, 89% of all women who attended a menopause clinic had depressive symptoms (11). Thus, it would seem that, whereas the occurrence of depressive symptoms is far from a ubiquitous phenomenon at the time of menopause, many women do, in fact, develop these symptoms particularly during the perimenopause. Moreover, some evidence suggests that vulnerability toward the development of depressive symptoms may be greater in women who undergo a surgical menopause.

Although a paucity of empirical evidence links cognitive functioning to changes in circulating levels of estrogen, complaints of memory and concentration difficulties are frequently voiced around the time of menopause. The inclusion of items to assess memory and concentration abilities in one of the earliest menopausal symptom

B. B. Sherwin: Departments of Psychology and Obstetrics and Gynecology, McGill University, Montreal, Quebec, Canada H3A 1B1.

checklists (1) serves as acknowledgment that changes in cognitive functioning have long been associated with the menopause. Unfortunately, no epidemiologic studies are available to shed light on the frequency and severity of these changes around the time of menopause.

Survey data point out the considerable frequency of a variety of sexual problems in menopausal women. In a nonclinical sample, Kinsey et al. (12) documented a 53% and a 48% decrease in the frequencies of coitus and orgasm, respectively. Longitudinal studies of menopausal women in Sweden, which found a 52% decrease in sexual interest and a 20% decrease in orgasm frequency, also established statistically that these decrements in sexual functioning were related to menopause and not to aging per se (13). Numerous survey studies of menopausal women have confirmed decreases in sexual interest of 33% (14), 85% (15), and 39% (16). These epidemiologic data serve to point out that between one-third and one-half of menopausal women recruited from the general population complain of a problem in one or more aspects of sexual functioning.

NEUROBIOLOGIC EFFECTS OF ESTROGEN, ANDROGEN, AND PROGESTIN

To account for changes in sex hormone production as determinants of psychologic symptoms in menopausal women, it is necessary to review briefly some of the known effects of these hormones on the brain. Estrogen has both direct and inductive effects on neurons. Direct effects of estrogen on the brain take place fairly rapidly. For example, estrogens alter the electrical activity of the hypothalamus (17). On the other hand, inductive effects of estrogen are both delayed in onset and prolonged in duration. Its mode of action here is assumed to occur via its induction of RNA and protein synthesis by means of genomic mechanisms, which, in turn, cause changes in levels of specific gene products such as neurotransmitter synthesizing enzymes (18).

Autoradiographic studies have demonstrated that neurons that contain specific nuclear receptors for estrogen are found in specific areas of the brain, predominantly in the pituitary, hypothalamus, limbic forebrain (including the amygdala and lateral septum), and the cerebral cortex (19). Specific cytosolic receptors for testosterone are found mainly in the preoptic area of the hypothalamus, with smaller concentrations in the limbic system and in the cerebral cortex (19).

Within the past decade, the direct modulation of neural development and neural circuit formation by estrogen has been demonstrated in both neonatal and in adult brain. Specifically, estrogen has a facilitatory effect on synapse formation in the hypothalamus in both adult and aged female rats (20), and it also increases the density of dendritic spines on neurons in the CA1 area of the hippocampus (21), a limbic system structure known to be important for memory functions. Estrogen also increases the production of the neurotransmitter acetylcholine, a deficit of which is pathognomonic of Alzheimer's disease (22); estrogen accomplishes this by increasing the concentration of choline acetyltransferase (CHAT), the synthetic enzyme for acetylcholine (23). Finally, estrogen enhances adrenergic function, which has also been linked to cognitive abilities. In one study, the administration of clonidine, an α-adrenergic agonist, was associated with a dose-dependent decreases in plasma norepinephrine levels and with reduced mental performance scores (25). Therefore, estrogen has beneficial effects on both neurochemical functions and neuroanatomic structures important for memory.

The idea that estrogen interacts with genomic mechanisms to regulate levels of specific gene products led to discoveries of numerous neurochemical effects of this sex steroid. Among the most relevant of its mechanisms of action with respect to the development of depression at the time of menopause is that estrogen increases the rate of degradation of monoamine oxidase (MAO), the enzyme that catabolizes the neurotransmitter serotonin (24), whose deficiency is thought to be one causal factor in depression.

In summary, neurophysiologic studies undertaken to localize function of estrogen and testosterone provide evidence that both sex steroids are found in areas of the brain that are thought to subserve emotion, memory, and sexuality. Moreover, findings from neurochemical investigations show that estrogen can profoundly affect the concentration of neurotransmitter synthesizing and catabolizing enzymes, which, in turn, influence the brain concentrations and synaptic availability of certain neurotransmitters. These mechanisms of estrogenic action on brain chemistry provide possible explanations for the purported influence of this hormone on mood, memory, and sexual functioning.

In contrast to the stimulatory effects of estrogen on various brain mechanisms, progestins have potent anesthetic properties (26). Indeed, the administration of large doses of progestins to humans induces dizziness, drowsiness, and even deep sleep (27). Moreover, whereas estrogen decreases MAO activity in the amygdala and hypothalamus (24), progestins increase it (28), thereby resulting in lower concentrations of brain serotonin, which may predispose to dysphoric moods. Indeed, these neurochemical effects of progestins may explain why some women on estrogen–progestin replacement regimens experience unpleasant behavioral side effects, as will be discussed in a subsequent section.

SEX STEROIDS AND MOOD

The most common strategy for investigating possible effects of estrogen on mood is to test menopausal women before and after a trial of hormone replacement therapy. The findings of many early studies are difficult to interpret because of their methodologic shortcomings; some studies were not blinded (29) or they contained women who had malignant disease (30) or concurrent psychiatric illness (31). Moreover, none of these studies had measured circulating levels of the sex hormones coincident with psychologic testing.

Several investigations undertaken in nonpsychiatric populations of postmenopausal women have reported changes in affect as a function of circulating sex hormone levels. In a prospective crossover study (32), premenopausal women who were scheduled for total abdominal hysterectomy (TAH) and bilateral salpingo-oophorectomy (BSO) for benign disease were tested 1 month before surgery. Following TAH and BSO, these women received either estrogen, androgen, an estrogen–androgen combined preparation, or placebo intramuscularly once a month for 3 months. During the fourth postoperative month all women received placebo, and 1 month later were crossed over to another treatment they had not already received for an additional 3 months. In addition to the placebo group, another group of women who required TAH only were included to control for the surgical procedure itself. Blood was sampled at each test time for assay of circulating levels of the sex hormones. In both treatment phases, women who received placebo had higher depression scores when compared with both those treated with any of the active hormone preparations and with those in the ovary-intact group (Fig. 16.1). Furthermore, depression scores of the hormone-treated women increased during the placebo month between the two treatment phases coincident with their significant decrease in plasma estradiol and testosterone levels at that time.

In a second study, Sherwin (33) investigated otherwise healthy women who had undergone TAH and BSO for benign disease approximately 4 years earlier. Women who had been receiving estrogen or an estrogen–testosterone combined drug intramuscularly once a month for the previous 2 years had more positive moods than a matched control group of women who had remained untreated since their TAH and BSO 4 years earlier. These findings confirmed the association between positive moods and plasma levels of estradiol and testosterone in healthy, nondepressed women.

It is important to note that the positive association between mood and sex hormone levels seen in these studies (32,33) occurred when the two variables fluctuated within the normal range. That is, when hormones were withdrawn during the placebo month, depression scores increased in all women, indicating more dysphoric moods. However, these patients did not become clinically depressed at that time as indicated by their scores on the depression measure. What they complained of subjectively when their hormone levels were low were

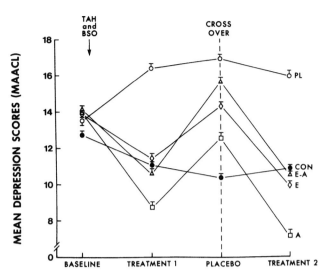

FIG. 16.1. Mean depression scores ± SEM. The treatment groups are: E–A(△), E(◇), A(□), PL(○), and hysterectomy CON(●). BSO, bilateral salpingo-oophorectomy; CON, hysterectomized control group with intact ovaries; PL, placebo group; TAH, total abdominal hysterectomy. (From Sherwin B, and Gelfand, MM. Sex steroids and affect in the surgical menopause: a double-blind cross-over study. *Psychoneuroendocrinology* 1985;10:325–335.)

feelings of sadness or being "blue." The findings of another study serve to underline this distinction. Affective responses to exogenous estrogen were investigated in postmenopausal women who had different levels of severity of depression. Nine of 10 women whose pretreatment depression scores were in the "mildly depressed" range improved after treatment with 1.25 mg conjugated equine estrogens daily. However, six of 10 women who were clinically depressed before treatment actually became more depressed on the same estrogen replacement regimen (34). Another recent prospective study found that depression scores decreased in postmenopausal women given either 0.625 or 1.25 mg conjugated equine estrogens for 3 months, whereas no mood changes occurred in patients who had received placebo (35). However, in that study of asymptomatic women, mood scores fell within the normal range of values during both the pretreatment and the posttreatment test times. On the other hand, when women with severe, refractory depression were given very large pharmacologic doses of conjugated estrogens (15 to 25 mg daily), depression scores decreased in 90% of patients after 3 months of treatment (36). Together, the findings from our own studies on healthy women (32,33) and those on severely depressed women (34,35) suggest that a conventional dose of estrogen given to treat menopausal symptoms enhances mood in nondepressed women but is therapeutically ineffective for mood disturbances of a clinical magnitude.

Recently, a metaanalysis of the effect of hormone replacement therapy on depressed mood in postmenopausal women was undertaken on 26 such studies (37). In most studies, subjects were dysthymic and few included women who would have met diagnostic criteria for a major depressive disorder. In these investigations which had pretreatment to posttreatment comparisons and treatment to control comparisons, estrogen replacement therapy (ERT) exerted a moderate to large effect on depressed mood in these dysthymic postmenopausal women; the overall effect size for ERT was 0.68, which indicated that the average treatment patient had lower levels of depressed mood than 76% of the control patients.

Results of a cross-sectional study of middle-aged and healthy women suggested that ERT might actually prevent episodes of depression in older women. Between 1984 and 1987, more than 1,100 white middle-class women from Rancho Bernardo, California aged more than 50 years were administered the Beck Depression Inventory (BDI) (38). A cut-point of 13 on the BDI was used to define cases of mild to severe depression on 18 scale items. In estrogen nonusers, mean depressive symptom scores increased steadily and significantly with age, whereas depression scores remained stable with increasing age in the women who took estrogen. Of course, it cannot be determined to what degree a self-selection bias in this sample may have influenced these findings.

Some suggest (but little empirical evidence) that estrogen might augment the efficacy of antidepressant drugs for the treatment of postmenopausal women with a major depressive disorder. In a recent multicenter trial of fluoxetine (20 mg/day)(39), 72 of these older women with a unipolar major depression were estrogen-users and 286 women were nonusers. All women were aged more than 60 years (mean age 67.9 years). The estrogen-users had a significantly greater responsiveness to fluoxetine than the depressed nonusers. In large part, however, the difference between the groups in their responsiveness to the antidepressant was due to the significantly lower responsiveness to placebo in subjects who used estrogen. Although it is possible to speculate that the better clinical response of the hormone-users was caused by an interactive effect between estrogen and fluoxetine, why estrogen-users had a much lower placebo response compared with the nonusers remains unexplained.

A fair amount of anecdotal and clinical evidence indicates that some considerable proportion of menopausal women on combined or sequential estrogen–progestin replacement regimens complain of dysphoric moods and irritability, which is thought to be causally related to the progestin. Indeed, women who received subcutaneous implants of estradiol and norethisterone (40), percutaneous estradiol plus lynestrenol (41), and ethinyl estradiol plus levonorgestrel (42) all experienced a dampening of mood compared with those treated with the same dose of estrogen alone. In a prospective study, we recently compared the effect of adding 5 mg medroxyprogesterone acetate (MPA) or placebo from days 15 to 25 to either 0.625 or 1.25 mg conjugated equine estrogen (CEE) taken from days 1 to 25 of the month (43). Women who received 0.625 mg CEE and 5 mg MPA had more negative moods (Fig. 16.2) and more psychologic symp-

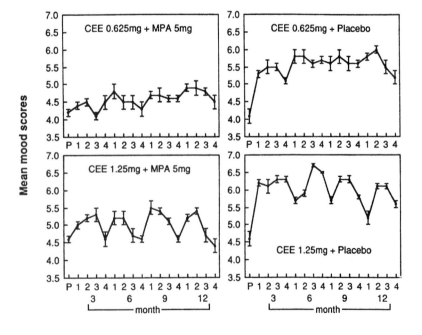

FIG. 16.2. Mean psychological symptom scores (±SD). CEE, conjugated equine estrogen; MPA, medroxyprogesterone acetate; P, pretreatment. (From Sherwin, B. The impact of different doses of estrogen and progestin on mood and sexual behavior in postmenopausal women. *J Clin Endocrinol Metab* 1991;72:336–343.)

tomatology during treatment compared with those who were taking 1.25 mg CEE and placebo. These findings suggest that the effects of progestin on the central nervous system are reflected in an increase in psychologic symptomatology and are attenuated by a higher estrogen:progestin dose ratio.

ESTROGEN AND COGNITIVE FUNCTIONING

Despite the fact that menopause is a universal phenomenon in the female life cycle and that impairment in cognitive functioning, particularly in memory, is frequently reported at that time, only a paucity of studies have attempted to investigate this relationship empirically. Several researchers have reported improvements in memory following estrogen replacement therapy but these findings were based solely on patients' subjective self-report (44,45). Results of several other studies that used psychometric measures to evaluate estrogenic effects on cognitive functions are inconsistent (46,47). This may have occurred because different estrogen preparations in various doses were administered in these studies and different psychometric tests were used to measure aspects of cognitive functioning. More recently, in a prospective study of surgically menopausal women, Sherwin (48) demonstrated that those who were given estrogen postoperatively maintained their scores on several tests of memory and abstract reasoning, whereas the performance of oophorectomized, placebo-treated women decreased. In another prospective study of oophorectomized women, those treated with estrogen postopera-

tively had higher scores on a paired-associates task (thought to indicate the capacity for new learning) and on immediate paragraph recall (a measure of short-term memory) compared with scores of patients who were given placebo (49). A recent replication of these findings (50) has allowed us to conclude that estrogen plays an important role in the maintenance of short-term memory in women, whereas the capacity for long-term memory does not seem to be substantially influenced by the hormonal milieu.

The estrogenic enhancement and memory we have consistently found in postmenopausal women was recently confirmed using an entirely different experimental paradigm. Women aged 34 years who were infertile because of a uterine myoma received a gonadotopin releasing-hormone analog (GnRH-a) for 12 weeks (51), which suppressed ovarian hormone production. Then, they were randomly given either the GnRH-a plus 0.625 mg CEE daily or the GnRH-a plus a placebo daily for an additional 8 weeks. Scores on neuropsychologic tests of verbal memory decreased from pretreatment to 12 weeks posttreatment in both groups, together with a dramatic decrease in plasma estradiol levels. These memory deficits were reversed in the group that subsequently received the GnRH-a plus CEE for 8 weeks coincident with an increase in their plasma estradiol levels, whereas verbal memory scores remained depressed in the group that received the GnRH-a plus placebo (Fig. 16.3). These results provide further compelling evidence that estrogen plays a role in maintaining verbal memory in women.

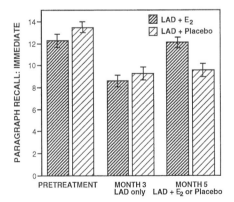 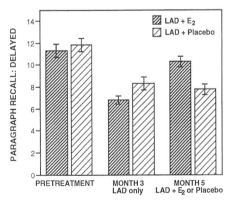

FIG. 3. Mean ± standard error of mean (SEM) scores for the immediate and delayed paragraph recall tests from the Wechsler Memory Scale at the three test times. LAD, leuprolide acetate depot. (From Sherwin BB, Tulandi T. "Add-back" estrogen reverses cognitive deficits induced by a gonadotropin-releasing hormone agonist in women with leiomyomata uteri. *J Clin Endocrinol Metab* 1996;81: 2545–2549.)

SEX STEROIDS AND SEXUALITY

In the attempt to assess the impact of changing sex hormone levels on sexuality in postmenopausal women, it is important to consider that human sexual behavior is composed of identifiably distinct but interrelated processes. Davidson et al. (52) have suggested that the components of human sexual behavior could be conceptualized under two major headings. The first category subsumes those behaviors associated with libido or sexual motivation, such as sexual desire, sexual fantasies, and satisfaction or pleasure, whereas potency refers to pelvic vasocongestion, orgasmic contractions, and possible extragenital responses. In humans, sexual dysfunctions are usually limited to one distinguishable aspect of the behavioral sequence.

It is also important to recall that during reproductive life, the ovary produces approximately 25% of total circulating testosterone, 60% of androstenedione, and 20% of dehydroepiandrosterone (53). Several investigators have reported that plasma testosterone levels are lower in naturally postmenopausal women compared with younger women whose blood was sampled during the follicular phase of the menstrual cycle (53,54). A more definitive determination of residual ovarian production of steroids after the menopause has been accomplished by measuring the concentration of steroids in blood samples taken from the ovarian artery and the ovarian vein at the time of abdominal surgery. The presence of a concentration gradient across the ovary indicates that the ovary is secreting steroids. In two such studies, it was found that the ovary continues to secrete appreciable amounts of testosterone in approximately 50% of postmenopausal women (55,56). In a third investigation, the ovarian vein values of testosterone were significantly lower in postmenopausal women than in a control group of young women during the periovulatory phase of the cycle (57). The available evidence, therefore, suggests that, whereas the postmenopausal ovary continues to secrete testosterone in approximately 50% of women, the concentrations produced are significantly lower than menstrual cycle values in younger women. Moreover, ovarian production of testosterone is negligible in 50% of naturally menopausal women. Of course, plasma testosterone levels decrease significantly within 24 to 48 hours following TAH and BSO (52,54).

Because the integrity of the tissues of the female reproductive tract is dependent on estrogen, degenerative changes in these structures ensue when levels of estrogen decrease after the menopause. It is to be expected, therefore, that some of these changes may adversely affect sexual functioning. For example, decreased vaginal lubrication and atropic vaginitis can result in dyspareunia. Moreover, low levels of estrogen may decrease blood flow to the reproductive organs, resulting in diminished pelvic vasocongestion. Indeed, blood flow to the vulva increased by 50% as measured by Doppler technology when estrogen was administered to postmenopausal women (58). Thus, the known effects of estrogen on peripheral tissues make it likely that the decrease in circulating estrogen at the time of menopause may cause specific averse effects on sexual functioning such as decreased vaginal lubrication and vasocongestion, and dyspareunia. These are functions related to sexual potency as defined by Davidson et al. (51). and they are usually reliably relieved by the administration of exogenous estrogen.

On the other hand, compelling evidence now indicates that libido, or sexual motivation, in women is dependent on androgens. Early evidence for this notion came from clinical reports of the libido-enhancing effects of testosterone given to women who had breast cancer (59,60). Similarly, a radical decrease in libido was also observed in women who were deprived of endogenous androgen production following their bilateral oophorectomies and adrenalectomies undertaken in the attempt to halt the course of metastatic breast cancer (61,62). During the past decade, androgenic effects on female sexuality have been investigated using more rigorous methodology. Prospective studies of subcutaneous implantation of pellets containing estradiol and testosterone to postmenopausal women have been carried out in Great Britain and Australia. When women who were preselected for the complaint of loss of libido received implants of both sex steroids, the symptom was reversed in two-thirds of them after 3 months (63,64). In another double-blind implant study, postmenopausal women who complained of loss of libido that had not been relieved by oral estrogen reported significant symptomatic relief following treatment with a combined estrogen–testosterone implant (65). In contrast, no change in libido occurred in the groups that had received implants of estrogen alone. In a recent prospective 2-year, single-blind randomized trial, 34 postmenopausal women received either estradiol (50 mg) implants or estradiol (50 mg) plus testosterone (50 mg) implants administered every 3 months (66). Sexual activity, satisfaction, and pleasure increased significantly in women treated with the combined estrogen–testosterone implants compared both with their pretreatment baseline scores and compared also with the group given estrogen alone.

Several prospective investigations of the intramuscular administration of an estrogen–androgen preparation to surgically menopausal women provide additional support for the androgenic enhancement of libido in women (67). Patients who received a combined estrogen–androgen drug reported higher levels of sexual desire and arousal and a greater frequency of sexual fantasies compared with those treated with estrogen alone or placebo following their surgery. These findings were subsequently confirmed in surgically menopausal women who had been treated with the estrogen–androgen combination long term, compared with matched groups treated long term with estrogen alone and a third group that remained untreated following their TAH and BSO at least 2 years earlier (68).

Together, the findings from both the subcutaneous implant pellet studies and the prospective investigations that used intramuscular hormonal preparations allow the conclusion that the addition of testosterone to an estrogen replacement regimen is associated with an enhancement of sexual desire, interest, and enjoyment of sex in postmenopausal women. These findings also support the contention that in women, as in men (69), testosterone has its major impact on the motivational or libidinal aspects of sexual behavior, such as desire and fantasies, and not on peripheral physiologic response. Studies on nonhuman primates support the conclusion that testosterone exerts this effect on sexual desire via mechanisms that impact directly on the brain rather than by an effect on peripheral tissues (70).

SUMMARY AND CLINICAL IMPLICATIONS

Although the intent of this chapter was to elucidate possible psychologic consequences of endocrine changes at the menopause, it is important to mention that nonbiologic factors also influence symptomatology at menopause. For example, cross-sectional studies have found that women of lower socioeconomic status are more likely to have more psychologic symptomatology around the time of menopause (6,8,71). Moreover, negative attitudes about the menopause, poor social support, poor marital relations, stressful life events, and recent bereavements also correlate positively with degree of psychologic symptoms (72,73). It is, therefore, extremely important that the physician make a reasonable effort to determine whether the psychologic symptoms presented by a given patient can be more rightfully ascribed wholly, or in part, to the hormonal changes she is experiencing rather than to concurrent stresses in her personal life for which hormone replacement therapy will be largely ineffective. As with all other patients whose psychologic distress is substantially influenced by adverse personal and social factors, menopausal women with such a history should be referred for psychiatric or psychologic evaluation. On the other hand, research findings reviewed here provide considerable evidence that sex steroids alter brain neurotransmitter activity in several ways to affect mood (18–25). Although the specific mechanisms of estrogenic action on neurochemical and neurophysiologic function have not been clearly elucidated, sufficient empirical grounds exist to conclude that estrogen enhances mood, whereas its relative absence dampens mood in many women. Thus, it is important to recall that the administration of estrogen in doses that are conventionally used to treat postmenopausal women will likely alleviate "minor psychiatric symptoms" such as irritability, short-

lasting mood swings, crying spells, and feelings of sadness that typically appear during the perimenopause. However, currently no reason is found to believe that these same doses of estrogen will have a significant beneficial effect on mood disorders that are of a clinical magnitude. As during all other life stages, major affective disorders in menopausal women usually need to be treated with psychotropic medications. Interestingly, evidence suggests that estrogen potentiates the effect of some antidepressants (74) so that estrogen-treated postmenopausal women may respond to lower doses of antidepressant drugs. A corollary of this observation is that postmenopausal women whose depression is refractory to antidepressant treatment may benefit by the addition of estrogen to their psychopharmacologic regimen.

Recent evidence that estrogen maintains or enhances aspects of short-term memory in postmenopausal women (47–49) has considerable potential importance. So too do preliminary findings showing that exogenous estrogen maintains or perhaps even slightly improves aspects of memory and general functions in postmenopausal women with early Alzheimer's disease (75–76), and it may actually protect elderly women against the development of Alzheimer's disease (77–79). However, the fact that this line of inquiry is still in its infancy suggests that judgment concerning the efficacy of exogenous estrogen with respect to protection against Alzheimer's disease in women ought to be suspended until more evidence becomes available.

Finally, with respect to disturbances in sexual functioning that are frequently reported by menopausal women, the simplest and most direct approach is to reverse, by means of estrogen administration, the genital tissue and vascular changes that inevitably ensue under conditions of estrogen deprivation. Estrogen replacement therapy ought to restore the integrity of the vaginal tissues and, concomitantly, alleviate symptoms such as decreased vaginal lubrication and dyspareunia. However, compelling evidence now indicates that testosterone and not estrogen is primarily responsible for the maintenance of sexual interest and desire in women. When it can be determined that the onset of this complaint was associated in time with the perimenopausal phase in a naturally menopausal woman or with the postoperative period in a surgically menopausal woman, treatment with a combined estrogen–testosterone preparation is highly effective in restoring sexual desire (63–68). However, when lack of sexual desire has been life-long or when this symptom considerably predated the menopause, the expectation that combined estrogen–testosterone therapy itself will reverse the symptom is doubtful and sexual counseling should be sought.

Historically, both gynecologists and menopausal women have attributed an astonishing array of psychologic symptoms to the endocrine changes that characterize the menopause. In large part, this was because of faculty logic that the occurrence of two events in temporal contiguity implies a cause and effect relationship. Two things have happened during the past decade that allow for more refined and precise formulations concerning the relationships between changing gonadal hormone levels and psychologic symptoms. First, recent advances in neuroscience have described mechanisms whereby the sex hormones influence brain morphology and function that serve to explain hormonal influences on specific symptoms such as mood. Second, increased methodologic rigor applied to clinical studies of hormone–behavior relationships has enhanced the reliability of these research findings and, consequently, has served to clarify possible associations between specific hormones and specific symptoms. New theoretical knowledge that bears on the manner in which sex hormones affect brain function is being used, as this chapter hopefully points out, to provide empirically based clinical guidelines for the evaluation and treatment of specific psychologic symptoms that may be associated with the menopause.

Finally, it should be acknowledged that the development of psychologic symptoms at the time of menopause is neither universal nor inevitable. The fact that several epidemiologic studies of nonclinical populations failed to find any increase in psychologic symptomatology at the time of menopause attests to the fact that some women do not experience any symptoms at all, or perhaps only to a trivial extent (1–4). On the other hand, overwhelming evidence suggests that most women who seek medical help around the time of menopause from family practitioners (7), gynecologists (10), or menopause clinics (11) have prominent psychologic symptomatology. It is these substantial numbers of women who stand to benefit from our increasing knowledge of the psychotropic properties of the sex hormones.

ACKNOWLEDGMENTS

The preparation of the manuscript for this chapter was supported by a grant from the Medical Research Council of Canada (No. MA-11623) awarded to B. B. Sherwin.

REFERENCES

1. Neugarten BL, Kraines RJ. Menopausal symptoms in women of various ages. *Psychosom Med* 1965;27:266–273.
2. McKinlay SM, Brambilla DJ, Pasner JG. The normal menopausal transition. *Maturitas* 1992;14:103–115.
3. Hallström T, Samuelsson S. Mental health in the climacteric: the longitudinal study of women in Gothenburg. *Acta Obstet Gynecol Scand* 1985;130:13–18.
4. McKinlay SM, Jeffreys M. The menopausal syndrome. *Br J Prev Soc Med* 1974;28:108–115.
5. Bungay GT, Vessey MP, McPherson CK. Study of symptoms in middle-life with special reference to the menopause. *Br Med J* 1980;2:181–183.
6. Greene JG, Cooke DJ. Life stresses and symptoms at the climacteric. *Br J Psychiatry* 1980;136:486–491.
7. Ballinger CB. Psychiatric morbidity and the menopause: screening of a general population sample. *Br Med J* 1975;3:344–346.
8. Hunter M, Battersby R, Whitehead M. Relationships between psychological symptoms, somatic complaints, and menopausal status. *Maturitas* 1986;8:217–228.
9. McKinlay JB, McKinlay SM, Brambilla D. The relative contribution of endocrine changes and social circumstances to depression in mid-aged women. *J Health Soc Behav* 1987;28:345–363.
10. Anderson E, Hamburger S, Liu JG, Rebar RW. Characteristics of menopausal women seeking assistance. *Am J Obstet Gynecol* 1987;156:428–433.
11. Montgomery JC, Brincat M, Tapp A, et al. Effect of oestrogen and testosterone implants on psychological disorders in the climacteric. *Lancet* 1987;(Feb. 7): 297–299.
12. Kinsey AC, Pomeroy WB, Martin CE, Gebhard PH. *Sexual behavior in the human female.* Philadelphia: WB Saunders, 1953.
13. Hallström T. Sexuality in the climacteric. *Clin Obstet Gynecol* 1977;4:227–239.
14. Hallström T, Samuelsson S. Changes in women's sexual desire in middle life: the longitudinal study of women in Gothenburg. *Arch Sex Behav* 1990;19:259–268.
15. McCoy NL, Davidson JM. A longitudinal study of the effects of menopause on sexuality. *Maturitas* 1985;7:203–210.
16. Sarrel PM, Whitehead MI. Sex and menopause: defining the issues. *Maturitas* 1985;7:217–224.
17. Kelly MJ, Moss RL, Dudley CA, Fawcett CP. The specificity of the response of preoptic-septal area neurons to estrogen: 17-β estradiol vs 17α-estradiol and the response of extrahypothalamic neurons. *Exp Brain Res* 1977;30:43–52.
18. O'Mally BW, Means AR. Female steroid hormones and target cell nuclei. *Science* 1974;183:610–620.
19. McEwen BS. The brain as a target organ of endocrine hormones. In: Kreiger DT, Hughes JS, eds. *Neuroendocrinology.* Sunderland, MA: Sinauer Associates, 1980: 33–42.
20. Matsumoto A, Arai Y, Osanai M. Estrogen stimulates neuronal plasticity in the deafferentated hypothalamic arcuate nucleus in aged female rats. *Neurosci Res* 1985;2:412–418.
21. Wooley CS, McEwen BS. Roles of estradiol and progesterone in regulation of hippocampal dendritic spine density during the estrous cycle in the rat. *J Comp Neurol* 1993;336:293–306.
22. Bartus RT, Dean RL, Beer B, Lippa AS. The cholinergic hypothesis of gyeriatric memory dysfunction. *Science* 1982;217:408–417.
23. Luine VN, Khylchevskaya RI, McEwen BS. Effect of gonadal steroids on activities of monoamine oxidase and choline acetylase in rat brain. *Brain Res* 1975;86: 293–306.
24. Luine VN, McEwen BS. Effect of estradiol on turnover of type A monoamine oxidase in brain. *J Neurochem* 1977;28:1221–1227.
25. Kugler J, Seus R, Krauskopf R, Brecht HM, Raschig A. Differences in psychic performance with guanfacine and clonidine in normotensive subjects. *Br J Clin Pharmacol* 1980;10:795–805.
26. Holzbauer M. Physiological aspects of steroids with anesthetic properties. *Med Biol* 1976;54:227–242.
27. Merryman W, Boidman R, Barnes L, Rothchild I. Progesterone ïanesthesiaî in human subjects. *J Clin Endocrinol Metab* 1954;14:1567–1569.
28. Holzbauer M, Yondin MBH. The oestrous cycle and monoamine oxidase activity. *Br J Pharmacol* 1973;48:600–608.
29. George GCW, Bearemont PVJ, Beardwood CJ. Effects of exogenous estrogen on minor psychiatric symptoms in postmenopausal women. *S Afr Med J* 1973;47: 2337–2344.
30. Chakravarti S, Collens WP, Newton JR. Endocrine changes and symptomatology after oophorectomy in premenopausal women. *Br J Obstet Gynaecol* 1977;84: 769–775.
31. Strickler RC, Booth R, Cecutti A. The role of estrogen replacement in the climacteric syndrome. *Psychol Med* 1977;7:631–639.
32. Sherwin BB, Gelfand MM. Sex steroids and affect in the surgical menopause: a double-blind cross-over study. *Psychoneuroendocrinology* 1985;10:325–335.
33. Sherwin BB. Affective changes with estrogen and androgen replacement therapy in surgically menopausal women. *J Affect Disord* 1988;14:177–187.
34. Schneider MA, Brotherton PL, Hailes J. The effect of exogenous oestrogens on depression in menopausal women. *Med J Aust* 1977;2:162–170.
35. Ditkoff EC, Crary WG, Cristo M, Lobo RA. Estrogen improves psychological function in asymptomatic postmenopausal women. *Obstet Gynecol* 1991;78:991–995.
36. Klaiber EL, Broverman DM, Vogel W, Kobayashi Y. Estrogen therapy for severe persistent depression in women. *Arch Gen Psychiatry* 1979;36:742–744.
37. Zweifel JE, O'Brien WH. A meta-analysis of the effect of hormone replacement therapy upon depressed mood. *Psychoneuroendocrinol* 1997;22:189–212.
38. Palinkas LA, Barrett-Connor E. Estrogen use and depressive symptoms in postmenopausal women. *Obstet Gynecol* 1992;80:30–36.
39. Schneider LS, Small GW, Hamilton SH, et al. and the Fluoxetine Collaborative Study Group. Estrogen replacement and response to fluoxetine in a multicenter geriatric depression trial. *Am J Geriatr Psychiatr* 1997;5:97–106.
40. Magos AL, Brewster E, Singh R, O'Dowd T, Bruncat M, Studd JWW. The effects of norethisterone in menopausal women on oestrogen replacement therapy: a model for the premenstrual syndrome. *Br J Obstet Gynaecol* 1986;93:1290–1296.
41. Holst J, Backström T, Hammerbäch S, von Schoultz B. Progestogen addiction during oestrogen replacement therapy—effects on vasomotor symptoms and mood. *Maturitas* 1989;11:13–19.
42. Dennerstein L, Burrows GD, Hyman G, Sharpe K. Hormone therapy and affect. *Maturitas* 1979;1:247–254.
43. Sherwin BB. The impact of different doses of estrogen and progestin on mood and sexual behavior in postmenopausal women. *J Clin Endocrinol Metab* 1991;72: 336–343.
44. Campbell S, Whitehead M. Oestrogen therapy and the menopausal syndrome. *Clin Obstet Gynecol* 1977;4:31–47.

45. Schneider HPG. Oestriol and the menopause: clinical results from a prospective study. In: Fioretti P, Martini L, Melis GB, Yenn SSC, eds. *The menopause: clinical, endocrinological and pathophysiological aspects.* New York: Academic Press, 1982:523–533.
46. Rauramo L, Langerspetz K, Engblom P, Punnonen R. The effects of castration and peroral estrogen therapy on some psychological functions. *Frontiers of Hormone Research* 1975;3:94–104.
47. Hackman VW, Galbraith D. Six-month study of estrogen therapy with piperazine oestrone sulphate and its effect on memory. *Curr Med Res Opin* 1974;4:21–27.
48. Sherwin BB. Estrogen and/or androgen replacement therapy and cognitive functioning in surgically menopausal women. *Psychoneuroendocrinology* 1988;10:325–335.
49. Sherwin BB, Phillips S. Estrogen and cognitive functioning in surgically menopausal women. *Ann NY Acad Sci* 1990;592:474–475.
50. Phillips S, Sherwin BB. Effect of estrogen on memory function in surgically menopausal women. *Psychoneuroendocrinology* 1992;17:485–495.
51. Sherwin BB, Tulandi T. "Add-back" estrogen reverses cognitive deficits induced by a gonadotopin releasing-hormone agonist in women with leiomyomata uteri. *J Clin Endocrinol Metab* 1996;81:2545–2549.
52. Davidson JM, Gray GD, Smith ER. The sexual psychoendocrinology of aging. In: Meites J, ed. *Neuroendocrinology of aging.* New York: Plenum Press, 1983:221–258.
53. Longcope C. Adrenal and gonadal steroid secretion in normal females. *J Clin Endocrinol Metab* 1986;15:213–228.
54. Vermeulen A. The hormonal activity of the postmenopausal ovary. *J Clin Endocrinol Metab* 1976;42:247–253.
55. Longcope C, Hunter R, Franz C. Steroid secretion by the postmenopausal ovary. *Am J Obstet Gynecol* 1980;138:564–568.
56. Lucisano A, Acampora MG, Russo N, Maniccia E, Montemurro A, Dell'Acqua S. Ovarian and peripheral plasma levels of progestogens, androgens and oestrogens in postmenopausal women. *Maturitas* 1984;6:45–53.
57. Botella-Llusia J, Oriol-Bosch A, Sanchez-Garrido F. Testosterone and 17b-estradiol secretion of the human ovary. *Maturitas* 1979;2:7–12.
58. Sarrel PM. Progestogens and blood flow. *Int Proc J* 1989;1:266–271.
59. Foss GL. The influence of androgens on sexuality in women. *Vitam Horm* 1947;5:317–321.
60. Kennedy BJ. Effects of massive doses of sex hormones on libido. *Med Aspects Hum Sex* 1973;7:67–75.
61. Drellich MG, Waxenberg SE. Erotic and affectional components of female sexuality. In: Masserman J, ed. *Science and psychoanalysis.* New York: Grune & Stratton, 1966:192–217.
62. Waxenberg SE, Drellich MG, Sutherland AM. Changes in female sexuality after adrenalectomy. *J Clin Endocrinol* 1959;19:193–202.
63. Burger HG, Hailes J, Menelaus M, Nelson J, Hudson B, Balazs N. The management of persistent menopausal symptoms with oestradiol-testosterone implants: clinical, lipid and hormonal results. *Maturitas* 1984;6:351–358.
64. Cardozo L, Gibb DMF, Tuck SM, Thom MH, Studd JWW, Cooper DJ. The effects of subcutaneous hormone implants during the climacteric. *Maturitas* 1984;5:177–184.
65. Burger H, Hailes J, Nelson J, Menelaus M. Effect of combined implants of oestradiol and testosterone on libido in postmenopausal women. *Lancet* 1987;294:936–937.
66. Davis SR, McClaud P, Strauss BJG, Burger H. Testosterone enhances estradiol's effect on postmenopausal bone density and sexuality. *Maturitas* 1995;21:227–236.
67. Sherwin BB, Gelfand MM, Brender W. Androgen enhances sexual motivation in females: a prospective cross-over study of sex steroid administration in the surgical menopause. *Psychosom Med* 1985;7:339–351.
68. Sherwin BB, Gelfand MM. The role of androgen in the maintenance of sexual functioning in oophorectomized women. *Psychosom Med* 1987;49:397–409.
69. Bancroft J, Wu FCW. Changes in erectile responsiveness during androgen replacement therapy. *Arch Sex Behav* 1983;12:59–66.
70. Everitt BJ, Herbert J. The effects of implanting testosterone propionate in the central nervous system on the sexual behavior of female rhesus monkeys. *Brain Res* 1975;86:109–120.
71. Polit D, Larocco S. Social and psychological correlates of menopausal symptoms. *Psychosom Med* 1980;42:335–345.
72. Schneider M, Brotherton P. Physiological, psychological and situational stresses in depression during the climacteric. *Maturitas* 1979;1:153–158.
73. Greene JG. Bereavement and social support at the climacteric. *Maturitas* 1983;5:115–124.
74. Price WA, Giannini AJ. Antidepressant effects of estrogen. *J Clin Psychiatry* 1985;46:506–510.
75. Honjo H, Ogino Y, Tanaka K et al. An effect of conjugated estrogen to cognitive impairment in women with senile dementia—Alzheimer's type: a placebo-controlled double blind study. *J Japan Menopause Soc* 1993;1:167–171.
76. Asthana S, Craft S, Baker LD, et al. Transdermal estrogen improves memory in women with Alzheimer's disease [Abstract]. *Soc Neurosci Abstr* 1996;22:200.
77. Paganini-Hill A, Henderson VW. Estrogen deficiency and risk of Alzheimer's disease in women. *Am J Epidemiol* 1994;140:256–261.
78. Tang M-X, Jacobs D, Stern Y, et al. Effect of estrogen during menopause on risk and age at onset of Alzheimer's Disease. *Lancet* 1996;348:429–432.
79. Kawas C, Resnick S, Morrison A, et al. A prospective study of estrogen replacement therapy and the risk of developing Alzheimer's disease. *The Baltimore Longitudinal Study of Aging Neurology* 1997;48:1517–1521.

Treatment of the Postmenopausal Woman: Basic and Clinical Aspects, Second Edition, edited by Rogerio A. Lobo, Lippincott Williams & Wilkins, Philadelphia © 1999.

CHAPTER 17

Estrogens and Depression in Women

David R. Rubinow, Catherine A. Roca, and Peter J. Schmidt

A role of estrogen in the regulation of mood can be inferred from descriptions of the neuromodulatory effects of estrogens, reports of the onset of depression or other mood disorders in association with the perimenopause and menopause, and observations by several authors of antidepressant-like effects of estrogen in hormone replacement regimens.

During the late 19th century early medical observers such as George Savage of the Bethlem Hospital in England reported the appearance of depression in association with the perimenopause (1,2). Contemporaneously, organotherapists have reported the beneficial effects of the extract of ovarian tissue in women with perimenopause-related hot flushes (3) and in some (but not all) women with perimenopause-related psychiatric illness (4). Subsequently, several investigators have examined the effects of estrogen replacement on mood with mixed results (see review by Rosenthal) (5). Although the role of estrogen in the treatment of hot flushes (also referred to as flashes) has been consistently documented, the relationship between perimenopause-related changes in estrogen and depression (as well as estrogen's therapeutic role in depression) remains to be established. In contrast, a considerable literature documents the widespread and important neuroregulatory effects of estrogen in animals, suggesting a neurobiologic basis for several recent reports of the salutary effects of estrogen on mood (alone or in combination with traditional antidepressants).

In this chapter we review the following: (a) the effects of estrogen on the central nervous system (CNS); (b) the relationship between perimenopause or postmenopause and depression; (c) the effect of estrogen on mood in humans; and (d) the clinical evaluation and management of depression during the perimenopause.

D. R. Rubinow, C. A. Roca, P. J. Schmidt: Behavioral Endocrinology Branch, National Institute of Mental Health, Bethesda, Maryland 20892.

EFFECTS OF ESTROGEN ON THE CENTRAL NERVOUS SYSTEM

As is the case with other members of the steroid hormone family (e.g., progesterone, androgen, glucocorticoid, and mineralocorticoid), estrogen is synthesized from cholesterol by a relatively small group of enzymes with multiple sites of action along the hormone synthetic cascade. On arrival at its target cell, estrogen diffuses into the cell and binds its receptor, which is located in the nucleus. The estrogen receptor is a member of a group of structurally related transcriptional factors (i.e., proteins that bind DNA or interact with one another to regulate transcription of m-RNA). Amino acid sequence and structure–function analyses of steroid receptors have identified a number of domains (i.e., sequences of amino acids) within the receptor protein, each with a particular function related to ligand binding or activation of the target genes (6–8). Two separate isoforms of the estrogen receptor have been identified: alpha (α) and beta (β) (9,10). In contrast to identified isoforms of progesterone and androgen receptors, which are posttranscriptional products, α and forms of the estrogen receptor are encoded by two separate genes, located on chromosomes 6 and 14, respectively (11). Structurally, both the α and β estrogen receptors share considerable amino acid sequence homology in both DNA (96%) and ligand binding (58%) domains (9). The two forms of the estrogen receptor are differentially distributed in a tissue-specific manner throughout the body, including the CNS (12–14) where estrogen receptor is abundant. The significance of the presence of these different forms of the estrogen receptor is revealed, in part, by observations that they are differentially modulated by estradiol, elicit different transcriptional responses, and modify each other's activity (15,16). In humans, region-specific concentrations of estradiol in brain have been observed in postmortem studies of women (17), with the highest concentrations in the hypothalamus, preoptic area, and substantia nigra.

Therefore, it is presumed that estrogen receptors are also present in the CNS of humans; however, they have yet to be demonstrated.

The actions of estrogen within the CNS are potent and widespread. As transcriptional regulators, activated estrogen receptors direct or modulate the synthesis of the synthetic and metabolic enzymes as well as the receptor proteins for many neurotransmitters and neuropeptides (18). Additionally, estrogen influences the levels of several critical enzymes involved in signal transduction. For example, Mobbs et al. (19) have shown that estrogen induces an isoform of phospholipase C-α in rat brain, and we have demonstrated that estrogen in women both decreases the level and increases the inactivation of the G protein G_i α-2 (Manji et al., unpublished data), consistent with the observed ability of estrogen to uncouple the D2 receptor from its signal transduction mechanisms (20). These actions permit gonadal steroids to potentially influence several aspects of neurotransmitter activity. For example, estrogen may modulate the synthesis of serotonin (21), serotonin uptake (by regulation of the serotonin transporter) (22,23), serotonin receptor transcription (24) and density (25), and the response to serotonin stimulation (26). The manifold action of estrogen and its receptor, therefore, provide the means by which the response of the CNS to incoming stimuli can be altered.

The neuroregulatory potential of estrogen and its receptor(s) is only partially conveyed by consideration of classical, activated receptor-mediated effects. First, many of the transcriptional actions of estrogen are directed by the presence or absence of tissue-specific transcriptional coactivators or corepressors (27). Second, several compounds have been observed to activate the estrogen receptor in the absence of estrogen: phytoestrogens (e.g., genistein and daidzein); selective estrogen receptor modulators (e.g., raloxifene [28]); and classical neurotransmitters (e.g., dopamine, activating the estrogen receptor via the D1 receptor (8,29). Third, in some tissues the unoccupied estrogen receptor may repress genomic transcription (30), perhaps through protein–protein interactions (27). Fourth, estrogen may have acute modulatory effects on the activity of membrane receptors (i.e., nongenomic actions). Thus, estradiol has been shown to acutely modulate non–N-methyl-D-aspartate (NMDA) receptor function in the hippocampus (31). Fifth, some actions of estrogen on brain appear to be context and developmental stage dependent. Toran-Allerand (32) has shown that estrogen has reciprocal interactions with CNS growth factors that can mediate, throughout development, the response to estrogen stimulation: estradiol stimulates its own receptor early in development, inhibits it during adulthood, and stimulates it again in the context of brain injury. These interactions between estradiol and growth factors are of further interest given recent reports that brain-derived neurotrophic factor (BDNF) levels are decreased by stress and are elevated by antidepressants (33–35).

The extent to which these effects underlie or contribute to differential effects of estrogen on brain physiology, behavior, and mood across individuals is unclear, but it is of considerable potential importance in the cause and treatment of depression during the perimenopause.

Data from several studies in humans have been adduced to propose candidate neural systems (e.g., serotonergic system) through which estradiol can impact on mood. First, a number of sexual dimorphisms have been reported in serotonergic measures in humans, including increased cerebral spinal fluid (CSF) 5-hydroxyindoleacetic acid (5-HIAA) (increased in pain syndromes and depression in women) (36–38), 5-hydroxytryptamine$_2$ (5-HT$_2$) receptor binding capacity in brain (decreased in women) (39), whole brain serotonin synthesis (decreased in women) (40), and response to tryptophan depletion (increased in women) (41–43). Second, the neuroendocrine response to stimulation with serotonin agonists has been reported to vary, albeit inconsistently, according to menstrual cycle phase. For example, stimulated prolactin secretion during the luteal phase has been observed to be augmented following m-chlorophenylpiperazine (m-CPP) (44) and buspirone (45), blunted following L-tryptophan (46), and unaffected following d-fenfluramine (41). Third, several serotonergic measures have been studied following estrogen replacement. Sherwin et al. (47) reported the upregulation of platelet ^{3}H-imipramine binding sites (a measure of the serotonin transporter) when estrogen was administered to hypogonadal women. These data parallel observations of estradiol-stimulated upregulation of the serotonin transporter m-RNA in the raphé of rats (48) but not macques (22). In contrast, an earlier study by Best et al. (49) did not observe an estrogen-related change in imipramine binding sites or 5-HT$_2$ receptor binding in hypogonadal women. Estrogen replacement increased the prolactin response to m-CPP (but not significantly) in postmenopausal women (50), although no effect of estradiol replacement was observed on m-CPP-stimulated neuroendocrine response in young women compared with the response seen during gonadotropin-releasing hormone agonist-induced hypogonadism (Schmidt et al., unpublished manuscript). Clearly, the nature (indirect) and multiplicity (e.g., serotonin synthesis, receptor concentration, and re-uptake; response to agonist) of the serotonergic measures employed in an already scanty literature preclude any inference about the role of serotonin in possible psychotropic effects of estrogen.

RELATIONSHIP BETWEEN PERIMENOPAUSE AND DEPRESSION

Community-based studies monitoring self-reports of menstrual cycle status and depressive symptom severity have uniformly observed that most postmenopausal women do not experience prominent symptoms of depression (51–55). Although the menopause itself has not been identified as a major cause of mood destabilization in women, perimenopause-related changes in mood have been observed in up to 10% of the women participating in some longitudinal, community-based studies (55,56).

Similarly, a higher than expected prevalence of depressivelike symptoms has been observed in perimenopausal and postmenopausal women attending gynecology clinics (57–60), with one study observing that up to 45% of the sample had high scores (consistent with clinically significant depression) on standardized rating scales for depression (60). In two additional studies, perimenopausal women were observed to report significantly more symptoms than postmenopausal women (58,59). Thus, both clinic-based surveys and epidemiologic studies suggest the relevance of the perimenopause in disturbances of mood in a substantial number of women.

Community-based surveys of the prevalence of affective *syndromes* (conditions meeting standardized diagnostic criteria, such as major or minor depression) have observed patterns of morbidity consistent with those reported in the surveys examining mood *symptoms*. Several epidemiologic studies examining gender and age-related differences in the 6-month to 1-year prevalences of major depression (but not minor depression) reported the absence of an increase in the prevalence of major depression in women at midlife (age range approximately 45 to 55 years) (61,62). Nevertheless, these studies also identified an increase during midlife in the female:male sex ratio for major depression from approximately 2:1 to approximately 3 to 4:1 (61,62). It is possible, therefore, as suggested by Bancroft (personal communication), that the perimenopause may differentially alter the effect of aging on mood stability in women. Alternatively, as suggested by Kessler et al. (62), the sample sizes employed within this age range may be too small to reliably estimate gender differences in the prevalence rate of depression. Finally, in contrast to the findings of previous epidemiologic studies, a recent multinational study by Weissman et al. identified an increased hazard rate for the onset of depression in a cohort of women (but not men) aged between 45 and 50 years.

To date, only Hay et al. (60) have examined the incidence rates of major and minor depression in endocrinologically confirmed perimenopausal women within a gynecologic clinic-based setting. These investigators employed a structured diagnostic interview and reported that 45% of the sample of women studied met criteria for major or minor depression. The report by Hay et al. (60), confirms suggestions (58,59) that clinic samples contain a greater proportion of perimenopausal women with clinically significant affective disorders.

In summary, epidemiologic studies examining the prevalence of both affective symptoms and syndromes have uniformly shown that most postmenopausal women do not experience a major depression associated with this phase of life. Additionally, although most epidemiologic studies of major depression conclude that the perimenopause is irrelevant to the development of affective disorders, a potential relationship is nonetheless suggested by the reports of gender differences in the age-related declines in major depressive illness. Moreover, gynecologic clinic-based surveys (58,60) suggest that a substantial number of perimenopausal women do, in fact, experience a clinically significant depression.

EFFICACY OF ESTROGEN IN MOOD DISORDERS

A 1934 report of one of the first controlled trials of estrogen (theelin injections) was published in the *Journal of the American Medical Association* that described the superior efficacy of estrogen compared with placebo. Subsequently, some (63–66), but not all (67,68), clinic-based, placebo-controlled trials have demonstrated the salutary effects of estradiol replacement on mood symptoms in perimenopausal women with high scores on depressive symptom rating scales. These studies in perimenopausal women are consistent with reports that estradiol replacement enhances mood in women after the surgical menopause (69–71). Additionally, Ditkoff et al. (72) reported estradiol to have an acute mood-enhancing effect in relatively asymptomatic postmenopausal women. (Of note, traditional antidepressants do not generally elevate mood in asymptomatic subjects.) Thus, the report by Ditkoff et al. (72) suggests that the mood-elevating effects of estrogen can be mediated by mechanisms other than those thought to be involved in the traditional antidepressant response. Finally, preliminary results of one study (73) as well as several case reports (74,75) suggest that estradiol replacement in some women augments the mood-stabilizing and antidepressant effects of traditional psychotropic medications. It is noteworthy, however, that the superior efficacy of estradiol augmentation in the study by Schneider et al. is seen relative to results with estradiol and placebo, not with antidepressant alone.

Two major confounds exist in studies attempting to assess the mood-enhancing effects of estrogen: the intimate relationship between estrogen deficiency-related vasomotor symptoms and mood disturbance, and the failure to study women meeting standardized diagnostic criteria for the syndrome of depression. For example, the salutary effects of estrogen on mood symptoms in the studies cited above could simply reflect the elimination of thermoregulatory dyscontrol and accompanying sleep disturbances. Moreover, depressive symptoms may be multidetermined, whereas depression, the syndrome, has specific biologic concomitants and treatment response characteristics. To eliminate these confounds, we performed a double-blind, placebo-controlled trial of estrogen administration in perimenopausal women (serial follicle-stimulating hormone [FSH] levels > 20 IU/L) meeting research diagnostic criteria for major or minor depression in the absence of a history of hot flushes. Preliminary results in 18 women studied to date demonstrate the superior efficacy of estradiol to placebo after 3 weeks of administration in the remediation of a variety of symptoms of depression including tearfulness, sadness, and social isolation. No significant additional improvement was noted following three additional weeks of estradiol. These data provide further indirect evidence for the role of alterations in estradiol levels in the development of depressions occurring in the context of the perimenopause and, additionally, suggest that the psychotropic effects of estrogen are not epiphenomenal to the remediation of thermoregulatory disturbance.

Despite evidence for an acute antidepressant effect of estradiol in hypogonadal women, the therapeutic role of estrogen in perimenopause-related depression remains to be determined. The possibility that estrogen's acute antidepressant effects may not be maintained long term has been described by Butler and Lewis (76). In their report, a woman with first onset depression during the perimenopause responded initially to estrogen replacement; however, she later experienced a relapse of her depression on estrogen that required treatment with traditional antidepressants (76). Trials evaluating the long-term efficacy of estrogen in the maintenance therapy of depression are required prior to recommending estrogen as a specific therapeutic agent for perimenopause-related depression. Similarly, no study has evaluated the efficacy of traditional antidepressants in women with depression during the perimenopause.

SUGGESTED EVALUATION AND MANAGEMENT OF PERIMENOPAUSE-RELATED DEPRESSION

The management of mood and behavioral disturbances during the perimenopause requires determination of the symptoms experienced and the hormonal context in which they appear. As a complement to a careful evaluation, longitudinal monitoring of symptoms on a daily basis can provide valuable information about the severity, stability, and pattern of symptom experience. Both affective and somatic (e.g., vaginal dryness, hot flashes, urinary incontinence) symptoms should be followed. If not done previously, the presence of the perimenopause and hypoestrogenism should be documented with FSH and estradiol measures. As part of our operational criteria, we have required three of four serial FSH levels greater than 20 IU/L for the perimenopause. Although estradiol levels less than 60 pg/mL are consistent with decreased ovarian function, levels greater than 60 pg/mL may appear, nonetheless, in the presence of markedly elevated FSH levels that suggest ovarian insensitivity.

The therapy selected for a major depressive disorder during the perimenopause depends on the nature and severity of the somatic symptoms and the type of hormone replacement therapy (if present). In perimenopausal women presenting with depression, the presence of distressing signs of estrogen deficiency (e.g., vaginal dryness, stress incontinence, or flushes) should lead to consideration of a trial of hormone replacement as the first approach, unless relative contraindications to estrogen replacement exist. Alternatively, if perimenopausal somatic symptoms are minimal despite laboratory evidence of hypoestrogenism and mood symptoms are moderate to severe, then the choice of hormone replacement versus antidepressant therapy may best be informed by such factors as past personal history of depression, family history of affective disorder, severity of affective symptoms, or the presence of contraindications to estrogen replacement. Finally, clinicians should appreciate that perimenopausal depression may present in the absence of typical perimenopause-related somatic symptoms, such as hot flushes or vaginal dryness. Thus, somatic symptoms are neither necessary nor sufficient for the production of depression during the perimenopause. Moreover, as demonstrated above, the absence of hot flushes in endocrinologically confirmed perimenopausal depressed women does not predict the lack of efficacy of estrogen in the treatment of depression.

The relationship between the onset of mood symptoms and the initiation of hormone replacement therapy should be determined for at least two reasons. First, mood and behavioral symptoms may appear with inadequate estrogen replacement, and they can remit with appropriate dosage adjustments or with a change to an alternative form of estrogen replacement. Adjustment of hormone replacement therapy, therefore, is recommended before considering adjunctive psychopharmacotherapy. Second, mood and behavioral symptoms may directly result from the hormone replacement therapy. Specifically, cyclic mood and behavioral symptoms have been reported in association with sequential hormone replacement in some (77–79) but not all (80,81) studies and may remit with a change in the replacement regimen from sequential to continuous combination therapy. Alternatively, if the addition of progesterone consistently precipitates adverse mood changes, estrogen replacement alone may be attempted if accompanied by appropriate monitoring of the endometrium. Symptoms of depression and loss of libido consequent to ovarian failure may, nonetheless, be responsive to antidepressant therapy, and this option should be considered (particularly in patients with more severe or disabling symptoms) irrespective of the strength of the association between ovarian dysfunction and affective disorder.

REFERENCES

1. Savage GH. Some mental disorders associated with the menopause. *Lancet* 1893;ii:1128–1128.
2. Savage GH. Some neuroses of the climacteric and summary of climacteric cases at Bethlem, from July 1, 1888, to June 30, 1893. *Tr Med Soc Lond* 1893;xvii:31–47.

3. Fosbery WHS. Severe climacteric flushings successfully treated by ovarian extract. *Br Med J* 1897;1:1039–1039.

4. Easterbrook CC. Organo-therapeutics in mental diseases. *Br Med J* 1900;2: 813–823.

5. Rosenthal S. The involutional depressive syndrome. *Am J Psychiatry* 1968;124: 21–35.

6. Williams GR, Franklyn JA. Physiology of the steroid-thyroid hormone nuclear receptor superfamily. *Baillieres Clin Endocrinol Metab* 1994;8:241–266.

7. Evans RM. The steroid and thyroid hormone receptor superfamily. *Science* 1988;240:889–895.

8. Tsai M-J, O'Malley BW. Molecular mechanisms of action of steroid/thyroid receptor superfamily members. *Annu Rev Biochem* 1994;63:451–486.

9. Mosselman S, Polman J, Dijkema R. ERb: identification and characterization of a novel human estrogen receptor. *FEBS Lett* 1996;392:49–53.

10. Kuiper GGJM, Enmark E, Pelto-Huikko M, Nilsson S, Gustafsson J-A. Cloning of a novel estrogen receptor expressed in rat prostate and ovary. *Proc Natl Acad Sci U S A* 1996;93:5925–5930.

11. Enmark EP-HM, Grandien K, Lagercrantz S, et al. Human estrogen receptor β-gene structure, chromosomal localization, and expression pattern. *J Clin Endocrinol Metab* 1997;4258–4265.

12. Jones BM, Jones MK. Women and alcohol: intoxication, metabolism and the menstrual cycle. In: Greenblatt M, Schuckit M, eds. *Alcoholism problems in women and children.* New York: Grune & Stratton, 1976.

13. Li X, Schwartz PE, Rissman EF. Distribution of estrogen receptor-β-like immunoreactivity in rat forebrain. *Neuroendocrinology* 1997;63–67.

14. Shughrue PJ, Komm B, Merchenthaler I. The distribution of estrogen receptor-β mRNA in the rat hypothalamus. *Steroids* 1996;61:678–681.

15. Pettersson K, Grandien K, Kuiper GGJM, Gustafsson J-A. Mouse estrogen receptor β forms estrogen response element-binding heterodimers with estrogen receptor α. *Mol Endocrinol* 1997;1486–1496.

16. Clarke CH, Cunningham KA, Bland DA, Steinsland OS. Sex hormone regulation of estrogen receptor (ERa and ERb) mRNA in female rat brain. *Abstracts of the 27th Annual Meeting, Society of Neuroscience* 1997;1501–1501.

17. Bixo M, Backstrom T, Winblad B, Andersson A. Estradiol and testosterone in specific regions of the human female brain in different endocrine states. *J Steroid Biochem Molec Biol* 1995;55:297–303.

18. Ciocca DR, Vargas Roig LM. Estrogen receptors in human nontarget tissues: biological and clinical implications. *Endocr Rev* 1995;16:35–62.

19. Mobbs CV, Kaplitt M, Kow LM, Pfaff DW. At the cutting edge: PLC-a: a common mediator of the action of estrogen and other hormones? *Mol Cell Endocrinol* 1991;80:C187–C191.

20. Maus M, Bertrand P, Drouva S, et al. Differential modulation of D1 and D2 dopamine-sensitive adenylate cyclases by 17β-estradiol in cultured striatal neurons and anterior pituitary cells. *J Neurochem* 1989;52:410–418.

21. Cohen IR, Wise PM. Effects of estradiol on the diurnal rhythm of serotonin activity in microdissected brain areas of ovariectomized rats. *Endocrinology* 1988;122: 2619–2625.

22. Pecins-Thompson M, Brown NA, Bethea CL. Regulation of serotonin re-uptake transporter mRNA expression by ovarian steroids in rhesus macaques. *Mol Brain Res* 1998;53:120–129.

23. Fink G, Sumner BEH. Oestrogen and mental state. *Nature* 1996;383:306–306.

24. Sumner BEH, Fink G. Estrogen increases the density of 5-hydroxytryptamine$_{2A}$ receptors in cerebral cortex and nucleus accumbens in the female rat. *J Steroid Biochem Molec Biol* 1995;54:15–20.

25. Fischette CT, Biegon A, McEwen BS. Sex differences in serotonin 1 receptor binding in rat brain. *Science* 1983;222:333–335.

26. Matsuda T, Nakano Y, Kanda T, Iwata H, Baba A. Gonadal hormones affect the hypothermia induced by serotonin$_{1A}$ (5-HT$_{1A}$) receptor activation. *Life Sci* 1991; 48:1627–1632.

27. Katzenellenbogen JA, OiMalley BW, Katzenellenbogen BS. Tripartite steroid hormone receptor pharmacology: interaction with multiple effector sites as a basis for the cell- and promoter-specific action of these hormones. *Mol Endocrinol* 1996; 10:119–131.

28. Yang NN, Venugopalan M, Hardikar S, Glasebrook A. Identification of an estrogen response element activated by metabolites of 17β-estradiol and raloxifene. *Science* 1996;273:1222–1225.

29. Power RF, Mani SK, Codina J, Conneely OM, OiMalley BW. Dopaminergic and ligand-independent activation of steroid hormone receptors. *Science* 1991;254: 1636–1639.

30. Tzukerman M, Zhang X, Hermann T, Wills KN, Graupner G, Pfahl M. The human estrogen receptor has transcriptional activator and repressor functions in the absence of ligand. *New Biologist* 1990;2:613–620.

31. Wong M, Moss RL. Long-term and short-term electrophysiological effects of estrogen on the synaptic properties of hippocampal CA1 neurons. *J Neurosci* 1992;12:3217–3225.

32. Toran-Allerand CD. Developmental interactions of estrogens with the neurotrophins and their receptors. In: Micevych P, Hammer RP, eds. *Neurobiological effects of sex steroid hormones.* Cambridge: Cambridge University Press, 1994: 391–411.

33. Smith MA, Cizza G. Stress-induced changes in brain-derived neurotrophic factor expression are attenuated in aged Fischer 344/N rats. *Neurobiol Aging* 1996;17: 859–864.

34. Duman RS, Heninger GR, Nestler EJ. A molecular and cellular theory of depression. *Arch Gen Psychiatry* 1997;54:597–606.

35. Siuciak JA, Lewis DR, Wiegand SJ, Lindsay RM. Antidepressant-like effect of brain-derive neurotrophic factor (BDNF). *Pharmacol Biochem Behav* 1997;56: 131–137.

36. Knorring Lv, Oreland L, Häggendal J, Magnusson T, Almay B, Johansson F. Relationship between platelet MAO activity and concentrations of 5-HIAA and HVA in cerebrospinal fluid in chronic pain patients. *J Neural Transm [Gen Sect]* 1986; 66:37–46.

37. Young SN, Gauthier S, Anderson GM, Purdy WC. Tryptophan, 5-hydroxyindoleacetic acid and indoleacetic acid in human cerebrospinal fluid: interrelationships and the influence of age, sex, epilepsy and anticonvulsant drugs. *J Neurol Neurosurg Psychiatry* 1980;43:438–445.

38. Agren H, Mefford IN, Rudorfer MV, Linnoila M, Potter WZ. Interacting neurotransmitter systems. A non-experimental approach to the 5-HIAA-HVA correlation in human CSF. *J Psychiatr Res* 1986;20:175–193.

39. Biver F, Lotstra F, Monclus M, et al. Sex difference in 5HT$_2$ receptor in the living human brain. *Neurosci Lett* 1996;204:25–28.

40. Nishizawa S, Benkelfat C, Young SN, et al. Differences between males and females in rates of serotonin synthesis in human brain. *Proc Natl Acad Sci U S A* 1997;94:5308–5313.

41. Ellenbogen MA, Young SN, Dean P, Palmour RM, Benkelfat C. Mood response to acute tryptophan depletion in healthy volunteers: sex differences and temporal stability. *Neuropsychopharmacology* 1996;15:465–474.

42. Anderson IM, Parry-Billings M, Newsholme EA, Fairburn CG, Cowen PJ. Dieting reduces plasma tryptophan and alters brain 5-HT function in women. *Psychol Med* 1990;20:785–791.

43. Walsh AES, Oldman AD, Franklin M, Fairburn CG, Cowen PJ. Dieting decreases plasma tryptophan and increases the prolactin response to d-fenfluramine in women but not men. *J Affective Disord* 1995;33:89–97.

44. Su T-P, Schmidt PJ, Danaceau M, Murphy DL, Rubinow DR. Effect of menstrual cycle phase on neuroendocrine and behavioral responses to the serotonin agonist m-chlorophenylpiperazine in women with premenstrual syndrome and controls. *J Clin Endocrinol Metab* 1997;82:1220–1228.

45. Yatham L, Barry S, Dinan TG. Serotonin in psychobiology of premenstrual syndrome. *Lancet* 1989;i:1447–1448.

46. Bancroft J, Cook A, Davidson D, Bennie J, Goodwin G. Blunting of neuroendocrine responses to infusion of L-tryptophan in women with perimenstrual mood change. *Psychol Med* 1991;21:305–312.

47. Sherwin BB, Suranyi-Cadotte BE. Up-regulatory effect of estrogen on platelet 3H-imipramine binding sites in surgically menopausal women. *Biol Psychiatry* 1990;28:339–348.

48. McQueen JK, Wilson H, Fink G. Estradiol-17β increases serotonin transporter (SERT) mRNA levels and the density of SERT-binding sites in female rat brain. *Mol Brain Res* 1997;45:13–23.

49. Best NR, Barlow DH, Rees MP, Cowen PJ. Lack of effect of oestradiol implant on platelet imipramine and 5-HT2 receptor binding in menopausal subjects. *Psychopharmacology* 1989;98:561.

50. Halbreich U, Rojansky N, Palter S, Tworek H, Hissin P, Wang K. Estrogen augments serotonergic activity in postmenopausal women. *Biol Psychiatry* 1995;37: 434–441.

51. McKinlay JB, McKinlay SM, Brambilla D. The relative contributions of endocrine changes and social circumstances to depression in mid-aged women. *J Health Soc Behav* 1987;28:345–363.

52. Kaufert PA, Gilbert P, Tate R. The Manitoba project: a re-examination of the link between menopause and depression. *Maturitas* 1992;14:143–155.

53. Avis NE, Brambilla D, McKinlay SM, Vass K. A longitudinal analysis of the association between menopause and depression: results from the Massachusetts Womenís Health Study. *Ann Epidemiol* 1994;4:214–220.

54. Matthews KA, Kuller LH, Wing RR, Meilahn EN. Biobehavioral aspects of menopause: lessons from the healthy women study. *Exp Gerontol* 1994;29:337–342.

55. Matthews KA. Myths and realities of the menopause. *Psychosom Med* 1992; 54:1–9.

56. Hunter M. The South-East England longitudinal study of the climacteric and postmenopause. *Maturitas* 1992;14:117–126.

57. Anderson E, Hamburger S, Liu JH, Rebar RW. Characteristics of menopausal women seeking assistance. *Am J Obstet Gyn* 1987;156:428–433.

58. Stewart DE, Boydell K, Derzko C, Marshall V. Psychologic distress during the menopausal years in women attending a menopause clinic. *Int J Psychiatry Med* 1992;22:213–220.

59. Dennerstein L, Smith AMA, Morse C, et al. Menopausal symptoms in Australian women. *Med J Aust* 1993;159:232–236.

60. Hay AG, Bancroft J, Johnstone EC. Affective symptoms in women attending a menopause clinic. *Br J Psychiatry* 1994;164:513–516.

61. Weissman MM, Leaf PJ, Tischler GL, et al. Affective disorders in five United States communities. *Psychol Med* 1988;18:141–153.

62. Kessler RC, McGonagle KA, Swartz M, Blazer DG, Nelson CB. Sex and depression in the National Comorbidity Survey I: lifetime prevalence, chronicity and recurrence. *J Affective Disord* 1993;29:85–96.

63. Dennerstein L, Burows GO, Hyman GJ. Hormone therapy and affect. *Maturitas* 1979;1:247–259.

64. Zohar J, Shapira B, Oppenheim G, Ayd FJ, Belmaker RH. Addition of estrogen to imipramine in female-resistant depressives. *Psychopharmacol Bull* 1985;21: 705–706.

65. Brincat M, Studd JWW, O'Dowd T, et al. Subcutaneous hormone implants for the control of climacteric symptoms: a prospective study. *Lancet* 1984;i:16–18.

66. Montgomery JC, Brincat M, Tapp A, et al. Effect of oestrogen and testosterone implants on psychological disorders in the climacteric. *Lancet* 1987;1:297–299.
67. Strickler RC, Borth R, Cecutti A, et al. The role of oestrogen replacement in the climacteric syndrome. *Psychol Med* 1977;7:631–639.
68. Coope J. Is oestrogen therapy effective in the treatment of menopausal depression? *Jr Coll Gen Prac* 1981;31:134–140.
69. Sherwin BB, Gelfand MM. Sex steroids and affect in the surgical menopause: a double-blind, cross-over study. *Psychoneuroendocrinology* 1985;10:325–335.
70. Sherwin BB. The impact of different doses of estrogen and progestin on mood and sexual behavior in postmenopausal women. *J Clin Endocrinol Metab* 1991;72:336–343.
71. Sherwin BB. Affective changes with estrogen and androgen replacement therapy in surgically menopausal women. *J Affective Disord* 1988;14:177–187.
72. Ditkoff EC, Crary WG, Cristo M, Lobo RA. Estrogen improves psychological function in asymptomatic postmenopausal women. *Obstet Gynecol* 1991;78:991–995.
73. Small GW, Schneider LS, Holman S, Brystritsky A, Meyers BS, Nemeroff CB. Estrogen plus fluoxetine for geriatric depression. *Abstracts of the APA 147th Annual Meeting* 1994;203–203.
74. Vogel W, Klaiber EL, Broverman DM. Roles of the gonadal steroid hormones in psychiatric depression in men and women. *Prog Neuropsychopharmacol* 1978;2:487–503.
75. Chouinard G, Steinberg S, Steiner W. Estrogen-progesterone combination: another mood stabilizer? *Am J Psychiatry* 1987;144:826–826.
76. Butler RN, Lewis MI. Late-life depression: when and how to intervene. *Geriatrics* 1995;50:44–55.
77. Smith RNJ, Holland EFN, Studd JWW. The symptomatology of progestogen intolerance. *Maturitas* 1994;18:87–91.
78. Hammarback S, Backstrom T, Holst J, Von Schoultz B, Lyrenas S. Cyclical mood changes as in the premenstrual tension syndrome during sequential estrogen-progestagen postmenopausal replacement therapy. *Acta Obstet Gynecol Scand* 1985;64:393–397.
79. Magos AL, Brewster E, Singh R, OíDowd T, Brincat M, Studd JWW. The effects of norethisterone in postmenopausal women on oestrogen replacement therapy: a model for the premenstrual syndrome. *Br J Obstet Gynaecol* 1986;93:1290–1296.
80. Kirkham C, Hahn PM, VanVugt DA, Carmichael JA, Reid RL. A randomized, double-blind, placebo-controlled, cross-over trial to assess the side effects of medroxyprogesterone acetate in hormone replacement therapy. *Obstet Gynecol* 1991;78:93–97.
81. Prior JC, Alojado N, McKay DW, Vigna YM. No adverse effects of medroxyprogesterone treatment without estrogen in postmenopausal women: double-blind, placebo-controlled, crossover trial. *Obstet Gynecol* 1994;83:24–28.

Treatment of the Postmenopausal Woman: Basic and Clinical Aspects, Second Edition, edited by Rogerio A. Lobo, Lippincott Williams & Wilkins, Philadelphia © 1999.

CHAPTER 18

Vulvovaginal Complaints

Gloria A. Bachmann, Gary A. Ebert, and Irina D. Burd

Estrogen loss from follicular depletion in the menopausal ovary is the major cause of vulvovaginal dysfunction in the older woman, and it accounts for most of the anatomic, cytologic, and bacteriologic genital changes that occur. As the overall life expectancy of women increases, so does the amount of time that women will spend in the postmenopausal phase of their lives. Although hot flushes (also referred to as flashes) and night sweats can dramatically herald the loss of estrogen production by the ovaries, these symptoms usually abate over time even without treatment. Vulvovaginal symptoms, in contrast to vasomotor disturbances, are usually progressive in nature. Urogenital symptoms can result in years of suffering with a significant impact on quality of life. Women may start to experience subtle signs of declining estrogen levels such as vaginal dryness as early as the perimenopausal years. Although the atrophic changes of the vulva, vagina, and lower urinary tract are unlikely to resolve spontaneously, they are effectively reversed when estrogen therapy is instituted. Systemic and local estrogens result in significant improvements in genitourinary symptoms, physiology, and function.

Other transient states of decreased estrogen stimulation (e.g., lactation, anorexia, intense athletic training, and medications such as gonadotropin-releasing hormone agonists and danazol) can cause vulvovaginal symptoms because of temporary hypoestrogenic effects on the genitalia. Atrophic changes of the vulva, vagina, and lower urinary tract are the most frequent causes of vulvovaginal complaints in the menopausal woman, but other causes should be considered. Similar symptoms can be experienced by postmenopausal women suffering from infection, trauma, foreign body, inflammatory con-

ditions of the vulva, and benign and malignant tumors (Table 18.1).

VULVOVAGINAL SYMPTOMS

Although effective treatments for the symptoms associated with urogenital atrophy were lacking until recently, estrogen-related vulvovaginal symptoms have been accurately described, albeit dismally, in both professional and lay publications for centuries. More than 100 years ago, Kellogg reported postmenopausal genital symptoms as a distressing leukorrheal discharge accompanied by violent itching, which often makes its appearance just after the change of life (1). Postmenopausal women report numerous vulvar, vaginal, and lower urinary tract symptoms ranging in severity from annoying to debilitating (Table 18.2).

Studies have been done to determine the prevalence of vulvovaginal symptoms in the general, noninstitutionalized elderly population. Using anonymous questionnaires, Stenberg et al. studied 1,280 women living in Uppsala County, Sweden who were 61 years of age. Of these women, 43% reported suffering from vaginal dryness and 10% vaginal burning. Of the 59% who were sexually active, 41% complained of dysparunia and 22% tried to avoid intercourse because of this discomfort. Urinary incontinence was reported by 73% of the respondents with 33% rating their incontinence as severe. Thirteen percent reported nocturia, 8% had frequency of urination, and 4% had experienced more than two urinary tract infections in the preceding year. Interestingly, only 47% of the respondents had asked their clinician for help with their symptoms (2).

Diokno et al. published a report of household interviews of senior citizens aged 60 years or older in Washtenaw County, Michigan. Of the 1,150 women interviewed, 38% reported urinary incontinence and 17% reported irritative bladder symptoms. An additional 12% of the women

G. A. Bachmann, G. A. Ebert, I. D. Burd: Department of Obstetrics, Gynecology and Reproductive Sciences, University of Medicine and Dentistry of New Jersey—Robert Wood Johnson Medical School, New Brunswick, New Jersey 08901.

TABLE 18.1. *Vulvovaginal complaints: differential*

Atrophy
Microbial infection
Trauma
Foreign body
Allergic reaction
Sebaceous, Bartholin's, and Skene's duct occlusions
Benign and malignant tumors
Vulvar dystrophy
Desquamative vaginitides
Chronic antibiotic, analgesic, and laxative use
Medical disorders (e.g., diabetes, lupus erythematosus)
Psychological cause

complained of frequency and 7% nocturia (three or more voids per night). Only 41% of the incontinent women had told their doctor about their urine loss problems (3).

During the perimenopausal and early menopausal years, vulvovaginal symptoms may be attributed to infectious, chronic inflammatory, or even psychologic causes. Women may go through several treatment regimens with various antifungal agents, antibiotics, steroids, vitamins, and antidepressants without significant relief of symptoms. Many older women will self-medicate with home remedies for relief of symptoms and seek medical assistance only at the point where the vulva is excoriated from the chronic scratching. This is especially true of the inflammatory conditions of the vulva such as contact dermatitis, squamous hyperplasia, or lichen sclerosus, which produce symptoms of severe pruritis, soreness, pain, and dyspareunia. Vaginal pressure in the older woman may result from atrophic changes in the genital region alone or in conjunction with uterine prolapse, cystocele, or rectocele. Although vaginal dryness can be bothersome to sexually abstinent women, it is most often voiced as a significant problem in sexually active women who find coital activity uncomfortable because of inadequate lubrication. As the atrophic changes worsen over time and the number and severity of symptoms increase, the association with estrogen deficiency becomes clearer and the symptom complex is referred to as "atrophic vaginitis."

TABLE 18.2. *Vulvovaginal complaints: common presentations*

Vaginal dryness and irritation
Vulvovaginal pruritis
Vaginal pressure
Malodorous vaginal discharge
Dyspareunia
Postcoital bleeding
Dysuria
Urinary frequency and urgency
Frequent urinary tract infections
Urinary stress incontinence

VALVOVAGINAL CHANGES CAUSED BY ESTROGEN LOSS

The atrophic vulva loses most of its collagen, adipose, and water-retaining ability and becomes flattened and thin with epithelial glands (eccrine and apocrine) attenuating (4). Although the sebaceous glands remain prominent, their secretions diminish. The prepuce of the clitoris often atrophies more than the glans, such that the clitoral glans loses its protective covering and is irritated more readily with any type of contact (e.g., clothing, pressure from prolonged sitting, and contact during sexual exchange, especially when lubrication is inadequate).

With estrogen loss, the vagina shortens and narrows and the vaginal walls become thinner, less elastic, and pale in color. The vaginal walls become progressively smoother as rugation decreases. Less secretions are produced in general and the onset of lubrication during sexual stimulation is delayed. The vaginal surface becomes friable, with petechiae, ulcerations, and bleeding often occurring after minimal trauma (e.g., speculum insertion). With repeated ulceration and bleeding, healing adhesions may develop between touching surfaces, especially in the sexually abstinent woman.

Histologically the vagina consists of three layers: the inner layer, composed of stratified squamous epithelium containing no true glands, a middle muscular layer, and an outer fibrous layer, which has evolved from the pelvic fascia (5). Vaginal epithelium growth is influenced by estrogen stimulation. Vaginal epithelial cells contain the greatest number of nuclear estrogen binding sites of any genital structure, with higher levels noted in the postmenopausal vagina as compared with the premenopausal vagina (6). When estrogenic stimulation is present, the vaginal epithelium matures and more superficial cells than parabasal cells are seen on vaginal cytology. When estrogen is progressively depleted during the postmenopausal years, the ratio of superficial cells to intermediate and parabasal cells decreases.

After the cessation of ovarian estrogen production, the quantity and character of the vaginal secretions change. The secretions, which are made up mainly of vaginal wall transudate, with lesser amounts of desquamated vaginal epithelial cells, cervical mucus, and fluid from the fallopian tubes and endometrium, decrease in amount and change in composition (i.e., the ratio of proteins, carbohydrates, and fatty acids) (7–9).

In the reproductive age woman, the acidic pH of the vaginal fluid is an important component of the nonspecific host defense against urogenital pathogens. Under the influence of estrogen stimulation the mature vaginal epithelium produces glycogen, which is broken down into glucose in the vagina. Lactobacillus species metabolize this glucose and produce lactic acid, which is responsible for the acidic pH of the vagina (10). When estrogenic stimulation is lacking, the population of lactobacilli decreases and an upward shift of the vaginal pH toward alkalinity occurs. The higher pH allows colonization of the vagina by fecal flora and other pathogens (11). Lactobacilli have also been shown to control the growth of vaginal pathogens through the production of hydrogen peroxide (12,13).

URINARY TRACT CHANGES CAUSED BY ESTROGEN LOSS

Historically, practitioners' attention to hypoestrogenism of the urogenital tract was directed mainly toward vaginal symptoms. Today, not only are the vaginal changes and complaints addressed by practitioners but urinary tract changes are addressed as well. The epithelium of the lower urinary tract, including the urethra and the trigone of the bladder, undergoes atrophic changes similar to those observed in the vagina. Estrogen receptors have been identified in the epithelium of the bladder, the trigone, and the urethra, as well as in the deeper muscle and fascial layers (14,15). Estrogen replacement therapy stimulates the growth of the urethral mucosa and results in a maturation of the squamous epithelium of the urethra (16). This finding is consistent with the dramatic improvement in lower urinary tract symptoms, including dysuria and urgency, noted after local estrogen replacement therapy (17–21).

Anatomic changes caused by estrogen loss also play a role in lower urinary tract symptoms. As a result of the atrophy of the vagina, the urethral meatus often changes its axis to the symphysis pubis from 90 degrees to 180 degrees. With the urethral opening closer to the introitus, any type of vaginal manipulation or pressure such as coitus, douching, or insertion of a vaginal preparation can cause irritation to the urethra. Repeated trauma in this way can contribute to lower urinary tract symptoms and the increased risk of urinary tract infection.

In addition to the irritative bladder symptoms, the postmenopausal period is also associated with an increased incidence of urinary tract infections. The changes in the vaginal microbial flora from estrogen deficiency provide a reservoir of pathogenic bacteria that can infect the urinary tract. In a randomized, double-blind, placebo-controlled trial, Raz and Stamm (22) found that postmenopausal women with a history of recurrent urinary tract infections treated with a local estrogen therapy had significantly less recurrences than control patients. They also found that, although none of the menopausal subjects had lactobacilli in their vaginas prior to treatment, lactobacillus was found in 22 of 36 patients after 8 months of estrogen therapy. As expected, the patients in the treatment arm had a significant decrease both in their vaginal pH and in the vaginal colonization by *Enterobacteriaceae*. Estrogen therapy strengthens nonspecific antimicrobial host defenses by increasing vaginal and urethral mucosal integrity and by supporting the growth of *Lactobacillus* species which results in a decrease in the presence of uropathogens, and a decrease in the rate of urinary tract infections.

SEXUAL COMPLAINTS

Although the incidence of sexual problems in the general population is high and increases with aging, older people are often reluctant to seek medical services for their sexual difficulties (23,24). In one large series of 2,550 patients evaluated for sexual problems by a psychiatric service over a 10-year period, only 192 (7.5%) were aged more than 50 years; and of these, only 42 (22%) were women (25). Although psychologic and sociocultural factors play an important role in the cause of many sexual problems, in the older population anatomic and physiologic causes of sexual dysfunctions are more common. Most sexual problems that the physician evaluates in the postmenopausal female are related to estrogen loss to the genitals, with the most common being lack of adequate vaginal lubrication with sexual arousal, dyspareunia, and postcoital bleeding. Although some women have a decrease in sexual desire, most women continue to want sexual relations well into their menopausal years; however, they may be reluctant to pursue these desires because of fear of coital pain from local atrophic changes.

Dyspareunia is usually of the insertional type in aging women. Although Hällström (26) reported coital pain in only 8% of 231 postmenopausal women he studied, Eskin noted that dyspareunia was the second most frequent presenting complaint of postmenopausal women requesting gynecologic services (27). Bachmann et al. (28) found that 30% of postmenopausal women not on hormone replacement therapy experience dyspareunia. These subjects also reported wanting less coital exchange than subjects without dyspareunia.

Vaginal dryness plays a significant role in sexual dysfunction in the menopausal woman. Vaginal dryness has not only been associated with painful intercourse, but also with a decrease in sexual desire (29). Because the postmenopausal vagina has decreased basal levels of vaginal capillary blood flow and oxygen it does not reach the level of engorgement that the estrogen-primed vagina does during sexual arousal. Estrogen replacement therapy results in an increase in vaginal lubrication, blood flow, and oxygen levels (9,30,31).

Menopausal patients should be given supportive guidance and factual information about changes in sexual function. Even when urogenital factors have been reversed by estrogen therapy, the loss of sexual desire and arousal may persist. Some women, especially those who have been oophorectomized, may need the addition of an androgen to improve sexual desire (32–35).

The level of sexual function for many older women will be determined by the activity of their partner. Vulvovaginal changes and associated symptoms of the woman may affect the sexual performance of the man as well. Medical problems and cancer become more prevalent during the later years and the impact of these diseases on sexual function also need to be addressed. When couples experience problems that are chronic and not improved by hormonal therapy, more extensive counseling and education, such as information on alternative sexual activities or referral to a sex specialist should be considered (36).

SURGERY AND VULVOVAGINAL FUNCTION

Vulvar or vaginal surgery, especially when done for malignancy, can further exacerbate genital dysfunction in the older woman as these procedures can also decrease the size of the introitus and vaginal barrel. The prevalence of hysterectomy with or without oophorectomy increases during the menopausal years. Although a simple hysterectomy usually does not interfere with the size and function of the vaginal vault, the vaginal anatomy and physiology can be adversely affected by radical procedures, in which a large portion of the vaginal barrel is excised or when radiation therapy to the pelvis precedes or follows the surgery. If vaginal problems are reported after a nonradical hysterectomy, they are usually related to loss of estrogen either from concomitant oophorectomy or surgical compromise of ovarian blood flow (37). It is interesting to note that a recent US trial studying the efficacy and safety of the estrogen-releasing vaginal ring versus vaginal estrogen cream reported a large percentage of the subjects (49% of the ring subjects and 40% of the cream subjects) were hysterectomized (18). Although some data suggest a role of the cervix in maintaining vaginal function and orgasmic ability, this relationship remains controversial.

Vulvectomy, especially when radical dissection is necessary, can affect genital appearance but usually does not cause vulvovaginal symptoms. Sexual complaints after vulvar surgery such as insertional dyspareunia, postcoital bleeding, or vaginismus may result from decreased introital size, scarring, or pressure against the perineum with intromission. If the vulvar excision compromises the cushioning effect of the vulva, the woman may note perineal discomfort with the use of snug undergarments or when sitting in a straddle position. Although it can impact on sexual comfort in some coital positions, vulvectomy with preservation of the clitoris should have no adverse effect on sexual desire, arousal, or orgasmic ability.

EVALUATION

In the reproductive-aged woman, most vulvovaginal complaints are assumed to be caused by an infectious process; in the menopausal woman, these complaints are assumed to occur because of atrophy from estrogen loss. A complete evaluation should be performed to rule out other causes as well. Often the most probable cause can be obtained from the medical history. The earliest symptoms of vulvovaginal dysfunction will be a gradual slowing in the onset and a decline in the amount of vaginal secretions during sexual exchange. The acute onset of vulvovaginal complaints accompanied by discharge and pelvic or abdominal pain, especially if associated with a recent change in sexual partner, would infer an infectious cause. Rapid swelling of the external genitalia would be suggestive of a sebaceous, Bartholin's, or Skene's gland cause. The growth of any lesion on the vulva or vagina should prompt the suspicion of a benign or malignant tumor. Although vulvar and vaginal cancers are uncommon, any suspicious lesions, new growths, plaques, ulcerations, sites of induration, or changes in color should be biopsied and histologically evaluated. Multiple biopsies may be necessary to differentiate the inflammatory lesions of the vulva such as squamous cell hyperplasia and lichen sclerosus (formerly the vulvar dystrophies) from vulvar intraepithelial neoplasia and squamous cell carcinoma.

The pelvic examination of menopausal patients should include assessment of vulvovaginal atrophy even if the patient has not offered these complaints. The visual inspection of the vaginal epithelium should assess its integrity including friability, pallor, and the presence of petechiae. Bleeding from minimal trauma such as speculum insertion should be noted. The amount and character of the vaginal fluid should be assessed because of its association with hormonal status. The vaginal pH has been shown to be a simple and reliable method of assessing estrogen influence, with the loss of the acidic vaginal pH corresponding to atrophic changes in vaginal cytology (11,38). Following the patient through the perimenopausal and postmenopausal years with a vaginal health index is often useful in determining current and future treatment (Table 18.3) (39). Estrogen-dependent maturation of the vaginal epithelium

TABLE 18.3. Vaginal health index

Condition	1	2	3	4	5
Overall elasticity	None	Poor	Fair	Good	Excellent
Fluid secretion, type, and consistency	None	Scant, thin, yellow	Superficial layer of thin white	Moderate layer of thin white	Normal (white, flocculent)
pH	6.1 or above	5.6–6.0	5.1–5.5	4.7–5.0	4.6 or below
Epithelial integrity	Petechiae noted before contact epithelium	Petechiae noted after contact	Bleeds with scraping	Not friable, thin epithelium	Not friable, normal
Moisture	None, epithelium inflamed	None, epithelium not inflamed	Minimal	Moderate	Normal

Note: the lower the score, the greater the atrophy.

can also be assessed using vaginal cytology. The Maturation Index (MI), Maturation Value (MV), and Karyopyknotic Index (KPI), are based on the relative proportions of superficial, intermediate, and parabasal cell types on vaginal cytology. Although these numeric values are mainly used in clinical research trials, they can also be used to evaluate an individual patient's response to treatment.

TREATMENT

Physician intervention in the care of women with vulvovaginal complaints should be individualized, and it should depend on the pattern and severity of symptoms, the medical history, and the lifestyle of the patient. Estrogen therapy, which is effective at reversing the atrophic changes of the menopause, will improve or eliminate the vulvovaginal symptoms these patients experience (17–21, 40–42). Although improvement in subjective complaints and objective signs can occur within a few weeks, other physiologic parameters of vaginal function can take months to reach maximal benefit (9). Semmens was the first to study scientifically postmenopausal vaginal physiology and the effect of estrogen (31). This work confirmed that with estrogen replacement therapy, vaginal blood flow and vaginal electropotential difference increased, vaginal pH decreased, and vaginal cytology returned to the premenopausal pattern (9,31). Of interest, menopausal women who are sexually active have been found to have a lower baseline vaginal pH and with estrogen use they had a greater decrease in vaginal pH than sexually abstinent women (9,43).

Local therapy can provide some patients with quicker or more complete relief of genitourinary complaints than systemic preparations (17,44). Women taking systemic estrogen therapy who have not had satisfactory resolution of vulvovaginal changes may benefit from use of local vaginal treatment as well. Vaginal estrogen creams are consistently effective at reversing the atrophic changes and relieving the local symptoms these women experience. Treatment should commence with a loading dose of 2 to 4 g (one-half to one-full applicator) of vaginal estrogen cream daily for 2 weeks. After the initial therapeutic response is achieved with the vaginal cream, the frequency and dose can be titrated to meet the requirements of the patient. Smaller doses used one to three times per week are usually sufficient to maintain the beneficial results. It is important to note that the systemic absorption of vaginally applied estrogen cream is significantly greater when the vagina is atrophic than when the normal physiology of the vagina has been restored (45).

An estradiol-releasing silicone vaginal ring has recently become available for the local delivery of estrogen to the vulvovaginal tissues. The estrogen ring, when placed in the top of the vaginal vault, continuously releases 5 to 10 µg/day of estradiol for up to 90 days (46). The estradiol-releasing ring has been shown to improve significantly patient symptoms such as vaginal dryness, vaginal pruritis, dyspareunia, frequency, and urgency. Ring use also results in improvement of vaginal cytology maturation, decrease in vaginal pH to premenopausal levels, and improvement in physician assessment of vaginal epithelial integrity (17–21).

Systemic estrogen therapy and high-dose vaginal estrogen therapies are known to have a stimulatory effect on the endometrium. Whenever unopposed estrogen replacement therapy is given, there should be concern about its trophic effects on the endometrium which can result in proliferation, hyperplasia, or carcinoma. Low-dose vaginal therapies have been studied in an attempt to find a way of providing relief of vulvovaginal symptoms without endometrial effects. In one study, estradiol 25 µg vaginal tablets given twice weekly relieved vaginal symptoms with only 6% (2 of 31) of patients demonstrating an endometrial response (e.g., a prestudy atrophic endometrium changing to a poststudy weakly proliferative one) (41). In another study, 109 menopausal women were given 3.5 mg estriol vaginal tablets twice weekly for 3 weeks, then once per week for 6 months; their vaginal symptoms improved without evidence of endometrial stimulation (42). One study using the low-dose estradiol-releasing vaginal ring showed no vaginal bleeding (20), whereas another showed no sign of stimulation on progestagen challenge test and endometrial stipe thickness as assessed by pelvic sonogram (21). Two other studies using the estrogen ring showed the rate of endometrial stimulation, as evidenced by progestagen challenge test and endometrial biopsy, to be equivalent to low-dose conjugated estrogen vaginal cream (17,18).

In patients who cannot use or choose not to use estrogen therapy, nonhormonal vaginal preparations can be of benefit, especially for the relief of coital discomfort. Water-based vaginal lubricating jellies are well tolerated. During sexual activity they provide relief of vaginal dryness with decreased friction on atrophic vulvovaginal structures. Longer lasting benefits may be achieved with a nonhormonal bioadhesive moisturizing gel (47,48). It is essential for the patients to be educated about urogenital atrophy as many may not be aware of therapies available, and may be reluctant to talk to their physicians about this problem. Improvement in vaginal dryness and dyspareunia can allow the return to the premenopausal level of sexual function for many older patients.

Treatment of the inflammatory conditions of the vulva starts with the removal of local irritants and improved hygiene. Soaps, bath lotions, deodorant powders, and laundry detergents should be carefully selected as these products can contain perfumes and dyes to which the patient is sensitive. If the onset of contact dermatitis is temporally associated with a new product, then removal may be curative. Prolonged exposure to moisture can also lead to vulvar irritation. Patients should be encouraged to avoid tight layers and synthetic garments that prevent evaporation of external genital moisture. Patients should thoroughly dry the genital area with towels or a blow dryer after bathing or swimming. Low-potency topical steroids will provide relief of symptoms and decrease inflammation while the conservative measures are being instituted.

Squamous cell hyperplasia of the vulva, formerly called "hyperplastic dystrophy," requires a medium strength steroid cream in addition to the avoidance of irritants. Fluocinolone acetonide (0.01%) or triamcinolone acetonide (0.1%) should be applied twice per day until symptoms start to improve and then treatment can be decreased to once per day. After 2 to 3 weeks, clinical improvement is usually complete and the steroid can be discontinued.

When vulvar biopsy indicates lichen sclerosis, treatment requires the use of a super-high potency steroid cream. Clobetasol propionate (0.05%) cream is effective at relieving the vulvar pruritis and discomfort these women experience, and it improves the gross and histologic features of the effected skin (49). Initial therapy should include application twice per day for 1 month and then daily for 2 months. A maintenance regimen consisting of twice weekly application has been shown to be effective for an additional 12 weeks (50).

Atrophic changes of the vulva, vagina, and lower urinary tract can detract from the quality of life of menopausal women. The patient may initially attribute the symptoms of atrophy to other vulvovaginal conditions. Embarrassment arising from cultural or religious beliefs can prevent the patient from openly discussing problems related to sexual function. Sensitive questioning and thorough evaluation will correctly identify the pattern of changes as those caused by the loss of estrogen. Hormonal and nonhormonal treatments can provide patients with relief and a return to their previous level of function. Because these atrophic changes respond favorably to estrogen therapy, no reason exists for older women to suffer from urogenital atrophy symptoms.

REFERENCES

1. Kellogg JH. Hygiene for women in advanced life. In: Kellogg JH, ed. *Plain facts for old and young: embracing the natural history and hygiene of organic life.* Burlington, IA: IF Segner; 1888:453–456.
2. Stenberg Å, Heimer G, Ulmsten U, Cnattingius S. Prevalence of genitourinary and other climacteric symptoms in 61-year-old women. *Maturitas* 1996;24:31–36.
3. Diokno AC, Brock BM, Brown MB, Herzog AR. Prevalence of urinary incontinence and other urological symptoms in the noninstitutionalized elderly. *J Urol* 1986;136:1022–1025.
4. Oriba HA, Maibach HI. Vulvar transepidermal water loss (TEWL) decay curves. Effect of occlusion, delipidation, and age. *Acta Derm Venereol* 1989;69(6):461–465.
5. Kaufman RH, Friedrich EG, Gardner HL. *Benign diseases of the vulva*, 3rd ed. Chicago: Year Book Medical Publishers, 1989.
6. Gould SG, Shannon JM, Cunha GR. The autoradiographic demonstration of estrogen binding in normal human cervix and vagina during the menstrual cycle, pregnancy, and the menopause. *Am J Anat* 1983;168(2):229–238.
7. Itoh I, Manaka M. Analysis of human vaginal secretions by SDS-polyacrylamide gel electrophoresis. *Forensic Sci Int* 1988;37:237–242.
8. Paavonen J. Physiology and ecology of the vagina. *Scand J Infect Dis Suppl* 1983; 40:31–35.
9. Semmens JP, Tsai CC, Curtis Semmens E, Loadholt CB. Effects of estrogen therapy on vaginal physiology during menopause. *Obstet Gynecol* 1985;66:15–18.
10. Steward-Tule DES. Evidence that vaginal lactobacilli do not ferment glycogen. *Am J Obstet Gynecol* 1964;88:676–679.
11. Milsom I, Arvidsson L, Ekelund P, Molander U, Eriksson O. Factors influencing vaginal cytology, pH and bacterial flora in elderly women. *Acta Obstet Gynecol Scand* 1993;72:286–91.
12. Eschenbach DA, Davick PR, Williams BL, et al. Prevalence of hydrogen peroxide-producing lactobacillus species in normal women and women with bacterial vaginosis. *J Clin Microbiol* 1989;27:251–256.
13. Klebanoff SJ, Hillier SL, Eschenbach DA, Waltersdorph AM. Control of the microbial flora of the vagina by H₂O₂-generating lactobacilli. *J Infect Dis* 1991;164:94–100.
14. Heimer G, Samsioe G. Effects of vaginally delivered estrogens. *Acta Obstet Gynecol Scand Suppl* 1996;163:16–25.
15. Iosif CS, Batra S, Ek A, Åstedt B. Estrogen receptors in the human female lower urinary tract. *Am J Obstet Gynecol* 1981;141:817–820.
16. Bhatia NN, Bergman A, Karram MM. Effects of estrogen on urethral function in women with urinary incontinence. *Am J Obstet Gynecol* 1989;160:176–181.
17. Ayton RA, Darling GM, Murkies AL, et al. A comparative study of safety and efficacy of continuous low dose oestradiol released from a vaginal ring compared with conjugated equine oestrogen vaginal cream in the treatment of postmenopausal urogenital atrophy. *Br J Obstet Gynecol* 1996;103:351–358.
18. Bachmann G, Notelovitz M, Nachtigall L, Birgerson L. A comparative study of a low-dose estradiol vaginal ring and conjugated estrogen cream for postmenopausal urogenital atrophy. *Prim Care Update Ob/Gyns* 1997;4:109–115.
19. Barentsen R, van de Weijer PHM, Schram JHN. Continuous low dose estradiol released from a vaginal ring versus estriol vaginal cream for urogenital atrophy. *Eur J Obstet Gynecol Reprod Biol* 1997;71:73–80.
20. Henriksson L, Stjernquist M, Boquist L, Ålander U, Selinus I. A comparative multicenter study of the effects of continuous low-dose estradiol released from a new vaginal ring versus estriol vaginal pessaries in postmenopausal women with symptoms and signs of urogenital atrophy. *Am J Obstet Gynecol* 1994;171:624–632.
21. Smith P, Heimer G, Lindskog M, Ulmsten U. Oestradiol-releasing vaginal ring for treatment of postmenopausal urogenital atrophy. *Maturitas* 1993;16:145–154.
22. Raz R, Stamm WE. A controlled trial of intravaginal estriol in postmenopausal women with recurrent urinary tract infections. *N Engl J Med* 1993;329:753–756.
23. Bachmann GA, Leiblum SR, Grill J. Brief sexual inquiry in gynecologic practice. *Obstet Gynecol* 1989;73:425–427.
24. Frank E, Anderson C, Rubinstein DR. Frequency of sexual dysfunction in normal couples. *N Engl J Med* 1978;299:111–115.
25. Wise TN, Rabins PV, Gahnsley J. The older patient with a sexual dysfunction. *J Sex Marital Ther* 1984;10:117–121.
26. Hällström T. Sexuality in the climacteric. *Clin Obstet Gynecol* 1977;4:227.
27. Eskin B. Sex and the gynecologic patient. In: Oaks WW, Melchiode GA, Ficher I, eds. *Sex and the life cycle.* New York: Grune & Stratton, 1976.
28. Bachmann GA, Leiblum SR, Kemmann E, et al. Sexual expression and its determinants in the post-menopausal woman. *Maturitas* 1984;6:19–29.
29. Bachmann GA, Leiblum SR, Bernard S, et al. Correlates of sexual desire in postmenopausal women. *Maturitas* 1985;7:211–216.
30. Hoon PW. Physiologic assessment of sexual response in women: the unfulfilled promise. *Clin Obstet Gynecol* 1984;27:767–779.
31. Semmens J, Wagner G. Estrogen deprivation and vaginal function in postmenopausal women. *JAMA* 1982;248:445.
32. Sherwin BB, Gelfand MM, Brender W. Androgen enhances sexual motivation in females: a prospective, crossover study of sex steroid administration in the surgical menopause. *Psychosom Med* 1985;47:339–351.
33. Sherin BB, Gelfand MM. Differential symptom response to parenteral estrogen and/or androgen administration in the surgical menopause. *Am J Obstet Gynecol* 1985;151:153–160.
34. Sherwin BB. Affective changes with estrogen and androgen replacement therapy in surgically menopausal women. *J Affect Disord* 1988;14:177–187.
35. Burger H, Hailes J, Nelson J, Menelaus M. Effect of combined implants of oestradiol and testosterone on libido in postmenopausal women. *Br Med J* 1987;295:936–937.
36. Schover LR, Evans RB, von Eschenbach AC. Sexual rehabilitation in a cancer center: diagnosis and outcome in 384 consultations. *Arch Sex Behav* 1987;16:445–461.
37. Seidenschnur G, Beck H, Uplegger H, et al. Attitude and sex behavior following hysterectomy. *Zentralbl Gynakol* 1989;111(1):53–59.
38. Nilsson K, Risberg B, Heimer G. The vaginal epithelium in the postmenopause—cytology, histology and pH as methods of assessment. *Maturitas* 1995;21:51–56.
39. Bachmann GA, Notelovitz M, Gonzalez SJ, Thompson C, Morecraft BA. Vaginal dryness in menopausal women: clinical characteristics and nonhormonal treatment. *Clin Prac Sexual* 1991;7:25–32.
40. Good WR, John VA, Ramirez M, Higgins JE. Double-masked, multicenter study of an estradiol matrix transdermal delivery system (Alora™) versus placebo in postmenopausal women experiencing menopausal symptoms. *Clinical Therapeutics* 1996;18(6):1093–1105.
41. Mettler L, Olsen PG. Long-term treatment of atrophic vaginitis with low-dose oestradiol vaginal tablets. *Maturitas* 1991;14:23–31.
42. Foidart JM, Vervliet J, Buytaert P. Efficacy of sustained-release vaginal oestriol in alleviating urogenital and systemic climacteric complaints. *Maturitas* 1991;13: 99–107.
43. Tsai CC, Semmens JP, Semmens EC, Lam CF, Lee FS. Vaginal physiology in postmenopausal women: pH value, transvaginal electropotential difference, and estimated blood flow. *South Med J* 1987;80(8):987–990.
44. Gabrielsson J, Wallenbeck I, Birgerson L. Pharmacokinetic data on estradiol in light of the estring concept. *Acta Obstet Gynecol Scand Suppl* 1996;163:26–31.
45. Pschera H, Hjerpe A, Carlstrom K. Influence of the maturity of the vaginal epithe-

lium upon the absorption of vaginally administered estradiol-17 beta and progesterone in postmenopausal women. *Gynecol Obstet Invest* 1989;27:204–207.

46. Schmidt G, Andersson SB, Nordle Ö, Johansson CJ, Gunnarsson PO. Release of 17-beta-oestradiol from a vaginal ring in postmenopausal women: pharmacokinetic evaluation. *Gynecol Obstet Invest* 1994;38:253–260.

47. Bygdeman M, Swahn ML. Replens versus dienoestrol cream in the symptomatic treatment of vaginal atrophy in postmenopausal women. *Maturitas* 1996;23: 259–263.

48. Nachtigall LE. Comparative study: replens versus local estrogen in menopausal women. *Fertil Steril* 1994;61(1):178–180.

49. Bracco GL, Carli P, Sonni L, et al. Clinical and histologic effects of topical treatments of vulval lichen sclerosus, a critical evaluation. *J Reprod Med* 1993;38(1): 37–40.

50. Cattaneo A, Carli P, De Marco A, et al. Testosterone maintenance therapy, effects on vulvar lichen sclerosus treated with clobetasol propionate. *J Reprod Med* 1996; 41:99–102.

Treatment of the Postmenopausal Woman: Basic and Clinical Aspects, Second Edition, edited by Rogerio A. Lobo, Lippincott Williams & Wilkins, Philadelphia © 1999.

CHAPTER 19

Collagen

The Significance in Skin, Bone, and Carotid Arteries

Mark P. Brincat and Ray Galea

Collagen is the major protein component of most connective tissues in vertebrates. It constitutes approximately 25% to 35% of total protein in mammals. It is present in virtually every animal tissue, providing an extracellular framework for all metazoan animals. It is a highly conserved, evolutionarily ancient family of molecules.

Collagens are a large family of proteins, which includes at least 19 different members found in human tissues. These members of the collagen family are made up of various combinations of approximately 30 distinct polypeptide chains. The polypeptide chains are all encoded by specific genes.

Collagen molecules are characterized by the formation of three left-handed polypeptide helical chains tightly coiled around each other in a ropelike fashion to form a right-handed super coil. The collagen helix is more extended than an alpha helix because it has three amino acid residues per turn with a pitch of 0.94 nm giving a rise of 0.31 nm per residue. All collagens contain greater or lesser stretches of this triple helix.

Two basic alpha-chains have been identified in collagen (α-1 and α-2) each consisting of over 100 amino acid in groups of three in the basic collagen triple helix configuration. The triple helix domains of the collagens consist of repeats of the amino acid sequence Gly-X-Y. Position X is usually filled by proline, whereas position Y is usually occupied by hydroxyproline. The ring structure of the latter amino acids is responsible for the stabilization of the helical conformations of the polypeptide chains. Hydroxy proline is usually formed in the endoplasmic reticulum by alteration of the proline residues by means of the enzyme, prolyl hydroxylase. These proline residues would have

already been incorporated into collagen polypeptide chains. Further stabilization of the triple helix is achieved because the hydroxyl groups of these modified amino acids tend to form hydrogen bonds between the polypeptide chains. This very stable structure forms the basic building unit of collagenous structures. Proline and hydroxyproline constitute 20% to 25% of total amino acids in collagen.

The biosynthesis of collagen has several unusual features. One is the extensive use of the principle of spontaneous self-assembly seen in the formation of crystals. The three polypeptide chains of the protein fold into a triple helical conformation by a process that begins with the formation of a small nucleus of triple helix at the C-terminal of the molecule, after which occurs propagation of the nucleus in a zipperlike fashion. The self-assembly of the collagen monomers into fibrils is an entropy driven, crystallization-like process.

Collagens can also be divided into two main groups: the fibrillar and the nonfibrillar collagens. Other smaller groups, such as the network forming and the anchoring filaments, exist. In the form of fibers, collagen acts to transmit forces, dissipate energy, and prevent mechanical failure in normal tissues. Deformation of collagen fibers involves molecular stretching and slippage, fibrillar slippage, and, ultimately, defibrillation.

Type I collagen, which constitutes 90% of the total collagen in the body, is the most important one (1). It is predominant in skin and bone. Skin also contains some of the very similar, type III, collagen.

CONNECTIVE TISSUE

Connective tissue consists of other cellular and extracellular elements in addition to collagen. The extracellular matrix contains three major classes of biomolecules:

M. P. Brincat, R. Galea: Department of Obstetrics and Gynaecology, St. Luke's Hospital Medical School, Gwardamangia, Malta.

- Structural proteins such as collagen, elastin, and fibrillin
- Specialized proteins such as fibronectin, fibrillin, and laminin
- Proteoglycans, consisting of long chains of repeating disaccharides (what were formerly called "mucopolysaccharides" and now known as "glycosaminoglycans" [GAG]) attached to specific core proteins

Glycosaminoglycan chains allow rapid diffusion of water molecules, and they are responsible for the turgor in the compressive forces. Collagen fibrils, on the other hand, resist stretching of the tissues. By weight, GAG amount to less than 5% of the fibrous protein; the rest are composed largely of collagen with some elastin (2). Although the bulk of the body collagen is remarkably stable, a fraction of the collagen in all tissues is continuously degraded and replaced even in old age. Such change in overall collagen metabolism can be followed by assaying excretion of peptide-bound hydroxyproline in urine (3) because excretion of these substances is largely caused by collagen degradation (4). Changes in collagen metabolism can also be assessed by urinary assay of pyridinium cross-links. Bone collagen markers are now becoming widely used to assess collagen turnover. Several studies now seem to show that bone collagen markers in combination with bone mass measurement may be useful in detecting the risk for osteoporosis and for fractures and in monitoring closely the efficacy of antiresorptive drugs in postmenopausal women (5).

COLLAGEN CHANGES WITH AGE

Quality, type, and amount of collagen change with age. For example, type III collagen is found in a greater amount in the skin of young animals than in that of older animals. This may indicate gene switching comparable to the switch from fetal and embryonic hemoglobin to hemoglobin A, the adult form. Growth of connective tissue involves an increased rate of collagen biosynthesis, which is reflected in an increased tissue level of intracellular posttranslational enzymes. Both the rates of translation and the levels of these enzymes decrease with age (6).

Collagen decrease in the skin and bone after the menopause gives rise to osteoporosis and decreased skin thickness. This decrease can be prevented with estrogen replacement therapy (ERT) (7). This finding suggests that the collagen decrease after the menopause is caused by estrogen deficiency (8). Although estrogen therapy prevents and also may reverse postmenopausal bone loss, it is still not clear whether this effect is mediated only via estrogens or if a progesterone deficiency also plays a part. Recent work has shown, however, that progesterone can increase osteoclast number, but with no apparent increase in osteoclast function. In the rat, progesterone did not prevent bone loss (9,10).

The menopause is a period in a woman's life characterized by a lack of estrogen. This hypoestrogenic state gives rise to profound effects on all organs containing connective tissue. Albright et al. (11) speculated that postmenopause

osteoporosis was part of a generalized connective tissue disorder, having observed that the skin of women with this disorder was noticeably thin. McConkey et al. (12) showed that transparent skin on the back of the hand was common in women aged more than 60 years, and they found that the incidence of osteoporosis in women with transparent skin was 83% versus 12.5% in women with opaque skin. In fact, because of the decrease in ovarian steroids, mainly estrogens, in the menopause a decline in skin thickness and skin collagen occurs, causing skin deterioration as evidenced by dry, wrinkled, flaky, and easily bruised skin. A concomitant decline also occurs in bone mass.

Evidence suggests that postmenopausal bone loss and the decrease in skin thickness share a common cause, that is, an overall decline in connective tissues affecting these organs. These changes occur as a result of estrogen deficiency. The organs affected include bone, skin, the vascular system, and the urogenital system, among others.

Bone and skin together contain approximately 80% of all the connective tissues found in the human body. Both show a deterioration with estrogen deficiency. This deterioration can be prevented and even reversed with appropriate and adequate estrogen replacement (13–16).

BONE

Bone is a dynamic structure. It is made up of both organic and inorganic material. Studies in postmenopausal women have concentrated primarily on the inorganic component. The main organic matter is protein of which there are two main types, the collagens and the noncollagen proteins.

Of the collagens, type I is the main collagen with type V being a minor component. The noncollagen proteins include plasma proteins, proteoglycans, osteocalcin, osteopontin, osteonectin, and bone sialoprotein. Collagen makes up the greatest proportion of bone as approximately 35% of dry defatted bone mass contains collagen. The organic matrix of bone acts rather like internal girders and confers on bone its tensile strength. It has been suggested that the decline in this organic matrix is the primary pathologic event leading to osteoporosis (17,18).

Because bone is a living structure, it is being remodeled throughout the lifespan. This remodeling is brought about at the cellular level by bone-resorbing cells (osteoclasts) and bone-forming cells (osteoblasts). The osteoclasts and osteoblasts remove and replace small quantities of bone at certain points throughout the skeleton. Bone mass at any point in life represents the balance attained between the peak bone mass laid down by the fourth decade of life and the amount of bone lost with aging. This loss of bone is an age-related loss in both sexes; however, in women bone loss accelerates following the menopause. It has been shown (19) that by the age of 70 years women lose up to 50% of their bone mass, whereas a man would be expected to lose only 25% by the age of 90 years.

To investigate the relationship between age, bone mass, and skin thickness, our group conducted a study of postmenopausal women. This was a biophysical study in which we looked at differences in various bone density measurements and in skin thickness. Bone was measured using a dual energy x-ray absorptiometer (between lumbar vertebra 2 and 4, at the femur neck, and at Ward's triangle), and skin thickness was measured using high frequency (22 MHz) ultrasound, which correlates with the collagen content in skin. These measurements were carried out on a group of untreated postmenopausal women and a group of untreated postmenopausal women who had sustained an osteoporotic fracture. The results showed that the skin thickness and bone density parameters were much lower in women who had sustained osteoporotic fractures compared with controls (Fig. 19.1).

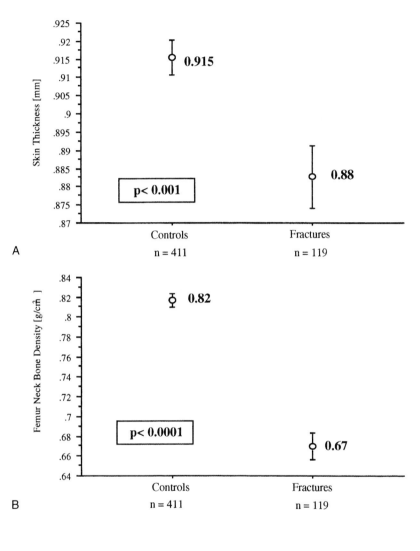

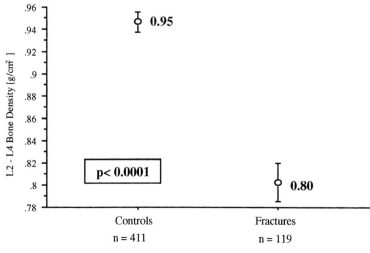

FIG. 19.1. Mean plot of skin thickness in patients with osteoporotic fractures and controls (**A**); femur neck bone density in patients with osteoporotic fractures and controls (**B**); and L2-L4 bone density in patients with osteoporotic fractures and controls (**C**).

Women with fractures had mean bone mass values that were approximately 20% below the mean values of controls. Skin thickness varied within a narrower range (mean difference 4%), but significant differences between controls and women who had sustained an osteoporotic fracture were also consistently noted. When the skin thickness measurements were combined with bone density parameters, the accuracy of predicting an osteoporotic fracture was increased as shown in Fig. 19.2 (20).

Bone has been shown to be an estradiol-responsive tissue. In women, a hypoestrogenemic state leads to increased bone loss, especially in the first few years of estrogen deprivation. This increased loss is probably caused by an increase in the number and activity of the osteoclasts. In fact, at the cellular level estrogen has been shown to inhibit the differentiation of osteoclasts, which results in a decrease in the numbers and activity of osteoclasts. The mechanism of action is probably mediated via some cytokines, most probably interleukin 1 (IL-1) and 6

(IL-6). It is known that estrogen regulates the expression of IL-6 in the bone marrow cells, although the modality of action is not known. On the other hand, the effect of estrogen on osteoblasts (the bone forming cells) may either be a direct effect or it may rely on an alteration of the coupling phenomenon of bone metabolism (21).

Estrogen replacement therapy affects osteoporosis in two ways: it can either prevent it or else it can treat it once it has occurred. It has been postulated that ERT led to an increase in bone mass by increasing collagen levels in bone. Indeed, the observation that women on ERT had a higher dermal skin collagen content than those who were not has led to the belief that a similar increase in bone collagen content in women on ERT occurred. It was possibly this increase in collagen content that was leading to an increase in bone strength and, thus, to a diminution of osteoporotic fractures. When estrogens are started in the menopausal period and continued into late life, the best result *vis-á-vis* bone density are obtained. If estrogen

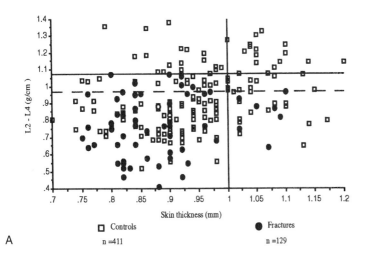

	Sensitivity	Accuracy
Skin Thickness	91.8%	38.7%
L2 - L4	100.0%	39.6%
Box L2 - L4	91.8%	50.1%

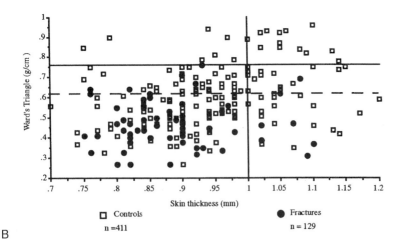

	Sensitivity	Accuracy
Skin Thickness	91.7%	39.2%
Ward's Triangle	100.0%	50.9%
Box Ward's Triangle	91.7%	59.1%

FIG. 19.2. A: Scattergram for L2-L4 versus skin thickness. **B:** Scattergram for Ward's triangle versus skin thickness.

therapy is initiated later on in life, however, the benefits obtained are also good (22)

To look at the collagen changes occurring with estrogen therapy, our group undertook another study (23). This was a biophysical–biochemical study between a group of untreated postmenopausal women and a group of women who were on estrogen replacement therapy. Apart from having the same bone density and skin thickness measurements as in the previous study mentioned above, the women in this study also had collagen marker estimations. In this study we looked at the excretion of procollagen I C-end terminal peptides (PCICP), a marker for bone formation and pyridinium crosslinks, a marker for bone resorption.

When the untreated postmenopausal controls were compared with women who had been on hormone replacement therapy, the latter showed a drastic decrease in osteoclastic activity (pyridinium crosslinks excretion). The mean decrease was 27.2%. A decrease was also seen in bone formation, and osteoblastic activity (serum PCICP) was decreased by a mean of 11.3%. All these differences ($p < 0.001$) indicated that bone remodeling had readjusted in patients on estrogen. The women in this study who were taking hormone replacement therapy had only been on this treatment for a short time (mean 6 months), which may imply that changes occur rapidly. It is interesting to note, according to the above calculations based on bone collagen markers, that a mean positive change of 15.9% occurred in bone remodeling in women on ERT. This value is of the same order as the mean percentage change in bone mass of the same women, measured using biophysical method, which showed a mean positive change at the L2–L4 region of 16.1% (Fig. 19.3) (23).

The finding could indicate that these markers are indeed sensitive and can be used in monitoring postmenopausal bone loss as well as accurately titrating response to treatment, both when such treatment is prophylactic and when used therapeutically in the management of established osteoporosis. The excretion of pyridinium crosslinks of collagen in the first morning void urine samples shows some intraindividual variation (24), which may be a limitation of their usefulness. Some authors (25) claim that the intact amino terminal propeptide of type I procollagen, a protein set free from the other end on the same procollagen molecule, is a more dynamic marker for bone metabolism than PCICP. According to these authors, therefore, it is recommended that PCICP be used as a marker reflecting the effect of estrogen on bone collagen formation during ERT. Increasing evidence (26) shows that collagen markers can be a useful tool in predicting osteoporosis and fracture risks, more so than bone mineral density measurements alone. It remains to be shown just how soon after treatment these collagen markers will change, although crosslink excretion has been shown characteristically to decrease after 6 months of treatment.

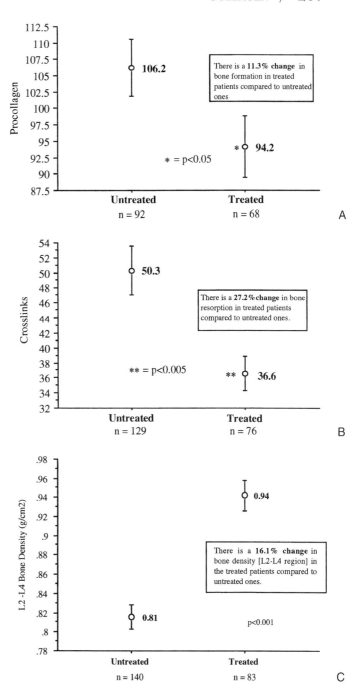

FIG. 19.3. A: Plot of mean procollagen in untreated patients an in patients with hormone replacement. B: Plot of mean crosslinks in untreated patients and in patients with hormone replacement. C: Plot of mean L2-L4 bone density in treated patients and in patients with hormone replacement.

The end result is that lack of estrogen present in women in the postmenopausal years causes this loss of bone mass, and clinically it results in osteoporosis with subsequent related osteoporotic fractures of the spine or hip. Such conditions are now both preventable and treatable and they should no longer be accepted as a part of the normal aging process. Physicians must be aware of this and they should strive to prevent or at least to treat osteoporosis.

SKIN

Skin is one of the largest organs in the body containing a sizable proportion of total body collagen. This organ is composed of a population of cells of diverse embryonic origin which under normal conditions exist side by side in complete harmony, forming a complex mosaic. Anatomically skin is made up of two main layers: the epidermis and dermis.

The epidermis, which forms a thin outer layer, is composed of keratinocytes (keratin-producing cells) of ectodermal origin intermingled with melanin-producing cells, the melanocytes, which arise from a specialized embryonic ectodermal tissue, the neural crest.

The other deeper layer is the dermis, a stroma that forms the main bulk of the skin. It is intimately bound with the overlaying epidermis; fingerlike processes or dermal papillae project upward into corresponding recesses in the epidermis. In contrast to the epidermis, the dermis is predominantly fibrous and contains blood vessels. It is of mesodermal origin as are all connective tissue (including bone). It also contains several structures derived from the embryonic ectoderm (e.g., sweat glands and hair follicles). The fibers present in the dermis consist of two main types of fibrous protein: collagen (97.5%) and elastin (2.5%) (27). Collagen fibers are responsible for the main mass and the resilience of the dermis. This collagen is disposed mainly in a parallel arrangement to the skin surface. The elastin fibers, on the other hand, form a subepidermal network, and they are only thinly distributed. Collagen is produced by fibroblasts. These cells contain abundant endoplasmic reticulum where secreted proteins such as collagen are synthesized from the main types of collagen found in connective tissues, types I, II, III, V, and XI.

Dermis atrophy after the menopause is caused by a decrease in the collagen content of the dermis. The amounts of hydroxyproline and glycosylated hydroxylysine (28,29) in type I collagen and of immature and reducible crosslinks decrease with age (30). To what extent these changes are fundamental to the aging process is still unknown. This decrease is not only arrested but reversed by hormone replacement therapy (31). Strong evidence as from the National Health and Nutrition Examination Survey (32) now indicates that estrogen use prevents dry skin and skin wrinkling, thus extending the potential benefits of postmenopausal estrogen therapy to include protection against selected age- and menopause-associated dermatologic conditions. In fact, estrogens have been shown to enhance the dermal content of water, GAG, and collagen. Both estrogen and androgen receptors have been identified on dermal fibroblasts (33). In a study to identify specific estrogen-sensitive structures (34), normal human skin was examined for the binding of the estrogen receptor (ER) D5 antibody, which is associated with p29, a 29 kd protein found in the cytoplasm of normal estrogen-sensitive cells. Strong and specific staining was seen to exert a specific effect on these tissues in the epidermis, with a gradient showing the most intense staining in the granular layer. Similar positive staining was seen in the hair follicles and sebaceous glands. Variable staining was seen in the eccrine glands and vessels. These findings demonstrate p29 to be present in these structures, and hence, that estrogens can exert a specific effect on these tissues.

Estrogen could increase the rate of collagen production (35) by altering the degree of polymerization of GAG. Estrogens increase the hydroscopic qualities (36), probably through enhanced synthesis of dermal hyaluronic acid (37). Collagenous fibrils were found to be less fragmented in the dermis of women treated with estrogens (38).

Studies have been carried out on skin changes in various connective tissue and endocrine disorders. Black (39) and Shuster et al. (40) looked at the relationship between skin thickness and skin collagen in systemic sclerosis, osteoporosis of mixed cause, and hirsute women and found a good correlation between the two. In a small study, Black (39) demonstrated changes in the collagen content and thickness of the skin of osteoporotic patients (mixed cause) treated with androgens, when compared with osteoporotic patients who had not been on this treatment. Shuster et al. (40) found an increase in skin collagen in hirsute women, but the increase was not statistically significant. Reports on the skin collagen changes with age are conflicting. Shuster and Bottoms (41,42) showed that the best way of expressing skin collagen content was by measuring the collagen content of a skin biopsy per square millimeter of skin surface. This method takes into account the possibility of changes in the total mass of the dermis. They reported a reduction in total skin collagen with age, but this was not confirmed by Reed and Hall (43). Shuster and Black found that the amount of collagen present in skin at all ages was greater in men than in women (40). Hall et al. (44) confirmed that skin collagen was greater in men than in women, but once again could not significantly confirm the decline of skin collagen with age. With increasing age past the menopause, the skin tends to get thinner, but this thinning can be reversed with adequate estrogen replacement therapy (17). This was first noted by Albright et al. (11) in 1940 who reported that elderly women with osteoporotic fractures had a higher incidence of thin skin. McConkey et al. (12) also showed that osteoporosis was more common in women with transparent skin then in women with thick opaque skin.

The dermal skin thickness is composed of connective tissue, including the predominant protein, collagen, elastin (small amounts), and glycoaminoglycans; it also has more than one variable that is affected by estrogen lack or its replacement. In the rat model, for example (35), castrated rats that were given estrogens had a 70% increase in their glycosaminoglycans content in 2 weeks. Similar glycosaminoglycan increases in women could lead to skin thickness increases beyond that which would be expected from collagen content increases alone.

Most of the studies have measured the thickness of dermis because it is the layer that is mainly composed of connective tissue. Subcutaneous tissue, which also includes subcutaneous fat, is an added variable and studies using Harpenden's calipers have been conflicting (45,46). Ultrasound can now be used to measure skin thickness. Ultrasound examination has been used by dermatologists when assessing dermal malignancies. Good reproducibility has been obtained by using high frequency (22 MHz) ultrasound to determine the thickness of the skin, excluding the subcutaneous tissues. Various studies have now shown that skin thickness increases with ERT. Skin and bone changes are linked with estrogen use at the menopause (17,18).

In animals, estrogen use appears to alter the vascularization of the skin (47). A change in the connective tissue of the dermis occurs, which is reflected by increased mucopolysaccharide incorporation, hydroxyproline turnover, and alterations in ground substance. In addition to increased dermal turnover of hyaluronic acid, the dermal water content is enhanced with estradiol therapy (37). Rauramo and Punnonen (48) observed that oral estrogen therapy in castrated women caused thickening of the epidermis for 3 months and persisted for 6 months.

Punnonen (49), using two different strengths of estrogens in castrated women, showed a statistically significant thickening of the epidermis after 3 months with both strengths, but this thickness persisted only with the lower dose. A third of the patients on the higher dose started getting significant thinning of the epidermis, possibly because the dosage and treatment was too strong and, therefore, was exerting a corticosteroid effect. Other authors were also able to show beneficial skin changes using both topical (18,50) and estradiol implants (51). Topical estradiol gel has also been shown to increase skin collagen content as measured by skin hydroxy proline. Skin blister fluids were assayed and an increase of both the C- and N-terminal peptides of procollagen I occurred with the gel.

In comparing a group of patients who had been on estradiol and testosterone implants from 2 to 10 years with a group of untreated postmenopausal women it was shown that the treated group had a highly significant greater skin collagen content than the untreated group. Optimal skin collagen was obtained after 2 years of an optimal estrogen regimen. A level too high or too low results in lower levels of collagen (52). The same conclusion was also reported in relation to the epidermis (53).

The decline in skin collagen content after the menopause occurs at a much more rapid rate in the initial postmenopausal years than in the later ones. Some 30% of skin collagen is lost in the first 5 years after the menopause (52) with an average decline of 2.1% per postmenopausal year over a period of 20 years. The increase in skin collagen content after 6 months of sex hormone therapy depends on the collagen content at the start of treatment (52). In women with a low skin collagen content, estrogens are initially of therapeutic value and later of prophylactic value, whereas in those with mild loss of collagen content in the early menopausal years estrogens are only of prophylactic value. Thus, a deficiency in skin collagen can be corrected but not over corrected.

Skin collagen content has been shown to have a strong correlation with skin dermal thickness measured radiologically (52). Using 100 mg subcutaneous estradiol implants, significant increases in skin thickness and metacarpal index occurred over a 1-year period. Most of the increase occurred in the first 6 months.

Brincat et al. (50–52, 54) and Castelo-Branco et al. (55,56) have shown that following the menopause skin collagen content and skin thickness are increased in women on estrogen replacement therapy compared with age-matched women on no treatment. Prospective studies have shown that skin thickness, skin collagen, and bone mass increase in postmenopausal women who start estrogen replacement therapy. Estrogen has been shown to reduce collagen turnover and improve collagen qualities (55,57). When postmenopausal women were treated with topical estrogens (58), after 6 months it was found that elasticity and firmness of the skin had markedly improved and the wrinkle depth and pore sizes had decreased by 61% to 100%. Furthermore, skin moisture also increased and the measurement of wrinkles using skin profilometry revealed significant, or highly significant, decreases in wrinkles. Immunohistochemistry of the same study group showed significant increases of type III collagen labeling were combined with increased numbers of collagen fibers at the end of the treatment period. This was also confirmed in a study by Creidi et al. (59).

The mechanical properties of the skin have been shown to be improved with ERT in other studies (60). In these studies, the mechanical properties were defined by ostensibility and elasticity measurements using a computerized device. Computerized measurements of skin deformability and viscoelasticity revealed differences between women on estrogen therapy, postmenopausal women on no treatment, and nonmenopausal controls. This parallels the changes noted elsewhere with skin collagen. A steep increase in skin extensibility was evidenced during the perimenopause in untreated women. Estrogen replacement therapy appeared to limit the age-related increase in cutaneous extensibility, thereby exerting a preventive effect on skin slackness. No effect of ERT was found on other parameters of skin viscoelasticity. Estrogen replacement therapy has a beneficial effect on some mechanical properties of skin and, thus, may slow the progress of intrinsic cutaneous aging.

Brincat et al. (51,61,62) found significant correlations between the skin (dermal) collagen, skin thickness (measured radiologically), and metacarpal index, both in postmenopausal women who had been on ERT and in untreated postmenopausal women. The common factor is the connective tissue present in all three sites. These findings were irrespective of the woman's age, number of years since the menopause, original skin thickness, or metacarpal index.

Attempts to identify the correct value of skin thickness measurement that could be used as a screening for menopausal osteoporosis have been underway for some time (63).

CAROTID ARTERIES

The cardioprotective effect of hormone replacement therapy has been proved (64). This effect has been attributed to the favorable serum lipoprotein profile brought

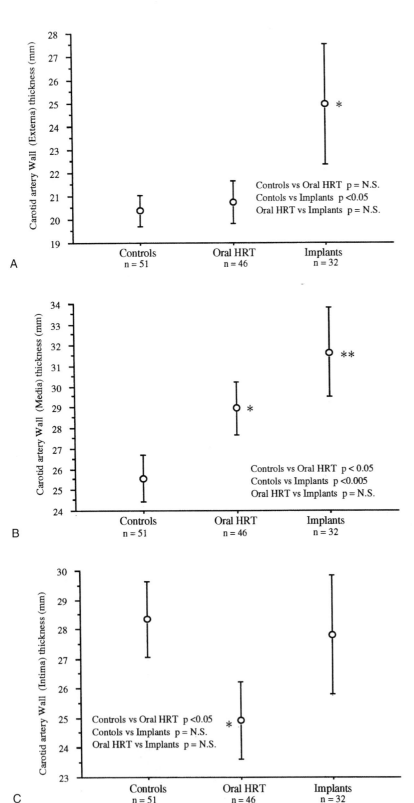

FIG. 19.4. A: Plot of artery wall (external [mean ± SE]) thickness in postmenopausal women on no treatment, on oral HRT, and estradiol implants. **B**: Plot of artery wall (media [mean ± SE]) thickness in postmenopausal women on no treatment, on oral HRT, and estradiol implants. **C**: Plot of artery wall (intima [mean ± SE]) thickness in postmenopausal women on no treatment, on oral HRT, and estradiol implants. HRT, hormone replacement therapy.

about by this treatment on postmenopausal women (65). Only 20% to 25% reduction in coronary artery plaque formation, however, can be accounted for (66); therefore, other mechanisms of cardioprevention are present. One such mechanism could result from postmenopausal connective tissue changes that mimic those in skin and bone. Using high-frequency ultrasound, our group looked at the differences in the layers of one of the major blood vessels, the carotid artery. One study investigated differences in the externa and media of the carotid artery in two groups of postmenopausal women on ERT and an untreated group, and also assessed the intima. The results showed that the media, the layer containing the greatest amount of collagen, was thicker in the estrogen treated group when compared with the untreated group. The intima of the untreated group was also shown to be significantly thicker than that of the treated group (Fig. 19.4). This finding signifies that less atherosclerotic plaque formed in the treated than in the untreated group. However, in women on a higher dose of estrogen (e.g., estradiol implant), the intima was as thick as in the untreated group. This was postulated as being caused by the collagen portion of the intima following the media and increasing in size at the expense of thinning of the atherosclerotic plaque as it is lost (67,68). Thus, it is postulated that these changes are brought about by estrogens. If these arterial changes induced by hormone replacement therapy also occur in the coronary arteries, which has been suggested (69), then such changes may partially explain the cardioprotective effect this treatment has on postmenopausal women.

CONCLUSIONS

The connective tissue component in the body represents a complex mass of intimately related cells and extracellular matrix that provides a mileau in which all the other cells are able to perform their functions and relate to each other. This tissue is acutely sensitive to sex steroids whose role has so far indicated that turnover of virtually every cell and of the extracellular matrix itself is modified by estrogen. Modifications in the noncollagenous extracellular matrix is outside the scope of this chapter, but the scanty evidence that exists suggests profound rapid changes in molecules such as GAG, hyaluronic acid, and other such mucopolysaccharides and noncollagenous molecules. The collagen components itself, so vitally important to the organism, undergoes measurable changes with estrogen deprivation, but fortunately this is preventable and, to a degree, replaceable with appropriate estrogen therapy. Early evidence suggests that selective estrogen receptors modulators (SERMS) do the same and raloxifine has been shown to have the same effect on estrogen markers as do estrogens (70).

Our conclusion is that sex steroids play a vital role in the integrity of the tissues of an individual and this con-

stitutes yet another strong argument for the use of long-term hormone (or SERMS) replacements.

REFERENCES

1. Murry RK, Keeley FW. The extracellular Matrix. In: Murray RK, Granner DK, Mayes PA, Rodwell VW, eds. *Harper's biochemistry*, 24th ed. London: Appleton & Lange, 1996:667–685.
2. Alberts B, Bray D, Laws J, Raff M, Roberts M, Watson D. Cell-cell adhesion and the extracellular matrix. In: Alberts B, et al. eds. *Molecular biology of the cell*, Vol 12. New York: Garland Publishing, 1983:673–718.
3. Kivirikko KI. Urinary excretion of hydroxyproline in health and disease *Int Rev Connect Tissue Res* 1973;5:93–163.
4. Krane SM, Kontrwitz FG, Byrne M, et al. Urinary excretion of hydroxylysine and its glycosides as an index of collagen degradation. *J Clin Invest* 1977;59:819–827.
5. Garnero P, Delmas PD. Biochemical markers of bone turnover. Applications for osteoporosis. *Endocrinol Metab Clin North Am* 1988;27(2):303–323.
6. Antinnen H, Orava S, Ryhänen L, Kivirikko KI. Assay of protocollagen lysyl hydroxylase activity in the skin of human subjects and changes in the activity with age. *Clin Chim Acta* 1973;47:289–294.
7. Skin thickness and skin collagen mimic an index of osteoporosis in the postmenopausal woman. In: Christiansen C, ed. *Osteoporosis*. Proceedings of the Copenhagen International Symposium on Osteoporosis, 1984:323–326.
8. Hall D. Gerontology: collagen disease. *Clin Endocrinol Metab* 1981;2:23.
9. Roux C, Kolta S, Chappard C, Morieux C, Dougados M, De Vernejoul MC. Bone effects of dydrogesterone in ovariectomized rats: a biologic, histomorphometric, and densitometric study. *Bone* 1996;19(5):463–468.
10. Yamamoto Y, Kurabayashi T, Tojo Y, Yahata T, Honda A, Tomita M, Tanaka K. Effects of progestins on the metabolism of cancellous bone in aged oophorectomized rats. *Bone* 1998;22(5):533–537.
11. Albright F, Bloomberg E, Smith PH. Postmenopausal osteoporosis. *Tram Assoc Amer Phys* 1940;55:298–305.
12. McConkey B, Fraser G R, Bligh A S, Whitely M. Transparent skin and osteoporosis. *Lancet* 1963;1:693–695.
13. Punnonen R, Vilska S, Rauramo L. Skinfold thickness and long-term post-menopausal hormone therapy. *Maturitas* 1984;5(4):259–262.
14. Dunn LB, Damesyn M, Moore AA, Reuben DB, Greendale GA. Does estrogen prevent skin aging? Results from the First National Health and Nutrition Examination Survey (NHANESI). *Arch Dermatol* 1997;133(3):339–342.
15. Schmidt JB, Binder M, Demschik G, Bieglmayer C, Reiner A. Treatment of skin aging with topical estrogens. *Int J Dermatol* 1996;35(9):669–674.
16. The Writing Group for the PEPI. Effects of hormone therapy on bone mineral density: results from the postmenopausal estrogen/progestin interventions (PEPI) trial. *JAMA* 1996;276(17):1389–1396.
17. Brincat M, Moniz CF, Kabalan S, et al. Decline in skin collagen content and metacarpal index after the menopause and its prevention with sex hormone replacement. *Br J Obstet Gynaecol* 1987;94:126–129.
18. Brincat M, Kabalan S, Studd JWW, et al. A study of the relationship of skin collagen content, skin thickness and bone mass in the postmenopausal woman. *Obstet Gynecol* 1987;70:840–845.
19. Gordan GS. Prevention of bone loss and fractures in women. *Maturitas* 1984;6(3):225–242.
20. Brincat M, Galea R, Muscat Baron Y. Italian menopause Society, Keynote Lecture, Rome, 1994.
21. Väänänen HK, Härkönen PL. Estrogen and bone metabolism. *Maturitas* 1996;23 (Suppl):S65–S69.
22. Schneider DL, Barrett Connor EL, Morton DJ. Timing of postmenopausal estrogen for optimal bone mineral density. The Rancho Bernardo Study. *JAMA* 1997;277(7):543–547.
23. Brincat M, Galea R, Muscat Baron Y, Xuereb A. Changes in bone collagen markers and in bone density in hormone treated and untreated postmenopausal women. *Maturitas* 1997;27(2):171–177.
24. Ginty F, Flynn A, Cashman K. Inter and intra-individual variations in urinary excretion of pyridinium crosslinks of collagen in healthy young adults. *Eur J Clin Nutr* 1998;52(1):71–73.
25. Suvanto Luukkonen E, Risteli L, Sundström H, Penttinen J, Kauppila A, Risteli J. Comparison of three serum assays for bone collagen formation during postmenopausal estrogen-progestin therapy. *Clin Chim Acta* 1997;266(2):105–116.
26. Melton LJ 3rd, Khosla S, Atkinson EJ, O'Fallon WM, Riggs BL. Relationship of bone turnover to bone density and fractures. *J Bone Miner Res* 1997;12(7):1083–1091.
27. Bailey AJ, Etherington DJ. Metabolism of collagen and elastin. In: Florkin M, Neuberger A, Van Dienen LLM, eds. *Comprehensive biochemistry*. New York: Elsevier, 1980:408–431.
28. Barnes MJ, Constable BJ, Morton LF, et al. Age-related variations in hydoxylation of lysine and proline on collagen. *Biochem J* 1974;139:461–468.
29. Murai A, Miyahara T, Shiozawa S. Age-related variations in glycosylation of hydroxyproline in human and rat skin collagens. *Biochim Biophys Acta* 1975;404:345–348.
30. Risteli J, Kivirikko KI. Intracellular enzymes of collagen biosynthesis in rat liver as a function of age and in hepatic injury induced by dimethylnitrosamine:

changes in prolyl hydoxylase, lysyl hydroxylase, collagen galactosyltransferase and collagen glucosyltransferase activities. *Biochem J* 1976;158:361–367.

31. Hall DA, Reed FB, Noki G, Vince JD. The relative effects of age and corticosteriod therapy on the collagen profiles of dermis from subjects with rheumatoid arthritis. *Age Ageing* 1974;3:15–22.

32. Dunn LB, Damesyn M, Moore AA, Reuben DB, Greendale GA. Does estrogen prevent skin aging? Results from the First National Health and Nutrition Examination Survey (NHANES I). *Arch Dermatol* 1997;133(3):339–342.

33. Stumpf WE, Sur M, Joshi SE. Estrogen target cells in the skin. *Experimentia* 1976;30:196.

34. Jemec GB, Wojnarowska F. The distribution of p29 protein in normal human skin. *Br J Dermatol* 1987;117(2):217–224.

35. Boucek RJ, Noble NL, Woessner JF Jr. Properties of fibroblasts. In: Page IH, ed. *Connective tissue thrombosis and atherosclerosis*. New York: Academic Press, 1959:193–211.

36. Danforth DN, Vies A, Breen M, Weinstein HG, Buckingham JC, Manalo P. The effect of pregnancy and labor on the human cervix: changes in collagen, glycoproteins and glucosaminoglycans. *Am J Obstet Gynecol* 1974;120:641–651.

37. Grosman N, Hindberg E, Schen J. The effect of oestrogenic treatment on the acid mucopolysaccharide pattern in skin of mice. *Acta Pharmacol Toxicol* 1971;30:458–464.

38. Goldzieher MA. The effects of estrogens on the senile skin. *J Gerontol* 1946;1:196.

39. Black MM. A modified radiographic method for measuring skin thickness. *Br J Dermatol* 1969;1:661.

40. Shuster J, Black MM, McVitie E. The influence of age and sex on skin thickness, skin collagen and density. *Br J Dermatol* 1975;93:639.

41. Shuster S, Bottoms E. Senile degeneration of skin collagen. *Clin Sci* 1963;25:487–491.

42. Shuster S, Bottoms E. Effect of ultraviolet light on skin collagen. *Mature* 1963;199:192–193.

43. Reed VB, Hall DA. In: Frische R, Hartmann F, eds. *Connective tissues—biochemistry and pathophysiology*. Berlin: Springer Verlag, 1974:290.

44. Hall DA, Reed FB, Noki G, Vince JD. The relative effects of age and corticosteriod therapy on the collagen profiles of dermis from subjects with rheumatoid arthritis. *Age Ageing* 1974;3:15–22.

45. Varila E, Rantala I, Ikarinem A, et al. The effect of topical oestriol on skin collagen of postmenopausal women. *Br J Obstet Gynaecol* 1995;102:985–989.

46. Tan CY, Stratham B, Marks R, Payne PA. Skin thickness measurements by pulsed ultrasound: its reproducibility, validation and variability. *Br J Dermatol* 1994;96:1392–1394.

47. Goodrich SM, Wood JE. The effect of estradiol 17B on peripheral venous distensibility and velocity of venous blood flow. *Am J Obstet Gynecol* 1966;96:407–412.

48. Rauramo L, Punnonen R. Wirking einer oralen estrogentherapie mit oestriolsuccinat auf die haut hastierter. *Frauen Haut Gerchluts Kr* 1969;44(13):463–470.

49. Punnonen R. Effect of castration and peroral therapy on skin. *Acta Obstet Gynaecol Scand* 1973;21(Suppl):1–4.

50. Brincat M, Moniz CJ, Studd JWW, et al. Long term effects of the menopause and sex hormones on skin thickness. *Br J Obstet Gynaecol* 1985;92:256–259.

51. Brincat M, Moniz CJ, Kabalan S, et al. Decline in skin collagen content and metacarpal index after the menopause and its prevention with sex hormone replacement. *Br J Obstet Gynaecol* 1987;94:126–129.

52. Brincat M, Moniz CF, Studd JWW, et al. Sex hormones and skin collagen content in postmenopausal women. *Br Med J* 1983;287:1337–1338.

53. Shahrad P, Marks RA. Pharmacological effect of oestrone on human epidermis. *Br J Dermatol* 1977;97:383–386.

54. Brincat M, Moniz CJ, Studd JWW, et al. Long term effects of the menopause and sex hormones on skin thickness. *Br J Obstet Gynecol* 1985;92:256–259.

55. Castelo-Barcia C, Pons F, Gratacos E, Fortuny A, Panrell JA, Gonzalez Merlo J. Relationship between skin collagen and bone changes during ageing. *Maturitas* 1994;18:199–206.

56. Castelo-Branco C, Duran M, Gonzalez-Merlo J. Skin collagen changes related to age and hormone replacement therapy. *Maturitas* 1992;15:113–119.

57. Holland EFN, Studd JWW, Mansell JP, Leather AT, Bailey AJ. Changes in collagen composition and cross-links in bone and skin of osteoporotic postmenopausal women treated with percutaneous estradiol implants. *Obstet Gynecol* 1994;83:180–183.

58. Schmidt JB, Binder M, Demschik G, Bieglmayer C, Reiner A. Treatment of skin aging with topical estrogens. *Int J Dermatol* 1996;35(9):669–674.

59. Creidi P, Faivre B, Agache P, Richard E, Haudiquet V, Sauvanet JP. Effect of a conjugated oestrogen (Premarin) cream on ageing facial skin. A comparative study with a placebo cream. *Maturitas* 1994;19:211–223.

60. Pverard GE, Letawe L, Dowlati A, Pierard-Franchimant L. Effect of hormone replacement therapy for menopause on the mechanical properties of skin. *J Am Soc* 1995;43(6):662–664.

61. Brincat M, Studd JWW, Moniz CF, Parsons V, Darby AJ. Skin thickness and skin collagen mimic an index of osteoporosis in the postmenopausal woman. In: Christiansen C, et al., eds. *Osteoporosis 1*, Proceedings of the Copenhagen International Symposium on Osteoporosis, 1984, 353–355.

62. Brincat M, Studd JWW, Moniz CF, Parsons V, Darby AJ. Skin thickness measurment. A simple screening method for determining patients at risk of postmenopausal osteoporosis. In: Christiansen C, et al., eds. *Osteoporosis 1*, Proceedings of the Copenhagen International Symposium on Osteoporosis, 1984:323–326.

63. Brincat M, Galea R, Muscat Baron Y. A screening model for osteoporosis using dermal skin thickness and bone densitometry. *In:* Wren BG, ed. *Progress in management of the menopause*. Cranforth, UK: Parthenon Publishing, 1997:175–178.

64. Stampfer MJ, Colditz GA, Willem WC, et al. Postmenopausal estrogen therapy and cardiovascular disease. Ten year follow-up from the Nurses Health Study. *N Engl J Med* 1991;325:756–762.

65. PEPI Trial Writing Group. Effects of estrogen and estrogen/progesterone regimens on heart disease risk factors in postmenopausal women. The postmenopausal estrogen/progestogen intervention (PEPI) trial. *JAMA* 1995;273:199–208.

66. Adams MR, Kaplan JR, Mauck SB. Inhibition of coronary artery atherosclerosis by 17b-estradiolin ovariectomised monkeys: lack of an effect of added progesterone. *Atherosclerosis* 1990;10:1051–1057.

67. Muscat Baron Y, Brincat M, Galea R. Carotid artery wall thickness in women treated with hormone replacement therapy. *Maturitas* 1997;27:47–53.

68. Muscat Baron Y, Galea R, Brincat M. Carotid artery wall changes in estrogen treated and untreated postmenopausal women. *Obstet Gynecol* 1998;91(6):982–986.

69. Wagner JD, St. Clair RW, Schwenke DC, Shirely CA, Adams MR, Clarkson TB. Regional difference in arterial low density lipoprotein in surgically postmenopausal cynomologous monkeys. Effects of oestrogen and progesterone replacement therapy. *Arterioscler Thromb Vasc Biol* 1992;12(16):717–726.

70. Delmas PD, Bjarnason NH, Mitlak BH, et al. Effects of raloxifene on bone mineral density, serum cholesterol concentrations and uterine endometrium in postmenopausal women. *N Engl J Med* 1997;337:1641–1647.

Treatment of the Postmenopausal Woman: Basic and Clinical Aspects, Second Edition, edited by Rogerio A. Lobo, Lippincott Williams & Wilkins, Philadelphia © 1999.

CHAPTER 20

Urinary Tract Disorders in Perimenopausal and Postmenopausal Women

Eileen F. DeMarco

Although urinary tract disorders can occur throughout a woman's life, their incidence rises during perimenopause, menopause, and the years beyond. Urogenital atrophy resulting from estrogen deficiency is an important factor contributing to urinary tract infection (UTI) and urinary incontinence in postmenopausal women (1). Other age-related physiologic changes in the female urinary tract also play a role in decreased infection resistance and impaired continence, including the shortened urethra, weakened sphincter, decreased bladder capacity, reduced urethral and bladder compliance, increased postvoid residual (PVR) urine volume, and increased uninhibited detrusor contractions (2,3). Relaxation of pelvic fascia and musculature secondary to vaginal childbirth, trauma, or aging can also compromise continence.

More than one-third of US women have already reached menopause, and the number of menopausal women will further increase during the next 20 years as increasing numbers of "baby boomers" approach their 50s. Because female life expectancy is nearing 80 years, huge numbers of women will spend more than a third of their lives postmenopausally. Consequently, the incidence of urinary tract symptomatology in postmenopausal women will increase in magnitude over time. Although generally not life-threatening, urinary tract disorders can have a severe impact on quality of life, producing physical debility, decreased physical activity, morbidity from infectious complications, psychologic stress, and social isolation.

Most women with urinary symptoms can be successfully treated. For UTI, simpler diagnostic tests have been developed, antibiotic treatments have improved, and preventive strategies for patients can be recommended. Regarding

incontinence disorders, technologically advanced diagnostic evaluations, including urodynamic studies, help to assess bladder and urethral function and help clinicians accurately classify the type of incontinence and institute appropriate medical or surgical treatment.

This chapter focuses on the pathophysiology, diagnosis, and management of urinary incontinence and urinary tract infection in older women.

URINARY INCONTINENCE

Epidemiology

Urinary incontinence affects 10% to 35% of all adults in the United States (4). In women aged 50 to 64 years, the incidence is approximately 10% to 30%, compared with 1.5% to 5% in men (5,6). Of ambulatory women aged 65 to 74 years, some 5% experience incontinence, whereas 15% of those older than 75 are affected (7). Among female nursing home residents, an estimated 50% have urinary incontinence (7). Families often cite urinary incontinence as the major consideration leading to the decision to place an elder in a nursing home.

Whether the increased incidence of incontinence is caused by the aging process or menopause itself has been questioned. The age-related urogenital atrophic changes attributed to postmenopausal estrogen loss, including atrophy of the bladder trigone, diminished sensitivity of the α-adrenergic receptors of the bladder neck and urethral sphincter, and thinning of the urethral mucosa (8), would seem to infer a plausible biologic relationship between menopause and urinary incontinence. However, one large epidemiologic study demonstrated that the prevalence of incontinence increased with age but not specifically at the time of the menopause (9). Another investigation, on the other hand, found that 70% of incontinent elderly women related its onset to their last men-

E. F. DeMarco: Department of Obstetrics and Gynecology, Columbia University College of Physicians & Surgeons, New York, New York 10032.

strual period (10). Other, more recent studies have also demonstrated conflicting results (11,12). In any event, female sex is considered one of the major independent risk factors for incontinence (along with neurologic impairment and immobility) (13).

The direct health care cost of incontinence for patients in the community as well as nursing home residents is $16.2 billion annually (based on 1994 dollars) (14), an amount 60% greater than a 1990 estimate (15). The increasing financial cost of incontinence may reflect the growth of our older population as well as rising health care costs.

Physiology of the Lower Urinary Tract

The urethra, distal vagina, and vestibule are derived from a common embryologic source, the urogenital sinus (16,17). In addition, these structures share a common network of vessels and tissue (18). Large concentrations of high-affinity estrogen receptors are present in the urethra, with lower concentrations in the trigone region and posterior neck of the bladder and in the pelvic floor (17), making these urinary tract structures as estrogen sensitive as the vagina.

The continence mechanism in women is formed predominantly by the bladder neck and proximal urethra (Fig. 20.1). The urethral submucosal tissues contribute to the continence mechanism by creating a "seal" effect in the urethra. Estrogen enhances this seal by two proposed mechanisms: by permitting maintenance and proliferation of the urethral submucosal vascular plexus and by promoting the function of the adrenergic receptors that exist in this structure and play a key role in urethral mucosal closure (19). At menopause, decreased estrogen levels result in urogenital atrophy and an increased incidence of urinary symptoms, including urgency, frequency, nocturia, and incontinence.

For continence to exist, the detrusor muscle of the urinary bladder and the sphincter muscles must be structurally intact and functional. Intraurethral resistance must exceed intravesical pressure at all times except during voiding. Although the onset of urinary incontinence is not considered a normal part of aging, a number of age-related physiologic changes (in addition to decreased estrogen levels) may predispose to it. These include *decreases* in bladder capacity, ability to postpone voiding, urethral and bladder compliance, maximal urethral closing pressure, and urinary flow rate, as well as *increases* in postvoid residual urine volume and uninhibited detrusor contractions. Any of these factors combined with comorbidity (such as congestive heart failure), medication use (such as diuretics), diminished ambulatory capability (limiting the ability to toilet), or cognitive impairment can contribute to the loss of continence (7). It is important to recognize that the causes of urinary incontinence in older women, especially those living in long-term care facilities, are likely to be multifactorial. Additional nonage-related risk factors associated with various types of urinary incontinence include diabetes, smoking, and high-impact physical activities (20–22).

Lower urinary tract performance depends greatly on the normal function of the autonomic nervous system. Figure 1 depicts the innervation of the bladder and urethra. Parasympathetic cholinergic fibers that emerge from the spinal cord at the S2–S4 level and travel via the pelvic splanchnic nerves innervate the detrusor muscle and sphincter, whereas sympathetic noradrenergic fibers innervate these structures via the paraaortic sympathetic chain. Sympathetic stimulation inhibits contraction of the detrusor and increases sphincter tone, thereby promoting

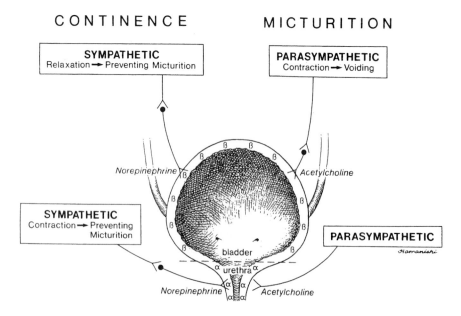

FIG. 20.1. The innovation of the bladder and urethra. Parasympathetic fibers arising in S2 through S4 have long preganglionic fibers and pelvic ganglia close to the bladder and urethra. These parasympathetic fibers excrete acetylcholine. Sympathetic fibers that have long postganglionic fibers discharge norepinephrine to β-receptors, primarily in the bladder, and α-receptors, primarily in the urethra. (Adapted from Stenchever MA. *Gynecologic urology, comprehensive gynecology.* St. Louis: CV Mosby, 1987.)

the urine storage. Parasympathetic stimulation results in detrusor contraction, sphincter relaxation, and micturition. The considerable neuronal connections between the motor nuclei of the detrusor and sphincter enable continuous interaction and balance between them.

Several "micturition centers," located in the lower spinal cord, brain stem, and cerebral cortex, mediate the coordination between the sympathetic and parasympathetic nervous systems and, hence, control the micturition reflex. The cerebral cortex is the site of voluntary control. There, voluntary restraint is exercised by synchronous inhibition of the detrusor and contraction of the sphincter and perineal muscles.

Dysfunction caused by injury, disease, or pharmacologic side effects at any point in the neurologic circuit can produce a loss of micturition regulation.

Types of Urinary Incontinence

This discussion will focus on the incontinence syndromes that commonly affect women in the menopausal and postmenopausal years: urge and stress incontinence.

Urge incontinence is characterized by the patient experiencing a sudden, strong desire to void and doing so involuntarily, being unable to suppress the urinary loss. The warning sensation can occur seconds to minutes before the involuntary voiding, and the amount of urine leaked can be moderate to large. The patient may note that the urine loss is related to a particular activity or exposure or may recognize no provoking factors. Increased urinary frequency and nocturnal incontinence commonly occur in patients with urge incontinence. Urge incontinence is the most common type of incontinence in elderly populations (19).

Patients with symptoms of urgency and frequency of urination who can control their urine until they reach a bathroom are said to have "overactive bladder." Urge incontinence is the far end of the spectrum of overactive bladder.

Urge incontinence is caused by an abnormality in detrusor muscle function characterized by overactivity, or hyperreflexia, of the detrusor and resultant uncontrollable bladder contractions. Based on cause, two subtypes of overactive detrusor contractions are seen (13):

- Primary detrusor hyperreflexia, or detrusor instability, in which no known neurologic basis is found for the unstable contractions
- Secondary detrusor hyperreflexia, caused by a neurologic disease, such as stroke, multiple sclerosis, parkinsonism, or spinal cord injury

Urge incontinence is also associated with local bladder disorders, such as outlet obstruction, infection, and carcinoma *in situ*.

Stress incontinence is characterized by intermittent leakage of small amounts of urine associated with sudden increases in abdominal pressure, as in coughing, sneezing, lifting, and abrupt changes of position. Stress incontinence occurs when intraabdominal pressure plus bladder pressure exceed urethral closure pressure. The cause is usually related to inadequate support of the bladder neck, base of the bladder, and the proximal urethra. This can result from a separation of the supports that hold the upper vagina and urethra to the pubic symphysis, from a relaxation of pelvic fascia and musculature secondary to childbearing or the aging process, or from trauma (23). When the bladder neck and sphincter descend from their normal intraabdominal position, increased intraabdominal pressure, which would normally reinforce the resting tone of the urinary sphincter, overwhelms it instead and urine expulsion results. This type of stress incontinence is termed "genuine stress incontinence."

Stress urinary loss can also be caused by failure of the urethral closure mechanism. This type, which is known as "intrinsic (urethral) sphincteric deficiency," occurs when the outlet mechanism fails to remain closed during urinary storage or to open in a coordinated way during voiding. Urine loss occurs continuously across the sphincteric mechanism without bladder contraction (19).

The postmenopausal decrease in estrogen levels, with subsequent atrophy and thinning of the urinary sphincter, pelvic floor muscles, and related pelvic supports, is associated with stress incontinence.

Detailed evaluation is necessary to distinguish urge incontinence from stress incontinence, because the overlap in urinary symptoms is great. In addition, many women present with mixed stress-urge incontinence. In the variant known as stress-induced detrusor instability, coughing, lifting, or other stress maneuvers that produce a sudden rise in intraabdominal pressure trigger uninhibited bladder contractions. Symptoms distinguishing this condition from simple stress incontinence include moderate to large volume leaked, more common occurrence of nighttime incontinence, and a slight delay between the stress maneuver and the passage of urine. The patient might also experience urgency. In such cases, both components must be treated to increase the likelihood of therapeutic success.

Transient Versus Established Incontinence

Transient incontinence usually has a definable, sudden onset and is most likely to have a reversible cause. Except for inflammatory or irritative conditions, such as urinary tract infection, the cause is not usually referable to the urinary tract. Common causes of transient incontinence, using the DIAPPERS mnemonic coined by Resnick (24), include:

- Delirium
- Infection, urinary
- Atrophic vaginitis
- Pharmacologic (drugs)

- Psychologic (e.g., depression)
- Endocrine
- Restricted mobility
- Stool impaction

Established incontinence is of a chronic nature. A careful patient history helps determine the onset and duration as well as the type of symptoms. It should be noted that transient incontinence can become established if the underlying cause or causes are not identified and managed in a timely fashion. Although established incontinence is less likely to be completely reversible, treatment can alleviate symptoms and reduce social limitations for many patients.

DIAGNOSTIC EVALUATION

Valuable data on the nature of a patient's bladder dysfunction can be obtained in the office workup, which includes a complete history taking, physical and pelvic examinations, and routine laboratory tests. More sophisticated urologic tests that require specialized diagnostic equipment can then be scheduled if necessary to formulate an accurate diagnosis.

History

A detailed history of the patient's urinary symptoms should be obtained, with each symptom characterized and quantified as accurately as possible. The onset and duration of symptoms should be noted. Symptoms of recent onset can signify a potentially reversible cause of bladder dysfunction or incontinence. When the patient has more than one symptom, her determination of the relative severity of each should be recorded. The following factors should be assessed as part of the urologic history:

- Frequency of urination during the day and night
- Painful or difficult urination or pain with bladder filling
- Time the patient can comfortably wait between urinations
- Reason patient voids so often (severe urge, convenience, attempt to avoid incontinence)
- Amount of urine lost during a wetting accident (a few drops, enough to saturate clothing)
- Use of protective pads and frequency of changing
- Patient awareness of the act of incontinence as it occurs
- Presence of a sense of urgency before the incontinent episode
- If urgency is felt, duration patient can postpone voiding
- Occurrence of urge incontinence (involuntary urine loss associated with sudden, strong desire to void)
- Urinary loss during coughing, sneezing, lifting, or rising from sitting to standing position
- With stress urinary loss, is urine lost for an instant during the stress or is voiding uncontrollable?

- Occurrence of incontinence in the lying or sitting position
- Difficulty initiating the urine stream
- Weak or interrupted urine stream
- Feeling of incomplete urine emptying
- Presence of postvoid dribbling

A chart or diary used by the patient at home to record incontinence episodes can be useful to help ascertain the relative severity of the urinary loss. Recording the pattern of incontinence and urinary frequency for 24 hours, which is a common approach, is depicted in Figure 20.2. Compliance is often difficult with more prolonged periods of recording. When the patient is elderly, family members can be helpful in providing history information.

Inquiry should be made regarding the amount and types of the patient's fluid intake, because many products (e.g., caffeine, alcoholic drinks, carbonated beverages, and certain food ingredients) act as dietary irritants .

Careful review of all medications the patient is taking and their indications is important to the evaluation. Many prescription and nonprescription drugs can affect bladder control. Antihypertensives, including antiadrenergics, calcium channel blockers, and angiotensin-converting enzyme (ACE) inhibitors, which can affect the autonomic nervous system or smooth muscle tone directly, are frequently implicated (13). The increased urine volume produced by diuretic therapy can challenge an older patient's decreased storage capacity. Over-the-counter cold medications that contain sympathomimetics or antihistamines with significant anticholinergic effects can also adversely affect detrusor and sphincter function. In addition, many of these agents can cause subtle degrees of delirium and cognitive dysfunction that can contribute to toileting problems, especially in older patients; sedative-hypnotics, tricyclic antidepressants, neuroleptics, narcotic analgesics, and alcohol can also be detrimental to cognition (13). The medication history, therefore, should note all drugs the patient is taking, the doses, and whether they appear related to the onset of the urinary symptoms (19).

A thorough medical history should be obtained. Neurologic conditions that specifically affect bladder and sphincter function, such as multiple sclerosis, spinal cord injury or neoplasm, myelodysplasia, stroke, and Parkinson's disease, should be inquired into. The patient should be asked about muscular weakness, paralysis or poor coordination, gait disturbance, tremor, tingling sensation, numbness, and double vision, symptoms suggestive of neuropathology. The presence of systemic diseases such as diabetes mellitus and autonomic neuropathy as well as any renal disorders should be recorded. It is important to elicit any history of cancer and its treatment so potential metastases or adverse effects of radiotherapy or chemotherapy on the urinary system can be investigated.

The patient's gynecologic and obstetric history should be documented. The number of pregnancies and births

VOIDING DIARY

NAME: _____   DATE: _____

TIME OF URGE TO VOID	STRENGTH OF PAIN OR URGE	TIME OF ACTUAL OF VOID	VOIDED VOLUME	INCONTINENCE (S,U, OR W) See below	AMOUNT OF LEAKAGE (LARGE=L, MEDIUM=M SMALL=S)

Urgency is the feeling that you have to urinate badly.

Incontinence is the loss of urine control before reaching the bathroom.

Stress Incontinence is wetting or leakage at times of coughing, sneezing, or with physical activity, etc.

Urge Incontinence is wetting or leakage because of urgency

Unaware Incontinence is wetting without conscious awareness of when it happens.

FIG. 20.2. Voiding diary. (Adapted from Blaivas, J. Personal communication, with permission).

and any prior gynecologic surgery clearly have special significance with regard to mobility of the pelvic organs and support structures. Postmenopausal women should be asked about the presence of any symptoms of urogenital atrophic changes and whether they are taking hormone replacement therapy.

It is essential to ascertain any previous surgical history. When performed for uterine or cervical cancer, hysterectomy can sometimes cause detrusor denervation (19). Prior surgical repair for incontinence may suggest the possibility of sphincter injury. In general, any prior urologic or gynecologic surgical procedure can contribute to the patient's current symptoms. Additionally, neurosurgical operations involving the back or cranium can affect bladder function.

Physical Examination

Because urogenital structural abnormalities and neurologic defects often coexist with and contribute to incontinence disorders, particular attention should be given to the neurologic and abdominopelvic aspects of the physical examination.

The neurologic examination can begin by observing the patient's gait, balance, and demeanor. A limp, uncoordinated movement, abnormal speech pattern, or facial asymmetry can be subtle indications of a neurologic condition. If systemic neurologic disease is suspected, examination of the cranial nerves and upper extremity function helps assess gross abnormalities. Reflexes of the knee and ankle are tested. The presence of Babinski's sign or clonus indicates upper motor neuron disease. Motor function and sensory evaluation of the lower extremities should be assessed and any weakness or deficits noted.

Anal sphincter tone and control, perianal sensation, and the bulbocavernosus reflex are checked during the rectal examination to evaluate the sacral dermatomes. The bulbocavernosus reflex, which reflects the integrity of the S2 to S4 levels of the sacral cord, is elicited by suddenly compressing the clitoris. The anal sphincter and perineal muscles will contract if the sacral cord is intact. However, up to 30% of neurologically normal women do not demonstrate this reflex.

The abdomen and flanks should be palpated for masses, tenderness, and bladder distention. Similarly, the adnexal structures should be evaluated for masses or tenderness during the pelvic examination.

Vaginal examination is performed to assess the pelvic organs and to check for incontinence and prolapse. Skin irritation and fungal infestation of the genitalia suggest the presence of prolonged incontinence. Atrophic changes in the vagina's epithelial lining may be observed in postmenopausal women who are not receiving hormone replacement therapy. The vulva and cervix should be checked for evidence of malignant changes.

The patient should have a full bladder and be examined first in the supine position. Speculum examination of the anterior wall of the vagina is performed, with the patient instructed to strain, in order to evaluate bladder, urethral, and cervical mobility and stress urinary incontinence. Protrusion of the anterior vaginal wall, which is accentuated when the patient strains, indicates the presence of a cystocele, prolapse of the bladder base and proximal urethra. Often seen as a component of the hypermobility associated with uncomplicated stress incontinence, this defect results from weakness of the supporting fascia of the bladder base. If stress incontinence is not observed, the patient should again strain or cough while the clinician manually reduces the cystocele in an attempt to demonstrate stress urinary loss.

The posterior vaginal wall is examined for a rectocele, herniation of the rectum into the vagina. This type of prolapse results from a defect in the pubococcygeus muscles, permitting anterior protrusion of the rectum. A rectocele can be accentuated by the Valsalva maneuver. The vaginal vault should be checked for an enterocele (intestinal protrusion), especially in patients who have undergone hysterectomy.

If pelvic organ prolapse or urinary incontinence is not demonstrated with the patient supine, she should be reexamined in the standing position, with one foot elevated on a small stool. The degree of uterine prolapse, if present, is more accurately assessed this way. The clinician should be sensitive to the patient's anxiety at being provoked to leak urine while someone is watching and reassure her that this is an essential part of a complete evaluation of her incontinence problem.

Mobility of the urethra and bladder can be further assessed by the so-called "Q-Tip test." With the patient supine, a lubricated, sterile cotton swab or tube is inserted through the urethra to the bladder, then withdrawn to the point of resistance (the level of the vesical neck). The resting angle from the horizontal is noted. The patient is instructed to strain, and the degree of rotation is assessed. A resting or straining angle of greater than 30 degrees from the horizontal indicates hypermobility. Initially, the

Q-Tip test was developed to differentiate the types of stress incontinence. Later investigations, however, found that although this test can quantify mobility of the bladder neck and proximal urethra, it is not sufficiently sensitive to elucidate a specific urologic diagnosis.

A postvoid residual (PVR) urine test is a simple, useful procedure that can be easily performed in the office. After the patient voids, a catheter is inserted and the remaining urine withdrawn and measured. Urinalysis and culture can be done to test for urinary tract infection. Normally, the amount of residual urine (after the patient has voided 100 to 150 mL) would be less than 50 mL. A large amount of PVR urine suggests inadequate bladder emptying because of detrusor hypocontractility or bladder outlet obstruction. If difficulty passing the urethral catheter is encountered, a urethral stricture or other abnormality may be present.

Bladder storage function can also be evaluated in the office without the use of sophisticated equipment. After the PVR test, the catheter is left in place and a graduated syringe (without the piston) is attached to the end of the catheter. Sterile water or saline is poured into the syringe in premeasured volumes and drips into the bladder by gravity. Filling is continued until the drip rate slows down or the column of fluid in the syringe rises, indicating a change in vesical pressure that may be caused by a detrusor contraction, an increase in abdominal pressure, or low bladder wall compliance. In addition, the patient is instructed to report when she first feels the urge to void, and the examiner notes the amount of fluid instilled. The urge normally occurs when approximately 150 to 200 mL has been instilled, but women with normal bladder capacity can maintain continence until 400 to 500 mL has been instilled, when a strong, normally uncontrollable urge to void occurs.

A sudden rise in pressure accompanied by the voiding urge or by incontinence suggests an involuntary detrusor contraction. If no involuntary detrusor contractions occur, the bladder is filled until the patient feels comfortably full, and the catheter is removed. The patient is then asked to cough or strain with increasing force. If urine immediately spurts from the urethra and stops as soon as the stress is over, stress incontinence may be present. The clinician should then manually elevate the bladder neck with a finger or instrument (being cautious not to compress and thereby occlude the urethra) and ask the patient to cough again. If urine loss no longer occurs, bladder neck separation from the pubic symphysis may be the underlying cause of the incontinence, and surgical repair may reestablish continence. Leakage that occurs without descent of the bladder base or that occurs with minimal provocation suggests the patient has intrinsic sphincteric deficiency.

These tests should be repeated with the patient standing if incontinence has not been provoked while she is supine.

Laboratory Tests

Urgency or urge incontinence can be the main symptom of urinary tract infection. Urinalysis and culture of a catheterized or clean-voided urine sample should be ordered. Microscopic examination of the urine may reveal hematuria, pyuria, or bacteriuria. Positive results of urine culture should prompt treatment with culture-specific antibiotics. Persistent bacteriuria or recurrent infections may require invasive testing. Because transitional carcinoma can also cause urgency and frequency, urine cytologic studies should be performed to identify malignant cells.

Blood chemistries to evaluate the patient's renal function (e.g., serum creatinine) and metabolic status (e.g., serum glucose and calcium) should be ordered as appropriate.

Specialized Urologic Tests

Often the information provided by the patient's history, physical examination, laboratory tests, and in-office urologic evaluation enable the clinician to arrive at a diagnosis and formulate an initial treatment plan. However, more formal urologic testing, including urodynamics, requiring special equipment and training may be necessary to determine the cause of urinary incontinence.

Urethroscopy and Cystoscopy

Use of urethroscopy and cystoscopy studies is based on diagnostic suspicions. Inflammation, diverticula, and other anatomic defects can be visualized with urethroscopy. Effects of estrogen deficiency and urethral tone can also be assessed. Cystoscopy permits visual inspection of the bladder's interior. Overt pathology such as an inflammatory process, tumor, or stone can be observed.

Cystometry

Multichannel cystometrography (CMG) graphically depicts the volume-related pressure changes (compliance) of the bladder during bladder filling, cough and stress maneuvers, and voiding. Detrusor activity, sensation, and capacity—indicators of bladder storage function—are evaluated.

As with the office procedure described earlier, fluid is instilled into the patient's bladder via a urethral catheter at a constant rate. Sensor-equipped catheters placed in the bladder (measuring urethral and bladder pressure) and in the vagina or rectum (representing measurements of intraabdominal pressure) continuously monitor pressure. This phase of the study identifies failure to store urine appropriately. During monitoring, the patient's first urge to void is identified, along with the sensation of bladder fullness. Detrusor contractions that occur involuntarily during bladder filling are noted and classified as detrusor instability (no known neurogenic cause) or detrusor

hyperreflexia (in the presence of nervous system pathology), as discussed earlier. In "normal" patients, the detrusor does not contract even though the patient may have an intense urge to urinate.

The next phase of the study evaluates the failure to store urine because of outlet dysfunction. As CMG monitoring continues, the patient is instructed to perform Valsalva and stress maneuvers, which may elicit stress urinary incontinence. The simultaneous monitoring of bladder and bladder outlet events can also help determine when defects in both bladder storage and outlet resistance combine to produce a failure-to-store condition.

Characteristics of the patient's voiding can be assessed by having the patient urinate while pressure and flow monitoring is continued. In this phase, poor bladder contraction that results in failure to empty can be identified. Alternatively, high-pressure or low-flow voiding will indicate outlet obstruction as the cause of failure to empty. Voiding cystourethrography (VCUG), which radiologically visualizes the lower urinary tract during bladder filling and voiding, is sometimes performed to determine the site of bladder outlet obstruction, integrity of the sphincteric mechanism, and the presence of vesicoureteral reflux or other abnormality. Fluoroscopic monitoring is generally preferable to static films.

Synchronous, multichannel videourodynamic investigation, which measures and displays a number of urodynamic parameters while radiographically imaging the lower urinary tract, is the most sophisticated and accurate tool for diagnosing micturition disturbances. It can document bladder outlet dysfunction and, because it records the act of micturition, can reveal continuous urine loss across the sphincteric mechanism in the absence of bladder contraction, which occurs in intrinsic sphincteric deficiency. Multichannel videourodynamics provide the best clinical insight into the underlying pathophysiologic process.

TREATMENT APPROACHES

Management of urinary incontinence involves a complex array of medical and surgical modalities as well as behavioral and lifestyle modifications. A treatment plan can be developed once the diagnosis is clear. Mixed stress-urge incontinence presents a particular therapeutic challenge. Although medical therapy may be ineffective for many women with mixed incontinence, surgery offers a good potential for resolution of the stress incontinence component, with 40% to 60% of women also experiencing improvement in concurrent urgency.

Urge Incontinence

Ideally, treatment of urinary incontinence caused by involuntary detrusor contractions would involve eliminating the underlying cause. This is rarely possible, however, when the cause is neurologic or idiopathic. When urethral obstruction is the cause, cure of the obstruction ameliorates the symptoms of detrusor instability. Urethral obstruction in women, however, is rare; it usually occurs because of previous pelvic surgery. Treatment generally involves urethrolysis and sometimes resuspension of the vesical neck. Therapy is reportedly effective in approximately 60% of women who develop detrusor instability after surgery for stress incontinence.

As discussed, causes of transient incontinence should be investigated and managed. It has been estimated that 50% to 75% of new-onset incontinence probably has a reversible cause, such as urinary tract infection, drug interactions, or cognition-related phenomena (13,19).

Treatment of urge incontinence is aimed at abolishing the involuntary detrusor contractions. Drug therapy, behavior modification, biofeedback techniques, and electrical neurostimulation are employed.

Drug Therapy

Anticholinergic drugs (e.g., propantheline bromide), which suppress parasympathetically mediated detrusor contractions, are used to treat detrusor instability or hyperreflexia. Common side effects include dry mouth, decreased sweating, blurred vision, constipation, palpitations, and tachycardia. Urinary hesitancy and retention have also been reported.

Musculotropic relaxants, or antispasmodics (e.g., oxybutynin chloride, flavoxate hydrochloride, dicyclomine hydrochloride, hyoscyamine), suppress detrusor contractility by virtue of their direct smooth-muscle relaxing effects and they may possess local anesthetic effects. A number of musculotropic agents also have some anticholinergic properties. Side effects are similar to those of anticholinergic agents.

Treatment success with anticholinergics or antispasmodics can be enhanced with behavior modification, such as timed voiding.

Tricyclic antidepressants (e.g., imipramine hydrochloride), which have a direct relaxant effect on bladder smooth muscle, as well as sympathomimetic and central effects, are used to treat detrusor instability. Anticholinergic and antihistaminic (e.g., drowsiness) side effects are commonly seen. Tricyclics should be used cautiously in elderly patients, because the risk of orthostatic hypotension and cardiac conduction abnormalities is particularly increased in this group. In addition, if the drug must be discontinued, it should be tapered over several weeks to avoid rebound depression.

Calcium channel blockers (e.g., nifedipine, verapamil) have recently been used in the treatment of urge incontinence, but their role is still under study. They may prove useful in patients who require treatment for angina or hypertension plus incontinence.

When bladder outlet dysfunction is present, drug therapy can be used to augment outlet resistance. α-Adrenergic agonists (e.g., ephedrine, phenylpropanolamine hydrochloride) provide excitation to the smooth muscle of the bladder neck and proximal urethra and increase closure.

Adequate dosage of these medications must be given for them to be effective. The dosage can be increased approximately every 3 to 5 days until the patient experiences clinical improvement or adverse side effects. The usual cautions should be exercised when prescribing for elderly patients who may have comorbid conditions being treated with various pharmacologic therapies.

Estrogen Therapy

Evidence is limited regarding the success of estrogen treatment for urinary urgency or urge incontinence in postmenopausal women. However, estrogen's physiologic effects on the urinary tract would suggest that replacing the hormone may have an adjunctive role in the treatment of urinary incontinence. For example, a high concentration of estrogen receptors is found in the urethra (25). Estrogens exert trophic effects on the urethral mucosa, submucosa, and pelvic floor and periurethral collagen, contributing to improved urethral sphincter function (26). In estrogen deficiency, thinning occurs in both the vaginal and urinary tract epithelium (25,27). Estrogen deficiency thus compromises the urethra's ability to maintain an adequate mucosal seal, thereby contributing to the development of urinary incontinence. Administration of estrogens to postmenopausal women has been shown to increase urethral pressure, mucosal thickness, and blood vessel engorgement (28).

Estrogen therapy in postmenopausal women also improves the vasculature of the bladder neck as well as the mucosa of the trigone. Estrogen's α-adrenergic stimulating capacity may contribute to overall urinary control.

Further, it has been proposed that estrogen deficiency reduces the sensory threshold of the lower urinary tract (29). In that study, the clinical and urodynamic variables of postmenopausal women treated with estrogen were compared with those of a nontreated group. The women who did not take supplements experienced significantly more urge incontinence and nocturia than the estrogen-treated group. Interestingly, the investigators found that the measures of urethral function, maximal urethral closure pressure and functional urethral length, did not differ between the two groups (29).

Other investigators have also reported estrogen's favorable therapeutic effect on women with urinary frequency, urgency, and urge incontinence. In one double-blind, placebo-controlled crossover study, 34 women aged 75 years took oral estriol (3 mg daily for 3 months) (30). Urge incontinence and mixed incontinence were improved by estriol therapy; no difference was found between estriol and placebo in women with stress incontinence. In a later investigation, researchers conducted a randomized, double-blind, placebo-controlled multicenter study of oral estriol (3 mg/day) in the treatment of 64 postmenopausal women with either sensory urgency or detrusor instability (31). Patient compliance was demonstrated by a significant improvement in the maturation index of vaginal wall smears in the estriol-treated women compared with those who took placebo. Although lower urinary tract function was both subjectively and objectively improved with estriol treatment, it was not significantly better than with placebo (31).

Although intervention studies using estrogen for urge incontinence have had mixed results, many physicians feel sufficient favorable evidence exists to support a treatment trial for postmenopausal women with symptoms of urinary urgency and urge incontinence. Estrogen supplementation is often used in conjunction with other pharmacologic and nonpharmacologic modalities.

As whenever prescribing hormone therapy, the risks and benefits of treatment must be weighed for each individual. Absolute and relative contraindications must be investigated. Choices must be made regarding the type of estrogen preparation, route of administration (oral, vaginal, transdermal), dosage, and need for concomitant progestin therapy. The side effect profile should be considered. With the numerous therapeutic options and delivery systems available, hormonal treatment can be tailored to the needs of each patient and adjusted as necessary. In addition, some women may have other indications, such as vasomotor symptoms or osteoporosis risk factors, that would benefit from hormone therapy. Such patients would be candidates for systemic therapy (oral, transdermal patch); a local estrogen (vaginal cream, estradiol-releasing vaginal ring) would be appropriate for women who have urogenital symptoms but no other indications for systemic therapy.

In addition to oral or transdermal therapy, local (intravaginal) hormone therapy is an option for women who have a contraindication to systemic therapy or react adversely to systemic preparations. Formulations are available as an estrogen-containing creams and an estradiol-releasing vaginal ring. Estrogen is well absorbed through the vaginal mucosa. In the low doses used for urogenital atrophy and urinary symptoms, its therapeutic effect is mainly local, and systemic absorption is minimal. Intravaginal estrogen stimulates the maturation of both vaginal and urethral endothelia, but it avoids the induction of endometrial proliferation and breakthrough bleeding. However, low-dose local therapy has little or no effect on nonurogenital menopausal symptoms and does not protect against osteoporosis.

Other Modalities

Behavior modification, electrical stimulation, and biofeedback techniques can be employed to help patients control detrusor contractility. These measures are often used as adjuncts to pharmacologic therapy or as primary modalities for patients who are not candidates for drug intervention.

Some simple changes in behavior can help many patients improve urinary control. Timed voiding and control of fluid intake are often successful. Patients should avoid foods or beverages, such as caffeine, spicy foods, and citrus fruits or juices, that irritate their bladder and cause a severe urge to void, urinary frequency, incontinence, or pain. Any medications the patient is taking should be evaluated for their effects on the urinary system. Bladder retraining may be useful. This involves a programmed, progressive lengthening of the period between urinations. Biofeedback techniques are sometimes used in this reeducation process. Whenever possible, incontinent women should plan to have bathroom facilities readily accessible. They should choose clothing that can be quickly and easily removed; elastic waists and self-stick closures are preferable to difficult buttons and belts. Assistive devices such as bedside commodes can help in managing nocturnal urinary symptoms.

Patients should be reminded to maintain good bowel habits, because constipation can produce adverse effects on the urinary process. Fiber and fluid intake should be adequate.

In patients with refractory urge incontinence that does not respond to behavioral therapy or medication, surgery may be indicated. Although some updated procedures are included for completeness including neural ablation by sacral rhizotomy or permanent subarachnoid block (19) and peripheral bladder denervation (modified Ingelman-Sundberg procedure), in refractory severe cases, augmentation cystoplasty or ileal vesicostomy (32,33) may be considered.

Stress Incontinence

As discussed, genuine stress incontinence is associated with lack of support of the bladder neck, bladder base, and proximal urethra, which can result from separation of vaginal and urethral supports, pelvic floor relaxation, or trauma. Many women ultimately require surgery to correct the anatomic relationships of these urinary tract structures. However, a variety of nonoperative management techniques can be used to help improve and sometimes even resolve mild to moderate stress incontinence in many patients.

Pelvic Strengthening

As illustrated in Figure 20.3, several pelvic structures are known to lend support to the method area. Isometric Kegel exercises strengthen the levator ani and pubococcygeal muscles of the pelvic floor. A strong pelvic muscle layer helps maintain the position of the bladder and prevents urine leakage during times of stress (coughing, sneezing). Several studies have demonstrated that

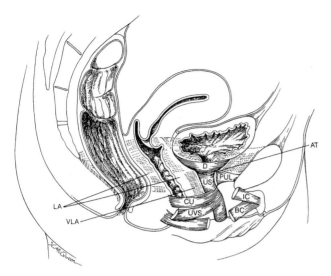

FIG. 20.3. Interrelationships of approximate location of periurethral structures. Levator ani muscles are shown as *light lines* running deep to the pelvic viscera. The vaginal levator attachment is shown as a *darker area*. VLA, vaginal levator attachment; LA, levator ani muscles; D, detrusor muscle; US, urethral sphincter; CU, compressor urethrae; UVS, urethrovaginal sphincter; AT, arcus tendineus fasciae pelvis; PUL, pubourethral ligament; IC, ischiocavernosus muscle; and BC, bulbocavernosus muscle. (Adapted from Stenchever MA. *Gynecologic urology, comprehensive gynecology.* St. Louis: CV Mosby, 1987).

patients who properly performed pelvic floor exercises experienced either resolution or improvement in stress urinary incontinence (34–36). Some urogynecology centers and physical therapy practices have on staff qualified specialists who are experts in pelvic floor strengthening. These experts can teach patients proper exercise methods, monitor their techniques, and provide technical and emotional support. Aids such as biofeedback techniques, vaginal cones, or electrical stimulation are sometimes used to help the patient better appreciate the pelvic floor and properly perform the exercises.

Lifestyle Changes

The behavioral, environmental, and dietary modifications discussed with regard to urge incontinence can also be used by patients with stress incontinence to improve bladder control.

Pharmacologic Therapy

Medical treatment for stress incontinence is limited to agents with α-adrenergic agonist activity, such as ephedrine, pseudoephedrine, and phenylpropanolamine. These agents provide stimulation of the smooth muscle of the bladder neck and proximal urethra, thereby increasing urethral closure. Imipramine's adrenergic activity makes it potentially useful in patients with stress incontinence.

This drug should be used with caution in elderly patients, because they are at higher risk of serious side effects.

Estrogen Therapy

Early studies of estrogen therapy in postmenopausal women with stress incontinence, although subjective and uncontrolled, demonstrated symptomatic improvement in many patients (37), and for years estrogens have been used in clinical practice to manage stress incontinence. Technologically advanced urodynamic studies have more recently permitted objective means of assessing outcome following estrogen therapy. Various studies have shown that estrogen therapy improved maximal urethral closure pressure (MUCP) and abdominal pressure transmission ratio and produced an objective decrease in urine loss, in addition to improving stress incontinence, urgency, and frequency symptoms (38–42). Other investigators, however, have reported that women taking estrogen for stress incontinence had no improvement in subjective response or objective urodynamic measures (30,43,44).

Interpreting the conflicting data from these studies is difficult, because only a limited number of prospective, double-blind, placebo-controlled trials have been conducted. Even they lack standardization concerning diagnosis, treatment regimens, and outcome measures. In a 1994 metaanalysis of 23 trials on estrogen therapy for urinary incontinence, however, the study authors concluded that an overall significant subjective improvement was seen with estrogen for the total group of all incontinent postmenopausal women as well as for the subgroup of women who had genuine stress incontinence alone (45). In addition, MUCP was significantly improved with estrogen, but no significant effect on quantitative urine loss was observed between the treated and nontreated groups. The authors theorized that estrogen's ability to enhance the overall quality of life, rather than directly improve urethral function, may account for its beneficial effects in women with urinary incontinence.

The combination of estrogen and phenylpropanolamine therapy for postmenopausal women with genuine stress incontinence has been shown more effective than either drug alone in improving both subjective and objective measures (46,47).

Estrogen administration appears to help maintain musculofascial support to the urethra and pelvic floor and improve pelvic floor tone and contractility (48–50). For some women, estrogen therapy plus pelvic strengthening exercises can correct their stress incontinence.

Pessaries

For women with stress incontinence related to pelvic organ prolapse who are not candidates for surgery, vaginal pessaries are an alternative approach. Pessaries specifically designed for incontinence can help prevent urinary leakage

---

associated with coughing, straining, and other stress maneuvers by lending support to the bladder neck.

Surgical Treatment

A number of operations have been developed to correct stress incontinence, with the choice of procedure depending on the cause. Women in whom pelvic organ prolapse is associated with stress incontinence should be evaluated for the appropriate surgical intervention. In women with stress incontinence associated with hypermobility of the proximal urethra and bladder neck but without significant vaginal wall relaxation, bladder neck suspension procedures are appropriate. The Marshall-Marchetti-Krantz suprapubic urethrovesical suspension operation and the Burch colposuspension are the most common procedures. Each has a 1-year success rate of approximately 90% to 95%; at 5 years, 75% continued success rates have been reported. Following these operations, some women experience delayed voiding for a few days or longer and require catheterization. Transvaginal procedures, which are less invasive and require a shorter recovery period than standard suspension operations, are also used in the surgical treatment of stress incontinence.

Pubovaginal sling procedures are appropriate for stress incontinence associated with intrinsic sphincteric deficiency, and they generally have an 80% success rate. This procedure is associated with a higher postoperative complication rate, with 30% of women having significant urgency-related symptoms and approximately 5% having permanent urinary retention (19). A fascial sling procedure may also be considered for urethral hypermobility when a Marshall-Marchetti-Krantz or Burch operation has failed and it is not deemed feasible to repeat a similar suspension. Using this procedure and creating an intraurethral pressure of 80 to 90 cm of water at the site of the sling, one group reported a 98.2% cure rate of stress incontinence (51). Delayed voiding was the most troublesome postoperative problem.

Intrinsic sphincteric deficiency has been treated with periurethral injection therapy to increase urethral resistance, with varying degrees of success. Injectable agents used include collagen, polytetrafluoroethylene (polytef), and autologous fat.

LOWER URINARY TRACT INFECTIONS

Incidence and Classification

Urinary tract infections (UTI) occur much more often in females than in males in all age groups except during the newborn period, when the incidence is much greater in males (52). Only occasionally does UTI develop in prepubertal girls; the incidence rises in late adolescence and during the second and third decades of life. It is more common in women who are sexually active and in those who use a diaphragm and spermicides for contraception.

The incidence of UTI increases as women age. Up to 20% of all women develop UTI at some point during their lifetime. By age 70, approximately 10% will have chronic UTI. Further, older patients hospitalized for other illnesses are at high risk for acquiring UTI because they often undergo urinary catheterization. An indwelling catheter in place for 24 hours leads to bacteriuria in up to 50% of patients; after 96 hours with a catheter, almost all patients have bacteriuria (23).

Urinary tract infections are usually classified as involving the lower urinary tract (cystitis, urethritis, and acute urethral syndrome) or the upper urinary tract (acute pyelonephritis, interstitial nephritis, and renal or perirenal abscess). The following discussion focuses on lower UTI, which occur much more commonly than upper tract infections.

Urinary tract infections are also categorized as being uncomplicated or complicated. Such classification depends on the absence or presence of host conditions that are known to promote infection, account for persistent infection, or favor recurrent infection. Complicated UTI, for example, occur in patients with structural or functional abnormalities of the urinary tract or who have had recent urinary catheterization or instrumentation; they are frequently hospital acquired. Patients with complicated infections often have a greater incidence of antimicrobial resistance, poorer therapeutic response, and greater risk of renal damage.

Symptoms

Typical symptoms of uncomplicated lower UTI include some combination of dysuria, frequency, urgency, nocturia, voiding small urine volumes, foul-smelling urine, pyuria, hematuria, and suprapubic or pelvic pain. Some women with recurrent UTI, especially older patients, have symptoms that are less apparent, such as a slight change in urinary frequency or vague abdominal pain. Incontinence can also be associated with acute and chronic infections. Fever is not usually present.

Clinical manifestations of complicated UTI, such as in hospitalized patients or patients with indwelling catheters, can range from asymptomatic bacteriuria to severe gram-negative sepsis with shock. Most catheter-associated UTIs are asymptomatic. Patients with complicated UTI may present with signs and symptoms of acute cystitis or acute pyelonephritis (flank or low back pain, fever, chills, sweats, nausea, vomiting). The key characteristic of complicated UTI is the broader spectrum of microorganisms involved. These tend to be more virulent, have a higher resistance to antibiotics, a lower clinical response rate to therapy, and they often recur.

Pathogenic Bacteria

The bacteria responsible for most UTI originate from flora in the lower intestine. Approximately 80% to 90%

of uncomplicated, community-based UTIs are caused by certain virulent strains of *Escherichia coli,* which is normally present in large quantities in feces. Other common uropathogens include such gram-negative organisms as *Klebsiella pneumoniae, Enterobacter aerogenes,* and *Proteus* species and gram-positive bacteria such as *Enterococcus faecalis, Staphylococcus epidermidis,* and *S. saprophyticus. S. saprophyticus* is the second most common pathogen, causing approximately 10% to 15% of uncomplicated lower UTI.

Bacteria presence in the urine does not necessarily indicate clinical infection. Contamination of urine samples by bacteria normally present in the anterior urethra or periurethra is common. To distinguish genuine bladder bacteriuria from contamination, therefore, certain values have been established. For women, significant bacteriuria is traditionally defined as the presence of more than 10^5/mL colonies of the same organism of clean-catch midstream urine. However, some women with recurrent UTI have had bacterial counts less than 10^5/mL that may have been responsible for symptoms. Further, some studies have shown that about one-third of women with acute lower UTI caused by *E. coli, S. saprophyticus,* and *Proteus* had colony counts of 10^2 to 10^4/mL of midstream urine.

Female Susceptibility

A number of factors make the female urinary tract vulnerable to infection. The most common route of infection is ascending transurethral infection, whereby fecal microorganisms colonize the periurethral area (vulva, vagina, rectum) and subsequently enter the bladder via the urethra. The shortness of the female urethra offers little impediment to the passage of these bacteria. Poor hygiene has been also implicated, including the practice of wiping toward the urethra after a bowel movement. Sexual intercourse provides easy transmission of bacteria to the entrance of the urethra and bladder. Indeed, several studies have shown that women with UTI are more likely to have had intercourse within the previous 24 to 48 hours than are women without a UTI. Engaging in both vaginal and anal intercourse also increases risk of infection. As mentioned, use of contraceptive diaphragms and spermicides increase the risk of UTI. Spermicides can destroy protective lactobacilli and alter the vaginal pH, thus promoting colonization by *E. coli,* which can then spread to the urethra. Diaphragms can introduce bacteria to the urethra during insertion or removal, cause a decreased sensation to urinate, and produce poor bladder emptying.

The following systemic and local urinary structural factors also increase susceptibility to UTI:

- Diabetes mellitus, malnutrition, a compromised immune system
- Local receptor characteristics of uroepithelial cells
- Presence of foreign bodies, such as stones, stent, catheter
- Urine stasis, caused by obstruction, overdistension of the bladder in neurogenic conditions, or pelvic relaxation
- Congenital or acquired abnormalities, such as ureterovesical reflux or bladder diverticula

Personal immunologic variations can also make one woman more susceptible to certain bacteria than another.

Estrogen Deficiency

Atrophic changes occur in the vagina and lower urinary tract as a result of postmenopausal estrogen loss (1). With decreased estrogen levels, the vaginal epithelium loses its glycogen content and, thus, its normal acidogenic bacterial flora. The vaginal pH rises from the normally acidic range of 4.5 to 5.5 to alkaline levels of 7 or higher (16), making the vagina more susceptible to colonization and infection with bacteria, fungi, viruses, and protozoa (53). Loss is also seen in muscle tone, contractility, and elasticity of the vagina because of understimulation of estrogen receptors in smooth muscle and connective tissue (16); this can result in shortening and narrowing of the vagina and friability of the tissue (54).

Estrogen loss leads to similar atrophic changes in the urinary structures. The urethral mucosa decreases in thickness and atrophies, with decreased urethral closure pressure. Increased urethral pH and consequent colonization by *E. coli* probably contribute to the greater susceptibility of postmenopausal women to UTI (55,56). In addition, the distance between the urethral and vaginal openings becomes shorter, and vaginal manipulation may therefore cause irritation and inflammation in the urethra (16).

Types of Lower Urinary Tract Infection

Cystitis is the most common of the urinary tract infections. Patients usually experience dysuria, frequency, urgency, and pain. Bacteria are present in the urine in a concentration of 10^5/mL organisms or more of clean-catch midstream urine. The urine usually also contains large numbers of white blood cells. Red blood cells are often present microscopically, and gross hematuria may occur. The bladder is noted to be reddened and inflamed if it is visualized.

Frequency and dysuria occur in 10% to 30% of women with sexually transmitted diseases or other forms of vaginitis. It is important to distinguish acute bacterial cystitis from vulvovaginitis caused by yeast, *Trichomonas,* or bacterial infections, as well as sexually transmitted infections involving the cervix and urethra, such as *Chlamydia trachomatis, Neisseria gonorrhoeae,* or herpes simplex virus. Patients with vulvovaginitis often have discomfort on voiding as urine flows over the inflamed labia (external dysuria). Other symptoms of vaginitis include soreness of the vulva, pruritus, foul vaginal discharge, and dyspareunia. Pus and blood in the urine are rare, and urine culture usually reveals less than 10^2/mL colonies of bacteria.

Urethritis generally presents with the typical findings of lower UTI, including dysuria, frequency, and urgency. The urethra is often tender to palpation. Significant pyuria is often noted in a clean-catch urine sample, especially that obtained early in the voiding. Urine samples should be obtained for culture. Pus can sometimes be expressed from the urethra; this is especially common in acute gonococcal or chlamydial infections. Culture of expressed pus often reveals *N. gonorrhoeae* or *Chlamydia*.

Urethritis caused by sexually transmitted organisms usually causes milder symptoms, with a more gradual onset of dysuria and absence of other urinary symptoms. Vaginal discharge or bleeding or lower abdominal pain may be present. Pyuria is usual, but hematuria is rare. Urine cultures demonstrate less than 10^2/mL bacterial colonies.

The acute urethral syndrome (also known as the "dysuria-pyuria syndrome") is characterized by signs and symptoms suggestive of lower UTI (dysuria, frequency, urgency, pain) but fewer than 10^5/mL bacteria in urine. The symptoms are generally of long duration, and no specific organism can be identified. Urethroscopic studies indicate a reddened, chronically inflamed urethra with spasm at the bladder neck. The acute urethral syndrome is common, with an estimated 30% to 50% of women with dysuria having this condition at one time or another (52). Although the cause is unknown, theories include allergic, immunologic, infectious, atrophic, neurologic, and psychogenic causes.

Asymptomatic bacteriuria is a term applied when greater than 10^5 of the same bacterial species/mL of urine are present in two consecutive midstream urine cultures, but signs and symptoms of UTI are absent. Up to 40% of elderly patients have asymptomatic bacteriuria, especially those residing in institutions (52). Asymptomatic bacteriuria only rarely leads to symptomatic infection.

Diagnostic Tests

Biochemical screening tests can be used in the office to detect significant bacteriuria. The Griess test is commonly used and is fairly reliable for detecting *Enterobacteriaceae*, but not gram-positive organisms or *Pseudomonas*. First-morning urine specimens are preferable for testing. This test, combined with the leukocyte esterase test on a single dipstick, can detect bacterial counts greater than 10^5/mL *Enterobacteriaceae* in urine with concomitant pyuria. The combination test has an overall sensitivity and specificity of approximately 85% and 75%, respectively.

To further support a diagnosis of UTI, centrifuged urine should be examined microscopically to detect significant pyuria (>4 white blood cells/high-power field) or hematuria (>4 red blood cells/high-power field). Pyuria is present in all patients who have UTI, but microscopic hematuria may be present in only half. Importantly, the presence of leukocyte casts points to a diagnosis of pyelonephritis.

Culture of clean-catch midstream urine samples is essential for documenting significant bacteriuria and the presence of UTI and to identify the pathogenic organism. The patient should be instructed regarding the proper collection technique. Suprapubic aspiration and bladder catheterization should only be used when it is impossible to obtain uncontaminated urine samples or in symptomatic patients who have low bacterial counts (10^2 to 10^4/mL).

Women with clear-cut signs and symptoms of a UTI associated with significant pyuria and bacteriuria who respond promptly to appropriate antibiotic treatment generally do not require urologic evaluation. Radiologic imaging techniques, such as computed tomography, ultrasound studies, and intravenous pyelography, and cystography are not routinely performed in the diagnosis and management of uncomplicated UTI. Such studies may be required, however, to investigate the cause of infection in the following circumstances: more than two UTIs in a 12-month period; infection with specific organisms (e.g., *Proteus mirabilus, Pseudomonas* sp.); symptoms suggestive of pyelonephritis; poor response to antibiotic therapy; kidney stones, obstruction, or stricture; or persistent hematuria.

Although cystoscopy is rarely indicated, it is part of the diagnostic workup of older patients with gross hematuria in whom bladder cancer is suspected. It may also be used in patients with recurrent or persistent unexplained urinary frequency and dysuria who have no bacteriuria on repeated testing.

Treatment

Women with a first episode of apparently uncomplicated cystitis are usually treated empirically with a short course of antibiotics. Short-course therapy (3 to 5 days) with the following agents are usually effective: trimethoprim (100 to 200 mg) every 12 hours; trimethoprim-sulfamethoxazole (TMP-SMZ) (160 mg/800 mg) every 12 hours; nitrofurantoin (100 mg) every 6 or 8 hours; amoxicillin (250 mg) every 8 hours; ciprofloxacin (250 to 500 mg) every 12 hours; or norfloxacin (500 mg) every 12 hours. TMP-SMZ is considered the drug of choice, because it reduces fecal, vaginal, and periurethral colonization. Nitrofurantoin should not be used in patients who have renal impairment.

Compared with longer (7 to 14 day) regimens, short-course therapy has fewer side effects, better patient compliance, less risk of emergence of resistant bacteria, and lower cost. Patients usually have improvement in symptoms within 1 to 2 days of treatment. Women whose symptoms recur after short-course therapy should provide a urine specimen for culture and be re-treated for 10 to 14 days, with antibiotic selection based on culture results. TMP-SMZ can be administered empirically until culture results become available.

With a view toward even greater patient convenience and compliance and reduced side effects and cost, much interest has recently focused on single-dose therapy. The following have been used as single-dose regimens, with reported cure rates of 85% to 90% or higher: TMP-SMZ (320 mg/1600 mg), two double-strength tablets; amoxicillin (3 g); cephaloridine (2 g); gentamicin (5 mg/kg), and doxycycline (300 mg). Urinary symptoms can persist for 1 to 2 days after single-dose therapy. In addition, a greater incidence of early recurrent infection occurs compared with short-course treatment using the same antibiotics.

Relapse Versus Reinfection

Approximately 20% of young women with a first episode of acute cystitis will develop recurrent UTI. Relapses with the same microorganism can occur because they are not adequately eradicated, because of either too low a dose of antibiotic, too short a period of treatment, or not taking the medication as prescribed. On the other hand, they may indicate that the source of bacteriuria is the upper urinary tract, which should be investigated for renal stones, scars, or polycystic kidneys. Repeat culture results demonstrating the same microorganism with the same antibiotic sensitivities suggest a relapse.

More than 90% of recurrent lower UTI in women is caused by reinfection. In a woman with one or two infections per year, each acute episode can be treated like a single infection, with short-course or a single-dose antibiotic. Three or more infectious episodes per year may be treated with short-course therapy plus a long-term (1 year), low-dose prophylactic antibiotic regimen. Drugs often used prophylactically include trimethoprim, TMP-SMZ, nitrofurantoin, norfloxacin, and cephalexin.

Women who tend to develop recurrent infection after sexual intercourse should void and take a single prophylactic dose of antibiotic after each intercourse. They should be counseled on the risks of diaphragms and spermicides as well.

Postmenopausal Urinary Tract Infection

As discussed, estrogen deficiency produces vaginal and urethral atrophic changes that predispose to bacterial colonization. In addition, the pelvic relaxation that often occurs after menopause can increase postvoid residual urine, which encourages bacterial growth. As a result of these changes, postmenopausal women may develop recurrent lower UTI.

Prophylactic antibiotic therapy can be used to prevent recurrences in these patients. However, the need for pro-phylactic antibiotics may be reduced in these women by estrogen replacement therapy. One study found that in a group of 12 postmenopausal women with a history of frequent UTI, estrogen treatment (either oral or vaginal) led to almost total eradication of recurrent UTI (57). In another trial that assigned women to oral estriol or placebo, 75% of patients receiving active treatment had a reduced rate of UTI after 12 weeks, whereas only 40% of those assigned to placebo improved (58). Results from a randomized, double-blind, placebo-controlled trial were also striking (56). Investigators studied 93 post-menopausal women with a history of recurrent UTI. Participants received either intravaginal estriol (0.5 mg) twice weekly or placebo and were followed by serial urine culture. The treated group experienced 0.5 UTI episodes per patient-year, whereas the corresponding rate in the control group was 5.9 UTI episodes. Improvements in pH and bacterial flora were noted in the treated groups in both these trials.

Estrogen replacement therapy in postmenopausal women may thus play an important role in preventing recurrent UTI, especially in view of the relative safety of estrogen (especially vaginal) compared with the morbidity of recurrent UTI.

Preventive Strategies

In an effort to prevent recurrent UTI, health care professionals often counsel patients on various voiding, hygiene, and dietary habits. Although research has not proved that these techniques prevent UTI, little risk or cost is involved in implementing these changes, and some patients may find them beneficial. These measures include voiding within 1 hour of the urge to urinate; drinking eight glasses of water per day; wiping from front to back after a bowel movement to prevent spreading bacteria; changing underwear daily; wearing cotton underwear; avoiding hot tubs and highly chlorinated pools; avoiding perfumed toilet paper, powders, and bubble baths; avoiding feminine hygiene products that can irritate the urethra; and avoiding food and beverage products believed to be bladder irritants.

CONCLUSION

Symptoms of urinary urgency, frequency, nocturia, or involuntary urine loss may lead a woman to seek medical evaluation when she can no longer tolerate their detrimental effects on her quality of life. Many women, however, do not complain of urinary problems because of embarrassment or unawareness of available therapies; they do not pursue treatment and may become increasingly debilitated and socially isolated. By asking post-menopausal patients who present for a routine gynecologic checkup or another gynecologic problem whether they are experiencing any urinary symptoms, gynecologists can help to bring bladder dysfunction "out of the closet" and help affected women regain their health, self-confidence, and an improved quality of life.

For many women, urinary tract infections are also a major health problem, producing adverse effects on the quality of life as well as leading to potentially life-threatening illnesses. Accurate diagnosis and appropriate antibiotic treatment often lead to cure. In cases of recurrent infection, prophylactic antibiotic therapy and, in postmenopausal women, estrogen replacement therapy, are often beneficial. Preventive practice strategies may also benefit some patients.

REFERENCES

1. Bachmann G. Urogenital ageing: An old problem newly recognized. *Maturitas* 1995;22(Suppl):S1–S5.
2. Resnick NM, Yalla SV. Management of urinary incontinence in the elderly. *N Engl J Med* 1985;313:300–305.
3. Resnick NM. An 89-year-old woman with urinary incontinence. *JAMA* 1996;276:1832–1840.
4. Urinary Incontinence in Adults Guideline Update Panel. *Clinical Practice Guideline on Urinary Incontinence in Adults.* Agency for Health Care Policy and Research, Public Health Service, US Department of Health and Human Services, 1996.
5. Burgio K, Matthews KA, Engel BT. Prevalence, incidence and correlates of urinary incontinence in healthy, middle-aged women. *J Urol* 1991;146:1255–1259.
6. Harrison GL, Memel DS. Urinary incontinence in women: its prevalence and its management in a health promotion clinic. *Br J Gen Pract* 1994;44(381):149–152.
7. Ouslander JG. Geriatric urinary incontinence. *Disease-A-Month* 1992;2:65–149.
8. Griebling TL, Nygaard IE. The role of estrogen replacement therapy in the management of urinary tract infection in postmenopausal women. *Endocrinol Metab Clin North Am* 1997;26:347–360.
9. Thomas TM, Plymat KR, Blannin J, Meade TW. Prevalence of urinary incontinence. *Br Med J* 1980;281:1243–1245.
10. Iosif CS, Bekassy Z. Prevalence of genito-urinary symptoms in the later menopause. *Acta Obstet Gynecol Scand* 1984;63:257–260.
11. Milsom I, Ekelund P, Molander U, Arvidsson L, et al. The influence of age, parity, oral contraception, hysterectomy, and menopause on the prevalence of urinary incontinence in women. *J Urol* 1993;149:1459–1462.
12. Rekers H, Drogendijk AC, Valkenburg HA, Riphagen F. The menopause, urinary incontinence and other symptoms of the genito-urinary tract. *Maturitas* 1992;15:101–111.
13. Levine SA, Barry PP, Eskew AH. The geriatric patient. In: Noble J, ed. *Textbook of primary care medicine,* 2nd ed. St. Louis: Mosby-Year Book, 1996.
14. Hu T. The cost impact of urinary incontinence on health care services. Presented at the Multi-Specialty Nursing Conference on Urinary Continence. Phoenix, AZ, January 1994.
15. Hu T. Impact of urinary incontinence on health-care costs. *J Am Geriatr Soc* 1990;38:292–295.
16. Forsberg JG. A morphologist's approach to the vagina—age-related changes and estrogen sensitivity. *Maturitas* 1995;22(Suppl):S7–S15.
17. Elia G, Bergman A. Estrogen effects on the urethra: beneficial effects in women with genuine stress incontinence. *Obstet Gynecol Surv* 1993;48:509–517.
18. Krantz KE. The human vagina. *J Clin Prac Sexual* 1990;(Special issue):4–10.
19. Dmochowski RR, Leach GE. Bladder dysfunction and urinary incontinence. In: Noble J, ed. *Textbook of primary care medicine,* 2nd ed. St. Louis: Mosby-Year Book, 1996.
20. Appell RA, Baum N. Neurogenic bladder in diabetes. *Pract Diabetol* 1990;9(4):1–4.
21. Bump RC, McClish DM. Cigarette smoking and pure genuine stress incontinence of urine: a comparison of risk factors and determinants between smokers and nonsmokers. *Am J Obstet Gynecol* 1994;170:579–582.
22. Nygaard IE, Thompson FL, Svengalis SL, Albright JP. Urinary incontinence in elite nulliparous athletes. *Obstet Gynecol* 1994;84:183–187.
23. Gynecologic urology. In: Mishell DR, et al., eds. *Comprehensive gynecology.* 3rd ed. St. Louis: Mosby, 1997;601–632.
24. Resnick NM, Yalla SV. Management of urinary incontinence in the elderly. *N Engl J Med* 1985;313:800–805.
25. Iosif CS, Butra SC, Ek A, et al. Estrogen receptors in the human female urinary tract. *Am J Obstet Gynecol* 1981;141:817.
26. Versi E, Cardozo LD, Brincat M, et al. Correlation of urethral physiology and skin collagen in postmenopausal women. *Br J Obstet Gynaecol* 1988;95:147–152.
27. Batra SC, Iosif CS. Female urethra: a target organ for estrogen action. *J Urol* 1983;129:418.
28. Miodrag A, Castleden CM, Vallance TR. Sex hormones and the female urinary tract. *Drugs* 1988;36:491.
29. Fantl JA, Wyman JF, Anderson RL, Matt DW, et al. Postmenopausal urinary incontinence: a comparison between non-estrogen-supplemented and estrogen-supplemented females. *Obstet Gynecol* 1988;71(6):833–838.
30. Samsioe G, Jansson I, Mellstrom D, Svandborg A. Occurrence, nature and treatment of urinary incontinence in a 70-year-old female population. *Maturitas* 1985;7:335–342.
31. Cardozo LD, Rekers H, Tapp A, Barnick C, et al. Oestriol in the treatment of postmenopausal urgency—a multicentre study. *Maturitas* 1993;18:47.
32. McGuire EJ, Ritchey ML, Wan JH. Surgical therapy of uncontrollable detrusor contractility. In: Kursh ED, McGuire EJ, eds. *Female urology.* Philadelphia: JB Lippincott, 1994:130–134.
33. Mundy AR, Stephenson TP. "Clam" ileocystoplasty for the treatment of refractory urge incontinence. *Br J Urol* 1985;57:641–646.
34. Henalla SM, Hutchins CJ, Robinson P, MacVicar J. Nonoperative methods in the treatment of female genuine stress incontinence of urine. *Br J Obstet Gynaecol* 1989;96:222.
35. Henalla SM, Kirwan P, Castleden CM, et al. The effect of pelvic floor exercises in the treatment of genuine urinary stress incontinence in women at two hospitals. *Br J Obstet Gynaecol* 1988;95:602.
36. Tchou DCH, Adams C, Varner RE, Denton B. Pelvic-floor musculature exercises in treatment of anatomical urinary stress incontinence. *Phys Ther* 1988;68:652.
37. Salmon UJ, Walter RI, Geist SA. The use of estrogens in the treatment of dysuria and incontinence in postmenopausal women. *Am J Obstet Gynecol* 1941;12:845.
38. Hilton P, Stanton SL. The use of intravaginal oestrogen cream in genuine stress incontinence. *Br J Obstet Gynaecol* 1983;90:940.
39. Caine M, Raz S. The role of female hormones in stress incontinence. *Proceedings of the 16th Congress of the International Society of Urology.* Amsterdam, 1973.
40. Rud T. The effects of oestrogens and gestagens on the urethral pressure profile in urinary continent and stress incontinent women. *Acta Obstet Gynecol Scand* 1980;59:265–270.
41. Walter S, Kjaergaard B, Lose G, Andersen JT, et al. Stress urinary incontinence in postmenopausal women treated with oral estrogen (estriol) and alpha adrenoceptor-stimulating agent (phenylpropanolamine): a randomised double-blind placebo-controlled study. *Int Urogynecol J* 1990;12:74–79.
42. Bergman A, Karram MM, Bhatia N. Changes in urethral cystometry following estrogen administration. *Gynecol Obstet Invest* 1990;20:211.
43. Walter S, Wolf H, Barlebo H, Jansen H. Urinary incontinence in postmenopausal women treated with oestrogens: a double-blind clinical trial. *Urol Int* 1978;33:135–143.
44. Wilson PD, Paragher B, Butler B, et al. Treatment with oral piperazine oestrone sulphate for genuine stress incontinence in post-menopausal women. *Br J Osbstet Gynaecol* 1987;94:568–574.
45. Fantl JA, Cardozo L, McClish DK. Estrogen therapy in the management of urinary incontinence in postmenopausal women: a meta-analysis. First report of the Hormones and Urogenital Therapy Committee. *Obstet Gynecol* 1994;83:12–18.
46. Beisland HO, Fossberg E, Moer A, Sander S. Urethral sphincteric insufficiency in postmenopausal females: treatment with phenylpropanolamine and estriol separately and in combination. *Urol Int* 1984;39:211–216.
47. Hilton P, Tweddel AL, Mayne C. Oral and intravaginal estrogens alone and in combination with alpha adrenergic stimulation in genuine stress incontinence. *Int Urogynecol J* 1990;12:80–86.
48. Cardozo LD. Role of estrogens in the treatment of female urinary incontinence. *J Am Geriatr Soc* 1990;38:326.
49. Rud T, Andersson KE, Asmussen M, Hunting A, et al. Factors maintaining the intaurethral pressure in females. *Invest Urol* 1980;17:343.
50. Bocho C, Winandy A. Etude preliminaire de l'influence hormonale sur les differents parametres du plancher pelvien chez la femme en activite genitale sans hormonotherapie et chez la femme menopausee. *Acta Urologica Belgica* 1992;60:45–60.
51. Beck RP, McCormick S, Nordstrom L. The fascia lata sling procedure for treating recurrent genuine stress incontinence of urine. *Obstet Gynecol* 1988;72:699.
52. Bastani B. Urinary tract infections. In: Noble J, ed. *Textbook of primary care medicine,* 2nd ed. St Louis: Mosby-Year Book, 1996:1236–1246.
53. Beard MK. Atrophic vaginitis: can it be prevented as well as treated? *Postgrad Med* 1992;91:257–260.
54. Bachmann GA. Impact of vaginal health on sexual function. *J Clin Prac Sexual* 1990;(Special issue):18–21.
55. Notelovitz M. Estrogen therapy in the management of problems associated with urogenital ageing: a simple diagnostic test and the effect of the route of hormone administration. *Maturitas* 1995;22(Suppl):S31–S33.
56. Raz R, Stamm WE. A controlled trial of intravaginal estriol in postmenopausal women with recurrent urinary tract infections. *N Engl J Med* 1993;329:753–760.
57. Privette M, Cade R, Peterson J, Mars D. Prevention of recurrent urinary tract infections in postmenopausal women. *Nephron* 1988;50:24–27.
58. Kirkengen AL, Andersen P, Gjersoe E, Johannessen GR, et al. Oestriol in the prophylactic treatment of recurrent urinary tract infections in postmenopausal women. *Scand J Prim Health Care* 1992;10:139–142.

The Brain and Dementia

In this edition, an expanded section on "The Brain and Dementia" is warranted due to the great deal of new information now available, and because this topic has relevance to the health and welfare of women as aging occurs.

The section begins with an overview of steroid action on the brain—and the multiple mechanisms now understood for these interactions—authored by Neil MacLusky, a researcher who has extensive experience in this area. Both classic receptor and genomic actions as well as nongenomic mechanisms are operative. Next, a clinical perspective on how this steroid action may influence physiology is offered by Vito Cela and Frederick Naftolin. Fred's group has contributed to our understanding of estrogen action in the brain for nearly three decades. Finally, two different groups will discuss the influence of estrogen on Alzheimer s disease risk: in the first chapter by Mary Sano, Diane Jacobs, and Richard Mayeux, the "Epidemiology of Alzheimer's" will be discussed briefly and followed by information on the effects of estrogen. This will be followed by a chapter by Victor Henderson who, together with Annlia Paganini-Hill, first described the protective effects of estrogen on Alzheimer's disease (AD) risk.

In order to put this into perspective, I will provide the following brief overview on dementia and AD: Dementia is diagnosed (DSM-IV criteria) if there are multiple cognitive deficits sufficiently severe to cause impairment in occupational or social functioning (1). The cognitive deficits have to involve memory and other cognitive domains without the presence of delirium. AD accounts for at least 56% of all dementia; vascular effects account for 14% of cases; multiple causes, Parkinson's, brain injury, and others account for 12%, 8%, 4%, and 6% of cases respectively.

AD is difficult to diagnose and ranges from early signs of impaired memory to the finding of severe cognitive loss. As will be discussed later, the prevalence is greater in women and increases with aging: after age 65, the prevalence doubles every five years (2). An important consideration is to potentially identify women at risk for AD. A large number of families with autosomal dominant AD have been described. Siblings have approximately twice the lifetime risk of developing Alzheimer's. There are three genes (on chromosomes 21, 14, and 1) where mutations may lead to AD. Polymorphisms of the apolipoprotein-E gene on chromosome 19 have been associated with the more typical sporadic and familial forms of AD (3). This also will be discussed in Victor Henderson's chapter on the "Role of Sex Steroids in AD." Another susceptibility gene may also occur on chromosome 12 (4).

While some of the specific issues related to AD are beyond the scope of this section, identifying women at risk is important. Potentially preventative strategies such as estrogen replacement, anti-inflammatory and antioxidant agents (5), the cessation of smoking (6), and close follow-up may prove to be important.

REFERENCES

1. American Psychiatric Association. Diagnostic and Statistical Manual of Mental Disorders, (DSM-IV). Washington, D.C: American Psychiatric Association; 1994:143–147.
2. Backman L, Ahlbom A, Winblad B. Prevalence of Alzheimer's disease and other dementia's in an elderly urban population, relationship with age, sex and education. Neurology 1991;41:1886–1892.
3. Mayeux R, Saunders AM, Shea S, Mirra S, Evans D, Roses AD, Hyman BT, Crain B, Tang M-X, Phelps CH. Utility of the APOE Genotype in the

Diagnosis of Alzheimer's Disease. The Alzheimer's Disease Centers Consortium on APOE and Alzheimer's Disease. New Engl J Med 1998;338:506–512.

4. McKeith IG, Ince P, Jaros EB, Fairbairn A, Ballard C, Grace J, Morris CM, Perry RH. What are the relations between Lewy body disease and AD? J Neural Transm Suppl 1998;54:107–16.

5. Stewart W, Kawas C, Corrada M, Metter E. The risk of Alzheimer's disease and duration of NSAID use. Neurology 1997; 48:626–632.

6. Merchant C, Tang M-X, Albert S, Manly J, Stern Y, Mayeux R. The influence of smoking on the risk of Alzheimer s disease. Neurology 1999; 52:1408–1412.

Treatment of the Postmenopausal Woman: Basic and Clinical Aspects, Second Edition, edited by Rogerio A. Lobo, Lippincott Williams & Wilkins, Philadelphia © 1999.

CHAPTER 21

Effects of Sex Steroids on the Brain

Neil J. MacLusky

The effects of gonadal steroids on the development and function of the central nervous system are powerful and pervasive. Their most obvious consequences are the patterns of neuroendocrine hormone release and behavior that subserve reproductive function (1). However, a wide variety of nonreproductive functions are also affected, including cerebral lateralization, responses of the brain to injury, and cognitive performance, particularly in tests of visuospatial and verbal abilities (1,2). In addition to effects on normal function, sex steroids also influence the development and expression of a number of neurologic disorders. Degenerative motor neuron diseases are more common in males, a problem associated in the case of Kennedy's disease with a defect in the androgen receptor (3,4). Many developmental cognitive problems, including dyslexia and autism, are more common and frequently more severe in boys (5). The incidence of schizophrenia exhibits a striking sexual dimorphism: on average, women become ill 3 to 4 years later than men but show a pronounced increase in incidence of the disease at around menopause (6,7). Tardive dyskinesia is also observed more commonly in postmenopausal women than in men of comparable age (8). Other neurologic diseases that do not show overt sex differences in their frequency may nevertheless be subject to effects of gonadal hormone secretions, as is the case with some forms of epilepsy. Epileptic girls who experience normal puberty may have increases in the frequency and severity of seizures at menarche (9). Fluctuations in epileptic seizure activity may also occur with stage of the menstrual cycle (i.e., "catamenial" epilepsy [10–13]).

The diversity and magnitude of steroid effects on the central nervous system (CNS) raise the possibility that hormonal therapy may be useful to ameliorate or prevent the occurrence of neurologic diseases that exhibit sensi-tivity to sex steroids. Several studies have already indicated the potential value of such an approach. The work of Herzog has shown that drugs that modify sex steroid signaling may be useful for treatment of epilepsy (14–16). Some investigators have suggested that the severity of schizophrenia and symptoms of dyskinesia may be improved by manipulation of sex steroid levels (8,17–19). Several studies have suggested that the incidence and severity of neurodegenerative diseases, such as Alzheimer's disease, in postmenopausal women may be reduced by hormone replacement therapy (20).

The mechanisms of action of steroids on the CNS have been the focus of considerable attention over the last few decades, resulting in a large volume of literature devoted to the effects of sex steroids on brain structure and function. Much of this work has emphasized studies on the pathways involved in regulating gonadotropin-releasing hormone (GnRH) release and the stereotyped patterns of sex behavior observed in laboratory animals. These data have been extensively reviewed (21–25); we do not attempt to recapitulate this information here. This chapter focuses instead on aspects of gonadal steroid action in the brain that may be particularly relevant to the proposed role of these steroids as neuroprotective agents in postmenopausal women.

SOURCES OF SEX STEROIDS IN THE CENTRAL NERVOUS SYSTEM

The CNS was first recognized as a target for the effects of sex steroids because of observations on the neuroendocrine and behavioral effects of gonadal secretions in animals. Models developed from these early studies remain the primary tools for investigation of the effects of gonadal steroids on the CNS; much of what we understand about the mechanisms of steroid action on the brain has been derived from them. However, there has been growing recognition that the exclusive emphasis of these models on the effects of steroids derived from the circu-

N. J. MacLusky: Center for Reproductive Sciences, Department of Obstetrics and Gynecology, Columbia University College of Physicians & Surgeons, New York, New York, 10032.

lation may be misleading. Studies during the last two decades have demonstrated that the brain itself is a steroidogenic organ, capable of synthesizing many if not all of the sex steroids found elsewhere in the body. The key enzymes involved in cholesterol side-chain cleavage, the conversion of pregnenolone and progesterone to androgens, and the aromatase enzyme necessary for conversion of androgens to estrogens are all expressed in different cells isolated from the central and peripheral nervous systems (26–32). These observations indicate that the classic view of the brain as a target for the effects of steroids synthesized elsewhere in the body is incomplete, because it ignores the potential contribution from locally synthesized steroids. Responses to gonadal steroids may be initiated through the actions of circulating hormones, through local steroidogenesis within the CNS itself, or through a combination of both mechanisms.

At first sight, this concept may appear counterintuitive. Although the idea that the brain can convert circulating prohormones such as testosterone to more biologically active molecules is consistent with conventional concepts of reproductive endocrinology, the notion that hormonal steroids can be synthesized *de novo* within the CNS does not appear to make sense. It raises the potential for confusion: how can the brain accurately respond to circulating steroid hormones, if those same hormones can be made locally within the brain itself? Although the answer to this question is not completely resolved, it seems likely that an important factor is the relative abundance of steroids derived from local and systemic sources. Under normal reproductive conditions, the quantities of the hormones generated by the gonads are greater than those derived from local biosynthesis within the brain itself, and gonadal feedback loops can operate successfully. This explanation, however, is not entirely satisfactory, because the question still remains of what possible function may be served by the locally synthesized steroids.

To understand the potential complementary roles of locally and systemically derived steroids in the CNS, it may be helpful to consider the way in which feedback loops between the gonads and the brain have evolved. Mechanisms by which gonadal function can be regulated through the pituitary and therefore the CNS offer enormous advantages for free-living multicellular organisms, because they create the opportunity for reproduction to be keyed to changes in the environment and coordinated with the behavior patterns of other members of the same species. Effective hormonal communication between the gonads and the neuroendocrine axis is an evolutionary development that seems to have emerged only with the development of true vertebrates. In the most primitive vertebrates (i.e., cyclostomes), the ovary appears to be relatively autonomous. In these species, although GnRH neurons are present in the hypothalamus and gonadotropins are found in the pituitary (33–35), hypophysectomy fails

to affect ovulation frequency and ovarian estrogen secretion (36). The ovary contains the enzymes necessary for conversion of cholesterol into all of the major classes of sex steroid (37), but circulating steroid hormone concentrations remain relatively low (36,38), suggesting that ovarian steroidogenesis primarily regulates local tissue differentiation rather than regulating the functions of distant target organs. Not until the evolution of the elasmobranchs does a serum luteinizing hormone (LH) surge occur before ovulation (39), and only in bony fishes does pituitary control over early gamete maturation finally emerge (40).

Steroidogenesis in the CNS, like that in the ovary, may therefore have initially evolved as a mechanism for local autocrine and paracrine cellular communication, a role that it probably still serves. As systems subsequently developed for neuroendocrine regulation of gonadal function, preexisting local response mechanisms were modified and expanded to provide for feedback control over gonadal function mediated through circulating hormone secretions. This concept has important physiologic implications. If steroidogenesis in the CNS is involved in normal developmental regulatory processes, it may be overly simplistic to consider the actions of the steroid hormones purely in terms of responses to changes in circulating hormonal levels. Conceptually, it may be more accurate to think of the effects of the gonadal steroids on the brain as representing one aspect of the normal mechanisms involved in maintaining tissue homeostasis, rather than purely in terms of the neuroendocrine regulation of gonadal function. An important corollary of this hypothesis is that local steroidogenic activity within the brain may have a considerable impact on the responses to declining circulating hormone levels. To take a simple hypothetical example, variations between women in the capacity of the brain for local androgen and estrogen biosynthesis could make a major contribution to individual differences in the behavioral and cognitive effects of menopause.

EFFECTS OF GONADAL STEROIDS ON CENTRAL NERVOUS SYSTEM STRUCTURE AND FUNCTION

Until recently, it was considered axiomatic that the brain had only a limited capacity for repair and regeneration in adulthood. Developmental mechanisms in the CNS, in which new neurons and glial cells are added and new cellular connections formed, were assumed to be largely or completely supplanted in the mature brain by a state in which structural remodeling could only occur to a very limited extent. Effects of gonadal steroids on the brain were considered within the context of a similar conceptual framework. During early life, sex steroids were viewed as exerting organizational effects, involved in the development of sex differences in behavior and neuroendocrine responses, which permanently altered the structure and function of certain regions within the CNS. Later in life, steroid effects were viewed as being primarily activational, modulating the function of preexisting, essentially rigidly organized pathways (1,41).

During the past few years, these simple models have had to be reevaluated. We now know that the mature CNS can undergo significant remodeling, including the generation of new neurons (42–44). Similarly, at least some aspects of the mechanisms involved in gonadal steroid-induced brain differentiation during development can also be activated in the mature brain (45). These observations raise the possibility that steroid-induced remodeling of the brain may contribute significantly to normal and pathophysiologic responses to alterations in the internal hormonal milieu.

Evidence for gonadal steroid-induced effects on the morphology of the brain emerged initially from studies of the mechanisms underlying CNS sexual differentiation. In many mammals, the organization of neural circuits controlling sexually differentiated neuroendocrine and behavioral functions is permanently modified as a result of exposure to sex-specific patterns of gonadal steroid secretion during early life. Testosterone exposure in the male induces permanent differentiation of the volume of certain hypothalamic and preoptic area cell groups, and it effects changes in the numbers, types, and topographic distribution of synaptic inputs (1,46,47). As in other androgen target tissues, the effects of testosterone on the developing brain depend heavily on conversion of the circulating hormone to locally active active metabolites. In contrast to the reproductive tract, however, in which formation of 5α-dihydrotestosterone is responsible for amplifying the response to the circulating steroid, in the brain, aromatization to estradiol appears to be of paramount importance (1). For example, testosterone-induced masculinization of the sexually dimorphic component of the medial preoptic area in rats is blocked by coadministration of the antiestrogen, tamoxifen (48).

Morphologic effects of gonadal steroid exposure, although most prominent in the hypothalamus and preoptic area, are by no means confined to this region of the brain. They also include structures known to be important for memory processing and cognitive function. During development, sex differences have been reported in the thickness of different regions of the cerebral cortex (49,50). In some strains of mice, males have more granule cell neurons in the hippocampal dentate gyrus than females (51). Likewise, male rats have a larger and more asymmetric dentate gyrus than females (52,53). In rats, sex differences have been demonstrated in the apical dendritic structure and the dendritic branching patterns of CA3 pyramidal neurons. Because the apical dendrites of CA3 pyramidal cells are the targets of afferent mossy fiber synapses from the granule cell layer of the dentate gyrus, these observations are consistent with the hypothesis that there is increased input from the dentate gyrus in

males (54). Additional evidence for functional differences in the innervation of the CA3 region has been provided by Galea et al. (55), who demonstrated a sex difference in the dendritic morphologic response observed in this region of the brain after repeated restraint stress.

Effects of gonadal steroids on hippocampal neuronal structure also occur in adulthood. The density of dendritic spines in the CA1 region of the hippocampus changes cyclically during the estrous cycle of the female rat, with a peak immediately after the proestrous estrogen surge (56). Estrogen treatment induces an increase in dendritic spine density in the CA1 region but is without effect in the CA3 region or dentate gyrus. Progesterone administration rapidly potentiates estrogen-induced spine formation, but this response is rapidly followed by downregulation of spine density. That this delayed effect of progesterone probably contributes significantly to the changes observed in the normal estrous cycle can be inferred from the fact that the downregulation of dendritic spines normally occurring between proestrous and estrus is blocked by administration of the progesterone antagonist RU486 (56).

Even more extensive hormone-induced remodeling processes are observed in adulthood in areas of the diencephalon. After surgical deafferentation of the rat mediobasal hypothalamus, estrogen treatment significantly enhances new synapse formation (57,58). In the hypothalamic arcuate nucleus, changes in neuronal membrane structure and in the density of inhibitory synaptic contacts occur sequentially across the ovarian cycle, reflecting opposing effects of estrogen and progesterone on these end points (59–62). In the same region of the brain, estradiol induces modifications in glial morphology, resulting in fluctuations in the nature and extent of contacts between arcuate neurons and glial processes (63,64).

HOW DO GONADAL STEROIDS EXERT THEIR EFFECTS ON THE BRAIN?

The effects of steroid hormones on the CNS are mediated through a number of distinct mechanisms, some quite well established and others still partly speculative. These mechanisms can be considered to fall into two broad categories: responses mediated through intranuclear receptors that comprise part of the steroid receptor superfamily and responses mediated through actions of the steroids at the cell membrane.

Nuclear Steroid Receptor Systems

Steroid receptors are members of a large family of ligand-activated transcription factors that also includes the thyroid hormone, vitamin D, and retinoic acid receptors; the *ERBA* oncogene; and a large number of other related transcription factors and nuclear proteins (65). All members of this gene family appear to be synthesized from single copy genes, each containing several exons. They all also appear to share certain specific structural features, comprising three principal molecular domains: the steroid-binding domain, comprising a section approximately 250 amino acids long at the C terminus of the receptor; a shorter, highly conserved section of about 70 amino acids that contains two zinc finger motifs that bind to specific base sequences (known as hormone response elements) in the DNA with high affinity; and a variable region at the N terminus that is involved in regulating transcriptional activation and that differs markedly between different receptors in terms of length and amino acid sequence. Binding of the steroid to its cognate receptor ligand binding domain initiates a cascade of molecular reactions involving binding of the receptor to the DNA, in concert with a number of other transcription factors and adapter proteins, culminating in activation or suppression of mRNA synthesis (66–69).

The actions of gonadal steroids on the brain appear to be mediated largely through nuclear receptor proteins similar to those found in nonneural steroid target tissues (70,71). Receptors for all of the major classes of hormonal steroid have been identified in the CNS. The phylogenetic conservation of these systems, from primitive fishes through primates (72,73), supports the view that the basic mechanisms of action of steroids on the brain have changed relatively little during vertebrate evolution. Estrogen and androgen receptors are found, with closely overlapping distributions, in several areas of the hypothalamus, preoptic area, amygdala, and septum. Lower concentrations of both receptors are found in other regions of the CNS, including the hippocampus, cerebral cortex, midbrain, brain stem, and spinal cord (73–77).

Much of the early work on estrogen receptor distribution used ligand-binding techniques that we now know preferentially detected only one of the two estrogen receptors found in target tissues: estrogen receptor-alpha (ERα). ERα was once believed to be the receptor responsible for mediating all of the transcriptional effects of estrogen on its target tissues. However, it has been shown that there are two distinct estrogen receptors (78,79). In addition to ERα, there is a second estrogen receptor (ERβ), encoded by a different gene that has extensive (>90%) sequence homology with ERα in the DNA binding domain but only partial homology in other regions of the molecule. ERα and ERβ have different estrogen-binding specificities and different distributions within the brain and in nonneural estrogen target tissues. Table 21.1 summarizes the distributions of ERα and ERβ gene expression in the brain of the rat (80). In many areas (e.g., the midbrain, amygdala, bed nucleus of the stria terminalis, medial preoptic area), the two receptors are coexpressed. However, in some structures, there appears to be preferential expression of one or other subtype. In the mediobasal hypothalamus, ERα expression predominates. In the olfactory bulb, cerebral cortex, hippocam-

TABLE 21.1. *Distribution of ERα and ERβ mRNA expression in the ovariectomized rat brain*

Region	ERα	ERβ
Olfactory bulb	−	++
Allocortex	+	++
Isocortex		
Layers 2–3	−	++
Layers 4–5	+/−	++++
Layer 6	+/−	+++
Hippocampus	+/−	++
Septum	+	++
Diagonal band	+	++
Bed nucleus of the stria terminalis	++++	++++
Amygdala	++++	+++
Medial preoptic area	++++	++++
Paraventricular nucleus	−	+++
Supraoptic nucleus	−	++++
Arcuate nucleus	+++	+
Ventromedial nucleus	++	−
Substantia nigra	−	+
Ventral tegmental nuclei	+	+
Raphe nuclei	−	+
Cerebellar cortex	−	+
Locus ceruleus	+	+
Nucleus of the solitary tract	++	++
Spinal cord	+	+

ER, estrogen receptor.
The intensity of the *in situ* hybridization signal in each region of the brain is represented on a 5-point scale from − (no detectable signal) to ++++ (strong labeling). For simplicity, an estimate of overall labeling intensities is indicated for each structure. In the original analysis from which these data are drawn (80), subdivisions within each of the major cell groups were sampled independently for numbers of labeled cells and overall labeling intensity. The data presented represent approximate overall labeling intensities for each structure, summarized from the more extensive and detailed data in the original publication (80).

pus, the hypothalamic paraventricular and supraoptic nuclei, and the cerebellum, ERβ is expressed with little or no ERα.

In some regions of the brain, estrogen induces the synthesis of progestin receptors (81,82). Particularly marked progestin receptor induction is observed within the hypothalamus and preoptic area, including the arcuate and ventromedial nuclei and the medial and periventricular preoptic area. These responses probably involve ERα and ERβ: studies using the ERα knockout mouse suggest that ERβ is capable of mediating at least partial induction of hypothalamic progestin receptor gene expression (83). Other regions of the brain, including the midbrain, amygdala, cerebral cortex, and hippocampus, also express progestin receptors, but the concentrations of these receptors are unaffected or are only slightly increased by treatment with estrogen (81,82).

Effects mediated by the nuclear gonadal steroid receptor systems on the CNS are functionally interrelated. Androgen receptor–mediated responses are important in the control of aromatase activity in the brain, and therefore contribute to the levels of estradiol available to the estrogen receptor system (84,85). Data from this and several other laboratories on interactions between the three main families of gonadal steroids indicate that androgens and progestins may antagonize the cellular effects of estrogens within the hypothalamus by downregulating the expression of the cognate receptor proteins (86–90). It is also possible that variant receptor isoforms may be involved in fine tuning cellular response mechanisms to different steroid hormone levels. Work using the ERα knockout mouse model suggests that normal expression and function of ERβ in some tissues may not occur unless ERα is present (91). A novel isoform of ERβ (ERβ-2) containing an additional in-frame 54 base pair insertion in the ligand binding domain of ERβ-1 has been identified in several estrogen target tissues of the rat, including the brain, bone, uterus, and ovary (92). The insertion causes loss of ligand binding activity without compromising interactions with the DNA. In a reporter gene experimental system, ERβ-2 dose-dependently suppressed ERα and ERβ-1–mediated transcriptional activation (92), suggesting that this receptor variant may function as a negative regulator of estrogen action.

The effects of the sex steroids may in some cases depend on coordinated interactions with effects mediated by other hormones or neurotransmitters. In nonneural steroid target tissues, numerous examples have been identified of heterologous interactions between nuclear transcription factors, including interactions between receptors for the sex steroids and other receptor proteins (67,93). In the rat brain, estrogen induction of female sexual behavior is inhibited by thyroid hormone (94). At the genomic level, estrogen induces expression of preproenkephalin mRNA in the hypothalamic ventromedial nucleus, a response that is attenuated by thyroid hormone (95). The mechanism of this effect appears to include direct interactions between liganded thyroid receptors and ERs at hormone response elements in the promoter region of the preproenkephalin gene (95).

Another type of coordinated response mechanism has been described with respect to the actions of growth factors and the neurotransmitter dopamine in the brain. In nonneural steroid target cells, phosphorylation of nuclear receptor proteins may, under some circumstances, activate transcriptional responses even when the normal steroid ligand is not present (96,97). Such mechanisms may serve as a means of modulating steroid responses, increasing or decreasing the sensitivity of the cell to steroids through the actions of other hormones or locally active autocrine or paracrine factors that operate through kinase-dependent receptor systems. In SK-ER3 neuroblastoma cells, insulin-like growth factor-1 (IGF-1) and insulin-like growth factor-2 (IGF-2) activate transcriptional responses mediated through the estrogen receptor to control cellular growth and differentiation (98). One of the factors recognized to

control the phosphorylation state of the progesterone receptor is the neurotransmitter dopamine (99). Studies using female sexual behavior in rodents as a progesterone-sensitive behavioral endpoint have demonstrated convergence of dopaminergic and steroid-mediated responses within progesterone target cells. Facilitation of female sexual behavior by activation of the D_1 receptor can be blocked by a D_1 antagonist, progesterone receptor antagonists, or antisense oligonucleotides to the progesterone receptor (100). Moreover, in mice with a null mutation for the progesterone receptor, the ability of dopamine to activate lordosis behavior is lost (101).

Membrane Receptor Systems

Steroids influence the electrical activity of the brain through effects that in some cases have latencies far too short to be mediated through changes in gene transcription initiated through intranuclear receptor proteins (102, 103). The mechanisms underlying these responses remain poorly defined. In the case of estrogens, there is growing evidence that there may be some form of neuronal membrane receptor, perhaps involving a G protein–coupled second messenger system (9,104). Evidence obtained using steroids coupled to albumin is consistent with the hypothesis that there may be membrane-associated receptors for estradiol, testosterone, and progesterone in the rat brain (105). The potential physiologic role of these putative receptor sites remains uncertain, although one of the estrogen binding sites has been characterized as the 23-kd oligomycin-sensitivity conferring protein subunit of adenosine triphosphate (ATP) synthase (106).

Progesterone and the corticosteroids also exert effects mediated through binding to γ-aminobutyric acid type A (GABA_A) receptors. Metabolism of steroids in this series through 5α-reduction and subsequent reduction of the 3-ketone to a 3α-hydroxyl results in compounds that have only a low affinity for the nuclear progestin and glucocorticoid receptors but that are capable at nanomolar concentrations of potentiating the actions of GABA on the GABA_A chloride channel (Fig. 21.1) (107–109). The two components of this metabolic pathway are localized in different cell types; 5α-reductase is found in neurons, oligodendrocytes, and type 2 astrocytes, and 3α-hydroxysteroid dehydrogenase is localized almost exclusively in type 1 astrocytes (110). These observations raise the possibility that cell-cell interactions may be important for progesterone's effects on the GABA system.

Steroid-Induced Changes in the Function of Neurotransmitter Systems

Gonadal steroids induce changes in the synthesis, release, and action of a large number of different neurotransmitters and neuromodulators within the CNS (22,23, 111). Many of these responses may contribute to the

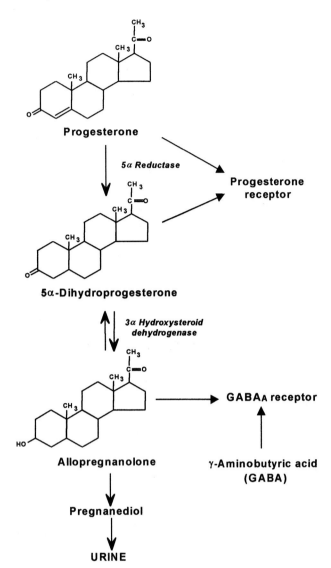

FIG. 21.1. Relationship between pathways of progesterone metabolism in the brain and activation of the progesterone and GABA_A receptors (Courtesy of Grace Erb Tavares, University of Toronto).

effects of gonadal steroids on cognitive function and the development of neurologic disease states. Some may also indirectly contribute to morphologic effects of the steroids on the brain. A complete review of these mechanisms is beyond the scope of this article. Some of the effects of gonadal steroids on cholinergic, catecholaminergic, serotonergic, and glutamatergic transmission are briefly summarized in view of their potential importance in the cause of CNS disorders and their relation to subsequent discussion of the possible neuroprotective effects of the ovarian steroids.

Cholinergic System

The forebrain cholinergic system is critically important for normal cognitive function. Alzheimer's disease patients exhibit marked deficits in cholinergic function, and the administration of cholinesterase inhibitors to reduce acetyl choline metabolism enhances cognitive performance (112). The first indication that estrogen might be important in the cause of age-related changes in cognitive function was provided by studies on the regulation of acetyl choline synthesis in the female rat. Experiments with ovariectomy and estrogen replacement therapy revealed an induction of choline acetyltransferase (ChAT), the rate-limiting enzyme for acetylcholine formation, within 6 to 24 hours in basal forebrain (113,114). Later studies showed that this response probably reflects a direct action of estrogen on forebrain cholinergic neurons (115,116) and at least in part reflects upregulation of ChAT mRNA expression (117, 2118). The trophic effects of estrogen on the cholinergic system are not confined to juvenile or young adult animals. Gibbs (119) reported that ChAT mRNA expression declines with time after ovariectomy in aging female rats, an effect that is partially reversed by short-term (3 days) estrogen treatment. Work by Singh et al. showed that long-term estrogen replacement slowed the normal age-related decline in high-affinity choline uptake and ChAT activity in the frontal cortex and hippocampus (120,121).

Aminergic Systems

Deficits in dopaminergic transmission are believed to underlie the movement disorders observed in Parkinson's disease and tardive dyskinesia. The serotonergic and noradrenergic systems have also been implicated in the regulation of cognitive function and mood state (122). Both of these systems appear to be sensitive to the effects of the ovarian steroids. Bethea (123) demonstrated the presence of estrogen-inducible progestin receptors in most serotonin (5-HT) neurons in the dorsal and ventral raphe of intact and ovariectomized, estrogen- and progesterone-treated macaques. Later studies demonstrated localization of ERs in neurons of the dorsal raphe in the rat, but curiously, these neurons appear not to be serotonergic, suggesting that estrogenic regulation of serotonergic function in rats may be indirect (124). Small numbers of estrogen target neurons are found in catecholaminergic cell groups in the midbrain and brain stem (80,125,126), but there is extensive colocalization of estrogen receptors with dopaminergic neurons in the hypothalamus (127). Studies have demonstrated marked upregulatory effects of estrogen on the levels of D_2 receptors in the striatum (128) and $5\text{-}HT_2$ receptors in several regions of the forebrain (129).

Ovarian steroids may also play an important role in the regulation of amine neurotransmitter concentrations through changes in the expression of the neurotransmitter transporters. Ovariectomy in rats results in upregulation of the striatal dopamine transporter, a response that is prevented by treatment with estradiol or estradiol plus progesterone but not by progesterone alone (130). Contrasting and opposite effects are observed with respect to the hypothalamic 5-HT transporter, which is downregulated by ovariectomy and restored to normal control levels by estrogen replacement (130).

Excitatory Amino Acids

There is abundant evidence that glutamatergic neurotransmission is important in the regulation of reproductive neuroendocrine function (131). The facilitatory effects of glutamate agonists, such as N-methyl-D-aspartic acid (NMDA), on GnRH secretion are dependent on the presence of estrogen (132,133), suggesting that estrogen exerts a stimulatory or permissive action on some component of the hypothalamic glutamate response mechanism. Attempts to demonstrate effects of estrogen on the levels of glutamate or of its receptors in the hypothalamus have yielded conflicting results. Hypothalamic glutamate release is not significantly different between ovariectomized and ovariectomized–estrogen replaced rats (134,135). These observations must be regarded as inconclusive because one of the problems of interpreting data on glutamate levels is that all cells also use this amino acid biosynthetically; it is therefore difficult to tease out changes that may be specifically associated with glutamate neurotransmitter function (22). Ovariectomy and estrogen replacement have been reported to have no significant effect on hypothalamic NMDA receptor levels (136). However, Diano et al. reported that estrogen might stimulate hypothalamic expression of a different glutamate receptor subtype, the so-called AMPA receptor (137). These findings are consistent with the hypothesis that the enhanced sensitivity of the GnRH pulse generator to glutamate after estrogen administration may at least in part be a consequence of upregulation of AMPA glutamate receptor expression (137).

In the hippocampus, there is clear evidence for estrogen-mediated upregulation of the NMDA glutamate receptor subtype. Estradiol induces NMDA receptor binding sites in the CA1 region of the rat hippocampus (138). Immunocytochemical studies using antibodies raised against the NMDA receptor R1 subunit have also demonstrated that treatment with estrogen elevates expression of receptor immunoreactivity in the cell bodies and dendrites of CA1 pyramidal neurons (Fig. 21.2) (139). These effects may be involved in mediating the changes in hippocampal structure occurring over the female reproductive cycle, as mentioned earlier (56). Surprisingly, estrogen induction of new spine synapses in the CA1 region is blocked by concurrent administration of NMDA receptor antagonists (140). These observations suggest that estrogen induction and, by extension, the progesterone-mediated inhibition of new spine synapses in the CA1 region may involve intermediary changes in the release of glutamate. How such changes may result in the initiation of changes in dendritic spine structure

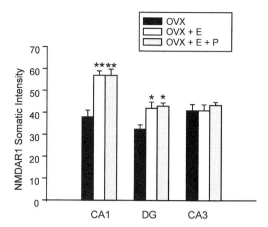

FIG. 21.2. Regulation of hippocampal N-methyl-D-aspartate (NMDA) receptor subunit 1 (NMDAR-1) by estrogen and progesterone. Ovariectomized (OVX) rats were treated with estrogen alone, estrogen plus progesterone, or the vehicle control. The intensity of NMDAR-1 immunostaining over the somata of neurons in the CA1, CA3, and dentate gyrus granule cell layers of the hippocampus was quantified by confocal laser scanning microscopy. Significant upregulation of NMDAR-1 staining intensity is observed over the CA1 and dentate gyrus cells (*$p < 0.05$; **$p < 0.0001$ versus the OVX group). (Adapted from ref. 139, with permission.)

remains obscure, but one possibility is that increases in calcium flux resulting from NMDA receptor activation may promote changes in the interactions between the major neuronal cytoskeletal proteins (56).

CELLULAR CONTROL OF NEURONAL GROWTH AND SURVIVAL

Although steroids can potentially modulate the structure of pathways in the CNS through alterations in neurotransmitter release and function, this is not the only available mechanism. Sex steroids may also affect neuronal differentiation and survival through several different local regulatory mechanisms. Just how powerful these systems can be has been demonstrated through studies using experimental models of CNS damage. Lesions placed in the fimbria decrease the numbers of medial septal neurons expressing choline acetyl transferase; the number of surviving cholinergic neurons is significantly augmented by estrogen treatment targeted to the brain (141). Administration of the neurotoxin 1-methyl-4-phenyl-1,2,3,6-tetrahydropyridine (MPTP) to mice results in significant damage to their nigrostriatal dopaminergic system, as evidenced by a marked reduction in dopamine levels. This response is attenuated by estrogen treatment (142,143). In animal models of stroke injury, estrogen treatment significantly reduces mortality and diminishes the volume of the infarct produced by vascular occlusion (144–147).

The various mechanisms through which gonadal steroids may regulate the growth and development of cells in the CNS can be considered under four main headings: regulation of proteins involved in neuronal survival, antioxidant effects, effects on neuronal energy metabolism, and induction of growth factor–mediated responses.

Metabolic Controls: Protection Against Cellular Metabolic Stress

Cell death can occur through one of two basic processes: apoptosis (i.e., programmed cell death [PCD]), or necrosis. The primary difference between these processes is that, whereas necrosis reflects an uncontrolled nonspecific event resulting from damage to the cell, PCD is a normal cellular function triggered through activation or release from suppression of a specific set of genes. An extensive body of evidence supports the hypothesis that PCD is important in the developing and the adult CNS (148). Cells dying through PCD often exhibit distinct morphologic and biochemical characteristics, including chromatin condensation and subsequent breakdown of the DNA into nucleosomal fragments, and cellular fragmentation. A delicate balance between several families of gene products appears to be involved in determining whether a cell enters into PCD (149). Indirect evidence supports the hypothesis that estrogens may regulate PCD in the brain. Estrogens regulate genes involved in PCD in hormone-dependent breast cancer (150–152). BCL2 related anti- and pro-apoptotic proteins play important roles in the initial decision step of the intracellular PCD pathway. Studies have demonstrated that BCL2 is upregulated by estrogen in the hypothalamic arcuate nucleus. The extent to which this protein is regulated in other regions of the brain, and the degree to which this regulation may affect the differential expression of other BCL2-related proteins, remain to be elucidated.

Another potential mechanism of protection involves the heat shock proteins (HSPs), the predominant forms of which have molecular weights of about 70 kd (HSP70) and about 90 kd (HSP90). These proteins are induced in mammalian cells in response to a wide variety of metabolic stressors. They are also important modulators of steroid responses, acting as molecular chaperons for the steroid receptor proteins (153). In the uterus, estrogen induces heat shock transcription factors (HTF) I and II (154). In the ventromedial nucleus of the hypothalamus, physiologic doses of estrogen induce the constitutive forms of HSP70 and HSP90 (155,156). Studies in the pheochromocytoma cell line PC-12 have demonstrated that heat shock partially protects these cells from cell death induced by addition of β-amyloid protein (157, 158). This raises the possibility that estrogens might protect nerve cells from death induced by mechanisms other than direct modulation of the PCD pathway.

Estrogens may affect neuronal survival by modulating the expression or metabolism of proteins that might otherwise present risk factors for neuronal function. One of the characteristic features of Alzheimer's disease is the accumulation of cerebral plaques containing β-amyloid peptides. Estrogen has been reported to decrease the production of β-amyloid by neuroblastoma cells and by primary cultures of mouse, rat, and human cerebral cortical neurons (159). There is also evidence that it may alter the secretory metabolism of the β-amyloid precursor protein, resulting in nonamyloidogenic processing (160). Epidemiologic studies have demonstrated a positive association between expression of the ε-4 variant of apolipoprotein E (apoE) and late-onset Alzheimer's disease (112). In C3H mice, estrogen treatment induces significant increases in the levels of brain apoE mRNA, but has no effect on the expression of the same gene in the liver (161). These observations raise the potential for interaction between estrogen exposure and apo-E expression in the pathology of late-onset Alzheimer's disease.

Estrogens as Antioxidants

Oxidative damage is a major risk factor for neuronal survival, during normal development and aging, as well under the specific circumstances of cellular damage resulting from transient hypoxia. Because estrogens have biologic antioxidant properties, these effects may also contribute significantly to the neuroprotective effects of this hormone.

The antioxidant effects of estrogens may involve a number of different mechanisms. Estrogens may indirectly protect cells against oxidative damage by altering the levels of cellular antioxidant defense systems, such as the levels of glutathione peroxidase (162) and ascorbic acid (163). They may also exert direct chemical antioxidant effects. Postmenopausal women taking estrogen replacement exhibit reduced levels of low-density lipoprotein (LDL) oxidation, an effect that has been linked to estrogen's protective effects with respect to atherosclerosis (164). Under *in vitro* conditions, a number of studies have shown that estrogens inhibit lipid peroxidation (165–167). The mechanisms involved are not completely understood. There is a considerable amount of evidence to support the view that nuclear estrogen receptors are not involved and that the feature of the molecule that is required for antioxidant activity is the phenolic ring, which can act as a source of hydrogen ions to terminate lipid peroxidation reactions (167). Estrogens such as 17α-estradiol and phytoestrogens such as equol and genistein, which have relatively low affinities for the estrogen receptor, also inhibit lipid oxidation *in vitro* (168,169). However, it is probably not valid to assume that estrogens act merely as chemical antioxidants. This is because the effects of the estrogens are clearly different under *in vitro* test conditions than they are *in vivo*. Under *in vitro* conditions, while estrogens have been shown to inhibit LDL oxidation, the concentrations of hormone required are in the micromolar range—well above the physiologic circulating levels of estradiol known to be adequate to significantly inhibit LDL oxidation *in vivo*.

An explanation for this apparent disparity has emerged from work carried out on the oxidation of LDL *in vitro* (170). Mechanisms exist in the blood, as well as potentially as in estrogen target tissues, that enhance the antioxidant properties of the estrogen molecule. Incubation of rat serum with a low physiologic concentration of 17β-estradiol (1 nM) resulted in significant protection against LDL oxidation (170). This was associated with apparent conversion of the estradiol to a C17 fatty acid ester. When esterification of the estradiol at C17 position was inhibited by coincubation with 5′,5′-dithiobis-(2-nitrobenzoic) acid (DTNB), the protective antioxidant effect of the hormone was lost (170). These findings suggest that C17 esterification of the estrogen molecule may result in the formation of lipophilic metabolites with enhanced antioxidant potency, an observation of considerable potential importance given the wide distribution and long biologic half-life of C17 estradiol esters in the body (171).

Whatever the basis for the antioxidant effects of estrogen, there is ample evidence to suggest that these effects may play an important role in the neuroprotective effects of this hormone, at least under some circumstances. *In vitro* cell culture studies have shown that estrogens protect rodent hippocampal neurons and human neuroblastoma cells from oxidative damage. Significantly, from the perspective of possible mechanisms involved in the development of Alzheimer's disease, β-amyloid (25–35) induced toxicity is attenuated in neurons exposed to high concentrations of estrogens (Fig. 21.3) (166). This effect is associated with decreased cellular lipid peroxidation.

The general impression of estrogen as a neuroprotective antioxidant must, however, be tempered with caution, because in some systems, long-term estrogen exposure may have exactly the opposite effect. In adult female rodents, reproductive senescence occurs primarily because of failure of the hypothalamic systems responsible for regulating GnRH secretion. This appears to be primarily the result of neurodegeneration in the arcuate nucleus resulting from repeated exposure to ovulatory levels of estradiol (172). Studies on the mechanisms underlying this effect have demonstrated that prolonged exposure to elevated estrogen concentrations damages the β-endorphin neurons in the mediobasal hypothalamus (173–175), possibly through an oxidative mechanism because the effects of estradiol are blocked by concurrent treatment with the antioxidant U74389F (176). There is not necessarily any disparity between these observations and the preceding discussion, because it is possible that at the cellular level the mechanisms involved may be quite different. Nevertheless, they illustrate the fact that the biochemical effects of estrogen on the CNS may vary considerably between one target structure and another.

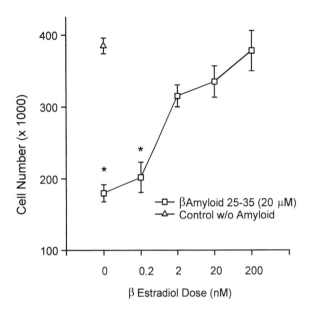

FIG. 21.3. HT-22 cells, a cell line derived from mouse hippocampus that lacks estrogen receptors, are killed by prolonged exposure to β-amyloid (25–35) peptide. Addition of 17β-estradiol exerts a dose-dependent protective effect against amyloid-induced cell death (*$p < 0.05$ versus the control group without amyloid). (Adapted from ref. 166, with permission.)

Estrogens and Brain Glucose Uptake

Under normal physiologic conditions, glucose is the brain's sole source of energy. Glucose cannot enter the brain by diffusion but must be carried across the blood-brain barrier by specific transporters—in particular, the GLUT-1 endothelial cell glucose transporter protein and the GLUT-3 neuronal glucose transporter. The activity of these transporter systems represents an important control point affecting overall cerebral function.

Studies have demonstrated correlations between glucose availability and cognitive performance. In animals, increasing circulating glucose levels enhances performance in tests of memory. A rise in glucose levels at the time of or after training enhances subsequent memory retention (177). In humans, deficits in glucose metabolism may be associated with the appearance of symptoms of neurodegenerative disease. Glucose metabolism and glucose transporter expression are decreased in the brains of Alzheimer's patients (178,179). A growing body of evidence suggests that abnormalities in mitochondrial function may contribute to the onset of neurodegenerative diseases (180,181), consistent with the hypothesis that deficiencies in mitochondrial oxidative metabolism may be an early step in the mechanism of these diseases. However, mutations in the mitochondrial genome have been found to segregate with only relatively few CNS disorders (180,181). Preliminary reports indicating that mutations in the mitochondrial glucose metabolizing enzyme, cytochrome oxidase *c*, may be associated with late onset

Alzheimer's disease (182) appear to be the result of an artifact resulting from polymerase chain reaction amplification of nuclear pseudogenes (183).

In view of the foregoing discussion, cerebral glucose metabolism has been shown to be profoundly sensitive to estrogen. Ovariectomy in female rats results in a significant reduction in brain glucose use, an effect that is reversed by estrogen replacement (184). Increased cerebral glucose use after estrogen could theoretically reflect the positive effects of this hormone on cerebral blood flow (185–187). However, estrogen also exerts specific effects on glucose transport across the blood-brain barrier. Physiologic doses of 17β-estradiol cause an increase in levels of endothelial GLUT-1 mRNA and protein (188). Replacement therapy with 17β-estradiol enhances GLUT-1 expression in the penumbral region surrounding experimental cerebral infarcts in rats, an effect that may contribute to the positive effect of the hormone on neuronal survival (144).

Steroidal Modulation of Growth Responses in the Central Nervous System

The recognition that testosterone and, hence, estradiol induce morphologic changes in the developing brain as part of the mechanisms involved in CNS sexual differentiation raised the possibility that these steroids might have neurotrophic effects. This hypothesis was first directly tested by Toran-Allerand, using an organotypic explant culture system. Estradiol and testosterone, but not the nonaromatizable androgen 5α-dihydrotestosterone, were found to enhance the growth and arborization of neuronal and astroglial processes from the rodent hypothalamus and cerebral cortex (189–191). This growth-stimulatory property of estrogen has subsequently been confirmed by a number of other laboratories in dissociated cell culture systems (192,193) and in fetal brain tissue transplanted into adult hosts (194).

The mechanisms responsible for these effects remain incompletely understood. Estrogen may directly upregulate expression of cytoskeletal and growth-related genes, such as tubulin (195), tau microtubule-associated protein (192), and growth-associated protein (GAP)-43 (196–198). It also increases the expression of a number of different growth factors that may contribute directly or indirectly to enhancement of the estrogen responses. Possible mechanisms are illustrated schematically in Fig. 21.4. According to this model, estrogen effects may be mediated through several interlinked pathways: through direct induction of estrogen-sensitive genes; through indirect effects mediated through changes in the expression of growth factors and growth factor receptors; and by intracellular crosstalk between different nuclear and membrane receptor-activated signaling cascades (45).

One of the first growth-promoting factors to be implicated in estrogen action in the brain was insulin. Several

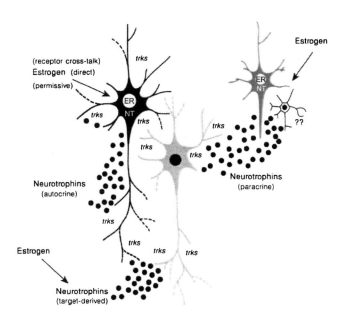

FIG. 21.4. Possible mechanisms of estrogen action in the developing central nervous system. Estrogen actions may be mediated directly through binding to estrogen receptors. Estrogen may regulate neurite growth and differentiation through modulatory interactions with endogenous peptide growth factors and their receptors through estrogen-induced autocrine, local paracrine, or target-derived mechanisms. Estrogen also may exert permissive effects by which the estrogen receptor may facilitate neurotrophin actions by means of genomic crosstalk with signaling cascades initiated through intracellular protein kinases. (From ref. 45, with permission.)

studies have suggested that there may be specific contributions of insulin and insulin-like growth factors to the development and expression of normal reproductive neuroendocrine function. In streptozotocin-induced female diabetic rats, reproductive function is impaired. This effect does not result from abnormal glucose levels, because even when glucose levels are normalized, the reproductive deficits remain, suggesting that hypoinsulinemia compromises normal responsiveness to circulating ovarian steroids (199). Under tissue culture conditions, insulin, alone or in combination with estrogen, induces morphologic responses in neurons and glia (27,189,190,200). Studies on the interactions between estrogens and IGF-1 suggest that IGF-1 release from astroglia may synergize with the effects of estrogen in promoting the survival and differentiation of hypothalamic neurons (62).

Some of the most dramatic evidence for growth factor–mediated effects of estrogen has emerged from studies of the effects of neurotrophins and neurotrophin receptors in the developing brain. In the CNS, a number of related neurotrophic factors have been identified, each with their own distinctive temporal and regional patterns of expression. These factors include nerve growth factor (NGF), brain-derived neurotrophic of factor (BDNF), neurotrophin-3, and neurotrophin-4/5 (NT-3 and NT4/5). Responses to the neurotrophins are mediated by two types of cell membrane receptors. One class is represented by members of the TRK family of tyrosine kinases (201,202). Three members of this family (TRKA, TRKB, and TRKC) are preferentially expressed in neural tissues and are required for signal transduction of NGF, BDNF, and NT-3, respectively. The other receptor, the p75 neurotrophin receptor (p75NTR) is a 75-kd transmembrane protein, previously referred to as the low-affinity NGF receptor. P75NTR, which is related to the TNF-CD40-FAS family of receptors (201,202), binds all of the neurotrophins and may act synergistically with TRK-mediated signaling in activating responses to NGF (203)

In rodents, estrogen receptor levels increase rapidly during early postnatal life in many areas of the brain, including the neocortex and hippocampus (204–209). Subsequently, receptor levels remain elevated in the hypothalamus, preoptic area, and amygdala but decline in the remainder of the brain to the relatively lower levels observed in adulthood. During early postnatal development, there is extensive colocalization of estrogen receptors with expression of the neurotrophins and their cognate membrane receptors, throughout the forebrain (210–212). That this relationship may be functional is suggested by the presence of putative estrogen response elements in the growth factor genes (45,213). In one of the classic models of NGF action, the rat pheochromocytoma PC-12 cell line, estrogen receptors are present only at relatively low levels in the undifferentiated cells. Treatment of the cells with NGF, however, increases the levels of estrogen receptor mRNA and protein. In these same cells, estrogen treatment transiently downregulates p75NTR mRNA and upregulates TRKA mRNA (214). A similar stimulatory effect of NGF on estrogen receptor expression has been reported for explant cultures of the developing rat cerebral cortex (215), suggesting that growth factor responses may be involved in regulating the transient expression of estrogen receptors observed in this region of the brain (205,208,209).

These studies, taken together, are consistent with the hypothesis that estrogen may regulate growth and differentiation processes in the developing CNS through modulation of growth factor synthesis and action. Moreover, the relationship may be reciprocal, in that growth factor action may play a role in regulating estrogen receptor levels. However, trophic effects of estrogen on the brain are not limited to early development but may be activated in adulthood by normal physiologic changes in steroid levels or by exposure to estrogens under conditions of neuronal damage and repair (141,144–147). To what extent can these effects also be explained on the basis of induction of growth factor–mediated responses?

The answer to this question is not entirely clear, but it seems likely that growth factor–mediated effects play at least some role in the responses of the adult nervous system to estrogen exposure. In the dorsal root ganglion, expression of mRNA transcripts for TRKA and the p75

neurotrophin receptor (p75NTR) is substantially higher (about 300%) in intact rats killed at proestrus compared with ovariectomized animals. Treatment of ovariectomized rats with estrogen rapidly downregulates p75NTR expression in the dorsal root ganglion and elicits a time-dependent upregulation of TRKA mRNA (211). In the olfactory bulbs and cerebral cortex of ovariectomized rats, estrogen rapidly upregulates levels of BDNF mRNA (213). Similar data have been reported by Gibbs et al. (216), who found that estrogen and progesterone hormone replacement in adult ovariectomized increases TRKA mRNA expression in the medial septum and BDNF mRNA in the dentate gyrus granule cell layer and the CA1 and CA3/4 regions of the hippocampus.

CONCLUSIONS

Little more than a decade ago, the focus of most work on the actions of gonadal steroids on the brain was directed toward the reproductive neuroendocrine and behavioral consequences of hormones delivered to the brain through the general circulation. In a remarkably short time, the emphasis of research in this field has changed. Although the reproductively oriented effects of the hormones remain as potent examples of steroid-induced CNS responses, there is a growing appreciation that nonreproductive functions of the CNS are also affected by gonadal steroids, throughout life. These effects may have a significant impact on the incidence and severity of human CNS disorders. Effects of gonadal steroids may be an integral part of the normal processes involved in development, maintenance, and repair of the brain. Interactions between the hormones and between the hormones and other cellular and intercellular signaling pathways may play critical roles in maintaining neurotransmitter receptor systems, in preventing irreversible cellular damage, and on potentiating processes involved in the remodeling of neural circuitry.

The effects of estrogens on the CNS are particularly powerful, affecting multiple systems involved in the neuroendocrine control of the pituitary, the expression of cognitive functions, and the regulation of mood. Of particular interest from the perspective of the potential use of estrogen replacement in the treatment of neurologic disease states, several of these effects involve mechanisms that may enhance the development and survival of neurons under conditions of metabolic stress. Experimental models of focal cerebral ischemia and neurotoxin exposure demonstrate the potency of estrogen as a neuroprotective agent. Whether these responses reflect all or only a subset of the effects of estrogen in the CNS remains uncertain. Estrogen may be effective in these model systems precisely because its actions involve a number of convergent and complementary mechanisms. Alternatively, there may be one or more individual pathways of estrogen action that are of primary importance as mediators of enhanced cell survival. There is insufficient information to distinguish between these possibilities.

The question of how estrogen exerts its neuroprotective effects is important for many reasons. An issue that has yet to be resolved is the extent to which the effects of estrogen on the brain are mimicked by partial estrogen antagonists, such as tamoxifen and raloxifene. These compounds have been called selective estrogen receptor modulators (SERMs) because of their capacity to selectively activate only some estrogen responses. SERMs have been proposed to represent an improved approach to hormone replacement therapy by virtue of the fact that they have estrogen-like effects on bone and the cardiovascular system but antagonize the growth-promoting effects of estradiol, particularly on the breast (217,218). There is also considerable interest in the potential for prophylactic use of these agents to reduce the risk of breast cancer (218). However, little is known about the CNS effects of these compounds, particularly in humans. If their actions on the brain are primarily antiestrogenic, chronic administration of SERMs could precipitate central estrogen withdrawal symptoms, potentially including an increased risk of neurodegenerative disease. The only information available on this point is equivocal. In general, the SERMs appear to exert weak estrogen-like negative feedback effects on the regulation of gonadotropin release (218), but whether these responses reflect an action at the level of the brain or the anterior pituitary remains uncertain. The CNS side effects of tamoxifen include increased incidence of hot flushes (also called hot flashes), nausea, mood disorders, and occasionally depression (218–221), all effects consistent with the hypothesis that tamoxifen's actions on the brain are primarily antiestrogenic. Preliminary data suggest that raloxifene has only minor CNS side effects, with an increased frequency of hot flushes observed with high-dose (600 mg/day) treatment (222). Animal data are in general concordant with the clinical observations. Tamoxifen inhibits estrogen-dependent reproductive behaviors, blocks the ovulatory LH surge, and inhibits neurochemical estrogen responses in the brain (223–226). Estrogen agonist responses are observed only with respect to changes in food intake (227). In relation to effects on neuronal growth responses, almost nothing is known because there have been no systematic studies of the effects of different SERMs on neuronal growth and differentiation. It seems possible that SERMs may exert at least some of the same beneficial effects as estrogen, but tamoxifen and its bioactive metabolite, 4-hydroxytamoxifen, have both been shown to protect human LDL from oxidative degradation, mimicking the antioxidant effects of estradiol (228).

An improved knowledge of the mechanism of estrogen action is also important from the perspective of anticipating the potential side effects of combining different therapeutic agents for long-term treatment of neurodegenerative diseases. In addition to estrogen, several different approaches to treatment of these diseases have been proposed, including the use of agents that block the early mitochondrial steps in the apoptotic cascade (229) and administration of drugs designed to enhance the function of specific neurotransmitter pathways (e.g., cholinesterase inhibitors for treatment of Alzheimer's disease). Lacking detailed knowledge of how estrogen exerts its effects, it is difficult to predict whether the effects of these drugs may be enhanced or suppressed by combination with hormone replacement therapy. In the case of cholinesterase inhibitors, the effects of combination therapy may be synergistic; a preliminary trial of the cholinesterase inhibitor tacrine demonstrated a significantly better tacrine response after 30 weeks of treatment in patients who were taking hormone replacement before the onset of the trial than in subjects who were not receiving estrogen (230).

Perhaps the most exciting prospect raised by the emerging new data on estrogen action in the brain is the possibility of developing agents capable of targeting individual cellular neuroprotective pathways. If a specific estrogen response mechanism is particularly important in terms of protection against neurodegeneration, it may be possible to design therapeutic agents with enhanced activity on this system. This could provide the opportunity for development of hormone replacement regimens with improved neuroprotective activity, without increasing the potential for unwanted side effects that might be observed with high doses of estrogen. There are already indications that this is a realistic possibility. Under *in vitro* conditions, the structural requirements for the antioxidant effects of estrogens appear to be very different from those required for nuclear receptor activation (167,168). Too many unanswered questions remain to allow rational design of new prospective neuroprotective estrogens. Data from studies on the oxidation of LDL illustrate the risks inherent in extrapolating from *in vitro* model systems to the situation *in vivo*. Although a wide range of phenolic steroids exhibits antioxidant properties *in vitro*, for physiologic concentrations in contact with plasma, Shwaery et al. reported that only 17β-estradiol significantly inhibited the oxidation of LDL because of the apparent dependence of this reaction on the intermediate formation of steroid C17 fatty acid esters; at the same concentrations, estrone and estriol are without effect (231).

Although estrogens can exert neuroprotective effects under a variety of experimental conditions, we still have too little information about the relative contributions made by different cellular mechanisms to the actions of the hormones *in vivo* to allow conclusions to be drawn about the likely outcome of long-term treatment. One of the challenges for future research will be to resolve this uncertainty.

ACKNOWLEDGMENTS

Financial Support for work in the author's laboratory has been provided by grants from the Natural Science and Engineering and the Medical Research Councils of Canada.

REFERENCES

1. MacLusky NJ, Naftolin F. Sexual differentiation of the central nervous system. *Science* 1981;211:1294–1303.
2. Witelson SF. Neural sexual mosaicism: sexual differentiation of the human temporo-parietal region for functional asymmetry. *Psychoneuroendocrinology* 1991; 16:131–153.
3. Danek A, Witt TN, Mann K, et al. Decrease in androgen binding and effect of androgen treatment in a case of X-linked bulbospinal neuronopathy. *Clin Invest* 1994;72:892–897.
4. MacLean HE, Choi W, Rekaris G, Warne GL, Zajac JD. Abnormal androgen receptor binding affinity in subjects with Kennedy's disease (spinal and bulbar muscular atrophy). *J Clin Endocrinol Metab* 1995;80:508–516.
5. Critchley M. *The dyslexic child.* Springfield, IL: Charles C Thomas, 1970.
6. Hafner H, an der Heiden W, Behrens S, et al. Causes and consequences of the gender difference in age at onset of schizophrenia. *Schizophr Bull* 1998;24:99–113.
7. Hafner H, an der Heiden W. Epidemiology of schizophrenia. *Can J Psychiatry* 1997;42:139–151.
8. Glazer WM, Naftolin F, Morgenstern H, Barnea ER, MacLusky NJ, Brenner LM. Estrogen replacement and tardive dyskinesia. *Psychoneuroendocrinology* 1985; 10:345–350.
9. Morrell MJ. Hormones and epilepsy through the lifetime. *Epilepsia* 1992;33 [Suppl 4]:S49–S61.
10. Duncan S, Read CL, Brodie MJ. How common is catamenial epilepsy? *Epilepsia* 1993;34:827–831.
11. Herkes GK, Eadie MJ, Sharbrough F, Moyer T. Patterns of seizure occurrence in catamenial epilepsy. *Epilepsy Res* 1993;15:47–52.
12. Bauer J, Wildt L, Flugel D, Stefan H. The effect of a synthetic GnRH analogue on catamenial epilepsy: a study in ten patients. *J Neurol* 1992;239:284–286.
13. Jacono JJ, Robertson JM. The effects of estrogen, progesterone, and ionized calcium on seizures during the menstrual cycle of epileptic women. *Epilepsia* 1987; 28:571–577.
14. Herzog AG. Reproductive endocrine considerations and hormonal therapy for women with epilepsy. *Epilepsia* 1991;32[Suppl 6]:S27–33.
15. Herzog AG, Klein P, Jacobs AR. Testosterone versus testosterone and testolactone in treating reproductive and sexual dysfunction in men with epilepsy and hypogonadism. *Neurology* 1998;50:782–784.
16. Herzog AG. Progesterone therapy in women with complex partial and secondary generalized seizures. *Neurology* 1995;45:1660–1662.
17. Bosse R, DiPaolo T. The modulation of brain dopamine and GABAA receptors by estradiol: a clue for CNS changes occurring at menopause. *Cell Mol Neurobiol* 1996;16:199–212.
18. Seeman MV. Clinical and demographic correlates of neuroleptic response. *Can J Psychiatry* 1985;30:243–245.
19. Lindamer LA, Lohr JB, Harris MJ, Jeste DV. Gender, estrogen, and schizophrenia. *Psychopharmacol Bull* 1997;33:221–228.
20. Yaffe K, Sawaya G, Lieberburg I, Grady D. Estrogen therapy in postmenopausal women: effects on cognitive function and dementia. *JAMA* 1998;279:688–695.
21. McEwen BS, Jones KJ, Pfaff DW. Hormonal control of sexual behavior in the female rat: molecular, cellular and neurochemical studies. *Biol Reprod* 1987;36: 37–45.
22. Herbison AE. Multimodal influence of estrogen upon gonadotropin-releasing hormone neurons. *Endocr Rev* 1998;19:302–330.
23. Kalra SP, Horvath T, Naftolin F, Xu B, Pu S, Kalra PS. The interactive language of the hypothalamus for the gonadotropin releasing hormone (GNRH) system. *J Neuroendocrinol* 1997;9:569–576.
24. Pfaff DW. Hormones, genes, and behavior. *Proc Natl Acad Sci USA* 1997;94: 14213–14216.
25. Mani SK, Blaustein JD, O'Malley BW. Progesterone receptor function from a behavioral perspective. *Horm Behav* 1997;31:244–255.
26. Naftolin F, Ryan KJ, Davies IJ, et al. The formation of estrogens by central neuroendocrine tissue. *Recent Prog Horm Res* 1975;31:295–319.
27. Jung-Testas I, Baulieu EE. Steroid hormone receptors and steroid action in rat glial cells of the central and peripheral nervous system. *J Steroid Biochem Mol Biol* 1998;65:243–251.
28. Baulieu EE, Schumacher M. Neurosteroids, with special reference to the effect of progesterone on myelination in peripheral nerves. *Multiple Sclerosis* 1997;3: 105–112.
29. Guennoun R, Fiddes RJ, Gouezou M, Lombes M, Baulieu E. A key enzyme in the biosynthesis of neurosteroids, 3beta-hydroxysteroid dehydrogenase/delta5-delta4-isomerase (3beta-HSD), is expressed in rat brain. *Mol Brain Res* 1995;30: 287–300.
30. Zwain IH, Yen SS, Cheng CY. Astrocytes cultured *in vitro* produce estradiol-17beta and express aromatase cytochrome P-450 (P-450 AROM) mRNA. *Biochim Biophys Acta* 1997;1334:338–348.
31. Compagnone NA, Mellon SH. Dehydroepiandrosterone: a potential signalling molecule for neocortical organization during development. *Proc Natl Acad Sci USA* 1998;95:4678–4683.
32. Baulieu EE, Robel P. Dehydroepiandrosterone (DHEA) and dehydroepiandrosterone sulfate (DHEAS) as neuroactive neurosteroids [Comment]. *Proc Natl Acad Sci USA* 1998;95:4089–4091.
33. Knox CJ, Boyd SK, Sower SA. Characterization and localization of gonadotropin-releasing hormone receptors in the adult female sea lamprey, *Petromyzon marinus.* *Endocrinology* 1994;134:492–498.
34. Ball JN. Hypothalamic control of the pars distalis in fishes, amphibians, and reptiles. *Gen Comp Endocrinoly* 1981;44:135–170.
35. Crim JW, Urano A, Gorbman A. Immunocytochemical studies of luteinizing hormone-releasing hormone in brains of agnathan fishes. I. Comparisons of adult Pacific lamprey (Entosphenus tridentata) and the Pacific hagfish (Eptatretus stouti). *Gen Comp Endocrinol* 1979;37:294–305.
36. Dodd JM. The ovary. In: Pang P, Schreibman MP, eds. *Vertebrate endocrinology: fundamentals and biological implications.* Boca Raton, FL: Academic Press, 1986;351–388.
37. Kime DE. The steroids. In: Chester-Jones PM, Ingleton PM, Philips JG, eds. *Fundamentals of comparative vertebrate endocrinology, I.* New York: Plenum Press, 1987;1–56.
38. Matty AJ, Tsuneki K, Gorbman A. Thyroid and gonadal function in hypophysectomized hagfish, Eptatretus stouti. *Gen Comp Endocrinol* 1976;30:500–516.
39. Callard IP, Klosterman LL, Sorbera LA, Fileti LA, Reese JC. Endocrine regulation of reproduction in vertebrates: archetype for terrestrial vertebrates. *J Exp Zool Suppl* 1998;2:12–22.
40. Nagahama Y. Endocrine regulation of gametogenesis in fish. *Int J Dev Biol* 1994; 38:217–229.
41. Goy RW, McEwen BS. *Sexual Differentiation of the Brain.* Cambridge: MIT Press, 1980.
42. Cameron HA, McEwen BS, Gould E. Regulation of adult neurogenesis by excitatory input and NMDA receptor activation in the dentate gyrus. *J Neurosci* 1995;15:4687–4692.
43. Gage FH. Stem cells of the central nervous system. *Curr Opin Neurobiol* 1998; 8:671–676.
44. Eriksson PS, Perfilieva E, Bjork-Eriksson T, et al. Neurogenesis in the adult human hippocampus. *Nat Med* 1998;4:1313–1317.
45. Toran-Allerand CD. The estrogen/neurotrophin connection during neural development: is co-localization of estrogen receptors with the neurotrophins and their receptors biologically relevant?. *Dev Neurosci* 1996;18:36–48.
46. Arnold AP, Gorski RA. Gonadal steroid induction of structural sex differences in the central nervous system. *Ann Rev Neurosci* 1984;7:413–442.
47. Toran-Allerand CD. On the genesis of sexual differentiation of the general nervous system: morphogenetic consequences of steroidal exposure and possible role of alpha-fetoprotein. *Prog Brain Res* 1984;61:63–98.
48. Dohler KD, Coquelin A, Davis F, et al. Pre- and postnatal influence of an estrogen antagonist and an androgen antagonist on differentiation of the sexually dimorphic nucleus of the preoptic area in male and female rats. *Neuroendocrinology* 1986;42:443–448.
49. Stewart J, Kolb B. The effects of neonatal gonadectomy and prenatal stress on cortical thickness and asymmetry in rats. *Behav Neural Biol* 1988;49:344–360.
50. Diamond MC, Dowling GA, Johnson RE. Morphologic cerebral cortical asymmetry in male and female rats. *Exp Neurol* 1981;71:261–268.
51. Wimer CC, Wimer RE. On the sources of strain and sex differences in granule cell number in the dentate area of house mice. *Brain Res Dev Brain Res* 1989; 48:167–176.
52. Roof RL, Havens MD. Testosterone improves maze performance and induces development of a male hippocampus in females. *Brain Res* 1992;572:310–313.
53. Roof RL. The dentate gyrus is sexually dimorphic in prepubescent rats: testosterone plays a significant role. *Brain Res* 1993;610:148–151.
54. Parducz A, Garcia-Segura LM. Sexual differences in the synaptic connectivity in the rat dentate gyrus. *Neurosci Lett* 1993;161:53–56.
55. Galea LA, McEwen BS, Tanapat P, Deak T, Spencer RL, Dhabhar FS. Sex differences in dendritic atrophy of CA3 pyramidal neurons in response to chronic restraint stress. *Neuroscience* 1997;81:689–697.
56. Woolley CS, McEwen BS. Roles of estradiol and progesterone in regulation of hippocampal dendritic spine density during the estrous cycle in the rat. *J Comp Neurol* 1993;336:293–306.
57. Matsumoto A, Arai Y, Osanai M. Estrogen stimulates neuronal plasticity in the deafferented hypothalamic arcuate nucleus in aged female rats. *Neurosci Res* 1985;2:412–418.
58. Matsumoto A, Arai Y. Synaptogenic effect of estrogen on the hypothalamic arcuate nucleus of the adult female rat. *Cell Tissue Res* 1979;198:427–433.
59. Derer P, Caviness VS Jr, Sidman RL. Early cortical histogenesis in the primary olfactory cortex of the mouse. *Brain Res* 1977;123:27–40.
60. Pérez J, Luquín S, Naftolin F, García-Segura LM. The role of estradiol and progesterone in phased synaptic remodelling of the rat arcuate nucleus. *Brain Res* 1993;608:38–44.
61. Baldazzi L, Baroncini C, Pirazzoli P, et al. Two mutations causing complete androgen insensitivity: a frame-shift in the steroid binding domain and a Cys→Phe substitution in the second zinc finger of the androgen receptor. *Hum Mol Genet* 1994; 3:1169–1170.

62. Fernandez-Galaz MC, Morschl E, Chowen JA, Torres-Aleman I, Naftolin FG, Garcia-Segura LM. Role of astroglia and insulin-like growth factor-I in gonadal hormone-dependent synaptic plasticity. *Brain Res Bull* 1997;44:525–531.

63. Garcia-Segura LM, Luquin S, Parducz A, Naftolin F. Gonadal hormone regulation of glial fibrillary acidic protein immunoreactivity and glial ultrastructure in the rat neuroendocrine hypothalamus. *Glia* 1994;10:59–69.

64. Garcia-Segura LM, Chowen JA, Duenas M, Torres-Aleman I, Naftolin F. Gonadal steroids as promoters of neuro-glial plasticity. *Psychoneuroendocrinology* 1994;19:445–453.

65. O'Malley BW, Tsai MJ. Molecular pathways of steroid receptor action. *Biol Reprod* 1992;46:163–167.

66. Landel CC, Kushner PJ, Greene GL. The interaction of human estrogen receptor with DNA is modulated by receptor-associated proteins. *Mol Endocrinol* 1994; 8:1407–1419.

67. Katzenellenbogen JA, O'Malley BW, Katzenellenbogen BS. Tripartite steroid hormone receptor pharmacology: interaction with multiple effector sites as a basis for the cell- and promoter-specific action of these hormones. *Mol Endocrinol* 1996; 10:119–131.

68. McInerney EM, Tsai MJ, O'Malley BW, Katzenellenbogen BS. Analysis of estrogen receptor transcriptional enhancement by a nuclear hormone receptor coactivator. *Proc Natl Acad Sci USA* 1996;93:10069–10073.

69. Burris TP, Nawaz Z, Tsai MJ, O'Malley BW. A nuclear hormone receptor-associated protein that inhibits transactivation by the thyroid hormone and retinoic acid receptors. *Proc Natl Acad Sci USA* 1995;92:9525–9529.

70. McEwen BS, Biegon A, Davis PG, et al. Steroid hormones: humoral signals which alter brain cell properties and functions. *Recent Prog Horm Res* 1982;38:41–92.

71. McEwen BS. Actions of sex hormones on the brain: "organization" and "activation" in relation to functional teratology. *Prog Brain Res* 1988;73:121–134.

72. Morrell JI, Pfaff DW. A neuroendocrine approach to brain function: localization of sex steroid concentrating cells in vertebrate brains. *Am Zool* 1978;18:447–460.

73. Stumpf WE, Sar M. Anatomical distribution of estrogen, androgen, progestin, corticosteroid and thyroid hormone target sites in the brain of mammals: phylogeny and ontogeny. *Am Zool* 1978;18:435–445.

74. Simerly RB, Chang C, Muramatsu M, Swanson LW. Distribution of androgen and estrogen receptor mRNA-containing cells in the rat brain: an in situ hybridization study. *J Comp Neurol* 1990;294:76–95.

75. Pfaff DW, Gerlach JL, McEwen BS, Ferin M, Carmel P, Zimmerman EA. Autoradiographic localization of estrogen-concentrating cells in the brain of the female rhesus monkey. *J Comp Neurol* 1976;170:279–293.

76. Puy L, MacLusky NJ, Becker L, Karsan N, Trachtenberg J, Brown TJ. Immunocytochemical detection of androgen receptor in human temporal cortex characterization and application of polyclonal androgen receptor antibodies in frozen and paraffin-embedded tissues. *J Steroid Biochem Mol Biol* 1995;55:197–209.

77. Brown TJ, Sharma M, Karsan N, Walters MJ, MacLusky NJ. in vitro autoradiographic measurement of gonadal steroid receptors in brain tissue sections. *Steroids* 1995;60:726–737.

78. Kuiper GGJM, Carlsson B, Grandien K, et al. Comparison of the ligand binding site specificity and transcript tissue distribution of estrogen receptors α and β. *Endocrinology* 1997;138:863–870.

79. Kuiper GG, Enmark E, Pelto-Huikko M, Nilsson S, Gustafsson JA. Cloning of a novel receptor expressed in rat prostate and ovary. *Proc Natl Acad Sci USA* 1996; 93:5925–5930.

80. Shughrue PJ, Lane MV, Merchenthaler I. Comparative distribution of estrogen receptor-alpha and -beta mRNA in the rat central nervous system. *J Comp Neurol* 1997;388:507–525.

81. Parsons B, Rainbow TC, MacLusky NJ, McEwen BS. Progestin receptor levels in rat hypothalamic and limbic nuclei. *J Neurosci* 1982;2:1446–1452.

82. MacLusky NJ, McEwen BS. Progesterone receptors in rat brain: distribution and properties of cytoplasmic progestin binding sites. *Endocrinology* 1980;106: 192–202.

83. Shughrue PJ, Lubahn DB, Negro-Vilar A, Korach KS, Merchenthaler I. Responses in the brain of estrogen receptor alpha-disrupted mice. *Proc Natl Acad Sci USA* 1997;94:11008–11012.

84. Roselli CE, Abdelgadir SE, Resko JA. Regulation of aromatase gene expression in the adult rat brain. *Brain Res Bull* 1997;44:351–357.

85. Roselli CE, Resko JA. Aromatase activity in the rat brain: hormonal regulation and sex differences. *J Steroid Biochem Mol Biol* 1993;44:499–508.

86. Brown TJ, Adler GH, Sharma M, Hochberg RB, MacLusky NJ. Androgen treatment decreases estrogen receptor binding in the ventromedial nucleus of the rat brain: a quantitative in vitro autoradiographic analysis. *Mol Cell Neurosci* 1994; 5:549–555.

87. Erskine MS, MacLusky NJ, Baum MJ. Effect of 5α-Dihydrotestosterone on sexual receptivity and neural progestin receptors in ovariectomized rats given pulsed estradiol. *Biol Reprod* 1985;33:551–559.

88. Brown TJ, MacLusky NJ. Progesterone modulation of estrogen receptors in microdissected region of the rat hypothalamus. *Mol Cell Neurosci* 1994;5: 283–290.

89. Feder HH, Marrone BL. Progesterone: its role in the central nervous system as a facilitator and inhibitor of sexual behavior and gonadotrophin release. *Ann N Y Acad Sci* 1977;286:331–354.

90. Fraser CL, Swanson RA. Female sex hormones inhibit volume regulation in rat brain astrocyte culture. *Am J Physiol Cell Physiol* 1994;267:C909–C914.

91. Couse JF, Lindzey J, Grandien K, Gustafsson JA, Korach KS. Tissue distribution and quantitative analysis of estrogen receptor-alpha (ERalpha) and estrogen receptor-beta (ERbeta) messenger ribonucleic acid in the wild-type and ERalpha-knockout mouse. *Endocrinology* 1997;138:4613–4621.

92. Maruyama K, Endoh H, Sasaki-Iwaoka H, et al. A novel isoform of rat estrogen receptor beta with 18 amino acid insertion in the ligand binding domain as a putative dominant negative regular of estrogen action. *Biochem Biophys Res Commun* 1998;246:142–147.

93. Pratt WB, Scherrer LC, Hutchison KA, Dalman FC. A model of glucocorticoid receptor unfolding and stabilization by a heat shock protein complex. *J Steroid Biochem Mol Biol* 1992;41:223–229.

94. Dellovade TL, Zhu YS, Krey L, Pfaff DW. Thyroid hormone and estrogen interact to regulate behavior. *Proc Natl Acad Sci USA* 1996;93:12581–12586.

95. Zhu YS, Yen PM, Chin WW, Pfaff DW. Estrogen and thyroid hormone interaction on regulation of gene expression. *Proc Natl Acad Sci USA* 1996;93:12587–12592.

96. Ignar-Trowbridge DM, Nelson KG, Bidwell MC, Curtis SW, Washburn TF, McLachlan JA, Korach KS. Coupling of dual signaling pathways: epidermal growth factor action involves the estrogen receptor. *Proc Natl Acad Sci USA* 1992; 89:4658–4662.

97. Ignar-Trowbridge DM, Teng CT, Ross KA, Parker MG, Korach KS, McLachlan JA. Peptide growth factors elicit estrogen receptor-dependent transcriptional activation of an estrogen-responsive element. *Mol Endocrinol* 1993;7:992–998.

98. Ma ZQ, Santagati S, Patrone C, Pollio G, Vegeto E, Maggi A. Insulin-like growth factors activate estrogen receptor to control the growth and differentiation of the human neuroblastoma cell line SK-ER3. *Mol Endocrinol* 1994;8:910–918.

99. Power RF, Mani SK, Codina J, Conneely OM, O'Malley BW. Dopaminergic and ligand-independent activation of steroid hormone receptors. *Science* 1991;254: 1636–1639.

100. Mani SK, Allen JMC, Clark JH, Blaustein JD, O'Malley BW. Convergent pathways for steroid hormone- and neurotransmitter-induced rat sexual behavior. *Science* 1994;265:1246–1249.

101. Mani SK, Allen JM, Lydon JP, et al. Dopamine requires the unoccupied progesterone receptor to induce sexual behavior in mice [published erratum appears in *Mol Endocrinol* 1997;11:423]. *Mol Endocrinol* 1996;10:1728–1737.

102. Wong M, Moss RL. Long-term and short-term electrophysiological effects of estrogen on the synaptic properties of hippocampal CA1 neurons. *J Neurosci* 1992;12:3217–3225.

103. Kelly MJ, Moss RL, Dudley CA. Effects of microelectrophoretically applied estrogen, cortisol and acetylcholine on medical preoptic-septal unit activity throughout the estrous cycle of the female rat. *Exp Brain Res* 1977;30:53.

104. Moss RL, Dudley CA. Molecular aspects of the interaction between estrogen and the membrane excitability of hypothalamic nerve cells. *Prog Brain Res* 1984;61: 3–22.

105. Ramirez VD, Zheng J. Membrane sex-steroid receptors in the brain. *Front Neuroendocrinol* 1996;17:402–439.

106. Ramirez VD, Zheng J, Siddique KM. Membrane receptors for estrogen, progesterone, and testosterone in the rat brain: fantasy or reality. *Cell Mol Neurobiol* 1996;16:175–198.

107. Hawkinson JE, Kimbrough CL, McCauley LD, Bolger MB, Lan NC, Gee KW. The neuroactive steroid 3alpha-hydroxy-5Beta-pregnan-20-one is a two-component modulator of ligand binding to the GABAA receptor. *Eur J Pharmacol Mol Pharmacol* 1994;269:157–163.

108. Gee KW, Bolger MB, Brinton RE, Coirini H, McEwen BS. Steroid modulation of the chloride ionophore in rat brain: structure-activity requirements, regional dependence and mechanism of action. *J Pharmacol Exp Ther* 1988;246:803–812.

109. Marrow AL, Pace JR, Purdy RH, Paul SM. Characterization of steroid interactions with gamma-aminobutyric acid receptor-gated chloride ion channels: evidence for multiple steroid recognition sites. *Mol Pharmacol* 1990;37:263–270.

110. Martini L, Melcangi RC, Maggi R. Androgen and progesterone metabolism in the central and peripheral nervous system. *J Steroid Biochem Mol Biol* 1993;47: 195–205.

111. Pfaff DW, Schwartz-Giblin S. Cellular mechanisms of female reproductive behaviors In: Knobil E, Neill J, eds. *The physiology of reproduction*. New York: Raven Press, 1988.

112. Cummings JL, Vinters HV, Cole GM, Khachaturian ZS. Alzheimer's disease: etiologies, pathophysiology, cognitive reserve, and treatment opportunities. *Neurology* 1998;51:S2–S17.

113. Luine VN, Khylchevskaya RI, McEwen BS. Oestrogen effects on brain and pituitary enzyme activities. *J Neurochem* 1974;23:925–934.

114. Luine VN. Estradiol increases choline acetyltransferase activity in specific basal forebrain nuclei and projection areas of female rats. *Exp Neurol* 1985;89:484–490.

115. Toran-Allerand CD, Miranda RC, Bentham WD, et al. Estrogen receptors colocalize with low-affinity nerve growth factor receptors in cholinergic neurons of the basal forebrain. *Proc Natl Acad Sci USA* 1992;89:4668–4672.

116. Gibbs RB. Expression of estrogen receptor-like immunoreactivity by different subgroups of basal forebrain cholinergic neurons in gonadectomized male and female rats. *Brain Res* 1996;720:61–68.

117. Gibbs RB. Fluctuations in relative levels of choline acetyltransferase mRNA in different regions of the rat basal forebrain across the estrous cycle: effects of estrogen and progesterone. *J Neurosci* 1996;16:1049–1055.

118. Gibbs RB, Wu D, Hersh LB, Pfaff DW. Effects of estrogen replacement on the relative levels of choline acetyltransferase, trkA, and nerve growth factor messenger RNAs in the basal forebrain and hippocampal formation of adult rats. *Exp Neurol* 1994;129:70–80.

119. Gibbs RB. Impairment of basal forebrain cholinergic neurons associated with aging and long-term loss of ovarian function. *Exp Neurol* 1998;151:289–302.

120. Singh M, Meyer EM, Simpkins JW. The effect of ovariectomy and estradiol replacement on brain-derived neurotrophic factor messenger ribonucleic acid expression in cortical and hippocampal brain regions of female Sprague-Dawley rats. *Endocrinology* 1995;136:2320–2324.

121. Singh M, Meyer EM, Millard WJ, Simpkins JW. Ovarian steroid deprivation results in a reversible learning impairment and compromised cholinergic function in female Sprague-Dawley rats. *Brain Res* 1994;644:305–312.

122. Mortola JF. Estrogens and mood. *J Soc Obstet Gynaecol Can* 1997;19[Suppl]:1–6.

123. Bethea CL. Regulation of progestin receptors in raphe neurons of steroid-treated monkeys. *Neuroendocrinology* 1994;60:50–61.

124. Alves SE, Weiland NG, Hayashi S, McEwen BS. Immunocytochemical localization of nuclear estrogen receptors and progestin receptors within the rat dorsal raphe nucleus. *J Comp Neurol* 1998;391:322–334.

125. Kritzer MF. Selective colocalization of immunoreactivity for intracellular gonadal hormone receptors and tyrosine hydroxylase in the ventral tegmental area, substantia nigra, and retrorubral fields in the rat. *J Comp Neurol* 1997;379:247–260.

126. Sar M, Stumpf WE. Central noradrenergic neurons concentrate 3H-oestradiol. *Nature (Lond)* 1981;289:500–502.

127. Sar M. Estradiol is concentrated in tyrosine hydroxylase-containing neurons of the hypothalamus. *Science* 1984;223:938–940.

128. Bosse R, DiPaolo T. The modulation of brain dopamine and GABAA receptors by estradiol: a clue for CNS changes occurring at menopause. *Cell Mol Neurobiol* 1996;16:199–212.

129. Fink G, Sumner BE, Rosie R, Grace O, Quinn JP. Estrogen control of central neurotransmission: effect on mood, mental state, and memory. *Cell Mol Neurobiol* 1996;16:325–344.

130. Attali G, Weizman A, Gil-Ad I, Rehavi M. Opposite modulatory effects of ovarian hormones on rat brain dopamine and serotonin transporters. *Brain Res* 1997;756:153–159.

131. Brann DW, Mahesh VB. Glutamate: a major neuroendocrine excitatory signal mediating steroid effects on gonadotropin secretion. *J Steroid Biochem Mol Biol* 1995;53:325–329.

132. Reyes A, Xia LN, Ferin M. Modulation of the effects of N-methyl-D,L-aspartate on luteinizing hormone by the ovarian steroids in the adult rhesus monkey. *Neuroendocrinology* 1991;54:405–411.

133. Arias P, Jarry H, Leonhardt S, Moguilevsky JA, Wuttke W. Estradiol modulates the LH release response to N-methyl-D-aspartate in adult female rats: studies on hypothalamic luteinizing hormone-releasing hormone and neurotransmitter release. *Neuroendocrinology* 1993;57:710–715.

134. Ping L, Mahesh VB, Wiedmeier VT, Brann DW. Release of glutamate and aspartate from the preoptic area during the progesterone-induced LH surge: in vivo microdialysis studies. *Neuroendocrinology* 1994;59:318–324.

135. Jarry H, Hirsch B, Leonhardt S, Wuttke W. Amino acid neurotransmitter release in the preoptic area of rats during the positive feedback actions of estradiol on LH release. *Neuroendocrinology* 1992;56:133–140.

136. Brann DW, Zamorano PL, Chorich LP, Mahesh VB. Steroid hormone effects on NMDA receptor binding and NMDA receptor mRNA levels in the hypothalamus and cerebral cortex of the adult rat. *Neuroendocrinology* 1993;58:666–672.

137. Diano S, Naftolin F, Horvath TL. Gonadal steroids target AMPA glutamate receptor-containing neurons in the rat hypothalamus, septum and amygdala: a morphological and biochemical study. *Endocrinology* 1997;138:778–789.

138. Weiland NG. Estradiol selectively regulates agonist binding sites on the N-methyl-D-aspartate receptor complex in the CA1 region of the hippocampus. *Endocrinology* 1992;131:662–668.

139. Gazzaley AH, Weiland NG, McEwen BS, Morrison JH. Differential regulation of NMDAR1 mRNA and protein by estradiol in the rat hippocampus. *J Neurosci* 1996;16:6830–6838.

140. Woolley CS, McEwen BS. Estradiol regulates hippocampal dendritic spine density via an N-methyl-D-aspartate receptor-dependent mechanism. *J Neurosci* 1994;14:7680–7687.

141. Rabbani O, Panickar KS, Rajakumar G, King MA, Bodor N, Meyer EM, Simpkins JW. 17-Beta-estradiol attenuates fimbrial lesion-induced decline of ChAT-immunoreactive neurons in the rat medial septum. *Exp Neurol* 1997;146:179–186.

142. Dluzen DE. Effects of testosterone upon MPTP-induced neurotoxicity of the nigrostriatal dopaminergic system of C57/B1 mice. *Brain Res* 1996;715:113–118.

143. Dluzen DE, McDermott JL, Liu B. Estrogen as a neuroprotectant against MPTP-induced neurotoxicity in C57/B1 mice. *Neurotoxicol Teratol* 1996;18:603–606.

144. Shi J, Zhang YQ, Simpkins JW. Effects of 17beta-estradiol on glucose transporter 1 expression and endothelial cell survival following focal ischemia in the rats. *Exp Brain Res* 1997;117:200–206.

145. Simpkins JW, Rajakumar G, Zhang YQ, et al. Estrogens may reduce mortality and ischemic damage caused by middle cerebral artery occlusion in the female rat. *J Neurosurg* 1997;87:724–730.

146. Toung TJ, Traystman RJ, Hurn PD. Estrogen-mediated neuroprotection after experimental stroke in male rats. *Stroke* 1998;29:1666–1670.

147. Dubal DB, Kashon ML, Pettigrew LC, et al. Estradiol protects against ischemic injury. *J Cereb Blood Flow Metab* 1998;18:1253–1258.

148. Raff MC, Barres BA, Burne JF, Coles HS, Ishizaki Y, Jacobson MD. Programmed cell death and the control of cell survival: lessons from the nervous system. *Science* 1993;262:695–700.

149. Steller H. Mechanisms and genes of cellular suicide. *Science* 1995;267:1445–1449.

150. Perry RR, Kang Y, Greaves B. Effects of tamoxifen on growth and apoptosis of estrogen-dependent and -independent human breast cancer cells. *Ann Surg Oncol* 1995;2:238–245.

151. Wilson JW, Wakeling AE, Morris ID, Hickman JA, Dive C. MCF-7 human mammary adenocarcinoma cell death in vitro in response to hormone-withdrawal and DNA damage. *Int J Cancer* 1995;61:502–508.

152. Bhargava V, Kell DL, van de Rijn M, Warnke RA. Bcl-2 immunoreactivity in breast carcinoma correlates with hormone receptor positivity. *Am J Pathol* 1994;145:535–540.

153. Smith DF, Toft DO. Steroid receptors and their associated proteins. *Mol Endocrinol* 1993;7:4–11.

154. Yang X, Dale EC, Diaz J, Shyamala G. Estrogen dependent expression of heat shock transcription factor: implications for uterine synthesis of heat shock proteins. *J Steroid Biochem Mol Biol* 1995;52:415–419.

155. Olazábal UE, Pfaff DW, Mobbs CV. Estrogenic regulation of heat shock protein 90 kDa in the rat ventromedial hypothalamus and uterus. *Mol Cell Endocrinol* 1992;84:175–183.

156. Olazábal UE, Pfaff DW, Mobbs CV. Sex differences in the regulation of heat shock protein 70 kDa and 90 kDa in the rat ventromedial hypothalamus by estrogen. *Brain Res* 1992;596:311–314.

157. Behl C, Davis JB, Klier FG, Schubert D. Amyloid beta peptide induces necrosis rather than apoptosis. *Brain Res* 1994;645:253–264.

158. Behl C, Schubert D. Heat shock partially protects rat pheochromocytoma PC12 cells from amyloid beta peptide toxicity. *Neurosci Lett* 1993;154:1–4.

159. Xu H, Gouras GK, Greenfield JP, et al. Estrogen reduces neuronal generation of Alzheimer beta-amyloid peptides. *Nat Med* 1998;4:447–451.

160. Jaffe AB, Toran-Allerand CD, Greengard P, Gandy SE. Estrogen regulates metabolism of Alzheimer amyloid beta precursor protein. *J Biol Chem* 1994;269:13065–13068.

161. Srivastava RA, Bhasin N, Srivastava N. Apolipoprotein E gene expression in various tissues of mouse and regulation by estrogen. *Biochem Mol Biol Int* 1996;38:91–101.

162. Massafra C, de Felice C, Gioia D, Buonocore G. Variations in erythrocyte antioxidant glutathione peroxidase activity during the menstrual cycle. *Clin Endocrinol (Oxf)* 1998;49:63–67.

163. Kume-Kick J, Ferris DC, Russo-Menna I, Rice ME. Enhanced oxidative stress in female rat brain after gonadectomy. *Brain Res* 1996;738:8–14.

164. Sack MN, Rader DJ, Cannon RO, 3rd. Oestrogen and inhibition of oxidation of low-density lipoproteins in postmenopausal women. *Lancet* 1994;343:269–270.

165. Ruiz-Larrea B, Leal A, Martin C, Martinez R, Lacort M. Effects of estrogens on the redox chemistry of iron: a possible mechanism of the antioxidant action of estrogens. *Steroids* 1995;60:780–783.

166. Simpkins JW. Estrogens and Memory Protection. *J Soc Obstet Gynaecol Can* 1997;19[Suppl]:14–20.

167. Sugioka K, Shimosegawa Y, Nakano M. Estrogens as natural antioxidants of membrane phospholipid peroxidation. *FEBS Lett* 1987;210:37–39.

168. Green PS, Bishop J, Simpkins JW. 17-Alpha-estradiol exerts neuroprotective effects on SK-N-SH cells. *J Neurosci* 1997;17:511–515.

169. Mitchell JH, Gardner PT, McPhail DB, Morrice PC, Collins AR, Duthie GG. Antioxidant efficacy of phytoestrogens in chemical and biological model systems. *Arch Biochem Biophys* 1998;360:142–148.

170. Shwaery GT, Vita JA, Keaney JF Jr. Antioxidant protection of LDL by physiological concentrations of 17-beta-estradiol: requirement for estradiol modification. *Circulation* 1997;95:1378–1385.

171. Hochberg RB. Biological esterification of steroids. *Endocr Rev* 1998;19:331–348.

172. Brawer JR, Schipper H, Naftolin F. Ovary-dependent degeneration in the hypothalamic arcuate nucleus. *Endocrinology* 1980;107:274–279.

173. Brawer JR, Beaudet A, Desjardins GC, Schipper HM. Pathologic effect of estradiol on the hypothalamus. *Biol Reprod* 1993;49:647–652.

174. Desjardins GC, Beaudet A, Brawer JR. Alterations in opioid parameters in the hypothalamus of rats with estradiol-induced polycystic ovarian disease. *Endocrinology* 1990;127:2969–2976.

175. Fuentes M, Sahu A, Kalra SP. Evidence that long-term estrogen treatment disrupts opioid involvement in the induction of pituitary LH surge. *Brain Res* 1992;583:183–188.

176. Schipper HM, Desjardins GC, Beaudet A, Brawer JR. The 21-aminosteroid antioxidant, U74389F, prevents estradiol-induced depletion of hypothalamic beta-endorphin in adult female rats. *Brain Res* 1994;652:161–163.

177. Messier C, White NM. Memory improvement by glucose, fructose, and two glucose analogs: a possible effect on peripheral glucose transport. *Behav Neural Biol* 1987;48:104–127.

178. Kennedy AM, Frackowiak RS, Newman SK, et al. Deficits in cerebral glucose metabolism demonstrated by positron emission tomography in individuals at risk of familial Alzheimer's disease. *Neurosci Lett* 1995;186:17–20.

179. Simpson IA, Chundu KR, Davies-Hill T, Honer WG, Davies P. Decreased concentrations of GLUT1 and GLUT3 glucose transporters in the brains of patients with Alzheimer's disease. *Ann Neurol* 1994;35:546–551.

180. Graeber MB, Muller U. Recent developments in the molecular genetics of mitochondrial disorders. *J Neurol Sci* 1998;153:251–263.

181. Beal MF. Mitochondrial dysfunction in neurodegenerative diseases. *Biochim Biophys Acta* 1998;1366:211–223.

182. Davis RE, Miller S, Herrnstadt C, et al. Mutations in mitochondrial cytochrome c oxidase genes segregate with late-onset Alzheimer disease. *Proc Natl Acad Sci USA* 1997;94:4526–4531.

183. Davis JN 2nd, Parker WD Jr. Evidence that two reports of mtDNA cytochrome

c oxidase "mutations" in Alzheimer's disease are based on nDNA pseudogenes of recent evolutionary origin. *Biochem Biophys Res Commun* 1998;244: 877–883.

184. Bishop J, Simpkins JW. Estradiol enhances brain glucose uptake in ovariectomized rats. *Brain Res Bull* 1995;36:315–320.

185. Alkayed NJ, Harukuni I, Kimes AS, London ED, Traystman RJ, Hurn PD. Gender-linked brain injury in experimental stroke. *Stroke* 1998;29:159–165.

186. Hurn PD, Littleton-Kearney MT, Kirsch JR, Dharmarajan AM, Traystman RJ. Postischemic cerebral blood flow recovery in the female: effect of 17-beta-estradiol. *J Cereb Blood Flow Metab* 1995;15:666–672.

187. Schmidt R, Fazekas F, Reinhart B, et al. Estrogen replacement therapy in older women: a neuropsychological and brain MRI study. *J Am Geriatr Soc* 1996;44: 1307–1313.

188. Shi J, Simpkins JW. 17-Beta-estradiol modulation of glucose transporter 1 expression in blood-brain barrier. *Am J Physiol* 1997;272:E1016–E1022.

189. Toran-Allerand CD. Neurite-like outgrowth from CNS explants may not always be of neuronal origin. *Brain Res* 1990;513:353–357.

190. Toran-Allerand CD, Pfenninger KH, Ellis L. Estrogen and insulin stimulation of neuritic growth *in vitro*. *Neurosci Abstr* 1984;10:455.

191. Toran-Allerand CD. Sex steroids and the development of the newborn mouse hypothalamus and preoptic area *in vitro*: implication for sexual differentiation. *Brain Res* 1976;189:413–427.

192. Ferreira A, Caceres A. Estrogen-enhanced neurite growth: evidence for a selective induction of Tau and stable microtubules. *J Neurosci* 1991;11:392–400.

193. Garcia-Segura LM, Canas B, Parducz A, et al. Estradiol promotion of changes in the morphology of astroglia growing in culture depends on the expression of polysialic acid of neural membranes. *Glia* 1995;13:209–216.

194. Matsumoto A, Murakami S, Arai Y. Neurotropic effects of estrogen on the neonatal preoptic area grafted into the adult rat brain. *Cell Tissue Res* 1988;252: 33–37.

195. Stanley HF, Borthwick NM, Fink G. Brain protein changes during development and sexual differentiation in the rat. *Brain Res* 1986;370:215–222.

196. Singer CA, Pang PA, Dobie DJ, Dorsa DM. Estrogen increases GAP-43 (neuromodulin) mRNA in the preoptic area of aged rats. *Neurobiol Aging* 1996;17: 661–663.

197. Shughrue PJ, Dorsa DM. Gonadal steroids modulate the growth-associated protein GAP-43 (neuromodulin) mRNA in postnatal rat brain. *Brain Res Dev Brain Res* 1993;73:123–132.

198. Lustig RH, Sudol M, Pfaff DW, Federoff HJ. Estrogenic regulation and sex dimorphism of growth-associated protein 43 kDa (GAP-43) messenger RNA in the rat. *Brain Res Mol Brain Res* 1991;11:125–132.

199. Karkanias GB, Morales JC, Li CS. Deficits in reproductive behavior in diabetic female rats are due to hypoinsulinemia rather than hyperglycemia. *Horm Behav* 1997;32:19–29.

200. Toran-Allerand CD, Bentham W, Miranda RC, Anderson JP. Insulin influences astroglial morphology and glial fibrillary acidic protein (GFAP) expression in organotypic cultures. *Brain Res* 1991;558:296–304.

201. Meakin SO, Shooter EM. The nerve growth factor family of receptors. *Trends Neurosci* 1992;15:323–331.

202. Chao MV, Hempstead BL. P75 and Trk: a two-receptor system. *Trends Neurosci* 1995;18:321–326.

203. Rossner S, Ueberham U, Schliebs R, Perez-Polo JR, Bigl V. Neurotrophin binding to the p75 neurotrophin receptor is necessary but not sufficient to mediate NGF-effects on APP secretion in PC-12 cells. *J Neural Transm Suppl* 1998;54:279–285.

204. Barley J, Ginsburg M, Greenstein BD, MacLusky NJ, Thomas PJ. A receptor mediating sexual differentiation. *Nature (Lond)* 1974;252:259–260.

205. MacLusky NJ, Chaptal C, McEwen BS. The development of estrogen receptor systems in the rat brain: postnatal development. *Brain Res* 1979;178:143–160.

206. O'Keefe JA, Pedersen EB, Castro AJ, Handa RJ. The ontogeny of estrogen receptors in heterochronic hippocampal and neocortical transplants demonstrates an intrinsic developmental program. *Brain Res Dev Brain Res* 1993;75:105–112.

207. O'Keefe JA, Handa RJ. Transient elevation of estrogen receptors in the neonatal rat hippocampus. *Brain Res Dev Brain Res* 1990;57:119–127.

208. Gerlach JL, McEwen BS, Toran-Allerand CD, Friedman WJ. Perinatal development of estrogen receptors in mouse brain assessed by radioautography, nuclear isolation and receptor assay. *Brain Res* 1983;313:7–18.

209. Miranda RC, Toran-Allerand CD. Developmental expression of estrogen receptor mRNA in the rat cerebral cortex: a nonisotopic in situ hybridization histochemistry study. *Cereb Cortex* 1992;2:1–15.

210. Toran-Allerand CD, Miranda RC, Bentham WD, et al. Estrogen receptors colocalize with low-affinity nerve growth factor receptors in cholinergic neurons of the basal forebrain. *Proc Natl Acad Sci USA* 1992;89:4668–4672.

211. Sohrabji F, Miranda RC, Toran-Allerand CD. Estrogen differentially regulates estrogen and nerve growth factor receptor mRNAs in adult sensory neurons. *J Neurosci* 1994;14:459–471.

212. Miranda RC, Sohrabji F, Toran-Allerand CD. Neuronal colocalization of mRNAs for neurotrophins and their receptors in the developing central nervous system suggests a potential for autocrine interactions. *Proc Natl Acad Sci USA* 1993;90: 6439–6443.

213. Sohrabji F, Miranda RCG, Toran-Allerand CD. Identification of a putative estrogen response element in the gene encoding brain-derived neurotrophic factor. *Proc Natl Acad Sci USA* 1995;92:11110–11114.

214. Miranda RC, Sohrabji F, Toran-Allerand D. Interactions of estrogen with the neurotrophins and their receptors during neural development. *Horm Behav* 1994;28: 367–375.

215. Miranda R, Sohrabi F, Singh M, Toran-Allerand CD. Nerve growth factor (NGF) regulation of estrogen receptors in explant cultures of the developing forebrain. *J Neurobiol* 1996;31:77–87.

216. Gibbs RB. Levels of trkA and BDNF mRNA, but not NGF mRNA, fluctuate across the estrous cycle and increase in response to acute hormone replacement. *Brain Res* 1998;787:259–268.

217. Tonetti DA, Jordan VC. Targeted anti-estrogens to treat and prevent diseases in women. *Mol Med Today* 1996;2:218–223.

218. Gradishar WJ, Jordan VC. Clinical potential of new antiestrogens. *J Clin Oncol* 1997;15:840–852.

219. Robinson E, Kimmick GG, Muss HB. Tamoxifen in postmenopausal women a safety perspective. *Drugs Aging* 1996;8:329–337.

220. Shariff S, Cumming CE, Lees A, Handman M, Cumming DC. Mood disorder in women with early breast cancer taking tamoxifen, an estradiol receptor antagonist. An expected or unexpected effect? *Ann N Y Acad Sci* 1995;761:365–368.

221. Cathcart CK, Jones SE, Pumroy CS, Peters GN, Knox SM, Cheek JH. Clinical recognition and management of depression in node negative breast cancer patients treated with tamoxifen. *Breast Cancer Res Treat* 1993;27:277–281.

222. Draper MW, Flowers DE, Huster WJ, Neild JA, Harper KD, Arnaud C. A controlled trial of raloxifene (LY139481) HCl: impact on bone turnover and serum lipid profile in healthy postmenopausal women. *J Bone Miner Res* 1996;11: 835–842.

223. Roy EJ, MacLusky NJ, McEwen BS. Antiestrogen inhibits the induction of progestin receptors by estradiol in the hypothalamus, pituitary and uterus. *Endocrinology* 1979;104:1333–1336.

224. Ferretti C, Blengio M, Ghi P, Racca S, Genazzani E, Portaleone P. Tamoxifen counteracts estradiol induced effects on striatal and hypophyseal dopamine receptors. *Life Sci* 1988;42:2457–2465.

225. Ferretti C, Ghi P, Blengio M, Gaietta G, Genazzani E. Tamoxifen specifically inhibits oestrogen-induced dopaminergic striatal supersensitivity. *Pharmacol Res* 1989;21:93–94.

226. Petersen SL, Barraclough CA. Suppression of spontaneous LH surges in estrogen-treated ovariectomized rats by microimplants of antiestrogens into the preoptic brain. *Brain Res* 1989;484:279–289.

227. Wade GN, Heller HW. Tamoxifen mimics the effects of estradiol on food intake, body weight, and body composition in rats. *Am J Physiol Regul Integr Comp Physiol* 1993;264:R1219–R1223.

228. Wiseman H, Paganga G, Rice-Evans C, Halliwell B. Protective actions of tamoxifen and 4-hydroxytamoxifen against oxidative damage to human low-density lipoproteins: a mechanism accounting for the cardioprotective action of tamoxifen? *Biochem J* 1993;292:635–638.

229. Tatton WG, Chalmers-Redman RM. Mitochondria in neurodegenerative apoptosis: an opportunity for therapy? *Ann Neurol* 1998;44:S134–S141.

230. Schneider LS, Farlow MR, Henderson VW, Pogoda JM. Effects of estrogen replacement therapy on response to tacrine in patients with Alzheimer's disease. *Neurology* 1996;46:1580–1584.

231. Shwaery GT, Vita JA, Keaney JF, Jr. Antioxidant protection of LDL by physiologic concentrations of estrogens is specific for 17-beta-estradiol. *Atherosclerosis* 1998;138:255–262.

Treatment of the Postmenopausal Woman: Basic and Clinical Aspects, Second Edition, edited by Rogerio A. Lobo, Lippincott Williams & Wilkins, Philadelphia © 1999.

CHAPTER 22

Clinical Effects of Sex Steroids on the Brain

Vito Cela and Frederick Naftolin

Improved quality of life has resulted in an increased life expectancy for women. Over the past century, improved medical, economic, and sociocultural conditions in our society have doubled the average life span of women to 82 years. This increase will continue into the next century, and the cases of brain dysfunction and disease will rise as this population ages. Health care implications will become increasingly important.

Menopause is an important period of transition in every woman's life. Relatively constant, low estrogen levels derived from peripheral conversion (extragonadal, including brain) of estrogen precursors replace the high cycling estradiol levels from the cycling ovary. The decrease in circulating estrogen concentration is most often reflected by signs of brain dysfunction. The common early symptoms of menopause are hot flushes (i.e., vasomotor episodes [VME]), mood and cognition changes, and sleep disorders. Although hot flushes (also called hot flashes) are often transient (3 to 5 years), they indicate a clinically relevant estrogen deficiency. Relief reported by women who take estrogen is evidence of the effects of estrogen on the brain's cells. It appears that the new hormone balance may lead to brain changes that involve brain function and brain cells.

The central and peripheral nervous systems, which are estrogen target tissues, undergo anatomic and biochemical remodeling throughout life. Until recently, symptoms after the expected loss of ovarian follicle development had been only vaguely related to actual brain changes, and the symptomatology tended to be ascribed to vague effects on other organs. Few appreciated the breadth of functional changes as a result of brain responses to low estrogens during the climacteric. However, it has become increasingly evident that sex hormones—estrogen, progesterone, and androgen—have important roles in the modulation of brain function. These hormones affect neurons, glia, and microglia (i.e., brain macrophages) in many areas in the brain, not just in the portions of the hypothalamus and preoptic area involved solely with reproductive function. Hormonal decline, particularly estrogen decline, during menopause is accompanied by changes in autonomic function, behavior, mood, sexuality, locomotor activity, immune response, memory, and cognitive function, and the list continues to grow (1).

Although these brain changes originate in the central nervous system (CNS), there are reports that hormonal changes also influence peripheral nervous system (PNS) functions such as sensory function, fine-touch perception, two-point discrimination, hearing, smell, and vision (2). These are less well documented and do not exclude primary effects of sex steroids on the tissues and organs in which the PNS is embedded and from which it derives its blood supply.

For completeness, we have listed the major groups of brain functions that may deteriorate during the menopause (Table 22.1). This table gives a powerful demon-

TABLE 22.1. *Brain functions affected during menopause*

Autonomic
  Gonadotrophins (125)
  Sleep
  Vasomotor episodes
  Libido (126)
  Mood
  Metabolic regulation (127)
Cognition
Sensory perception (128)
Memory
Voluntary motor function (1)
Immunologic function (129)
Sexually dimorphic function and dysfunction (presumed
  to be sex steroid related)

V. Cela: Department of Reproductive Medicine and Child Development, and Department of Obstetrics and Gynecology, University of Pisa, Pisa, Italy, 56123.

F. Naftolin: Department of Obstetrics and Gynecology, Yale University School of Medicine, New Haven, Connecticut 06520-8063.

stration of the brain's integrative function and estrogen's role. Because of space limitations, the remainder of this chapter concentrates on brain functions in which sex steroids are best known to play a role and that may be preserved by hormone replacement therapy (HRT). An overview of the brain, its functional construction, and the mechanism of sex steroid actions on the brain precede these considerations.

THE BRAIN AND SEX STEROIDS

Anatomic-Functional Correlations

The brain is a linear ensemble of structures that develop along the neural tube and that are roughly proportional in size to the functional requirements of individual species (Fig. 22.1). Humans have a large cortical area, which serves to develop and use cognition, memory, and mood. The frontal cognitive cortical area and the central, sensory cortical areas are linked with other regions through axonal connections running along the area beneath the original neural tube (i.e., adult ventricular system). These axons form "tracts" that connect distant areas of the brain, allowing signals to be processed between brain areas and eventually stored, used, or discarded (Fig. 22.2). The hippocampus, which primarily processes and stores short-term memory, is located in and connected to the temporal cortex. There are also major reciprocal connections with the hypothalamus and cortical areas in which long-term memory is stored and other cognitive functions occur. There are memory and cognitive centers along the visual pathway that contribute to the final inflow path to the hippocampus. The interaction of all of these structures results in optimal function of the

brain. Evidence for this arrangement shows that age-related dystrophy affecting the hippocampal neurons first results in a deficit of short-term memory and then is generalized to most brain functions (3). Many important other examples of hormone-affected brain areas are plentiful. Because the brain is an active metabolic tissue, it requires a massive blood flow, which is also hormone sensitive (4).

The brain is mainly composed of glial cells, particularly astroglia, which outnumber neurons 9 : 1. Discordance in size and in areas of the brain most likely reflects glial differences. Moreover, neurons interact through arborization of their axonal (afferent) processes, which connect to the dendritic (efferent) tree or receive processes that carry messages to the neuronal cell body or perikarya. The cellular actions in the perikarya are not much different from other cells. The main difference is in the widely arborized communicating axons and dendrites, which allows local and long distance communication rather than the usual local geometric interactions between cells in other parts of the body. The astroglia, like the neurons, are sex steroid sensitive and can form metabolites through the steroid degradation process; androgens are aromatized by neurons (5) and ring-A reduced by astroglia (6).

Neuronal processes connect through myriad synapses, cell-cell interfaces that perform the specialized function of furnishing neurotransmitters to the synaptic cleft and passing them back and forth (uptake and reuptake). Neurotransmitter expression is regulated by many substances, including sex steroids (7). The formation and maintenance of synapses is estrogen regulated (8), especially in the areas where there are estrogen receptors (ERs). Sex steroids also regulate the number and function of the neurotransmitter receptors that translate the messages carried into the synapses by the neurotransmitters. With aging, there is a shift in the balance between circulating steroids and locally formed steroids; with menopause, the follicular estrogen decreases, leaving a greater burden of steroid supply to peripheral conversion by brain and other tissues.

The glial cells are far from passive in all of these activities. The astroglia are the embedment of the neurons. Synapses must penetrate sheets of glial process to make their connections. The glia respond to neuronal products in the area of the neuronal cell bodies and along the neurites (neural processes) and synapses (6). The glia buffer the leaking of neural products (e.g., neurotransmitters, cytokines, free radicals). In this way, the glia cells form a protective or reparative barrier between neurons. We and others have shown that the astroglia are extremely physically active, slinging out processes and shuttering the space vacated by changing synapses (9).

A specialized form of glia, the oligodendroglia, is present in CNS and PNS. These glial cells wrap axons with myelin, ensuring efficient neurotransmission. In animals,

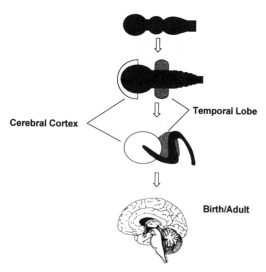

FIG. 22.1. Brain development along the neural tube results in functional and anatomic mini-organs linked by tracts. The adult brain is the result of folding the neural tube and its derivatives to fit the cranium.

Cerebral Cortex

Temporal Lobe

Birth/Adult

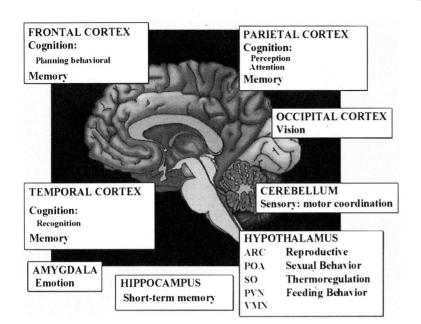

FRONTAL CORTEX
Cognition:
Planning behavioral
Memory

PARIETAL CORTEX
Cognition:
Perception
Attention
Memory

OCCIPITAL CORTEX
Vision

TEMPORAL CORTEX
Cognition:
Recognition
Memory

CEREBELLUM
Sensory: motor coordination

AMYGDALA
Emotion

HIPPOCAMPUS
Short-term memory

HYPOTHALAMUS
ARC   Reproductive
POA   Sexual Behavior
SO   Thermoregulation
PVN   Feeding Behavior
VMN

FIG. 22.2. Each region of the brain has an important role in specific brain functions. Optimal brain activity is maintained by means of the integration of different areas by neural tracts. ARC, arcuate nucleus; POA, preoptic area; SO, supraoptic nucleus; PVN, paraventricular nucleus; VMN, ventromedial nucleus.

the oligodendroglia have also been shown to metabolize cholesterol and its other Δ5 (unsaturated B-ring) steroids (10). Chief among their metabolic products is allopregnanolone (THP), which is presently being studied as a sedative, anxiolytic neuroactive compound (11).

Another type of glia, the microglia, constitutes the brain's macrophages. The microglia contain ERs and aromatase and are regulated by estrogen. We have proposed that the microglia form the (estrogen-sensitive) immunologic brain barrier and regulate free radical formation and clearance in the brain. This may play a role in estrogen's regulation of brain function and dystrophy (12).

Estrogen and Brain Function

Estrogen appears to affect all brain cells. It does this by direct cellular effects in addition to indirect effects (estrogen-sensitive cells regulating connected non–ER–bearing cells). Estrogen affects neurons and glia. Estrogen also regulates the brain's blood vessels. Estrogen has been shown to influence most brain functions, regulating biochemical and anatomic parameters and modulating the uptake and turnover of neurotransmitters, neuronal enzyme activity, and the expression of steroid receptors on the brain. This is a sweeping statement, but true. It is therefore necessary to discuss what we know about the mechanism of estrogen action on brain cells. Most estrogen actions on brain cells are ER mediated. Because there has been an important discovery of a second ER in the brain (13,14), we concentrate on ER-mediated estrogen actions on brain cells, commenting on non–receptor-mediated actions such as direct ion channel or enzyme effects as they pertain to specific brain functions.

Estrogen, Estrogen Receptors, and the Brain

Since Doisy and Butenandt identified and determined the formula for estrogen (15), the term *estrogen* has many times been redefined because of the discovery of many classes of compounds that are estrogenic and because of the broadening description of specific biochemical actions of estrogenic compounds.

After the development of the primary steroidal estrogens (e.g., estradiol, estrone, estriol), the first nonsteroidal, synthetic estrogen, diethylstilbestrol (DES), was produced. Description of estrogenic effects of plant estrogen (i.e., phytoestrogen) soon followed, and a large group of nonsteroidal compounds were also found to have estrogenic actions. Shortly thereafter, estrogen became clinically available. The stage was then set for commercial development: steroidal estrogens, nonsteroidal estrogens, estrogen agonists or antagonists, and antiestrogens were drawn from the previously described compounds or their congeners. Researchers became interested in studying differences in mechanism of action of these classes of compounds. The development of compounds with new agonist or antagonist properties was accompanied by descriptive terms that appear to add little to the fundamental understanding of estrogen action: phytoestrogens, xenoestrogens, estrogen-like endocrine disrupters, and selective estrogen receptor modulators (SERMs) (16).

With increased knowledge of estrogen actions on the brain, quantitative and qualitative inconsistencies were apparent in clinical situations. This may be resolved by the discovery of a second, specific ER (ER-β) (13,14), which has a regional distribution and specificity of action in the brain that differs from ER-α, although ER-α and ER-β may be found together in specific brain areas (Fig. 22.3). Comparing Figs. 22.1 and 22.3, it is possible to

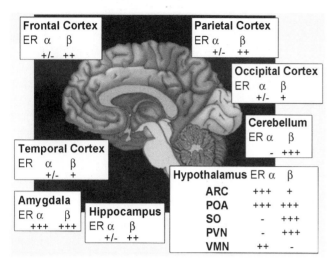

FIG. 22.3. Distribution of estrogen receptors ERα and ERβ mRNA in the rat brain.

develop a functional map of the brain and possible roles of specific ERs (17,18).

Estrogen regulation of neural activity can largely be explained by genomic effects regulated by intracellular ERs. As with other steroids, the control of gene expression requires liganding of estrogen and binding the liganded receptor in apposition to the DNA in the nucleus. DNA binding regulates transcription of RNA for new protein synthesis and expression. Because the liganded ERs dimerize before DNA binding and there are two individual ERs (ER-α and ER-β), the formation of homodimers or heterodimers is possible (19). This and the qualitatively different effects of liganding specific estrogenic compounds further increase the complexity. The resulting transcription and the effect can be agonistic or antagonistic to transcription depending on the ligands (20), the receptor type (21), and possible effects of homodimer or heterodimer formation (Fig. 22.4) (19). For the sake of brevity, we have included a table of possible ligands, ER

combinations, and functional outcomes (transcriptional products) that may be expected (Table 22.2).

Although receptors mediate the bulk of steroid actions in the brain, some actions appear to not require receptors. These have been shown experimentally to include changes in cell membrane channel permeability (22). Other, rapid actions of sex steroids may be cause by direct effects. However, several possibilities such as early-intermediate gene activation (e.g., *FOS, JUN*) or neurotrophin-driven actions have yet to be excluded (23).

Studies mapping estrogen and progestin receptors (PRs) in the brain have shown that ERs and PRs are located in many areas, including the hypothalamus, hippocampus, amygdala, and limbic forebrain system (24, 25). Studies showing that ER-β is present in areas previously thought to be devoid of ERs, such as the cortex, are especially promising for explaining effects of estrogen (17,18). The distribution of steroid receptors is regionalized in a manner similar to the regionalization of function in the brain (Figs. 22.2 and 22.3). For example, ER levels are high in the hypothalamus, where estrogen-dependent actions regulate neuroendocrine functions such as reproduction, feeding behavior, sexual behavior, and vasomotor stability. Although synaptic transmission is the main form of cell-cell communication in the brain, unlike more homogeneous organs (e.g., liver, muscles), the brain has only a few cells that are neurons. The number of neurons in a synaptic network may be disproportional to their effects because of the synapses that their axons form with other neurons. For example, a small number of acetylcholine neurons under the control of estrogen send axons throughout the brain, allowing indirect effects of estrogen on distant neurons. The obverse is that areas receiving innervation (e.g., acetylcholine) are actually estrogen dependent even though their neurons may not have ERs (26). It also follows that cell death or dystrophy among neurons will have widely felt consequences.

Sex Steroids and Brain Phenotype

The presence of morphologic or functional sexual dimorphism in brain areas could give clues to estrogen action on the brain. In animals, hormonal effects during early prenatal and postnatal development induce sexual differentiation of many organ systems, including the brain (27). These sex differences carry over into adulthood, when estrogen effects females and males differently. In addition to classic signs of menopause in women (e.g., hot flushes), the incidence of depression (28) and Alzheimer's dementia (AD) are higher among women (29–31), supporting the hypothesis that gender or hormonal balance is involved.

In monkey models, neurite formation and synaptogenesis have been proven to be targets of estrogen in developing and adult subjects (32,33). The hypothalamus (autonomic centers) and limbic system (memory, cogni-

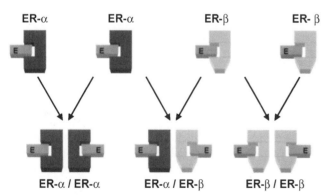

FIG. 22.4. Possibilities for dimerization of liganded receptors as they regulate DNA transcription.

TABLE 22.2. *Estrogen receptors and possible functions*

Ligands	Steroidal estrogens
	Nonsteroidal estrogens (agonists/antagonists)
	   Syntetics (DES and others)
	   Naturally (phytoestrogens)

Receptors	ER-α, ER-β
Possible dimerization groupings	ER-α–ER-α; ER-β–ER-β; ER-α–ER-β
Possible transcriptional outcomes in the brain (estrogenic/antiestrogenic effects)	
Morphologic effect	Neurons, regulation of fiber growth and branching, synaptic plasticity, dendritic spines, synaptogenesis, glial cell function, blood flow regulation
Biochemical effect	Neurotransmitters/neuropeptides, neurotransmitter receptors, neurotrophic factors, clearance of proteins (e.g., β-amyloid)

tion, and emotion centers) have been most widely studied and shown to be steroid responsive. The enzyme aromatase (i.e., estrogen synthetase) is present in many brain areas (34). During the normal reproductive cycle, physiologically important levels of estrogen enter the circulation and reach the brain, thereby being the important regulator as opposed to locally formed estrogen. In the postreproductive years, the circulating estrogen falls and androgens are relatively maintained. This emphasizes local estrogen formation in specific brain areas as having functional dominance. Because of the geographic disparity between ER and aromatase in brain areas, this should result in complex effects of local estrogen formation during menopause. The presumed disparities would be overshadowed by systemic estrogen replacement. We therefore consider local estrogen formation as being mainly important to untreated agonadal or climacteric individuals and rarely a reason to avoid HRT. In a similar manner, in the absence of clinical studies, it is not suggested that brain androgen or progestin formation can obviate clinical treatment.

HORMONES AND BRAIN FUNCTIONS OF CLINICAL IMPORTANCE

Vasomotor Episodes

Figure 22.5 is the first of a series of accompanying figures as we begin to address individual functions associated with estrogen action. Each condition is accompanied by a similar figure highlighting the anatomic brain regions involved.

The hypothalamus is where thermoregulatory centers are located and is the region responsible for the control of vasomotor tone and VMEs. VMEs are the most common symptom reported by climacteric women and are the primary cause for them seeking medical advice. A previous chapter extensively discussed VMEs. Our purpose is to underline the role of estrogen in VME. VMEs arise from dysfunction in the hypothalamus. They appear to be strongly linked to race or nationality, because reported incidence varies dramatically between cultures, with 50% to 85% of women in North America and Europe reporting VMEs (35,36). The impact of VMEs on a woman's life is

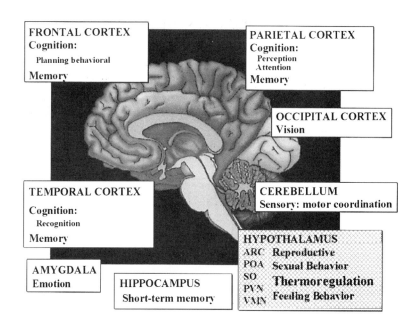

FIG. 22.5. The hypothalamus is where thermoregulatory centers are located and is the region responsible for the control of vasomotor tone and the ventromedial nucleus.

important. There are marked effects on personal and professional performance. These may be associated with other estrogen deficiency symptoms such as sleep cycle disintegration (37), cognitive disorders (38), and neuroendocrine dysfunction (39,40). Most women have VMEs only for a limited time, 3 to 5 years, although estrogen levels remain low. Some compensatory changes in the brain or elsewhere must cause this loss of symptoms. To explore this link, we studied VMEs in postpartum women and found that suckling-related VMEs continued past the reestablishment of ovarian cycles, indicating the presence of an intermediary neuronal network such as oxytocin in the chain of VME events (41). In any case, the role of estrogen cannot be doubted, because any time women (or men) undergo estrogen withdrawal, they have VMEs (42,43). Perhaps the most important clinical function of VMEs is to act as the "canary in the tunnel," indicating estrogen deficiency and that long-term effects are likely to follow, such as heart disease and fractures.

The therapy for VMEs is estrogen. Although other approaches have been tried, they are largely unsuccessful and do not act to avoid the long-term consequences of ovarian failure. Although phytoestrogens or other forms of estrogen have been used, their efficacy and usefulness against long-term estrogen deficiency remains to be proven (44).

Sleep

The hypothalamus contains nuclei involved in sleep regulation (Fig. 22.6). This hypothalamic area is associated with the circadian clock located in the suprachiasmatic nucleus. The periaqueductal gray matter is near and is involved in sleep regulation. In addition to ERs, the periaqueductal gray matter has a high PR content.

Sleep is a reparative brain function. Sleep architecture is influenced by internal and external signals, including estrogen and progesterone. Loss of these hormones results in disintegrating sleep patterns, as measured clinically and by electroencephalogram recordings (45). Sleep is clinically divided into two major states: rapid eye movement (REM) sleep and non–rapid eye movement (NREM) sleep. During sleep, NREM and REM alternate or cycle. The average individual falls asleep within 10 minutes. The first part of sleep normally is an NREM phase, which is followed after 70 to 90 minutes by REM. The onset of sleep and the first REM period is defined as REM latency. Sleep can be disturbed by many external and internal factors. For example, sleep disturbances may be associated with VMEs in menopausal women (37). Associated complaints include sleeplessness, sweating to the point of needing to change clothes during the night, and impairment of one's daily life because of a lack of rest.

Our group has shown that another cause of failed sleep, sleep apnea, occurs in menopausal women and responds to HRT. Sleep apnea is important because, in addition to lost sleep, it is thought to be a precursor to nocturnal cardiac arrhythmias and myocardial infarction (46).

REM latency is increased and sleep efficiency decreased in menopausal women experiencing VMEs compared with those without VMEs (47,48). Because VMEs and sleep disorders go hand in hand, estrogen is the first-line pharmacologic approach for both disorders (37), and earlier studies showed that estrogen was effective for reducing sleep disorders in menopausal women and reducing hot flushes (49). A pilot study investigated the effects of estrogen replacement therapy (ERT) on the rates of cycling alternate patterns of sleep (CAPS) and nocturnal hot flushes in postmenopausal women. It confirmed the previously described findings. Estrogen less-

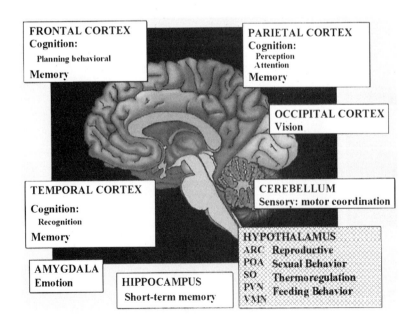

FIG. 22.6. The hypothalamus contains nuclei involved in sleep regulation. This hypothalamic area is associated with the circadian clock located in the suprachiasmatic nucleus. The periaqueductal gray matter is near and is also involved in sleep regulation. In addition to estrogen receptors, the periaqueductal gray matter has high progestin receptor content.

ened the hot flushes and sleep disturbances, decreasing the rate of CAPS (50). Moreover, estrogen treatment of hypogonadal women decreased sleep latency, reduced waking episodes, and prolonged REM sleep (51). Others investigators' analyses of hot flushes and night sweats as the cause of psychosocial, behavioral, and health factors have suggested nonpharmacologic therapy (48), but this should only be tried in cases of failed HRT. The key issues are the long-term effects of estrogen deficiency.

Mood

Many brain regions are involved in mood. The highlighted brain areas in Fig. 22.7 are most directly associated; however, many brain areas subserve mood and cognition simultaneously. Mood is a generic term with many aspects such as feeling of worth, aggression, and depression. Mood is often summarized in normal individuals as their "feeling of well-being." Mood disorders are designated "dysphorias." Despite an apparent continuum, it is important to distinguish between mood changes, dysphorias, and true depression. We divide the entities in this chapter.

The climacteric and premenstrual syndrome (PMS) are associated with symptoms such as irritability, anxiety, fatigue, depression, and sleep disturbances, which raises the consideration of hormonal causes. Depression also is more prevalent among women than men (52), a discordance that could be related to developmental sex differences but more likely reflects the neurotransmitter and hormonal environment. Cyclic affective disorders seem to be more often expressed by females (53) after puberty the rate increases rapidly in girls compared with boys (28). Despite these variations, there is no evidence that depression in women is related only to abnormalities of gonadal function.

Women are subject to changes in mood and to hormonal shifts. It is therefore not surprising that the two have been associated and many therapeutic attempts have been made at connecting the two. However, the results of these treatments are equivocal and appear to be specific to the individual being treated. Moreover, these patients often receive mood-altering drugs and HRT, further complicating the issue.

Anatomic Basis for Sex Steroids and Mood

Our understanding of the anatomic basis of CNS function is an amalgam of animal studies and clinical observations. The main anatomic areas related to the regulation of mood are limbic brain structures including the amygdala, hippocampus, parahippocampal gyrus (part of the temporal lobe), thalamus, mamillary body, septum pellucidum, cingulate cortex, and cingulum. The hypothalamus has many connections to these areas and is considered by some to be part of the limbic system. However, because of its neuroendocrine activity, we prefer to consider it a distinct region that contributes to limbic function. All of these structures interact by neural networks, together affecting brain functions related to emotion and mood. Similarly, areas of the temporal cortex, including the amygdala, have been related to specific emotions such as joy, fear, and anger. Sex steroids directly affect all of these areas. Estrogen receptors are very dense in regions of the limbic system and hypothalamus. ER-α and ER-β have been localized in these regions and may be involved in estrogen's regulation of mood (17,18).

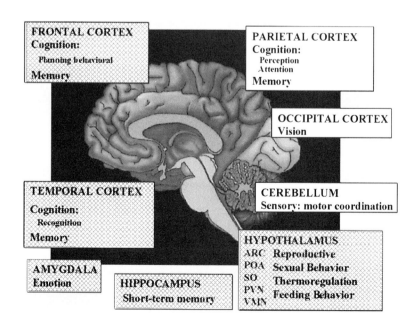

FIG. 22.7. Many brain regions are involved in mood. The highlighted brain areas are most directly associated; however, many brain areas are involved in mood and cognition simultaneously.

Functional Basis for Mood

The problem of composing a mechanistic description or even a solution based on anatomic or neuroendocrine differences in clinical subjects or patients is extraordinarily complex. Animal models are very poor substitutes for human mood or behavior. Our own work with postpartum depression underscores (54) the lack of demonstrable endocrinopathies or neurotransmitter changes in clinical depressions. Most studies have required grossly (i.e., clinically diagnosable) abnormal mood to even show effects of hormone treatment. Less disturbed mood is often identified after its correction, when HRT is employed for some other reason. Because of this we have considered that there is a "substrate" of brain function on which is laid the effects of many neurotransmitter and neuroregulatory substances, including sex steroids. Although the complex equation that is represented by "mood" may well respond to hormone replacement (55), especially when the hormone deficiency is direct and abrupt (56,57), numerous psychotropic agents, especially the selective serotonin reuptake inhibitors (SSRIs), may have effects on the same substrate. These effects may be direct or indirect. For example, the SSRIs have been shown to cause rapid changes in serotonin metabolism, but only gradual improvement in dysphoria. Some intermediate shift in the substrate seems likely; in such cases, catecholamines may be the final pathway of positive results. In a similar manner, sex steroids may shift the substrate, improving dysphoria and other moods.

Hormonal fluctuations have been associated with mood changes and perhaps mood disorders. In this context, hormonal decline during the climacteric often symptomatic. The effects of changing estrogen levels are likely through changes in neurotransmitter systems. For example, when an estrogen deficit is evident, changes have been reported in the cholinergic, catecholaminergic, and serotoninergic systems (58). Variations in serotonin function are related to mood and depression. This focused interpretation of serotonin's role may be an overinterpretation of the clinical response to SSRIs instead of resulting from serotonin's general importance in neural function in these areas. However, the clinical observations have been supported by low levels of serotonin in postmortem cerebrospinal fluid and brains of some depressed patients. Antiserotonin drugs have been shown to induce depression in some humans (59).

Estrogen has been shown to influence the midbrain serotoninergic system. Serotonin activity and serotonin receptors are increased by estrogen while monoamine oxidase (MAO) levels are decreased. This relation between estrogen and serotonin has become prominent because HRT and serotonin reuptake inhibitors are commonly coprescribed. Menopause may be accompanied by a decrease in serotonin levels, which is reversed by HRT (60). Other neurotransmitter systems may be involved in estrogen's effect on SSRI efficacy. For example, estrogen has also been shown to have a dose-dependent effect on the dopamine system. Estrogen increases dopamine transmission and D_2 dopamine receptors. Estrogen action on the neurotransmitters' receptors and synapses involved in all of these systems is quite rapid. Although estrogen action and its relationship to mood altering situations (e.g., menopause, PMS) and therapy (e.g. SSRIs and MAO inhibitors) is becoming increasingly accepted, the precise effects and balance that estrogen adds is not yet understood.

Effects of Sex Steroids on Mood

The role of individual sex steroids in mood is of great interest and a mystery. Extreme deficiencies of androgens or estrogens respond well to replacement therapy. Little or nothing is known about progestin deficiency, although recent work (primarily in animals) indicates that ring-A reduced progestins, especially THP, may be useful in clinical anxiety, mood disorders, and dysphorias.

Less clear are the effects of progesterone or the 19-norprogestins, both of which are employed in HRT for their antiestrogenic actions on the endometrium. Every gynecologist can easily recall anecdotes regarding depression and dysphorias apparently related to the use of systemic progestins. However, blinded, cross-over studies employing controls have not confirmed this clinical impression (61,62). With the exception of clinically disturbed subjects or a strong history, it appears that the substrate defines outcomes in normal subjects.

Placebo-controlled clinical studies have tested the effects of ERT on mood symptoms in women during the postpartum period and in natural and surgical menopause. Generally, women treated with high-dose estrogen therapy have reported improved symptoms, particularly an improved sense of well-being (55). On the other hand, contradicting studies have reported no effects of hormone replacement on women's mood (51,63). These studies evaluated various estrogen regimens: estrogen alone and combined sequentially with progestin. Negative moods and psychologic symptoms were expressed by women in therapy with low-dose estrogen plus progestin compared with estrogen and placebo (64). Studies in hysterectomized women also reported a decrease in depressive symptoms after treatment with estrogen therapy (56,57).

Mood is a complex term that should be distinguished from clinical mania, depression, and other disorders. The basis of mood disorders is not clear, but they often are related to or affected by hormone status. Estrogen generally is most often helpful if the patient is androgen deficient, usually associated with ovariectomy. Progestins, although anecdotally depressants, have not been proven to depress apparently normal women when the progestin is given for less than 2 weeks per month as a counter balance to the effect of estrogen on the uterus. However, nothing is known prospectively of the long-term effect of repeated progestin administration regarding such chronic conditions as the neural dystrophies. Considerations for treatment should follow these guidelines:

1. Treatment should only be for indications.
2. All drugs have side effects and patients should be accordingly monitored.
3. All efforts made to minimize dosage have thus far been rewarded.
4. Because the basis for success and failure of sex steroids in affecting "mood" is unclear, other possible underlying causes may appear during treatment.

Depression

Although mood disorders may be troublesome, clinical depression is recognized because of its disabling nature. Severely disordered sleep, psychomotor retardation, and feelings of worthlessness characterize depression and may be associated with suicidal ideation. Clinical depression is a severe dysphoria and requires a rigorous evaluation, follow-up, and treatment plan.

Although there has been considerable evaluation of the possible relation between thyroid status and adrenocorticoid status and depression, less attention has been given to sex steroids and clinical depression. Despite dropping the diagnosis of "postmenopause melancholia," longitudinal studies continue to report increased rates of mild clinical depression during the perimenopause period (65–67). Most postmenopausal women do not experience prominent symptoms of depression (68).

Mood changes are influenced by various factors, such as a history of depression or PMS. However, it is hard to evaluate the role of the clinical history, and the literature is ambiguous (69). In any case, it seems that severe psychiatric illnesses are prone to recurrences (70,71).

Since the report of improvement in clinically depressed postmenopausal women on treatment with 5 to 25 mg/daily of conjugated equine estrogen (72), many attempts at hormonal treatment of depressive symptoms have been undertaken. Most of the studies showed positive results in patients with depressed mood or mild depressive symptoms but do not provided new information about the effect of HRT on major depression (55). A report appeared regarding women affected by "postpartum depression," a clinical depression marked by psychomotor retardation and sleep disorder. High doses of transdermal estradiol were administered. In this preliminary study, a striking improvement in depression was reported compared with those receiving placebo. During the first month of therapy, about 50% of women reported beneficial effect on depressive symptoms. Those are encouraging results because one-half of the patients reported a rapid effect on mood symptoms in contradistinction to the usual 2-week delay seen with SSRIs (73).

Unfortunately, the researchers did not disclose the previous treatment status of their patients. Further and better described studies are needed. Patient selection and the test instruments play important roles in the outcomes and interpretation of studies on depression. It seems unlikely that depression will ever be treated solely with hormones. Because improvement of depression with psychotropic agents, especially the SSRIs, has been dramatic, it is likely that hormones will remain an adjunct therapy.

The first diagnostic measures must distinguish between mood disorders and major depressive illnesses. A dysphoric mood can be treated with estrogens at the outset. Psychotropic agents may then be added. It is important to add tricyclics or SSRIs slowly. Their effects may take some time to be fully felt. Estrogen may synergize with antidepressants. In the case of major depression, because ERT has not been shown to regularly or sufficiently improve the symptoms, we consider ERT as second-line adjunctive therapy. Possible synergistic actions between ERT and psychotropic drugs must be kept in mind (74). In all cases of major depression, a psychiatric consultation must be attained. No evidence supports a role for progestins or androgens in the treatment of major depression.

Cognitive Function

Many brain regions are involved in the cognitive process. Although this section focuses on memory and the limbic system, other cognitive functions may bypass the limbic system (Fig. 22.8). For example, the visual cognitive system apparently has multiple memory and cognitive way stations that contribute to the complete cognitive process. Cognition is the mental process by which knowledge is acquired or used, and it depends on several elements of the brain functioning harmoniously. These include the intake of information, processing, and distribution of action (including autonomic function) and memory.

Anatomic Basis for Sex Steroids' Effects on Cognition

The areas of the brain involved in cognition are mainly the cerebral cortex, the temporal lobes, and the limbic system. New information enters the brain through the sensory system (i.e., peripheral and cranial nerves) and is processed through the sensory cortex. Each of these areas has been shown to contain ERs (ERβ > ER-α) (17,18) and therefore can be expected to be estrogen sensitive. Study results have supported the effect of estrogen on cognition (75); however, because ER distribution is selective, it is reasonable to expect that estrogens can affect even small numbers of cells in specific regions of cortex. This high degree of selectivity results in a multitude of cognitive functions that may respond to estrogen. It also complicates evolution of estrogen effects on cognition.

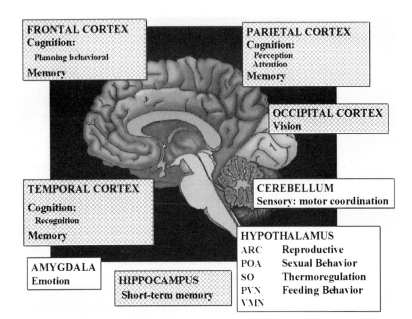

FRONTAL CORTEX
Cognition:
   Planning behavioral
Memory

PARIETAL CORTEX
Cognition:
   Perception
   Attention
Memory

OCCIPITAL CORTEX
Vision

TEMPORAL CORTEX
Cognition:
   Recognition
Memory

CEREBELLUM
Sensory: motor coordination

AMYGDALA
Emotion

HIPPOCAMPUS
Short-term memory

HYPOTHALAMUS
ARC   Reproductive
POA   Sexual Behavior
SO   Thermoregulation
PVN   Feeding Behavior
VMN

FIG. 22.8. Many brain regions are involved in the cognitive process. Although this section focuses on memory and the limbic system, other cognitive functions may bypass the limbic system. For example, the visual cognitive system apparently has multiple memory and cognitive way stations that contribute to the complete cognitive process.

Normal aging in healthy women is often accompanied by a gradual decline in cognition. Many factors, including genetics, lifestyle, and social status, are important aspects of aging. Differences in estrogen concentrations during normal reproduction and the climacteric may be related to the brain's substrate of neurons, glia, and other cells. For example, estrogen has been shown to have an effect on regions of the brain related to memory and cognition (76), much of whose functions center in the hippocampus, which controls information flow and the processing of short-term memory before the distribution of information to the cortex, limbic system, hypothalamus, and other areas. Estrogen's regulation of these processes has been shown in animal models to be associated with changes in neurotransmitters, their receptors, and even in the number of synapses in the involved areas (76,77).

Functional Basis for Cognition

The functional basis for cognition is a very active area of clinical research. For example, levels of choline acetyltransferase (ChAT) and the numbers of acetylcholine receptors are decreased in women affected by AD (78) and increased in the presence of estrogen (79). The acetylcholine system is important to brain function, especially in the temporal lobe. From a small enclave of acetylcholine cells, there are widely distributed axons that support memory in many areas of the cortex (Fig. 22.9). The hippocampus itself functions in a manner analogous to a computer processor that receives messages from cortical and other sensory inputs plus hypothalamic connections, all of which it processes into memory and cognition. A main key to this juncture between the hippocampal processor and the inflow tract is the entry at CA1 of synapses from receiving stations in the brain (Fig.

22.10). These synapses interact with the dendrites of the hippocampus, sending information to cell bodies and then to the outflow tract (e.g., cortex, hypothalamus, limbic system). The transactions of information occur in real time; they are constantly incoming, and unless they are successfully captured by the hippocampal dendritic spines, they are lost. The number and efficiency of synapses at this point regulates the information flow.

Synaptogenesis in the hippocampus and other brain areas is estrogen regulated. Morphologic studies have shown that, under the influence of estrogen, neurons in the CA1 region of the hippocampus increase the number and length of dendrite spines (80). In one such study, ovariectomized rats were treated with estradiol, which facilitated the formation of a greater number of spine synapses on treatment with estrogen (81). The length of

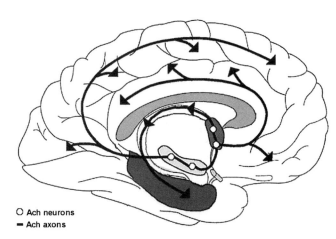

O Ach neurons
— Ach axons

FIG. 22.9. Illustration of the widespread influence of few acetylcholine- and estrogen-receptor–containing neurons on the brain.

Inflow tracts from
Sensory System, etc.

Outflow tracts to
Cerebral Cortex, etc.

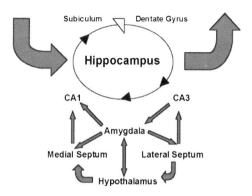

FIG . 22.10. Functional associations between elements of the memory-encoding system. The hippocampus serves the role of a processor, receiving and sending information. Several other such systems in the brain process memory during sensory intake and passage (e.g., toward the hippocampus).

the dendrite spines also regulates the passage of ionic calcium (Ca^{2+}) into the dendrites for processing (i.e., long-term potentiation), which prepares for information processing in the brain. We have shown that in the limbic system there also are greater numbers of glutamate receptors expressed during estrogen's peak (77). As the climacteric begins, it is not surprising that function of the estrogen-dependent memory unit deteriorates.

More than just the estrogenic environment plays a role in cognitive decline related to aging. For example, from the endocrine side, neuronal loss has been associated with stress, possibly through adrenocorticosteroids (82). Much work remains to complete the understanding of the process and derailment of memory and estrogen replacement represents a disproportionately large clinical therapeutic area that will shrink as more information appears.

Effect of Sex Steroids on Cognition and Memory

Verbal memory has also been positively correlated with endogenous estrogen levels during the luteal phase of the ovarian cycle and in HRT-treated menopausal women (83). Menopausal women undergoing estrogen treatment often remark on the beneficial effects on memory and cognitive functions, even though they did not initially complain of deficits. Several studies have evaluated the effects of estrogen replacement therapy on cognitive function in menopausal women. Although these studies are heterogeneous in their experimental designs and evaluations, in general they support a role for HRT, specifically ERT, in maintaining several types of short-term memory and cognition (75,84,85). Other investigators have evaluated treatments using estrogen or estrogen plus androgen versus placebo in total abdominal hysterectomy (TAH) and bilateral salpingo-oophorectomy (BSO) women, showing beneficial effects of the drugs on mem-

ory (38,86). Similarly, causing pharmacologic menopause with a gonadotropin-releasing hormone (GnRH) analogue to induce artificial menopause showed a decline in verbal memory score during the GnRH treatment that was reversed by treatment with conjugated equine estrogen (83). In our own double-blind, cross-over study, we have shown (unpublished data) that ERT improves verbal and cognitive reading skills dramatically.

Evaluating cognition and memory is a complex task in the usual clinical situation. Most often, the improvement is noticed in retrospect. We suggest simple memory tests as surrogates for cognitive and memory test banks. The recollection of strings of numbers is useful, as is the evaluation of recollected information. Based on our current work, the speed, accuracy, and comprehension of a simple patient-read paragraph, which the physician furnishes, may be a good tool in this evaluation (unpublished data). Although the picture of estrogen's effect on memory is promising, further studies comparing like aspects of memory and excluding confounding side effects of estrogen, such as improved sleep, are needed.

Dementia

Severe loss of intellectual function and short-term memory in aging subjects are the hallmarks of dementia. AD and vascular dementia are the most frequent diagnoses; the former is more common in the United States. Dementia is estimated to increase approximately 5% per year in women older than 65 years of age, reaching 50% in women older than 85 (87).

AD is a neurodegenerative disease associated with neuronal cell loss and with development of degenerative lesions called amyloid plaques and neurofibrillary tangles. These lesions are present in relatively larger numbers than seen in normal aging. It is critical to distinguish AD from vascular dementia, because neuronal death from vascular insufficiency is not replaceable. The two conditions may coexist. As in AD, the occurrence of repeated small strokes results in short-term memory loss. On the contrary, long-term memory is more durable and continues to function when not required for storage or retrieval of impaired of short-term memory and cognition loss. The dementia is progressive and distinguished mainly by a decline in memory followed by a gradual disintegration of intellectual function and orientation, language, judgment, and problem solving. Ultimately, other vital functions begin to fail, leaving the patient unable to care for herself or himself and subject to terminal wasting or intercurrent illness.

With worsening of the dementia, the patient becomes unable to live alone, and the family inevitably becomes enmeshed with her care or must arrange a supervised environment (88). This stage of AD is the most trying and destructive to the family. All treatment should aim to avoid late progress of AD. Prevention of early AD can also accomplish the same objective (89). It is critical to understand this end point's importance: anything that delays the transition from self-sufficiency is of greater importance than improvement of individual brain activities such as cognitive skill scores. This is the therapeutic goal in AD cases, not complete rehabilitation.

Vascular dementia is caused by multiple small infarctions but may occur without a major stroke. Although only preliminary results are available, they indicate that there is vasodilatatory effect of estrogen and a vasoconstrictive effect of progestins on cerebral vessels (90).

Estrogen and Dementia

Several factors support a protective role of estrogen in dementia, and there is evidence that diminished estrogen, as found in menopausal women, may contribute to the neurodegenerative process associated with dementia (Chapters 23 and 24). AD has been shown to have an age-corrected rate between 1.4 to 3 times higher in women than in men (29–31). Women with AD weigh less than those without AD, and obese women have a higher production rate of estrogen from endogenous androgen in adipose tissue (91).

Animal studies also support a protective role for estrogen. In 1998, evidence regarding a possible mechanism through which estrogen exerts an antineurodegenerative role in the brain was reported in a multicenter study. It showed that the metabolism of the Alzheimer β-amyloid precursor protein may be regulated by 17β-estradiol in neuroblastoma cells and in primary cell cultures derived from human and rat neocortex (92). These data emphasize the possible role that estrogen replacement therapy may play in the prevention and delay of the onset of AD.

Table 22.3 reviews a group of commonly quoted epidemiologic studies (89,93–96), largely supporting lower dementia (AD) incidence in women taking estrogen. Among these, the ongoing prospective study of Tang et al. is the most interesting. This group of about 1,200 women received neurologic examinations before beginning the study. Although their estrogen usage was not controlled and the case-control method was being used, the study strongly supports a delay by HRT of AD diagnosis, which may be dose related. In the Tang study of ERT patients, the diagnosis of AD was delayed by about 2 years. However, once diagnosed, the progression of AD of the cases apparently was similar to the progress of the control subjects (89). We have already pointed out the importance of even a short delay of the onset and course of dementia in this elderly population. The apparent similarity in disease progress between HRT users and controls is consistent with a collateral protective effect by estrogen.

Not all researchers agree that estrogen delays the incidence of AD. Brenner et al. reported that several oral estrogen preparations were not related to the risk of AD. A negative correlation between ERT and cognitive function was evaluated. They compared women who never used estrogen with women currently under treatment or treated in the past, showing no evident difference on cog-

TABLE 22.3. *Epidemiologic studies on estrogen use and dementia*

Study	Year	Type of Study	Number of patients	Follow-up	Outcome
Henderson et al.	1994	Case-control study of community elderly women	143 with AD; 7% taking ERT; 92 controls; 18% taking ERT	No report	Postmenopausal ERT may be associated with decreased risk of AD.
Paganini-Hill et al.	1994	Case-control study of retirement community	138 with AD or other dementia; 38% taking ERT; 550 controls; 46% taking estrogens	9 years	Increase incidence of AD in elderly women may correlate with estrogen deficiency.
Mortel et al.	1995	Case-control study of friends and relatives	93 with AD; 12% taking ERT; 65 with VD; 11% taking ERT; 148 controls whom 20 taking ERT.	14 years	Lack of ERT is associated with increased risk of dementia.
Tang et al.	1996	Prospective cohort study of community-based study of aging northern Manhattan, New York	167 women developed AD from 1124 women, 13% taking estrogens.	1–5 years	AD onset was later in women who had taken estrogen compared with women who never used it.
Kawas et al.	1997	Prospective cohort of community-dwelling women	34 women developed AD from 472 post/perimenopause women, 34% taking ERT	16 years	Reduced risk of AD for women who had reported the use of estrogen

AD, Alzheimer's disease; ERT, estrogen replacement therapy; VD, vascular dementia.

nitive performance (97). Although studies using animal models support estrogen's reduction of degenerative processes of aging in the CNS, further clinical prospective evaluation of the role played by estrogen on the onset of AD-like lesions must be accomplished.

Effects of Sex steroids on Dementia

Only a few small studies exist regarding the treatment of AD with estrogen. In the main, these reports encourage the use of estrogen to improve cognitive functions in AD patients. Honjo et al. showed that six of seven women treated for 6 weeks with ERT, after which ERT was stopped (ERT was stopped after 3 weeks for two women), reported an improvement in cognitive functions compared with nontreated women (98). Later, these results were supported by the only placebo-controlled study reported (99). It was performed using 14 subjects. Other, uncontrolled studies also reported benefits of ERT for AD. Fillit et al. conducted a short trial performed with seven women affected by AD. Four patients reported an increased in cognitive performance, especially attention and orientation, after 6 weeks of ERT (100). Okura et al., using conjugated equine estrogen for 5 to 45 months (101), reported an improvement in performance on psychometric tests of cognitive functions for four of seven affected patients.

Further studies, especially prospective controlled trials, are needed to confirm these first positive findings before confirmation of the beneficial effects of estrogen therapy in AD. However, the available results are encouraging. Because the effects of progestins and androgens are not proven to be directly salutary in AD and they are antiestrogens, we do not use them in treatment of AD. Because we are using ERT only, appropriate periodical evaluation of the uterus is necessary.

Effects of Progesterone and Progestins on the Brain

Progesterone is a 21-carbon steroid normally formed during the metabolic transformation of cholesterol to androgens and estrogens. Because of pharmacodynamic problems, the clinical formulations often use progesterone substitutes (i.e., progestins), which are 19-nor-androgens. Several progesterone-containing patches, creams, and other formulations have become available and are expected to replace the use of progestins, because many progestins have untoward effects because of their origin as androgens. Progesterone and progestins interact with the androgen progesterone and adrenocortical receptors; it is easy for progestins to affect the brain. We furnish an abbreviated review of this topic because it is in a state of flux and new reports often disagree, perhaps because of the previously mentioned differences in progestin compounds and the lack of progesterone usage.

It is important to understand that the chief reason to employ progesterone or progestins is because of their antiestrogen qualities (102), although increasing evidence documents direct effects on neurons by progesterone or progestins. The onset of menopause is characterized by a marked reduction of estrogen accompanied by the lack of the luteal (progesterone) phase. As a result, most postmenopausal progesterone comes from the adrenal cortex. The balance of their effects is to antagonize estrogen action. We view progesterone or progestin as a "necessary evil" and something to be avoided or at least minimized to local treatment whenever possible.

The main use of progesterone or progestins is to antagonize the effect of estrogen on reproductive tissues. We are skeptical about this use (103). The use of progesterone or progestins may be a disadvantage if the (beneficial) effects of estrogen are opposed throughout the body. However, because estrogen treatment has been associated with an increased rate of endometrial cancer and breast tenderness, progesterone or progestins are prescribed to downregulate the ER-mediated actions.

Receptor-mediated and non–receptor-mediated progesterone effects are not confined to the reproductive organs (104). For example, progesterone crosses the blood-brain barrier. Robel and Baulieu indicated that progesterone and its metabolites may also be formed in the brain (105), but this remains work in progress for women. Brain progesterone levels can be reduced by 5α-reductase and then formed into active metabolites among which THP has been shown to interact with γ-aminobutyric acid (GABA) receptors in animal brain studies (11). Specific glia cells (i.e., oligodendroglia) perform this metabolism. Other glia (i.e., astrocytes) and some neurons contain 5α-reductase, which may contribute to THP formation and action (106). Regional differences in brain steroid concentrations have been shown in postmortem women, emphasizing the local role that may be played by progesterone, its metabolites, and THP in brain function. Brain THP variations have been found during autopsies on fertile women during the luteal phase compared with postmenopausal control women (107). Moreover, high plasma levels of progesterone and THP have been correlated with increased fatigue and confusion in healthy women taking an oral dose of micronized progesterone (108).

Additional mechanisms by which progesterone and its metabolites can act on the brain have been proposed, largely on the basis of studies in rats. Neuroendocrine and behavioral function can be mediated by progesterone receptors and protein synthesis (109). This action of progesterone may also downregulate ER (102). However, progesterone and its ring-A reduced metabolites may also effect areas of the CNS where PR expression is low or absent, indicating non–receptor-mediated progesterone actions. Rapid alterations of CNS excitability, producing behavioral effects not attributable to intracellular receptors, have been reported seconds after the parenteral introduction of many steroids (22). This emphasizes the possible sedative roles played by these steroids in physiologic conditions such as pregnancy and stress (110), perhaps through increased GABA-inhibitory synaptic neurotransmission in the brain. This effect is mediated by the interaction between reduced progesterone and the GABA$_A$ receptor complex through activation of receptor-gated Cl$^-$ channels.

In humans, progesterone has been reported to cause sedative and anesthetic effects (111). In this regard, administered progesterone, had anxiolytic and hypnotic properties (108). These actions are similar to those of the benzodiazepines and barbiturates that are known to interact with GABA$_A$ receptors (112). Although progesterone or progestins have been reported to have similar effects on mood when used in contraception (113–115), such effects remain less documented in postmenopausal women during HRT.

Despite widely held beliefs, contradictory findings have been reported in the assessment of the effects of progesterone/progestins during HRT. Two double-blind, placebo-controlled, cross-over trials with postmenopausal women reported no psychologic effects of medroxyprogesterone administered alone (62) or sequentially with transdermal estrogen (61) Absence of negative effects in anxiety and depression have been found in other studies during sequentially and combined HRT (116). When synthetic progestins were used in sequentially combined transdermal therapeutic systems no adverse affects were found regarding mood (117). However, most gynecologists' bias is that mood changes are often associated with progesterone or progestins during HRT. This problem is often one of the major causes of nonacceptability and noncompliance in HRT. This bias is a serious issue, because it obstructs the use of ERT. It is important to develop objective findings of negative effects of progesterone or progestins on mood. Some studies have confirmed negative effects of progestin added sequentially to estrogen during HRT (64,118). However, because negative psychologic changes are not reported by all women, a relation between the dose of progesterone or progestin preparations and rate of mood disturbances has been suggested as an explanation (117).

Despite a growing body of evidence indicating that circulating or locally formed progestins may act through the GABA receptor system to affect mood or alertness, the picture remains unclear in HRT. In practice we employ minimum systemic progestin treatment, favoring local progestins for protection of reproductive tissue hyperplasia. Although women continue to have the bias agonist progestins, more evidence is required before this is justified.

Effects of Androgen on the Brain

There seems to be little value in treating women who retain their ovaries after menopause; the corpora atretica furnish measurable testosterone and androstenedione. These plus the adrenal androstenedione furnish precursors for estrogen formation elsewhere in the body. The unconverted androgens may directly act to masculinize the phenotype or to block estrogen action and, although plentiful data exists to show local estrogen formation in the brain or elsewhere (119), evidence that this peripheral conversion has clinical significance remains to be adduced. Such studies are needed.

There are numerous reports that the feeling of well-being and sexual desire are improved in postovariectomy (57) subjects who receive ERT plus androgens. This is the subject of another chapter in this book.

Attention has turned toward the possible benefits of dehydroepiandrosterone (DHEA) and dehydroepiandrosterone sulfate (DHEAS), which are the major 19-carbon secretions from the adrenal gland. Although animal data indicate that DHEA and DHEAS may also play a role in the brain (120), but this remains to be shown in humans. There are many experiments using animal models that support roles for DHEA, its metabolites and congeners acting in the brain, tissues (120,121); but these await confirmation in clinical situations (122). These compounds are not overtly androgenic, however they may be peripherally converted into androstenedione and then into the potent androgens testosterone and dihydrotestosterone. DHEA-derived androstenedione and testosterone may also be converted into estrogen. DHEA and DHEAS decrease gradually in men and women after a peak in early adulthood (123). Beneficial effects on energy, longevity, cardiovascular diseases, cancer and immunoresponse, have been reported (124). In the absence of a proven DHEA receptor in humans, and pharmacologic regimens that have excluded transformation to active androgens and estrogens, it is difficult to consider DHEA or DHEAS are primary preventive or therapeutic agents in hormone replacement and brain function.

REFERENCES

1. Backstrom T. Symptoms related to menopause and sex steroid treatments. In: Ciba Foundation Symposium, ed. *Non-reproductive actions of sex steroids.* London: J Wiley & Sons, 1995:171–180.
2. Zimmerman E, Parlee M. Behavioral changes associated with the menstrual cycle: an experimental investigation. *J Appl Psychol* 1973;3:335–344.
3. Morrison J, Hof P. Life and death of neurons in the aging brain. *Science* 1997;278:412–418.
4. Ohkura H, Eshima Y, Isse K, et al. Estrogens increases cerebral and cerebellar blood flows in postmenopausal women. *Menopause* 1994;2:13–18.
5. Naftolin S. Brain aromatization of androgens. *J Reprod Med* 1994;39:257–261.
6. Garcia-Segura L, Chowen J, Naftolin F. Endocrine glia: roles of glial cells in the brain actions of steroid and thyroid hormones and in the regulation of hormone secretion. *Front Neuroendocrinol* 1996;17:180–211.
7. Reichlin S. Neuroendocrinology. In: Wilson J, Foster D, eds. *Williams textbook of endocrinology,* 8th ed. Philadelphia: WB Saunders, 1995:135–219.
8. Naftolin F, Leranth C, Horvath T, Garcia-Segura L. Potential neuronal mechanisms of estrogen actions in synaptogenesis and synaptic plasticity. *Cell Mol Neurobiol* 1996;16:213–223.
9. Olmos G, Naftolin F, Perel J, Tranque P, Garcia-Segura L. Synaptic remodeling in the rat arcuate nucleus during estrus cycle. *Neuroscience* 1989;32:663–667.
10. Negri-Cesi P, Poletti A, Celotti F. Metabolism of steroids in the brain: a new insight into the role of the 5alpha-reductase and aromatase in the brain differentiation and functions. *J Steroid Biochem Mol Biol* 1996;58:455–466.

11. Paul S, Purdy R. Neuroactive steroids. *FASEB J* 1992;6:2311–2322.
12. Mor G, Naftolin F. Estrogen, menopause and immune system. *J Br Menopause Soc (in press)*.
13. Mosselman S, Polman J, Dijekema R. ERbeta: identification and characterization of a novel human estrogen receptor. *FEBS Lett* 1996;392:49–53.
14. Kuiper G, Enmark E, Pelto-Huikko M, Nilsson S, Gustafsson J. Cloning of a novel estrogen receptor expressed in rat prostate and ovary. *Proc Natl Acad Sci USA* 1996;93:5925–5930.
15. Korak KS, Migliaccio S, Davis VL. Estrogens. In: Munson P, Mueller R, Breese G, eds. *Principles of pharmacology: basic concepts and clinical implications.* New York: Chapman & Hall, 1994:809–826.
16. MacGregor J, Tonetti D, Craig Jordan V. The complexity of selective estrogen receptor modulation: the design of a postmenopausal prevention maintenance therapy. In: Linsday R, Dempster D, Craig Jordan V, eds. Estrogens and antiestrogens. Philadelphia: Lippincott-Raven Publishers, 1997.
17. Shughrue P, Lane M, Merchenthaler I. Comparative distribution of estrogen receptor-alpha and -beta mRNA in the rat central nervous system. *J Comp Neurol* 1997;388:507–525.
18. Laflamme N, Nappi R, Drolet G, Labrie C, Rivest S. Expression and neuropeptidergic characterization of estrogen receptor (ER alpha and beta) thought the rat brain: anatomical evidence of district role of each subtype. *J Neurobiol* 1998;36:357–378.
19. Giguere V, Tremblay A, Tremblay G. Estrogen receptor beta: re-evaluation of estrogen and antiestrogen signaling. *Steroids* 1998;63:335–339.
20. Kuiper G, Carlsson B, Grandien K, et al. Comparison of the ligand binding specificity and transcript tissue distribution of estrogen receptors alpha and beta. *Endocrinology* 1997;3:863–869.
21. Peach K, Webb P, Kuiper G, et al. Differential ligand activation of estrogen receptors ER alpha and ER beta at AP1 sites. *Science* 1997;277:1508–1510.
22. McEwen B. Non-genomic and genomic effects of steroids on neural activity. *Trends Pharmacol Sci* 1991;12:141–147.
23. Landers J, Spelsberg T. New concepts in steroid hormone action: transcription factors, proto-oncogenes and the cascade model for steroid regulation of gene expression. In: Stein G, Stein J, Lian L, eds. *Critical review of eukaryotic gene expression.* Boca Raton, FL: CRC Press, 1992.
24. MacLusky N, McEwen B. Progestin receptors in the developing rat brain and pituitary. *Brain Res* 1980;189:262–268.
25. McEwen B, Davis P, Gerlach J, et al. Progestin receptors in the brain and pituitary gland. In: Bardin C, Milgrom E, Mauvais-Jarvis P, eds. *Progesterone and progestin.* New York: Raven Press, 1983.
26. Honjo H, Tamura T, Matsumoto Y, et al. Estrogen as a growth factor to central nervous cells: estrogen treatment promotes development of acetyl-cholinesterase-positive basal forebrain neurons transplanted in the anterior eye chamber. *J Steroid Biochem Mol Biol* 1992;41:633–635.
27. MacLusky N, Naftolin F. Sexual differentiation of central nervous system. *Science* 1981;211:1294–1302.
28. Kessler R, McGonagle R, Swartz M, et al. Sex and depression in the National Comorbidity Survey: lifetime prevalence, chronicity and recurrence. *J Affect Disord* 1993;29:85–96.
29. Rocca W, Amaducci L, Schoenberg B. Epidemiology of clinically diagnosed Alzheimer's disease. *Ann Neurol* 1986;19:415–418.
30. Jorm A, Korten A, Henderson A. The prevalence of dementia: a quantitative integration of the literature. *Acta Psychiatr Scand* 1987;76:465–479.
31. Hofman A, Rocca W, Brayne C, et al. The prevalence of dementia in Europe: a collaborative study of 1980–1990 findings—Eurodem Prevalence Research Group. *Int J Epidemiol* 1991;20:736–748.
32. Witkin J, Ferin M, Popilskis S, Silverman A. Effects of gonadal steroids on the ultrastructure of GnRH neurons in the rhesus monkey: synaptic input and glial apposition. *Endocrinology* 1991;128:1083–1092.
33. Naftolin F, Leranth C, Perez J, Garcia-Segura L. Estrogen induces synaptic plasticity in adult primate neurons. *Neuroendocrinology* 1993;57:935–939.
34. Jakab R, Horvath T, Leranth C, Harada N, Naftolin F. Aromatase immunoreactivity in the rat brain: gonadectomy sensitive hypothalamic neurons and an unresponsive "limbic ring" of the lateral septum-bed nucleus-amygdala complex. *J Steroid Biochem Mol Biol* 1993;44:481–498.
35. Rybo G, Westemberg H. Symptoms in the postmenopause a population study: a preliminary report. *Acta Obstet Gynecol Scand* 1971;50:25.
36. Thompson B, Hart S, Durno D. Menopausal age and symptomatology in general practice. *J Biosoc Sci* 1973;5:71–82.
37. Erlik Y, Tataryn I, Meldrum D, Lomax P, Bajorek J, Judd H. Association of waking episodes with menopausal hot flash. *JAMA* 1981;245:1741–1744.
38. Phillips S, Sherwin B. Effects of estrogen in memory function in surgically menopausal women. *Psychoneuroendocrinology* 1992;17:485–495.
39. Rosenberg J, Larsen S. Hypothesis: pathogenesis of postmenopausal hot flush. *Med Hypotheses* 1991;35:349–350.
40. Meldrum D, Tataryn I, Frumar A, Erlik Y, Lu K, Judd H. Gonadotropins, estrogens, and adrenal steroids during the menopausal hot flash. *J Clin Enocrinol Metab* 1980;50:685.
41. Greene R, Kletzky O, Cabus E, Naftolin F. Similarities between peripheral perfusion augmentation changes induced by postpartum lactation and postmenopausal hot flushes. Presented at the 41st Annual Meeting of the Society for Gynecologic Investigation; Chicago, IL, 1994.
42. Smith J. Management of hot flushes due to endocrine therapy for prostate carcinoma. *Oncology* 1996;10:1319–1322.
43. Hardt W, Schmidt-Gollwitzer M. Sustained gonadal suppression in fertile women with the LHRH agonist buserelin. *Clin Endocrinol* 1983;19:613–617.
44. Tham D, Gardner C, Haskell W. Potential health benefit of dietary phytoestrogens: a review of the clinical, epidemiological and mechanistic evidence. *J Clin Endocrinol Metab* 1998;83:2223–2235.
45. Kupfer D. The sleep EEG in diagnosis and treatment of depression. In: Rush A, Altshuler L, eds. *Depression, basic mechanisms, diagnosis and treatment.* New York: Guilford, 1986.
46. Keefe D, Watson R, Naftolin F. Hormone replacement therapy alleviates sleep apnea in menopausal women. *Menopause (in press)*.
47. Shaver J, Giblin E, Lentz M, Lee K. Sleep patterns and stability in perimenopausal women. *Sleep* 1988;11:556–561.
48. Avis N, Crawford S, McKinlay S. Psychosocial, behavioral, and health factors related to menopause symptomatology. *Womens Health* 1997;3:103–120.
49. Thomson. J. Double blind study on the effect of estrogen on sleep, anxiety and depression in perimenopausal women: preliminary results. *Proc R Soc Med* 1976, 69:829–830.
50. Scharf M, McDonnold MD, Stover R, Zaretsky N, Berkovitz DV. Effects of estrogen replacement therapy on rates of cyclic alternating patterns and hot-flush events during sleep in postmenopausal women: a pilot study. *Clin Ther* 1997;19:304–311.
51. Schiff I, Regestein Q, Tulchinisky D, et al. Effects of estrogens on sleep and psychological state of hypogonadal women. *JAMA* 1979;242:2405.
52. Weissman M, Bland R, Canino G. Cross-national epidemiology of major depression and bipolar disorder. *JAMA* 1996;276:293–299.
53. Parry B. Reproductive factors affecting the course of affective illness in women. *Psychiatr Clin North Am* 1989;12:207–220.
54. Saks B, Frank J, Lowe T, Berman W, Naftolin F, Cohen D. Depressed mood during pregnancy and the puerperium: clinical recognition and implication for clinical practice. *Am J Psychiatry* 1985;142:728–731.
55. Zweifel J, O'Brien W. A meta-analysis of the effect of hormone replacement therapy upon depressed mood. *Psychoneuroendocrinology* 1997;22:189–212.
56. Sherwin B, Gelfand M. Sex steroids and affect in surgical menopause: a double-blind crossover study. *Psychoneuroendocrinology* 1985;10:325–335.
57. Sherwin B, Gelfand M. Differential symptoms response to parenteral estrogen and/or androgen administration in surgical menopause. *Am J Obstet Gynecol* 1985;151:153–160.
58. Genazzani A, Cela V, Spinetti A, et al. Neuroendocrine aspects of the menopause and hormone replacement therapy. *J Cardiovasc Pharmacol* 1996;28[Suppl 5]:S58–S60.
59. Keefe D, Naftolin F. Brain neurochemistry and mood. In: Smith S, Schiff I, eds. *Modern management of premenstrual syndrome.* New York: WW Norton, 1992; 55–70.
60. Gonzales G, Carrillo C. Blood serotonin levels in postmenopausal women: effects of age and serum estradiol levels. *Maturitas* 1993;17:23–29.
61. Kirkham C, Hahn P, Van Vugt D, et al. A randomized, double blind, placebo-controlled, cross-over trial to assess the side effects of medroxyprogesterone acetate in hormone replacement therapy. *Obstet Gynecol* 1991;78:93–97.
62. Prior J, Alojado N, McKay D, et al. No adverse effects of medroxyprogesterone treatment without estrogen on postmenopausal women: double blind, placebo-controlled, crossover trial. *Obstet Gynecol* 1994;83:24–28.
63. Myers L, Dixen J, Morissette D, et al. Effects of estrogen androgen and progestin on sexual psychobiology and behavior in postmenopausal women. *J Clin Endocrinol Metab* 1990;70:1124–1130.
64. Sherwin B. The impact of different doses of estrogen and progestin on mood and sexual behavior in postmenopausal women. *J Clin Endocrinol Metab* 1991;72:336–343.
65. Avis N, Brambilla D, McKinlay S, et al. A longitudinal analysis of the association between menopause and depression: result from the Massachusetts Women's Health Study. *Ann Epidemiol* 1994;4:214–220.
66. Hunter M. Somatic experience of the menopause: a prospective study. *Psychosom Med* 1990;52:357–367.
67. Hay A, Bancroft J, Johnstone E. Affective symptoms in women attending a menopause clinic. *Br J Psychiatry* 1994;164:513–516.
68. Schmidt P, Roca C, Ribinow D. Perimenopausal depression. In: Lobo R, ed. *Perimenopause.* New York: Springer, 1997:246–254.
69. Blehar M, Oren D. Women's increased vulnerability to mood disorders: integrity psychobiology and epidemiology. *Depression* 1995;3:3–12.
70. Parry B. Reproductive related depression in women: phenomena of hormonal kindling? In: Hamilton J, Harberger P, eds. *Postpartum psychiatric illness: a picture puzzle.* Philadelphia: University of Pennsylvania Press, 1992.
71. Yorkers K. The association between premenstrual dysphoric disorder and other mood disorder. *J Clin Psychiatry* 1997;58[Suppl]:19–25.
72. Klaiber E, Brovermen D, Vogel V, Kobayashi Y. Estrogen therapy for severe persistent depression in women. *Arch Gen Psychiatry* 1979;36:742–744.
73. Henderson A, Gregorie A, Kumar R, Studd J. Treatment of severe postnatal depression wish estradiol skin patches. *Lancet* 1991;338:816–817.
74. Schneider L, Small G, Hamilton S, Bystritsky A, Nemeroff C, Meyers B. Estrogen replacement and response to fluoxetine in a multicenter geriatric depression trial: fluoxetine collaborative study group. *Am J Geriatr Psychiatry* 1997;5:97–106.
75. Wickelgren J. Estrogen stakes claim to cognition. *Science* 1997;27:675–678.
76. McEwen B, Alves S, Bulloch K, Welland N. Ovarian steroids and the brain: implications for cognition and aging. *Neurology* 1997;48[Suppl 5]:S8–S15.
77. Diano S, Naftolin F, Horvath T. Gonadal steroids target AMPA glutamate recep-

tor-containing neurons in the rat hypothalamus, septum and amygdala: a morphological and biochemical study. *Endocrinology* 1997;138:778–789.

78. Bartus R, Dean R, Beer B, Lippa A. The cholinergic hypothesis of memory dysfunction. *Science* 1982;217:208–217.

79. Luine V. Estradiol increases choline acetyltransferase activity in specific basal forebrain nuclei and projection areas of female rats. *Exp Neurol* 1985;80:484–490.

80. Woolley C, McEwen B. Roles of estradiol and progesterone in regulation of hippocampal dendritic spine density during the estrus cycle in the rat. *J Comp Neurol* 1993;336:293–306.

81. McEwen B, Wolley C. Estradiol and progesterone regulate neuronal structure and synaptic connectivity in adult as well as developing brain. *Exp Gerontol* 1994;29:431–436.

82. Lupien S, McEwen B. The acute effects of corticosteroids on cognition: integration of animal and human studies. *Brain Res Rev* 1997;24:1–27.

83. Sherwin B, Tulandi T. "Add back" estrogen reverses cognitive deficits induced by gonadotropin release-hormone agonist in women with leiomyomatosis uteri. *J Clin Endocrinol Metab* 1996;81:2545–2549.

84. Haskell R, Richardon E, Horwitz R. The effects of estrogen replacement therapy on cognitive function in women: a critical review of the literature. *J Clin Epidemiol* 1997;50:1249–1264.

85. Sherwin B. Estrogen and cognitive functioning in women. *Proc Soc Exp Biol Med* 1998;217:17–22.

86. Sherwin B. Estrogen and/or androgen replacement therapy and cognitive functioning in surgically menopausal women. *Psychoneuroendocrinology* 1988;10:325–335.

87. Bechman D, Wole P, Linn R. Prevalence of dementia and probable senile dementia of Alzheimer type in the Framinghan study. *Neurology* 1992;42:115–119.

88. Holey W. The family caregiver's role in Alzheimer's disease. *Neurology* 1997;48:S25–S29.

89. Tang M, Jacobs D, Stern Y, et al. Effect of estrogen during menopause on risk age at onset of Alzheimer's disease. *Lancet* 1996;348:429–432.

90. Schneck MJ, Sarrel PM, Albakri E, et al. Oral progesterone therapy impairs cerebrovascular reactivity. *Stroke* 1995;26:724.

91. Beringer W, Potter J. Low body mass index in demented outpatients. *J Am Geriatr Soc* 1991;39:973–978.

92. Xu H, Gouras G, Greenfield J, et al. Estrogen reduces neuronal generation of Alzheimer β-amyloid peptides. *Nat Med* 1998;4:447–451.

93. Henderson V, Paganini-Hill A, Emanuel C. Estrogen replacement therapy in older women. *Arch Neurol* 1994;51:896–900.

94. Paganini-Hill A, Henderson V. Estrogen deficiency and risk of Alzheimer's disease in women. *Am J Epidemiol* 1994;140:256–261.

95. Mortel K, Meyers J. Lack of postmenopausal estrogen replacement therapy and the risk of dementia. *J Neuropsychiatry Clin Neurosci* 1995;7:334–337.

96. Kawas C, Resnick S, Morrison A, et al. A prospective study of estrogen replacement therapy and the risk of developing Alzheimer's disease: the Baltimore Longitudinal Study of Aging. *Neurology* 1997;48:1517–1521.

97. Brenner D, Kukull W, Stergachis A, van Belle G, Bowen J, McCormick W. Postmenopausal estrogen replacement therapy and risk of Alzheimer's disease: a population based case-control study. *Am J Epidemiol* 1994;140:262–267.

98. Honjo H, Ogino Y, Naitoh K, et al. In vivo effects by estrone sulfate on the central nervous system-senile dementia (Alzheimer's type). *J Steroid Biochem* 1989;34:521–525.

99. Honjo H, Ogino Y, Naitoh K, et al. An effect of conjugated estrogen to cognitive impairment in women with senile dementia Alzheimer's type: a placebo-controlled double blind study. *J Jpn Menopause Soc* 1993;1:167–171.

100. Fillit H, Weinreb H, Cholst I, et al. Observation in a preliminary open trial of estradiol therapy for senile dementia Alzheimer's type. *Psychoneuroendocrinology* 1986;11:337–345.

101. Ohkura T, Isse K, Akazawa K, et al. Evaluation of estrogen treatment in female patient with dementia of the Alzheimer's type. *J Endocrinol* 1994;41:361–371.

102. Clarke C, Sutherland R. Progestin regulation of cellular proliferation. *Endocr Rev* 1990;11:266–301.

103. Naftolin F, Rutherford T, Chambers J, Carcangiu M. More evidences on whether estrogen replacement causes cancer. *J Soc Gynecol Invest* 1997;4:57.

104. Graham J, Clarke C. Physiological action of progesterone in target tissues. *Endocr Rev* 1997;18:502–519.

105. Robel P, Baulieu E. Neurosteroids. Biosynthesis and function. *Crit Rev Neurobiol* 1995;9:383–394.

106. Poletti A, Rabuffetti M, Celotti F. The 5α-reductase in the rat brain. In: Genazzani A, Petraglia P, Purdy R, eds. *The brain source and target of sex steroids hormones.* London: The Parthenon Publishing Group, 1996.

107. Bixo M, Andersson A, Winblad B, Purdy R, Backstrom T. Progesterone, 5α-pregnane-3,20-dione and 3α-hydroxy-5α-pregnane-20-one in specific regions of the human female brain in different endocrine states. *Brain Res* 1997;764:173–178.

108. Freeman E, Purdy R, Coutifaris C, Rickels K, Paul S. Anxiolytic metabolites of progesterone: correlation with mood and performance measures following oral progesterone administration to healthy female volunteers. *Neuroendocrinology* 1993;58:478–484.

109. Yamamoto K. Steroid receptor regulated transcription of specific genes and gene networks. *Annu Rev Genet* 1985;19:209–252.

110. Purdy R, Morrow A, Moore P, Paul S. Stress-induced elevations of aminobutyric acid type A receptor-active steroids in the rat brain. *Proc Natl Acad Sci USA* 1991;88:4553–4557.

111. Selye H. The anesthetic effect of steroid hormones. *Proc Soc Exp Biol Med* 1941;46:116–121.

112. Majewska M, Harrison N, Schwartz R, Barker J, Paul S. Steroids hormone metabolites are barbiturate-like modulators of GABA receptor. *Science* 1986;232:1004–1007.

113. Kane F. Evaluation of emotional reactions to oral contraceptive uses. *Am J Obstet Gynecol* 1976;126:968–972.

114. Wagner K. Major depression and anxiety disorder associated with Norplant. *J Clin Psychiatry* 1996;57:152–157.

115. Jensvold M. Nonpregnant reproductive-age women. Part II. Exogenous sex steroid hormones and psychopharmacology. In: Jensvold M, Halbreich U, Hamilton J, eds. *Sex, gender and hormones.* Washington, DC: American Psychiatric Press, 1996.

116. Siddle N, Fraser D, Whitehead M, et al. Endometrial, physical and psychological effects of postmenopausal estrogen therapy with added dydrogesterone. *Br J Obstet Gynaecol* 1990;97:1101–1107.

117. Whitehead M, Hillard T, Crook D. The role and use of progestogens. *Obstet Gynecol* 1990;75:S59–S76.

118. Holst J, Backstrom T, Hammarback S, et al. Progestogen addition during estrogen replacement therapy-effects on vasomotor symptoms and mood. *Maturitas* 1989;11:13–20.

119. Abrahm G. Ovarian and adrenal condition to peripheral androgens during the menstrual cycle. *J Clin Endocrinol Metab* 1974;39:340–345.

120. Robel P, Baulieu E. Dehydroepiandrosterone (DHEA) is a neuroactive neurosteroid. *Ann N Y Acad Sci* 1997;774:82–109.

121. Majewska M. Neuronal actions of Dehydroepiandrosterone. Possible roles in brain development aging, memory and affect. *Ann N Y Acad Sci* 1995;774–782.

122. Morales A, Nolan J, Nelson J, Yen S. Effect of replacement dose of dehydroepiandrosterone in men and women of advancing age. *J Clin Endocrinol Metab* 1994;78:1360–1367.

123. Ravaglia G, Forti P, Maioli F, et al. The relationship of DHEAS to endocrine-metabolic parameters and functional status in the oldest-old: results from an Italian study on healthy free-living over-ninety-year-olds. *J Clin Endocrinol Metab* 1996;81:1173–1778.

124. Casson P, Hornsby P, Ghusn H, Buster J. Dehydroepiandrosterone (DHEA) replacement in postmenopausal women: present status and future promise. *Menopause* 1997;4:225–231.

125. Horvath T, Garcia-Segura L, Naftolin F. Control of gonadotropin feedback: the possible role of estrogen-induced hypothalamic synaptic plasticity. *Gynecol Endocrinol* 1997;11:139–143.

126. Sherwin B. Sex hormones and psychological functioning in postmenopausal women. *Exp Gerontol* 1994;29:423–430.

127. Grady C, Rapoport S. Cerebral metabolism in aging and dementia. In: Birren J, Sloane R, Cohen G, eds. *Handbook of mental health and aging.* San Diego: Academic Press, 1992:53–65.

128. Marsh G. Perceptual changes with aging. In: Busse E, Blorer D, eds. *Textbook of geriatric psychiatry.* Washington DC: American Psychiatric Press, 1996:49–59.

129. Reder A. Neural regulation of the immune system. In: Antel J, Birnbaum G, Hartung H, eds. *Clinical neuroendocrinology.* Boston: Blackwell Science, 1998:55–71.

Treatment of the Postmenopausal Woman: Basic and Clinical Aspects, Second Edition, edited by Rogerio A. Lobo, Lippincott Williams & Wilkins, Philadelphia © 1999.

CHAPTER 23

The Epidemiology of Alzheimer's Disease and the Role of Estrogen Replacement Therapy in the Prevention and Treatment of Alzheimer's Disease and Memory Decline in Older Women

Mary Sano, Diane M. Jacobs, and Richard Mayeux

Alzheimer's disease (AD), the most common form of dementia, is characterized by profound loss of memory and other cognitive functions sufficient to interfere with social and occupational functioning. The prevalence and incidence of AD, as well as the cost to society, increases exponentially with age. It has been estimated that, starting at age 65, the prevalence of AD doubles with every 5 years of age, with prevalence estimates reaching 20% for those older than 90 (1). It has been recognized that even before the diagnosis of AD, cognitive deficits—in particular significant memory impairment, occurs. Although the impact of this prodromal state is not well documented, it is easy to imagine the potential for significant functional problems in an increasingly technologic society. Without considering the impact of this prodromal state, estimates of the total cost of AD range from 60 to 90 billion dollars annually (2).

A growing interest in women's health and an awareness of the aging of society has spurred many research initiatives to explore the relationship of estrogen and dementia. Evidence from epidemiologic, clinical, and laboratory investigations suggests that postmenopausal estrogen replacement therapy (ERT) may play a role in ameliorating the devastation of AD and memory loss in aging. Epidemiologic studies suggest that ERT may reduce the risk of dementia and age-associated memory decline. A growing number of studies suggest that estrogen may improve memory in elderly women. Clinical studies also have suggested that estrogen replacement may have some role in the treatment of AD and other dementias. This chapter reviews the research suggesting a link between estrogen replacement and AD, discusses its strengths and limitations, and defines potential directions to maximize our knowledge about the role estrogen may play in the treatment and prevention of AD.

EPIDEMIOLOGY OF REDUCING THE RISK OF ALZHEIMER'S DISEASE WITH ESTROGEN REPLACEMENT THERAPY

There have been a number of epidemiologic investigations of the effects of ERT and risk of dementia in postmenopausal women. In a review of this literature and metanalysis, Yaffe et al. (3) cited contradictory findings, with some studies demonstrating a reduced risk of AD among women who were current or past users of ERT and others demonstrating no such effect. Despite these mixed findings, a metanalysis of the 10 observational studies published between 1984 and 1997 (eight case-control and two prospective cohort studies) suggested that women who had used ERT had an overall 29% decreased risk of developing AD.

M. Sano and D.M. Jacobs: Department of Neurology, the Gertrude H. Sergievsky Center, and Taub Center for Alzheimer's Disease Research, Columbia University College of Physicians and Surgeons, New York, New York 10032.

R. Mayeux: Departments of Neurology and Psychiatry, the Gertrude H. Sergievsky Center, and Taub Center for Alzheimer's Disease Research, Columbia University College of Physicians and Surgeons, New York, New York 10032.

TABLE 23.1. *Summary of case-control studies of estrogen use and dementia*

Study	Comparison	Odds ratio (95% CI)
Heyman et al., 1984[4]	Current v. no current use	2.4 (0.7–7.8)
Amaducci et al., 1986[5]	Ever v. never use	1.6 (0.4–5.9)
Broe et al., 1990[30]	≥6 mo v. never use	0.7 (0.4–1.6)
Graves et al., 1990[6]	Use at the time of dementia onset v. no use	1.2 (0.5–2.6)
Brenner et al., 1994[31]	Ever v. never use	1.1 (0.6–1.8)
Henderson et al., 1994[7]	Current v. no current use	0.3 (0.1–0.7)
Paganini-Hill et al., 1994[8]	Ever v. never use	0.7 (0.5–1.0)
Mortel et al., 1995[32]	Current v. no current use	0.6 (0.3–1.2)
Paganini-Hill et al., 1996[9]	Ever v. never use	0.7 (0.5–0.9)
Baldereschi et al., 1998[10]	Ever v. never use	0.2 (0.1–0.8)

Tables 23.1 and 23.2 list the epidemiologic investigations that have been completed. A review of the details of these studies provides an illustration of the benefits and limitations of observational studies.

Case-Control Studies

Table 23.1 lists 10 case-control studies that have compared exposure to ERT in AD cases and nondemented control subjects. Two early studies assessed estrogen use along with other risk factors in AD (4,5). Both of these case-control studies had relatively small sample sizes of patients and controls. In the study by Heyman et al. (4), 28 community-dwelling women with onset of AD before age 70 were identified through clinical practice and were matched to community-dwelling controls by age and race. The nonsignificant trend toward increased risk of AD among estrogen users reported in this study is difficult to interpret, because the sample size is small and the presence of another risk factor in a single case could change the direction of this trend. In a second study, consisting of clinically diagnosed patients with AD and hospital and community controls, an in-person interview was conducted with next of kin to determine a series of possible risk factors. ERT, defined as "use of estrogens in menopause," was more common among women with AD than controls, although the difference was not significant (5). Information about estrogen use was unavailable for nearly one-half the participants in this cohort, illustrating a serious limitation of this method of capturing ERT use; an informant may have little knowledge of the perimenopausal period, which might have occurred decades earlier.

In another case-control study of 130 patients with AD, a telephone survey was used to ask an informant about estrogen use by patients at the time of symptom onset (6). A friend or nonblood relative was used as a control subject, and an informant was asked about ERT use for a similar period. No significant difference in exposure to ERT was found between AD cases and control subjects.

In contrast, in their comparison of 143 community-dwelling women who had AD with 92 nondemented volunteer controls, Henderson et al. (7) found that AD patients were significantly less likely than control subjects to use ERT. Women with dementia who were receiving ERT scored significantly higher on cognitive testing than demented women who were not receiving hormone replacement, despite comparable age, education, and dementia duration.

In a nested case-control study of women in the Leisure World retirement community, Paganini-Hill and Henderson (8) compared estrogen use among those who died of AD or related dementias with those who died of other causes. This report used death certificates to identify cases rather than clinical populations, and estrogen use was assessed by review of prescriptions. A significantly lower risk of AD or related dementia was found among women who used estrogen than among women who had not use estrogen during the postmenopausal period. Similar results were obtained when the analysis was restricted to include only those patients with a diagnosis of AD. In an update of this investigation that included a higher number of deaths, these results seem unaltered (9). A history of longer duration of estrogen use, higher estrogen dose, and an early age at menarche also were associated with a lower risk of death from AD.

TABLE 23.2. *Summary of prospective cohort studies of estrogen use and dementia*

Study	Cohort	Comparison	Risk ratio (95% CI)
Tang et al., 1996[12]	1124 community-dwelling women in New York City	Ever v. never use	0.4 (0.2–0.9)
Kawas et al., 1997[13]	472 community-dwelling women in Baltimore	Ever v. never use	0.5 (0.2–1.0)

Large Population-Based Case-Control Studies

Since the comprehensive summary report and met-analysis of Yaffe et al. (3), two large case-control cohort studies have been published demonstrating a significantly decreased risk of AD among women with history of estrogen use. A large, multicenter, population-based study of more than 1,500 women in Italy found ERT was significantly more common among nondemented women (10). This study ascertained cases of AD by examination and ERT use by interview with the participant or an informant in the case of a demented participant. History of postmenopausal estrogen use was associated with a 76% decreased risk of AD. Estrogen use was associated with younger age and higher education, but the effect remained significant when analyses controlled for these variables. The overall duration of ERT use was 3 years, but only three women with dementia ever used ERT, making it impossible to assess the effect of duration of use. The results of this study support the notion that ERT protects against AD.

A case-control study from Rochester, Minnesota, examined medical records from the Rochester Epidemiology Project records linkage system (11). Cases were defined as individuals with a diagnosis of AD during the period 1980 to 1984. These cases were matched with nondemented individuals based on age and length of time in the record system. Estrogen exposure included oral, parenteral, topical, or suppository use and was defined as use after the onset of menopause and before the onset of dementia. The length of exposure and the demographic and other clinically relevant variables were extracted from medical records. Cases and controls were comparable on education, age at menarche, age at menopause, and percent with hysterectomies. Estrogen use was associated with a 60% decreased risk of AD.

Limitations of Case-Control Studies

Case-control investigations of the association between ERT and AD have yielded disparate results, with some studies reporting a significantly decreased risk of AD associated with ERT and others finding no such difference. In part, these contradictory findings may result from methodologic differences between the studies. Investigations differed in the methods of case ascertainment, selection and matching of controls subjects, methods of obtaining information about estrogen use (e.g., from the participant, a proxy, or medical records), and exposure of interest (e.g., current or lifetime use of ERT).

Limitations inherent in case-control studies also may have contributed to the disparate results. For example, the way in which cases and controls are recruited may result in selection bias. In a likely scenario in which selection bias may be a problem, control subjects are not adequately screened for dementia, and participants with AD are included as control subjects. Recall bias, or the influence having a disease exerts on the likelihood of recalling exposure to an agent such as ERT, also may have affect the outcome of case-control studies. This is particularly true for a disease such as AD; patients may not remember whether they took ERT, and caregivers or informants may not know or remember whether the patient used ERT at menopause, which probably occurred decades earlier.

For studies investigating the effects of current estrogen use, prescribing practices may differ for patients and controls. For example, some practitioners may discontinue ERT when a women becomes demented because of fear that she will not be able to comply with the treatment regimen.

Any of these biases may affect the direction or strength of an association between ERT and AD. Prospective cohort studies are less susceptible to these methodologic biases.

Prospective Cohort Studies

Two community-based, prospective cohort studies have investigated the association of ERT and risk of developing AD. These studies provide strong support for a protective effect of estrogen against AD.

Tang et al. examined the effect of a history of estrogen use on the development of AD among elderly women residing in a New York City community (12). This cohort illustrates several advantages of epidemiologic investigation. Participants were demographically representative of the multiethnic population from which they were drawn, and they were followed for as long as 5 years. In-person, standardized medical, neurologic, and cognitive assessments were used to establish the diagnosis of AD.

The effect of ERT on risk of AD was examined in more than 1,100 nondemented women with a mean age at baseline of 74 years. Approximately 14% of women reported that they had received postmenopausal ERT. The average duration of estrogen use was 6.8 years (range, 2 months to 49 years). Women who used estrogen were younger and better educated than those who had not used estrogen. African-American women were less likely to have used ERT than Caucasian or Hispanic women. Women who took estrogen were also more likely to have had a hysterectomy and to have begun menopause at an earlier age. During follow-up, 14.9% of the women developed AD. Women who developed AD were older and had fewer years of education than those who did not, illustrating typical confounding variables. Oral estrogen use during the postmenopausal period significantly delayed the onset of AD and lower reduced the risk of disease by 60%. Women who reported having used estrogen for more than 1 year had a lower risk of AD compared with women who had used estrogen for less than 1 year. Twenty-three women were still taking estrogen at the time they entered the study, and none have developed AD over the study period. The reduction in risk of AD associated with ERT remained significant after adjusting for group differences in age, education, ethnicity, and apolipoprotein E genotype.

Kawas et al. reported a similar reduction in AD risk associated with estrogen use (oral, transdermal, or both forms) in the Baltimore Longitudinal Study of Aging, a prospective cohort study of women living in Baltimore, Maryland (13). In this study, subjects were evaluated every 2 years with a multidiciplinary evaluation, including medical history, medication use, and physical, neurologic, neuropsychologic, and functional assessments. Duration of follow-up ranged from 1 to 16 years. Data analysis was conducted on 472 women. This cohort was primarily a white (92%), highly educated group (63% had college or graduate degrees), and 29% had undergone hysterectomy. Among the 472 women, 230 (48.7%) reported estrogen use, with 95% of the use in the form of oral estrogen and 5% in the form of transdermal estrogen. There were 34 incident cases of AD during follow-up. After adjustment for education, a reduction in risk for AD by about 54% was found among users compared with nonusers. These investigators did not find a significant effect of duration of ERT usage.

Although these studies provide important evidence of a link between ERT and risk of AD, the presence of confounding variables limits the conclusions that can be drawn from them. Confounding variables are factors that are associated with the risk factor (e.g., ERT use) and with the outcome (e.g., AD). Age and educational attainment are two common confounding variables in this line of research. When these variables can be identified and assessed directly, their effects can be controlled statistically. However, other variables that may be less evident (e.g., access to medical care, exposure to other risk or protective factors, healthy lifestyle) may not be apparent or cannot be measured reliably, resulting in misleading interpretations. To definitively determine whether ERT reduces the risk of developing AD, randomized, double-blind, placebo-controlled trials must be performed. Two such trials are underway.

EFFECTS OF ESTROGEN REPLACEMENT THERAPY ON COGNITIVE FUNCTION

There is evidence that estrogen use has a beneficial role on cognitive function in nondemented women, particularly on tests of memory. Sherwin (14) found improved performance on tests of attention (digit span), abstract reasoning, clerical speed and accuracy, and immediate paragraph recall among women receiving ERT among after hysterectomy. In a later report, Phillips and Sherwin (15) demonstrated preservation of verbal paired-associate learning and improved immediate paragraph recall among surgically postmenopausal women treated with ERT.

Effects of ERT on cognitive function in elderly women have not been examined in clinical trials; however, reports from population-based observational studies suggest that estrogen may help to maintain or improve cognitive abilities older women as well. For example, Resnick et al. (16) found better performance on a visual memory test in women using estrogen compared with those not receiving estrogen replacement in the Baltimore Longitudinal Study of Aging. In the study, 116 women currently using ERT were compared with 172 nonusers. Women using ERT made significantly fewer errors in recalling a series of geometric designs than nonusers. Repeated measures analyses examined a small sample of women (n = 18 per group) at two time periods. Those who were never treated with estrogen had a greater change in scores (i.e., poorer performance at time 2 compared with time 1) than those receiving estrogen, whose scores remained essentially unchanged.

Data from a community-based sample in New York City also suggest that ERT may help to maintain cognitive function in nondemented postmenopausal women (17). Women included in these analyses were free of dementia or significant cognitive impairment at their initial evaluation and had no history of stroke or Parkinson's disease. Women who had a history of postmenopausal estrogen use scored higher on measures of verbal memory, abstract reasoning, and language. The performance of women who had used estrogen improved on a measure of verbal memory over an average of 2.5 years of follow-up. Women who used estrogen for longer than 1 year tended to perform higher than those who had used estrogen for less than 1 year. The effect of estrogen on cognition was independent of age, education, ethnicity, and apolipoprotein E genotype.

Although these studies suggest that there is a cognitive benefit from estrogen use in elderly women, particularly in the area of memory, other similar investigation have failed to observe a beneficial effect of ERT on cognitive function or consider the effects too small to be meaningful (18). Randomized, double-blind, placebo-controlled clinical trials are needed to definitively establish this effect.

Clinical Trials of Estrogen in Alzheimer's Disease and Related Disorders

The effects of estrogen as a treatment for AD have not been rigorously assessed. Several small, uncontrolled clinical trials of estrogen therapy in AD patients showed improvement in measures of cognition and mood (19,20). Improvement in attention, orientation, mood, social interaction, and memory occurred in most women. The greatest response was observed among women who were depressed and had low scores on the a mental status examination. Fillit et al. (19) emphasized the correlation between estrogen blood levels and cognitive performance, revealing a performance decline in all responders after discontinuation of estrogen; this was consistent with falling estrogen levels. Similar results were obtained by Honjo et al., with most subjects demonstrating improved performance on measures of memory, orientation, and calculation, although only seven women were studied (20). Ohkura and colleagues (14) reported improvement in a global ratings, mental status examination, and depression scales and found increases of the mean cerebral blood flow in the lower frontal regions and the primary motor areas in seven patients with AD using estrogen.

Other evidence of a benefit from estrogen use comes from a clinical trial of an antidementia drug (21). Patients were randomly assigned to receive a cholinesterase inhibitor or a placebo. Concomitant medication use revealed that a small portion of women were also taking estrogen. In this *post hoc* analysis, it appeared that women taking estrogen and the cholinesterase inhibitor had a greater benefit than those taking the cholinesterase inhibitor alone.

Laboratory Investigation of Estrogen

Several lines of basic research support a role for estrogen in the prevention of AD. The loss of tropic support has been proposed as a mechanism contributing to the pathogenesis of AD and cognitive decline among elderly women. The natural reduction in gonadal steroid levels, particularly among women, may contribute to the loss of neurons and neuronal systems vital to cognitive functions. Whether this occurs in AD, with the onset of the postmenopausal state, or as a manifestation of normal aging is unknown. The cellular and molecular mechanisms and the signaling pathways mediating the growth-promoting actions of estrogen in the brain and the means by which estrogen prevents AD are also unknown. Estrogen enhancement of neuron growth in the developing rodent forebrain and in the estrogen-deprived aging brain may result from the actions of the estrogen alone or interactions with endogenous growth factors (e.g., neurotrophins) and their receptors (22,23). However, estrogen has direct effects on amyloid, the protein found in the neuritic plaques in brains of patients with AD. Estrogen may also be capable of reducing the toxic effects of amyloid on neurons (24).

Estrogen modulates levels of neurotrophic factors, particularly in the hippocampus and basal forebrain. These regions, which have long been associated with learning and memory, degenerate in AD and may be responsible for the severe loss of memory and other cognitive functions. Toran-Allerand et al. found that estrogen receptors are colocalized with mRNA for the nerve growth factor family of neurotrophins and their receptors in developing neurons of the rodent basal forebrain (22,23). Ovariectomized rats treated with 17β-estradiol performed better than those deprived of estrogen on a memory task, and they showed preservation of neurons in the basal fore-

brain and a return of neurotrophin mRNA levels to near normal (25–27). These findings imply that estrogen may influence neurotrophin synthesis and release or may promote survival by other mechanisms.

Because AD is associated with neuronal cell loss, neurofibrillary tangle formation, and deposition of amyloid plaques, factors that affect amyloid β peptide (Aβ) metabolism are important. Estrogen protects hippocampal neurons in culture that are exposed to excitotoxins, oxidative stress, or Aβ and could reduce neuronal Aβ generation (25,26). Cells cultured in the presence of 17β-estradiol accumulate a soluble form of the Aβ precursor protein. Other studies (28) show that, in mouse neuroblastoma cell lines and in primary rat cortical neuronal cultures, 17β-estradiol diminishes the release of Aβ peptide, which is believed to play a major role in the cause of AD.

Mechanisms involving oxidative stress also may contribute to the pathogenesis of neuronal degeneration in AD. Free radicals generated by inefficient metabolism appear to be the source of this oxidative stress. Goodman et al. (29) examined the degree of protection by estrogen from toxicity associated with oxidative stressors, glutamate (excitotoxic), $FeSO_4$, and glucose deprivation. In these models, estradiol and progesterone protected neurons. Estradiol, with and without progesterone, also favorably affected lipid peroxidation and glutamate-induced elevation of intracellular free calcium ions, both indicators of oxidative stress. These data suggest that estrogen, with or without progesterone, may protect against a wide variety of insults to the aging brain.

CONCLUSIONS

Taken together, these data provide strong support for the hypothesis that estrogen delays the onset of AD; however, each line of inquiry has limitations. The observational epidemiologic studies cannot identify all of the risks and benefits associated with the use of estrogen nor identify the possible confounding variables. The clinical trials using patients with AD have not included the necessary rigor of randomization, using a placebo control, or blinding participants and investigators to group assignment. The available laboratory studies represent theoretically plausible models of mechanisms of the disease, which may or may not apply to human beings.

Future research on the benefits of estrogen will include randomized, double-blind, placebo-controlled clinical trials to determine if estrogen is a safe and effective agent for preventing or treating AD and age-associated cognitive decline. Research to determine whether estrogenic receptors in the central nervous system can be selectively activated without peripheral activation will permit us to explore the potential benefits of estrogen in men and women.

ACKNOWLEDGMENTS

This work was supported by federal grants AG07370, AG07232, AG08702, MH44176, and MH50038; The Taub Foundation; and the Charles S. Robertson Memorial Gift for Alzheimer's Disease Research from the Banbury Fund.

REFERENCES

1. Jorm AF. *The epidemiology of Alzheimer's disease and related disorders.* New York: Chapman & Hall, 1990.
2. Ernst RL, Hay JW. The US economic and social costs of Alzheimer's disease revisited. *Am J Public Health* 1994;84:1261–1264.
3. Yaffe K, Sawaya G, Lieberburg I, Grady D. Estrogen therapy in postmenopausal women. *JAMA* 1998;279:688–695.
4. Heyman A, Wilkinson WE, Stafford JA, Helms MJ, Sigmon AH, Weinberg T. Alzheimer's disease: a study of epidemiological aspects. *Ann Neurol* 1984;15:335–341.
5. Amaducci LA, Fratiglioni L, Rocca WA, et al. Risk factors for clinically diagnosed Alzheimer's disease: a case-control study of an Italian population. *Neurology* 1986;36:922–931.
6. Graves AB, White E, Koepsell TD, et al. A case-control study of Alzheimer's disease. *Ann Neurol* 1990;28:766–774.
7. Henderson VW, Paganini-Hill A, Emanuel CK, Dunn ME, Buckwalter JG. Estrogen replacement therapy in older women: comparisons between Alzheimer's disease cases and nondemented control subjects. *Arch Neurol* 1994;51:896–900.
8. Paganini-Hill A, Henderson VW. Estrogen deficiency and risk of Alzheimer's disease in women. *Am J Epidemiol* 1994;140:256–261.
9. Paganini-Hill A, Henderson VW. Estrogen replacement therapy and risk of Alzheimer's disease. *Arch Intern Med* 1996;156:2213–2217.
10. Baldereschi MDA, Lepore V, Bracco L, et al. Estrogen-replacement therapy and Alzheimer's disease in the Italian Longitudinal Study on Aging. *Neurology* 1998;50:996–1002.
11. Waring SC, Rocca WA, Petersen RC, Kokmen E. Postmenopausal estrogen replacement therapy and Alzheimer's disease: a population-based study in Rochester, Minnesota. *Neurology* 1997;48:A79.
12. Tang M-X, Jacobs D, Stern Y, et al. Effect of oestrogen during menopause on risk and age at onset of Alzheimer's disease. *Lancet* 1996;348:429–432.
13. Kawas C, Resnick S, Morrison A, et al. A prospective study of estrogen replacement therapy and the risk of developing Alzheimer's disease: the Baltimore Longitudinal Study of Aging. *Neurology* 1997;48:1517–1521.
14. Ohkura T, Isse K, Akazawa K, Hamamoto M, Yaoi Y, Hagino N. Long-term estrogen replacement therapy in female patients with dementia of the Alzheimer type: 7 case reports. *Dementia* 1995;6:99–107.
15. Phillips SM, Sherwin BB. Effects of estrogen on memory function in surgically menopausal women. *Psychoneuroendocrinology* 1992;17:485–495.
16. Resnick SM, Metter EJ, Zonderman AB. Estrogen replacement therapy and longitudinal decline in visual memory: a possible protective effect? *Neurology* 1997;49:1491–1497.
17. Jacobs DM, Tang M-X, Stern Y, et al. Cognitive function in nondemented older women who took estrogen after menopause. *Neurology* 1998;50:368–373.
18. Barrett-Connor E, Kritz-Silverstein D. Estrogen replacement therapy and cognitive function in older women. *JAMA* 1993;269:2637–2641.
19. Fillit H, Weinreb H, Cholst I, et al. Observations in a preliminary open trial of estradiol therapy for senile dementia—Alzheimer's type. *Psychoneuroendocrinology* 1986;11:337–345.
20. Honjo H, Ogino Y, Naitoh K, et al. In vivo effects by estrone sulfate on the central nervous system—senile dementia (Alzheimer's type). *J Steroid Biochem* 1989;34:521–525.
21. Schneider LS, Farlow MR, Henderson VW, Pogoda JM. Effects of estrogen replacement therapy on response to Tacrine in patients with Alzheimer's disease. *Neurology* 1996;46:1580–1584.
22. Miranda RC, Sohrabji F, Toran-Allerand CD. Presumptive estrogen target neurons express mRNAs for both the neurotrophins and neurotrophin receptors: a basis for potential developmental interactions of estrogen with the neurotrohpins. *Mol Cell Neurosci* 1993;4:510–525.
23. Toran-Allerand CD, Miranda RC, Bentham WD, et al. Estrogen receptors colocalize with low affinity nerve growth factor receptors in cholinergic neurons of the basal forebrain. *Proc Natl Acad Sci USA* 1992;89:4668–4672.
24. Jaffee AB, Toran-Allerand CD, Greengard P, Gandy SE. Estrogen regulates metabolism of Alzheimer amyloid beta precursor protein. *J Biol Chem* 1994;269:13065–13068.
25. Singh M, Meyer EM, Simpkins JW. The effect of ovariectomy and estradiol replacement on brain-derived neurotrophic factor messenger ribonucleic acid expression in cortical and hippocampal brain regions of female Sprague-Dawley rats. *Endocrinology* 1995;136:2320–2324.
26. Singh M, Meyer EM, Huang FS, Millard WJ, Simplkins JW. Ovariectomy reduces ChAT activity and NGF mRNA levels in the frontal cortex and hippocampus of the female Sprague Dawley rat. *Abstr Soc Neurosci* 1993;19:1254.
27. Simpkins JW, Singh M, Bishop J. The potential role for estrogen replacement therapy in the treatment of the cognitive decline and neurodegeneration associated with Alzheimer's disease. *Neurobiol Aging* 1994;15[Suppl 2]:S195–S197.
28. Xu H, Sweeney D, Wang R, et al. Generation of Alzheimer beta-amyloid protein in the trans-Golgi network in the apparent absence of vesicle formation. *Proc Natl Aca Sci USA* 1997;94:3748–3752.
29. Goodman Y, Bruce AJ, Cheng B, Mattson MP. Estrogens attenuate and corticosterone exacerbates excitotoxicity, oxidative injury and amyloid beta-peptide toxicity of hippocampal neurons. *J Neurochem* 1996;66:1836–1844.
30. Broe GA, Henderson AS, Creasey H, et al. A case-control study of Alzheimer's disease in Australia. *Neurology* 1990;40:1698–1707.
31. Brenner DE, Kukull WA, Stergachis A, et al. Postmenopausal estrogen replacement therapy and the risk of Alzheimer's disease: a population-based case-control study. *Am J Epidemiol* 1994;140:262–267.
32. Mortel KF, Meyer JS. Lack of postmenopausal estrogen replacement therapy and the risk of dementia. *J Neuropsychiatry Clin Neurosci* 1995;7:334–337.

Treatment of the Postmenopausal Woman: Basic and Clinical Aspects, Second Edition, edited by Rogerio A. Lobo, Lippincott Williams & Wilkins, Philadelphia © 1999.

CHAPTER 24

The Role of Sex Steroids in Alzheimer's Disease: Prevention and Treatment

Victor W. Henderson

Dementia is among the most feared accompaniments of aging. Representing a loss of mental abilities that substantially interferes with the ability to conduct one's daily affairs, dementia can be caused by a number of different specific diagnoses. Of these, Alzheimer's disease (AD) is by far the most common (1,2). In AD, cognitive loss begins insidiously and progresses gradually over a period of about a decade. The inability to learn and recall new information is an early and consistent feature. Most patients also show difficulties with language, visuospatial skills, judgment, and abstract reasoning. Behavioral symptoms such as depression, apathy, agitation, or delusions are at times prominent.

Key histopathologic features of AD include neurofibrillary tangles within vulnerable neurons and neuritic plaques (3). Plaques, which accumulate in the neuropil between neuronal cell bodies, often contain a central core of β-amyloid, a polypeptide proteolytically derived from the larger amyloid precursor protein. Within the plaque, the presence of microglia and reactive astrocytes, together with cytokines, complement proteins, and acute phase reactants suggests an inflammatory process (4).

The pathogenesis of AD is unknown, although it is apparent that different genetic and nongenetic factors—only some of which have been identified—can in isolation or combination culminate in the characteristic symptoms and neuropathology of AD. Point mutations in genes on chromosomes 14, 1, and 21 are expressed as autosomal dominant traits and lead to dementia symptoms before about 60 years of age (5). These mutations do not play an important role in later-onset illness, in which it is likely that a number of "susceptibility" genes influence

risk. The best described of these is the chromosome 19 gene that encodes apolipoprotein E. This lipid transport protein exists in three common variants, or polymorphisms, with an increased susceptibility to AD conferred by possession of one or two copies of the ε4 allele (6). Gender appears to modify risk, with the ε4 allele acting to increase risk particularly for women carriers (7,8).

Alzheimer's disease is more common with advancing age (9), but other exogenous factors may also modify risk, as reviewed by Graves and Kukull (10). Risk may be elevated by low educational attainment, female gender, prior head injury, or prior episodes of depression. Although controversial, there is also evidence that risk is decreased by antiinflammatory medications, nicotine, and estrogen.

Of these putative protective factors, estrogen exposure is the best studied. Although other steroid hormones may be relevant to AD, few data directly consider this possibility. A separate but related issue concerns AD treatment, and some studies indicate that estrogen may ameliorate symptoms of this disorder. The following sections describe the potential estrogen effects on brain and behavior before addressing specific issues of AD prevention and treatment.

RELEVANCE OF ESTROGEN TO COGNITION AND MOOD

Menopause, with the loss of ovarian estrogen production (11), occurs on average at age 51. In the absence of hormone replacement, a women spends about 40% of her adult life in a state of relative estrogen deprivation. Consequences of estrogen deprivation on the brain, an important target organ for estrogen and other sex steroids, remains an area of intense study and some controversy.

Men and women perform similarly on most cognitive tasks, but on average, men tend to score better on visuo-

V. W. Henderson: Departments of Neurology, Gerontology, and Psychology, University of Southern California, Los Angeles, California 90033.

spatial and mathematical reasoning tasks, and women tend to score better on verbal tasks (12). Estrogen modulates neural activity that occurs during cognitive processing (13). Moreover, in performing a given cognitive task, there may be gender-associated differences in patterns of neuronal activation, suggesting a difference in functional organization within the brain (14). Such differences may in part be mediated by long-term and short-term effects of exposures to sex steroids.

Partial support for an estrogen role in human behavior comes from analyses in large cohorts of older women. Cross-sectional analyses in a population-based cohort in Austria indicate that estrogen users outperform nonusers in a number of cognitive domains (15), and in an American cohort, estrogen appeared to protect against longitudinal decline, as measured by a task involving visual memory and visuoconstruction (16). Two other American studies found no compelling evidence that estrogen replacement preserved cognitive function, although some estrogen users in these cohorts scored better on tasks assessing verbal fluency (17,18).

Putative estrogen effects on cognition are also implied by performance fluctuations during a woman's menstrual cycle (19–22), by neuropsychologic dysfunction after the suppression of endogenous estrogen production (23), by enhanced test scores in women receiving estrogen replacement after the menopause (24–26), and by changes in test performance in transsexual men and women given cross-gender hormone therapy (27). A common interpretation of these studies is that estrogen maintains skills at which women tend to excel (e.g., certain verbal abilities), although not all analytic results are consistent with this simple formulation.

Estrogen can affect mood in healthy women. Among older postmenopausal women, estrogen users typically endorse fewer depressive symptoms than nonusers (28). Estrogen replacement given during the perimenopausal or postmenopausal period can diminish anxiety and can enhance mood and subjective well-being (29–32). Although mood can impact test performance when cognitive abilities are being measured, estrogen effects on cognition appear to be independent of effects mood (26,33).

RELEVANCE OF ESTROGEN TO BRAIN FUNCTION AND ALZHEIMER'S DISEASE

A number of estrogen actions are potentially relevant to AD (Table 24.1) (34). Within the brain, estrogen interacts with specific intranuclear receptors to regulate protein synthesis and with pharmacologically characterized membrane receptors where genomic interactions are not implicated (35–37). Estrogen modulates growth proteins (38,39), enhances the outgrowth of nerve processes (40,41), and promotes the formation of synaptic connections (42,43). Estrogen may protect against neuronal

TABLE 24.1. *Estrogen actions that may be relevant to Alzheimer's disease*

Effects on neuronal growth, differentiation, and survival
Effects on glial cells
Effects on neurotransmitter systems: acetylcholine, noradrenalin, serotonin, dopamine, glutamate, γ-aminobutyric acid, and others
Decreased formation of β-amyloid
Increased expression of apolipoprotein E in the brain
Antioxidant effects
Antiinflammatory effects
Blunted stress response
Increased cerebral blood flow
Increased cerebral metabolism

Adapted from ref. 34.

death due to oxidative stress, excitatory neurotoxicity, or other insults (44–47). Estrogen also promotes glia cell plasticity (48).

Estrogen influences several neurotransmitter systems of the brain. A coherent body of experimental and clinical evidence indicates the importance of acetylcholine in memory and attention (49), and a popular approach to AD therapy targets this neurotransmitter. In the United States, medications currently approved for AD treatment inhibit the enzyme acetylcholinesterase, leading to elevated brain levels of acetylcholine. Neurofibrillary tangle formation prominently involves cholinergic neurons of the basal forebrain area (50), and these neurons, which possess receptors for estrogen (51), project widely to the hippocampus and neocortex. Experimentally, estrogen treatment can elevate cholinergic markers in the basal forebrain and in projection target areas (52,53). Cholinergic neurons within the basal forebrain also have receptors for neurotrophins, proteins that promote growth and help maintain cell viability, and estrogen may modulate neurotrophin effects in this region (38,51,54).

Estrogen interacts with monoaminergic neurotransmitters, which are thought to be important in mood regulation. Neurons in the locus ceruleus (origin of noradrenergic fibers) and the raphe region of the brain stem (origin of serotonergic fibers) are affected by AD. Estrogen influences both of these transmitters (55–58).

Estrogens may reduce the formation of β-amyloid, a key biochemical abnormality of AD. Estradiol promotes the degradation of the amyloid precursor protein to polypeptide fragments less likely to accumulate as β-amyloid (59). There may also be an important link between estrogens and apolipoprotein E. Apolipoprotein E levels are reduced in AD in the cerebrospinal fluid (60) and brain (61). Estrogen increases the expression of central nervous system apolipoprotein E (62), which could facilitate neuronal repair (63).

Other estrogen actions on inflammation, free radicals, and the stress hormone cortisol may also favorably influence the course of AD. Antiinflammatory medications are postulated to reduce Alzheimer's risk (64) and to improve dementia symptoms (65). Estrogen may moderate some aspects of the inflammatory process (66,67).

There is prominent indication of oxidative damage in AD brain (68), and the antioxidant α-tocopherol (vitamin E) may slow decline in AD patients (69). Neuronal damage attributed to β-amyloid may be mediated or potentiated by free radicals (70,71). Antioxidant properties of estrogens (72,73) may therefore have some role in AD.

Basal cortisol levels are reported to be increased in AD (74). Corticosteroid secretion that occurs in response to behavioral stress can deleteriously affect neurons in the hippocampus (75), and estrogen therapy may mitigate the stress response in older women (76).

ESTROGEN THERAPY AND THE PREVENTION OF ALZHEIMER'S DISEASE

Epidemiologic studies of estrogen and AD have been reviewed (77). Early case-control studies considered estrogen as one of many possible factors influencing the risk of AD (78–81). No significant effect of estrogen exposure was found, although the number of estrogen users in these studies was small, and the statistical power to detect a significant effect was low. In 1994, as part of a longitudinal study of aging and dementia, Henderson et al. (82) in Los Angeles studied 143 women with AD and 92 healthy women without dementia (mean age of both groups = 76 years). Eighteen percent of controls but only 7% of patients used oral estrogens. The two groups were comparable in terms of the total number of prescription medications, the most commonly prescribed medication, and surgical procedures likely to influence the prescription of estrogen. Differences in estrogen usage were significant (estimate of relative risk, or odds ratio [OR] = 0.33, 95% confidence interval [CI] = 0.15 to 0.74.) Similar results were subsequently described by Birge in St. Louis (83), Mortel and Meyer in Houston (84), Baldereschi et al. in Italy (85), and Lerner et al. (86) in Cleveland. In these case-control studies, estimates of relative risk for AD among current estrogen users or among women who had ever received estrogen ranged from 0.07 to 0.58.

In some of these studies, the temporal sequence between estrogen exposure and the onset of AD was unclear (82–84), and analyses based on current estrogen use may lead to biased estimates of the extent of estrogen exposure before the onset of dementia symptoms. Moreover, recall bias could occur when information on estrogen exposure is obtained differently for an Alzheimer's patient (e.g., from a proxy informant) than for a control subject (e.g., from the woman herself) (82–84,86).

Van Duijn et al. (87) identified 124 Alzheimer's cases in a European population-based study of early-onset disease. Based on an informant interview for cases and matched controls, a history of estrogen usage was found less often among cases (OR = 0.40, 95% CI = 0.19 to 0.91). Other analyses have used information on post-menopausal estrogen use collected prospectively, before the onset of dementia symptoms (88–93). The largest such study is from the Leisure World retirement community, an upper-middle-class cohort in southern California that was established by postal survey in the early 1980s (88,90). Detailed information on hormone use in this defined cohort was collected at the time of enrollment from each woman. Death certificates were subsequently obtained for deceased participants. From records of female cohort members who died before 1996, Paganini-Hill and Henderson (90) identified AD and other diagnoses likely to represent AD (i.e., senile dementia, dementia, or senility). Two hundred and forty-eight female cases were matched by year of birth and death to 1198 controls without mention of these disorders. In this nested case-control study, estrogen users had a one-third lower risk of an AD or related diagnosis (OR = 0.65, 95% CI = 0.49 to 0.88). Similar risk estimates were obtained in *post hoc* analyses that were based solely on AD diagnoses and excluded other dementia diagnoses (88). When considered individually, different routes of estrogen administration (i.e., oral, oral plus injection or cream, injection or cream) were each associated with significantly lower risks of AD (90). In Leisure World, cases were identified from death certificate records, and some cases were almost certainly missed. Misclassification in this cohort, however, was most likely nondifferential with respect to estrogen exposure, and the resulting risk estimate was therefore likely to be a conservative estimate of the true association between estrogen and the risk of AD.

Findings similar to those observed in Leisure World are reported from New York, Baltimore, and Rochester, Minnesota. In a community-based cohort in the northern Manhattan section of New York City, Tang et al. (91) identified 167 incident cases of AD. The risk of AD was reduced by one-half among women who had ever used oral estrogen (OR = 0.5, 95% CI = 0.25 to 0.9). For women who developed AD, the age at onset was significantly higher among women who used estrogen.

Kawas et al. (92) identified 34 incident cases of AD from among 472 older women in the Baltimore Longitudinal Study of Aging. The risk of this illness was reduced by more than one-half when women who had used oral or transdermal estrogen were compared with never-users (OR = 0.46, 95% CI = 0.209 to 0.997). Waring et al. (93) analyzed medical records of 222 women in Rochester who developed AD during a 5-year interval. Nondemented matched controls were significantly more likely to have used estrogen for at least 6 months than AD cases (OR = 0.4, 95% CI = 0.2 to 0.8).

In contrast to these positive studies, no protective effect of estrogen was observed in a case-control analysis of subjects derived from a health maintenance organization cohort in Seattle, Washington. Brenner et al. (89)

compared estrogen exposures between 107 incident cases of AD and 120 controls. Using computerized pharmacy records, they found no association between AD and having received a prescription for estrogen (OR = 1.1, 95% CI = 0.6 to 1.8), although in *post hoc* analyses, the risk estimate was somewhat less when just oral estrogen use was considered (OR = 0.7, 95% CI = 0.4 to 1.5).

If estrogen does help to protect against AD, greater estrogen exposure would be expected to lead to larger risk reductions. In Leisure World, risk estimates for AD did decrease significantly with increasing dose of the longest used oral estrogen preparation (90). Similarly, significant associations between the duration of estrogen use and the degree of risk reduction were observed in the Leisure World (90) and New York City (91) cohorts, but no significant trend was discerned in the Baltimore study (Fig. 24.1) (92). A significant relation between the extent of estrogen exposure and the degree of risk reduction was also reported from Rochester (93), and in Seattle, women who filled the largest number of estrogen prescriptions experienced the lowest AD risk (89).

Several factors are postulated to modify the putative protective effect of estrogen. In a study of early-onset AD, estrogen replacement appeared to protect only women who carried the apolipoprotein E ε4 allele (87), but Tang et al. (91), found that estrogen protected women with and without the ε4 allele. One study found estrogen effects to be more evident among women who smoked cigarettes (86).

ESTROGEN THERAPY IN WOMEN WITH ALZHEIMER'S DISEASE

Observational analyses of Henderson et al. (94) imply that women with AD who receive hormone therapy per-

form better on cognitive tasks than other women with this diagnosis (Fig. 24.2). Differences favoring estrogen users were greatest on a semantic memory, or naming, task (94), suggesting that estrogen could differentially affect discrete cognitive domains in AD. Naming abilities in AD are more impaired in women than men (95,96), even though healthy women ordinarily perform as well as or better than men on this type of task. Body weight after the menopause is associated with higher estrogen levels (97), and in an analysis that adjusted for age, education, symptom duration, and height, greater body weight in women with AD was significantly linked to better cognitive test scores (98).

Several clinical trials have examined the effects of oral or transdermal estrogen on symptoms of women with AD, and most results suggest a beneficial effect of estrogen therapy (99–108). Oral estrogen doses employed in most clinical trials have been in the range of those used in clinical practice (e.g., 0.625 to 1.25 mg/day of conjugated estrogens [100–104,107]). In general, women with more severe dementia symptoms may be less likely to improve than mildly demented women (99,102).

Interventional trials reported have been small, with no more than 30 subjects (99–107). Four studies were conducted as randomized, placebo-controlled trials (101, 105–107), although only one of these has yet been published as a peer-reviewed article (101). In the only full report, a 3-week study conducted in Japan, Honjo et al. (101) randomized 14 women with AD (mean age, 84 years) to receive 1.25 mg/day of oral conjugated estrogens or an oral placebo. Outcome was assessed with three psychometric tests, the Mini-Mental State examination, the revised Hasegawa Dementia Scale, and the New

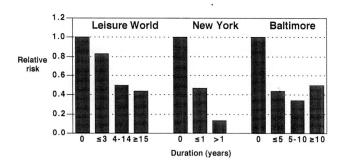

FIG. 24.2. Psychometric performance in Alzheimer's patient by estrogen status. In this observational analysis, current estrogen users (n = 9) and nonusers (n = 27) were matched by age, education, and duration of dementia symptoms. Test scores were significantly different between groups at the $p < 0.05$ level for semantic memory (naming), verbal fluency, language comprehension, picture drawing, and forward digit span tasks but not for the word list recall or forward visual span tasks. The effect size was largest for the semantic memory task, for which $p = 0.003$. (Data from ref. 94, with permission.)

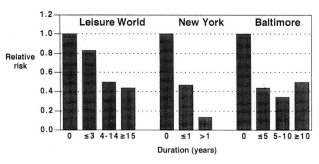

FIG. 24.1. Duration of estrogen use and estimates of relative risk for Alzheimer's disease. Women who never used estrogen constitute the reference group, for whom the relative risk is 1.0. Significant trends for increasing duration of estrogen use to be associated with lower Alzheimer's risk were found in the Leisure World ($p < 0.001$) and New York City ($p = 0.003$) cohorts but not in the Baltimore cohort. (Leisure World data from ref. 90, New York data from ref. 91, and Baltimore data from ref. 92, with permission.)

Screening Test for Dementia. On each task, mean scores of women in the active treatment arm improved significantly over baseline scores; mean scores did not change significantly in the placebo group. *Post hoc* analyses of individual test items suggested that estrogen users showed specific improvements in memory.

Partial or preliminary results are reported for three other randomized estrogen trials (105–107). In a placebo-controlled, cross-over study, Fillet (105) treated eight women with low-dose transdermal estradiol (0.05 mg, twice each week) or placebo for 21 days per month; cognitive scores did not differ between estrogen and placebo phases of the trial, each of which lasted 3 months. Asthana et al. (106) also used transdermal estradiol (0.05 mg), but on a daily basis. In this 8-week parallel group trial, five women with AD received the estrogen patch, and five received a placebo patch. Significant differences favoring the estrogen group were found on two verbal memory measures (106), and a separate preliminary report from the same study also suggested improvements on an attentional measure (109). Birge (107) announced results of an interim analysis of a 9 month trial using oral conjugated estrogens, 0.625 mg/day. Five of 10 estrogen-treated women improved on the clinician's impression of overall change, but none of the 10 women in the parallel placebo group improved on this measure.

There are many reasons why estrogen may have a favorable impact on AD symptoms, but interactions with the cholinergic system of the brain are especially intriguing. Retrospective analyses of data from a multicenter trial of a cholinesterase inhibitor found that women using oral estrogen at the time of study enrollment and subsequently randomized to the active treatment arm performed significantly better on the primary cognitive outcome measure than women randomized to placebo; AD patients in the anticholinesterase arm who were not taking estrogens performed comparably to those in the placebo group (110). The number of estrogen users in this trial was small, and estrogen use was not itself randomized, but these observations are consistent with the hypothesis that estrogen effects in AD are mediated in part through cholinergic mechanisms.

OTHER SEX STEROIDS AND ALZHEIMER'S DISEASE

A woman with a uterus cannot be treated indefinitely with unopposed estrogen. Depending on the experimental model, progesterone can enhance, modify, or oppose estrogen actions in the brain. Limited clinical data raise the possibility that the addition of a progestogen adversely influences putative benefits of estrogen in AD (110,111). Nevertheless, positive results are reported in longer estrogen trials of AD patients to whom progestogens have also been administered (104,107).

Women, like men, have androgen receptors in the brain. Like estrogens, androgens can modify nervous system structures (35), human cognition (112,113), and mood (114). In contrast to levels of estrogen, testosterone levels do not decline after menopause in women with intact ovaries, but oophorectomy removes a major source of androgen production. However, no published study has yet examined effects of testosterone therapy on AD symptoms in either sex.

Dehydroepiandrosterone and dehydroepiandrosterone sulfate are of potential interest in AD. Although produced primarily by the adrenal glands and therefore not classified as sex steroids, one of the principal metabolites is testosterone. Levels of these adrenal steroids decline with aging (97). Dehydroepiandrosterone sulfate can enhance memory performance in aging rodents (115), and reduced serum levels of were associated with functional limitations in a large cohort of older women (116). In a randomized cross-over trial of dehydroepiandrosterone (50 mg/day), active treatment of healthy women increased serum androgens and enhanced feelings of psychologic well-being (117). However, levels of dehydroepiandrosterone sulfate are probably not reduced in AD patients (118,119) [but see Yanase et al. (120)], and low levels do not predict incipient dementia (116). There are no convincing studies—positive or negative—on dehydroepiandrosterone or its sulfate for the prevention or treatment of AD.

CONCLUSIONS

Most clinicians acknowledge that potential benefits of postmenopausal estrogen replacement compare favorably with potential risks (121), even in if postulated effects in AD are discounted. A strong biologic rationale supports the hypothesis that postmenopausal estrogen usage reduces a woman's risk of developing AD and palliates symptoms of women who have developed this illness. However, relevant clinical data are not compelling. Analytic studies since 1994 imply that the risk of AD among women who received estrogen replacement may be reduced by about one-half, an effect equivalent to postponing the onset of AD by 5 years (9). If confirmed, this reduction in risk would be of enormous public health importance. However, in the absence of randomized, controlled trials, there remains the possibility that undetected bias or residual confounding could account for the reported associations in these epidemiologic analyses.

Consistent findings in future cohort studies—especially those that are population based—would strengthen the argument for a causal link between estrogen therapy and reduced AD risk. Adequately powered randomized, placebo-controlled intervention trials could provide the strongest support for this contention. For example, the Memory Study, part of the Women's Health Initiative sponsored by the National Institutes of Health in the United States, involves the randomized use of oral conjugated estrogens (with or without a progestogen, depending on the presence or absence of a uterus). This long-term study of AD and dementia is underway, but results will not be available for years.

Results of clinical trials are still inconclusive with respect to the role of estrogen in ameliorating AD symptoms. Most trials report better scores for at least some estrogen-treated women on at least some test measures. Ancillary measures of regional cerebral blood flow and electroencephalographic activity in demented women given estrogen (103) support these clinical data. Given small sample sizes, the short treatment durations in most trials, and especially the lack of subject randomization or experimenter blinding in some trials, these encouraging results must be interpreted cautiously. Results of larger randomized, controlled trials, now underway, could clarify the issue before the next millennium.

REFERENCES

1. Schoenberg BS, Kokmen E, Okazaki H. Alzheimer's disease and other dementing illnesses in a defined United States population: incidence rates and clinical features. *Ann Neurol* 1987;22:724–729.
2. Evans DA, Funkenstein HH, Albert MS, et al. Prevalence of Alzheimer's disease in a community population of older persons: higher than previously reported. *JAMA* 1989;262:2551–2556.
3. Mirra SS, Heyman A, McKeel D, et al. Consortium to Establish a Registry for Alzheimer's Disease (CERAD). Part II: Standardization of the neuropathologic assessment of Alzheimer's disease. *Neurology* 1991;41:479–486.
4. McGeer PL, McGeer EG. The inflammatory response system of brain: implications for therapy of Alzheimer and other neurodegenerative diseases. *Brain Res Rev* 1995;21:195–218.
5. Pericak-Vance MA, Haines JL. Genetic susceptibility to Alzheimer disease. *Trends Genet* 1995;11:504–508.
6. Strittmatter WJ, Saunders AM, Schmechel D, et al. Apolipoprotein E: high-avidity binding to β-amyloid and increased frequency of type 4 allele in late-onset familial Alzheimer disease. *Proc Natl Acad Sci USA* 1993;90:1977–1981.
7. Poirier J, Davignon J, Bouthillier D, Kogan S, Bertrand P, Gauthier S. Apolipoprotein E polymorphism and Alzheimer's disease. *Lancet* 1993;342:697–699.
8. Payami H, Zareparsi S, Montee KR, et al. Gender difference in apolipoprotein E–associated risk for familial Alzheimer disease: a possible clue to the higher incidence of Alzheimer disease in women. *Am J Hum Genet* 1996;58:803–811.
9. Jorm AF, Korten AE, Henderson AS. The prevalence of dementia: a quantitative integration of the literature. *Acta Psychiatr Scand* 1987;76:465–479.
10. Graves AB, Kukull WA. The epidemiology of dementia. In: Morris JC, ed. *Handbook of dementing illnesses*. New York: Marcel Dekker, 1994:23–69.
11. Jaffe RB. The menopause and perimenopausal period. In: Yen SSC, Jaffe RB, eds. *Reproductive endocrinology*, 3rd ed. Philadelphia: WB Saunders, 1991: 389–408.
12. Halpern DF. *Sex differences in cognitive abilities*. Hillsdale, NJ: Lawrence Erlbaum, 1992.
13. Berman KF, Schmidt PJ, Rubinow DR, et al. Modulation of cognition-specific cortical activity by gonadal steroids: a positron-emission tomography study in women. *Proc Natl Acad Sci USA* 1997;94:8836–8841.
14. Shaywitz BA, Shaywitz SE, Pugh KR, et al. Sex differences in the functional organization of the brain for language. *Nature* 1995;373:607–609.
15. Schmidt R, Fazekas F, Reinhart B, et al. Estrogen replacement therapy in older women: a neuropsychological and brain MRI study. *J Am Geriatr Soc* 1996;44: 1307–1313.
16. Resnick SM, Metter EJ, Zonderman AB. Estrogen replacement therapy and longitudinal decline in visual memory: a possible protective effect? *Neurology* 1997;49: 1491–1497.
17. Barrett-Connor E, Kritz-Silverstein D. Estrogen replacement therapy and cognitive function in older women. *JAMA* 1993;269:2637–2641.
18. Szklo M, Cerhan J, Diez-Roux AV, et al. Estrogen replacement therapy and cognitive functioning in the Atherosclerosis Risk in Communities (ARIC) study. *Am J Epidemiol* 1996;144:1048–1057.
19. Hampson E. Variations in sex-related cognitive abilities across the menstrual cycle. *Brain Cogn* 1990;14:26–43.
20. Phillips SM, Sherwin BB. Variations in memory function and sex steroid hor-

mones across the menstrual cycle. *Psychoneuroendocrinology* 1992;17: 497–506.
21. Krug R, Stamm U, Pietrowsky R, Fehm HL, Born J. Effects of menstrual cycle on creativity. *Psychoneuroendocrinology* 1994;19:21–31.
22. Bibawi D, Cherry B, Hellige JB. Fluctuations of perceptual asymmetry across time in women and men: effects related to the menstrual cycle. *Neuropsychologia* 1995;33:131–138.
23. Varney NR, Syrop C, Kubu CS, Struchen M, Hahn S, Franzen K. Neuropsychologic dysfunction in women following leuprolide acetate induction of hypoestrogenism. *J Assist Reprod Genet* 1993;10:53–57.
24. Kampen DL, Sherwin BB. Estrogen use and verbal memory in healthy postmenopausal women. *Obstet Gynecol* 1994;83:979–983.
25. Robinson D, Friedman L, Marcus R, Tinklenberg J, Yesavage J. Estrogen replacement therapy and memory in older women. *J Am Geriatr Soc* 1994;42:919–922.
26. Phillips SM, Sherwin BB. Effects of estrogen on memory function in surgically menopausal women. *Psychoneuroendocrinology* 1992;17:485–495.
27. Van Goozen SHM, Cohen-Kettenis PT, Gooren LJG, Frijda NH, Van de Poll NE. Gender differences in behaviour: activating effects of cross-sex hormones. *Psychoneuroendocrinology* 1995;20:343–363.
28. Palinkas LA, Barrett-Connor E. Estrogen use and depressive symptoms in postmenopausal women. *Obstet Gynecol* 1992;80:30–36.
29. Fedor-Freybergh P. The influence of oestrogens on the well-being and mental performance in climacteric and postmenopausal women. *Acta Obstet Gynecol Scand* 1977;64[Suppl]:1–91.
30. Montgomery JC, Appleby L, Brincat M, et al. Effect of oestrogen and testosterone implants on psychological disorders in the climacteric. *Lancet* 1987;1:297–299.
31. Sherwin BB. Affective changes with estrogen and androgen replacement therapy in surgically menopausal women. *J Affect Disord* 1988;14:177–187.
32. Ditkoff EC, Crary WG, Cristo M, Lobo RA. Estrogen improves psychological function in asymptomatic postmenopausal women. *Obstet Gynecol* 1991;78: 991–995.
33. Kimura D. Estrogen replacement therapy may protect against intellectual decline in postmenopausal women. *Horm Behav* 1995;29:312–321.
34. Henderson VW. Estrogen, cognition, and a woman's risk of Alzheimer's disease. *Am J Med* 1997;103[Suppl 3A]:11–18.
35. Kawata M. Roles of steroid hormones and their receptors in structural organization in the nervous system. *Neurosci Res* 1995;24:1–46.
36. Wong M, Thompson TL, Moss RL. Nongenomic actions of estrogen in the brain: physiological significance and cellular mechanisms. *Crit Rev Neurobiol* 1996;10: 189–203.
37. Kuiper GGJM, Enmark E, Pelto-Huikko M, Nilsson S, Gustafsson J-A. Cloning of a novel estrogen receptor expressed in rat prostate and ovary. *Proc Natl Acad Sci USA* 1996;93:5925–5930.
38. Miranda RC, Sohrabji F, Toran-Allerand CD. Presumptive estrogen target neurons express mRNAs for both the neurotrophins and neurotrophin receptors: a basis for potential developmental interactions of estrogen with neurotrophins. *Mol Cell Neurosci* 1993;4:510–525.
39. Shughrue PJ, Dorsa DM. Estrogen modulates the growth-associated protein GAP-43 (neuromodulin) mRNA in the rat preoptic area and basal hypothalamus. *Neuroendocrinology* 1993;57:439–447.
40. Toran-Allerand CD. Organotypic culture of the developing cerebral cortex and hypothalamus: relevance to sexual differentiation. *Psychoneuroendocrinology* 1991;16:7–24.
41. Brinton RD, Tran J, Proffitt P, Montoya M. 17β-Estradiol enhances the outgrowth and survival of neocortical neurons in culture. *Neurochem Res* 1997;22: 1339–1351.
42. Chung SK, Pfaff DW, Cohen RS. Estrogen-induced alterations in synaptic morphology in the midbrain central gray. *Exp Brain Res* 1988;69:522–530.
43. Woolley CS, McEwen BS. Estradiol mediates fluctuation in hippocampal synapse density during the estrous cycle in the adult rat. *J Neurosci* 1992;12:2549–2554.
44. Goodman Y, Bruce AJ, Cheng B, Mattson MP. Estrogens attenuate and corticosterone exacerbates excitotoxicty, oxidative injury, and amyloid β-peptide toxicity in hippocampal neurons. *J Neurochem* 1996;66:1836–1844.
45. Singer CA, Rogers KL, Strickland TM, Dorsa DM. Estrogen protects primary cortical neurons from glutamate toxicity. *Neurosci Lett* 1996;212:13–16.
46. Behl C, Skutella T, Lezoualc'h F, et al. Neuroprotection against oxidative stress by estrogens: structure-activity relationship. *Mol Pharmacol* 1997;51:535–541.
47. Regan RF, Guo Y. Estrogens attenuate neuronal injury due to hemoglobin, chemical hypoxia, and excitatory amino acids in murine cortical cultures. *Brain Res* 1997;764:133–140.
48. Garcia-Segura LM, Chowen JA, Dueñas M, Parducz A, Naftolin F. Gonadal steroids and astroglial plasticity. *Cell Mol Neurobiol* 1997;16:225–237.
49. Bartus RT, Dean RL, Beer B, Lippa AD. The cholinergic hypothesis of geriatric memory dysfunction. *Science* 1981;217:208–217.
50. Coyle JT, Price DL, DeLong MR. Alzheimer's disease: a disorder of cortical cholinergic innervation. *Science* 1983;219:1184–1190.
51. Toran-Allerand CD, Miranda RC, Bentham WDL, et al. Estrogen receptors colocalize with low-affinity nerve growth factor receptors in cholinergic neurons of the basal forebrain. *Proc Natl Acad Sci USA* 1992;89:4668–4672.
52. Luine V. Estradiol increases choline acetyltransferase activity in specific basal forebrain nuclei and projection areas of female rats. *Exp Neurol* 1985;89: 484–490.
53. Gibbs RB, Pfaff DW. Effects of estrogen and fimbria/fornix transection on

p75[NGFR] and ChAT expression in the medial septum and diagonal band of Broca. *Exp Neurol* 1992;116:23–39.

54. Salehi A, Verhaagen J, Dijkhuizen PA, Swaab DF. Co-localization of high-affinity neurotrophin receptors in nucleus basalis of Meynert neurons and their differential reduction in Alzheimer's disease. *Neuroscience* 1996;75:373–387.

55. Greengrass PM, Tonge SR. The accumulation of noradrenaline and 5-hydroxytryptamine in three regions of mouse brain after tetrabenazine and iproniazid: effects of ethinyloestradiol and progesterone. *Psychopharmacologia* 1974;39:187–191.

56. Sar M, Stumpf WE. Central noradrenergic neurones concentrate ³H-oestradiol. *Nature* 1981;289:500–502.

57. Biegon A, Reches A, Snyder L, McEwen BS. Serotonergic and noradrenergic receptors in the rat brain: modulation by chronic exposure to ovarian hormones. *Life Sci* 1983;32:2015–2021.

58. Sumner BEH, Fink G. Estrogen increases the density of 5-hydroxytryptamine$_{2A}$ receptors in cerebral cortex and nucleus accumbens in the female rat. *J Steroid Biochem Mol Biol* 1995;54:15–20.

59. Jaffe AB, Toran-Allerand CD, Greengard P, Gandy SE. Estrogen regulates metabolism of Alzheimer amyloid β precursor protein. *J Biol Chem* 1994;269:13065–13068.

60. Blennow K, Hesse C, Fredman P. Cerebrospinal fluid apolipoprotein E is reduced in Alzheimer's disease. *Neuroreport* 1994;5:2534–2536.

61. Bertrand P, Poirier J, Oda T, Finch CE, Pasinetti GM. Association of apolipoprotein E genotype with brain levels of apolipoprotein E and apolipoprotein J (clusterin) in Alzheimer disease. *Mol Brain Res* 1995;33:174–178.

62. Stone DJ, Rozovsky I, Morgan TE, Anderson CP, Hajian H, Finch CE. Astrocytes and microglia respond to estrogen with increased apoE mRNA *in vivo* and *in vitro*. *Exp Neurol* 1997;143:313–318.

63. Poirier J. Apolipoprotein E in animal models of CNS injury and in Alzheimer's disease. *Trends Neurosci* 1994;17:525–530.

64. Rich JB, Rasmusson DX, Folstein MF, Carson KA, Kawas C, Brandt J. Nonsteroidal anti-inflammatory drugs in Alzheimer's disease. *Neurology* 1995;45:51–55.

65. Rogers J, Kirby LC, Hempelman SR, et al. Clinical trial of indomethacin in Alzheimer's disease. *Neurology* 1993;43:1609–1611.

66. Pacifici R, Brown C, Puscheck E, et al. Effect of surgical menopause and estrogen replacement on cytokine release from human blood mononuclear cells. *Proc Natl Acad Sci USA* 1991;88:5134–5138.

67. Josefsson E, Tarkowski A, Carlsten H. Anti-inflammatory properties of estrogen. *Cell Immunol* 1992;142:67–78.

68. Smith MA, Harris PLR, Sayre LM, Beckman JS, Perry G. Widespread peroxynitrite-mediated damage in Alzheimer's disease. *J Neurosci* 1997;17:2653–2657.

69. Sano M, Ernesto C, Thomas RG, et al. A controlled trial of selegiline, alpha-tocopherol, or both as treatment for Alzheimer's disease. *N Engl J Med* 1997;336:1216–1222.

70. Sagara Y, Dargusch R, Klier FG, Schubert D, Behl C. Increased antioxidant enzyme activity in amyloid β protein-resistant cells. *J Neurosci* 1996;16:497–505.

71. McDonald DR, Brunden KR, Landreth GE. Amyloid fibrils activate tyrosine kinase-dependent signaling and superoxide production in microglia. *J Neurosci* 1997;17:2284–2294.

72. Mooradian AD. Antioxidant properties of steroids. *J Steroid Biochem Mol Biol* 1993;45:509–511.

73. Sack MN, Rader DJ, Cannon ROI. Oestrogen and inhibition of oxidation of low-density lipoproteins in postmenopausal women. *Lancet* 1994;343:269–270.

74. Davis KL, Davis BM, Greenwald BS, et al. Cortisol and Alzheimer's disease. *Am J Psychiatry* 1986;143:442–446.

75. McEwen BS, Sapolsky RM. Stress and cognitive function. *Curr Opin Neurobiol* 1995;5:205–216.

76. Lindheim SR, Legro RS, Bernstein L, et al. Behavioral stress responses in premenopausal and postmenopausal women and the effects of estrogen. *Am J Obstet Gynecol* 1992;167:1831–1836.

77. Henderson VW. The epidemiology of estrogen replacement therapy and Alzheimer's disease. *Neurology* 1997;48[Suppl 7]:27–35.

78. Heyman A, Wilkinson WE, Stafford JA, Helms JJ, Sigmon AH, Weinberg T. Alzheimer's disease: a study of epidemiological aspects. *Ann Neurol* 1984;15:335–341.

79. Amaducci LA, Fratiglioni L, Rocca WA, et al. Risk factors for clinically diagnosed Alzheimer's disease: a case-control study of an Italian population. *Neurology* 1986;36:922–931.

80. Broe GA, Henderson AS, Creasey H, et al. A case-control study of Alzheimer's disease in Australia. *Neurology* 1990;40:1698–1707.

81. Graves AB, White E, Koepsell TD, et al. A case-control study of Alzheimer's disease. *Ann Neurol* 1990;28:766–774.

82. Henderson VW, Paganini-Hill A, Emanuel CK, Dunn ME, Buckwalter JG. Estrogen replacement therapy in older women: comparisons between Alzheimer's disease cases and nondemented control subjects. *Arch Neurol* 1994;51:896–900.

83. Birge SJ. The role of estrogen deficiency in the aging central nervous system. In: Lobo RA, ed. *Treatment of the postmenopausal woman: basic and clinical aspects*. New York: Raven Press, 1994:153–157.

84. Mortel KF, Meyer JS. Lack of postmenopausal estrogen replacement therapy and the risk of dementia. *J Neuropsychiatry Clin Neurosci* 1995;7:334–337.

85. Baldereschi M, Di Carol A, Maggi S, et al. Estrogen replacement therapy and the risk of dementia in the Italian longitudinal study on aging. *Eur J Neurol* 1996;3 [Suppl 5]:85–86(abst).

86. Lerner A, Koss E, Debanne S, Rowland D, Smyth K, Friedland R. Smoking and oestrogen-replacement therapy as protective factors for Alzheimer's disease [Letter]. *Lancet* 1997;349:403–404.

87. van Duijn C, Meijer H, Witteman JCM, et al. Estrogen, apolipoprotein E and the risk of Alzheimer's disease. *Neurobiol Aging* 1996;16[Suppl]:S79–S80(abst).

88. Paganini-Hill A, Henderson VW. Estrogen deficiency and risk of Alzheimer's disease in women. *Am J Epidemiol* 1994;140:256–261.

89. Brenner DE, Kukull WA, Stergachis A, et al. Postmenopausal estrogen replacement therapy and the risk of Alzheimer's disease: a population-based case-control study. *Am J Epidemiol* 1994;140:262–267.

90. Paganini-Hill A, Henderson VW. Estrogen replacement therapy and risk of Alzheimer's disease. *Arch Intern Med* 1996;156:2213–2217.

91. Tang M-X, Jacobs D, Stern Y, et al. Effect of oestrogen during menopause on risk and age at onset of Alzheimer's disease. *Lancet* 1996;348:429–432.

92. Kawas C, Resnick S, Morrison A, et al. A prospective study of estrogen replacement therapy and the risk of developing Alzheimer's disease: the Baltimore Longitudinal Study of Aging. *Neurology* 1997;48:1517–1521.

93. Waring SC, Rocca WA, Petersen RC, Kokmen E. Postmenopausal estrogen replacement therapy and Alzheimer's disease: a population-based study in Rochester, Minnesota. *Neurology* 1997;48[Suppl 2]:A79(abst).

94. Henderson VW, Watt L, Buckwalter JG. Cognitive skills associated with estrogen replacement in women with Alzheimer's disease. *Psychoneuroendocrinology* 1996;21:421–430.

95. Henderson VW, Buckwalter JG. Cognitive deficits of men and women with Alzheimer's disease. *Neurology* 1994;44:90–96.

96. Ripich DN, Petrill SA, Whitehouse PJ, Ziol EW. Gender differences in language of AD patients: a longitudinal study. *Neurology* 1995;45:299–302.

97. Meldrum DR, Davidson BJ, Tataryn IV, Judd HL. Changes in circulating steroids with aging in postmenopausal women. *Obstet Gynecol* 1981;57:624–628.

98. Buckwalter JG, Schneider LS, Wilshire TW, Dunn ME, Henderson VW. Body weight, estrogen and cognitive functioning in Alzheimer's disease: an analysis of the tacrine study group. *Arch Gerontol Geriatr* 1997;24:261–267.

99. Fillit H, Weinreb H, Cholst I, et al. Observations in a preliminary open trial of estradiol therapy for senile dementia–Alzheimer's type. *Psychoneuroendocrinology* 1986;11:337–345.

100. Honjo H, Ogino Y, Naitoh K, et al. In vivo effects by estrone sulfate on the central nervous system—senile dementia (Alzheimer's type). *J Steroid Biochem* 1989;34:521–525.

101. Honjo H, Ogino Y, Tanaka K, et al. An effect of conjugated estrogen to cognitive impairment in women with senile dementia–Alzheimer's type: a placebo-controlled double blind study. *J Jpn Menopause Soc* 1993;1:167–171.

102. Ohkura T, Isse K, Akazawa K, Hamamoto M, Yaoi Y, Hagino N. An open trial of estrogen therapy for dementia of the Alzheimer type in women. In: Berg G, Hammar M, eds. *The modern management of the menopause: a perspective for the 21st century*. Carnforth, UK: Parthenon, 1994:315–333.

103. Ohkura T, Isse K, Akazawa K, Hamamoto M, Yaoi Y, Hagino N. Evaluation of estrogen treatment in female patients with dementia of the Alzheimer type. *Endocr J* 1994;41:361–371.

104. Ohkura T, Isse K, Akazawa K, Hamamoto M, Yaoi Y, Hagino N. Low-dose estrogen replacement therapy for Alzheimer disease in women. *Menopause* 1994;1:125–130.

105. Fillit H. Estrogens in the pathogenesis and treatment of Alzheimer's disease in postmenopausal women. *Ann N Y Acad Sci* 1994;743:233–238.

106. Asthana S, Craft S, Baker LD, et al. Transdermal estrogen improves memory in women with Alzheimer's disease. *Soc Neurosci Abstr* 1996;22:200(abst).

107. Birge SJ. The role of estrogen in the treatment of Alzheimer's disease. *Neurology* 1997;48 [Suppl 7]:S36–S41.

108. Henderson VW. Estrogen replacement therapy for the prevention and treatment of Alzheimer's disease. *CNS Drugs* 1997;8:343–351.

109. Baker LD, Craft S, Avery E, et al. Transdermal estrogen improves attention in postmenopausal women with Alzheimer's disease. *J Int Neuropsychol Soc* 1997;3:35–36(abst).

110. Schneider LS, Farlow MR, Henderson VW, Pogoda JM. Effects of estrogen replacement therapy on response to tacrine in patients with Alzheimer's disease. *Neurology* 1996;46:1580–1584.

111. Ohkura T, Isse K, Akazawa K, Hamamoto M, Yaoi Y, Hagino N. Long-term estrogen replacement therapy in female patients with dementia of the Alzheimer type: 7 case reports. *Dementia* 1995;6:99–107.

112. Sherwin BB. Estrogen and/or androgen replacement therapy and cognitive functioning in surgically menopausal women. *Psychoneuroendocrinology* 1988;13:345–357.

113. Janowsky JS, Oviatt SK, Orwoll ES. Testosterone influences spatial cognition in older men. *Behav Neurosci* 1994;108:325–332.

114. Sherwin BB, Gelfand MM. Sex steroids and affect in the surgical menopause: a double-blind cross-over study. *Psychoneuroendocrinology* 1985;10:325–335.

115. Flood JF, Roberts E. Dehydroepiandrosterone sulfate improves memory in aging mice. *Brain Res* 1988;448:178–181.

116. Berr C, Lafont S, Debuire B, Dartigues J-F, Baulieu E-E. Relationships of dehydroepiandrosterone sulfate in the elderly with functional, psychological, and

mental status, and short-term mortality: a French community-based study. *Proc Natl Acad Sci USA* 1996;93:13410–13415.

117. Morales AJ, Nolan JJ, Nelson JC, Yen SSC. Effects of replacement dose of dehydroepiandrosterone in men and women of advancing age. *J Clin Endocrinol Metab* 1994;78:1360–1367.

118. Schneider LS, Hinsey M, Lyness S. Plasma dehydroepiandrosterone sulfate in Alzheimer's disease. *Biol Psychiatry* 1992;31:205–208.

119. Birkenhager-Gillesse EG, Derksen J, Lagaay AM. Dehydroepiandrosterone sulphate (DHEAS) in the oldest old, aged 85 and over. *Ann N Y Acad Sci* 1994;719:543–552.

120. Yanase T, Fukahori M, Taniguchi S, et al. Serum dehydroepiandrosterone (DHEA) and DHEA-sulfate (DHEA-S) in Alzheimer's disease and in cerebrovascular dementia. *Endocr J* 1996;43:119–123.

121. Lobo RA. Benefits and risks of estrogen replacement therapy. *Am J Obstet Gynecol* 1995;173:982–990.

SECTION VI

Osteoporosis

It has been estimated that 4 to 6 million white postmenopausal women in the United States have osteoporosis. Hip fracture is the most devastating consequence of osteoporosis, which may result in 10%–20% excess mortality within 1 year. In 1995 direct medical expenditures for osteoporotic fractures was $13.8 billion. As the population ages, this figure is likely to increase.

This section addresses the epidemiology, detection, pathophysiology, and treatment of osteoporosis and each chapter is authored by a true expert in the field. Epidemiology is discussed by Charles Slemenda and Conrad Johnston. In the next chapter Cornelis van Kuijk and Harry Genant describe the imaging techniques for the detection of low bone mass and osteoporosis. Recently there has been a trend to measure biochemical indices of bone loss; this topic will be critically assessed by Richard Eastell and Rosemary Hannon. Typically more than one bone marker is necessary to measure, and there are several markers of bone resorption and bone formation. In the following chapter, Bob Lindsay and Felicia Cosman discuss the pathophysiology of bone loss and osteoporosis. As with most diseases, there are multiple mechanisms involved; several mechanisms can contribute to the accelerated loss of bone after menopause. Finally Claus Christiansen will discuss various treatment options. Many more products and doses are available today

Since the last edition, the National Osteoporosis Foundation has published a Physician's guide to the prevention and treatment of osteoporosis (1). Some of these statements will be summarized here.

1. Physician Recommendations

- Urge every postmenopausal women to consider her risk of osteoporosis.
- Ensure that skeletal health is addressed and recorded for at-risk women at each office visit.
- Evaluate for osteoporosis using bone mineral density (BMD) in all women with fractures.
- Recommend BMD to women <65 years who have osteoporosis or key risk factors.
- Recommend BMD to women >65 years.
- Recommend weight bearing and muscle strengthening exercises.
- Consider treatment for all postmenopausal women with vertebral or hip fractures.
- Initiate treatment to reduce fracture risk with BMD T-scores below 2 without risk factors and in women with T-scores below 1.5 if there are risk factors.
- Options for treatment include HRT, alendronate, raloxifene, and calcitonin.

2. Key Risk Factors for Determining Risk of Hip Fracture Independent of BMD

- *Nonmodifiable:* personal history of fracture; history of fracture in first degree relative.
- *Modifiable:* cigarette smoking; low body weight (<127 lbs. or 57 kg).

REFERENCE

1. National Osteoporosis Foundation, 1999; 1150 17th Street, NW, Suite 500, Washington, D.C. 20036.

Treatment of the Postmenopausal Woman: Basic and Clinical Aspects, Second Edition, edited by Rogerio A. Lobo, Lippincott Williams & Wilkins, Philadelphia © 1999.

CHAPTER 25

Epidemiology of Osteoporosis

Charles W. Slemenda and C. Conrad Johnston, Jr.

Each year in the United States, at least 250,000 hip fractures result from osteoporosis. Although this is the most devastating of the consequences of a weakened skeleton, hip fractures represent only a small fraction of the fractures attributable to osteoporosis. It has been shown that reduced bone mass is associated with increased fracture risk in the hip (1,2), the spine (3), and virtually all other skeletal sites (4–6). Reduced skeletal mass alone does not, however, totally account for the exponential rise in fracture rates among older women. Falls (7) and other factors (e.g., impaired protective reflexes) must also play a role.

GEOGRAPHIC AND RACIAL PATTERNS

Fracture rates are generally highest among women in the United States and Europe, particularly Scandinavia, and lowest in developing nations (8). In developed countries, the fracture rates for men are usually about one-half the rates for women, but in developing nations this ratio is closer to 1:1. Black women in the United States have hip fracture rates that are one-third of the rates of white women (9). It has been assumed that this difference is largely attributable to the difference in skeletal density between blacks and whites in the United States, which averages 10% to 15% in most studies (10). Black women in Africa have still lower hip fracture rates (as low as 5% to 10% of U.S. white rates), even allowing for the possibility of substantial underreporting (8). However, no study has yet demonstrated that Africans have substantially higher bone mass than Europeans or Americans. The few completed studies suggest similar (11) or slightly lower bone mass in African women (12) compared with American whites and much lower bone mass than American blacks. It seems likely that nonskeletal factors play an important role in international differences in fracture rates, although within populations bone mass is clearly the most critical, modifiable influence on fracture risk.

FRACTURE PATTERNS

Low bone mass is a risk factor for fractures at nearly all skeletal sites (4–6). Fractures of the hip, which have the most severe consequences in terms of health and health care costs, rise almost exponentially with age after midlife, at least through the ninth decade of life (13). Colles' fractures of the distal radius appear to peak in incidence between the ages of 60 and 70, at least for women, and then level off. This probably reflects nonskeletal factors, such as a declining frequency of the type of fall (forward) that usually produces these fractures (14). Less is known about vertebral fractures for several reasons: the uncertain proportion of cases that come to medical attention; the lack of widely accepted, uniformly applied standards for defining such fractures; and the inability to distinguish between prevalent and incident fractures without sequential radiographs because of the permanent changes in vertebral shape that result from fracture.

Despite these problems, it is believed that the peak in vertebral fracture incidence precedes that for hip fractures. Riggs and Melton proposed the terms *type I and II osteoporosis* to describe, respectively, the rapid, early menopausal loss of primarily trabecular bone (leading to vertebral crush fractures) and the steady, long-term loss of cortical and trabecular bone (leading to other fractures such as those of the hip).

PATTERNS OF GAIN AND LOSS OF BONE MASS

Skeletal mass increases steadily through childhood. At puberty, there is an acceleration of mineral accretion in the spine and to a lesser extent in the hip, but gain in the

C. W. Slemenda: Department of Medicine, Indiana University, Indianapolis, Indiana 46202-5200.

C. C. Johnston, Jr.: Division of Endocrinology and Metabolism, Department of Medicine, Indiana University School of Medicine, Indianapolis, Indiana 46202-5124.

radius (and perhaps in other long bones) appears to proceed at about the same rate as before puberty (15). In the late teens, there is a dramatic slowing of skeletal mineral accumulation (at about age 16 in girls and 18 in boys) (16). Although a matter of some dispute, data demonstrate the potential for further bone mineral accumulation, despite the lack of longitudinal growth, for women in their 20s (17). Near age 30, the accumulation of skeletal mineral ends, bone mass is at its peak, and a period of relative stability probably ensues. Peak bone mass is on average higher in men than women, with larger differences in the cortical skeleton and much smaller differences in trabecular bone (e.g., spine) (18). Bone loss may begin at different ages, depending on the skeletal site and an individual's lifestyle, but it affects men and women from middle age until at least age 80.

Bone loss in women is accelerated by estrogen deficiency, regardless of the cause (e.g., menopause, athletic amenorrhea) (19,20). Hypogonadism in men probably causes bone loss as well, but this affects only a minority of hypogonadal individuals (21) and is therefore a less important factor in causing osteoporosis among men than is menopause for women. Because of menopausal bone loss, which is most severe in the immediate postmenopausal period and slows thereafter, women lose more bone than men, and combined with their lower peak bone mass, they achieve markedly lower bone mass in old age. Combined with their longer life spans, this accounts for much of the higher fracture risk of women in developed countries.

Genetic Effects on Peak Bone Mass and Bone Loss

Genetic factors are unquestionably the single most important factor in the determination of peak adult skeletal mass. Studies of adult twins have indicated that perhaps 60% to 80% of the variability in bone mass may be attributed to genetic factors (22–24). Investigations of adolescent and younger twins yield similar estimates of genetic effects on bone mass (22). However, there is also evidence that differences within identical twin pairs increase with aging (25), suggesting that genetic effects may be less important in bone loss. Longitudinal studies of middle-aged men have demonstrated that there are reasonably strong familial, but not genetic, effects on bone loss over a 15- to 20-year period (26,27). These familial effects are probably attributable to shared environmental influences on bone loss (which are discussed later). Long-term studies of the role of genetic effects on bone loss in women are under way and may yield different answers from the studies on men, particularly if the menopausal bone loss because of estrogen deficiency is controlled by genetic factors.

Family studies (e.g., parent and offspring) have yielded slightly lower estimates of genetic influences on bone mass (28,29). The differences between twin and family

studies in part may be related to the assumptions of the models used for making these estimates and in part to the mechanisms of inheritance. Studies that have examined the assumptions of these genetic models have found evidence suggestive of gene interaction in the determination of bone mass (23). The presence of several major genes in the determination of skeletal mass would account for several of the observations made.

Daughters of postmenopausal women with fractures have lower bone mass than similarly aged women of mothers without fractures, but these differences are relatively small (28). However, many studies have failed to find family fracture histories valuable in identifying women with low bone mass (30,31). In part this is because fractures in older women reflect skeletal fragility, longevity, and the likelihood of falling, perhaps because of the loss of protective reflexes and other factors.

Efforts have been made to find the gene or genes that are responsible for variation in bone mass. A number of candidate genes have been investigated, including those for vitamin D receptor (32), estrogen receptor (33), interleukin-6 (34), and collagen Iα1 (35). many of these have been association studies and the effect sizes generally were small, and in some cases, they were not reproducible in other populations. True linkage has not been established. Genome searches that are underway show promise of finding new genes that may be involved.

Environmental Factors Influencing Peak Bone Mass

Peak bone mass is achieved in most people near the end of the third decade of life (17), although some researchers have suggested that accumulation of bone mineral ends with adolescence (16). Regardless of the resolution of this issue, there is no doubt that approximately 90% of skeletal mineral is present by age 18. Maximizing skeletal mineral growth in this period is critical. The influences on this process, beyond genetics, are being studied.

The dominant influences on skeletal mineral in pubertal children are probably hormonal, although direct studies of sex steroids, growth hormone, and other similar factors have not been carried out for this age group. However, when there are disturbances in normal hormonal function, skeletal deficits appear. Amenorrhea in adolescents, regardless of the cause, results in reduced bone mass (19,36). In some circumstances, factors causing the amenorrhea (e.g., nutritional inadequacies associated with anorexia nervosa) may also contribute to the skeletal deficit (36), but in other circumstances (e.g., athletic amenorrhea), it is probable that the hormonal deficit itself is the sole cause of the bone loss. Prompt correction of menstrual irregularities in young women is probably crucial to allowing this group to achieve their genetic potential.

Physical activity is associated with higher bone mass in children and adolescents (37), which is similar to the findings for adult populations. Those who participated in weight-bearing activities (e.g., basketball, soccer, baseball, softball) had an additional 5% to 7% bone mass for each extra hour per day of weight-bearing activity. Swimming and cycling showed no beneficial effects. These same patterns have also been observed for rates of gain in bone mass (15). However, as with all observational studies, the possibility cannot be excluded that children with larger, more dense skeletons are more inclined to participate in athletics. Intense physical activity may also be associated with diminished bone mass in young women with amenorrhea (19). There are reports of some elite athletes apparently escaping the negative skeletal consequences of athletic amenorrhea, perhaps as a result of extremely intense training (38,39). For these rare individuals, the intensity and duration of training are well beyond that undertaken by most athletes, even those competing at the collegiate level, and athletic amenorrhea should always be viewed as a potentially serious problem in young women.

The role of dietary factors in skeletal development has not been well studied. In parts of the world where osteoporosis is a problem, nutrition is generally very good compared with the developing countries, where osteoporosis is uncommon. This has led some researchers to conclude that diet, particularly dietary calcium, is of little importance in the development of peak bone mass.

However, several studies indicate that calcium and other factors probably play an important role in developing maximum skeletal mass. In a study of well-nourished children (diets contained on average 900 mg of calcium daily; the recommended dietary allowance [RDA] is 800 mg/day), an additional 700 mg of calcium daily resulted in prepubertal children gaining significantly more bone mass over 3 years than did their placebo-supplemented identical twin siblings (40). The magnitudes of the differences were 3% to 5%, depending on the skeletal site, which if maintained throughout adult life, would reduce fracture risk by 30% to 40% (1,2). Previous, smaller studies had suggested that such an effect might exist but had not achieved statistical significance (42). For children going through puberty, the importance of additional dietary calcium, beyond the 1,200 mg/day RDA, has not been established. Nevertheless, Matkovic and Heaney (43) reviewed most of the calcium balance studies done over the last 50 years and concluded that positive calcium balance in young children may continue to increase up to a total intake of about 1,500 to 1,600 mg/day.

A study addressing the issue of additional calcium in teenage girls is underway. Preliminary results suggest that additional calcium during adolescence may also be beneficial. Calcium also appears to have a positive effect on the accumulation of skeletal mineral during the third decade of life. One report found the dietary calcium to protein ratio to be positively associated with the rate of gain in spine bone mass during the third decade of life

(17). This ratio reflects the positive association of calcium intake with change in bone mass and the negative correlation between protein intake and bone mass. Dietary protein intake has previously been shown to increase urinary calcium excretion (43). A higher ratio of calcium to protein intake appears to be a favorable dietary pattern in terms of skeletal mineralization.

The effects of other dietary factors on skeletal growth and mineralization have not been well studied. Caffeine, for example, has been suggested as a potentially negative skeletal influence, given its effect, albeit weak, on increasing urinary calcium excretion (43). However, many studies have been unable to find significant caffeine effects on bone mass or changes in bone mass in the range of usual intakes for coffee, tea, and other caffeine-containing drinks (30,44). It is therefore unlikely that caffeine has any substantial effects in this area, although at extremely high intakes this remains a possibility.

For children and young adolescents, genetics, hormonal influences (some likely to be genetically determined), diet, and physical activity are the primary factors influencing rates of skeletal mineral growth. These same factors appear to be important for women between the ages of 20 and 30. It is also possible, but unproven, that in young adulthood, cigarette smoking and other factors may influence rates of bone mineral growth.

INFLUENCES ON SKELETAL HEALTH AFTER PEAK MASS IS ACHIEVED

Studies examining factors affecting bone mass in older people include prospective studies of bone loss and, more commonly, cross-sectional or retrospective investigations of factors associated with low bone mass or fractures. The precise timing and rates of bone loss at various skeletal sites are not well understood. Although bone loss in women is probably more important in terms of influencing ultimate fracture risk, it is perhaps simpler to first consider men, because of the seemingly simpler processes involved. Middle-aged men lose bone mass at a rate of about 0.5% per year from the radius (26) between the ages of 44 and 59. The known influences on these rates of loss include cigarette smoking, alcohol consumption (both detrimental), and physical activity (beneficial) (27).

Genetics

To address the question of genetic influences, studies of twins have been completed. Although there are highly significant correlations between members of twin pairs, these correlations are similar for identical and fraternal pairs, suggesting that a common environment, rather than genetic factors, plays the major role in this bone loss (26,27). Adjusting for known influences on bone loss (e.g., cigarettes), which are also elements of a shared environment, reduces these within-twin-pair correlations somewhat, although they remain about 0.4. These data suggest that there are major, unaccounted for elements of common environment that contribute to bone loss in middle-aged men (27).

Cigarette Smoking

It is likely that environmental influences on bone loss do not differ greatly between men and women. Women smokers have been shown to have lower bone mass around the time of menopause (45) and greater rates of bone loss after menopause (46). Women with vertebral crush fractures are also more likely to be smokers than nonsmokers (47). The mechanism for the detrimental effect of smoking on the skeleton is unknown, but several reports have indicated that smoking probably interferes with aspects of estrogen metabolism, rendering postmenopausal estrogen therapy less effective (48) and altering estrogen metabolism premenopausally (see Chapters 11 and 13) (49).

Alcohol Consumption

The effect of moderate alcohol consumption on the female skeleton is not as clear as that of smoking. Many studies of volunteers have shown no apparent detrimental effect of moderate alcohol consumption (30), but the levels of alcohol consumption in these groups are quite low, about one-third of the level of the men cited earlier (27). Besides lower alcohol consumption among women generally, heavier drinkers are less likely to volunteer for or remain in long-term studies. Case-control studies of hip fracture patients have shown alcoholics to have an elevated risk (50), but whether this risk reflects lower bone mass or an increased propensity for falling is unknown.

Physical Activity

Physical activity plays a clear role in the development and maintenance of skeletal mass. These effects are most noticeable at the extremes of activity. Prolonged bed rest and space travel, situations in which the skeleton is almost completely relieved of loading forces, result in rapid bone loss (51,52), which is at least partially reversible in the short term. Hemiplegia results in significant bone loss on the affected side of the body, demonstrating the specificity of this effect (53). Conversely, professional and elite amateur athletes demonstrate markedly increased skeletal densities in the areas stressed by their particular endeavors. Tennis players, for example, have much greater densities in their playing than their nonplaying limbs (54). Similarly, Olympic-caliber figure skaters have higher skeletal densities in the legs and pelvis than age-matched inactive women; densities at other skeletal sites apparently do not differ (39).

Studies such as these, however, do not address the question of how much activity is necessary or useful for the average person and whether increases in activity should be recommended for the prevention of osteoporosis. Several frequently recommended forms of exercise, including swimming and walking, have not been shown to slow bone loss or to be associated with higher bone mass in menopausal women (55,56). Theoretical models and experiments with animals (57,58) have indicated that greater strain rates rather than more repetitions of lower strains are necessary to positively affect bone. Although swimming and walking may be recommended for cardiovascular benefits, it is probable that more intense skeletal loading is required to slow bone loss. Studies of children during skeletal growth support this view.

Nonrandomized exercise studies generally suggest the benefits of physical activity, at least on the skeletal sites stressed by the activity, although this may reverse when the activity is stopped (59). However, randomized exercise trials have been notoriously difficult to complete primarily because of noncompliance with the prescribed regimens. In contrast to the studies of walking on bone loss, a few studies have demonstrated slower bone loss in older women, randomly assigned to forms of exercise that involved loading the skeletal sites of interest (60,61). Nevertheless, it remains to be shown that there are forms of exercise that can effectively load the hip and spine, which are the sites of the most serious and most common fractures, respectively.

Hormones

Although bone loss probably begins before the menopause, there is an acceleration of loss that accompanies the cessation of ovarian hormone production. This corresponds to the period of most rapid skeletal loss in women, amounting to several percent per year in the spine and 1% or more per year in predominantly cortical sites (e.g., the midshaft radius) (20,62). These rates are roughly twice as great as those seen in similarly aged men (26,27). The rates of bone loss in the late perimenopausal and early postmenopausal years are primarily determined by endogenous estrogen concentrations; studies have suggested that mean serum estradiol concentrations near 100 pg/mL prevent bone loss (20). Higher serum androgen concentrations also appear to be associated with slower rates of bone loss (20). Crush fracture patients have been shown to have lower androgen concentrations (63).

Among the causes of menopausal bone loss, serum estrogen deficiency is the most important, but it is also probably the best understood and the most easily altered. The more rapid rates of skeletal turnover and bone loss typical of postmenopausal women (20) are almost immediately returned to premenopausal levels with estrogen therapy (64,65). The addition of a progestin to estrogen replacement therapy does not appear to diminish the beneficial skeletal effects of this therapy (66) while apparently protecting against the increased risk of endometrial cancer, which accompanies unopposed estrogen use.

Calcium Intake

Bone loss slows as time from the menopause increases, and as loss slows, the effects of nonhormonal influences are more easily observed. The influence of calcium intake on rates of bone loss has been the subject of considerable debate. Although there is little to suggest that additional calcium can slow the bone loss driven by estrogen deficiency immediately after the menopause, data have shown that supplemental calcium can slow bone loss a few years later (67). However, these effects were seen primarily in women who had quite low dietary calcium intake (<400 mg/day). Whether additional calcium beyond the 800 mg/day RDA figure can be useful remains to be shown. It has been suggested that older women may require as much as 1,500 mg of calcium daily, but clinical trials demonstrating the utility of such intake have not yet been completed.

Fluoride

Although mainly thought of as an experimental, therapeutic agent, nontherapeutic exposures to fluoride are common. Several studies have suggested that these exposures may not be benign. High concentrations of fluoride (about 4 ppm) in drinking water supplies have been associated with increased hip fracture rates in these communities (68). Similarly, communities with fluoridated water (about 1 ppm) have had higher hip fracture rates than nonfluoridated communities (69). This finding parallels an earlier study, which found higher hospital discharge rates for hip fracture in cities with fluoridated water (70).

Ecologic studies such as these cannot associate an individual's fluoride intake with fracture and are therefore subject to cautious interpretation. However, it has also been shown in a clinical trial that those randomized to receive 75 mg/day of fluoride had higher fracture rates than subjects randomized to receive placebo (71). Although the dose in this clinical trial was substantially higher than that which people drinking normally fluoridated water supplies might consume in a day, it does add to the body of evidence warranting further investigation into the role of fluoride in fracture risk. There have been contrary findings to those cited earlier (72). Further studies, which can quantify fluoride exposures and fracture occurrences for individuals, are necessary before conclusions are reached regarding the role of fluoridated water supplies in the cause of hip and other fractures.

The potential importance of fluoride in causing fractures also introduces one difficulty with the use of bone mass measurements for assessing fracture risk. Fluoride can produce significant increases in bone mass, particu-

larly at more trabecular sites, such as the spine (72). However, the bone produced may not be normal; its strength may be less than that predicted by its mass because of the presence of fluoride crystals in the mineral structure. The extent to which "abnormal" bone is formed by fluoride in drinking water is unknown, but this may explain in part the observed differences in fracture rates. The issue of bone quality, in the context of the effects of therapeutic agents and environmental exposures, remains poorly understood but potentially important. Methods for the assessment of bone quality in epidemiologic studies do not yet exist.

NONSKELETAL FACTORS INFLUENCING THE RISK OF OSTEOPOROTIC FRACTURES

Reduced bone mass alone cannot account for all osteoporotic fractures. Although some hip fractures may be truly spontaneous (i.e., without any trauma), more than 90% result from falls. The trauma associated with a fall from standing height or less (e.g., on rising from a chair) is adequate to fracture an osteogenic hip, but many falls in older osteoporotic women do not result in fractures. It has been shown that the nature of the fall may be critical to determining whether or not a fracture occurs. Falls to the side and those that result in an impact on the hip increase the risk of hip fracture by more than 10-fold (7). There is also an increased fracture risk with the self-reported absence of protective reflexes (7). Falling forward or backward was associated with a much lower fracture risk.

Other fractures also involve trauma. Although some vertebral deformities may occur gradually, many normal activities, such as coughing, sneezing, and lifting small objects, involve energies adequate to fracture an osteogenic vertebra (7).

Colles' fractures of the distal radius are most frequently associated with a fall forward, such as may occur when someone walking quickly, trips, and lands on an outstretched arm. It has been suggested that the early plateau in the incidence of Colles' fractures (age 60 to 70) reflects a decline in the frequency of such falls, thereby reducing the exposure of the wrist to the type of trauma that yields fractures.

Other nonskeletal factors (e.g., soft tissue energy absorption during falls and diminishing vision) may also be important, although it is clear that an osteogenic skeleton is the central element in the cause of osteoporotic fractures. Interventions directed at reducing fracture incidence are difficult to evaluate because fractures occur very late in life, and interventions are probably most effective many years earlier. For example, estrogen replacement therapy is generally applied near the time of the menopause, but hip fracture incidence peaks 30 years later. However, it is clear that interventions that increase peak bone mass or diminish bone loss are likely to be effective. Studies underway will address questions regarding nonskeletal influences on fracture incidence. For example, can exercise help maintain balance and reduce falls in the elderly, or can certain types of padding (worn inside the clothing over the greater trochanter) diminish the skeletal impact of some falls?

CONCLUSIONS

Osteoporotic fractures are the product of skeletal changes during midlife and beyond; processes influencing peak bone mass during childhood, adolescence, and young adulthood; and nonskeletal factors affecting risk for trauma. Activities aimed at the prevention of such fractures, which now are focused on postmenopausal women, should be expanded to include younger women and, to a lesser extent, men. Diet and exercise during childhood and into the third decade of life appear to influence peak bone mass and are modifiable factors, in contrast to the strong and predetermined influences of a person's genetic makeup.

Smoking and higher levels of alcohol consumption have negative influences on the skeleton, probably by diminishing peak skeletal mass during the later stages of skeletal growth and by accelerating bone loss. Diet and exercise appear to influence rates of bone loss during periods of life, but the effects of sex steroids are primary around the time of the menopause, making it difficult to observe effects of nonhormonal influences at this time.

In old age, when most osteoporotic fractures occur, risk factors for low bone mass and increased exposure to trauma need to be considered. Diet (including calcium, protein, and perhaps other nutrients) and physical activity appear to be important factors in maintaining the skeleton. Whether physical activity increases the risk of trauma among the elderly or reduces it by maintaining functional abilities has not been studied.

REFERENCES

1. Hui SL, Slemenda CW, Johnston CC Jr. Baseline measurement of bone mass predicts fracture in white women. *Ann Intern Med* 1989;111:355–361.
2. Cummings SR, Black DM, Nevitt MC, et al. Appendicular bone density and age predict hip fracture in women. *JAMA* 1990;263:665–668.
3. Ross PD, Davis JW, Epstein RS, Wasnich RD. Pre-existing fractures and bone mass predict vertebral fracture incidence in women. *Ann Intern Med* 1991;114:919–923.
4. Hui SL, Slemenda CW, Johnston CC Jr. Age and bone mass as predictors of fracture in a prospective study. *J Clin Invest* 1988;81:1804–1809.
5. Gardsell P, Johnell O, Nilsson BE. Predicting fractures in women by using forearm bone densitometry. *Calcif Tissue Int* 1989;44:235–242.
6. Seeley DG, Browner WS, Nevitt MC, Genant HK, Scott JC, Cummings SR. Which fractures are associated with low appendicular bone mass in elderly women? *Ann Intern Med* 1991;115:837–842.
7. Hayes WC, Piazza SJ, Zysset PK. Biomechanics of fracture risk prediction of the hip and spine by quantitative computed tomography. *Radiol Clin North Am* 1991;29:2–18.
8. Chesnut CH III. Osteoporosis: a world-wide problem? In: Christiansen C, Overgaard K, eds. *Osteoporosis 1990*, vol 1. Copenhagen: Osteopress, 1990:33–35.
9. Melton LJ III. Epidemiology of fractures in North America. In: Christiansen C, Overgaard K, eds. *Osteoporosis 1990*, vol 1. Copenhagen: Osteopress, 1990:36–41.
10. Trotter MN, Broman GE, Peterson RR. Densities of bones of white and negro skeletons. *J Bone Joint Surg Am* 1960;41:50–58.
11. Solomon L. Bone density in aging Caucasian and African populations. *Lancet* 1979;3:1326–1329.
12. Lo CW, Jarjou LM, Poppitt S, Cole TJ, Neer R, Prentice A. Delayed development of bone mass in West African adolescents. In: Christiansen C, Overgaard K, eds. *Osteoporosis 1990*, vol 1. Copenhagen: Osteopress, 1990:73–77.
13. Melton LJ. A "Gompertzian" view of osteoporosis. *Calcif Tissue Int* 1990;46:285–286.
14. Cummings SR, Nevitt MC. Epidemiology of hip fractures and falls. In: Kleerekoper M, Krane SM, eds. *Clinical disorders of bone and mineral metabolism.* Amsterdam: Elsevier Scientific Publishers, 1989:231–236.
15. Slemenda CW, Hui SL, Miller JZ, Johnston CC Jr. The effects of physical activity, sexual maturation, and weight gain on bone growth in children. *J Bone Miner Res* 1992;[Suppl 1];7:93.
16. Bonjour JP, Theintz G, Buchs B, Slosman D, Clavien H, Rozzoli R. Critical years and pubertal stages for spinal and femoral bone mass accumulation during adolescence. In: Christiansen C, Overgaard K, eds. *Osteoporosis 1990*, vol 1. Copenhagen: Osteopress, 1990:394–395.
17. Recker RR, Davies KM, Hinders SM, Heaney RP, Stegman MR, Kimmel DB. Bone gain in young adult women. *JAMA* 1992;268:2403–2408.
18. Kelly PJ, Twomey L, Sambrook PN, Eisman JA. Sex differences in peak adult bone mineral density. *J Bone Miner Res* 1990;5:1169–1175.
19. Drinkwater BL, Nilson K, Chestnut CH, Brenner WJ, Shainholtz S, Southworth MD. Bone mineral content of amenorrheic and eumenorrheic athletes. *N Engl J Med* 1984;311:277–281.
20. Slemenda CW, Hui SL, Longcope C, Johnston CC. Sex steroids and bone mass: a study of changes about the time of menopause. *J Clin Invest* 1987;80:1261–1269.
21. Greenspan SL, Neer RM, Ridgway EC, Klibanski A. Osteoporosis in men with hyperprolactinemic hypogonadism. *Ann Intern Med* 1986;104:777–782.
22. Smith DM, Nance WE, Kang KW, Johnston CC Jr. Genetic factors in determining bone mass. *J Clin Invest* 1973;52:2800–2808.
23. Slemenda CW, Christian JC, Williams CJ, Norton JA, Johnston CC Jr. Genetic determinants of bone mass in adult women: a reevaluation of the twin model and the potential importance of gene interaction on heritability estimates. *J Bone Miner Res* 1991;6:561–567.
24. Pocock NA, Eisman JA, Hopper JL, Yeates MG, Sambrook PN, Ebert L. Genetic determinants of bone mass in adults: a twin study. *J Clin Invest* 1987;80:706–710.
25. Slemenda CW, Christian JC, Williams CJ, Johnston CC Jr. The changing relative importance of genetics and environment in adult women. In: Cohn DV, Glorieux FH, Martin TJ, eds. *Calcium regulation and bone metabolism.* Amsterdam: Elsevier Scientific Publishers, 1990:491–496.
26. Christian JC, Yu P-L, Slemenda CW, Johnston CC Jr. Heritability of bone mass: a longitudinal study in aging male twins. *Am J Hum Genet* 1989;44:429–433.
27. Slemenda CW, Christian JC, Reed T, Reister TK, Williams CJ, Johnston CC Jr. Long-term bone loss in men: effects of genetic and environmental factors. *Ann Intern Med* 1992;117:286–291.
28. Seeman E, Hopper JL, Bach LA, et al. Reduced bone mass in daughters of women with osteoporosis. *N Engl J Med* 1989;320:554–558.
29. Tylavsky FA, Bortz AD, Hancock RL, Anderson JJ. Familial resemblance of radial bone mass between premenopausal mothers and their college-age daughters. *Calcif Tissue Int* 1989;45:265–269.
30. Slemenda CW, Hui SL, Longcope C, Wellman H, Johnston CC Jr. Predictors of bone mass in perimenopausal women. *Ann Intern Med* 1990;112:96–101.
31. Stevenson JC, Lees B, Devenport M. Determinants of bone density in normal women: risk factors for future osteoporosis? *BMJ* 1989;298:924–928.
32. Morrison NA, Qi JC, Tokita A, et al. Prediction of bone density from vitamin D receptor alleles. *Nature* 1994;367:284–287.
33. Smith EP, Boyd J, Frank GR, et al. Estrogen resistance caused by a mutation in the estrogen-receptor gene in a man. *N Engl J Med* 1994;331:1056–1061.
34. Murray RE, McGuigan F, Grant SFA, Reid DM, Ralston SH. Polymorphisms of the interleukin-6 gene are associated with bone mineral density. *Bone* 1997;21:89–92.
35. Uitterlinden AG, Burger H. Huang Q, et al. Relation of alleles of the collagen type Iα1 gene to cone density and the risk of osteoporotic fractures in postmenopausal women. *N Engl J Med* 1998:338:1016–10212.
36. Rigotti NA, Nussbaum SR, Herzog DB, et al. Osteoporosis in women with anorexia nervosa. *N Engl J Med* 1984;311:1601–1606.
37. Slemenda CW, Miller JZ, Hui SL, Reister TK, Johnston CC Jr. Role of physical activity in the development of skeletal mass in children. *J Bone Miner Res* 1991;6:1227–1233.
38. Snyder AC, Wenderoth MP, Johnston CC, Hui SL. Bone mineral content of elite lightweight amenorrheic oarswomen. *Hum Biol* 1986;58:863–869.
39. Slemenda CW, Johnston CC Jr. High intensity activities in young women: site specific bone mass effects among female figure skaters. *Bone Miner* 1993;20:125–132.
40. Johnston CC, Miller JZ, Slemenda CW, et al. Calcium supplementation in increases in bone mineral density in children. *N Engl J Med* 1992;327:82–87.
41. Matkovic V, Fontana D, Tominac C, Goel P, Chestnut CH III. Factors that influence peak bone mass formation: a study of calcium balance and the inheritance of bone mass in adolescent females. *Am J Clin Nutr* 1990;52:878–888.
42. Matkovic V, Heaney RP. Calcium balance during human growth: evidence for threshold behavior. *Am J Clin Nutr* 1992;55:992–996.
43. Heaney RP, Recker RR. Effects of nitrogen, phosphorus, and caffeine on calcium balance in women. *J Lab Clin Med* 1982;99:46–55.
44. Cooper C, Atkinson EJ, Wahner HW, et al. Is caffeine consumption a risk factor for osteoporosis? *J Bone Miner Res* 1992;7:465–471.
45. Slemenda CW, Hui SL, Longcope C, Johnston CC Jr. Cigarette smoking, obesity, and bone mass. *J Bone Miner Res* 1989;4:737–741.

46. Krall E, Dawson-Hughes B. Smoking and bone loss among postmenopausal women. *J Bone Miner Res* 1991;4:331–338.
47. Daniell HW. Osteoporosis of the slender smoker. *Arch Intern Med* 1976;136: 298–304.
48. Kiel DP, Baron JA, Anderson JJ, Hannan MT, Felson DT. Smoking eliminates the protective effect of oral estrogens on the risk for hip fracture among women. *Ann Intern Med* 1992;116:716–721.
49. Michnovicz JJ, Hershcopf RJ, Naganuma H, Bradlow HL, Fishman J. Increased 2-hydroxylation of estradiol as a possible mechanism for the anti-estrogenic effect of cigarette smoking. *N Engl J Med* 1986;315:1305–1309.
50. Nilsson BE. Conditions contributing to fracture of the femoral neck. *Acta Chir Scand 1970;*136:383–384.
51. Globus RK, Bikle DD, Morey-Holton E. The temporal response of bone to unloading. *Endocrinology* 1986;118:733–742.
52. Nicogossian AE. Overall physiological response to space flight. In: Nicogossian AE, Huntoon CL, Pool SL, eds. *Space physiology and medicine.* Philadelphia: Lea & Febiger, 1989:139.
53. Prince RL, Price RI, Ho S. Forearm bone loss in hemiplegia: a model for the study of immobilization osteoporosis. *J Bone Miner Res* 1988;3:305–310.
54. Huddleston AL, Rockwell D, Hulund DN, et al. Bone mass in lifetime tennis athletes. *JAMA* 1980;224:1107–1109.
55. Sandler RB, Canley JA, Hom DL, Sashim D, Kriska AM. The effects of walking on the cross-sectional dimensions in postmenopausal women. *J Bone Miner Res* 1987;41:65–69.
56. Cavanaugh DJ, Cann CE. Brisk walking does not stop bone loss in post-menopausal women. *Bone* 1988;9:201–204.
57. Lanyon LE, Goodship AE, Pye CJ, MacFie JH. Mechanically adaptive bone remodelling. *J Biomech* 1982;15:141–154.
58. Carter DR, Orr TE, Fyhrie DP, Schurman DJ. Influences of mechanical stress on prenatal and postnatal skeletal development. *Clin Orthop* 1987;219:237–250.
59. Dalsky GP, Stocke KS, Ehsani AI, Slatopolsky E, Lee W, Birge SJ. Weight-bearing exercise training and lumbar bone mineral content in postmenopausal women. *Ann Intern Med* 1988;108:824–828.
60. Chow R, Harrison JE, Notarius C. Effect of two randomized exercise programs on bone mass of healthy postmenopausal women. *BMJ* 1987;295:1441–1444.
61. Simkin A, Ayalon J, Leichter I. Increased trabecular bone density due to bone loading exercises in post-menopausal osteoporotic women. *Calcif Tissue Int* 1987; 40:59–63.
62. Harris S, Dawson-Hughes B, Rates of change in bone mineral density of the spine, heel, femoral neck and radius in healthy postmenopausal women. *Bone Miner* 1992;17:87–95.
63. Longcope C, Baker RS, Hui SL, Johnston CC Jr. Androgen and estrogen dynamics in women with vertebral crush fractures. *Maturitas* 1984;6:309–318.
64. Lindsay R, Hart DM, Forrest C, Baird C. Prevention of spinal osteoporosis in oophorectomized women. Lancet 1980;2:1151–1153.
65. Ettinger B, Genant HK, Cann C. Long-term estrogen therapy prevents fractures and preserves bone mass. *Ann Intern Med* 1985;102:319–324.
66. Christiansen C, Rils BJ, Nilas L, Rodbro P, Deftos L. Uncoupling of bone formation and resorption by combined oestrogen and progestogen therapy in postmenopausal osteoporosis. *Lancet* 1987;1:1105–1108.
67. Dawson-Hughes B, Dallal GE, Krall EA, Sadowski L, Sahyoun N, Tannenbaum S. A controlled trial of the effect of calcium supplementation on bone density in postmenopausal women. *N Engl J Med* 1990;323:878–883.
68. Sowers MR, Clark MK, Jannasch ML, Wallace RB. A prospective study of bone mineral content and fracture in communities with differential fluoride exposure. *Am J Epidemiol* 1991;133:649–660.
69. Danielson C, Lyon JL, Egger M, Goodenough GK. Hip fractures and fluoridation in Utah's elderly population. *JAMA* 1992;268:746–748.
70. Jacobsen SJ, Goldberg J, Miles TP, Brody JA, Stiers W, Rimm AA. Regional variation in the incidence of hip fracture: US white women aged 65 and older. *JAMA* 1990;264:500–502.
71. Riggs BL, Hodgson SF, O'Fallon WM, et al. Effect of fluoride on the fracture rate in postmenopausal women with osteoporosis. *N Engl J Med* 1990;322: 802–809.
72. Simoen O, Laitinen O. Does fluoridation of drinking-water prevent bone fragility and osteoporosis? *Lancet* 1985;2:432–434.

Treatment of the Postmenopausal Woman: Basic and Clinical Aspects, Second Edition, edited by Rogerio A. Lobo, Lippincott Williams & Wilkins, Philadelphia © 1999.

CHAPTER 26

Detection of Osteopenia

Cornelis van Kuijk and Harry K Genant

The term *osteopenia* is a nonspecific term used to describe a decreased quantity of bone regardless of the cause (1). *Osteoporosis* is defined as a condition of diminishing bone mass, deteriorating bone architecture, and subsequent fracturing of skeletal parts. Osteopenia can therefore be regarded as the precursor or early stage of osteoporosis. Osteoporotic fractures cause considerable morbidity, mortality, and public health expenditure. Vertebral, hip, and wrist fractures are the most common fractures associated with osteoporosis. The risk of a 50-year-old American woman fracturing her hip in her remaining lifetime is estimated to be 16%; fracturing her wrist, 15%; and sustaining a vertebral fracture, 32% (2). The number of osteoporotic patients is expected to increase in the future because of increased life expectancy. As the world's population rapidly increases from an estimated 5.3 billion people in 1990 to 8.3 billion in 2025, the number of osteoporotic fractures will increase dramatically worldwide (3). The annual cost burden of osteoporosis was estimated at $13.8 billion in the United States for 1995 (4).

Clinical management in osteoporosis can be discussed in terms of prevention and treatment. In the normal aging process, bone mass increases until approximately the third decade of life. The maximum bone mass achieved is called the *peak bone mass.* With further aging, bone mass is gradually diminishing. Postmenopausal women experience an accelerated bone loss in the first years after menopause (5,6).

Prevention in osteoporosis means intervention that creates an environment and basic lifestyle that ensures a high peak bone mass and its preservation for the individual. Adequate nutrition and exercise are recommended, as is omitting risk factors such as smoking and alcohol abuse.

Treatment of osteoporosis means an intervention in patients with osteoporotic fractures. The aim is to reduce the risk of further fractures and to decrease the morbidity associated with the fracture. Early detection of low bone density or osteopenia and early initiation of treatment can possibly prevent osteoporosis. This reduces the cost burden of osteoporosis and improves the quality of life in the elderly.

Several drugs have been useful in the prevention and treatment of osteoporosis. Hormonal replacement therapy (in several prescription formats), calcitonin, sodium fluoride, vitamin D analogues, several bisphosphonates, and parathyroid hormone analogs have been or are tested in clinical drug trials, and their availability for clinical use is widespread, although different from country to country.

Determination of bone mineral content (i.e., quantifying osteopenia) can predict future fracture risk (7,8). Anthropomorphic measurements, biomarkers of bone metabolism, and patient history cannot be used to identify women with osteopenia reliably (9,10). It is therefore a clinical challenge to determine the patients at risk of osteoporotic fractures and to select patients for preventive therapy. The clinician needs a tool to monitor and evaluate therapeutic intervention. Bone densitometry (i.e., measurement of the amount of bone in the skeleton) for assessment and monitoring of osteopenia and osteoporosis plays an important role in osteoporosis management, one of the key issues in postmenopausal women.

TECHNIQUES

Conventional Radiographic Reading

To the clinician, osteoporosis means a fragility fracture caused by low-impact trauma or without any history of trauma. Conventional radiographs are still the main clinical diagnostic tools in fracture assessment. More gener-

C. van Kuijk: University of Amsterdam, Department of Radiology, Academic Medical Center, 1105 AZ Amsterdam, The Netherlands.

H. K. Genant: Department of Radiology, University of California at San Francisco, San Francisco, California 94143-0628.

ally, however, osteoporosis means decreased bone mass (i.e., osteopenia) associated with an increased fracture risk. Cortical thinning and increased intracortical porosity in tubular bones is a well-known radiologic feature of osteopenia, as is loss of specific trabecular structures in the femoral neck and vertebral bodies. However, it has been estimated that at least 30% of the skeletal calcium is lost before osteopenia has become detectable on conventional radiographs (11–13). Some semiquantitative grading methods have been developed, such as the Singh index (14), in which the appearance of the trabecular structure in the femoral neck is graded. A grading method for osteopenia of the vertebral body also has been reported (15). Although these methods can give some information, the reproducibility of the results is disappointing, possibly because of the inherent subjectivity of the readings. Consequently, true objective techniques for quantifying bone mineral mass have been developed that are capable of detecting early bone loss.

Radiogrammetry

In radiogrammetry, the thickness of the cortex of the metacarpal or phalangeal bones is measured on standard radiographs of the hand. However, with this method, no information is obtained about trabecular bone, and intracortical porosity cannot be detected (16). For epidemiologic studies with large study populations, this method appears to be a valuable tool in predicting osteoporotic fractures (17). Although already published in the 1960s and since then superseded by more sophisticated methods, radiogrammetry has regained scientific interest, largely because of emerging reimbursement constraints threatening more sophisticated techniques and because of new computerized image processing capabilities (18–20). Bone dimensions, such as cortical width and cortical area, were usually measured with rulers and calipers. Computer-aided techniques have been developed that use image processing and analysis tools to perform these measurements in a semiautomated fashion.

An addition to this field is the measurement of the hip-axis length on standard radiographs of the hip and on images acquired by bone densitometers [i.e., dual-energy x-ray absorptiometry (DEXA) equipment]. The hip-axis length seems to be a prognostic factor for future hip fractures, independent of bone density at the hip (21,22).

Radiographic Absorptiometry

In radiographic absorptiometry, a standardized radiograph of the hand is made along with an aluminum reference wedge (23,24). The optical density of the phalanges or metacarpals is determined and compared with that of the wedge using a videodensitometric technique after digitizing the radiograph (25–26). The results are usually given in arbitrary units, aluminum equivalent values, or as calculated conversions to g/cm^3 bone equivalent values. No distinction is made between the cortical and trabecular compartments of bone. Like radiogrammetry, radiographic absorptiometry has regained broad interest. Several studies indicate the usefulness of this simple and cheap technique for the detection of osteopenia (26–28). Innovations using charge-coupled devices and other nonfilm techniques and improved computer technology have led to the possibility of the development of small table-top devices providing fast and easy accessible measurements.

Single-Energy X-ray Absorptiometry

In single-energy x-ray absorptiometry (SXA), a highly collimated photon beam from an x-ray source is used to measure the photon attenuation of the measurement site (usually the forearm or the heel), which is converted to bone mineral content (BMC) in grams or area bone mineral density (BMD) in grams per square centimeter using a known standard. SXA measurements are confined to the appendicular skeleton (29–30). As in radiographic absorptiometry, SXA cannot measure the cortical and trabecular compartments of bone separately.

Dual-Energy X-ray Absorptiometry

DEXA is used for bone mass measurements in the central skeleton (e.g., hip, spine), the peripheral skeleton (e.g., forearm, heel), and total-body bone mineral content and fat content assessment (18,26,29,31,32). A dual-energy spectrum is generated by rapid switching of the x-ray tube voltage supply or by K-edge filtering. The two measurements at the two different energies create the possibility to assess bone mass at axial skeletal sites, such as the spine. DEXA technology has gained widespread acceptance and distribution, especially because measurements can be done at all important fracture sites, most prominently the spine and the hip. Examples of DEXA scans are shown in Fig. 26.1.

In spinal DEXA (anteroposterior projection), the measurement can be confounded by spinal osteoarthritis (33). Spinal DEXA in the lateral projection has been suggested as a possible alternative. However, the reproducibility of lateral measurements is generally worse than measurements in the anteroposterior direction (29,31).

Quantitative Computed Tomography

Quantitative computed tomography (QCT) is the only method that can estimate bone density separately in the trabecular and cortical bone compartments and the only

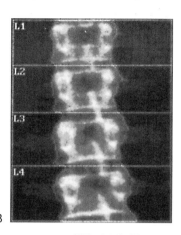
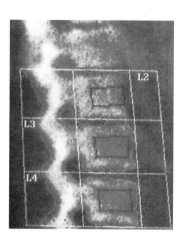
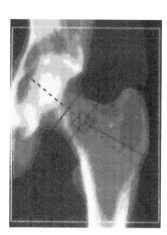
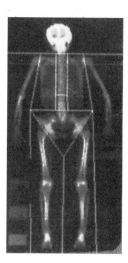

A,B   C,D

FIG. 26.1. Typical dual-energy x-ray absorptiometry (DEXA) examinations. **A:** Anteroposterior DEXA examination of the lumbar spine. **B:** Lateral DEXA examination of the lumbar spine. **C:** DEXA examination of the hip. **D:** Total-body DEXA examination.

method giving a true density (in g/cm^3) estimate. The vertebral body usually is the preferred site of measurement. The vertebral body has a high content of trabecular bone, which because of its high surface to volume ratio is known to have a high bone turnover. Measurements at this site are therefore sensitive to change in metabolic activity, such as increased bone resorption (34).

On a lateral scout view, a slice selection is made at the midvertebral levels of three to four consecutive vertebral bodies. A reference standard is placed under the lumbar spine of the patient and scanned simultaneously. The average attenuation value of the object of interest is measured in the image and compared with the attenuation values of the calibration standard (35). An example of a QCT examination is shown in Fig. 26.2.

Single-energy QCT is the technique most widely used and recommended. Dual-energy QCT has been used to improve the accuracy of the bone density assessments. However, decreased precision, increased radiation dose and technical difficulties has limited this technique to

research purposes (36). Although QCT is primarily used for bone mass measurements in the spine, femoral QCT has been used (37,38). Newer CT systems capable of spiral CT scanning allow a volumetric acquisition of imaging data from which a highly accurate three-dimensional reconstruction of vertebral bodies or femora can be made. With advanced image analysis tools, this allows sophisticated density measurements in several regions of interest and measurements of geometric dimensions of the object of interest.

Special purpose CT systems have been developed for peripheral QCT (pQCT) of the forearm and lower leg (39,40). The first generation of these pQCT systems used nuclear sources. Newer systems use x-ray sources.

Quantitative Ultrasound

Ultrasound velocity and attenuation measurements are used for noninvasive measurement of bone quantity and structure (41–44). Measurements are confined to the

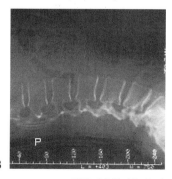
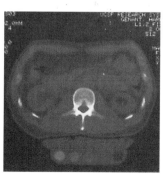
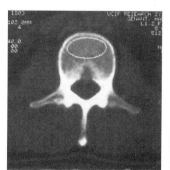
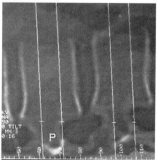

,B   C,D

FIG. 26.2. Typical quantitative computed tomography (QCT) examination. **A:** Lateral scout view of lower spine. **B:** Scanned volume in QCT of vertebral body. **C:** CT image of patient on calibration standard. **D:** Trabecular region of interest in vertebral body.

TABLE 26.1 *Techniques for the detection of osteopenia*

Technique	Anatomic site of interest	Precision *in vivo* (%)	Examination and analysis time (min.)	Estimated Effective dose equivalent (μSv)
Conventional radiographs	Spine, hip	NA	<5	2000
Radiogrammetry	Hand	1–3	5–10	<1
Radiographic absorptiometry	Hand	1–2	5–10	<1
Single x-ray absorptiometry	Forearm, heel	1–2	5–10	<1
Dual x-ray absorptiometry	Spine, hip, forearm, total body	1–3	5–20	1–10
Quantitative computed tomography	Spine, forearm, hip	2–4	10–15	50–100
Quantitative ultrasound	Heel, hand, lower leg	1–3	5–10	None

NA, not applicable.

peripheral skeleton, where the bone is close to the skin. Newer, more experimental equipment also provides the possibility to measure at more remote sites such as the hip. Equipment is available that measures at the heel, the fingers, and the lower leg. Parameters measured are ultrasound transmission velocity and broadband ultrasound attenuation or a combination of these, sometimes referred to as stiffness. These parameters are generally postulated to be determined by bone density and bone architecture, although the latter claim is still controversial, because different studies have shown that the output parameters of the various apparatus are highly correlated with BMD as measured with other modalities. The clear advantage of quantitative ultrasound is its absence of radiation exposure.

A summary of several features of the available techniques is given in Table 26.1. In this table, precision refers to reproducibility of the measurement technique *in vivo* and is given as coefficient of variation (%). For the clinical reading of radiographic films, the reproducibility is not given. Dose refers to the effective dose equivalent (in μSv). For comparison, the annual natural dose is approximately 2,500 μSv; a transatlantic flight between San Francisco and Amsterdam enhances this dose with approximately 55 μSv.

CLINICAL USE

The various techniques for bone densitometry are widely used. There is general consensus that low bone mass predicts fracture risk at least as well as high cholesterol levels predict the risk of heart disease. The following clinical applications are recommended (45–48).

Patients with metabolic diseases known to affect the skeleton should be assessed. Many metabolic disorders, such as Cushing's syndrome, malabsorption syndromes, and hypogonadism, adversely affect the skeleton. In these secondary forms of osteoporosis, bone densitometry is used to assess the bone mineral status of the patient and to monitor changes in bone mineral content over time, which can prompt therapeutic intervention (e.g., estrogen replacement therapy in hypogonadism).

Perimenopausal women should be assessed for initiation of preventive therapy. Because bone loss is accelerated in women after menopause and women achieve a lower peak bone mass compared with men, women are especially at risk for osteoporosis. Estrogen replacement therapy can preserve bone mass. It could be claimed that medication should be restricted to women with low bone mass and an increased fracture risk to maximize cost-effective use. The exact knowledge of bone status can enhance compliance with preventive therapy.

The elderly should be assessed for osteopenia. Osteoporosis is a continuum of increasing osteopenia eventually leading to fractures, most notably of the vertebral bodies in the spine and of the hip. Because the absolute level of bone mass is predictive for future fracture risk, bone densitometry is recommended for the elderly, especially if other risk factors are present, such as decreased mobility, bad nutrition, propensities to falls because of neurologic deterioration, or use of medications affecting coordination.

Bone density can be used to monitor the efficacy of treatment or disease course. If applied properly, modern bone densitometry techniques have a sufficient longitudinal reproducibility (1% to 2%) to justify follow-up measurements for an individual.

INTERPRETATION OF BONE MEASUREMENTS

Because bone density decreases with aging and differences in bone density exist between sexes and races, bone density measurements should be compared with those of age-, sex-, and race-matched controls. A normative data base is mandatory for interpreting the level of bone mineral content. Usually, the estimated bone density is given as a Z-score. The Z-score gives the patient's results as the deviation from the mean of age-matched controls divided by the standard deviation (SD) of this mean, which is an indication of the biologic variability. In addition to the Z-score, the bone density of a patient is compared with the peak bone mass of young normal adults. The estimation is given as the T-score. The T-score, similar to the Z-score, gives the patient's results as a deviation from the mean of young normal adults divided by the SD of the mean.

To provide some guidelines for the interpretation of bone density measurements, the World Health Organization (WHO) has generated a document with some working definitions (49):

Normal: a value for BMD/BMC not more than 1 SD below the average value of young adults

Low bone mass or osteopenia: a value for BMD/BMC of more than 1 SD deviation below the young adult average but not more than 2.5 SD deviations below

Osteoporosis: a value for BMD/BMC more than 2.5 SD below the young adult average

Severe osteoporosis: a value for BMC/BMD more than 2.5 SD below the young adult average value and the presence of one or more fragility fractures

There is some criticism concerning these threshold-based diagnoses. It is argued that as fracture risk increases with decreasing bone density in a linear fashion, the applicability of the WHO suggested classification and categorization of patients is limited. The use of the WHO criteria requires access to and availability of a normative database that is locally derived, because there are significant differences in normative values between geographic areas and between countries (50). The manufacturers of densitometers usually provide normative database acquired at a limited number of centers and geographic areas. Another problem is the dissimilarity in spinal and femoral scores. A patient classified as osteopenic using the hip as measurement site could still be normal in terms of her spine (51). It makes clinical sense to combine the bone densitometry result of a patient with the assessment of other risk factors for fracture such as maternal history of osteoporosis, loss of height, confounding medication (e.g., corticosteroids), premature menopause, low body mass index, prolonged immobilization, malnutrition and malabsorption syndromes. This combined information added to the wish of the patient to be treated should be sufficient to give the patient the appropriate advice.

A limited number of studies indicate that biochemical bone markers could be used to identify so-called fast bone losers. However, the reproducibility of such tests is relatively poor. Ongoing studies will probably give more information in the future concerning the role of biomarkers in the detection of subjects at risk for osteoporosis.

COMPARISON OF DIFFERENT TECHNIQUES

Because the clinician has a wide choice in techniques for bone densitometry, the question arises about which technique to use. Several researchers have tried to determine the distinct values of these techniques. When these techniques are compared in terms of their discriminative power between normal healthy patients and (spinal) osteoporotics or between mild and severe osteoporotics, QCT seems to be the better choice, followed by DEXA, SXA, and radiographic absorptiometry, although all techniques show a considerable overlap between normal subjects and osteoporotic patients (26,27,53–55). In several studies and at several conferences and meetings, it has been suggested that measurements should be performed at the suspected fracture site: spinal measurements (QCT or DEXA) for vertebral body fracture risk and hip measurements (DEXA) for hip fracture risk.

In large epidemiologic studies, it has been shown that measurements at various anatomic sites with a variety of techniques do equally well in predicting future osteoporotic fractures. Debate continues about whether the cheaper and more accessible peripheral measurement techniques (SXA, quantatative ultrasound, radiographic absorptiometry) should be regarded as first-line screening tools, while the measurement techniques capable of measuring the sites prone to osteoporotic fractures (DEXA, QCT) should be used for confirming diagnosis and for monitoring disease course and interventions.

The correlation between the different techniques is modest (typically, $r = 0.6$–0.7). This precludes prediction of bone mass at one site by bone mass measurement at another site because of technical differences between the techniques and the differences in measurement sites, which have a different composition (i.e., ratio of cortical to trabecular bone) and different metabolic activities. The various techniques are therefore complementary rather than competitive. For daily clinical practice, the choice of technique largely depends on the local availability of techniques and experts.

REFERENCES

1. Mayo-Smith W, Rosenthal DI. Radiographic appearance of osteopenia. *Radiol Clin North Am* 1991;29:37–47.
2. Cummings SR, Black DM, Rubin SM. Lifetime risk of hip, Colles', or vertebral fracture and coronary heart disease among white postmenopausal women. *Arch Intern Med* 1989;149:2445–2448.
3. Gullberg B, Johnell O, Kanis JA. World-wide projections for hip fracture. *Osteoporosis Int* 1997;7:407–413.
4. Fox Ray N, Chan JK, Thamer M, Melton LJ III. Medical expenditures for the treatment of osteoporotic fractures in the United States in 1995: report from the National Osteoporosis Foundation. *J Bone Miner Res* 1997;12:24–35.
5. Arlot ME, Sornay-Rendu E, Garnero P, Vey-Marty B, Delmas PD. Apparent pre- and postmenopausal bone loss evaluated by DEXA at different skeletal sites in women; the OFELY cohort. *J Bone Miner Res* 1997;12:683–690.
6. Elders PJM, Netelenbos JC, Lips P, Van Ginkel FC, Vander Stelt PF. Accelerated vertebral bone loss in relation to the menopause: a cross-sectional study on lumbar bone density in 286 women of 46–55 years of age. *Bone Miner* 1988;5:11–19.
7. Cummings SR, Black DM, Nevitt MC, et al. Bone density at various sites for prediction of hip fractures: the study of osteoporotic fractures. *Lancet* 1993;341:72–75.
8. Düppe H, Gärdsell P, Nilssson B, Johnell O. A single bone density measurement can predict fractures over 25 years. *Calcif Tissue Int* 1997;60:171–174.
9. Slemenda CW, Hui SL, Longcope C, Wellman H, Johnston CC. Predictors of bone mass in perimenopausal women. *Ann Intern Med* 1990;112:96–101.
10. Cooper C, Shah S, Hand DJ, et al. Screening for vertebral osteoporosis using individual risk factors. *Osteoporosis Int* 1991;2:48–53.
11. Adran GM. Bone destruction not demonstrable by radiography. *Br J Radiol* 1951; 24:107.
12. Kawashima T, Uhthoff HK. A pattern of bone loss of the proximal femur: a radiologic, densitometric and histomorphometric study. *J Orthop Res* 1991;9:634–640.
13. Finsen V, Anda S. Accuracy of visually estimated bone mineralization in routine radiographs of the lower extremity. *Skeletal Radiol* 1988;17:270–275.
14. Singh M, Nagrath AR, Maini PS. Change in trabecular pattern of the upper end of the femur as an index of osteoporosis. *J Bone Joint Surg Am* 1970;52;457–467.
15. Pogrund H, Makin M, Robin G, et al. Osteoporosis in patients with femoral neck fracture in Jerusalem. *Clin Orthop Rel Res* 1977;124:165–172.
16. Johnston CC. Noninvasive methods for quantitating appendicular bone mass In: Avioli LV, ed. *The osteoporotic syndrome.* Orlando: Grune & Stratton, 1983:73–84.

17. van Hemert AM, Vandenbroucke JP, Birkenhäger JC, Valkenburg HA. Prediction of osteoporotic fractures in the general population by a fracture risk score: a 9-year follow-up among middle-aged women. *Am J Epidemiol* 1990:132:123–135.
18. Aguado F, Revilla M, Hernandez ER, Villa LF, Rico H. Behavior of bone mass measurements: dual-energy x-ray absorptiometry total body bone mineral content, ultrasound bone velocity, and computed metacarpal radiogrammetry, with age, gonadal status, and weight in healthy women. *Invest Radiol* 1996;31:218–222.
19. Meema HE, Meindok H. Advantages of peripheral radiogrammetry over dual-photon absorptiometry of the spine in the assessment of prevalence of osteoporotic vertebral fractures in women. *J Bone Miner Res* 1992;7:897–903.
20. Heaney RP, Barger-Lux MJ, Davies KM, Ryan RA, Johnson ML, Gong G. Bone dimensional changes with age: Interactions of genetic, hormonal, and body size variables. *Osteoporosis Int* 1997;7:426–431.
21. Faulkner KG, Cummings SR, Black D, Palermo L, Glüer CC, Genant HK. Simple measurement of femoral geometry predicts hip fracture: the study of osteoporotic fractures. *J Bone Miner Res* 1993;8:1211–1217.
22. Glüer CC, Cummings SR, Pressman A, et al. Prediction of hip fractures from pelvic radiographs: the study of osteoporotic fractures. *J Bone Miner Res* 1994;9:671–677.
23. Cosman F, Herrington BS, Himmelstein S, Lindsay R. Radiographic absorptiometry: a simple method for determination of bone mass. *Osteoporosis Int* 1991;2:34–38.
24. Trouerbach WTH, Hoornstra K, Birkenhäger JC, Zwamborn AW. Roentgendensitometric study of the phalanx. *Diagn Imaging Clin Med* 1985;54:64–77.
25. Strid KG, Kalebo P. Bone mass determination from microradiographs by computer assisted videodensitometry. I. Methodology. *Acta Radiol* 1988;29:465–472.
26. Ravn P, Overgaard K, Huang C, Ross PD, Green D, McClung M, for the EPIC study group. Comparison of bone densitometry of the phalanges, distal forearm and axial skeleton in early postmenopausal women participating in the EPIC study. *Osteoporosis Int* 1996;6,308–313.
27. Yates AJ, Ross PD, Lydick E, Epstein RS. Radiographic absorptiometry in the diagnosis of osteoporosis. *Am J Med* 1995;98[Suppl 2A],41S–47S.
28. Bouxsein ML, Michaeli DA, Plass DB, Schick DA, Melton ME. Precision and accuracy of computed digital absorptiometry for assessment of bone density of the hand. *Osteoporosis Int* 1997;7:444–449.
29. Bjarnason K, Nilas L, Hassager C, Christiansen C. Dual energy x-ray absorptiometry of the spine—decubitus lateral versus anteroposterior projection in osteoporotic women: comparison to single energy x-ray absorptiometry of the forearm. *Bone* 1995;16:255–260.
30. Cheng S, Suominen H, Sakari-Rantala R, Laukkanen P, Avikainen V, Heikkinen E. Calcaneal bone mineral density predicts fracture occurrence; a five-year follow-up study in elderly people. *J Bone Miner Res* 1997;12:1075–1082.
31. Jergas M, Genant HK. Lateral Dual x-ray absorptiometry of the lumbar spine: current status. *Bone* 1997;20:311–314.
32. Yamada M, Ito M, Hayashi K, Ohki M, Nakamura T. Dual-energy x-ray absorptiometry of the calcaneus: comparison with other techniques to assess bone density and value in predicting risk of spine fractures. *Am J Roentgenol* 1994;163:1335–1440.
33. Rand TH, Seidl G, Kainberger F, et al. Impact of spinal degenerative changes on the evaluation of bone mineral density with dual energy x-ray absorptiometry (DEXA). *Calcif Tissue Int* 1997;60:430–433.
34. Genant HK, Cann CE, Ettinger B. Quantitative computed tomography of vertebral spongiosa: a sensitive method for detecting early bone loss after oophorectomy. *Ann Intern Med* 1982;97:699–705.
35. Kalender WA, Klotz E, Suess C. Vertebral bone mineral analysis: an integrated approach with CT. *Radiology* 1987;164:419–423.
36. Van Kuijk C, Grashuis JL, Steenbeek JCM, Schütte HE, Trouerbach WTH. Evaluation of postprocessing dual-energy methods in quantitative computed tomography. Part 2: Practical aspects. *Invest Radiol* 1990;25:882–889.
37. Kuiper JW, Van Kuijk C, Grashuis JL, Ederveen AHG, Schütte HE. Accuracy and the influence of marrow fat on quantitative CT and dual-energy x-ray absorptiometry of the femoral neck *in vitro. Osteoporosis Int* 1996;6:25.
38. Lang TF, Keyak JH, Heitz MW, Augat P, Lu Y, Mathur A, Genant HK. Volumetric quantitative computed tomography of the proximal femur: precision and relation to bone strength. *Bone* 1997;21:101–108.
39. Müller A, Rüegsegger E, Rüegsegger P. Peripheral QCT. A low risk procedure to identify women predisposed to osteoporosis. *Phys Med Biol* 1989;34:741–749.
40. Schneider P, Borner W. Peripheral quantitative computed tomography for bone mineral measurement with a new special purpose QCT-scanner. *Fortschr Rontgenstr* 1991;153:292–299.
41. Orgee JM, Foster H, McCloskey EV, Khan S, Coombes G, Kanis JA. A Precise method for the assessment of tibial ultrasound velocity. *Osteoporosis Int* 1996;6:1–7.
42. Ventura V, Mauloni M, Mura M, Paltrinieri F, de Aloysio D. Ultrasound velocity changes of the proximal phalanxes of the hand in pre-, peri- and postmenopausal women. *Osteoporosis Int* 1996;6:368–375.
43. Njeh CF, Boivin CM, Langton CM. The role of ultrasound in the assessment of osteoporosis: a review. *Osteoporosis Int* 1997;7:7–22.
44. Glüer CC for the International Quantitative Ultrasound Consensus Group. Quantitative ultrasound techniques for the assessment of osteoporosis: expert agreement on current status. *J Bone Miner Res* 1997;12:1280–1288.
45. Genant HK, Block JE, Steiger P, Glüer CC, Ettinger B, Harris ST. Appropriate use of bone densitometry. *Radiology* 1989;170:817–822.
46. Johnston CC Jr, Slemenda CW, Melton LJ III. Clinical use of bone densitometry. *N Engl J Med* 1991;324:1105–1109.
47. Miller PD, Bonnick SL, Rosen CJ, Consensus of an international panel on the clinical utility of bone mass measurements in the detection of low bone mass in the adult population. *Calcif Tissue Int* 1996;58:207–214.
48. Kanis JA, Delmas P, Burckhardt P, Cooper C, Torgerson D. Guidelines for diagnosis and management of osteoporosis. *Osteoporosis Int* 1997;7:390–406.
49. WHO. Assessment of osteoporotic fracture risk and its role in screening for postmenopausal women. WHO technical reports series. Geneva: World Health Organization, 1994.
50. Ahmed AIH, Blake GM, Rymer JM, Fogelman I. Screening for osteopenia and osteoporosis: do the accepted normal ranges lead to overdiagnosis. *Osteoporosis Int* 1997;7:432–438.
51. Bonnick SL, Nichols DL, Sanborn CF, et al. Dissimilar spine and femoral Z-scores in premenopausal women. *Calcif Tissue Int* 1997;61:263–265.
52. Consensus Development Statement. Who are candidates for prevention and treatment for osteoporosis. *Osteoporosis Int* 1997;7:1–6.
53. Grampp S, Genant HK, Mathur A, et al. Comparison of non-invasive bone mineral measurements in assessing age-related loss, fracture discrimination, and diagnostic classification. *J Bone Miner Res* 1997;12:697–711.
54. Ito M, Hyashi K, Ishida Y, et al. Discrimination of spinal fractures with various bone mineral measurements. *Calcif Tissue Int* 1997;60:11–15.
55. Genant HK, Engelke K, Fuerst T, et al. Noninvasive assessment of bone mineral and structure: state of the art. *J Bone Miner Res* 1996;11:707–730.

Treatment of the Postmenopausal Woman: Basic and Clinical Aspects, Second Edition, edited by Rogerio A. Lobo, Lippincott Williams & Wilkins, Philadelphia © 1999.

CHAPTER 27

Biochemical Markers of Bone Turnover

Richard Eastell and Rosemary A. Hannon

Over the past decade several new assays have been introduced for the measurement of biochemical markers of bone turnover. These new markers are specific to bone and are sensitive to the relatively small increases in bone turnover that occur at the menopause. As a result, there is growing interest in the use of these markers in the postmenopausal woman.

The major advantages of these methods are that they are noninvasive, relatively inexpensive, and can be measured repeatedly in one subject. In this chapter we review the most commonly used markers of bone turnover and discuss the use of these markers in the care of the postmenopausal woman.

MARKERS OF BONE TURNOVER

Biochemical markers of bone turnover are generally classified as markers of bone formation or markers of bone resorption (Table 27.1), reflecting osteoblast and osteoclast activity, respectively. The ideal marker is bone specific and reflects either bone formation or bone resorption, but not both. However, it must be borne in mind that bone formation and bone resorption are coupled events in most circumstances so that any marker of bone formation or bone resorption can be used to characterize both the high-turnover state after the menopause and the decrease in bone turnover resulting from hormone replacement therapy.

Markers of Bone Formation

Procollagen Propeptides

The procollagen propeptides, procollagen type I carboxy-terminal propeptide (PICP) and procollagen type I

R. Eastell and R. A. Hannon: Bone Metabolism Group, Section of Medicine, Division of Clinical Sciences, University of Sheffield, Northern General Hospital, Sheffield S5 7AU, United Kingdom.

amino-terminal propeptide (PINP), are released into the circulation during the extracellular conversion of procollagen to collagen. Type I collagen is a trimer comprising two identical $\alpha_1(I)$ polypeptide chains and one $\alpha_2(I)$ polypeptide chain and is the major protein of bone matrix (90%) (1). It is synthesized by osteoblasts as a precursor, procollagen, and secreted into the extracellular space, where it undergoes a series of posttranslational modifications including the cleavage of the propeptides by specific proteases (Fig. 27.1). The propeptides are released into the circulation, and the newly formed collagen molecules assemble as fibrils. PICP is a globular polypeptide with a molecular mass of 100 kd that contains both intra- and interchain disulfide bridges. PINP is a smaller polypeptide, molecular mass 35 kd, with intra- but no interchain disulfide bridges. It is primarily a globular peptide but contains a small amount of helix.

Intact PINP appears to be the more sensitive marker of bone formation than PICP: the increases in PINP during the pubertal growth spurt, at the menopause, and in Paget's disease are significantly greater than those for PICP (2).

TABLE 27.1. *Biochemical markers of bone formation and bone resorption*

Markers of bone formation	Markers of bone resorption
Serum	Serum
Total and bone-specific alkaline phosphatase	Tartrate-resistant acid phosphatase
Osteocalcin	Free pyridinium crosslinks
Propeptides of type I procollagen	Telopeptides of type I collagen
	Urine
	Hydroxyproline
	Calcium
	Pydridinoline and deoxypyridinoline
	Telopeptides of type I collagen
	Galactosyl hydroxylysine

PROCOLLAGEN MOLECULE

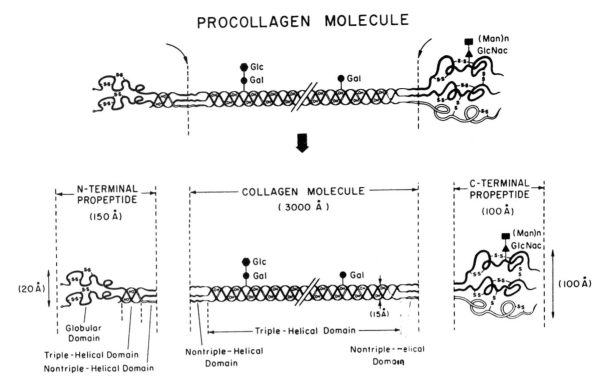

FIG. 27.1. Extracellular cleavage of the propeptides of type I collagen illustrating the origins of markers of bone formation, procollagen type I carboxy-terminal propeptide (PICP), and procollagen type I amino-terminal propeptide (PINP). (From ref. 110, with permission.)

Likewise, the percentage decrease in PINP after 1 year of hormone replacement therapy (HRT) was about 40% compared to about 20% in PICP in 47 postmenopausal women (3). There are several possible reasons for this difference in sensitivity. Although the contribution to circulating levels of the propeptides from nonosseous sources is thought to be small (4), differences in the patterns of cleavage of the propeptides from procollagen in different tissues may be responsible for intact PINP being more bone specific than PICP. PICP is completely cleaved and released in amounts equimolar to the amount of collagen synthesized in any tissue, whereas PINP is completely cleaved in collagen found in mineralized tissues but may be retained in fibers in soft tissues and released during fiber growth or collagen degradation in a degraded form (5) that is not detected by the intact PINP assay.

Differences in the clearance mechanisms of the two propeptides may also account for some of the difference in sensitivity. PICP is cleared by the mannose receptor of the liver endothelial cells, which is sensitive to hormones including estrogen, whereas PINP is cleared by the scavenger receptor of liver endothelial cells, which is thought not to be sensitive to circulating hormones (5–7).

Osteocalcin

Osteocalcin (bone Gla protein) is the most abundant noncollagenous bone matrix protein, also found in dentin. It is a small protein of 49 amino acid residues and molecular mass 58 kd that is synthesized almost exclusively by osteoblasts and is therefore bone specific, an important property for a marker of bone formation (8). The majority of newly synthesized osteocalcin is incorporated into the bone matrix, but about 10% to 30% is released into the circulation. Osteocalcin mRNA has recently been detected in bone marrow megakaryocytes and platelets in rats. However, osteocalcin levels in these cells are very low or undetectable, which suggests that the contribution from platelet osteocalcin to total circulating levels of osteocalcin is minimal (9). Osteocalcin is cleared by the kidneys and to a lesser extent by the liver. In renal failure, levels of osteocalcin and particularly its fragments are elevated (10).

The function of osteocalcin is not fully understood. It has been suggested that it is involved in the regulation of coupling of bone resorption and bone formation (11). In a recent study of osteocalcin knockout mice, bone formation was increased, but bone resorption was unaffected, which suggests that osteocalcin may be a limiting factor for bone formation (12).

A major feature of the primary structure of osteocalcin is the γ-carboxylated glutamic acid residues at positions 17, 21, and 24. The posttranslational γ-carboxylation of these residues is vitamin K dependent. Osteocalcin in bone is not completely carboxylated, and serum levels of the undercarboxylated form increase with age, especially in elderly women (13). The degree of carboxylation appears to be related to bone strength because Vergnaud et al. (14) have shown that increased serum levels of undercarboxylated osteocalcin predict hip fracture risk independently of femoral neck bone mineral density. Elderly women with hip fracture have lower levels of vitamin K_1 and menquinone 7 and 8, two major components of vitamin K_2 (15).

Although numerous immunoassays are available for the measurement of serum or plasma osteocalcin, comparability of the different assays is poor (16). This is probably because of the heterogeneity of the circulating fragments of osteocalcin and differences in the immunorecognition of these fragments by different assays. Intact osteocalcin is degraded in the circulation and *in vitro* (17). Only about 36% of circulating immunoreactive osteocalcin is the intact protein; a further 30% is a large N-midmolecule fragment (residues 1–43), and the remainder consists of smaller fragments. The six-amino-acid C terminal is the most easily cleaved fragment. The cleavage of the C-terminal fragment leaves a 1–43 N-midmolecule fragment, which appears to be relatively stable. The apparent stability (18) of immunoreactive osteocalcin is significantly greater when assays designed to measure the intact molecule and N-midmolecule fragment are used than when assays designed to measure only the intact molecule are used. Assays that measure the intact peptide and the N-midmolecule fragment are, therefore, to be recommended, particularly in clinical practice.

Alkaline Phosphatase

Total serum alkaline phosphatase has been used for many years as a marker of bone formation. Alkaline phosphatase is a membrane-bound orthophosphoric monoester phospho-2-hydrolase with optimum activity at alkaline pH. Several different isoenzymes of alkaline phosphatase exist, coded for by four different genes: tissue nonspecific, intestinal, placental, and germ-cell line. The tissue nonspecific gene codes for bone, liver, and kidney isoforms: the differences in these isoforms result from differences in the patterns of posttranslational glycosylation (19). In healthy adults, circulating alkaline phosphatase consists primarily of the bone isoform (about 50%) and the liver isoform (about 50%). Only trace amounts of the intestinal and placental isoenzymes are found in normal adult serum. Circulating placental isoenzyme is increased in pregnancy, and circulating placental-like isoenzymes are found in malignancy (20). The precise function of the bone isoform remains unclear, but it is thought to be associated with mineralization.

Total alkaline phosphatase is a useful marker of bone formation in diagnosis and monitoring of treatment of diseases characterized by major disturbances in bone turnover such as Paget's disease, and some would argue that in most clinical situations measurement of total alka-

line phosphatase provides sufficient information (21). However, there is evidence to support the contrary argument that the bone alkaline phosphatase is a more sensitive and more clinically useful marker in the measurement of more subtle changes in bone turnover, such as occur at the menopause (22,23). Garnero et al. (22) found a 77% increase in bone alkaline phosphatase after the menopause compared to a 24% increase in total alkaline phosphatase.

Until recently serum levels of bone and liver isoforms have been quantified using methods based on differences in the heat stability, urea and neuraminidase sensitivity, electrophoretic mobility, and affinity for wheat germ lectin of the two isoforms. However, immunoassays are now available that are specific for the bone isoform. The crossreactivity of these assays is between 7% and 16%, which should be a problem only in patients with liver disease (22,24).

Markers of Bone Resorption

Hydroxyproline

Hydroxyproline has been used extensively as a marker of bone resorption. It represents about 13% of the amino acid content of collagen and is released into the circulation during bone resorption but is not reincorporated into new collagen (25). It circulates either in the free form (90%) or in peptide-bound forms. Most of the free hydroxyproline is filtered and reabsorbed by the kidney. The remainder is excreted in the urine together with the dialyzable and nondialyzable peptide-bound forms. Only about 10% of the hydroxyproline released from collagen degradation is excreted in the urine. The nondialyzable form, which represents 10% of total urinary hydroxyproline, is thought to be derived from the degradation of the N-terminal procollagen propeptide (25) and to be a marker of bone formation (26). Urinary hyrdoxyproline suffers from three major disadvantages as a marker of bone resorption: (a) a significant fraction of it is derived from nonosseous sources (27); (b) hydroxyproline is absorbed from dietary sources, and diet must be restricted for 24 hours before samples are collected (28); and (c) most hydroxyproline is metabolized in the liver.

Tartrate-Resistant Acid Phosphatase

Acid phosphatase is found in several tissues including bone, platelets, erythrocytes, prostate, and spleen. These different isoenzymes can be distinguished by their different electrophoretic mobilities on polyacrylamide gels. The isoenzyme from bone migrates in the fastest band, band 5, which can be further resolved into bands 5a and 5b (29). Osteoclasts release an isoenzyme of acid phosphatase into the circulation that is indistinguishable from band 5b. Furthermore, this isoenzyme is resistant to L-

(+)-tartrate, unlike the prostatic isoenzyme (30). The precise function of this tartrate-resistant acid phosphatase (TRAP) during bone resorption is unclear. Serum and plasma TRAP are usually measured by kinetic assays. This method may lack specificity for osteoclastic TRAP (31) because TRAP from platelets, erythrocytes, and possibly osteoblasts may be present in the sample. Other disadvantages of the kinetic assays are the presence of enzyme inhibitors in the serum or plasma and the instability of frozen samples. Some of these problems may be resolved with the development of specific immunoassays for osteoclastic TRAP (32–34).

Pyridinium Collagen Crosslinks and Related Telopeptides

The markers of bone resorption that have been developed most in the last decade are pyridinium collagen crosslinks and the related telopeptides. Figure 27.2 shows the origins of these markers in collagen. The pyridinium crosslinks, pyridinoline and deoxypyridinoline, are nonreducible crosslinks found in mature collagen. They are formed by the condensation of lysine and hydroxylysine residues in the telopeptide regions and specific lysine or hydroxylysine residues in the helical regions of adjacent collagen molecules. The ratio of pyridinoline to deoxypyridinoline varies according to tissue; in bone the ratio is 3.5:1 (35). Although present in smaller amounts than pyridinoline, deoxypyridinoline is more specific to bone; deoxypyridinoline is not found in skin or cartilage, whereas large amounts of pyridinoline are found in cartilage. Small amounts of deoxypyridinoline are found in other tissues, but turnover in these tissues is limited, so the contribution to serum or urinary levels of deoxypyridinoline will be small.

During bone resorption crosslinks are released into the circulation and excreted in the urine. Free and peptide-bound forms of crosslinks are detectable in both serum and urine (36). In adult urine 40% to 50% are free, and 50% to 60% are bound (37), but the ratio of free to bound in both serum and urine may depend on the level of bone turnover: the higher the rate of bone turnover, the smaller the ratio of free to bound crosslinks (36,38). Whether crosslinks are released from the bone matrix by the osteoclasts in the free and/or peptide-bound form is debatable. An in vitro study of the action of osteoclasts on human bone suggests that osteoclasts release only peptide-bound forms (39). The peptide-bound crosslinks may be partially degraded to the free form in the kidney, by a putative saturable enzymatic process (36). The effect of rate of turnover on the ratio of free to bound crosslinks in serum and on renal handling of peptide-bound crosslinks may account, in part, for the smaller changes in free urinary crosslinks compared to the changes in bound crosslinks after antiresorptive treatment (38,40,41).

Pyridinium crosslinks are measured as free crosslinks, peptide-bound crosslinks, and total crosslinks (free plus peptide bound). Until recently urinary free and total crosslinks were usually measured by HPLC. Increased sensitivity of the method now means that crosslinks can also be measured in serum, where they are 100-fold less concentrated than in urine (36). This method probably represents the gold standard method, but immunoassays for free crosslinks and the related telopeptides have been developed that have been validated against the HPLC method and are much more convenient to use.

The immunoassays for the free pyridinolines measure either urinary pyridinoline-deoxypyridinoline or deoxypyridinoline alone (42,43). The urinary peptide-bound crosslinks can be assessed by measuring either the N-telopeptide of type I collagen (NTx) or C-telopeptide (crosslaps, CTx). The NTx assay is a competitive enzyme-linked immunosorbent assay (ELISA) that uses monoclonal antibodies raised against the N-telopeptide crosslinking domain of type I collagen extracted from adolescent urine (44). The CTx assay is also a competitive ELISA assay and uses polyclonal antibodies raised against a synthetic eight-amino-acid sequence that corre-

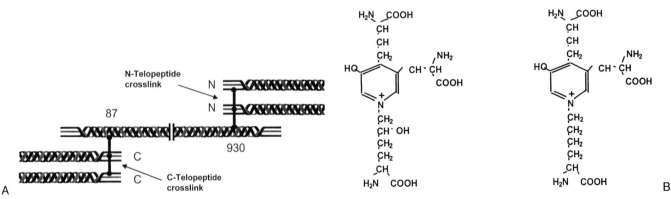

FIG. 27.2. A: Schematic diagram illustrating the location of the N- and C-telopeptide crosslinks in type I collagen and **(B)** the structures of pyridinoline **(left)** and deoxypyridinoline.

sponds to the region of the C telopeptide of the $\alpha_1(I)$ chain, the second residue of which is involved in the pyridinoline and deoxypyridinoline crosslinks (45). These assays measure both pyridinoline and deoxypyridinoline peptide-bound crosslinks.

One of the major disadvantages of measuring urinary crosslinks is the large intraindividual variability of urinary markers (46). This problem may be overcome by measuring crosslinks in serum. One serum marker of collagen degradation, carboxy-terminal telopeptide ICTP, has been in use for some time. It has proved to be a useful marker in the study of metastatic bone diseases, but in studies where smaller changes in bone turnover are observed, it lacks specificity as a marker of bone resorption and is probably best regarded as a marker of overall bone turnover (47,48). More recently, sensitive HPLC methods discussed above and immunoassays for NTx and CTx have been developed (49,50) to measure crosslinks in serum.

Urinary Hydroxylysyl Glycosides

The galactosyl hydroxylysines, β-1-glactosyl-O-hydroxylysine (GH) and β-1,2-glucosyl-galactosyl-O-hydroxylysine (GGH), like the pyridinium crosslinks, are products of collagen degradation and are excreted in the urine. The ratio of GGH/GH is 1.61 and 0.15 for human adult skin and bone, respectively; hence, GH may be regarded as a fairly specific marker for bone collagen (51). Urinary GH and GGH are measured by conversion of the amino groups of hydroxylysine into fluorescent dansyl derivatives before their separation by reverse-phase HPLC (52). Bettica et al. (53), in a small comparative study, suggest that GH is comparable to urinary deoxypyridinoline and pyridinoline as a marker of bone resorption, although in a recent study of postmenopausal women, GH did not respond to HRT (54). Use of GH as a marker of bone resorption still requires further evaluation.

Summary

Thus, many markers are currently available. In clinical research we recommend measuring two markers of bone formation and two markers of bone resorption, and in clinical practice one marker of bone formation and one marker of bone resorption. We would choose bone alkaline phosphatase (immunoassay), osteocalcin (intact plus N-midfragment assay), or PINP as a marker(s) of bone formation and free deoxypyridinoline, NTx, or CTx as a marker(s) of bone resorption.

VARIABILITY OF MARKERS

Although biochemical markers are useful noninvasive tools that can be used repeatedly in the same patient to assess bone turnover, one of the major confounding factors for their use is their variability. There are numerous sources of variability such as age, gender, pubertal stage, menopausal status, diseases, drugs, fractures, and menstrual, seasonal, day-to-day, and circadian cycles. The main components of overall intraindividual variability are analytic and biologic. Analytic variability is small compared to biologic variability for most assays (55,56). In the normal healthy adult, the strongest influences on the intraindividual variability are circadian, menstrual, and seasonal variability.

The intraindividual variability is greater for the urinary markers than for the serum markers. The intraindividual variability for serum markers is in the order of 10%, whereas for urinary markers it may be as much as 35% (46,55). This difference may result from difficulties in timing and completeness of urine collections or day-to-day changes in renal clearance or the renal conversion of peptide-bound to free crosslinks. Variability may also be affected by osteoporosis, tending to be higher for all markers in women with postmenopausal osteoporosis than in normal postmenopausal women (57).

Intraindividual variability has considerable impact on the use of markers in research and in clinical practice. A useful concept that accounts for the intraindividual variability when deciding if there has been a true biologic change in a marker is that of the least significant change. The least significant change is calculated from the intraindividual variation and represents a cutoff point. Any change between two measurements must be greater than this cutoff point to be biologically significant.

Circadian rhythms can have a major impact on variability of the markers. Both markers of bone resorption and bone formation exhibit circadian rhythms, reaching a peak between 2300 and 0800 and falling to a nadir between 1200 and 1700. The greatest circadian changes are seen in the urinary markers of bone resorption. In young women, the amplitude of the variation, i.e., the difference from peak to trough, is 70% of the mean value for 24 hours for total deoxypyridinoline (DPD) (Fig. 27.3) and 63% for NTx (58). The amplitude of the circadian rhythm of free deoxypyridinoline appears to be smaller than that of crosslinked telopeptides (46), and the amplitude of the variation for bone formation markers ranges from 5% to 30% (59–62).

These circadian rhythms are maintained into old age (63). In late postmenopausal women with osteopenia or osteoporosis, the circadian rhythm of some biochemical markers of bone turnover appears to be disturbed. The peak in total DPD excretion is extended into the morning in women with osteoporosis compared to healthy age-matched women (64). However in women with osteopenia (forearm BMC more than 2 SD below premenopausal mean BMC), the circadian rhythm in total DPD is the same as that for age-matched women (65). The nocturnal peak in PICP, but not in osteocalcin or bone alkaline phosphatase, is higher and extended in the osteopenic women (60).

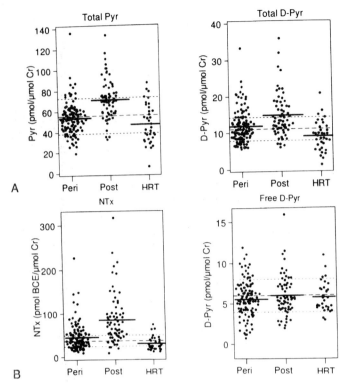

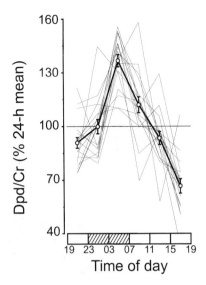

FIG. 27.4. Circadian variation in excretion of deoxypyridino-line (DPD) in 18 healthy premenopausal women. Results are shown as percentages of the 24-hour mean excretion in each subject. Each thin line represents one individual. The solid lines represent the mean ± SEM of the normalized values. Data are plotted at the midpoint of each 4-hour collection period. Subjects were recumbent with the lights off during the period indicated by the shaded bar. (Modified from ref. 58, with permission.)

FIG. 27.3. Individual values for four biochemical markers of bone resorption in 221 perimenopausal women and post-menopausal women, and postmenopausal women on hormone replacement therapy. For each marker, the solid line represents the group mean; the dashed line and dotted lines in the background represent, respectively, the mean ± 1 SD for premenopausal women. **A:** Total pyridinoline and total deoxypyridinoline. **B:** NTx and free deoxypyridinoline. (From ref. 78, with permission.)

The implications of these circadian rhythms are considerable both in investigative studies and in clinical practice. For example, if NTx is measured in a urine sample collected in the early morning (0700) and in a second sample collected in the afternoon (1500), there could be a difference in the measurements of 50%, which is comparable to the change in NTx expected after 6 months of HRT (Fig. 27.4).

Menstrual and seasonal variations in markers are much weaker than the circadian variations. Markers of bone formation have been shown to be 15% higher in the luteal phase than in the follicular phase (66). Urinary levels of markers of resorption, NTx and total pyridinium crosslinks, are somewhat higher during the earlier parts of follicular and luteal phases than in the later parts of the phases (67). ICTP, a serum marker of bone resorption, is 17% higher in the luteal phase than in the follicular phase (68).

Seasonal variation in markers of bone turnover has been observed in several but not all studies (69–72). In most studies that have demonstrated a significant seasonal rhythm, bone turnover tends to be lower in the summer than in the winter (70,72). Woigte et al. (72) have recently suggested that the seasonal variation may account for as much as 12% of the variability of markers of bone turnover.

The impact of fractures and drugs on intraindividual variability of markers is particularly important for post-menopausal women. They have an increased risk of fracture and are more likely to be taking drugs that affect bone metabolism than premenopausal women. Biochemical markers of bone formation and bone resorption increase up to 30% during the healing of a Colles fracture, a characteristic osteoporotic fracture (73). Furthermore, the markers can remain elevated for up to 1 year after the fracture.

In addition to drugs taken to prevent bone loss, such as hormone replacement therapy and bisphosphonates, other drugs can affect levels of biochemical markers. Corticosteroids suppress bone formation without having a direct effect on bone resorption. Consequently, markers of bone formation, in particular osteocalcin, are reduced during corticosteroid treatment. There may be a small increase in markers of bone resorption as a result of a secondary hyperparathyroidism induced by the effect of the corticosteroid on calcium absorption. Thiazide diuretics reduce bone turnover (74). Conversely, treatment with anticonvulsant drugs results in threefold increases in markers of bone resorption (75) and increases of up to 33% in markers of bone formation in women (76).

Summary

A number of strategies can be followed to minimize variability: (a) samples, particularly for resorption markers, should be collected at a fixed time of day; (b) two or more samples can be collected on different days within a given period, and the mean level of the marker reported; (c) patients should be asked about previous fractures and use of drugs.

CHANGES IN MARKERS AT MENOPAUSE, IN OSTEOPOROSIS, AND IN RESPONSE TO THERAPY

Menopause

Estrogen deficiency caused by amenorrhea or drug therapy, such as GnRH agonist therapy, results in a rapid increase in the levels of markers of bone turnover (54). Similarly, the menopause is marked by an increase in levels of markers. The magnitude of the increase varies for the different markers, probably reflecting their specificity for bone or differences in their metabolism in low- and high-turnover states. The markers probably start to increase in the perimenopausal period before menstruation has ceased. Premenopausal women over the age of 40 years have higher levels of CTx and osteocalcin than younger women (77), which may be weakly associated with lower BMD. In women with altered menstrual patterns, where FSH is elevated but estradiol is still at premenopausal levels, NTx is increased by 20%, but formation markers are unchanged, compared to premenopausal levels (Fig. 27.3) (78). Once the estradiol levels decrease, markers of bone resorption and formation increase (79).

In the first years of the menopause, mean levels of pyridinium crosslinks excretion significantly increase and may even be doubled (44,80,81), but there is still considerable overlap with levels in premenopausal women. The increases in the telopeptides and in total crosslinks are greater than the increase in the free pyridinolines, possibly for reasons discussed above (78,82). Garnero et al. (38) found increases of 80% to 100% in total crosslinks measured by HPLC, 100% to 130% in telopeptides, and 50% in free deoxypyridinoline in a comparative study of 14 premenopausal women aged 33 to 44 years and 29 postmenopausal women aged 46 to 53 years who were within 3 years of the menopause. There is a considerably smaller increase in the serum markers of bone resorption, TRAP and ICTP, of the order of 20% to 25% (83,84).

The differences in the increases in markers of bone formation in postmenopausal women may be related to the different aspects of bone formation that each marker reflects. They may also reflect a difference in tissue specificities of the markers. The increases in bone alkaline phosphatase and osteocalcin are of the order of 50% to 100% but may be as high as 150%. The increase in PICP is considerably less, around 20%. PINP, which may be the most bone-specific propeptide, shows the greatest increase at the menopause (85).

Whether the increase in bone turnover that occurs at the menopause is maintained into old age has been questioned (86), but we have found elevated levels of bone turnover in women into their eighth decade (87). More recently Garnero et al. have shown that NTx and CTx and markers of bone formation remain elevated in women for 40 years after the menopause (88).

Osteoporosis

Markers of bone resorption are significantly elevated in osteoporotic postmenopausal women as compared to normal postmenopausal women, but the markers of bone formation are much less elevated and may indeed be decreased (89,90). This pattern of changes suggests that a degree of imbalance between bone resorption and bone formation occurs in osteoporosis. We found a mean increase of 40% in the level of total deoxypyridinoline in a group of 63 women with postmenopausal osteoporosis compared to a group of 67 normal postmenopausal women (91). However, there was a considerable overlap of individual levels in the two groups. The heterogeneity of bone resorption in the osteoporotic group probably indicates different causes of the disease or may represent differences in the stage observed in the individuals in the study. Single measurements of total and free crosslinks are unlikely to be useful in identifying osteoporosis in an individual postmenopausal woman. However, a recent study suggests that NTx can discriminate among normal postmenopausal, osteopenic, and osteoporotic women, as defined by the WHO criteria (92). Further work is required in this area, especially with the newer markers of bone turnover.

Response to Therapy

Antiresorptive therapy, such as HRT or bisphosphonate, reduces markers of bone turnover to premenopausal levels, and indeed, it has been suggested that the therapeutic goal should be the premenopausal mean.

In general, the markers of resorption decrease rapidly and reach a plateau between 3 and 6 months, whereas the markers of formation do not decrease for the first 6 to 8 weeks and then decrease steadily for at least 4 months (Fig. 27.5). In the first 6 months of treatment, the timing of the measurement is critical in the interpretation. After 6 months of HRT, the decrease in markers of bone resorption ranges from 10% for the serum markers to 80% for the urinary telopeptides (41). The change in the telopeptide markers is greater than that of the free crosslinks, and the decrease in the total crosslinks is intermediate between the telopeptides and the free. The decreases in osteocalcin, bone alkaline phosphatase, and PICP are

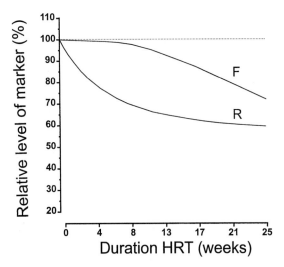

FIG. 27.5. Schematic illustration of the time course of response to hormone replacement therapy for markers of bone formation (F) and markers of bone resorption (R). (From ref. 111, with permission.)

25% to 30% (93). PINP, on the other hand, decreases by 40%, which is in keeping with the differences in specificity and clearance between PICP and PINP (3). Similar decreases in markers are found after bisphosphonate treatment, although Garnero et al. found that free crosslinks responded significantly to estrogen therapy but not to alendronate (94). The response of markers to alendronate is dose dependent (95). The responses of the markers to another bisphosphonate, cyclic etidronate, although significant, are not quite as great as those in alendronate therapy (96).

PREDICTION OF BONE LOSS, FRACTURE, AND RESPONSE TO THERAPY

Bone Loss

Bone mineral density in the postmenopausal woman is determined by peak bone mass and the amount of bone lost since the menopause. With increasing age, the contribution of bone loss to the resultant BMD becomes more significant (97). Furthermore, increased bone turnover becomes an increasingly important determinant of BMD as women grow older (88). In several studies bone loss has been shown to correlate with markers of bone turnover, although this is not a universal finding. In 1977, Christiansen et al. (98) estimated the rate of bone loss from four parameters—calculated fat mass, alkaline phosphatase, fasting urinary hydroxyproline, and fasting urinary calcium—in early postmenopausal women and identified so-called fast and slow losers (i.e., bone loss ≥3% per year and <3% per year). After 12 years the fast losers had lost 26.6%, and the slow losers 16%, bone mineral content at the forearm (99). In other studies of

women in the first 7 years after the menopause, a combination of resorption and formation markers or a combination of pyridinoline with estradiol glucuronide and body mass index can predict up to 59% of the variance of bone loss at the forearm (100,101). Change in BMD at the spine and hip, the clinically relevant sites, can be only poorly predicted, if at all (102,103). In women over the age of 70 years, the correlation between baseline levels of biochemical markers and annual rate of change of BMD over a 3-year period, at the total hip, was at best moderate (104). A combination of osteocalcin, NTx, and serum PTH predicted only 43% of the variance of rate of change in BMD at the total hip.

Fracture

Although biochemical markers of bone turnover may be able to predict bone loss and hence fracture risk, they may also predict fracture risk independently of bone mineral density. High bone turnover per se can disrupt the trabecular architecture by increasing the incidence of trabecular perforation and buckling, thus reducing bone strength, without necessarily affecting bone mineral density significantly. In retrospective and prospective studies, fracture risk is associated with increased levels of markers of bone resorption but not bone formation, although in one study decreased levels of ICTP significantly increased the risk of fracture (105). This may be an example of ICTP acting not as a typical marker of bone resorption but more as a general marker of bone turnover. In a short prospective study of elderly French women, a 1 SD increase in CTx and free deoxypyridinoline, adjusted for femoral neck BMD and gait, above the upper limit for premenopausal women, resulted in a two- or 1.7-fold increase, respectively, in risk of hip fracture over a 22-month follow-up period (106). Increased pyridinolines have also been shown to predict a history of fracture independent of BMD, age, and other markers of bone turnover (107).

However, there is little convincing evidence to indicate that a single measurement of a biochemical marker of bone turnover can predict fracture risk in an individual woman, even over a short period of time. The combination of a biochemical marker and BMD may be a much more powerful predictor of fracture than BMD alone. Women with a low hip BMD (<2.5 SD below premenopausal mean) and high CTx (>2 SD above premenopausal mean) have a considerably higher risk of hip fracture than those who have only one of these independent risk factors (106).

For the individual early postmenopausal woman, a single measurement of a biochemical marker of bone turnover is unlikely to be of much use in predicting bone loss (108) or fracture risk over her postmenopausal life. A better prediction may result from the use of several markers combined with each other or with other measurements, such as body mass index or hormone levels. Biochemical markers of bone turnover cannot subsitute for serial bone mineral density measurements but may be useful when considered in conjunction with BMD measurement.

Response to Therapy

Antiresorptive therapy, HRT and bisphosphonate therapy, reduce markers of bone resorption and bone formation to premenopausal levels (Fig. 27.3). The response to antiresorptive treatment may be greater in those with higher initial levels of bone turnover. Every increase of 30 nM BCE/mM creatinine in NTx increased fivefold the odds of a gain in BMD at the lumbar spine after 1 year of HRT (109). Markers may therefore have a role in predicting and monitoring response to therapy.

MONITORING THERAPY

For the individual woman the change in bone mineral density in the first year of antiresorptive treatment is not large enough, relative to the precision of the measurements, to determine whether she has responded to the treatment. So it is often normal clinical practice to wait for 1 to 2 years before repeating the bone density measurement. The advantage of using markers of bone turnover to monitor response is that a significant change may be seen between 3 and 6 months after initiation of treatment. If markers are to be used in monitoring therapy, it is important to remember that the magnitude of the observed change per se may yield very little and possibly misleading information if it is not considered relative to the intraindividual variability of the marker concerned. For a woman who has two single measurements at baseline and after 6 months of treatment, for example, the change must be greater than the LSC (described above) for that marker for her to be classified as a responder. An understanding of the time course of the changes in markers, particularly in the first 6 months, is also important in making decisions based on monitoring response with markers. Figure 27.5 illustrates that although a marker of bone resorption may have almost reached its nadir at 3 months, and a measurement at this time may yield useful information, a measurement of bone formation should be made at 6 months.

CONCLUSION

Biochemical markers of bone turnover have proved to be useful, noninvasive, and relatively inexpensive tools for studying bone metabolism in population studies, but they do not as yet have an established role in the management of the individual postmenopausal woman. The most likely role will probably be in monitoring response to therapy. However, full evaluation of biochemical markers of bone turnover in clinical practice has yet to be carried out.

REFERENCES

1. Burgeson RE. New collagens, new concepts (review). *Annu Rev Cell Biol* 1988;4:551–577.
2. Naylor KE, Blumsohn A, Hannon RA, Peel NFA, Eastell R. Different responses of carboxy and amino terminal propeptides of type I collagen. *J Bone Miner Res* 1996;11:S194.
3. Suvanto-Luukkonen E, Risteli L, Sundstrom H, Penttinen J, Kauppila A, Risteli J. Comparison of three serum assays for bone collagen formation during postmenopausal estrogen-progestin therapy. *Clin Chim Acta* 1997;266:105–116.
4. Risteli J, Melkko J, Niemi S, Risteli L. Use of a marker of collagen formation in osteoporosis studies. *Calcif Tissue Int* 1991;49:S24–S25.
5. Risteli J, Niemi S, Kauppila S, Melkko J, Risteli L. Collagen propeptides as indicators of collagen assembly. *Acta Orthop Scand* 1995;66:1–6.
6. Melkko J, Hellevik T, Risteli L, Risteli J, Smedsrod B. Clearance of NH2-terminal propeptides of types I and III procollagen is a physiological function of the scavenger receptor in liver endothelial cells. *J Exp Med* 1994;179:405–412.
7. Smedsrod B, Melkko J, Risteli L, Risteli J. Circulating C-terminal propeptide of type I procollagen is cleared mainly via the mannose receptor in liver endothelial cells. *Biochem J* 1990;271:345–350.
8. Price PA, Otsuka AS, Poser JW, Kristaponis J, Raman N. Characterization of a gamma-carboxyglutamic acid-containing protein from bone. *Proc Natl Acad Sci USA* 1976;73:1447–1451.
9. Thiede MA, Smock SL, Petersen DN, Grasser WA, Thompson DD, Nishimoto SK. Presence of messenger ribonucleic acid encoding osteocalcin, a marker of bone turnover, in bone marrow megakaryocytes and peripheral blood platelets. *Endocrinology* 1998;135:929–937.
10. Delmas PD, Wilson DM, Mann KG, Riggs BL. Effect of renal function on plasma levels of bone gla-protein. *J Clin Endocrinol Metab* 1983;57:1028–1030.
11. Skjodt H, Gallagher JA, Beresford JN, Couch M, Poser JW, Russell RGG. Vitamin D metabolites regulate osteocalcin synthesis and proliferation of human bone cells *in vitro*. *J Endocrinol* 1985;105:391–396.
12. Ducy P, Desbois C, Boyce B, et al. Increased bone formation in osteocalcin-deficient mice. *Nature* 1996;382:448–452.
13. Cairns JR, Price CA. Direct demonstration that the vitamin K-dependent bone gla protien is incompletely γ-carboxylated. *J Bone Miner Res* 1994;9:1989–1998.
14. Vergnaud P, Garnero P, Meunier PJ, Breart G, Kamihagi K, Delmas PD. Undercarboxylated osteocalcin measured with a specific immunoassay predicts hip fracture in elderly women: the EPIDOS study. *J Clin Endocrinol Metab* 1997;82:719–724.
15. Hodges SJ, Pilkington MJ, Stamp TC, et al. Depressed levels of circulating menaquinones in patients with osteoporotic fractures of the spine and femoral neck. *Bone* 1991;12:387–389.
16. Masters PW, Jones RG, Purves DA, Cooper EH, Cooney JM. Commercial assays for serum osteocalcin give clinically discordant results. *Clin Chem* 1994;40:358–363.
17. Garnero P, Grimaux M, Segain P, Delmas PD. Characterisation of immunoreactive forms of human osteocalcin generated *in vivo* and *in vitro*. *J Bone Miner Res* 1994;9:255–264.
18. Blumsohn A, Hannon RA, Eastell R. Apparent instability of osteocalcin in serum as measured with different commercially available immunoassays. *Clin Chem* 1995;41:318–319.
19. Fishman WH. Alkaline phosphatase isozymes: Recent progress. *Clin Biochem* 1990;23:99–104.
20. van Hoof VO, De Broe ME. Interpretation and clinical significance of alkaline phosphatase isoenzyme patterns. *CRC Crit Rev Clin Lab Sci* 1994;31:197–293.
21. Woitge HW, Seibel MJ, Ziegler R. Comparison of total and bone-specific alkaline phosphatase in patients with nonskeletal disorders or metabolic bone diseases. *Clin Chem* 1996;42:1796–1804.
22. Garnero P, Delmas PD. Assessment of the serum levels of bone alkaline phosphatase with a new immunoradiometric assay in patients with metabolic bone disease. *J Clin Endocrinol Metab* 1993;77:1046–1053.
23. Takahashi M, Kushida K, Hoshino H, Miura M, Ohishi T, Inoue T. Comparison of bone and total alkaline phosphatase activity on bone turnover during menopause and in patients with established osteoporosis. *Clin Endocrinol* 1997;47:177–183.
24. Price CP, Milligan TP, Darte C. Direct comparison of performance characteristics fo two immunoassays for bonr isoform of alkaline phosphatase in serum. *Clin Chem* 1997;43:2052–2057.
25. Prockop DJ, Kivirikko KI, Tudermann L, Guzman NA. The biosynthesis of collagen and its disorders. *N Engl J Med* 1979;301:12–23.
26. Haddad JG, Couranz S, Avioli LV. Nondializable urinary hydroxyproline as an index of bone collagen formation. *J Clin Endocrinol* 1970;30:282–287.
27. Deacon AC, Hulme P, Hesp R, Green JR, Tellez M, Reeve J. Estimation of whole body bone resorption rate: a comparison of urinary total hydroxyproline excretion with two radioisotopic tracer methods in osteoporosis. *Clin Chim Acta* 1987;166:297–306.
28. Gasser A, Celada A, Courvoisier B, et al. The clinical measurement of urinary total hydroxyproline excretion. *Clin Chim Acta* 1979;95:487–491.
29. Yam LT. Clinical significance of the human acid phosphatases. *Am J Med* 1974;56:604–616.
30. Lam W, Eastlund DT, Li CY, Yam LT. Biochemical properties of tartrate-resistant acid phosphatase in serum of adults and children. *Clin Chem* 1978;24:1105–1108.
31. Ballanti P, Minisola S, Pacitti MT, et al. Tartrate-resistant acid phosphatase activity as osteoclastic marker: sensitivity of cytochemical assessment and serum

assay in comparison with standardised osteoclast histomorphometry. *Osteoporosis Int* 1997;7:39–43.

32. Kraenzlin ME, Lau KHW, Liange L, et al. Development of an immunoassay for human serum osteoclastic tartrate-resistant acid phosphatase. *J Clin Endocrinol Metab* 1990;71(2):442–451.

33. Halleen J, Hentunen TA, Hellman J, Vaananen HK. Tartrate-resistant acid phosphatase from human bone: purification and development off an immunoassay. *J Bone Miner Res* 1996;11:1444–1452.

34. Cheung CK, Panesar NS, Haines C, Masarei J, Swaminathan R. Immunoassay of a tartrate-resistant acid phosphatase in serum. *Clin Chem* 1995;41:679–686.

35. Eyre DR, Koob TJ, Van Ness KP. Quantitation of hydroxypyridinium crosslinks in collagen by high performance liquid chromatography. *Anal Biochem* 1984;137:380–388.

36. Colwell A, Eastell R. The renal clearance of free and conjugated pyridinium crosslinks of collagen. *J Bone Miner Res* 1996;11:1976–1980.

37. Seibel MJ, Woitge H, Scheidt-Nave C, et al. Urinary hydroxypyridinium crosslinks of collagen in a population-based screening for overt vertebral osteoporosis: results of a pilot study. *J Bone Miner Res* 1994;9:1433–1440.

38. Garnero P, Gineyts E, Arbault P, Christiansen C, Delmas P. Different effects of bisphosphonates and estrogen therapy on free and peptide bound bone crosslinks excretion. *J Bone Miner Res* 1995;10:641–649.

39. Apone S, Lee MY, Eyre DR. Osteoclasts generate cross-linked collagen N-telopeptides (NTx) but not free pyridinolines when cultured on human bone. *Bone* 1997;21:129–136.

40. Blumsohn A, Naylor KE, Assiri AM, Eastell R. Different responses of biochemical markers of bone resorption to bisphosphonate therapy in Paget disease. *Clin Chem* 1995;41:1592–1598.

41. Rosen CJ, Chesnut CH III, Mallinak NJS. The predictive value of biochemical markers of bone turnover for bone mineral density in early postmenopausal women treated with hormone replacement or calcium supplementation. *J Clin Endocrinol Metab* 1997;82:1904–1910.

42. Seyedin SM, Kung VT, Daniloff YN, et al. Immunoassay for urinary pyridinoline—the new marker of bone resorption. *J Bone Miner Res* 1993;8:635–641.

43. Robins SP, Woitge H, Hesley R, Ju J, Seyedin S, Seibel M. Direct, enzyme-linked immunoassay for urinary deoxypyridinoline as a specific marker for measuring bone resorption. *J Bone Miner Res* 1994;9:1643–1649.

44. Hanson DA, Weis MAE, Bollen A, Maslan SL, Singer FR, Eyre DR. A specific immunoassay for monitoring human bone resorption: Quantitation of type 1 collagen cross-linked n-telopeptides in urine. *J Bone Miner Res* 1992;7:1251–1258.

45. Bonde M, Qvist P, Fledelius C, Riis BJ, Christiansen C. Immunoassay for quantifying type I collagen degradation products in urine evaluated. *Clin Chem* 1994;40:2022–2025.

46. Ju HJ, Leung S, Brown B, et al. Comparison of analytical performance and biological variability of three bone resorption assays. *Clin Chem* 1997;43:1570–1576.

47. Hassager C, Jensen LT, Podenphant J, Thomsen K, Christiansen C. The carboxy-terminal pyridinoline cross-linked telopeptide of type I collagen in serum as a marker of bone resorption: the effect of nandrolone decanoate and hormone replacement therapy. *Calcif Tissue Int* 1994;54:30–33.

48. Prestwood KM, Pilbeam CC, Burleson JA, et al. The short term effects of conjugated estrogen on bone turnover in older women. *J Clin Endocrinol Metab* 1994;79:366–371.

49. Clemens JD, Herrick MV, Singer FR, Eyre DR. Evidence that serum NTx (collagen-type I N-telopeptide) can act as an immunochemical marker of bone resorption. *Clin Chem* 1997;43:2058–2063.

50. Bonde M, Garnero P, Fledelius C, Qvist P, Delmas PD, Christiansen C. Measurement of bone degradation products in serum using antibodies reactive with an isomerized form of an 8 amino acid sequence of the C-telopeptide of type I collagen. *J Bone Miner Res* 1997;12:1028–1034.

51. Segrest JP. Urinary metabolites of collagen. *Methods Enzymol* 1982;82:398–410.

52. Moro L, Modricky C, Stagni N, Vittur F, de Bernard B. High-performance liquid chromatographic analysis if urinary hydroxylysyl glycosides as indicators of collagen turnover. *Analyst* 1984;109:1621–1622.

53. Bettica P, Moro L, Robins SP, et al. Bone resorption markers galactosyl hydroxylysine, pyridinium crosslinks and hydroxproline compared. *Clin Chem* 1992;38:2313–2318.

54. Marshall LA, Cain DF, Dmowski WP, Chesnut CHI. Urinary N-telopeptides to monitor bone resorption while on GnRH agonist therapy. *Obstet Gynecol* 1996;87:350–354.

55. Panteghini M, Pagani F. Biological variation in urinary excretion of pyridinium crosslinks: recommendations for the optimum specimen. *Ann Clin Biochem* 1996;33:36–42.

56. Panteghini M, Pagani F. Biological variation in bone-derived biochemical markers in serum. *Scand J Clin Lab Invest* 1995;55:609–616.

57. Beck Jensen J, Sorensen HA, Kollerup G, Jensen LB, Sorensen OH. Biological variation of biochemical bone markers. *Scand J Clin Lab Invest* 1994;54:36–39.

58. Blumsohn A, Herrington K, Hannon RA, Shao P, Eyre DR, Eastell R. The effect of calcium supplementation on the circadian rhythm of bone resorption. *J Clin Endocrinol Metab* 1994;79:730–735.

59. Neilsen HK, Brixen K, Mosekilde L. Diurnal rhythm in serum activity of wheat-germ lectin alkaline phosphatase: temporal relationships with the diurnal rhythm of serum osteocalcin. *Scand J Clin Lab Invest* 1990;58:851–856.

60. Pedersen BJ, Schlemmer A, Rosenquist C, Hassager C, Christiansen C. Circadian rhythm in type I collagen formation in postmenopausal women with and without osteopenia. *Osteoporosis Int* 1995;5:472–477.

61. Eastell R, Simmons PS, Colwell A, et al. Nyctohemeral changes in bone turnover assessed by serum bone gla-protein concentration and urinary deoxypyridinoline excretion: effects of growth and ageing. *Clin Sci* 1992;83:375–382.

62. Hassager C, Risteli J, Risteli L, Jensen SB, Christiansen C. Diurnal variation in serum markers of type I collagen synthesis and degradation in healthy premenopausal women. *J Bone Miner Res* 1992;7:1307–1311.

63. Greenspan SL, Dresner-Pollak R, Parker RA, London D, Ferguson L. Diurnal variation of bone mineral turnover in elderly men and women. *Calcif Tissue Int* 1997;60:419–423.

64. Eastell R, Calvo MS, Burritt MF, Offord KP, Russell RGG, Riggs BL. Abnormalities in circadian patterns of bone resorption and renal calcium conservation in type-I osteoporosis. *J Clin Endocrinol Metab* 1992;74:487–494.

65. Schlemmer A, Hassager C, Pedersen BJ, Christiansen C. Posture, age, menopause, and osteoporosis do not not influence the circadian variation in the urinary excretion of pyridinium crosslinks. *J Bone Miner Res* 1994;9:1883–1888.

66. Nielsen HK, Brixen K, Bouillon R, Mosekilde L. Changes in biochemical markers of osteoblastic activity during the menstrual cycle. *J Clin Endocrinol Metab* 1990;70:1431–1437.

67. Gorai I, Chaki O, Nakayama H, Minaguchi H. Urinary biochemical markers for bone resorption during the menstrual cycle. *Calcif Tissue Int* 1995;57:100–104.

68. Schlemmer A, Hassager C, Risteli J, Risteli L, Jensen SB, Christiansen C. Possible variation in bone resorption during the normal menstrual cycle. *Acta Endocrinol* 1993;129:388–392.

69. Vanderschueren D, Gevers G, Dequeker J, et al. Seasonal variation in bone metabolism in young healthy subjects. *Calcif Tissue Int* 1991;49:84–89.

70. Thomsen K, Eriksen EF, Jorgensen JCR, Charles P, Mosekilde L. Seasonal variation of serum bone GLA protein. *Scand J Clin Lab Invest* 1989;49:605–611.

71. Douglas AS, Miller MH, Reid DM, Hutchison JD, Porter RW, Robins SP. Seasonal differences in biochemical parameters of bone remodelling. *J Clin Pathol* 1996;49:284–289.

72. Woitge HW, Scheidt-Nave C, Kissling C, et al. Seasonal variation of biochemical indexes of bone turnover: results of a population-based study. *J Clin Endocrinol Metab* 1998;83:68–75.

73. Mallmin H, Ljunghall S, Larsson K. Biochemical markers of bone metabolism in patients with fracture of the distal forearm. *Clin Orthop* 1993;295:259–263.

74. Perry HMI, Jensen J, Kaiser FE, Horowitz M, Perry HM Jr, Morley JE. The effects of thiazide diuretics on calcium metabolism in the aged. *J Am Geriatr Soc* 1993;41:818–822.

75. Ohishi T, Kushida K, Takahashi M, et al. Urinary bone resorption markers in patients with metabolic bone disorders. *Bone* 1994;15:15–20.

76. Valimaki MJ, Tiihonen M, Laitinen K, et al. Bone mineral density measured by dual-energy x-ray absorptiometry and novel markers of bone formation and resorption in patients on antiepileptic drugs. *J Bone Miner Res* 1994;9:631–637.

77. Ravn P, Fledelius C, Rosenquist C, Overgaard K, Christiansen C. High bone turnover is associated with low bone density in bone pre- and postmenopausal women. *Bone* 1996;19:291–298.

78. Ebeling PR, Atley LM, Guthrie JR, et al. Bone turnover markers and bone density across the menopausal transition. *Clin Endocrinol Metab* 1996;81:3366–3371.

79. Griesmacher A, Peichl P, Pointinger P, Mateau R, Broll H. Biochemical markers in menopausal women. *Scand J Clin Lab Invest* 1998;57:64–72.

80. Hassager C, Colwell A, Assiri AM, Eastell R, Russell RG, Christiansen C. Effect of menopause and hormone replacement therapy on urinary excretion of pyridinium cross-links: a longitudinal and cross-sectional study. *Clin Endocrinol (Oxf)* 1992;37:45–50.

81. Uebelhart D, Gineyts E, Chapuy M, Delmas PD. Urinary excretion of pyridinium crosslinks: a new marker of bone resorption in metabolic bone disease. *Bone Miner Res* 1990;8:87–96.

82. Gorai I, Taguchi Y, Chaki O, Nakayama K, Minaguchi H. Specific changes of urinary excretion of cross-linked N-telopeptides of type I collagen in pre- and postmenopausal women: correlation with other markers of bone turnover. *Calcif Tissue Int* 1997;60:317–322.

83. Scarnecchia L, Minisola S, Pacitti MT, et al. Clinical usefulness of serum tartrate-resistant acid phosphatase activity determination to evaluate bone turnover. *Scand J Clin Lab Invest* 1991;51:517–524.

84. Hassager C, Risteli J, Risteli L, Christiansen C. Effect of the menopause and hormone replacement therapy on carboxy-terminal pyridinoline cross-linked telopeptide of type I collagen. *Osteoporosis Int* 1994;4:349–352.

85. Melkko J, Kauppila S, Niemi S, et al. Immunoassay for intact amino-terminal propeptide of human propeptide of human type I collagen. *Clin Chem* 1996;42:947–954.

86. Kelly PJ, Pocock NA, Sambrook PN, Eisman JA. Age and menopause-related changes in indices of bone turnover. *J Clin Endocrinol Metab* 1989;69(6):1160–1165.

87. Eastell R, Delmas PD, Hodgson SF, Eriksen EF, Mann KG, Riggs BL. Bone formation rate in older normal women: concurrent assessment with bone histomorphometry, calcium kinetics, and biochemical markers. *J Clin Endocrinol Metab* 1988;67:741–748.

88. Garnero P, Sornay-Rendu E, Chapuy MC, Delmas PD. Increased bone turnover in late postmenopausal women is a major determinant of osteoporosis. *J Bone Miner Res* 1996;11:337–349.

89. Valimaki MJ, Tahtela R, Jones JD, Peterson JM, Riggs BL. Bone resorption in healthy and osteoporotic postmenopausal women: comparison markers for serum carboxy-terminal telopeptide of type 1 collagen and urinary pyridinium crosslinks. *Eur J Endocrinol* 1994;131:258–262.

90. Kushida K, Takahashi M, Kawana K, Inoue T. Comparison of markers for bone formation and resorption in premenopausal and postmenopausal subjects, and osteoporosis patients. *J Clin Endocrinol Metab* 1995;80:2447–2450.

91. Eastell R, Robins SP, Colwell T, Assiri AM, Riggs BL, Russell RG. Evaluation of bone turnover in type I osteoporosis using biochemical markers specific for both bone formation and bone resorption. *Osteoporosis Int* 1993;3:255–260.

92. Schneider DL, Barrett-Connor EL. Urinary N-telopeptide levels discriminate normal, osteopenic, and osteoporotic bone mineral density. *Arch Intern Med* 1997;157:1241–1245.

93. Hassager C, Fabbri-Marbelli G, Christiansen C. The effect of the menopause and hormone replacement therapy on serum carboxy-terminal propeptide of type I collagen. *Osteoporosis Int* 1993;3:50–52.

94. Garnero P, Gineyts E, Arbault P, Christiansen C, Delmas PD. Different effects of bisphosphonate and estrogen therapy on the excretion of free and peptide-bound crosslinks. *J Bone Miner Res* 1994;9:S154.

95. Harris ST, Gertz BJ, Genant HK, et al. The effect of short term treatment with alendronate on vertebral density and biochemical markers of bone remodeling in early postmenopausal women. *J Clin Endocrinol Metab* 1993;76:1399–1406.

96. Meunier JP, Confavreux E, Tupinon I, Hardouin C, Delmas PD. Prevention of early postmenopausal bone loss with cyclical etidronate therapy (a double-blind, placebo-controlled study and 1-year follow-up). *J Clin Endocrinol Metab* 1997;82:2784–2791.

97. Hui SL, Slemenda CW, Johnston CC Jr. The contribution of bone loss to post-menopausal osteoporosis. *Osteoporosis Int* 1990;1:30–34.

98. Christiansen C, Riis BJ, Rodbro P. Prediction of rapid bone loss in post-menopausal women. *Lancet* 1987;1:1105–1108.

99. Hansen MA, Overgaard K, Riis BJ, Christiansen C. Role of peak bone mass and bone loss in postmenopausal osteoporosis—12 year study. *BMJ* 1991;303:961–964.

100. Uebelhart D, Schlemmer A, Johansen JS, Gineyts E, Christiansen C, Delmas PD. Effect of menopause and hormone replacement therapy on the urinary excretion of pyridinium crosslinks. *J Clin Endocrinol Metab* 1991;72:367–373.

101. Mole PA, Walkinshaw MH, Robins SP, Paterson CR. Can urinary pyridinium crosslinks and urinary oestrogens predict bone mass and rate of bone loss after the menopause. *Eur J Clin Invest* 1992;22:767–771.

102. Cosman F, Nieves J, Wilkinson D, Schnering D, Shen V, Lindsay R. Bone density change and biochemical indices of skeletal turnover. *Calcif Tissue Int* 1996;58:236–243.

103. Keen RW, Nguyen T, Sobnack R, Perry LA, Thompson PW, Spector TD. Can biochemical markers predict bone loss at the hip and spine? A 4-year prospective study of 141 early postmenopausal women. *Osteoporosis Int* 1996;6:399–406.

104. Dresner-Pollak R, Parker RA, Poku M, Thompson J, Seibel MJ, Greenspan SL. Biochemical markers of bone turnover reflect femoral bone loss in elderly women. *Calcif Tissue Int* 1996;59:328–333.

105. Akesson K, Ljunghall S, Jonsson B, et al. Assessment of biochemical markers of bone metabolism in relation to the occurence of fracture: a retrospective and prospective population-based study of women. *J Bone Miner Res* 1995;10:1823–1829.

106. Garnero P, Hausherr E, Chapuy M, et al. Markers of bone resorption predict hip fractures in elderly women: the EPIDOS prospective study. *J Bone Miner Res* 1996;11:1531–1538.

107. Melton LJ III, Khosla S, Atkinson EJ, O'Fallon WM, Riggs BL. Relationship of bone turnover to bone density and fracture. *J Bone Miner Res* 1997;12:1083–1091.

108. Blumsohn A, Eastell R. The performance and utility of biochemical markers fo bone turnover: do we know enough to use them in clinical practice? *Ann Clin Biochem* 1997;34:449–459.

109. Chestnutt III, Bell NH, Clark GS, et al. Hormone replacement therapy in post-menopausal women: urinary N-telopeptide of type I collagen monitors theraputic effect and predicts response of bone mineral density. *Am J Med* 1997;102:29–37.

110. Prockop DJ, Kivirikko KI, Tuderman L, Guzman NA. The biosynthesis of collagen and its disorders—First of two parts. *N Engl J Med* 1979;301:13–23.

111. Blumsohn A, Hannon RA, Eastell R. Biochemical assessment of skeletal activity. *Phys Med Rehabil Clin North Am* 1995;6:483–505.

Treatment of the Postmenopausal Woman: Basic and Clinical Aspects, Second Edition, edited by Rogerio A. Lobo, Lippincott Williams & Wilkins, Philadelphia © 1999.

CHAPTER 28

Pathophysiology of Bone Loss

Robert Lindsay and Felicia Cosman

The introduction of techniques that allow the noninvasive measurement of bone mass has made it possible to evaluate the changes that occur in the skeleton as a function of age or menopause. It is now clear that a prolonged period of bone loss precedes osteoporotic fracture. This phenomenon of bone loss is generally considered to be asymptomatic. Loss of bone tissue is accompanied, in cancellous bone, by changes in the architecture of the skeleton that further exacerbate fracture risk (1). However, because bone mass is inversely related to fracture risk, this gradual decline in bone mass produces an invariable increase in fracture risk. It is now clear that a major determinant of skeletal status among aging women is ovarian function. Loss of ovarian function at any time in a woman's life results in fundamental alterations in skeletal homeostasis that cause net loss of bone tissue (2). The fact that loss of ovarian function at menopause occurs in all women at the average age of 51 years contributes to the importance of menopause in the population of aging women. Postmenopausal women will live an average 30 years past the time of menopause, so the consequence of loss of bone mass is a gradual increase in the risk of fracture with increasing age or years from menopause (3).

Osteoporosis is now defined in terms of bone mass. A report issued by a working group of the World Health Organization defined osteoporosis as a bone mass below the range expected in young healthy adults of the same sex (statistically stated to be BMD that is more than 2.5 standard deviations below the mean for peak bone mass) (4). Those at risk of osteoporosis can then be categorized as those having bone mass that is in the low range expected in young adult life (i.e., between 1 and 2.5 standard deviations below average), with all above that being

categorized as normal. The presentation of a patient who has osteoporosis with fractures represents a complication of the disease, just as a stroke represents a complication of hypertension.

Osteoporotic fractures are now recognized as a major public health problem occurring globally but currently affecting mostly Western countries. However, as the demographics of the population change, with increasing age of the population occurring in all countries, the current public health epidemic seen in the Western countries might be expected to have a major global impact during the early part of the next century (5). Currently, the financial cost of osteoporotic fractures is enormous, exceeding $13.8 billion in the United States in 1991 for the acute care of the predominant fracture, which is fracture of the hip. Increasing health care cost and the increasing number of individuals in the "at-risk" age groups continues to assure escalation of the dollar cost of hip fracture (6). In addition, there appears, at least in some countries, to be a secular change in fracture frequency (7). The cause of this age-specific increase in fractures is not clear, but it adds further to the estimates of future costs for the disease (5).

In addition to their dollar costs, osteoporotic fractures contribute much to the chronic disability of the aging female population, and hip fractures are a major cause of death and disability among the aged (8). Hip fractures represent one of the most common causes for entry to nursing homes among the aging female population, and in that population, who can be considered to be the frail elderly, there is an even higher incidence of hip fracture than occurs in the general population. More than 50% of those individuals who fracture their hip never function again in society in the way in which they did previously. Other osteoporotic fractures such as those of the spine (vertebral crush fractures), wrist, pelvis, humerus, or other bones are also significant contributors to disability among the aging population. Because of the effects of menopause and consequent estrogen deficiency, women are at greatest risk of this disease.

A. R. Lindsay and F. Cosman: Departments of Internal Medicine and Endocrinology, Helen Hayes Hospital, West Haverstraw, New York 10993.

BONE MASS AND SKELETAL HOMEOSTASIS

The skeleton consists of two different types of bone (9). Cortical bone forms the shafts of the long bones and is a close-packed series of structures called osteons. The arrangement of cortical bone is such that it most effectively resists bending forces. Its surface area is limited primarily to an external surface (the periosteum) and an internal surface (the endosteum), on which remodeling processes can be initiated. Cancellous bone forms the internal structure of the metaphyses of long bones and the vertebral bodies and constitutes an intricate network of trabeculae, which interconnect and are designed to resist compressive stress. The surface-to-volume ratio is considerably greater for cancellous bone, and although by mass this type of bone contributes only some 20% of the skeleton, it contributes about 80% of the available surface area. Consequently, trabecular bone is considerably more metabolically active than cortical bone because the processes involved in bone remodeling are primarily surface phenomena. However, there are considerable variations among sites, perhaps in part related to the constituency of the marrow surrounding the skeletal structures. Thus, cancellous bone in the vertebral bodies has a higher rate of remodeling than the same type of bone in the hip or in the distal radius.

Bone remodeling is the process by which old bone is replaced by new bone and functions at least in part as a type of preventive maintenance program (10). In the adult, following the cessation of linear growth and under most normal circumstances, this is the major mechanism by which new bone is formed. The other process of bone formation, modeling, is the process by which the entire shape of a bone can be altered. In the adult, modeling mostly occurs in pathologic circumstances. For example, following a fracture, if the bone is set in a position of malalignment, the process of modeling will attempt to improve the alignment. A small amount of bone formation occurs throughout life on the periosteal surfaces of the long bones. Thus, as individuals age, long bones become generally larger cylinders.

The process of remodeling is discrete in both time and place (9,10). It is initiated by a poorly understood process called activation in which multinucleate giant cells called osteoclasts are recruited to the resting surface of bone (Fig. 28.1). During this process, the resting osteoblasts on the surface of bone appear to separate and allow osteoclasts to migrate to the bone surface, to which they attach securely. Osteoclasts then begin to resorb bone by forming an acid microenvironment between the cell and the tissue, which allows removal of mineral. Secretion of enzymes into this environment, including metaloproteinases and collagenase, results in removal of the organic component. By this process, a team of osteoclasts gradually moves in cancellous bone along the surface of the bone, removing preset volumes

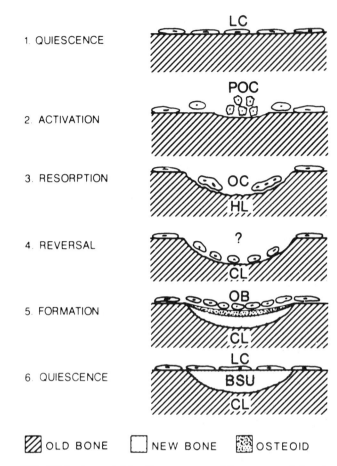

FIG. 28.1. A model for the process of bone remodeling in cancellous bone. The description is found in the text. Note the key features: POC/OC, osteoclast; HL, Howship's lacuna; CL, cement lin'e; OB, osteoblast.

of bone tissue, and in cortical bone, the osteoclast team burrows through the bone, creating an anatomic structure known as a cutting cone. In cancellous bone, the equivalent is the resorption cavity or Howship's lacuna. Osteoclasts work relatively rapidly and are followed by mononuclear cells whose function is still poorly understood but that seem to be important in preparing the bone surface for the formation of new bone tissue. These cells may also provide an important function in attracting active osteoblasts to the site of bone formation. Osteoblasts synthesize new bone by secreting collagen, which is laid down in the lamellae on the surface of the eroded bone. The process of mineralization of the collagen follows as an extracellular process by which crystals of hydroxyapatite are arranged between the collagen fibrils. Under conditions of normal homeostasis, the amount of bone that is formed is exactly equal to the amount of bone that has been removed. In other words, there is a balance across the remodeling cycle in which the net change is zero. This remodeling process is thought to be important in maintaining the vitality of the skeleton and its capacity to resist stress by ensuring that the tissue itself does not become of excessive age or rigidity. Thus, the average age of bone tissue within the skeleton is thought to be around 8 years. Increasing the age would increase the likelihood of fatigue damage and subsequent failure or fracture (11). This remodeling process also contributes to calcium homeostasis being one of the more chronic mechanisms by which calcium can be removed from the skeleton to maintain calcium levels in serum within a very tight range (9). Acute changes in serum calcium are probably not mediated by this mechanism but rather by relocation of calcium across the surfaces of cells such as the resting osteoblast population on the surface of bone and perhaps also the osteocyte population.

In order for there to be loss of bone tissue, changes must occur in the remodeling cycle. Several possibilities exist by which there could be net loss of bone. First, the osteoclast population might simply increase their capacity for bone resorption, creating larger Howship's lacunae or moving more rapidly through cortical bone. A second possibility might be disruption in the linkage between bone resorption and bone formation such that bone formation failed to follow the process of bone resorption. A third possibility might be that the osteoblast population failed to completely refill the hole created by the osteoclasts. In each of those scenarios, there would be a net loss of bone across the remodeling cycle that would be permanent at that site until another remodeling cycle was initiated at the same location, when the process could be repaired. It seems entirely feasible that each of these mechanisms contributes to bone loss, although the relative importance of each varies, perhaps with age and type of insult. A final possibility that would result in a transient reversible loss of bone would be an increase in the frequency with which new remodeling sites are activated. In this situation, when the increase in remodeling occurs, there would be a temporary increase in the proportion of bone within the skeleton that was undergoing the process of resorption. As the remodeling activation frequency attained a new steady state, assuming that there is no net change across each individual remodeling cycle, there would be no further loss of bone. If the activation of bone remodeling were to be slowed again, then there would be a transient apparent increase in bone mass until once again the process reached a new steady state.

A wide variety of insults can modify bone remodeling as individuals age. In 1941, Fuller Albright pointed out that osteoporosis was more common among women who had lost ovarian function before the average age of menopause and that there was a high frequency of surgical ovariectomy in his patients presenting with osteoporotic fractures (12). This focused attention on the role of ovarian failure and the pathophysiology of osteoporosis. However, it was not until techniques for evaluating skeletal mass or density using noninvasive technology became available that this process could be studied in detail. It is now apparent that estrogen deficiency at any time during adult life causes changes within the skeletal remodeling system that result in net loss of bone mass. If this is prolonged, loss of bone mass is accompanied by architectural changes that, in combination, result in a dramatic increase in the likelihood of skeletal fracture (1).

As women become estrogen deficient, irrespective of the cause, specific disturbances occur in the remodeling system (13). First, there is an increase in the frequency with which new remodeling sites are activated. As noted above, this results in an increase in the volume of bone undergoing remodeling at any time point. This causes a rapid reduction in the mass of the skeleton that equates to about 5% in cancellous bone but a significantly smaller increase in cortical bone. Because bone loss continues longitudinally with prolonged estrogen deficiency, it is assumed, but has never been rigorously proven, that with estrogen deficiency the balance between resorption and formation at each remodeling site alters in such a way that more bone is removed than is synthesized (14). The available data are suggestive of an increase in the size of each individual resorption cavity in cancellous bone, without an accompanying increase in the new bone formation. Thus, at the end of each remodeling cycle, there is less bone than at the start, with a consequent permanent deficit, which again, as noted above, can be repaired only when remodeling begins again at that site. Indeed, for that particular damage to be reversed, the opposite situation would need to be in effect. That is, the amount of bone formed in the new remodeling unit would have to be greater than the amount that had been removed.

The combination of the increase in frequency of remodeling sites and the likelihood that the resorption cavity is enlarged results in an increased likelihood that osteoclasts may be able to completely penetrate a single trabecula. When this occurs, there is complete loss of the template on which new bone might be formed, creating the situation in which bone formation cannot logically follow resorption. The consequence is that, in this situation, there is rapid loss of bone with alterations in trabecular architecture that make it impossible for the damage to be repaired. It is noteworthy that there is a gender difference in the pattern of bone loss such that in men trabecular penetration is seen considerably less frequently (1). Consequently, loss of bone in men tends to be associated with trabecular thinning, whereas in women trabecular loss dominates. Potentially, therefore, osteoporosis in men might be more amenable to reversal than the disease in estrogen-deficient women.

In histologic specimens of bone from women with osteoporosis, trabeculae are first converted from three-dimensional plates of bone into thin, friable-looking rods of bone and then eventually disappear (1). In addition to loss of mass, the loss of connectivity among trabeculae adds to increased vulnerability of the skeleton (Fig. 28.2).

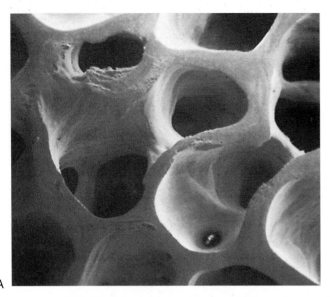
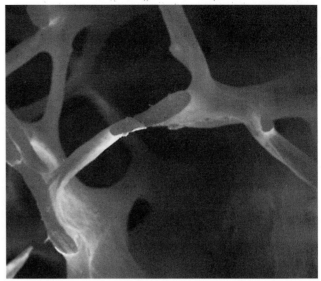

A

B

FIG. 28.2. Low-power scanning electron micrographs of iliac crest biopsies from normal **(A)** and osteo-porotic **(B)** individuals. Note the thin rod-like trabeculae, with loss of plate structure. Field width, 2.6 mm. (From ref. 1, with permission.)

In the spine, there appears to be selective loss of trabeculae subject to the least stress—that is, the horizontal trabeculae—which leads to a much greater loss of strength that would be predicted from the change in mass. Imagine a ladder or scaffolding without any cross struts, and imagine that structure attempting to support a vertical load. This gives a picture of the situation within vertebral bodies after loss of horizontal trabeculae.

CONSEQUENCES OF ESTROGEN DEPRIVATION

Metabolic studies support the changes in mineral homeostasis that occur across the menopause. There is a decrease in calcium economy with increased urinary calcium loss and decreased calcium absorption across the intestine (15,16). Consequently, at least in the early years after menopause, there is an apparent calcium drain that appears dependent on estrogen withdrawal and can be reversed by estrogen intervention but not simply by increasing the nutritional calcium supply.

Biochemical markers of both bone formation and bone resorption increase in serum and urine as women transition across the menopause (17). Originally this was observed as increased urinary calcium, urinary hydroxyproline, and serum levels of alkaline phosphatase (18). Within the last few years, more specific markers of bone resorption and formation have been developed, and here again the changes confirm the metabolic alterations within the skeleton as a consequence of estrogen deficiency (17). New markers of bone resorption include pyridinoline, deoxypyridinoline, or small peptide chains linked to either of these cross-linking molecules measured in urine and corrected for creatinine. Because the

majority of deoxypyridinoline in the body is present as a molecule linking C- or N-termini of type I collagen, the predominant collagen in bone, measurement of these entities has superseded the less specific and more difficult to measure hydroxyproline (19). For bone formation, measurement of osteocalcin, the most common protein in bone after collagen, which is also synthesized by the osteoblast, and by assays more specific for the bone isoenzyme of alkaline phosphatase, have replaced total alkaline phosphatase assays for bone formation. These more specific measures have confirmed that there is increased metabolic activity within the skeleton following estrogen deficiency, leading to increased bone resorption coupled with increased bone formation. This suggests an increase in the frequency of activation of new remodeling sites, but it is the continued loss of bone demonstrated by measurements of bone mass that implies an imbalance between resorption and formation within each remodeling focus.

The distribution of bone mass in the young adult population is essentially normal with a standard deviation equal to approximately 10% to 12% of the mean value, irrespective of the site of measurement (20). Bone loss after cessation of ovarian function occurs at an average rate of 2% to 3% per year (21). Thus, after very few years, average bone mass will have fallen by 1 standard deviation (i.e., 10% to 12%), but the change in architecture that accompanies this is sufficiently serious that it amplifies the effect on fracture risk, which increases by approximately twofold for each standard deviation reduction in bone mass (22).

Although it is generally stated that there is an accelerated phase of bone loss that occurs in the immediate postmenopausal year (probably related to increased activation frequency), it is now clear that bone loss continues into very old age and that bone loss may accelerate in older age. In part, this may be related to those with the lowest production of sex steroids as they age, but it is clearly modified by a variety of other factors that impinge on the skeleton with increasing age, such as impaired calcium absorption, decreasing mobility, intercurrent illness, etc.

MECHANISM OF ESTROGEN ACTION

Although the relationship between loss of ovarian function and osteoporosis was described almost 60 years ago (12), the mechanism by which estrogen influences bone remodeling is still not entirely clear. An original hypothesis by Heaney suggested that the absence of estrogen rendered the skeleton more sensitive to the bone-resorbing effects of parathyroid hormone (23). We recently demonstrated that the increase in markers of bone resorption following infusion of the amino-terminal peptide of parathyroid hormone (PTH) (hPTH$_{1-34}$) is significantly less in estrogen-replete women than in those who are estrogen deficient (24). Because estrogen loss increases the activation of bone-remodeling sites, and estrogen intervention reverses this phenomenon, the altered response to parathyroid hormone could mean simply that there are fewer osteoclasts present during the infusion in the estrogen-replete individuals to respond to PTH. It is thought that parathyroid hormone is responsible for recruitment of new remodeling sites (25); however, and increased activation of remodeling in estrogen deficiency could be a manifestation of greater skeletal sensitivity to PTH. It is noteworthy in this regard that the disease primary hyperparathyroidism is more frequently observed in postmenopausal women than in premenopausal women (26). This may simply be an observation related to a change in skeletal sensitivity to parathyroid hormone rather than to a real increase *de novo* in the disease incidence.

Irrespective of whether increased sensitivity for parathyroid hormone is a mechanism for the actions of estrogen on the skeleton, it seems likely that estrogen, for which there are two recognized receptors on a large number of cell types in many tissues, can have multiple effects on the skeleton (27,28). Recently, specific receptors for estrogen have been identified in cells of the osteoblast lineage (29,31). In addition, it has been suggested that osteoclasts, particularly from studies of avian osteoclasts, may also have estrogen receptors (30). Physiologic responses of osteoblast cell lines have been demonstrated in response to incubation with biologically meaningful concentrations of 17β-estradiol (32). However, in some situations, this has not been the case. It is now clear that osteoblasts *in vitro* lose functional estrogen receptors rapidly if they are incubated in completely estradiol-free circumstances. In part, this may explain the

fact that variable responses *in vitro* have been demonstrated, including both positive and negative changes in growth, alterations in synthesis and secretion of potential second messengers, as well as changes in collagen and noncollagenous protein synthesis. Riggs et al. could find no effects of estrogen on growth, bone Gla protein (BGP), or alkaline phosphatase production (33). In one other cell line, estrogen effects were demonstrable only after transfection of the cells with the estrogen receptor (34). Thus, it is still not entirely clear whether estrogens *in vivo* directly affect osteoblast function.

Other cell types within bone marrow are also putative sites of estrogen action. For example, mononuclear cells obtained from circulation appear to have an increased capacity to synthesize interleukin-1 (IL-1) after menopause, a phenomenon that is reversed by estrogen therapy (35). In studies in mice, estrogen deficiency increased secretion of interleukin-6 (IL-6), and bone loss was inhibited by infusion of an antibody blocking the IL-6 receptor, suggesting a causal interrelationship (36). Both IL-1 and IL-6 can be shown in some *in vitro* systems to stimulate osteoclast activity or recruitment (37), but again the results are not consistent (D. W. Dempster, *personal communication*). Prostaglandin E$_2$ is a potent stimulator of bone resorption *in vitro* and has been found to be increased in rats after ovariectomy (38). However, the role of prostaglandins in bone resorption following menopause in humans is not known. Prostaglandin synthetase inhibitors appear to have very little effect on bone loss in postmenopausal women (39). Finally, estrogens may also control the synthesis and secretion of a variety of growth factors within bone, particularly transforming growth factor-β (TGF-β) and the insulin-like growth factors (IGF-1 and IGF-2), as well as their regulatory proteins (40). TGF-β or a member of the TGF-β superfamily has been suggested as being the messenger responsible for the linking of bone formation to resorption in the remodeling cycle, the so-called coupling factor (41). Both IGF-1 and IGF-2 have been linked to bone formation in humans by a variety of *in vitro* experiments. Short-term administration of IGF-1 appears to increase bone remodeling in the adult (42). Several attempts have been made to integrate the known effects of the cytokines and growth factors into estrogen effects on the skeleton, but at present those remain merely models or hypotheses.

It is noteworthy that in addition to effects on skeletal remodeling, estrogen status may also independently affect calcium homeostasis. The elegant work of Heaney has demonstrated that calcium economy deteriorates after menopause. The efficiency with which calcium is absorbed across the intestine declines, and calcium loss from the kidney increases (15,16). Indeed, a primary renal leak of calcium could well be a mechanism by which the increased bone remodeling is stimulated in an attempt to maintain the constancy of serum calcium.

PEAK SKELETAL MASS

Peak skeletal mass is achieved at the end of linear growth. The heavier skeleton of the man is achieved during puberty (43). However, although by two-dimensional non-invasive techniques such as dual-energy x-ray absorptiometry (DEXA), the skeleton of the man appears to be denser, this is probably not true and is simply a reflection of the larger size of the male skeleton. After puberty, a further small increase in bone mass occurring particularly in cortical bone has been described, but this appears to increase total bone mass by a modest amount. At this point in life, the amount of bone in the skeleton is primarily under genetic control (44), although influenced somewhat by factors during growth such as nutrition and lifestyle (45,46). A diet deficient in protein and calcium, for example, a lifestyle in which the skeleton is not used to its full extent, and chronic ill health can all impact negatively on bone during growth, reducing the capacity to reach maximum genetic potential. The achievement of adequate sex hormone production during the pubertal years appears to be particularly important in ensuring maximum peak skeletal mass (47). Because the amount of bone that is present in the skeleton in later life is influenced by this initial mass, it is important to ensure that during childhood and adolescence conditions are such that growth will be maximized. A potential public health approach to osteoporosis prevention requires modification of diet and lifestyle in the growing pediatric population, whereby modifications of peak bone mass by as much as 5% to 10% might be achieved by inexpensive changes in protein and calcium intake and exercise.

Cross-sectional data in premenopausal women generally find no evidence of bone loss, at least in the spine or peripheral skeleton. However, some bone loss does appear to occur in the femoral neck between the ages of 20 and 50 (20,47,48). The reasons why this site may behave differently from the others in not clear. In the healthy premenopausal ovulatory woman, manipulations of diet and lifestyle appear to produce modest if any effects. Nonetheless, loss of ovarian function at any age produces the expected increase in skeletal remodeling and loss of bone mass that is seen in the postmenopausal population. Thus, lower bone mass has been demonstrated in situations of hyperprolactinemia associated with amenorrhea (49), anorexia (50), exercise-induced amenorrhea (51,52), or following the use of gonadotropin-releasing hormone (GnRH) agonists (53). Irregular ovarian function of sufficient severity to produce amenorrhea appears to lower bone mass. One recent study that suggested that ovulatory disturbances were also associated with low bone mass has not been confirmed (54,55). Women with Turner's syndrome have low bone mass and predisposition to fracture at an early age, probably at least in part because of the failure to develop adequate ovarian function (56), but also related to the phenotypic characteristics of Turner's syndrome. In men, bone loss and osteoporosis are associated with reduction in testicular supply of testosterone and Klinefelter's syndrome (57). Thus, at all ages in both sexes, the loss of sex hormone disturbs skeletal homeostasis and results in loss of bone mass.

OTHER FACTORS MODIFYING BONE LOSS WITH AGE

As in other circumstances associated with chronic disease, epidemiologists have identified a large number of risk factors for osteoporotic fracture that operate in the population in addition to the loss of sex hormones (58). The fact that there appear to be many such risk factors implies perhaps that each is relatively trivial by itself, either within individuals or on a population basis. These risk factors can be roughly divided into risk factors for bone loss and risk factors for osteoporotic fractures that are independent of bone mass or loss (Table 28.1). Some risk factors may feature in both lists. Thus, immobility or chronic ill health, by themselves, will produce loss of bone mass, but in addition, the reduced strength and protective reflexes produce an increase in the likelihood of falls and osteoporotic fractures. Risk factors that increase the likelihood of falling are perhaps more likely to be associated with hip fracture and fractures of the distal radius than with fractures of the vertebrae. Consequently, there may be considerable site specificity in these risk factors. For example, it has been suggested that in younger individuals, gait speed, which is generally more rapid than in older individuals, results in increased likelihood of falling on the outstretched hand, thereby producing a fracture of the distal radius (59). As individuals age and become more frail, slower gait in these individuals is more likely to be associated with a fall toward the side and consequently with a direct trauma to the hip and an accompanying fracture at that site.

Factors that specifically affect skeletal remodeling with increasing age can be roughly be divided into nutritional, lifestyle, and endocrine factors and secondary causes of bone loss. Lifestyle and nutritional factors that affect the skeleton have a fairly high prevalence among the aging population, and it is important that the clinician address these in ascertaining individual susceptibility and in counseling individuals about prevention and therapy.

TABLE 28.1. *Proposed risk factors for osteoporosis*

Factor	Example
Genetic	Race, sex, familial prevalence
Nutritional	Low calcium intake, high alcohol intake, high caffeine intake, high sodium intake, high animal protein intake
Life-style	Cigarette use, low physical activity
Endocrine	Menopausal age (oophorectomy), body composition

Nutritional Factors

The most frequently cited and commonly recognized nutritional risk factor is calcium. It is clear that calcium deficiency can cause osteoporosis in animal models and increases the rate of bone loss in adults (60). The precise level of calcium intake at which osteoporosis risk increases in any individual is impossible to assess clinically, as there is no specific marker that can be used to indicate calcium deficiency (analogous to ferritin for iron).

However, over the past several years, information has accumulated from epidemiologic studies as well as controlled clinical trials with both BMD and fractures as outcome. These studies have confirmed the importance of calcium insufficiency in the pathogenesis of bone loss and fractures.

It is perhaps self-evident that calcium is important in skeletal development and growth. Calcium intake at this stage in life must be sufficient to allow a positive calcium balance. During growth there is some evidence that the efficiency with which calcium is absorbed and retained is greater than at any other period in life. However, it is still important to ensure a reasonable intake of calcium, particularly during the prepubertal growth spurt (47).

During adult life, maintenance of adequate calcium intake ensures that skeletal calcium is not utilized to maintain serum calcium within its tightly controlled limits. In older adults the efficiency of calcium absorption across the intestine declines. The consequence is increased endogenous production of parathyroid hormone. The effects of PTH are to reduce urinary calcium losses and increase the 1-hydroxylation of vitamin D in the kidney to its active metabolite 1,25-dihydroxyvitamin D. This hormone stimulates the active transport of calcium across the intestine, a physiologic response to declining calcium supply. However, with age, the response of the intestine to 1,25-dihydroxyvitamin D also falls. Thus, there is incomplete adaptation to the falling calcium supply and continued increased PTH production. This chronic state of secondary hyperparathyroidism leads to increased bone resorption and consequent loss of bone mass. Much of this can be offset by ensuring increased calcium intake.

Several general recommendations can be made regarding calcium intake. First, calcium is a nutrient and should be obtained from nutritional sources as part of a good diet. However, given dietary habits in the Western world, that is difficult for most adults, as the main source of calcium is usually dairy products, avoided because of calories or fat content. Bioavailable supplements are an alternative and reasonable source of calcium when food sources are inadequate.

The information available in the literature suggests that most (90%) adults will be close to calcium balance if total intake can be maintained at 1,000 to 1,500 mg/day (15). Dietary surveys in the United States suggest that average intake is 400 to 600 mg/day (61). Therefore, provision of 500 to 1,000 mg as a daily supplement would bring most individuals to an adequate intake. This is easily accomplished by supplementing calcium at mealtimes by 200 to 300 mg. The addition of a single chewable tablet of calcium carbonate supplies this. The data available suggest that calcium supplementation to those whose intake is clearly inadequate (below 400 mg/day) will have some effect on bone loss, with the exception of the period immediately following menopause, when bone loss is driven by sex hormone deficiency (62). Finally, there is no evidence that such advice applied to the general population will be hazardous in any way.

Recently, some attention has been paid to the issue of vitamin D and the importance of undersupply of vitamin D in the pathogenesis of osteoporosis. Although all the answers are not yet available, it is simple and inexpensive to ensure adequate vitamin D status. Among the young and healthy, vitamin D supply from endogenous sources is sufficient to ensure adequacy, with compensatory supply made in the skin. However, with age and illness, the capacity to synthesize sufficient cholecalciferol in the skin declines, as does vitamin D absorption, creating another stimulus for secondary hyperparathyroidism. Provision of vitamin D in daily amounts of 200 to 800 IU/day is sufficient to ensure adequate vitamin D status. Such amounts can be obtained in multivitamin preparations or in certain calcium supplements.

Other nutrients that are considered as possible risk factors include protein (especially animal protein), caffeine, sodium, and perhaps phosphate (60). The evidence linking each of these to osteoporosis is considerably less secure than for calcium (which some would still debate), and dietary advice should be limited to ensuring moderation in intake.

Lifestyle Factors

Alcohol consumption links nutrition and lifestyle. There seems little doubt that excess alcohol consumption is a risk factor for this disorder as it is for others, and again, moderation should be encouraged (63). The precise level at which alcohol intake increases the risk of osteoporosis is not well established. Some evidence suggests that those with low or moderate alcohol intakes have greater skeletal mass than those who abstain or those whose alcohol intake is excessive. Because most individuals underestimate personal intake when discussing this with their physicians, I assume that any individual who admits to alcohol consumption should be warned about this potential concern.

The other two lifestyle factors that appear to alter risk are cigarette consumption and physical activity. Because there are no health advantages to cigarette use and clear disadvantages of which osteoporosis is but one (64), elimination of this habit is to be encouraged for this reason also.

The recommendations for physical activity are more complex. Complete disuse is clearly detrimental to the skeleton (68) (if you don't use it, you'll lose it). However, the level of activity, as well as the type of activity, that is necessary to maintain skeletal health is still debated. For younger individuals, I adopt the criteria for good cardiovascular health (summarized as 30 minutes of aerobic activity three times per week, minimum). For premenopausal women, excessive activity, to the point at which ovarian function is impaired, is clearly detrimental (51,52). But aside from that caveat, for the bones most exercise appears beneficial (65). Weight-bearing activities that supply an impact to the important skeletal sites appear most beneficial, however. For those with established osteoporosis, care must be employed in providing recommendations because there is a risk of fracture. An experienced physical therapist can provide a supervised program that does not appear to increase risk and provides considerable benefit by increasing strength, decreasing pain, and reducing risk of recurrent fracture, although hard data to support that assertion are difficult to find (66). For all, advice about exercise must include the necessity to persist, and failure to comply with any recommendations is commonplace and well recognized by clinicians experienced in preventive medicine. In providing exercise advice, I tell my patients that there are two simple rules: make it a priority and make it fun. Positive effects of exercise programs in the elderly are probably related more to reduction in falling frequency than to increased bone mass per se.

SECONDARY CAUSES OF BONE LOSS

Postmenopausal osteoporosis is a diagnosis made by exclusion. The diagnosis is relatively simple to make in the otherwise healthy postmenopausal women presenting with an acute vertebral fracture, but the careful physician must be aware of those disorders that can masquerade as osteoporosis and ensure that these are excluded. Of particular concern is multiple myeloma, which occasionally presents as a fracture syndrome with generalized osteoporosis on radiographs and without the typical punched-out lesions characteristic of the disease. Other malignancies may also present as apparent osteoporotic fractures. Many other chronic diseases such as rheumatoid arthritis, inflammatory bowel disease, and neurologic diseases such as multiple sclerosis and Parkinson's disease have been associated with increased osteoporosis even when not treated with steroids. This may be in part related to decreased mobilization as well as other factors.

Excess glucocorticoids also cause osteoporosis. The mechanisms by which adrenal steroids increase bone loss include reduction in intestinal calcium absorption, decreased osteoblast activity, increased renal calcium wasting, and increased osteoclast activity, in part at least consequent on secondary hyperparathyroidism from the impaired calcium absorption (67). Because steroids are commonly used as therapeutic agents in postmenopausal women, they often compound the effects of estrogen loss. Bone loss occurs early and rapidly in some individuals, and there is great variability in skeletal response to steroids. Rarely, Cushing's syndrome presents with osteoporotic fracture, but therapeutic use of steroids is a far more common reason for referral to an osteoporosis clinic.

The use of thyroid hormone also can impact on the skeleton (68). Where thyroid hormone is used for replacement, the dose should be titrated by measuring circulating thyroid-stimulating hormone (TSH). With age there is a decline in the requirement for thyroid, and those on long-term replacement presenting for evaluation for osteoporosis should have TSH levels tested. Levels of thyroid hormone that do not suppress TSH probably have no negative impact.

IDENTIFICATION OF THOSE AT RISK

If any preventive intervention is being considered for protection against osteoporosis specifically, it is often of value to the clinician and patient to have some estimate of risk. Although many risk factors for osteoporotic fracture have been described, these are of limited use clinically because they fail to provide an accurate profile of risk when applied to the individual patient. A similar situation exists with hypertension and stroke. In the latter case, the clinician always measures blood pressure, but especially notes to do so when several of the suspected risk factors are found in the patient. We now know that a similar situation exists with osteoporotic fracture. The presence of several risk factors can be used to raise the level of suspicion about the disease, but because the aim in prevention is to treat the decline in bone mass, it is necessary to estimate skeletal mass before initiating therapy.

Bone mass is related to the prevalence and incidence of osteoporotic fracture (55–57). In prospective studies, the level of fracture risk is related to the initial measure of bone mass. Bone mass cannot be predicted from assessment of risk factors. Thus, measurement of bone mass is a useful investigation for the estrogen-deficient patient who indicates a willingness to take estrogen but will do so only if the physician can inform her about her future risk of osteoporosis. Because menopause is the point at which (roughly speaking) bone loss begins in the aging female population, this becomes a useful time marker at which to determine individual risk. In this category we use bone mass measurement to assess risk and use the result to guide the patient in discussing the appropriateness for intervention. As agents other than estrogen become available in the future, this strategy will become more important, as the pharmacologic agents in development target the skeleton specifically and do not have the other features of estrogens. The National Osteoporosis Foundation has developed clinical guidelines for the use of these tests (58).

INTERVENTION STRATEGY

In general, the lower the bone mass the more likely is the necessity for intervention. A bone mass above the mean value for young normal individuals generally allows the opportunity for conservative management and future reevaluation. Bone mass below average implies earlier consideration for treatment. For each patient, after assessment of bone mass, we employ a risk assessment and management strategy in addition to the consideration of therapy. Some risk factors for hip fracture have been found to be independent of bone mass, including previous adult fractures, family history, smoking, being very thin, and recurrent falling. If any of these factors is present in a patient, it should increase the bone mass level at which pharmacologic treatment is recommended.

From the clinician's standpoint, those risk factors requiring attention are those that are more amenable to change. In addition to estrogen deficiency, those are generally the nutritional and life-style factors outlined earlier. Superimposed on these are a variety of insults that are often not easily changed. The latter include chronic diseases known to accelerate bone loss or to increase the risk of falling. Examples include Cushing's syndrome, which by virtue of the excess of glucocorticoids increases bone loss, and Parkinson's disease, which increases the risk of falling. Many other examples exist and are included in the list of proposed risk factors in Table 28.1. Adequate and successful treatment for the primary condition assists in prevention of osteoporosis. For patients who require glucocorticoid therapy, there is often no alternative, and intervention with a strategy to reduce the risk of osteoporotic fracture is often mandatory.

REFERENCES

1. Dempster DW, Shane E, Horbert W, Lindsay R. A simple method for correlative light and scanning electron microscopy of human iliac crest bone biopsies: qualitative observations in normal and osteoporotic subjects. *J Bone Miner Res* 1986;1:15–21.
2. Lindsay R. Estrogen deficiency. In: Riggs BL, Melton LJ, eds. *Osteoporosis: etiology, diagnosis and management, 2nd ed.* New York: Raven Press, 1995:133–160.
3. Melton LJ III. Epidemiology of fractures. In: Riggs BL, Melton LJ, eds. *Osteoporosis: etiology, diagnosis and management, 2nd ed.* New York: Raven Press, 1995:133–160.
4. World Health Organization. *Assessment of fracture risk and its application to screening for ostmenopausal osteoporosis. Report of a WHO study group.* Geneva: WHO, 1994.
5. Cooper C, Campion G, Melton LJ II. Hip fractures in the elderly: a world-wide projection. *Osteoporosis Int* 1992;6:285–290.
6. Ray NF, Chan JK, Thamer M, Melton LJ III. Medical expenditures for the treatment of osteoporotic fractures in the United States in 1995: report from the National Osteoporosis Foundation. *J Bone Miner* 1997;12:24–35.
7. Bengner U, Ekbom T, Johnell O, Nilsson BE. Incidence of femoral and tibial shaft fractures. Epidemiology 1950–1983 in Malmo, Sweden. *Acta Orthop Scand* 1990;61:251–254.
8. US Congress, Office of Technology Assessment. *Hip fracture outcomes in people age 50 and over (background paper).* Washington, DC: US Government Printing Office.
9. Dempster DW. Bone remodeling. In: Coe FL, Favus MJ, eds. *Disorders of bone and mineral metabolism.* New York: Raven Press, 1992:355–382.
10. Frost HM. The skeletal intermediary organization. A. synthesis. In: Peck WA, ed. *Bone and mineral research, 3rd ed.* Amsterdam: Elsevier, 1985:49–107.
11. Kleerekoper M, Villanueva AR, Stanciu J, Rao DS, Parfitt AM. The role of three-dimensional trabecular microstructure in the pathogenesis of vertebral compression fractures. *Calcif Tissue Int* 1985;37:594–597.
12. Albright F, Smith PH, Richardson AM. Postmenopausal osteoporosis. *JAMA* 1941;116:2465–2474.
13. Recker RR, Kimmel DB, Parfitt AM. Static and tetracycline-based bone histomorphometric data from 34 normal postmenopausal females. *J Bone Miner Res* 1988;3:133–144.
14. Parfitt AM. Bone remodeling: relationship to the amount and structure of bone, and the pathogenesis and prevention of fractures. In: Riggs BL, Melton LJ, eds. *Osteoporosis: etiology, diagnosis, and management.* New York: Raven Press, 1988:45–93.
15. Heaney RP, Recker RR, Saville PD. Menopausal changes in calcium balance performance. *J Lab Clin Med* 1978;92:953–963.
16. Heaney RP, Recker RR, Saville PD. Menopausal changes in bone remodeling. *J Lab Clin Med* 1978;92:964–970.
17. Seibel MJ, Cosman F, Shen V, et al. Urinary hydroxypyridinium crosslinks of collagen as markers of bone resorption and estrogen efficacy in postmenopausal osteoporosis. *J Bone Min* 1993;9:881–889.
18. Nordin BEC, Polley KJ. Metabolic consequences of the menopause. A cross-sectional, longitudinal, and intervention study on 557 normal postmenopausal women. *Calcif Tis* 1987;41(S):51–58.
19. Delmas PD. Biochemical markers for the assessment of bone turnover. In: Riggs BL, Melton LJ, eds. *Osteoporosis: etiology, diagnosis and management, 2nd ed.* New York: Raven Press, 1995:319–333.
20. Looker AC, Wahner HW, Dunn WL, et al. Proximal femur bone mineral levels of US adults. *Osteoporosis Int* 1995;5:389–409.
21. Slemenda C, Hui SL, Longcope C, Johnston CC. Sex steroids and bone mass; a study of changes about the time of the menopause. *J Clin Invest* 1987;80:1261–1269.
22. Cummings SR, Black DM, Nevitt MC, et al. Appendicular bone density and age predict hip fracture in women, The Study of Osteoporotic Fractures Research Group. *JAMA* 1990;263:665–668.
23. Heaney RP. A unified concept of osteoporosis. *Am J Med* 1965;39:377–380.
24. Cosman F, Shen V, Xie F, et al. A mechanism of estrogen action on the skeleton: protection against the resorbing effects of (1–34)hPTH infusion as assessed by biochemical markers. *Ann Intern Med* 1992;118:337–343.
25. McGuire JL, Marks SCJ. The effects of PTH on bone cell structure and function. *Clin Orthop* 1974;100:392–405.
26. Horowitz M, Nordin BEC. *Metabolic bone and stone disease, 3rd ed.* Edinburgh: Churchill Livingstone, 1993.
27. Kuiper G, Enmark E, Pelto-Huikko M, Nilsson S, Gustafsson J-A. Cloning of a novel estrogen receptor expressed in rat prostate and ovary. *Proc Natl Acad Sci USA* 1996;93:5925–5930.
28. Enmark E, Pilto-Huikko M, Grandien K, et al. Human estrogen receptor β-gene structure, chromosomal localization, and expression pattern. *J Clin Endocrinol* 1997;82:4258–4265.
29. Komm BS, Terpening CM, Benz DJ. Estrogen binding, receptor mRNA, and biologic response in osteoblast-like osteosarcoma cells. *Science* 1988;241:81–84.
30. Eriksen EF, Colvard DS, Berg NJ, et al. Evidence of estrogen receptors in normal human osteoblast-like cells. *Science* 1988;241:84–86.
31. Oursler MJ, Osdoby P, Pyfferoen J, Riggs BL, Spelsberg TC. Avian osteoclasts as estrogen target cells. *Proc Natl Acad Sci USA* 1991;88:6613–6617.
32. Ernst M, Heath JK, Rodan GA. Estradiol effects on proliferation, messenger ribonucleic acid for collagen and insulin-like growth factor-I, and parathyroid hormone-stimulated adenylate cyclase activity in osteoblastic cells from calvariae and long bones. *Endocrinology* 1989;125:825–833.
33. Keeting PE, Scott RE, Colvard DS, Han IK, Spelsberg TC, Riggs BL. Lack of a direct effect of estrogen on proliferation and differentiation of normal human osteoblast-like cells. *J Bone Miner Res* 1991;6:297–304.
34. Watts CKW, Parker MG, King RJB. Stable transfection of the oestrogen receptor gene into a human osteosarcoma cell line. *J Steroid Biochem* 1989;34:483–490.
35. Pacifici R, Brown C, Puscheck E, et al. Effect of surgical menopause and estrogen replacement on cytokine release from human blood mononuclear cells. *Proc Natl Acad Sci USA* 1991;88:5134–5138.
36. Jilka RL, Hangoc G, Girasole G, et al. Increased osteoclast development after estrogen loss: mediation by interleukin-6. *Science* 1992;257:88–91.
37. Raisz LG. Local and systemic factors in the pathogenesis of osteoporosis. *N Engl J Med* 1988;318:818–828.
38. Feven JHM, Raisz LG. Prostaglandin production by calvariae from sham-operated and oophorectomized rats: effect of 17β-estradiol *in vivo. Endocrinology* 1987;121:819–821.
39. Sibonga JD, Bell NH, Turner RT. Evidence that ibuprofen antagonizes selective actions of estrogen and tomoxifen on rat bone. *J Bone Miner Res* 1998;13:863–870.
40. Canalis E, McCarthy TL, Centrella M. Growth factors and cytokines in bone cell metabolism. *Annu Rev Med* 1991;42:17–24.
41. Linkhart TA, Mohan S, Baylink DJ. Growth factors for bone growth and repair: IGF, TGF beta and BMP. *Bone* 1996;19(1S):1S–12S.
42. Kassem M, Okazaki R, Harris SA, Spelsberg TC, Conover CA, Riggs BL. Estrogen effects on insulin-like growth factor gene expression in a human osteoblastic cell line with high levels of estrogen receptor. *Calcif Tis* 1998;61:60–66.
43. Garn SM. The phenomenon of bone formation and bone loss. In: DeLuca HF, et al, eds. *Osteoporosis: recent advances in pathogenesis and treatment.* Baltimore: University Park Press; 1981:1–16.
44. Pocock NA, Eisman JA, Hopper JL, Yeates MG, Sambrook PM, Ebers S. Genetic determinants of bone mass in adults. *J Clin Invest* 1987;80:706–710.

45. Nieves JW, Golden AL, Kelsey JL, Siris E, Lindsay R. Teenage and current calcium intake are related to bone mineral density of the hip and forearm in women age 30–39. *Am J Epidemiol* 1995;141:342–351.

46. Nieves JW, Rekola K, Nelson L, et al. Weight bearing physical activity is beneficial to bone mineral density of the hip in women age 30–39. *Am J Epidemiol* (in press).

47. Bonjour J-P, Rizzoli R. Bone acquisition in adolescence. In: Marcus R, Feldman D, Kelsey J, eds. *Osteoporosis.* San Diego: Academic Press, 1996:465–476.

48. Stevenson JC, Lees B, Devenport M, Cust MP, Ganger KF. Determinants of bone density in normal women: risk factors for future osteoporosis? *Br Med J* 1989; 298:924–928.

49. Klibanski A, Neer RM, Beitins IZ, Ridgway C, Zervas NT, MacArthur J. Decreased bone density in hyperprolactinemic women. *N Engl J Med* 1980;303: 1511–1514.

50. Rigotti NA, Nussbaum SR, Herzog DB, et al. Osteoporosis in women with anorexia nervosa. *N Engl J Med* 1984;311:1601–1606.

51. Drinkwater BD, Nilson KL, Chestnut CH III. Bone mineral content of amenorrheic and eumenorrheic athletes. *N Engl J Med* 1984;311:277–281.

52. Marcus R, Cann C, Madorg P, et al. Menstrual function and bone mass in elite women distance runners. *Ann Intern Med* 1988;102:158–163.

53. Cann CE, Henzl MR, Burrk K, et al. Reversible bone loss is produced by the GnRH agonist nafarelin. In: Cohn DV, Martin TJ, Meunier PJ, eds. *Calcium regulation and bone metabolism: basic and clinical aspects.* Amsterdam: Elsevier; 1987:123–127.

54. Prior JC, Vigna YM, Schecter MT, Burgess AE. Spinal bone loss and ovulatory disturbances. *N Engl J Med* 1990;323:1221–1227.

55. Waller K, Reim J, Fenster L, et al. Bone mass and subtle abnormalities in ovulatory function in healthy women. *J Clin Endocrinol* 1996;81(2):663–668.

56. Park E. Cortical bone measurements in Turner's syndrome. *Am J Phys Arthropol* 1977;46(3):455–461.

57. Smith DAS, Walker MS. Changes in plasma steroids and bone density in Klinefelter's syndrome. *Calcif Tissue Res* 1976;22:225–228.

58. Slemenda CW, Johnston CC, Hui SL. Assessing fracture risk. In: Marcus R, Feldman D, Kelsey J, eds. *Osteoporosis.* San Diego: Academic Press, 1996:623–633.

59. Grisso JA, Capequti E, Schwartz A. In: Marcus R, Feldman D, Kelsey J, eds. *Osteoporosis.* San Diego: Academic Press, 1996:599–611.

60. Heaney RP. Nutrition and risk for osteoporosis. In: Marcus R, Feldman D, Kelsey J, eds. *Osteoporosis.* San Diego: Academic Press, 1996:483–509.

61. Carrol MD, Abraham S, Dresser CM. Dietary intake source data: US, 1976–1980. *Vital and health statistics, Ser 11-No. 231, DHHS publication No. (PHS) 83-PHS.* Washington, DC: US Government Printing Office, 1983.

62. Elders PJ, Netelenbos JC, Lips P, et al. Calcium supplementation reduces vertebral bone loss in perimenopausal women: a controlled trial in 248 women between 46 and 55 years of age. *J Clin Endocrinol* 1991;73:533–540.

63. Seeman E. The effects of tobacco and alcohol use on bone. In: Marcus R, Feldman D, Kelsey J, eds. *Osteoporosis.* San Diego: Academic Press, 1996:577–597.

64. Minare P, Meunier P, Edouard C, Bernard J, Courpron P, Bournet J. Quantitative histological data on disuse osteoporosis. Comparison with biological data. *Calcif Tissue Res* 1974;17:57–63.

65. Gutin B, Kasper MJ. Can vigorous exercise play a role in osteoporosis prevention? A review. *Osteoporosis Int* 1992;55:69.

66. Morey MC, Cowper PA, Feussner JR, et al. Evaluation of a supervised exercise program in a geriatric population. *J Am Geriatr Soc* 1989;37:348–354.

67. Lukert B. Glucocorticoid-induced osteoporosis. In: Marcus R, Feldman D, Kelsey J, eds. *Osteoporosis.* San Diego: Academic Press, 1996:801–820.

68. Ross DS. Subclinical hyperthyroidism: possible danger of overzealous thyroxine replacement therapy. *Mayo Clin Proc* 1988;63:1223–1228.

69. Melton LJ III, Riggs BL. Epidemiology of age-related fractures. In: Avioli LV, ed. *The osteoporotic syndrome.* New York: Grune & Stratton; 1983:45–72.

Treatment of the Postmenopausal Woman: Basic and Clinical Aspects, Second Edition, edited by Rogerio A. Lobo, Lippincott Williams & Wilkins, Philadelphia © 1999.

CHAPTER 29

Treatment of Osteoporosis

Claus Christiansen

Osteoporosis is a systemic skeletal disease characterized by low bone mass and microarchitectural deterioration of bone tissue, with a consequent increase in bone fragility and susceptibility to fracture (1). Although both men and women experience some degree of bone loss as a natural part of the aging process, bone loss progresses rapidly in postmenopausal women, and the disorder has become a major health problem in Western countries (2), where increased life expectancy has placed new emphasis on aging-related disorders.

Bone mass increases rapidly in growing children and adolescents, reaching a peak in adults between the second and third decades. After age 35 to 40, bone mass begins to decline. Men lose bone mass at approximately the same rate over their lifetime; in women, however, the rate of bone loss increases dramatically after menopause (or oophorectomy) (3). It is also important to note that bone mass in women after the age of 50 is only two-thirds of that found in men (4). These two factors—lower initial adult bone mass and a more rapid rate of bone loss—combine to produce a high incidence of osteoporosis in older women.

Significant morbidity and mortality are attributed to osteoporosis-related fractures, and new therapeutic and preventive modalities must be evaluated and applied in high-risk populations. In postmenopausal women with low bone mass or osteoporosis, there are today several options for therapy and preventive measures that may be implemented with positive results. Treatment of established osteoporosis in quite elderly women (>80 years) who have already suffered multiple nontraumatic fractures (e.g., vertebral crush fractures) is difficult, but in the past few years drugs have been developed that may also help this population.

In adult women before the onset of menopause, rates of bone formation and bone resorption are approximately equal; calcium balance is maintained, and no loss of bone mass occurs (3). But after menopause, although both bone formation and bone resorption rates increase, the rate of bone resorption increases more rapidly, resulting in calcium imbalance and a net loss of bone. The first goal of therapy for osteoporosis, therefore, should be the restoration of bone resorption and bone formation to premenopausal levels. Optimally, bone formation may be maintained at a slightly higher level than that of bone resorption, producing a positive calcium balance and preventing bone loss.

ESTROGEN AND ESTROGEN-PROGESTOGEN REPLACEMENT THERAPY

Replacement therapy with estrogen alone (without a progestogen) is often called unopposed estrogen therapy and is abbreviated ERT, whereas combined estrogen-progestogen therapy is abbreviated HRT. If estrogen is given alone to women with an intact uterus, the risk of developing endometrial hyperplasia and cancer is considerably increased. Therefore, estrogen is often given in combination with a progestogen either in a cyclic regimen or in a so-called continuous-combined regimen. In the cyclic regimen, a progestogen is added to a part of the cycle, perhaps 10 or 14 days of the estrogen cycle. This mimics the natural premenopausal cycle and thus provokes monthly menstrual-like bleeding. In the continuous combined therapy, the progestogen is given every day together with the estrogen. In this way, the endometrium is kept atrophic continuously, and bleeding is avoided in many, but not all, users (5). A completely new concept was recently reported (6) in which the progestogen is given in a cyclophasic regimen. The regimen is based on calculations of the endometrial estrogen receptor kinetic. It assumes that the optimal regimen for a constant atrophic endometrium, with the lowest possible dose of progestogen, is 3 days with estrogen alone followed by 3 days with combined estrogen-progestogen.

Estrogens: Definition

Estrogens (estradiol, 17β-estradiol, E_2) can be defined as compounds that are able to produce vaginal cornifica-

C. Christiansen: Center for Clinical and Basic Research, Ballerup, Denmark, DK-2750.

tion or uterotrophic effects in oophorectomized rats or mice (7). Estrogens can be divided into four main groups:

1. Synthetic estrogen analogs without a steroid skeleton, often stilbestrol derivatives.
2. Synthetic estrogen analogs with a steroid skeleton.
3. Nonhuman estrogens, produced from an equine source (conjugated estrogens).
4. Native human estrogens or compounds that are transformed to native estrogens in the body.

The potencies of different estrogens vary. The various bioassays used to determine potencies, however, do not give the same potency ratios. This indicates that, in addition to the differences in potency, estrogens have qualitative differences (7,8). Studies have thus indicated that nonsynthetic estrogens produce fewer metabolic side effects than do synthetic estrogens (9).

Synthetic estrogens without a steroid structure are now obsolete. Synthetic estrogens with a steroid structure (such as ethinyl estradiol) are still the most used estrogens in oral contraceptives.

For postmenopausal therapy, conjugated equine estrogens are the most commonly prescribed in the United States, whereas in Europe there has been a tradition of using native human estrogen (i.e., 17β-estradiol) or estradiol valerate.

Progestogen: Definition

Substances described as progestogens differ greatly in their additional properties, but they have at least one property in common: they are all able to cause secretory transformation of an estrogen-primed endometrium (10). In addition to this effect, progestogens may have estrogenic, antiestrogenic, androgenic, antiandrogenic, antigonadotropic, glucocorticoid-like, and adrenocorticotropic hormone (ACTH)-stimulating activities.

The classes of progestogens may be divided into three subgroups:

1. 19-Norethisterone (norethindrone) derivatives, with a relatively high androgenic effect.
2. 17-Hydroxyprogesterone derivatives, with less androgenic activity.
3. Natural human progesterone, which is available in a micronized form for oral therapy.

EFFECTS OF BONE REMODELING

Estrogens

Calcium reaches the extra- and intracellular volumes through intestinal absorption, which is mainly regulated by the active metabolite of vitamin D, 1,25(OH)$_2$D. Furthermore, calcium is transported from the skeleton to the extracellular volume (bone resorption) and in the opposite direction (bone formation) (11,12).

The metabolism of calcium changes dramatically when estrogen production declines in women. The main char-

acteristic is increased bone remodeling, which is reflected in high serum concentrations of biochemical indicators of bone resorption and bone formation. This increased bone turnover is maintained throughout life and is also seen in women with symptomatic postmenopausal osteoporosis (13).

All conditions of estrogen deprivation result in loss of bone. This includes natural or surgical menopause and drugs that inhibit estrogen production or its effects [luteinizing hormone-releasing hormone (LH-RH) agonists, antagonists, or antiestrogens]. Strenuous exercise or other conditions that provoke anovulation also may result in bone loss. Withdrawal of estrogen primarily affects bone resorption, as shown by a rapid increase in the biochemical indicators of bone resorption. Because of the coupling of bone resorption and formation, bone formation will show a secondary increase, reflected by a delayed elevation in the biochemical estimates of bone formation (Fig. 29.1) (14).

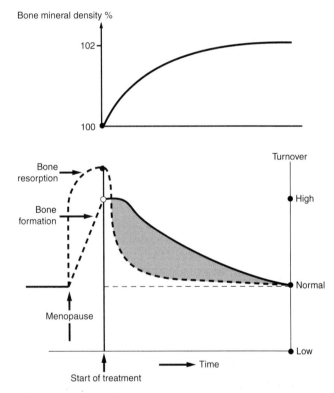

FIG. 29.1. The effect of hormone replacement therapy (HRT) on bone remodeling. Estrogen deficiency (menopause) primarily affects bone resorption, as shown by a rapid increase in the biochemical markers of bone resorption. Because of the coupling of bone resorption and formation, bone formation will show a secondary increase, reflected by a delayed elevation in the biochemical estimates of bone formation. The opposite sequence of events is seen when HRT is prescribed to an estrogen-deficient woman. Bone resorption is primarily normalized or at least decreased toward a premenopausal level, and only secondarily, bone formation is depressed. This phenomenon results in an increase in bone mass that may last several years but is transient by nature and will level off when the rates of bone resorption and formation approach each other.

It is self-evident that all types of bone loss are the result of an imbalance between bone resorption and bone formation, which implies, in the case of post-menopausal bone loss, that bone resorption is increased more than bone formation. The difference between the two processes seems to be greatest in the first years after menopause (where bone loss is largest), whereas in the long term it moves toward a new steady state at a higher level. Postmenopausal estrogen therapy rapidly normalizes both bone resorption and formation, leading to a reestablishment of bone balance (15,16).

Estrogen replacement therapy primarily decreases bone resorption and only secondarily decreases bone formation, which results in a temporary positive bone balance for some time. In this period, when the resorption lacunae are filled up, bone density will increase. After some time, when the rate of formation has picked up this difference, the increase in bone density will level off. Further treatment will result in a stabilization of bone density, but no further increase (Fig. 29.1).

Progestogens

Because the progestogens have such different qualities, the effects on bone and calcium metabolism of the various progestogens and progesterone itself need to be studied separately. Only a few studies have been published on the individual effects of progestogens on postmenopausal calcium metabolism. Apparently, however, gestronol hexanoate and norethisterone acetate (NETA) may prevent the loss of bone (17,18), whereas medroxyprogesterone does not have this effect.

Studies have suggested that NETA may have bone formation-stimulating effects. A short-term pathophysiologic investigation (19) studied the separate effects of E_2 alone and E_2 plus NETA on biochemical markers of bone turnover. The markers of bone resorption decreased relatively more than the markers of bone formation during E_2-NETA therapy than during E_2 alone.

The next study of the effect of NETA on bone density included a group of premenopausal women with endometriosis (20). To alleviate the endometriosis symptoms, women were treated with the LH-RH agonist Nafarelin. This compound blocks estrogen production and thereby relieves the pain around menstruation. However, the treatment has the severe adverse effect that bone density declines relatively rapidly, accompanied by significant increases in biochemical markers of bone turnover. When this endometriosis treatment was combined with a small dose of NETA, the bone loss was prevented. The biochemical markers of bone turnover also displayed a different response than those of the Nafarelin alone group, compatible with a relative high ratio of bone formation to resorption.

In a recently published study (21) of alendronate treatment of early postmenopausal women, a combination of E_2 and NETA was included for comparison. The study included a total of 1,460 women aged 45 to 59 years, and

of those, 110 received HRT. The optimum dose of alendronate appeared to be 5 mg (ALN5). After 2 years of treatment, bone mineral density in the spine had increased by 3.34% in the ALN5 group and by 5.14% in the Trisequens group ($p < 0.01$). The same numbers in the hip were 1.60% versus 3.21% ($p < 0.001$), in the forearm 1.14% versus 0.54%, and in the total body 0.64% versus 2.59% ($p < 0.001$), respectively.

Estrogen-Progestogen Combinations

A number of studies have been carried out with combined hormone therapy (15–17,22–24). Progestogens do not counteract the estrogenic effect on calcium metabolic parameters and may in some instances even add to the effect of the estrogen (25).

EFFECTS ON BONE

Both ERT and HRT prevent osteoporosis in postmenopausal women (22–24). Bone loss caused by estrogen deficiency is prevented by estrogen and estrogen-progestogen therapy, independent of age and menopausal age (25–28).

Hormone Replacement Therapy in Early Postmenopausal Women

In early postmenopausal women, numerous studies have demonstrated that oral estrogen and estrogen-progestogen regimens stop bone loss. This is true for use of both synthetic and nonsynthetic estrogens, although nonsynthetic estrogens should be preferred for postmenopausal therapy. The estrogenic effect on bone is dose dependent; if a sufficient serum concentration of estrogen is not obtained, bone loss will not be arrested completely. For oral estrogen and estrogen-progestogen therapy, studies have demonstrated that doses of 0.625 mg of conjugated estrogens and 2 mg of 17β-estradiol prevent early postmenopausal bone loss (Fig. 29.2) (29–31). However, recent studies (6,32–35)

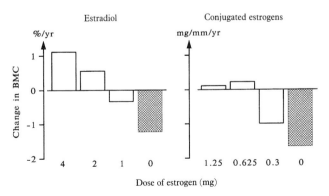

FIG. 29.2. The effect of different doses of estrogens on loss of bone mineral. The optimum bone-sparing dose of estradiol lies between 1 and 2 mg daily and is 0.625 mg daily for conjugated estrogens. (**Left** from ref. 30 and **right** from ref. 31, with permission.)

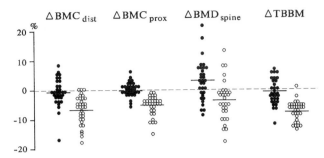

FIG. 29.3. Bone mass measured in different areas of the skeleton during HRT (○) or placebo (●). Note that the bone loss is prevented in all skeletal areas. (From ref. 23, with permission.)

suggest that lower doses may be sufficient to prevent bone loss, which is important because adverse effects are dose dependent.

The postmenopausal bone loss is a generalized phenomenon affecting all parts of the skeleton, that is, areas with mainly trabecular bone (e.g., the spine) as well as areas with mainly cortical bone (e.g., the forearm and the hip) (23,24). Postmenopausal estrogen therapy prevents bone loss from all skeletal areas (Fig. 29.3). Studies of total body bone mineral have thus demonstrated that estrogen therapy prevents the bone loss in the head, chest, arms, pelvis, and legs (36,37). Other studies, where the bone mass in the spine, hip, and forearm have been examined directly, have revealed that HRT definitely arrests bone loss in all skeletal areas (23,24).

In addition to oral HRT, other delivery systems are available. Percutaneous 17β-estradiol, that is, estradiol given in a gel applied every day on the skin, prevents skeletal bone loss as effectively as oral HRT (19). The same is the case with transcutaneous estradiol, that is, estradiol given in a patch that is changed two to three times per week. Studies have demonstrated that this delivery system also prevents bone loss (38).

Hormone Replacement Therapy Later in Life

The increased bone remodeling seems to be most pronounced in the early postmenopausal years. With increasing age postmenopausally, there may be a tendency toward a slowing down in bone turnover and thereby in the rate of bone loss. The greatest benefit from HRT is therefore obtained if it is instituted shortly after menopause. Indeed, it has been debated whether HRT in elderly postmenopausal women has an effect at all. However, the literature contains clear evidence that HRT prevents bone loss at all stages of postmenopausal life (25–28,39).

Lindsay et al. treated osteoporotic patients with estrogen and calcium or calcium alone (26). The mean number of years since menopause was 12, with a range of 4 to 35. At the end of 24 months, mean bone mass in the spine and hip was significantly higher in the estrogen-treated group than in the calcium-treated group. At both skeletal sites, bone loss was stopped, and bone density even increased moderately.

Christiansen et al. treated 65-year-old women who had their first osteoporotic fracture with a continuous combination of E₂ and NETA (25). After 12 months of treatment, bone density in skeletal areas with a high content of trabecular bone (spine and ultradistal forearm) had increased by 8% to 10% when compared to placebo. The total skeleton and the distal forearm, which contain approximately 80% cortical bone, increased on the average 3% to 5% (Fig. 29.4).

Riggs et al. treated 66 osteoporotic patients with transdermal estrogen, 0.1 mg, 25 days per month plus medroxyprogesterone acetate, 10 mg/day, for 10 days per month, or placebo (39). All subjects consumed 800 mg of dietary calcium per day. Estrogen-treated patients showed a sharp decrease in histologic features of osteoporotic bone resorption and bone formation, an increase in spinal bone density, and a decrease in fracture rate compared to placebo-treated patients. These anatomic changes were accompanied by a significant decrease in serum markers of bone turnover in treated patients: at 1 year, mean serum osteocalcin had decreased by approximately 20%, and bone alkaline phosphatase and urinary hydroxyproline both by approximately 40%.

A recent study suggested that bone loss may increase again in old women, especially in the hip region (40). If this holds true, treatment, also with HRT, may successfully be instituted even very late in life.

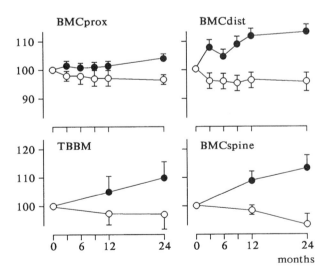

FIG. 29.4. Bone mass measurement in different areas of the skeleton during therapy of 65-year-old woman with hormones (○) or placebo (●). (From ref. 25, with permission.)

Effects of Hormone Replacement Therapy on Fractures

When HRT is stopped, bone loss recurs. The rate of bone loss after stopping HRT has been shown to be accelerated compared to average postmenopausal bone loss (41). However, others have shown that the rate of bone loss after cessation of HRT is similar to average bone loss (22). Several epidemiologic studies have shown that HRT provides protection against fractures (42,43). However, it is obvious that the treatment has to be continued for some years to be effective. It is difficult to suggest a definite treatment period, but 5 to 10 years is what may be necessary before this fracture protection can be observed if estrogens are prescribed in the immediate postmenopausal period. A number of case-control studies have demonstrated that HRT given for at least 6 years reduces the risk of hip fractures and Colles' fractures by 50%. Cohort studies have also shown that long-term HRT reduces the incidence of vertebral deformities in postmenopausal women by about 90% (1).

HORMONE REPLACEMENT THERAPY AND CALCIUM

It is still debated which role calcium intake plays in the development of a low bone mass and/or in susceptibility to fractures. In large parts of the Western world, the daily calcium intake approximates 500 mg. One cross-sectional study of calcium metabolism has indicated that a daily requirement of 1,000 mg of calcium for premenopausal women and 1,500 mg for postmenopausal women (44) is what is required. Moreover, the study indicated that a sufficiently high calcium intake can reverse a negative calcium balance and thereby suppress bone loss. However, this has not been confirmed in longitudinal studies of early postmenopausal women (45,46).

The adverse effects of estrogen therapy are dose dependent. It would, therefore, be of major importance if it were possible to reduce the dose of estrogen required to prevent bone loss and osteoporosis. A recent study suggested that the daily dose of estrogen could be reduced by 50% if it was combined with a daily calcium supplement of 1,000 mg (47). The study was not double-blind placebo-controlled and will thus have to be confirmed in future studies before final conclusions can be drawn. Another study has examined whether a calcium supplement could provide additional benefit to an already optimized estrogen regimen (48). In this study, estrogen alone prevented bone loss as effectively as estrogen combined with calcium.

ESTROGEN ANALOGS

Antiestrogens and Selective Estrogen Receptor Modulators

In 1973, McGuire and Chamness (48a) summarized their work on the estrogen receptor in animal and human breast tumors and, in so doing, described a target for therapeutic intervention. At that time there were no clinically useful antiestrogens, but the subsequent development of tamoxifen for breast cancer therapy has revolutionized the approach to treatment. In addition to breast cancer therapy with antiestrogens, a new strategy is being developed to exploit the target site for the beneficial actions of estrogen, that is, prevention of bone loss and cardiovascular disease (49).

Today, three so-called selective estrogen receptor modulators (SERMs) are being evaluated as a treatment for osteoporosis: raloxifene, levomeloxifene, and droloxifene.

Raloxifene is the compound that is in the most advanced stage of development, and the first reports from the first interim analysis of the first phase III studies have just been published (50). Raloxifene is a selective estrogen receptor modulator that in animal models acts as an estrogen receptor antagonist in breast and endometrial tissue but as an estrogen agonist in the skeletal and cardiovascular systems. The clinical trials have demonstrated that raloxifene is well tolerated and normalizes bone turnover and slows the bone loss in healthy early postmenopausal women without stimulating uterus and breast tissues. In contrast, preliminary data suggest that raloxifene may even decrease the risk of breast cancer (Fig. 29.5) (50).

In elderly women with osteoporosis, defined as more than one previous vertebral fracture, the same effects were seen as in the younger women: normalization of bone turnover and reduction and even an increase in bone mass (51). In this study, which was a preliminary fracture study, the effect on fracture incidence was of borderline statistical significance. There were overall multiple beneficial effects on bone, although, under the conditions of that study, they appear to be less prominent than have been reported with estrogen (51).

Raloxifene has been shown to reduce aortic atherosclerosis significantly in cholesterol-fed rabbits (52). In the clinical trails reported so far, raloxifene lowered serum cholesterol and LDL-cholesterol significantly in both early and late postmenopausal women (51). Raloxifene is expected to be available in several countries within the next year or so.

Levomeloxifene, another SERM compound, has previously been shown to inhibit bone loss and arterial cholesterol accumulation in estrogen-depleted animal models without stimulation of the endometrial glands or the epithelium. Different doses of levomeloxifene decrease bone turnover parameters and serum cholesterol and LDL-cholesterol in postmenopausal women (53).

Droloxifene, a third SERM compound, has been shown to decrease bone turnover, prevent bone loss, and reduce total serum cholesterol in ovariectomized rats without stimulating the endometrium (54).

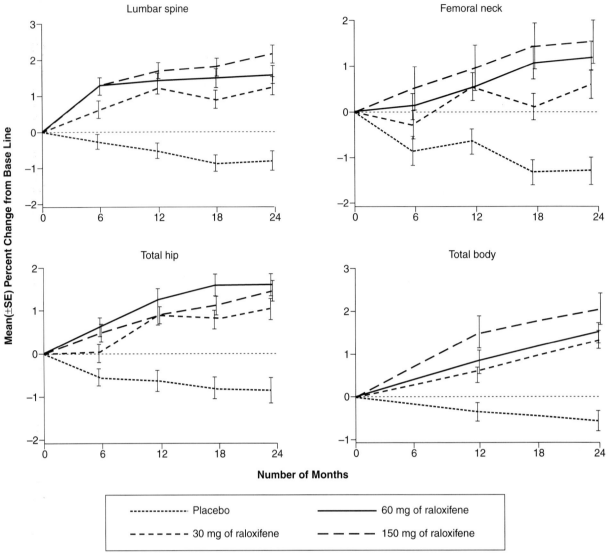

FIG. 29.5. Mean percentage change in bone mineral density in postmenopausal women given ralox-ifene or placebo for 2 years. (From ref. 50, with permission.)

Adverse Events

It may not be possible to summarize adverse effects of all known SERMs in one paragraph. The different SERMs may have different metabolic actions and short- and long-term adverse effects. However, at the present time, only raloxifene has been studied to an extent that makes it possible to reach any conclusion about side effects. Generally, the SERMs are well tolerated. The most annoying side effect may be an increased number of hot flushes, which seem to disappear after a few months' treatment (50). The big question is, of course, the effect on the endometrium and breast tissues, which

will be answered only at the end of the large, long-term clinical trials.

Other Antiestrogens

Tibolone is a synthetic steroid with estrogenic, androgenic, and progestogenic properties. It is approved in many countries for treatment of menopausal symptoms such as hot flushes. This compound also prevents bone loss (34) and reduces the bone turnover to normal levels (55). A recent study showed that the half of the normally recommended dose has the same effect on bone metabolism (34). Tibolone reduces serum cholesterol and triglycerides, although LDL-cholesterol is unaffected. However, it decreases HDL-cholesterol and apolipoprotein A₁ by about 30%. The overall effect on hemostatic factors tends toward increased fibrinolysis and unchanged coagulation. This may be beneficial and might theoretically counterbalance the potentially negative effect of the decrease in HDL-cholesterol (56).

BISPHOSPHONATES

The bisphosphonates are a class of drugs developed in the past two decades for use in various diseases of bone and teeth as well as in calcium metabolism. Bisphosphonates are compounds characterized by two carbon-phosphorus bonds. They are analogous to the physiologically occurring inorganic pyrophosphate in which an oxygen atom has been replaced by a carbon atom. The structure of the bisphosphonates allows a great number of variations. Each bisphosphonate has its own physicochemical and biologic characteristics. One should thus not speak generally about the effect of "the bisphosphonates" but rather consider each bisphosphonate on its own.

It is known that pyrophosphate impairs the crystallization as well as the dissolution of calcium phosphate crystals. This effect is apparently related to the strong surface adsorption of pyrophosphate on solid-phase calcium phosphate. Bisphosphonates act in a similar way and thus have the ability both to block the production of apatite crystals and to delay the dissolution of the crystals. Bisphosphonates, when given both parenterally and orally,

have been found to inhibit experimentally induced calcification of soft tissues such as arteries, kidney, skin, and heart. If administered in sufficiently high doses, certain bisphosphonates can also inhibit the normal calcification that occurs in bone, cartilage, and teeth. Bisphosphonates are resorption inhibitors, as are estrogen and calcitonin; that is, they decrease the rate of bone resorption.

Bisphosphonates have undergone a revolutionary development during the past 5 years, and they are now a reality as an option for osteoporosis prevention and treatment. In the Unites States, and in many other countries, alendronate (Fosamax) is now approved for both prevention and treatment of osteoporosis. The approval was based on a number of very large double-blind studies in both early and late postmenopausal women as well as in osteoporotic women.

Prevention of Bone Loss

For prevention of bone loss, a dose of 5 mg/day of alendronate is approved (Fig. 29.6) (57). This dose has now been studied for 5 years (58); in the spine there is an increase in bone density within the first 2 years of treatment by a total of approximately 4%. Thereafter, a plateau is reached, as would be expected for an antiresorptive agent (see above), and bone mass is thereafter kept constant. The same pattern is seen in the hip, forearm, and total body.

Other bisphosphonates are under development for prevention of bone loss, including ibandronate (Fig. 29.7) (59).

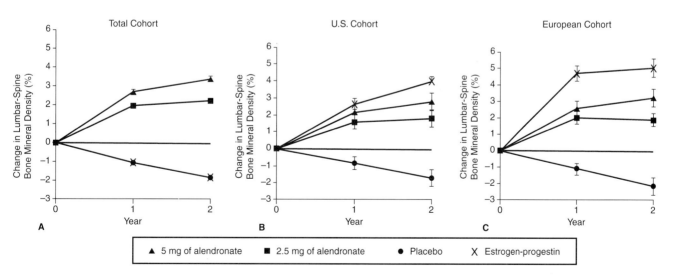

FIG. 29.6. Mean (±SE) percentage change from baseline in lumar spine bone mineral density after 1 and 2 years of treatment with placebo, 2.5 mg or 5 mg alendronate, or estrogen-progestin in the total cohort **(A),** the U.S. cohort **(B),** and the European cohort **(C).** (From ref. 21, with permission.)

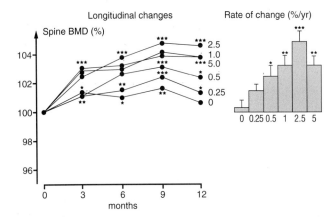

FIG. 29.7. Left: Serial measurements of bone mineral density (BMD) in the lumber spine (L1-4) expressed as percentage of baseline values and given as the mean percentage value in each group over the 12-month study period. ***p < 0.001; **p < 0.01; *p < 0.05 (compared to baseline). **Right:** Values of the slopes of the linear regression lines (%/year) between bone mineral density and time in each group. ***p < 0.001; **p < 0.01; *p < 0.05 (compared to placebo). (From ref. 59, with permission.)

Treatment of Osteoporosis and Prevention of Fractures

For treatment of women who already have osteoporosis, a dose of 10 mg/day of alendronate is approved. A very large study (60) showed that alendronate reduced the

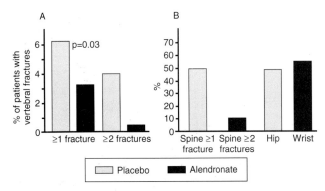

FIG. 29.8. A: Effect of the daily oral administration of either 5 mg or 10 mg for 3 years or 20 mg for 2 years followed by 5 mg for 1 year of alendronate (all mean data pooled) on new vertebral fractures in postmenopausal osteoporotic women with or without fractures. (Data from Liberman UA, et al. Effect of oral alendronate on bone mineral density and the incidence of fractures in postmenopausal osteoporosis. The alendronate phase III osteoporosis treatment study group. *N Engl J Med* 1995;333:1437–1443.) **B:** Effect of 5 mg alendronate orally daily for 2 years followed by 10 mg for approximately 1 year in postmenopausal osteoporotic women with at least one vertebral fracture. (Data from ref. 60.) Alendronate reduces the risk of vertebral and clinical fractures in women with existing vertebral fractures. (All data are expressed as percentage of patients who received placebo. All differences are statistically significant.) (From Fleish H. *Bisphosphonates in bone disease.* New York: Parthenon, 1997)

risk of the most common forms of osteoporotic fracture (spine, hip, wrist) by approximately 50% in women with low hip bone density and previous fracture. Also, women with no previous fracture at enrollment into the study had fracture incidence decreased by approximately 50% (Fig. 29.8) (61).

In many countries, but not in the United States, etidronate is approved for treatment. In two double-blind, placebo-controlled studies (62,63), etidronate was given orally at 400 mg/day for 2 weeks, followed by 10 to 13 weeks of calcium supplementation (a cyclic regimen). After 2 to 3 years of study, vertebral fractures in cyclical etidronate-treated patients were reduced by 50% compared to patients receiving calcium. The treatment regimen also produced increases in vertebral bone mass of 4% to 8% versus control over the 2 to 3 years. Furthermore, cyclic etidronate maintained cortical bone at the hip and wrist.

Adverse Effects

It is also difficult to say anything in common about the large number of bisphosphonates because they have very different profiles in terms of adverse effects. Bisphosphonates are generally absorbed very poorly from the gut, and the absorption is seriously disturbed by such factors as concomitant food ingestion. Bisphosphonates, therefore, in general have to be taken a certain amount of time before and after a meal. Calcium-containing food products are the worst because they will bind the bisphosphonates and avoid absorption.

The bisphosphonates already approved or in development seem to be associated with few adverse effects. The most discussed adverse affect is gastrointestinal irritation, which may occur for several reasons. However, one way to try to avoid it may be to stay up when the tablet has been taken. Going back to bed immediately may not be a good idea.

CALCITONIN

Calcitonin is a long-chain polypeptide hormone that is produced by the parafollicular cells of the thyroid gland. Its role in humans is uncertain, but its administration inhibits bone resorption by a direct inhibitory action on the activity of osteoclasts. Abundant calcitonin receptors are present on the surface of osteoclasts, and until now such receptors have not been detected on any other type of bone cell.

Long-term treatment with calcitonin seems not only to inhibit osteoclast activity but also to decrease the number of osteoclasts. To date, calcitonin has been isolated from humans and over 15 other species, but currently, only human, eel, porcine, and salmon calcitonins are in medical use. Salmon calcitonin has been used extensively in clinical studies. Calcitonin has been used for many years in the management of Paget's disease or malignant hypercalcemia. Because of its protein-like nature, calcitonin is degraded by the gastric juices if given by mouth. Calcitonin has therefore been administered subcutaneously, either daily or thrice weekly. The parenteral route, however, is not practical for long-term treatment. Calcitonin has now been developed for administration through the nasal mucosa, using a nasal spray.

Calcitonin-salmon has been approved by the United States Food and Drug Administration (FDA) for the treatment of Paget's disease of bone, hypercalcemia, and postmenopausal osteoporosis. Since the discovery of calcitonin in 1961, it has also been used effectively to reverse the bone loss observed in immobilized paraplegic patients, Sudeck's atrophy of bone, patients treated with glucocorticoid medications, and in malignant diseases such as multiple myeloma.

Calcitonin in Osteoporosis

Calcitonin has been evaluated in therapeutic trials in osteoporotic women for the past 13 to 15 years. Reports of therapeutic responses have been very variable.

Because calcitonin acts primarily to suppress osteoclastic activity in bone, one could anticipate that individuals with high-turnover forms of the osteoporotic process could respond much more rapidly to calcitonin therapy than those with less active disturbances in bone remodeling. In fact, this hypothesis has been substantiated with reports of larger effects in patients with high bone turnover (64). In 1987, Reginster et al. (65) provided early evidence that calcitonin therapy effectively counteracted the propensity for vertebral bone loss in women who had been menopausal for no more than 36 months and, as such, were most likely to have active or high-turnover bone remodeling. These findings, demonstrating a protective effect of calcitonin after ovarian failure, when active bone turnover dominates, were confirmed by Overgaard et al. in 1989 (66).

In a double-blind study, Overgaard et al. (67) demonstrated that 200 IU daily of nasal salmon calcitonin (plus 500 mg calcium) prevents further bone loss in postmenopausal women with low bone mass. The nasal administration form produced no metabolic, vascular, or gastrointestinal side effects, nor was there any local irritation. From this study it was concluded that nasal calcitonin might be a potential treatment for women with low bone mass 10 to 15 years after the menopause. Twelve months after withdrawal of therapy, a subgroup of the women resumed treatment with calcitonin, 200 IU, plus calcium, 500 mg, daily in an open design for an additional 1-year period (68). A control group of 19 age-matched women (no forearm fracture) did not receive any treatment. At the end of the 3 years, the control group had lost significantly more bone in the forearm and spine than had the group treated with intranasal calcitonin for 2 years. The group

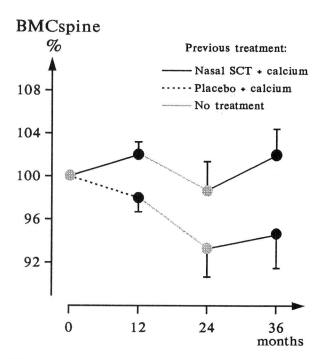

FIG. 29.9. Spinal bone mass in elderly osteoporotic women receiving either intranasal calcitonin (●) or placebo (○) for the first 12 months, no treatment in the second year (all women); and intranasal calcitonin in the third year (all women). (From ref. 68, with permission.)

receiving calcitonin for 1 year had intermediate bone mass values. In the year after withdrawal, the rate of bone loss was similar in the women who had received calcitonin and those who had received placebo (Fig. 29.9). Calcitonin was especially effective in women with initially high bone turnover and low bone mass. The bone response in the spine could thus be estimated by the changes in bone turnover. The data suggest that discontinuous treatment with intranasal calcitonin affects bone and calcium metabolism in established osteoporosis. In women with high-turnover osteoporosis, the therapy results in a net gain of bone in both the peripheral and axial skeleton.

Calcitonin and Fractures

A Mediterranean osteoporosis study (69) designed to examine the incidence of hip fracture in more than 5,000 men and women 50 years or older from six countries in southern Europe demonstrated that calcitonin, like estrogen therapy, significantly decreased the incidence of hip fractures. In a double-blind study of 400 women with osteoporosis treated with either 100, 200, or 400 IU/day nasal salmon calcitonin or placebo for 2 years, the vertebral fracture rate was reduced by two-thirds (70). These data have recently been confirmed in a large study including 1,175 osteoporotic women (71).

In both studies the increase in bone density was relatively modest. One may wonder about the mechanism behind a decreased incidence of vertebral fracture despite only a modest increase in spinal bone mass. One answer may be that in trabecular bone, the thin unprotected vertical trabeculae may be protected against buckling and perforation when the bone turnover rate is decreased, and this may stabilize bone structure.

Adverse Effects

Approximately 8% to 10% of patients treated with calcitonin have nausea and mild gastric discomfort. These symptoms characteristically occur at the initiation of therapy but either decrease in severity or disappear completely during treatment. Facial flushing and dermatologic hypersensitivity occur in 2% to 5% of patients, and local pruritic reactions are felt at injection sites in approximately 10% of patients. These latter symptoms are usually mild and respond to appropriate antihistaminic therapy such as diphenhydramine HCl (Benadryl), 50 mg orally 20 to 30 minutes before the subcutaneous injection of calcitonin. The dermatologic symptoms also tend to disappear with continued administration of the drug. Occasional gastrointestinal side effects, such as bloating or mild epigastric fullness, can be minimized if the drug is administered 4 to 5 hours after a meal, preferably at bedtime. Only rarely are urinary frequency and diarrhea encountered. As expected, the side effects of therapy are more severe when calcitonin is given parenterally and minimized when given subcutaneously because of the higher peak blood levels achieved after parenteral injections. The side effects observed in the past with injectable forms of calcitonin are substantially decreased when the drug is administered by nasal spray.

SODIUM FLUORIDE

Sodium fluoride (NaF) has been used for many years for the prevention of dental caries. A number of countries fluoridate their water for this purpose. It has been estimated that water fluoridation at one part per million results in a fluoride consumption of approximately 1 mg/day, a dosage that inhibits the formation of dental caries in children but does not exert an appreciable effect on bone structure (72).

It was the realization that moderate amounts of fluoride could produce osteosclerosis (abnormally increased bone density) that prompted the investigation of fluoride as a treatment of osteoporosis. This occurred in the 1950s, when it was noticed that moderate (5 to 10 ppm) concentrations of fluoride in the water supply of the population of Bartlett, Texas, had resulted in the development of osteosclerosis.

Mechanism of Action

The specific actions of fluoride on bone are complex and not completely understood. In the mineral phase of bone formation, fluoride substitutes for the hydroxyl radical in the hydroxyapatite crystal lattice to form fluoroapatite (73). Fluoride stimulates bone formation by causing an increase in both osteoblast activity and osteoblast number. The effect on osteoblast number is greater than that on activity (74). *In vitro* work suggests that the direct action of fluoride involves the stimulus for the proliferation of osteoblast precursors (74).

Effects of Fluoride on Bone

Treatment with fluoride increases trabecular bone mass, especially in the spine. Cortical bone volume (e.g., in the forearm or hip), however, is not increased and may even be decreased. The histomorphometric change resulting from fluoride treatment is a marked increase in the osteoid surfaces (formation surface) without a significant increase in resorption surfaces. The result of this increase in formation surfaces is an imbalance of the coupling of resorption to formation in favor of bone formation. This leads to a substantial increase in trabecular bone volume.

Fluoride stimulates osteoid formation but increases mineralization lag time, which may result in histologic osteomalacia. In addition to its stimulatory effect on bone formation, fluoride increases bone resorption, although to a lesser degree than bone formation. This effect results from increases in osteoclastic resorptive activity (75,76).

Fluoride Treatment of Osteoporosis

The ideal therapeutic program for osteoporosis should not just prevent further bone loss but should increase bone mass to a level that exceeds the fracture threshold. For this to occur, bone formation must be substantially greater than bone resorption. Although various regimens that have the potential for stimulating bone formation are currently under investigation, only therapy with sodium fluoride has been widely evaluated.

Sodium fluoride has been used to treat patients with osteoporosis for over 20 years. Despite its widespread and growing use, there are concerns about its safety and antifracture efficacy. The incidence of side effects is relatively high, particularly those relating to gastric irritation and pain in the lower extremities (77,78). Moreover, bone formed during the administration of fluoride may be structurally abnormal because of defective mineralization of the newly synthesized bone (79). Indeed, in some uncontrolled studies, fluoride therapy increased the occurrence of hip fractures (80), although this has not been confirmed in controlled studies (81–83).

Eventually, two ambitious double-blind studies were carried out to examine these issues in depth (77,78). The Mayo Clinic study (77) comprised 202 postmenopausal women and used a dose of sodium fluoride of 75 mg/day (equivalent to 33.9 mg of fluoride ion per day) and a calcium supplement of 1,500 mg/day. One hundred-thirty-five women completed the 4 years of treatment. Bone mass increased by +35% in the spine and by +12% in the femoral neck over 4 years (about 8% to 9% and 3% per year, respectively) but decreased by 4% in the radius. The trend for a decrease in vertebral fractures with fluoride was not significantly different from placebo, and the number of nonvertebral fractures tended to be even higher in the fluoride group (Fig. 29.10).

It was argued that the "negative" results of the Mayo Clinic study resulted from the dose. A daily dose of 75 mg was said to be so high that it would result in fluorosis. Consequently, expectations in the French study, using lower doses, were high. The French study (78) comprised 354 osteoporotic women who received either fluoride as sodium fluoride (50 mg/day, equivalent to 22.6 mg of fluoride ion per day) or monofluorophosphate (MFP, 150 or 200 mg, equivalent to 19.8 or 26.4 mg of fluoride ion per day, respectively) or placebo for 2 years. In this study, all the women received 1,000 mg of calcium plus 800 IU of vitamin D_2 per day. The results were disappointing. The BMD of the lumbar spine increased significantly by 10.8% (or about 5% per year) in the women treated with fluoride, but there was no reduction in the percentage of new vertebral fractures (assessed semiquantitatively) during the 2 years of the study. In fact, the incidence of women with one or more vertebral fractures was virtually identical in the two groups (33% in the fluoride group and 27% in the placebo group). The incidence of nonvertebral fractures was also similar between the groups.

A recent study reported the effect of combined fluoride therapy, given as MFP, equivalent to 20 mg/day of fluoride and HRT given as a 50-μg estradiol patch and 1 mg NETA per day (84). Treatment with HRT + MFP resulted in a pro-

nounced and almost linear increase in spinal BMD (11.8 ± 1.7% per year), which was statistically significantly greater than the increase in the HRT-alone group (4.0 ± 0.5% per year) ($p < 0.0001$). Treatment with MFP alone induced a smaller increase (2.4 ± 0.6% per year) in spinal BMD, and there was no change over time in the placebo group (0.0 ± 0.5% per year). In the femoral neck the changes were +3.4 ± 1.5% in the HRT + MFP group, +1.4 ± 0.4% in the HRT-alone group, -0.1 ± 0.4% in the MFP-alone group, and +0.1 ± 0.3% in the placebo group. A similar pattern was found in the forearm and the total skeleton.

Variation in Individual Responsiveness

Recent data suggest that responsiveness of individual patients to fluoride therapy varies. Riggs et al. (85) reported that 12 of 27 osteoporotic patients (44%) treated for 4 years or more failed to show a roentgenographic increase in trabecular bone thickening of the vertebrae. Briancon and Meunier (76) found that 7 of 28 osteoporotic patients (25%) who had iliac crest biopsies before and after 2 years of fluoride therapy failed to increase trabecular bone volume. Farley et al. (86) found that 23% of treated patients did not increase alkaline phosphatase activity significantly. For the group of fluoride-treated osteoporotic patients shown in Fig. 29.2, 13 of 40 (32%) failed to increase bone mass to a level significantly greater than baseline (87).

The cause of individual variability in responsiveness is unknown. It does not appear to involve noncompliance or other identifiable factors (88). Possibly there is a primary defect in osteoblast function that prevents response to fluoride therapy. It is noteworthy, however, that both Briancon and Meunier (76) and Lane et al. (89) found that pretreatment levels of bone turnover as assessed by tetracycline-based histomorphometry of iliac crest biopsy could not predict subsequent outcome. Whatever its cause, individual nonresponsiveness remains a problem in practical management.

Adverse Effects

Results of large series have reported that significant adverse effects occur in 30% to 50% of patients (72). These have been of two types: symptoms related to gastric irritation and a lower extremity pain syndrome.

The gastric symptoms are epigastric pain, nausea, vomiting, and occasionally blood-loss anemia. Minor gastric symptoms are even more common. These adverse effects result from the irritant effect of fluoride ions on gastric mucosa. The frequency of gastric adverse effects can be reduced by giving calcium supplements such as calcium carbonate, an effective antacid. Because an increase in calcium ions in the intestine lowers fluoride absorption, the dosage of sodium fluoride must be increased by approximately 25% to achieve the same

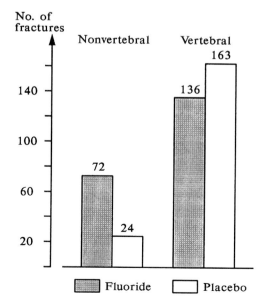

FIG. 29.10. Continuous NaF did not appear to be more effective than calcium carbonate in reducing vertebral fracture rate or height loss in white women with postmenopausal osteoporosis. (Adapted from ref. 82, with permission.)

amount of absorbed fluoride when calcium is given concomitantly (90). In patients with adverse effects that persist after the dosage is reduced, reduction in gastric acid secretion by administration of H_2-receptor blockers may be effective. Finally, Pak et al. (91) reported that gastric adverse effects could be reduced sharply by administering the fluoride in a delayed-release tablet.

The second major adverse effect is a syndrome of periarticular pain and tenderness at the large joints of the lower extremities or in the feet (88). These symptoms disappear within 2 to 6 weeks of discontinuing treatment and usually do not recur when therapy is reinstituted at a lower dosage. The symptoms most commonly involve a single region, although two or more regions are sometimes involved. If symptoms recur, the same area or another area may be involved. In order of decreasing frequency, the most commonly involved areas are the ankles and lower leg, the feet, the knees and lower femur, and the upper femur. Although the exact causal mechanism is not established, it is now apparent that the symptoms are of osseous rather than synovial origin, as was formerly believed. Schnitzler and Solomon (92) demonstrated the presence of trabecular stress fractures in the painful region of all five fluoride-treated patients who developed the syndrome. O'Duffy et al. (93) were able to document stress fractures in only 5 of 11 symptomatic patients. Because quantitative skeletal uptake of ^{99m}Tc-diphosphonate demonstrated that fluoride-treated osteoporotic patients with the pain syndrome had greater bone activity than did asymptomatic fluoride-treated patients or calcium-treated osteoporotic patients,

they concluded that the underlying mechanism might be intense skeletal remodeling, which may be complicated by development of stress fractures. Schultz et al. (94) failed to find stress fractures in symptomatic fluoride-treated patients and attributed the pain to the periosteal new bone formation, which they observed radiographically. Nonetheless, it may be premature to exclude stress fractures as the cause of pain in all cases because they are sometimes difficult to demonstrate, even by serial x-ray examination. Thus, although there is a high incidence of major adverse effects during fluoride therapy, these can be controlled in most patients.

ANABOLIC STEROIDS

Anabolic steroids are chemically related to natural androgens. They are distinguished from the latter by a powerful protein anabolic effect in doses that produce little androgen effect. Complete separation of the two activities is not possible because they differ only with respect to their treatment location: anabolic activity causes extragenital stimulation of protein synthesis, whereas androgen activity is expressed at the area of the sex organs. The dissociation of the anabolic from the androgen effects seems to be at least partly dependent on the serum concentration of the drug. It has been demonstrated for the anabolic steroid, nandrolone decanoate, that after an intramuscular injection, the dynamics of the release of nandrolone esters from the depots is responsible for the dominant anabolic to androgen effect ratio.

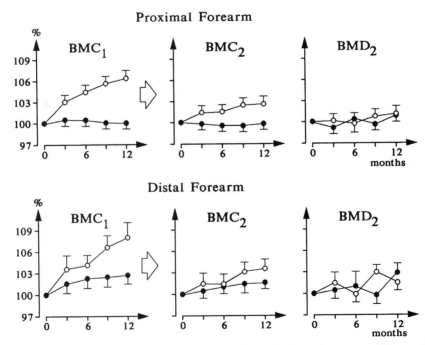

FIG. 29.11. Forearm bone mass during treatment with nandrolone decanoate (○) or placebo (●). BMC_1, uncorrected bone mineral content; BMC_2, fat-corrected bone mineral density. Proximal and distal refer to two different measurement sites (see text). Values are given as percentage of initial mass, mean ± 1 SEM. (From ref. 95, with permission.)

In spite of this dissociation, some untoward side effects might also be observed during treatment with nandrolone decanoate. There is a wide individual variation with respect to the doses producing side effects, which depends on an individual's sensitivity. Hoarseness or lowering of the voice, male-type growth of hair on arms, legs, and face, and with higher doses muscle enlargement and clitoromegaly, as well as increased libido, may occur. Retention of sodium chloride might result in edema. All such untoward side effects are reversible, perhaps with the exception of the voice disturbance. Liver toxicity has been observed in a few cases.

Anabolic steroids have been used for many years for the treatment of osteoporosis. Such therapy was based more on tradition than on scientific results. Recent clinical trials, however, have indicated that patients with established osteoporosis obtain a positive calcium balance during treatment with nandrolone decanoate (95) (Fig. 29.11). Furthermore, patients obtain an increased amount of muscle mass and a decreased fat mass (96).

PARATHYROID HORMONE

Parathyroid hormone (PTH) is one of the calcium-regulating hormones. The PTH secretion increases in response to decreased serum levels of calcium. The PTH then stimulates bone resorption and the production of 1,25-dihydroxyvitamin D, which in turn increases the intestinal absorption of calcium. In this way, the serum concentration of calcium tends to rise. The physiologic effect of PTH is therefore to stimulate bone resorption. Recent studies, however, have shown that injections of low doses of synthetic PTH stimulate bone formation. PTH is currently being investigated as a treatment for osteoporosis. The preliminary results look promising (97), but it is too soon to tell whether PTH will be an option in the future for osteoporosis therapy.

A recent study (98) of 34 postmenopausal women with osteoporosis compared the combination of PTH and HRT (n = 17) with HRT alone (n = 17). The authors found a significant increase in bone mass at all skeletal sites, most pronounced in the spine, where the increase was 13% over three years and 2.7% at the hip. The increase was most pronounced during the first year of PTH treatment. Calculations of vertebral fracture incidence showed a decreased incidence in the PTH + HRT group compared to the HRT-alone group.

REFERENCES

1. Consensus Development Conference. Diagnosis, prophylaxis and treatment of osteoporosis. *Am J Med* 1993;94:646–650.
2. Melton LJ. Epidemiology of fractures. In: Riggs BL, Melton LJ, eds. *Osteoporosis: etiology, diagnosis and management.* New York: Raven Press, 1988:133–154.
3. Nilas L, Christiansen C. Bone mass and its relationship to age and the menopause. *J Clin Endocrinol Metab* 1987;65:697–702.
4. Thomsen K, Gotfredsen A, Christiansen C. Is postmenopausal bone loss an age-related phenomenon? *Calcif Tissue Int* 1986;39:123–127.
5. Christiansen C, Riis B. Five years with continuous-combined oestrogen-progesto-

gen treatment. Effects on calcium metabolism, lipoproteins, and bleeding pattern. *Br J Obstet Gynecol* 1990;97:1087–1091.
6. Alexandersen P, Hassager C, Sandholdt I, Riis BJ, Christiansen C. The effect of cyclophasic hormone replacement therapy on postmenopausal bone mass and bone turnover. *J Bone Miner Res* 1997;12(Suppl 1):S499.
7. Hammond CB, Maxson WS. Current status of estrogen therapy for the menopause. *Fertil Steril* 1982;37:5–25.
8. Mashchak CA, Lobo RA, Dozono-Takono R, et al. Comparison of pharmacodynamic properties of various estrogen formulations. *Am J Obstet Gynecol* 1982;144:511–518.
9. Hammond CB, Maxson WS. Estrogen replacement therapy. *Clin Obstet Gynecol* 1968;29:407–430.
10. Neumann F. The physiological action of progesterone and the pharmacological effects of progestogen. A short review. *Postgrad Med* 1978;54:11–24.
11. Nordin BBC. Calcium. *J Food Nutr* 1986;42:67–82.
12. Parfitt AM. Quantum concept of bone remodeling and turnover: implications for the pathogenesis of osteoporosis. *Calcif Tissue Int* 1979;28:1–5.
13. Riggs BL, Mann KG. Assessment of bone turnover in osteoporosis using biochemical marker. In: Christiansen C, et al, eds. *Osteoporosis 1987, vol 2.* Copenhagen: Osteopress ApS, 1987:67–76.
14. Christiansen C, Rødbro P, Tjellesen L. Serum alkaline phosphatase during hormone treatment in early postmenopausal women. *Acta Med Scand* 1984;216:11–17.
15. Christiansen C, Christensen MS, NcNair P, Hagen C, Stocklund K-E, Transbøl I. Prevention of early postmenopausal bone loss. Controlled 2-year study in 315 normal females. *Eur J Clin Invest* 1980;10:273–279.
16. Riis BJ, Thomsen K, Strøm V, Christiansen C. The effect of percutaneous estradiol and natural progesterone on postmenopausal bone loss. *Am J Obstet Gynecol* 1987;156:61–65.
17. Lindsay R, Hart DM, Purdie D, Ferguson MM, Clark AS, Kraszewski A. Comparative effects of estrogen and a progestogen on bone loss in postmenopausal women. *Clin Sci* 1978;54:193–195.
18. Abdalla HI, Hart DM, Lindsay R, Leggate I, Hooke A. Prevention of bone mineral loss in postmenopausal women by norethisterone. *Obstet Gynecol* 1985;66:789–792.
19. Christiansen C, Nilas L, Riis BJ, R dbro P, Deftos L. Uncoupling of bone firmation and resorption by combined oestrogen and progestogen therapy in postmenopausal osteoporosis. *Lancet* 1985,2:800–801.
20. Riis BJ, Christiansen C, Johansen JS, Jacobsen J. Is it possible to prevent the bone loss in young women treated with LH-RH agonist? *J Clin Endocrinol Metab* 1990;70:920–924.
21. Hosking D, Chilvers C, Ravn P, et al. Prevention of bone loss with oral alendronate in postmenopausal women under age 60. *N Engl J Med* 1998;338:485–492.
22. Christiansen C, Christensen MS, Transbøl I. Bone mass in postmenopausal women after withdrawal of estrogen/gestagen replacement therapy. *Lancet* 1981;1:459–461.
23. Riis BJ, Jensen J, Christiansen C. Cyproteroneacetate, an alternative gestagen in postmenopausal oestrogen/gestagen therapy? *Clin Endocrinol* 1987;26:327–334.
24. Riis BJ, Thomsen K, Strøm V, Christiansen C. The effect of percutaneous estradiol and natural progesterone on bone loss. *Am J Obstet Gynecol* 1987;156:61–65.
25. Christiansen C, Riis BJ. 17β-Estradiol and continuous nor-ethisterone: a unique treatment of established osteoporosis in elderly women. *J Clin Endocrinol Metab* 1990;71:836–841.
26. Lindsay R, Aitken JM, Andersen JB, Hart DMM, MacDonald EB, Clarke AC. Long-term prevention of postmenopausal osteoporosis by oestrogen. *Lancet* 1976;1:1038–1040.
27. Jensen GF, Christiansen C, Transbøl I. Treatment of postmenopausal osteoporosis. A controlled therapeutic trial comparing oestrogen/gestagen, 1,25-dihydroxyvitamin D₃ and calcium. *Clin Endocrinol* 1982;16:515–524.
28. Quigley MET, Martin PL, Burnier AM, Brooks P. Estrogen therapy arrests bone loss in elderly women. *Am J Obstet Gynecol* 1987;156:1516–1523.
29. Horsman A, Jones M, Francis R, Nordin BBC. The effect of estrogen dose on postmenopausal bone loss. *N Engl J Med* 1983;309:1405–1407.
30. Christensen MS, Hagen C, Christiansen C, Transbøl I. Dose–response evaluation of cyclic estrogen/gestagen in postmenopausal women. Placebo-controlled trial of its gynecologic and metabolic actions. *Am J Obstet Gynecol* 1982;144:873–879.
31. Lindsay R, Hart CM, Clark DM. The minimum effective dose of estrogen for prevention of postmenopausal bone loss. *Obstet Gynecol* 1984;63:759–763.
32. Bjarnason NH, Hassager C, Christiansen C. 17β-Estradiol 1 mg and 2 mg in combinations with a new gestagen, gestodene are equally preventive on bone loss in early postmenopausal women. *Bone* 1997;20:93S.
33. Bjarnason NH, Hassager C, Christiansen C. Profile of a new substitution principle: Low dose 17β estradiol and gestodene. *Acta Obstet Gynecol Scand* 1997;76 (Suppl 167):S56.
34. Bjarnason NH, Bjarnason K, Haarbo J, Rosenquist C, Christiansen C. Tibolone: prevention of bone loss in late postmenopausal women. *J Clin Endocrinol Metab* 1996;81:2419–2422.
35. Stadberg E, Mattson L-C, Uvebrant M. Low doses 17-beta-estradiol and norethisterone acetate as continuous combined hormone replacement theraoy in postmenopausal women: Lipid metabolic effects. *Menopause* 1996;3:90–96.
36. Gotfredsen A, Nilas L, Riis BJ, Thomsen K, Christiansen C. Bone changes occurring spontaneously and caused by oestrogen in early postmenopausal women; a local or generalized phenomenon? *Br Med J* 1986;292:1098–1100.
37. Riis BJ, Christiansen C. Measurement of spinal or peripheral bone mass to estimate early postmenopausal bone loss? *Am J Med* 1988;84:646–653.
38. Ribot C, Tremollierés F, Pouillés JM. Cyclic Estraderm TTS 50 plus oral progestogen in the prevention of postmenopausal bone loss over 24 months. In: Chris-

tiansen C, Overgaard K, eds. *Osteoporosis 1990, vol 2*. Copenhagen: Osteopress ApS, 1990:1979–1984.

39. Lufkin EG, Wahner HW, O'Fallon WM, et al. Treatment of postmenopausal osteoporosis with transdermal estrogen. *Ann Intern Med* 1992;117:1–9.

40. Black DM. Why elderly women should be screened and treated to prevent osteoporosis. *Am J Med* 1995;98(2A):67S–75S

41. Lindsay R, Hart DM, Maclean A, Clark AC, Kraszewski A, Garnwood J. Bone response to termination of estrogen treatment. *Lancet* 1978;1:1321–1327.

42. Weiss NS, Ure CL, Ballard JH, Williams AR, Dalin JR. Decreased risk of fractures of the hip and lower forearm with postmenopausal use of estrogen. *N Engl J Med* 1980;303:1195–1198.

43. Kiel DP, Felson DT, Andersen JJ, Wilson PWF, Moskowitz MA. Hip fracture and the use of estrogens in postmenopausal women. The Framingham study. *N Engl J Med* 1987;317:1169–1174.

44. Heaney RP, Recker RR, Saville PD. Menopausal changes in calcium balance performance. *J Lab Clin Med* 1978;92:953–963.

45. Nilas L, Christiansen C, Rødbro P. Calcium supplementation and postmenopausal bone loss. *Br Med J* 1984;289:1103–1106.

46. Riis BJ, Thomsen K, Christiansen C. Does calcium supplementation prevent postmenopausal bone loss; a double-blind controlled clinical study. *N Engl J Med* 1987;316:173–177.

47. Ettinger B, Genant HK, Cann CE. Postmenopausal bone loss is prevented by treatment with low-dosage estrogen with calcium. *Ann Intern Med* 1987;104: 40–44.

48. Riis BJ, Nilas L, Christiansen C. Does calcium potentiate the effect of estrogen therapy on postmenopausal bone loss? *Bone Miner* 1987;2:1–5.

48a. McGuire WL, Chamness GC. In: O'Malley BW, Means AR, eds. *Receptors for reproductive hormones*. New York: Plenum Press, 1973.

49. Jordan VC. Third annual William L. McGuire memorial lecture. Studies on the estrogen receptor in breast cancer—20 years as a target for the treatment and prevention of cancer. *Breast Cancer Res Treat* 1995;36:367–385.

50. Delmas PD, Bjarnason NH, Mitlak BH, et al. The effects of raloxifene on bone mineral density, serum cholesterol, and uterine endometrium in postmenopausal women. *N Engl J Med* 1997;337:1641–1647.

51. Lufkin EG, Whitaker R, Argueta R, Caplan RH, Nickelsen T, Riggs BL. Raloxifene treatment of postmenopausal osteoporosis. *J Bone Miner Res* 1997;12 (Suppl 1):S150.

52. Bjarnason NH, Haarbo J, Byrjalsen I, Kauffman RF, Christiansen C. Raloxifene inhibits aortic accumulation of cholesterol in ovariectomized, cholesterol-fed rabbits. *Circulation* 1997;96:1964–1969.

53. Bjarnason K, Skrumsager BK, Kiehr B. Levomeloxifene, a new partial estrogen receptor agonist, demonstrates anti-resorptive and anti-atherogenic properties in postmenopausal women. *J Bone Miner Res* 1997;12(Suppl 1):S346.

54. Ke HZ, Chidsey-Frink KL, Oi H, et al. Droloxifene increases bone mass in ovariectomized rats with established osteopenia. *J Bone Miner Res* 1997;12 (Suppl 1):S349.

55. Bjarnason NH, Bjarnason K, Hassager C, Christiansen C. The response in spinal bone mass to tibolone treatment is related to bone turnover in elderly women. *Bone* 1997;2:151–155.

56. Bjarnason NH, Bjarnason K, Haarbo J, Bennink HJ, Christiansen C. Tibolone: influence on markers of cardiovascular disease. *J Clin Endocrinol Metab* 1997;6: 1752–1756.

57. Hosking D, Chilvers CED, Christiansen C, et al. Prevention of bone loss with alendronate in postmenopausal women under age 60 years of age. *N Engl J Med* 1998;338:485–492.

58. Weiss S, McClung M, Gilchrist N, et al. Five-years efficacy and safety of oral alendronate for prevention of osteoporosis in early postmenopausal women. *J Bone Miner Res* 1997;12(Suppl 1):S144.

59. Ravn P, Clemmesen B, Riis BJ, Christiansen C. The effect on bone mass and bone markers of different doses of ibandronate: a new bisphosphonate for prevention and treatment of osteoporosis: a 1-year, randomized, double-blind, placebo-controlled dose-finding study. *Bone* 1996;5:527–533.

60. Black DM, Cummings SR, Karpf DB, et al. Randomised trial of effect of alendronate on risk of fracture in women with existing vertebral fracture. Fracture intervention trial research group. *Lancet* 1996;348:1535–1541.

61. Cummings SR, Black DM, Thompson DE, for the FIT research group. Alendronate reduces the risk of vertebral fractures in women without pre-existing vertebral fractures: Results of the fracture intervention trial. *J Bone Miner Res* 1997;12(Suppl 1):S149.

62. Storm TM, Thamsborg G, Steiniche T, Genant HK, Sørensen OM. Effect of intermittent cyclical etidronate therapy on bone mass and fracture rate in women with postmenopausal osteoporosis. *N Engl J Med* 1990;322:1265–1271.

63. Nelson BW, Harris ST, Genant HK, et al. Intermittent cyclical etidronate treatment of postmenopausal osteoporosis. *N Engl J Med* 1990;323:73–79.

64. Civitelli R, Gonnelli S, Zacchei F, et al. Bone turnover in postmenopausal osteoporosis *J Clin Invest* 1988;82:1268.

65. Reginster JY, Denis D, Albert A, et al. One-year controlled randomized trial of prevention of early postmenopausal bone loss by intranasal calcitonin. *Lancet* 1987;2:1481–1483.

66. Overgaard K, Riis BJ, Christiansen C, Hansen MA. Effect of calcitonin given intranasally on early postmenopausal bone loss. *Br Med J* 1989;299:477–479.

67. Overgaard K, Riis BJ, Christiansen C, Pødenphant J, Johansen JS. Nasal calcitonin for treatment of established osteoporosis. *Clin Endocrinol* 1989;30: 435–442.

68. Overgaard K, Hansen MA, Nielsen VH, Riis BJ, Christiansen C. Discontinuous calcitonin treatment of established osteoporosis—effects on withdrawal of treatment. *Am J Med* 1990;89:1–6.

69. Kanis JA, Johnell O, Gullberg B, et al. Evidence for efficacy of drugs affecting bone metabolism in preventing hip fracture. *Br Med J* 1992;305:1124–1129.

70. Overgaard K, Hansen MA, Birk-Jensen J, et al. Effect of salcatonin given intranasally on bone mass and fracture rates in established osteoporosis: A dose-response study. *Br Med J* 1992;305:556–560.

71. Stock JL, Avioli LV, Baylink DJ, et al, for the PROOF study group. Calcitonin-salmon nasal spray reduces the incidence of new vertebral fractures in postmenopausal women: Three-year interim results of the PROOF study. *J Bone Miner Res* 1997;12(Suppl 1):S149.

72. Riggs BL. Treatment of osteoporosis with sodium fluoride: an appraisal. *Bone Miner Res* 1983;2:366–393.

73. Kanis JA, Meunier PJ. Should we use fluoride to treat osteoporosis? A review. *Q J Med* 1984;53:145–164.

74. Baylink DJ, Duane PB, Farley SM, et al. Monofluorophosphate physiology: the effect of fluoride on bone. *Caries Res* 1983;17(Suppl 1):56–76.

75. Vigorita VJ, Suda MK. The microscopic morphology of fluoride-induced bone. *Clin Orthop* 1983;July/Aug:274–282.

76. Briancon D, Meunier PJ. Treatment of osteoporosis with fluoride, calcium and vitamin D. *Orthop Clin North Am* 1982;12:629–648.

77. Kleerekoper M, Peterson EL, Nelson DA, et al. A randomized trial of sodium fluoride as a treatment for postmenopausal osteoporosis. *Osteoporosis Int* 1991;1: 155–161.

78. Lundy MW, Stauffer M, Wergedal JE, et al. Histomorphometric analysis of iliac crest bone biopsies in placebo-treated versus fluoride-treated subjects. *Osteoporosis Int* 1995;5:2–17.

79. Kanis JA. *Osteoporosis*. London: Blackwell Science, 1994:204.

80. Reginster J-Y, Zegels B, Meurmans L, et al. Monofluorophosphate decreases vertebral fracture rate in postmenopausal osteoporosis: a randomised, placebo-controlled, double-blind study. *Osteoporosis Int* 1996;6(Suppl 1):239.

81. Mamelle N, Meunier PJ, Netter P. Fluoride and vertebral fractures. *Lancet* 1990; 336:243.

82. Riggs BL, Hodgson SF, O'Fallon WM, et al. Effect of fluoride treatment on fracture rate in postmenopausal osteoporosis. *N Engl J Med* 1990;322:802–809.

83. Meunier PJ, Sebert JL, Reginster JY, et al, and the FAVOS Study Group. Fluoride salts compared to calcium–vitamin D in the treatment of established postmenopausal osteoporosis. *Osteoporosis Int* 1996;6(Suppl 1):251.

84. Alexandersen P, Hassager C, Sandholdt I, Riis B, Christiansen C. Synegistic effect of hormone repplacement therapy (HRT) combined with monofluorophosphate (MFP) on bone mass in late postmenopausal women. *J Bone Miner Res* 1997;12 (Suppl 1):S104.

85. Riggs BL, Seeman E, Hodgson SF, et al. Effect of the fluoride calcium regimen on vertebral fracture occurrence in postmenopausal osteoporosis: Comparison with conventional therapy. *N Engl J Med* 1982;306:446–450.

86. Farley SMG, Wergedal JE, Smith LC, et al. Fluoride therapy for osteoporosis: characterization of the skeletal response by serial measurements of serum alkaline phosphatase activity. *Metabolism* 1987;36:211–218.

87. Riggs BL, Hodgson SF, O'Fallon WM, et al. Effect of fluoride treatment on the fracture rate in postmenopausal women with osteoporosis. *N Engl J Med* 1990; 322:802–809.

88. Riggs BL. In: Peck WA, ed. *Bone and mineral research. Annual 2: a yearly survey of developments in the field of bone and mineral*. Amsterdam: Excerpta Medica, 1984:366–393.

89. Lane JM, Healy JH, Schwartz E, et al. Treatment of osteoporosis with sodium fluoride and calcium: effect on vertebral fracture incidence and bone histomorphometry. *Orthop Clin North Am* 1984;15:729–745.

90. Riggs BL, Hodgson SR, Hoffman DL, et al. Treatment of primary osteoporosis with fluoride and calcium. *JAMA* 1980;243:446–449.

91. Pak CYC, Sakhaee K, Gallagher C, Pariel C, Peterseon R. Safe and effective treatment of osteoporosis with intermittent slow release sodium fluoride: augmentation of vertebral bone mass and inhibition of fractures. *J Clin Endocrinal Metab* 1989;68:150–159.

92. Schnitzler CM, Solomon L. Trabecular stress fractures during fluoride therapy for osteoporosis. *Skel Radiol* 1985;14:276–279.

93. O'Duffy JD, Wahner HW, O'Fallon WH, et al. Mechanism of acute lower extremity pain syndrome in fluoride-treated osteoporotic patients. *Am J Med* 1986;80: 561–566.

94. Schultz EE, Engstrom H, Sauser DD, et al. Osteoporosis: radiographic detection of fluoride-induced extra-axial bone formation. *Radiology* 1986;159:457–462.

95. Johansen JS, Hassager C, Pødenphant J, et al. Treatment of postmenopausal osteoporosis: Is the anabolic steroid nandrolone decanoate a candidate? *Bone Miner* 1989;6:77–86.

96. Hassager C, Pødenphant J, Riis BJ, Johansen JS, Jensen J, Christiansen C. Changes in soft tissue body composition and plasma lipid metabolism during nandrolone decanoate therapy in postmenopausal osteoporotic women. *Metabolism* 1989;38:238–242.

97. Rosenthal DI, Slovik DM, Neer RM. Treatment of osteoporosis with parathyroid hormone. In: Gennant HK, ed. *Osteoporosis update, vol 1*. Amsterdam: Elsevier, 1987:297–299.

98. Lindsay R, Nieves J, Formica C, et al. Randomised controlled study of effects of parathyroid hormone on vertebral-bone mass and fracture incidence among postmenopausal women on oestrogen with osteoporosis. *Lancet* 1997;350:550–555.

Cardiovascular Disease

This section has been extensively revised and expanded due to the enormity of its importance to the health of postmenopausal women. Cardiovascular disease (CVD) is the leading cause of mortality in postmenopausal women in the United States, and accounts for twice the deaths annually (approximately 500,000) compared to cancer. That and other facets of the disease will be discussed extensively.

Since the last edition of this book, the results of Postmenopausal Estrogen/Progestin Interventions (PEPI) and the Heart and Estrogen/Progestin Replacement Study (HERS) have been published, and the primary prevention trial of the Women's Health Initiative (WHI) is well underway. Also the multiple direct actions of estradiol on the vascular system have been elucidated, defining which mechanisms are both estrogen receptor- (ERα and ERβ) and non receptor-mediated. As the results of the HERS were not available at the time that several chapters were being completed for this volume, the findings will be discussed in this introduction.

The first chapter in this section is a review of the epidemiology and risk factors of CVD by George Gorodeski and Wulf Utian. The evidence for a protective effect of estrogen on coronary artery disease will be discussed by Meir Stampfer and Francine Grodstein. Their data from the Nurses cohort has contributed greatly to our understanding of CVD in women. The next few chapters address the mechanisms of the protective effects of estrogen and the interactions between sex steroids and the CV system. Ron Krauss discusses lipids and lipoproteins and the effects of various types of hormones on these markers of CVD. Next Mike Adams, Scott Washburn, Janice Wagner, Koudy Williams, and Tom Clarkson describe the arterial changes of estrogen and progestogen in the cynomologus monkey. The monkey model of atherosclerosis and coronary artery disease has been extremely valuable to our understanding of the effects of estrogens and progestogens on CVD. Next, Peter Collins reviews blood flow and vasomotion from the vantage point of postmenopausal women. Peter has contributed greatly to our understanding of direct arterial effects of estrogen in women. His most recent work confirms an attenuating effect of added progestogen on estrogen's action. These data are important and may help to explain some of the findings in HERS discussed below. Physiological estrogen replacement improves insulin sensitivity. These data will be reviewed by Ian Godsland who covers the important topic of carbohydrate tolerance. The important issue of thrombosis and distinguishing venous from arterial thrombosis is the subject of the next chapter by Morris Notelovitz. For a long time we were emphatic in stating that estrogen replacement in normal postmenopausal women was not associated with a thrombosis risk. Now we are clear that there is a small but increased risk with oral estrogen. However, this risk is for venous thrombosis, and there is no excess mortality. The last chapter in this section discusses the evaluation and treatment of hypertension, and the effects of estrogen in particular. Our field has sustained a major loss in the recent death of Jay Sullivan who has contributed much to our understanding of CVD in women.

Some controversy has surrounded the publication of the HERS trial (1). HERS was a secondary intervention trial of 2763 women with established coronary disease. The regimen used was continuous estrogen (conjugated equine estrogen 0.625 mg) with continuous daily medroxy progesterone acetate, 2.5 mg. After 4.1 years, 172 women in the hormone group and 176 women in the placebo group had sustained a myocardial infarction or CV death for a relative hazard of 0.99 (0.8—1.22).

There was however a significant trend effect with more events in the first year and fewer events in years 4 and 5 among the hormone users. The fact that there was not a substantial beneficial effect is inconsistent with observational data and the cardioprotective mechanisms of estrogen action, that will be covered in this section. The observational data of Sullivan (2) addressed the issue of secondary prevention and a significantly lower relative risk (0.3) was found. Indeed women who had worse coronary disease benefited more. While there are many interpretations of the HERS findings, and it must be noted that these women were older and already receiving the standard of care treatment, many investigators, including myself, point to the daily progestogen exposure (medroxyprogesterone acetate, MPA) as a confounding variable. Progestogen, particularly MPA, has been shown—at least in animal studies—to induce vasospasm and reduce the benefits of estrogen on blood flow and coronary atherosclerosis (3,4). Clearly much more analysis and more data are needed. The data at hand suggest an initial deleterious or toxic effect of the progestogen combination regimen that decreases with time, allowing for an ultimate estrogen-induced benefit. While it might be a valid conclusion that a fixed daily estrogen-progestogen regimen may not be beneficial for coronary disease in women with existing preconditions, it does not negate the data or the findings we have for the beneficial effects of estrogen alone.

REFERENCES

1. Hulley S, Gradv D, Bush T, et al. For the Heart and Estrogen/progestin Replacement Study (HERS) Research Group: Randomized trial of estrogen plus progestin for secondary prevention of coronary heart disease in postmenopausal women. *JAMA* 1998; 280:605–613.
2. Sullivan JM, Vander Zwaag R, Hughes JP, et al. Estrogen replacement and coronary artery disease. Effect on survival in postmenopausal women. *Arch Intern Med* 1990;150:2557–2562.
3. Adams MR, Kaplan JR, Manuck SBI et al. Inhibition of coronary artery atherosclerosis by 17-β estradiol in ovariectomized monkeys: lack of an effect of added progesterone. *Arteriosclerosis* 1990; 10:1051–1057.
4. Miyagawa K, Rosch J, Stanczyk F, et al. Medroxyprogesterone interferes with ovarian steroid protection against coronary vasospasm. *Nat Med* 1997; 3:324–327.

Treatment of the Postmenopausal Woman: Basic and Clinical Aspects, Second Edition, edited by Rogerio A. Lobo, Lippincott Williams & Wilkins, Philadelphia © 1999.

CHAPTER 30

Epidemiology and Risk Factors of Cardiovascular Disease in Postmenopausal Women

George I. Gorodeski and Wulf H. Utian

Cardiovascular disease is the leading cause of morbidity and mortality in men and women, significantly outweighing other causes such as cancer, cerebrovascular disease, lung disease, infectious diseases, accidents, suicide, diabetes mellitus, and others (Fig. 30.1) (1–4). Cardiovascular disease in women has been traditionally dealt with by general practitioners, internists, and cardiologists. In the last decade, however, the subject of cardiovascular disease in women has become the focus of interest for gynecologists for two reasons. The first is the gender difference in the prevalence of cardiovascular disease between men and women. Life expectancy in the United States is constantly increasing for both men and women (Fig. 30.2), and historically the difference in life expectancy between the sexes, which widened from 1900 to 1972, has narrowed since 1979 (Fig. 30.3).

Sex differences in the rate of coronary artery heart disease (CAHD), which is the largest single component of fatal cardiovascular disease in women (54%) (5), were observed and reported almost two centuries ago (6), and World Health Organization (WHO) data show an overall ratio of male to female incidence of 2.24 ± 0.08 (7). In childhood, cardiovascular disease is rare and is attributed mostly to congenital heart disease, and the incidence in boys and girls is equal. As early as the second and third decades, the male to female risk ratio of cardiovascular disease increases and is maintained twofold higher in men than in women (Fig. 30.4) until the fourth and fifth decades of life, when it increases more steeply in women than in men, reaching an almost equal male and female incidence at the seventh to ninth decades of life (1–3,7). These observations

suggest, among other things, that young women have a protective factor that is lost after the fifth decade or that younger men have a risk factor that exposes them to earlier development of CAHD. Because most women become menopausal at this age, many have speculated that the protective factor is the female hormone estrogen or that the risk factor is increased levels of androgen (testosterone).

Among the following race and sex groups, white women continue to have the highest life expectancy at birth (79.2), followed by African-American women (73.5), white men (72.7), and African-American men (64.8 years). Overall, the largest gain in life expectancy between 1980 and 1989 was for white men (2.0 years), followed by white women (1.1 years) and African-American men and women (1.0 year). Parallel to the increase in life expectancy, there is a reciprocal decrease in death rates from heart disease. Mortality from heart disease increased more in men than in women between 1920 and the 1960s and began to decline earlier in women than in men (1950s vs. 1960s), but the absolute decline in men was greater than that in women (Fig. 30.3) (1,2).

In addition to the gender-related differences in the epidemiology of heart disease, a series of publications appeared in the literature in the last decade that indicated differences also in the management of cardiovascular disease between men and women (8–10). Conclusions from these studies are that women may have initial symptomatology of CAHD that is different from that in men, that women may undergo less invasive diagnostic and curative procedures than men, and that the overall morbidity and mortality following the initial ischemic heart event is worse in women than in men. These observations have drawn the attention of the general public and the medical community to the fact that ischemic heart disease in women has not been given the same attention as that in men, and that conclusions drawn from studies in men

G. I. Gorodeski and W. H. Utian: Department of Obstetrics and Gynecology, University MacDonald Women's Hospital, and Department of Reproductive Biology, Case Western Reserve University, Cleveland, Ohio 44106.

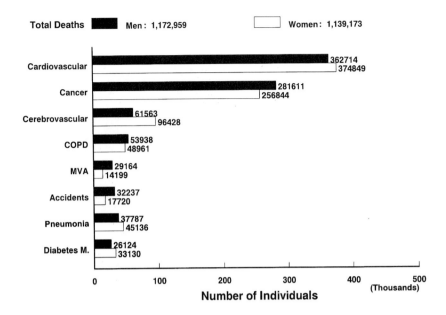

FIG. 30.1. Leading causes of death by sex in the United States, 1995. Accidents category also includes adverse effects. Pneumonia category includes also influenza. COPD, chronic obstructive pulmonary disease; MVA, motor vehicle accident. (Data from ref. 1.)

may not be relevant to the management of women with cardiovascular disease.

A second point of interest is concerned with the prevention of cardiovascular disease in women. Considerable effort and resources were devoted in the past to study risk factors and to establish programs to prevent cardiovascular disease in men, but until recently only few studies included women. Certainly, the most investigated risk factor in women is postmenopausal estrogen deficiency, and estrogen replacement therapy emerges as the single most significant factor that can be pharmacologically manipulated to decrease cardiovascular disease risk in women. These considerations have led to a surge of interest in female-gender-related cardiovascular disease risk factors and to study means of manipulating them in order to decrease the prevalence of CAHD in women.

The largest growing segment of the U.S. population is women over the age of 75; their increased life expectancy will change the demographics of women's health care. It

is estimated that at the turn of the century, more than one-third of the female population will be in their postreproductive years, compared to about 10% at present, and the impact of cardiovascular disease on women's health management will increase (11). Although certain forms of cardiovascular disease can be treated medically or surgically, the most effective means to decrease the impact of cardiovascular disease on woman's health is by modifying the contribution of specific factors that increase the risk of the disease. The major contribution to decreasing morbidity and mortality of cardiovascular disease in men was achieved by relatively simple measures such as

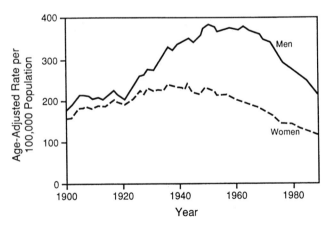

FIG. 30.3. Death rates for heart disease by sex in the United States, 1900–1989. Heart disease mortality rate increased more in men than in women between 1920 and the 1960s and began to decline earlier in women (1950s) than in men (1960s). The rise in mortality was steeper in nonwhites than in whites; rates remained higher in white men than in non-white men and higher in nonwhite women than in white women. (From ref. 2, with permission.)

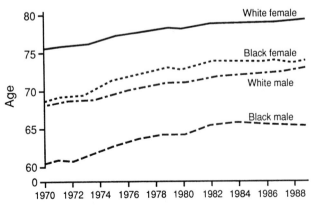

FIG. 30.2. Life expectancy by sex and race in the United States, 1970–1989. (From ref. 2, with permission.)

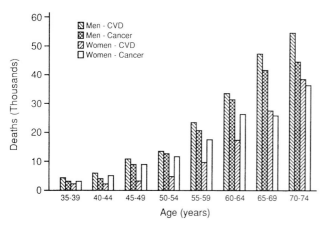

FIG. 30.4. Age- and sex-adjusted deaths from heart disease and cancer in the United States, 1989. (Data from ref. 3.)

changing lifestyle habits, eliminating cigarette smoking, and lowering plasma lipid levels.

The present chapter describes the epidemiology of cardiovascular disease in women, the pathogenesis of ischemic heart disease in women, and the risk factors involved, with special emphasis on the relation between estrogen deficiency and heart disease.

EPIDEMIOLOGY OF CARDIOVASCULAR DISEASE IN WOMEN

In women, 46% of deaths are from cardiovascular disease, and 50% of these are from coronary artery heart disease, indicating that in the United States, a woman has a 23% life chance of dying of ischemic heart disease (1,2). This is in contrast to 4% from breast cancer, 2.5% from osteoporotic fractures, and 2% from genital tract neoplasia (4,12). About one-third of deaths in women from CAHD are premature (age less than 65), accounting for over 100,000 cases of death per year (13).

As of 1983, cardiovascular disease caused death in a greater proportion of women (52%) than in men (46%). Age-adjusted mortality from cardiovascular disease shows that cardiovascular disease becomes the leading cause of death in men by approximately age 35, and in women by approximately age 70 (Fig. 30.4) (1–3,11). Although the risks of cardiovascular disease in general, and CAHD in particular, are higher in African-Americans than in whites, a similar pattern of age-adjusted risk between white and African-American men and women is apparent, as shown in Fig. 30.5, namely, that at approximately age 45 in African-Americans, and at age 55 in whites, the incidence of CAHD in women increases;

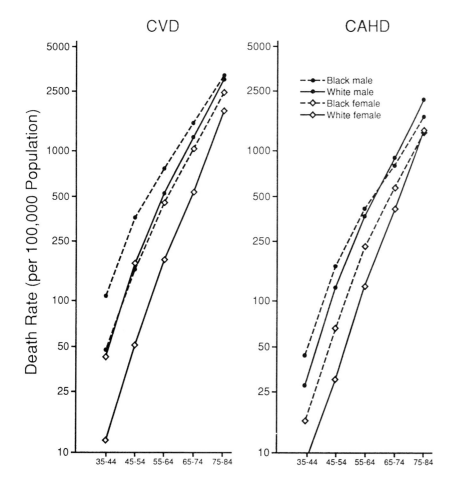

FIG. 30.5. Age-adjusted death rates by sex and race from all-cause heart disease and coronary artery heart disease in the United States, 1989. CVD, cardiovascular disease; CAHD, coronary artery heart disease. (Data from ref. 3.)

however, the incidence in men remains higher for any specific age group both in African-Americans and in whites. Because women on the average have a longer life expectancy than men by 7 to 8 years, ultimately more women than men die of cardiovascular disease.

Data on morbidity are more difficult to collect than data on mortality. At every age after early childhood, women report more symptoms, illness, short- and long-term disability, and poorer health than men. Women use preventive and curative medical services more frequently, including visits with doctors, over-the-counter and prescription medications, hospitalizations (even excluding childbirth), psychiatric treatment, diagnostic tests, and surgical procedures. Some of the differences reflect reporting bias (overreporting by women and underreporting by men), gender roles regarding illness behavior, and gender bias in diagnosis and in treatment. Despite these difficulties, it is possible to draw some conclusions on the prevalence of cause-specific morbidity, and based on self-reporting and hospital discharge diagnoses, it appears that cardiovascular disease is also the leading cause of morbidity in women (Figs. 30.6 and 30.7) (3).

Gender differences in the clinical presentation of patients with ischemic heart disease have an important epidemiologic role. More women than men have their initial manifestation of CAHD as angina pectoris (65% and 35%, respectively) (14,15), but fewer women than men (29% and 43%, respectively) will suffer an acute myocardial infarction as their first manifestation (11). Of all coronary heart disease in women, 36% present with sudden cardiac death or fatal myocardial infarction (16). More than 50% of women with angina pectoris undergoing coronary angiography will have normal coronary arteries, compared to fewer than 10% of men (17,18), a syndrome referred to as atypical angina, or syndrome X (severe angina, positive exercise-related electrocardiographic changes suggesting ischemia, and normal coronary arteries). Although these patients initially have a good prognosis with regard to myocardial infarction and cardiovascular mortality (19), many of them have signif-

icant limitations in daily activities because of pain (20), and some are erroneously diagnosed as having other vascular disorders such as hot flashes, Raynaud's phenomena, and migraine (21,22).

The gender-related differences in the initial manifestation of ischemic heart disease result in differences in the management of women with CAHD compared to men. Women have milder symptomatology despite more severe disease and are less likely to be referred for coronary artery angiography than men, even when they have a positive exercise test. Therefore, they are referred at a more advanced stage of disease, are less likely to be diagnosed initially as acute ischemic heart condition, and take longer to be admitted for observation and treatment (8–10,23). Initially, women are less likely to have invasive diagnostic procedures such as thrombolytic therapy, coronary artery angiography, and coronary angioplasty (9). In 1989, of the cardiovascular operations and procedures done in the United States (including valve replacements, angioplasty, coronary bypass, pacemaker installment, cardiac catheterization, and open heart surgery), more than 2,200,000 procedures were performed on men, compared to fewer than 1,500,000 in women (11).

Women with chest pain are less likely to have serious coronary artery stenosis, and their symptoms are probably related to reversible coronary vasospastic episodes (syndrome X) (24). Many physicians believe that angina pectoris in women is a benign disease and know that stress testing is less accurate for the diagnosis of coronary heart disease. The fact that women with acute myocardial infarction are 7 to 8 years older than men seems to contribute to the reluctance to perform invasive procedures. Overall, women who undergo coronary artery bypass have a twofold increased mortality, which remains significant even after age adjustment (25).

Gender-related differences were also observed in the outcome of the acute coronary event. Once CAHD is diagnosed in women, the case fatality rate for women exceeds that for men (15,26). Thirty-nine percent of women who have an acute myocardial infarction die within a year, com-

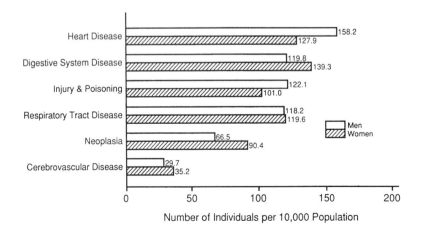

FIG. 30.6. Rate of patients discharged from short-stay hospitals, by sex and first-listed diagnosis in the United States, 1990. Rates of discharge of all conditions were 1,015.5 for men and 1,440.9 for women. (Data from ref. 3.)

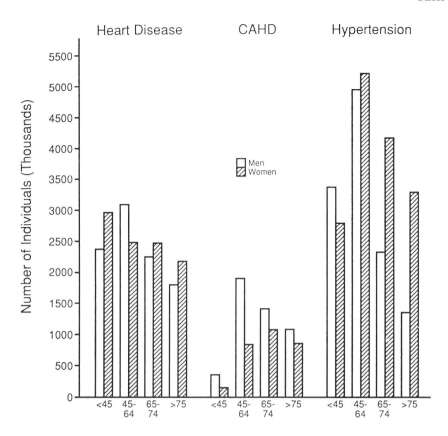

FIG. 30.7. Selected reported chronic conditions (heart disease, coronary artery heart disease, and hypertension) by sex and age, United States, 1990. (Data from ref. 3.)

pared to 31% in men (11). Although the age-adjusted hospital mortality in cases of acute myocardial infarction in women equals that in men, most (although not all) authors indicate that women have more prolonged angina pectoris, congestive heart failure, stroke, and reinfarction than men, even after age adjustment (8–10). Women with severe disease comparable in degree to men fare less well after coronary bypass than men (25).

Although most patients with repeat myocardial infarction are men (27) (80%; i.e., women are more likely to die after their first acute myocardial infarction), the rate of reinfarction in women is higher, a phenomenon that can be explained by more advanced age and severity of disease (28). During the first 3 to 4 years after acute myocardial infarction, 20% of women, versus 15% of men, will have repeat acute myocardial infarction (11).

Women are less likely than men to return to work during the first 2 years after acute myocardial infarction. Reasons proposed for this phenomenon are the more advanced age of women at their index event and gender-related differences in behavioral response to illness (29).

PATHOGENESIS OF CARDIAC ISCHEMIA

Proper function of the myocardium depends on a positive balance of oxygen and nutrient supply and demand. Decreased oxygen supply to the cardiac muscle is usually caused by decreased arterial blood flow as a result of

coronary artery occlusion. Understanding the chronic and acute processes of coronary artery occlusion is the key in identifying risk factors that cause, sustain, and augment cardiac ischemia.

Cardiac ischemia is most often associated with occlusion of the coronary arteries and is most often the end result of pathologic processes that begin as early as life *in utero* and end with the formation of atherosclerotic plaques in the proximal coronary arteries. Other pathologic processes that are important for the understanding of cardiac ischemia in women are abnormal vasoreactivity of the coronary arterioles, increased blood viscosity, and events related to ischemia-reperfusion. All these processes are dependent on sex hormones, and estrogen treatment can modify their occurrence.

The coronary arterial tree is susceptible to flow injuries because of its special branching pattern. Disturbances in the pattern of blood flow, which occur in bending points near branching vessels, cause microscopic intimal insult and attract circulating monocytes to reside as macrophages over the area of injury (30–32). Macrophages release toxic products and further augment macrophage and platelet residence. The cells release mitogenic factors, which stimulate proliferation and migration of smooth muscle cells, fibrointimal thickening, and formation of a capsule over an existing lesion (32). Accumulation of fat by the macrophage causes the fibrointimal thickening to become fat-laden, and the lesion is recognized as a fatty streak.

Coronary artery fatty streak lesions can be found in fetuses *in utero* and in 45% of infants under 1 year of age. Their incidence in male and female fetuses is the same, and most will reverse (33). In contrast, childhood lesions are not reversible (34,35). Some authors have found that coronary artery intimal layers are thicker in male than in female infants, suggesting an inborn sex difference in the structure of the coronary artery that renders men more susceptible to ischemic heart disease (36); others, however, have found no such sex difference in fetuses and children up to age 19 (7,37). In certain ethnic groups with unusually high prevalence of CAHD, coronary artery intimal layers are thicker in boys than in girls (36).

Between the second and fourth decades of life, the fibrointimal fatty streak lesions in women grow slowly compared to men. The growth of the lesion is the result of accumulation of fat-loaded macrophages, fibromuscular organization of the thrombus, and thickening of the cap that surrounds the lesion. During the second and fourth decades of life, the cap surrounds multiple lipid cores that, in later years, become confluent to a single extracellular core called an atheroma. The lesion surrounded by the cap is the atherosclerotic plaque (30,32).

The four key cells in the generation of the plaque are the macrophage, platelets, endothelial cells, and smooth muscle cells. All four interact to accentuate the formation of the atheroma. The molecular mechanisms that operate in plaque formation involve attraction of macrophages to the site of injury, secretion of cytokines that further attract macrophages and platelets, enhanced uptake of oxidized low-density lipoproteins (LDL) particles by the activated macrophages (a process that can be inhibited by high-density lipoprotein, HDL), enhanced production of oxygen reactive species (ORS, or free radicals), augmented lipid peroxidation, and enhanced secretion of proteases (elastase and collagenase) by macrophages (32–47). Once a plaque has been established, the interaction among the macrophages, endothelial and smooth muscle cells, and platelets results in a self-promoted growth (48). Increases in blood viscosity tend to contribute to plaque formation by enhancing platelet aggregation and adherence and formation of thrombi (46). The end result of plaque formation is narrowing of the coronary artery, stiffness, and dysfunction, resulting in stenosis.

Age-specific data on the incidence of coronary artery stenosis in women are lacking, although it appears that at all ages after puberty, the incidence in women is lower than in men (8–10,32,47). Even at an advanced age, women with coronary ischemia who undergo angiography have a lower incidence of stenosis than men (24), indicating that female-specific atherogenesis-protective processes operate from puberty onwards.

Clinically, coronary artery stenosis is a chronic process associated with maladaptation to exercise, resulting in negative oxygen balance, that is, stable angina pectoris. In contrast, acute coronary symptoms—unstable angina, acute myocardial infarction, and sudden ischemic death— are the result of acute narrowing of the lumen of the coronary artery. The precipitating factors of the acute coronary syndromes are two: disruption of the atherosclerotic plaque resulting in coronary thrombosis and acute coronary spasm (32).

Disruption of the atherosclerotic plaque (also referred to as complicated plaque) is the result of injury to the cap surrounding the plaque and exposing its raw surface to the blood. This results in platelet aggregation and thrombus formation. Beginning minutes after the injury, and completed within 24 hours, platelets aggregate, causing thrombin deposition and formation of thrombus. Depending on the extent of damage, the thrombus can either dislodge, stabilize, or, together with the exposed collagen, activate the clotting system and further organize. Adherent and activated platelets produce and locally secrete active agents such as thromboxanes and serotonin. These further stimulate platelet aggregation, thus promoting vasoconstriction and a neointimal proliferative response. Neighboring smooth muscle cells in the media undergo hypertrophy and proliferate in response to growth factors secreted by the platelets. Three to five days after the injury, smooth muscle cells migrate from the media into the intima and accumulate extracellular matrix. At this stage, small thrombi can organize and can be lysed or fragmented. Fragments can be dislodged from the site of injury to more distant parts of the artery, causing peripheral occlusion. Fourteen days to 3 months after the acute event, the injury site is healed by the formation of a thick fibromuscular tissue, which narrows the lumen and causes the coronary artery to lose its elasticity and become stiff (30,32).

Correlating plaque injury with clinical data and coronary angiography has revealed important conclusions with regard to the progression of CAHD in both men and women. Coronary angiography is helpful in assessing the severity of coronary artery disease and in predicting the risk of morbidity and mortality related to occlusive events. However, with the exception of its ability to detect an irregular and ulcerated lesion, which can be used to predict the site of impending thrombosis or rethrombosis, it cannot predict further sites of coronary occlusion (47,49). In many patients, and in women in particular, acute ischemic events are a complication not of the fibrotic and calcified stenosis but of the disruption of stenotic lipid-rich plaques (50). The latter are softer and more prone to disrupt because of their high fat content. Although the severity of coronary artery stenosis and the number of diseased vessels are prognostic markers for further cardiac morbidity and mortality (women less frequently having chronic coronary stenosis than men) (51), coronary lesions with less severe angiographic stenosis are more prone to rapid and total occlusion (32).

From a clinical point of view, plaque disruption followed by thrombosis can result in two different responses: (a) thrombotic occlusion of moderately atherotic vessels, which rarely progresses to total occlusion but frequently is associated with acute coronary syndrome, and (b) thrombotic occlusion of severely stenotic vessels, which leads to complete blockade and formation of collaterals (30,32,47). The latter is associated with chronic ischemia and less frequently with acute coronary syndromes. The incidence of these events in women is unknown; it appears that the incidence of the former process is less common in women than in men, and vice versa regarding the latter. It is also presently unknown whether women produce the same degree of collaterals as men. Collateral arterial circulation is the compensatory mechanism of providing arterial blood supply to the affected cardiac muscle in patients with chronic stenosis (52).

Spasm of the vessel wall may precipitate acute narrowing of the lumen of the coronary artery. The vasotonus of the coronary artery is determined by the interplay of several locally produced agents. Endothelial cells produce mediators of smooth muscle cell tone, which, under normal conditions and in the presence of an intact endothelium, result in relaxation of the coronary artery. Known endothelium-derived mediators are the relaxing factors prostacyclin, nitric oxide (previously referred to as the endothelium-derived relaxing factor, EDRF), and the hyperpolarization-dependent vasorelaxant. Endothelins are endothelium-dependent vasoconstrictors (53,54). Following an insult to the coronary artery, platelets aggregate and induce vasospasm by releasing vasoconstrictors such thromboxane A_2, serotonin, adenosine diphosphate (ADP), and adenosine triphosphate (ATP) (55). Factors released systemically and delivered to the coronary arteries may also affect the tonus of the coronary vessels and have a dual role, depending on the intactness of the coronary endothelium. In vessels with an intact endothelium, agents such as acetylcholine, bradykinin, angiotensin II, histamine, and norepinephrine usually stimulate vasorelaxation and cause vasodilation of the coronary artery. However, if the endothelium is damaged, some of these agents directly reach the smooth muscle cells and cause vasoconstriction (56,57). The net vasotonus of the coronary artery, therefore, is the result of a complex interplay between vasodilatory and vasoconstrictive agents produced locally by the vessel wall and by the aggregating platelets, and agents delivered to the coronary circulation from the periphery.

Increased viscosity of the blood can precipitate a decrease in coronary artery blood flow. Changes in the rheologic properties of the blood, in particular increased viscosity, can contribute to coronary and to total peripheral resistance and diminish blood flow in coronary vessels (58,59).

An additional mechanism that may damage the myocardium is reperfusion of a previously ischemized myocardium. With the progress made in diagnostic and surgical techniques, patients with cardiac ischemia are being diagnosed and managed earlier after the onset of the event; more patients undergo invasive procedures such as coronary bypasses, balloon angioplasty, coronary atherectomy, thrombolysis, and elective cardioplegia (during open heart surgery), which increase the incidence and prevalence of ischemia and reperfusion (60). These active interventions can salvage cardiac tissue from hypoxia and degeneration; however, reperfusion of previously anoxemic heart can lead to irreversible cell damage and cardiac death. During ischemia, vital organelles that operate at a high energy level or those that undergo rapid turnover may become damaged. Examples are ion transporters (e.g., calcium efflux mechanisms, which have to extrude calcium in order to maintain a 10^4 gradient of extracellular/intracellular concentration), enzymes involved in respiration and maintenance of transmembranal electrochemical gradients, and scavenger mechanisms including antioxidants. The ischemic cells are limited in their capacity to withstand the influx of blood-borne chemicals carried by the flow of fresh blood. As a result, the affected cells are subject to further injury and accelerated death.

Proposed mechanisms for the ischemia-reperfusion syndrome are impaired production of nitric oxide (61–70), impaired prostaglandin production, and rapid overproduction and release of free radicals (oxidants). As a result, cells become necrotic, they attract and activate polymorphonuclears and platelets (71–78). This may lead to impaired blood flow in the microvasculature, recurrent thrombosis, increased vascular resistance, accelerated necrosis, and cardiac death (79).

Relatively little is known about gender differences in the outcome of cardiac ischemia-reperfusion. Recent experimental data in animals suggest that estrogens may protect the hearts of female subjects from cardiac ischemia. These topics are discussed below.

To summarize, cardiac ischemia in women may be the result of a number of pathologic processes that act in concert and result in diminished blood supply to the heart. Chronic narrowing of the lumen of the coronary artery is the result of a continuous process of plaque formation, disruption, reorganization, and reformation that begins as early as life *in utero,* and it may lead to stable angina. Acute coronary syndromes are associated with diminished coronary blood flow as a result of acute disruption of the plaque followed by thrombus formation, or acute vasospasm of the vessel. Increased viscosity of the blood is a precipitating factor, and the ability of cardiac cells to adapt to reperfusion of blood after the anoxia may determine cardiac viability following the ischemic event. Direct studies on the incidence in women of the occurrence of these insults are lacking. Based on epidemiologic, clinical, and experimental studies, it appears that women, compared to men, have lower incidence of coronary artery stenosis and higher incidence of acute coronary ischemia because of vasoconstriction of the coronary artery (18). In addition, recent data suggest that estrogens may favorably modulate the clinical outcome of cardiac ischemia in women (80–85).

RISK FACTORS FOR CARDIAC ISCHEMIA IN WOMEN

Cardiac ischemia is the end result of genetic, constitutive, behavioral, and environmental factors that act in concert throughout life and result in progressive cardiac damage. In the past, most research interest regarding risk factors of cardiac ischemia focused on CAHD. The traditional list of risk factors for CAHD includes obesity, abnormal plasma lipid profile, hypertension, diabetes mellitus, cigarette smoking, sedentary life style, increased blood viscosity, augmented platelet aggregability, stress, and autonomic imbalance. An important risk factor in women is estrogen deficiency after spontaneous or medically induced menopause. In most patients with CAHD, more than one risk factor can be identified, making it difficult to isolate a single risk factor that precipitated the coronary event. However, some risk factors have a stronger impact on the prevalence of the disease and are therefore considered "independent" or even "causative."

To illustrate the difficulty of targeting a single risk factor for CAHD, obesity, a clinically recognized risk factor for CAHD, will be used an an example of the interdependence of the risk factors. Obesity can be genetically determined, and it increases adiposity (86). Leptin, a product of the *OB* gene, is secreted from adipose tissue and acts on central neuronal networks that regulate ingestive behavior and energy balance (87–89). Obese individuals have increased levels of leptin (90); assuming that leptin levels are regulated by negative feedback, these findings suggest resistance to the leptin effect. Thus, genetic factors that determine adiposity and *OB* gene expression may aggrevate obesity. Hypertension and diabetes mellitus are two pathologic constitutive conditions that may occur independent of obesity, although obesity usually increases their prevalence. Hypertension and diabetes mellitus may affect arteriosclerosis directly and are therefore causative factors for CAHD. Behavioral traits, such as sedentary life style and cholesterol-rich diet, can aggravate obesity; environmental factors, such as nicotine or stress-generating occupation, can modify behavioral patterns and can activate the stress response. These effects, in concert, may determine the onset and severity of CAHD.

Although oversimplified, such a model can be drawn for most other recognized risk factors of CAHD and may help in elucidating the cause–effect relationship between the index risk factor and the disease as well as in formulating intervention protocols. An example is the effect of hypercholesterolemia on CAHD in African-American women. Hypercholesterolemia is an independent risk factor for CAHD in both men and women. In the past, cholesterol-lowering interventional programs targeted populations at risk for CAHD, considering midlife as a starting point. More recent studies revealed that hypercholesterolemia begins in childhood and that it may have strong genetic basis. Furthermore, the incidence of hypercholesterolemia is significantly higher among young African-American girls than among Caucasians (91), and the differences persist among adults and postmenopausal women. The risk of CAHD is higher in African-American girls than in Caucasians, possibly because of a higher prevalence of hypercholesterolemia in the former (91). The clinical implications are that in order to modify risks of CAHD in older women, intervention with regard to hypercholesterolemia should begin in childhood!

Obesity

Obesity is the most frequently quoted risk factor for cardiovascular disease in men and women, and most studies report a positive correlation between obesity and CAHD (Fig. 30.8) (92,93). Seventy percent of CAHD in obese women, and 40% in all women, is attributed to overweight and is potentially preventable (94). In the United States, 25% of white and 44% of African-American women are >20% over their desirable weight (11). Middle-aged women tend to gain about 0.8 kg/year in their perimenopausal years, and the weight changes are not related to menopausal estrogen deficiency (95).

Obesity develops as a result of positive energy balance, an energy intake higher than energy expenditure. Women

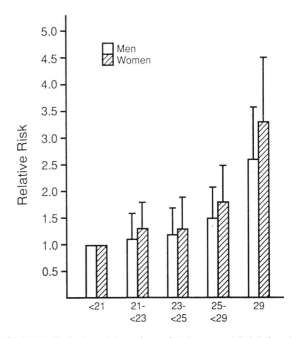

FIG. 30.8. Relative risks of nonfatal myocardial infarction and fatal coronary heart disease (combined), according to category of Quetelet index in a cohort of U.S. women 30 to 55 years of age in 1976. The highest Quetelet index (29) corresponds to a weight 30% of the desired. Quetelet index 25–28.9, mild to moderately overweight. (From ref. 94, with permission.)

have a greater prevalence of obesity than men, and the differences are accounted for by differences in the 24-hour energy expenditure, which is higher in men by 124 kcal/day; the basal metabolic rate is higher by 116 kcal/day, and sleeping metabolic rate is higher by 208 kcal/day (96). Of the three, basal metabolic rate is of the greatest significance because it accounts for 60% to 70% of total daily energy expenditure and increases with age.

Obesity, expressed either as body mass index (BMI, weight in kilograms divided by height in meters squared) or Quetelet index (weight in kilograms divided by the square root of height in meters), is not an independent risk factor for CAHD (94,97) but is associated with other coronary risk factors such as hypertension, dysplipidemia, hyperinsulinemia, insulin resistance, and diabetes mellitus. The age- and smoking-adjusted relative risk of coronary artery heart disease is 3.3 among severely obese women and 80% increased in mild to moderately obese women (94).

In women, body fat distribution is a better prognostic marker for obesity than weight (Fig. 30.9) (98,99). Centralized body fat, also termed androgenic obesity, is a strong prognostic factor for CAHD both in men and in women. It is better than gluteal body fat (also termed gynecoid obesity) (99,100) and is positively correlated with hypertension, dyslipidemia, and diabetes mellitus (99,101). Although obese premenopausal women tend to have gluteal-type obesity, after the menopause the fat distribution changes to centralized (waist) type obesity (99,102). The waist-to-hip and waist-to-thigh ratios (WHR and WTR) are the markers found to correlate best with CAHD in men and in women, and recent studies indicate that increased WHR remains positively correlated with CAHD even after controlling for hypertension, glucose intolerance, blood lipids, smoking, and BMI. The gender-associated risk disappears, however, after controlling for WHR (99).

Centralized-type obesity increases with age in both men and women and is the result of increased visceral fat, abdominal subcutaneous fat, or both (103). Men over 50 appear to accumulate more visceral, intraabdominal fat than comparable-aged women (99). The mechanism by which centralized obesity confers an increased CAHD risk is not completely understood, although it appears to be the result of differential response of upper body versus lower body adipocytes in free fatty acid mobilization (98,104).

The impact of weight reduction programs on lowering CAHD risk in women remains to be determined. It is estimated, however, that weight reduction, coupled with changes in life style such as participation in formal exercise programs, are beneficial in favorably modifying plasma lipids. Maintaining body weight at an ideal level is estimated to reduce the overall risk of CAHD by 35% to 55% (4).

Plasma Lipids

Unfavorable changes in plasma lipids are considered a causative factor for the development of CAHD both in men and in women (105,106). Studies have indicated that a 1% increase in plasma total cholesterol or LDL-C increases the risk of CAHD by 2%, and a 1% decrease in HDL-C increases the risk by 2% to 4.7% (4,16,107). Similar but opposite changes in plasma levels of the respective lipids are associated with reciprocal changes in the CAHD risk. Most of these studies were done in men, but some also included women, and more recent studies have reported similar trends in women (16,108,109).

Plasma total cholesterol is an independent risk factor for CAHD (Fig. 30.10) (4,5,106,110). The evidence is

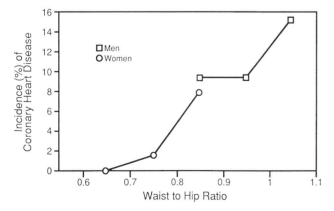

FIG. 30.9. Twelve-year incidence of coronary heart disease by waist : hip ratio and sex. Study included women aged 50, 54, and 60 years at baseline and men aged 54 at baseline, Gothenburg, Sweden (men, 1967–1979; women, 1968–1969 to 1980–1981). (From ref. 99, with permission.)

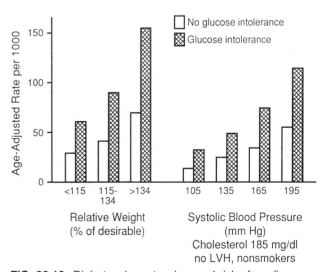

FIG. 30.10. Diabetes, hypertension, and risk of cardiovascular disease in women. Incidence of hypertension by diabetic status and relative weight (Metropolitan relative weight). Risk of cardiovascular disease by systolic blood pressure and diabetic status: women ages 45 years. LVH, left ventricular hypertrophy. (Data from ref. 127, with permission.)

clear in persons with cholesterol levels higher than 260 mg/dL (6.72 mM), who are at a high risk, and in patients with total cholesterol levels of 240 to 259 mg/dL (6.21 to 6.70 mM), who are at a moderate risk. Recent studies indicate that even subjects with low total cholesterol (160 to 190 mg/dL, 4.10 to 4.90 mM) have an increased risk in that a 1% increase in plasma total cholesterol is associated with a 2% increased risk of CAHD (4,5); the trends are similar in men and women and in adults and elderly. In the United States, 27% of all women aged 20 to 74 have plasma total cholesterol over 240 mg/dL (Table 30.1) (109).

Elevated plasma levels of triglycerides are also associated with increased risk of CAHD but are not an independent risk factor (111).

Plasma levels of LDL-C and HDL-C are independent and causative risk factors for CAHD both in men and in women (112). An LDL-C plasma level of 130 to 159 mg/dL (3.36 to 4.11 mM) is associated with moderately increased risk, and levels of 160 mg/dL (4.14 mM) and above are associated with high risk (4,5,113). Plasma levels of HDL-C are a better predictive factor than LDL-C, both for women and for men (4,5,113). In women, elevated HDL-C levels above the median level (55 mg/dL, 1.42 mM) can neutralize the adverse effects of high total cholesterol and LDL-C levels (114–116). One-third of postmenopausal women in the United States are at moderate risk, and one-fourth at high risk, of CAHD as indicated by HDL-C levels lower than 45 mg/dL (11).

Unfavorable plasma lipids are found in persons with congenital and acquired hyperlipidemias and dyslipidemias, and these individuals are at a significant risk to die of CAHD at a young age. More commonly, however, unfavorable changes in plasma lipids are found in the aging population, and the effect is positively correlated with advancing age. Several studies have dealt with the question of whether in women, the unfavorable changes in plasma lipids seen after the fifth decade of life are age-related or menopause-related. Previous studies, including the Framingham Study, have indicated that levels of HDL-C in women show little change after the fifth decade, whereas levels of LDL-C in women increase abruptly after the age of 50 to 55 (117). More recent studies show that postmenopausal women have greater increases in LDL-C and greater decreases in HDL-C than age-adjusted premenopausal controls (118). In a recent study, acute changes after the menopause (within 6 months after cessation of menstrual periods) were observed in total cholesterol levels (6% increase), in triglycerides (11% increase), and in LDL-C (10% increase). The HDL-C levels have decreased gradually by 6% 2 years after cessation of the menstrual periods (119).

Several studies have investigated the effect of cholesterol-lowering therapy on reducing the risk of CAHD, but only a few have included women as part of the trial, and the results in women are still inconclusive. Based on the results obtained in men, it is evident that decreasing plasma LDL-C and increasing plasma HDL-C, regardless of the absolute levels of the plasma lipids, can lower the total risk of CAHD (4). Normalization of elevated lipoprotein levels retards progression of coronary atherosclerotic lesions and may even regress existing plaques (115,120).

A few studies have addressed the mechanism of age-related and menopause-related changes in plasma lipids. With regard to LDL-C, it appears that the increase in the lipoprotein level is the result of age-related reduced capacity for its removal, mediated via reduced hepatic LDL receptor (121). Menopause-related changes are the result of estrogen deficiency (see below).

Women with chronic anovulation, such as polycystic ovarian syndrome, have increased levels of LDL-C and decreased levels of HDL-C. Some of these patients may also have insulin resistance and be at an increased risk of CAHD (122,123).

Hypertension

Hypertension is a risk factor for CAHD, and its impact in women is stronger than that in men (Table 30.2) (124,125). Both elevated systolic and diastolic blood pressure levels are independent risk factors, directly and positively associated with acute coronary events as well as mortality from all cardiovascular causes (4,5,125,126). Hypertension is the direct cause of death of 4.7% of white and 22.8% of African-American women (11). Twenty-four percent of white and 43% of African-American women aged 20 to 74 have blood pressure levels above 140/90 (11). The prevalence of hypertension increases with age; 27% of women 18 to 74 have blood pressure levels over

TABLE 30.1. *Estimated prevalence (%) of hypercholesterolemia in U.S. men and women by plasma cholesterol level at different ages*

Cholesterol	0–9 M	0–9 F	10–19 M	10–19 F	20–24 M	20–24 F	25–34 M	25–34 F	35–44 M	35–44 F	45–54 M	45–54 F	55–64 M	55–64 F	65–74 M	65–74 F
≥170 mg/dL	35	42	30	35												
≥200 mg/dL					27	30	43	36	61	52	72	75	74	87	67	84
≥240 mg/dL					6	7	15	12	28	21	37	41	37	53	32	52

Data modified from ref. 11, with permission.

TABLE 30.2. *Hypertension and the risks of cardiovascular disease (CVD), coronary artery heart disease (CAHD), and stroke*

	Age-adjusted RR		Estimated reductions in risk	
			Decline of 1 mm Hg diastolic blood pressure (mortality)	1% decline of systolic blood pressure (morbidity)
	35–64	65–94		
All CVD	3.4	1.8	4%	
CAHD	3.3	2.0	2–3%	2–6%
Stroke	3.0	3.0	7–8%	3.5%

Data compiled from refs. 4, 11, and 127.

140/90 compared to 53% of women aged 55 to 64 and 67.5% of women above 65 (11). In women, lowering the diastolic blood pressure is associated with a reduction in acute coronary events, even at levels of diastolic blood pressures that are considered normal (11,125).

Elevated levels of blood pressure are observed in patients who have other CAHD risk factors such as obesity, unfavorable lipid profile, and diabetes mellitus. The combination of hypertension and diabetes mellitus is of particular importance in women because diabetic patients frequently (50%) have hypertension, and the prevalence of diabetes mellitus in hypertension is also high (15% to 18%) (127); these patients have a higher incidence of other atherogenic risk factors including dyslipidemias, hyperuricemia, and elevated fibrinogen levels.

Because of its high prevalence in the population, the attributable risk of hypertension is the highest among the risk factors, and it reaches 55% compared to 5% of diabetes mellitus and 2.8% of cigarette smoking (109,127). Controlling hypertension significantly reduces the risk of cardiovascular disease, but the reductions in acute coronary risks are less than expected, indicating that hypertension has had a chronic interrelated effect with other factors (4).

Diabetes Mellitus

Hyperinsulinemia, chronic hyperglycemia, insulin resistance, and diabetes mellitus are independent risk factors for cardiovascular disease morbidity and mortality and are considered causative factors of premature mortality from CAHD (128–130). Diabetes mellitus accelerates atherosclerosis and increases the risk of acute coronary ischemia, particularly in women (127). Women with diabetes mellitus lose the female-gender-related advantage of cardiovascular disease over men (126). Age-adjusted relative risk for CAHD in patients with diabetes mellitus is 2 to 3 in men and 3 to 7 in women (4). Blood glucose levels are a graded independent risk factor for cardiovascular disease in women even within a relatively normal blood sugar range, and early-onset diabetes mellitus exposes the patient to a further increased risk (127).

The combination of impaired glucose tolerance, hypertension, insulin resistance, obesity, and unfavorable plasma lipid profile often occurs jointly and may act synergistically to predispose the patient to CAHD (127). Obesity and family history of diabetes mellitus are major determinants for the development of non–insulin-independent diabetes mellitus (NIDDM) (4). Both hypertension and diabetes mellitus share a strong relationship to obesity, but the excess of hypertension in diabetic women occurs in both lean and obese subjects (Fig. 30.10) (131).

Because of the association among diabetes mellitus, hypertension, and dyslipidemias, it has been suggested that there are preexisting genetic traits or metabolic factors in the causal pathway common to these conditions (132).

The exact mechanisms of increased risks in patients with diabetes mellitus are unclear. Hyperglycemia, hyperinsulinemia, or insulin resistance can adversely affect platelet function, resulting in increased risk for thrombosis, and can cause cardiac autonomic neuropathy and cardiomyopathy (4).

Whether regulating glucose levels in women with diabetes mellitus can decrease the risk of CAHD remains to be answered. Programs directed at reducing plasma glucose levels in patients with NIDDM have used measures that control obesity, promote exercise, and favorably affect plasma lipids; although these measures lowered the risk of CAHD, including in women, it was impossible to conclude whether the effect was solely through the control of blood glucose and/or insulin levels (133).

Cigarette Smoking

Cigarette smoking is the single most important preventable risk factor for cardiovascular disease in women (134–136). In women, cigarette smoking is directly responsible for 21% of all mortality from cardiovascular disease (136,137) and for 50% of all acute coronary events before the age of 55 (138). In women under 65, the proportion of deaths from CAHD directly attributed to smoking rose from 26% in 1965 to 41% in 1985 (137). Although the prevalence of smoking in the last decade in the United States decreased at 0.3% per year, the rate of smoking initiation increased by 1% per year (11). Currently 29% of women in the United States smoke, and in the next millennium women smokers will exceed male smokers (11).

The effect of cigarette smoking on the risk of fatal CAHD is dose related (Table 30.3) (138–141), and its

TABLE 30.3. *Age-adjusted relative and attributable risks of fatal and nonfatal coronary artery heart disease (combined) in women in relation to daily cigarette consumption*

	RR	Attributable risk (per 100,000 person years)
Nonsmokers	1.0	0
Ex-smokers	1.5	10
Smokers		
1–4[a]	2.4	32
5–14[a]	2.1	22
15–24[a]	4.2	67
25–34[a]	5.4	90
35–44[a]	7.1	120
≥45[a]	10.8	205

[a]Cigarettes per day.

effect is more than additive to other coronary risk factors such as diabetes mellitus, hypertension, and dyslipidemias (136,140). In addition, it is also strongly and directly linked to peripheral vascular arterial disease and can potentiate other risk factors in these patients (143).

Cigarette smoking exerts its adverse coronary effects via several known mechanisms. Nicotinic alkaloids release catecholamines, stimulate the sympathetic nervous system, and subsequently increase plasma levels of free fatty acids and LDL-C (144,145). Nicotine has been shown to increase platelet aggregability (144) and fibrinogen plasma levels (147,148). These three mechanisms can contribute to an increased risk of coronary thrombosis. Cigarette smokers have a higher incidence of insulin resistance than do nonsmokers, and their plasma lipids demonstrate an unfavorable profile: increased levels of total cholesterol and triglycerides, increased levels of the LDL-C, VLDL-C, and VLDL-TG, and decreased levels of HDL-C (139,141,149). Premenopausal women who smoke cigarettes are usually deficient in estrogen, and cigarette smoking eliminates the estrogen protective effect on cardiovascular disease (150,151). In addition, premenopausal cigarette smokers have a higher incidence of central (abdominal) adipose tissue distribution and lower incidence of the gluteal (gynecoid) adipose tissue distribution (150). As indicated before, a higher incidence of android adipose tissue distribution is associated with an increased risk of CAHD. Postmenopausal women on estrogen replacement therapy who smoke cigarettes have lower estrogen levels than nonsmokers (152). Cigarette smoking is also positively correlated with a risk of early natural menopause and with a greater prevalence of hirsutism, oligomenorrheas, and infertility in premenopausal women (153). These observations suggest that cigarette smoking in women may provoke a low-estrogenic, high-androgenic condition. This assumption is supported by several observations: pre- and postmenopausal smokers have a lower incidence of estrogen-dependent cancers such as endometrial cancer (154,155), and smoking eliminates the protective effect of oral estro-

gens on hip fracture in postmenopausal women (151). Nicotinic alkaloids directly inhibit human granulosa-cell aromatase activity and the conversion of androgens to estrogens (156). Cigarette smoking induces hepatic microsomal mixed-function oxidase systems that metabolize sex hormones; this effect enhances 2-hydroxylation, resulting in synthesis of nonagonistic estrogen metabolites (151,157).

In recent years, new forms of cigarettes have been introduced into the market claiming low yield of nicotine; it was found that there are no differences in the relative risk for CAHD in women who smoke high-yield nicotine (over 1.3 mg/cigarette) versus those who smoke the low-yield nicotine (less than 0.4 mg/cigarette); relative risks, respectively, were 4.2 and 4.7 (138,140). Cessation of smoking is associated with an estimated reduction of 50% to 70% in the risk of CAHD. Women who are ex-smokers have decreased their risk after 2 to 3 years of cessation of smoking, resulting in a risk comparable to that in nonsmokers (4,138,140,158).

Sedentary Life Style

The effect of physical exercise on risk of cardiovascular disease in women is not clear (159). The relative risk of death from CAHD is higher in sedentary men than in active controls by 1.9-fold (160). Cross-sectional studies report that middle-aged women who had higher levels of physical activity had lower weight, lower systolic and diastolic blood pressure levels, favorable lipid profile, and lower fasting glucose (161). Longitudinal observational studies in middle-aged women report conflicting results. Some report that leisure-time physical activity in women increased between 1980 to 1982 and 1985 to 1987 from 111 to 124 kcal/day (162), but others reported that in middle-aged women followed over 3 years the overall level of activity did not change (163). Women who increased their activity level gained less weight and had fewer adverse changes in their lipid profile compared to controls; the effects were more noticeable in postmenopausal women. Walking and aerobic exercise were the two types of exercise women chose. Reasons for participating in physical activity were "to maintain fitness," "to feel good," and to "lose or maintain weight." Reasons for not getting enough exercise were lack of motivation, lack of time, and dislike of exercise (163).

Although common thinking is that sedentary persons have higher body weight than active persons because of their lower energy expenditure, at least one recent publication has challenged that notion and indicated that in women of all ages, the current low physical activity is a result, rather than a cause, of higher body weight (164).

Potential mechanisms by which physical exercise can decrease incidence of CAHD include improvement of the functional work capacity, lowered heart rate and blood pressure, weight reduction, improvement in lipid profile, modulation of plasma leptin levels, decreased platelet adhesiveness and aggregability, enhanced fibrinolysis, and decreased adrenergic response to stress (4,165). In women, physical exercise can also reduce incidence of depression, which further contributes to a sedentary life style (163,165). Estimated reduction of acute coronary disease in men with the maintenance of an active life style is 35% to 55% (4,167,168).

Hematologic Factors

Changes in rheologic properties of the blood are associated with increased risk of CAHD. Plasma viscosity and fibrinogen levels are higher both in men and in women compared to controls following acute cardiovascular events such as stroke, myocardial infarction, or sudden cardiac death (47,59,169,170). Increased blood viscosity can be caused by abnormal changes in the red cell population such as increased hematocrit or increased red cell deformity or by increased plasma viscosity as a result of elevated levels of fibrinogen and other high-molecular proteins such as the coagulation factors, and dehydration.

The risk of CAHD correlates with increases in the activity of thrombogenic factors such as fibrinogen, procoagulants, and coagulation factors VII and VIII, and with decreased activity of thrombolytic and fibrinolytic factors such as antithrombin III and plasminogen activator (59). Factors that promote platelet aggregation and adherence also correlate with CAHD risk (47).

Stress and Autonomic Imbalance

Popular belief is that persons under stress are at an increased risk for cardiovascular disease, but very few studies have addressed this issue with regard to midlife changes in women. In men, the risk of CAHD in type A personalities (competitive, achievement oriented, time urgent, and hostile) is twofold higher than in type B personalities (those who lack type A characteristics) (171); however, no studies were reported in women. The onset of acute coronary syndromes is more prevalent in awakening hours, that is, 6 to 9 AM. Some authors have described a peak incidence of acute MI at these hours compared to a trough at 6 to 12 PM (172,173); interestingly, these data correlate with peak diurnal sympathetic activity (174). Similar to the previous studies, this one included mostly men. Evidence for gender-related differences in response to stress stimuli is derived from observations in animals and in humans. Women, compared to men, secrete sixfold higher amounts of norepinephrine in urine in response to an adrenergic stimulation, and the responses are unrelated to the phase of the cycle (171).

The mechanisms by which stress modulates the risk of CAHD are unclear. Stress can modify sympathetic neuroendocrine activity and the responses of the coronary vasculature to stimuli (171). In addition to the effect on vasotonus, sympathetic hormones and glucocorticoids can also promote arteriosclerosis (47). In women, stress can be related to estrogen production, and in animals there is an association between stress and hypoestrogenism (175). In women, psychosocial stress may exacerbate natural falls in estrogen during the menstrual cycle and reduce peak levels of estrogens, causing menstrual and fertility problems. Stressful life events have been found to be significant predictors of the premenstrual syndrome and menstrual irregularity, possibly as a result of defective folliculogenesis and relative hypoestrogenism (175–177).

Menopause occurs during a phase of life that includes many forms of stress such as retirement, illness and/or death of parents, problems with offspring, and increasingly apparent aging in a youth-oriented society (175). Evidence that menopause may be associated with the stress response and with enhanced sympathetic activity comes from recent studies that looked into the effects of menopause and estrogen replacement on heart rate variability and beat-to-beat blood pressure dynamics. Both parameters can yield important information about sympathetic tone; low variability of either parameters is considered causally related to CAHD (178,179). From indexes of heart rate variability calculated from 24-hour Holter monitoring, it was found that postmenopausal women have an increased sympathetic tone, which was improved following estrogen replacement therapy (180). Estrogen replacement therapy to postmenopausal women attenuated the low-frequency vasomotor response to posture change and meal digestion, compared to untreated postmenopausal women (179). In addition, a higher heart rate variability was found in physically active postmenopausal women than in less active postmenopausal women (181). Collectively, these data suggest that hypoestrogenism after menopause may increase the sympathetic tone and thereby increase the risk of CAHD.

Estrogen Deficiency and Estrogen Replacement Therapy

The observations that middle-aged women and older women have an increased risk for cardiovascular disease had raised a question whether the increased incidence is a result of aging or of estrogen deficiency. The age-related incidence of CAHD in women shows a higher increase after the fifth decade, and by extrapolation, it begins to be equal among men and women at the seventh to ninth decades. These observations indicate an additional factor to aging that increases the risk in women, and it is speculated to be estrogen deficiency.

Although there is no direct proof of this hypothesis, several lines of indirect evidence support it. First, the age-adjusted risk of CAHD in women with premature menopause is higher than in premenopausal women (Fig. 30.11) (7,182). Second, women with late menarche have an increased risk for CAHD (183,184). Third, most stud-

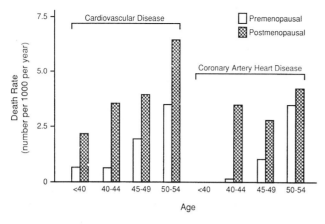

FIG. 30.11. Age-adjusted mortality rate in women from all-cause cardiovascular disease and from coronary artery heart disease by status of menopause. (Data from ref. 182, with permission.)

ies of estrogen replacement therapy in postmenopausal women show a lower risk of CAHD by about 50% in estrogen-treated women compared to controls (110, 185–218). Although most of these studies suffer from methodologic problems (5,218–221), the results appear to be consistent (185,189,218–221), indicating that the degree of putative estrogen protection is clinically significant and exceeds any other known risk factor in women. Fourth, in women with angiographically proven coronary stenosis, estrogen replacement therapy decreases the risk of cardiac death and may prolong life in patients with severe CAHD (203,204,207,222).

Collectively, these studies suggest that estrogen deficiency after the menopause is a risk factor for CAHD and that estrogen replacement therapy to postmenopausal women may attenuate the incidence of CAHD and favorably affect the outcome of the disease.

Mechanisms of Action for Estrogen in Cardiovascular Protection

Estrogens act on target cells by different mechanisms such as gene regulation via nuclear receptors (223–234), modulation of protein translation and processing (235, 236), modulation of ion transport mechanisms (237–240), and regulation of plasma membrane-related signal transduction mechanisms (241). Estrogens can also regulate cell homeostasis by affecting oxidation reactions. The latter reactions depend on the interaction of the hydroxyphenolic ring of estrogen with free radicals, thus modulating the exposure of plasma membrane and membranes of intracellular structures to potential oxidative reactions (242–250). Recent data suggest that estrogens may modulate cells of the cardiovascular system via most of these mechanisms (251).

The cardiovascular protective effects of estrogen are attributed to both extracardiac and cardiac actions of the hormone. Estrogens regulate plasma lipids, blood functions, and the autonomic and neuroendocrine systems. Estrogens modulate structure and function of vascular endothelial and smooth muscle cells; they control systemic vascular resistance and blood pressure and can modify pathologic processes, including arteriosclerosis. The cardiac effects of estrogen include modulation of structure and function of coronary vascular endothelial and smooth muscle cells and modulation of cardiac myocyte activity.

Lipid Metabolism

After menopause, and possibly as a result of hypoestrogenism, adverse changes in lipid profile occur: total cholesterol, tryiglycerides, HDL-C$_3$, lipoprotein(a), and LDL-C levels rise, and levels of HDL-C$_2$ fall (118). Low-dose estrogens reverse the menopause-related changes in lipid profile (4,5,185,252). Estrogens elevate levels of HDL-C$_2$, HDL-C$_3$, Apo-AI, and Apo-AII and decrease levels of LDL-C and lipoprotein(a) (118,253–259). Of interest is the finding that estrogens increase plasma levels of Apo-AI: this fraction decreases in postpubertal boys; it remains stable in postpubertal girls; and it decreases in women after the menopause (260). Apo-AI is considered to be a protective factor for coronary arteries; it stimulates cholesterol efflux from cells (261), and the gender- and age-related changes in its plasma levels suggest that estrogens regulate its activity (262). Estrogens also lower plasma lipoprotein(a) (56,263–266), but the clinical importance of these changes is unclear. Estrogens increase plasma triglycerides (174,267); these changes involve raising plasma levels of the VLDL-C, which has only mild impact on atherosclerosis (56,174). Estrogen modulates plasma leptin levels (268,269) and may affect adiposity. In secondary intervention trials, the effects of estrogen replacement on lipid profile are more significant than in primary trials, also when compared to the responses in men (51,270–274).

The intrahepatic lipid-related mechanisms of estrogen actions are the following:

1. Estrogens increase catabolism and clearance of LDL by increasing the number of LDL (Apo B/E) receptors in hepatocytes (275).
2. Estrogens decrease hepatic HDL receptors and thereby decrease HDL catabolism (276).
3. Estrogens reduce the activity of hepatic lipase, thereby raising levels of HDL-C (mostly HDL-C$_2$) (35–37,44).
4. Estrogens inhibit formation of regulatory oxysterols so that the increased uptake of LDL is not associated with reduced cholesterol synthesis (277).
5. Estrogens inhibit catabolism of cholesterol to bile acids, thus diminishing a major disposal path for hepatic free cholesterol (277); as a result, biliary secretion of cholesterol and cholesterol esterification are enhanced.

6. Estrogens increase the clearance of chylomicron remnants (277,278). The overall effect is to reduce cholesterol accumulation in peripheral tissues and to increase its concentration in the biliary fluid.

Rheologic and Hemostatic Effects

Menopause is associated with increased blood viscosity and with increased risk of thrombosis, and the effects are attributed in part to hypoestrogenism. After menopause, plasma levels and/or activities of thrombogenic factors such as fibrinogen, factor VII isoforms, and factor VIII and plasminogen activator inhibitor activity increase (169,170,267,279–291). Estrogens reduce plasma levels of fibrinogen and possibly decrease plasma activity of factor VII and enhance fibrinolysis by decreasing the activity of plasminogen activator inhibitor (267,282, 286,289–295). Oral preparations of estrogen replacement have more potent effects than transdermal preparations (292,296), suggesting that these effects are mediated by the liver. Estrogens inhibit platelet aggregation, reduce secretion of platelet-derived thromboxanes (potent stimulators of platelet aggregation), augment secretion of endothelium-derived prostacyclin (PGI_2, a vasodilator and an inhibitor of platelet aggregation), and reduce the reactivity of monocytes (297–305). Collectively, these data suggest that low-dose estrogen replacement decreases the risk of thrombosis.

Autonomic and Neuroendocrine Factors

Estrogens modulate the effects of the adrenergic system by peripherally downregulating the activity of monoamine oxidase and by potentiating the action of catecholamines (306). Estrogens and catecholestrogens sensitize arterial blood vessels to the effects of α- and β-adrenergic agents (306,307) and modulate their receptors (308,309). Low-dose estrogen replacement therapy to postmenopausal women lowers systolic blood pressure and mean blood pressure by decreasing the systemic vascular resistance (310). In most hypertensive or normotensive postmenopausal women, natural estrogens lower blood pressure; however, 5% to 7% of women may have an idiosyncratic reaction of elevated blood pressure, which is reversible on stopping the treatment (311). A possible mechanism by which estrogens lower blood pressure, in addition to their direct vasorelaxant effects (see below), is by modulating angiotensin-converting enzyme activity (312). Estrogen replacement therapy improves overall pancreatic β-cell function, decreases insulin and mean glucose levels, and improves insulin resistance (267,313). Estrogens affect plasma levels of other hormones that may have a direct or indirect relation to atherosclerosis (e.g., androgens) and stress (e.g., glucocorticoids) (313,314). The effects are mediated by increased liver production of the respective binding proteins and, therefore, decreasing plasma levels of the free hormones.

Treatment of women with estrogens usually increases cardiac output and decreases the systemic (or the local vascular bed, e.g., coronary) vascular resistance with only mild changes in mean arterial pressure (315–322). These effects are usually the result of estrogen-induced vasodilation of the resistance arterioles, which decrease, respectively, the systemic or the vascular-bed (e.g., coronary) resistance.

The Vascular System

The vascular system in women is a target for estrogen actions, and estrogens modulate functions of endothelial and of vascular smooth muscle cells. Estrogens promote angiogenesis by modulating endothelial cell migration, by inhibiting vascular smooth muscle cell migration, and by suppressing collagen secretion and assembly (323–332). These factors are essential for coordinated angiogenesis.

Estrogens are vasodilators and modulate reactivity of coronary arteries. The vasodilator effects of estrogens occur at all levels of the coronary arterial tree and involve large proximal epicardial vessels (331–333) as well as the microscopic arterioles that determine the coronary vascular resistance (319–322). In women and in animal models, estrogens can promote vasorelaxation even of atherosclerotic coronary vessels (334–336). The effects of estrogen on the vasculature may involve modulation of endothelium-dependent and endothelium-independent mechanisms. Estrogens upregulate endothelium-dependent mechanisms, e.g., nitric oxide synthase(s), prostacyclin production, and potassium-related hyperpolarizing mechanisms (338–340). All promote coronary vasodilation either directly (prostacyclin) or indirectly, by acting as distal messengers (e.g., nitric oxide) to stimuli originating from the endothelium (e.g., acetylcholine). Estrogens may also induce coronary vasodilation by downregulating endothelium-dependent vasoconstrictive mechanisms, notably the endothelins and their receptors (341). Furthermore, the vasodilatory effect of estrogens is not entirely mediated by the endothelium (342–345). These findings may be important for the understanding of estrogen vasorelaxation of coronary arteries in hearts of hypercholesterolemic women with moderate atherosclerosis (57,334–336). Hypercholesterolemia and early-stage atherosclerosis affect mainly the endothelium; normally this would lead to vasoconstriction and will diminish coronary blood flow. By acting on endothelium-independent vasorelaxing mechanisms, estrogens can maintain and even increase blood flow to the heart, even if the endothelium is damaged.

Additional mechanisms by which estrogens can modulate vasoreactivity are by regulating the sensitivity to adrenergic (mainly β) (308,346) and cholinergic stimuli (347,348) and by direct inhibition of smooth muscle cell contraction. The latter may involve inhibition of calcium influx, attenuation of platelet-dependent release of vasoconstrictors (serotonin and thromboxanes), and modulation of release of endothelial secretagogues and mediators of inflammatory reaction (349). Under normal conditions, the effect of platelets on the microvasculature is small. However, when flow in the vascular tree is impaired, or in the presence of arteriosclerosis, platelets may adhere and aggregate to loci of injury or stenosis, secrete vasoconstrictors, and aggravate the vasospasms.

These data suggest that estrogens play an important role in conferring vasorelaxation of the coronary vasculature in women. Estrogen deficiency, such as that after the menopause, may promote coronary vasoconstriction, even in normal (atherosclerosis-free) vessels. Support for this hypothesis includes clinical observations in estrogen-deficient postmenopausal women who have a higher incidence than men of nonstenotic angina. This syndrome, referred to as syndrome X (350,351), is believed to be the result of impaired coronary vasodilation caused by estrogen deficiency; replacement of estrogen alleviated some of the ensuing cardiac ischemia.

An interesting insight into the effects of estrogen deficiency on nonstenotic cardiac ischemia was recently provided by studies in female rabbits. It was shown that *in vivo*, the amount of estrogen necessary to confer coronary vasodilation is low and that maximal effects of estrogen occur at concentrations that are at the lower range of normal (322). On the basis of these observations, it was suggested that in women, estrogen deficiency after the menopause may aggravate an increase in coronary vascular resistance and decrease coronary blood flow.

Estrogens modulate arteriosclerosis of both peripheral and coronary vessels directly via a number of mechanisms (352–357). Estrogens inhibit influx of esterified cholesterol into the vessel wall and inhibit lipid accumulation; the hormones attenuate oxidative conversion of LDL in coronary arteries, even before affecting plasma lipids, and enhance efflux of cholesterol from the vessel wall (42–52,278). Estrogens inhibit endothelial cell and smooth muscle cell hyperplasia and collagen and elastin deposition (323,324), effects that slow coronary artery atherogenesis. Some of the beneficial antiatherogenic effects of estrogen may be related to the antioxidant properties of the hormone (358).

Recent studies indicate that estrogens modulate endothelial permeability by stabilizing endothelial tight junctions (359) and by increasing the tight junctional resistance to the movement of fluids and solutes across the endothelium. This finding may be important for understanding the protection conferred by estrogens for ischemia-reperfusion (see below) because hypoxia increases endothelial permeability, and after reperfusion, the augmented influx of solutes from the blood through the endothelium and into the cardiac parenchyma may lead to irreversible cell damage and cardiac death. By controlling the degree of endothelial permeability, estrogens can protect cardiac myocytes from sudden osmolar changes, such as those occurring during reperfusion.

Estrogen Effects on Cardiac Myocytes in Women

In addition to the regulation of coronary vasculature, estrogens also directly regulate cardiac myocytes in women (251). Estrogens can affect metabolism, signal transduction, contractility, and heart rate. Most of these studies were done on hearts of animals, but indirect data also suggest similar results in women.

Estrogens modulate activity of lysosomal enzymes in cardiac cells. Lysosomes are membranous bags of hydrolytic enzymes used for controlled intracellular digestion of macromolecules. In rats, ovariectomy increased the activities of cathepsin B and of acid phosphatase and decreased the activity of cathepsin D (360). Estrogen treatment decreased the activity of cathepsin B and restored activities of cathepsin D and acid phosphatase. At present the significance of the specific changes in cardiac-cell lysosomal enzyme activities is unclear; however, because lysosomal enzymes are important for cell homeostasis, such changes may alter the metabolic activity of cardiac cells.

Estrogens increase glycogen content in hearts of female mice (361). Glycogen is an intracellular source for glucose, which is an energy source for cardiac myocytes. Estrogens may therefore affect the bioenergetic condition of cardiac cells by regulating intracellular carbohydrate storage. Estrogens may regulate respiration of cardiac myocytes via effects on creatine kinase. The creatine kinases catalyze transfer of high-energy phosphates from ATP to creatine and shuttle energy-rich molecules across the mitochondria in a well-regulated manner. The B-type cytosolic creatine kinase isoenzyme and the mitochondrial creatine kinase (MtCK), both expressed in heart tissues, are estrogen-regulated proteins (362).

The nitric oxide pathway plays an important role in signal transduction of excitable cells. Cardiac cells express nitric oxide synthase(s), which stimulate the formation of nitric oxide from L-arginine and oxygen, and estrogens upregulate the expression of calcium-dependent nitric oxide synthase (eNOS) in female hearts (363).

Cardiac output is augmented in pregnancy, and the effect is attributed to the increased plasma activity of estrogens (315,316). Cardiac output is also increased in postmenopausal women treated with estrogens and in animals treated with the hormone (364–368). In contrast, it decreases 1% per year in men and in women after the age of 50 because of diminished stroke volume and increased peripheral resistance (30). These findings prompted investigators to determine if estrogen deficiency after the menopause may be a contributory factor for the decrease in cardiac performance.

Bolus administration of estrogen is associated with an increase in cardiac performance in women (368), and the most likely mechanism is augmented coronary blood flow. This effect was also reported in postmenopausal women with coronary atherosclerosis, indicating that estrogen preserves the vasodilatory response of both normal and atherosclerotic coronary arteries (57,320,336, 369–371). In contrast, longer-term estrogen replacement to postmenopausal women for 4 to 12 weeks had little effect on excercise performance (372,373), and estrogen therapy for more than 1 year abolished the acute estrogen-induced coronary flow augmentation in postmenopausal women (368). A possible explanation is that of tachyphylaxis of the coronary vascular response to estrogen (317). However, other studies in postmenopausal women showed that women treated with estrogen for 6 to 9 months had improved cardiac function both in rest and during excercise (374). These data are hard to interpret in terms of the direct effects of estrogens on cardiac cells. Estrogens may modulate different cardiovascular functions such as heart rate, blood pressure, and systemic vascular resistance and affect preload and afterload (251, 322), and it is possible that the responses vary in their time course and sensitivity to estrogens.

Studies in animal models provided the means to determine the direct cardiac effects of estrogens. In rodents, ovariectomy decreased stroke work by 20%, and estrogen replacement restored the effect. Interestingly, similar trends were found related to the activity of Ca-myosin ATPase, and actin-activated Mg-myosin ATPase. Biochemical analysis of cardiac myosin isoenzymes showed that ovariectomy reduced myosin isoenzyme type V_1 and increased types V_2 and V_3. In contrast, estrogen had opposite effects and tended to restore the biochemical profile of V_1, V_2, and V_3 myosin isoenzymes to control values. Because V_1 is associated with enhanced cardiac contractility, the estrogen-related changes in cardiac contractility may be the result of direct modulation by estrogen of the cardiac myocyte myosin apparatus (375–377). A less well understood phenomenon is the regulation of cardiac cell contractility by nitric oxide. In isolated contracting ventricular myocytes of rats, the inotropic effort of isoproterenol (a β-adrenergic agent) was augmented by the inhibition of nitric oxide synthase, suggesting that nitric oxide mediates a decrease in inotropy (378). This effect may be similar to the effect of nitric oxide in the vascular system (200).

The autonomic regulation of the cardiovascular system appears to differ between men and women (307–309, 380–382). The mechanisms of the gender-related differences are complex and not entirely clear. Some investigators showed that sex hormones modulate autonomic regulation of the peripheral vasculature. For instance, women are more sensitive than men to adrenergic stimulation of tachycardia (379). Two studies reported that estrogen decreases heart rate in both men (383) and women (384), suggesting that estrogens exert a direct negative chronotropic effect. Because nitric oxide mediates cardiac bradycardia (378), and estrogen upregulates nitric oxide activity in cardiac cells (363), it is possible that the estrogen-induced bradycardia is mediated by upregulation of nitric oxide mechanisms in cardiac myocytes.

Another mechanism of estrogen-related changes in heart rate is modulation of cardiac cell sensitivity to autonomic simuli. Estrogens increase cardiac content of epinephrine (306,307), augment release of adrenergic transmitters from nerve endings in the heart (308,346), and modulate the effects of adrenergic agents on coronary vascular reactivity (381,382). Estrogens modulate the effects of cholinergic agents on coronary vascular reactivity, possibly by regulating cardiac muscarinic receptors (308,309,347,348). However, only a few studies looked into effects in cardiac cells. In hearts of female rats *in vivo*, estrogen or progesterone alone had no significant effect on the binding affinities of [^{3}H]dihydroalprenolol (β-adrenergic agonist) and [^{3}H]quinuclidinyl (muscarinic agonist). Treatment with estrogen increased the density of adrenergic receptors in the heart, whereas progesterone had no effect. Combined estrogen plus progesterone treatment increased adrenergic receptors by twofold. Treatment with estrogen or with progesterone alone decreased the density of muscarinic receptors mildly, but combined estrogen plus progesterone treatment increased the density of muscarinic receptors significantly (385). These results suggest a complex mode of regulation of autonomic receptors in cardiac cells by the sex hormones in the rat.

Although it is difficult to draw definitive conclusions on the direct effects of estrogens on cardiac function, the above data suggest that cardiac myocytes are a target for estrogen actions. The data suggest that estrogens enhance inotropy and decrease chronotropy, thus lowering the cardiac respiratory and energetic demands. Hypoestrogenism may lead to nonadvantageous changes in cardiac function, and the effects can be reversed, to a degree, by estrogen replacement therapy.

Selective Estrogen Receptor Modulators

The controversy over the question of whether long-term estrogen replacement therapy increases the risk of breast cancer in postmenopausal women renewed the interest in medications that do not have stimulatory effects on the breast (or on the endometrium) but exert estrogen-like effects in other organs/tissues (386–388). One such group of chemicals are the selective estrogen receptor modulators (SERMs), and the prototype is raloxifene hydrochloride (389). At the present time, relatively little is known about cardiovascular-related effects of the drug in women. Raloxifene hydrochloride appears to have similar lipid-lowering effects on total cholesterol and on LDL-C as combined continuous estrogen-progestin hormone therapy, but it does not increase HDL-cholesterol. Compared to combined continuous estrogen-progestin treatment, it lowers triglycerides, it is more effective in lowering fibrinogen, but its effects on lipoprotein(a) and on plasminogen activator inhibitor-1 are weaker (390). Although no data were published about the long-term effects of raloxifene hydrochloride treatment on risks of cardiac ischemia in women, the effects on plasma lipids, fibrinogen, and plasminogen activator inhibitor-1 raise the question of whether the drug will have similar cardioprotective effects as estrogens.

Cardioprotective Effects of Estrogens from Ischemia and Reperfusion in Women

Cardiac ischemia may lead to arrhythmia, infarction, and death; in cases of reperfusion to previously ischemized areas, cardiac tissues may undergo additional injury leading to accelerated necrosis (391). Recent data suggest that estrogens can favorably affect the outcome of cardiac ischemia in women and salvage myocardial tissues from the consequences of reperfusion injury.

In female cats, bolus administration of 17β-estradiol (but not of 17α-estradiol) 60 minutes after occlusion of the left anterior ascending coronary artery and 30 minutes before its reperfusion resulted in a 50% reduction in cardiac necrosis and attenuated neutrophil adherence to *ex vivo* coronary vascular endothelium compared to control animals not treated with the hormone (81). Similar results were obtained in female rabbits (82). Studies in dogs showed that 2 weeks of treatment with 17β-estradiol protected cardiac function, preserved coronary flow and coronary vasorelaxation, and prevented arrhythmias after brief ischemia-reperfusion compared to placebo treatment; furthemore, the release of *n*-pentane gas *in vivo,* an index of lipid peroxidation, was attenuated in animals previously treated with estrogen (80,83,84,392). In isolated beating perfused hearts of female rabbits, short-term stunning reversibly stops heart beating and lowers left ventricular pressure; treatment with 17β-estradiol for 4 days before experiments hastened the recovery of peak left ventricular pressure (P_v) from stunning, induced by brief periods of repeated ischemia. The recovery time of cardiac contractility from repeated ischemia in control hearts tended to increase, whereas in estrogen-treated hearts it remained stable (i.e., estrogen facilitates preconditioning). In hearts obtained from estrogen-treated animals, coronary flow rates were increased by about 50%; stunning led to a postischemic increase in coronary flow, but the changes in flow were independent of the initial baseline coronary flow (85). Collectively, these data suggest that estrogen protects the hearts of female subjects from ischemia.

The molecular mechanisms by which estrogens protect the heart from the consequences of ischemia and reperfusion are unclear. Estrogens can modulate endothelial permeability by increasing the resistance of the tight junctions; this would tend to control the flow of solutes from the blood through the endothelium and into the cardiac parenchyma (359). An additional proposed mechanism is modulation of tissue damage from free radicals, notably an antioxidative effect. Oxidative damage to macromolecules such as lipo- and glycoproteins, and to nucleic acids, is the main effector of tissue degeneration and aging (392–396). *In vivo,* the main oxidants are free radicals, which are by-products of normal metabolism, including aerobic respiration, phagocytosis, leakage from peroxisomes, and reactions catalyzed by cytochrome P450 enzymes (393). Known defense mechanisms against oxidation are reductive enzymes (e.g., catalase and superoxide dismutase), DNA and protein repair enzymes, peroxisomes, plasma proteins (e.g., transferrin, ferritin, ceruloplasmin), and dietary antioxidants (vitamins C and E and carotenes) (391–396). Estrogens may have antioxidant properties *in vivo* because of their chemical structure, which contains a hydroxyphenolic ring, but little is known about the effects on the cardiovascular system. Another possible mechanism is the nitric oxide mechanism, which may act as a scavenger of free radicals. Most, although not all, studies suggest that endogenous nitric oxide protects against ischemia-reperfusion injury (397–412).

In summary, cardiac ischemia in postmenopausal women can be the result of stenosis of proximal coronary arteries, nonstenotic impaired coronary vasoreactivity, and ischemia-reperfusion syndrome. Estrogen deficiency after the menopause is a risk factor for all three mechanisms, and estrogen replacement therapy to postmenopausal women attenuates development of atherosclerosis of proximal coronary arteries, coronary stenosis, coronary thrombosis, and impaired vasoreactivity secondary to estrogen deficiency. Thus, estrogens are important for primary prevention and for risk reduction of cardiac ischemia in postmenopausal women. Epidemiologic studies indicate that current users of estrogen replacement therapy have a higher degree of protection from coronary artery heart disease than previous users by a factor of 3 to 1 (7). This also suggests that estrogens protect the ischemic heart in women.

Progesterone Effect

Postmenopausal women with an intact uterus who are treated with estrogen replacement therapy are usually also supplemented with progestins to oppose the effects of estrogen on the endometrium and to prevent endometrial hyperplasia and cancer (413). Because progesterone and the progestins are in many respects antagonistic in their action to estrogen, a concern was raised that add-on progestin can block the beneficial estrogenic effect on the cardiovascular system. The greatest concern was about effects on lipids and subsequently on coronary atherosclerosis, and about effects on coronary vasoreactivity. These assumptions are supported in part by experimental data in animals, but data in women are lacking.

Of the progestins, the androgenic derivatives, such as the 19-nortestosterone derivatives, have unfavorable effects on plasma lipids in women: they elevate LDL and Apo-B and decrease HDL-C, HDL-C$_2$, Apo-AI, and triglycerides. The 19-nortestosterone derivatives have particularly adverse effects on HDL-C and counteract the estrogen beneficial effect (414–420). For that reason, they are not recommended as an add-on progestin therapy. The C$_{21}$ derivatives such as medroxyprogesterone acetate are a better choice because their lipidogenic and atherogenic effects are minimal. Recent studies have shown that low-dose medroxyprogesterone acetate added to estrogen replacement therapy resulted in no change in the overall beneficial estrogen effect on plasma lipids; higher doses (10 mg vs. 5 mg), however, were associated with a smaller increase in the HDL-C compared to estrogen-only recipients. Natural progesterone has no effect on plasma lipids and is not considered an atherogenic substance (267,421,422).

Most studies in women on hormone (estrogen plus progestin) replacement therapy showed only mild attenuation of the estrogen-dependent favorable effects on CAHD (267). This is in contrast to studies in animals showing an attenuation of the estrogen effect (423). These discrepancies are at present unclear. Although the responses in women may differ from those in animal models, the duration of follow-up in women was effectively shorter than that in animals, and therefore, more data are needed to be able draw definitive conclusions.

Previous case reports described vasospasm of proximal coronary arteries in postmenopausal women induced by progesterone (424). In animals, progesterone and the progestins block the vasodilatory effect of estrogen, including that in the coronary vasculture (425,426). The vasospastic effects of the natural progesterone and the progestins may be mediated by antagonizing the estrogen-induced increase in prostacyclin levels (113,427) or in nitric oxide (322,426).

An additional concern was the potential of progesterone and the progestins to adversely affect other coronary risk factors by antagonizing estrogen effects on glucose metabolism, the sympathetic system, and the responsiveness of the peripheral vascular system to various stimuli (306,428–430). In contrast, progesterone and the progestins do not seem to antagonize the effects of estrogen on the structure of the vascular wall (431).

CONCLUSIONS

The desire to improve outcome of cardiac ischemia in women has met with difficulties. Analyses of morbidity and mortality trends in women reveal that cardiac ischemia, and notably CAHD, have the greatest impact after the seventh decade of life and that virtually every woman is prone to develop heart disease. Prevention of cardiac ischemia in women in the strict biologic sense is

impossible because of aging- and tissue-degeneration-related processes. Given the present state of knowledge, the objective should be to attenuate the impact of risk factors on the cardiovascular system in women in order to prevent the onset of cardiac ischemia at an early age (primary prevention) and to improve the quality of life. Secondarily, such efforts will also impact on other pathologic conditions because a deterioration of the cardiovascular system usually impairs the function of other systems and body mechanisms (432–444).

The risk factors for CAHD can be categorized into two major groups: those that promote plaque formation and those that promote plaque disruption and acute ischemia. Genetic predisposition, family history of CAHD, obesity, unfavorable lipid profile, and glucose intolerance relate primarily to the former group and are associated with increased risk of atherogenesis. Time of day (445), stress (446), presence of intercurrent systemic disease such as infection, high levels of plasma coagulation factors such as fibrinogen, and factors VII and VIII positively correlate with increased incidents of acute coronary ischemia. Some risk factors such as hypertension, cigarette smoking, estrogen deficiency, progesterone/progestins, and exercise may be associated with both plaque formation and disruption. Estrogen is of particular interest, as it seems to protect from atherogenesis, to regulate the vasotonus of the coronary artery, and to improve the performance of the heart.

There are several strategies to reduce the impact of CAHD in women (Table 30.4), and they all depend on early education from childhood on proper principles of health care. Postpubertal women have endogenous protection from CAHD compared to men, but potentially hazardous risk factors can be detected at an early age. For example, in the Bogalusa Heart Study, plasma triglycerides in both white and African-American girls and women began to increase at ages 11 to 12, VLDL at 7 to 8, LDL at 20, and HDL began to decrease at age 20. Plasma total cholesterol in white women began to increase at the age of 20, and that in African-American girls at the age of 5 to 6 (90). The early onset of hypercholesterolemia in African-American girls can explain the high incidence of cardiovascular disease in these individuals. Hypercholesterolemia is a potentially preventable risk factor with proper education to maintain a balanced low-fat diet. As shown in Table 30.5, the prevalence of potentially preventable CAHD risk factors, such as cigarette smoking, obesity, plasma total cholesterol, and hypertension, is high in young adult women in the United States.

Measures such as avoidance or cessation of cigarette smoking, proper active life style, balanced low-fat and low-salt diet, and early detection of unfavorable lipid profile and plasma glucose and insulin abnormalities should begin at an early age and be part of the routine medical care provided to postpubertal girls. In middle-aged and elderly women, additional preventive measures should be

TABLE 30.4. *Strategy for the prevention of coronary artery heart disease in women*

Risk factor	Goal	Strategy	Estimated reduction in risk
Weight	Maintenance of ideal body weight	Balanced diet	35–55% lower compared with obese (≥20% above desirable weight)
Lipids	Total cholesterol ≥200 mg/dL HDL-C ≥55 mg/dL LDL-C ≤130 mg/dL	Low-fat diet, lipid-lowering medications, weight reduction, modifications in life style	2–4.7% reduction per 1% decrease in total cholesterol or 1% increase in HDL-C
Hypertension	<140 mm Hg systolic and <90 mm Hg diastolic blood pressure	Weight reduction, salt-restricted diet, hypotensive drug therapy	2–3% decline in risk for each reduction of 1 mm Hg in DBP
Glucose intolerance	Normoglycemia and normoinsulinemia	Early detection of abnormality, weight reduction, controlled diet, hypoglycemic therapy	Unknown
Cigarette smoking	Cessation of smoking	Prevention, education	50–70% reduced risk, compared with current smokers
Sedentary life style	Active life style	Life style modifications	45% lower risk (data obtained in men)
Diet	Balanced diet, mild alcohol consumption	Life style modifications	25–45% lower risk for those who consume small amount of alcohol daily
Estrogen deficiency	Equivalent of plasma E_2, 50–200 pg/mL	Estrogen replacement after the menopause	50% lower risk in users compared to nonusers; effect of added progesterone is unknown
Progesterone or progestins	Reduce the risk of the add-on progesterone/ progestin to estrogen replacement in postmenopausal women	Use of C_{21} progesterone or progestin, lowest necessary dose to transform the endometrium to secretory type	Unknown; low-dose MPA does not seem to significantly reduce the beneficial effect of estrogen
Time of day	Decrease elevated risk of acute coronary events in awakening hours.	Life style modifications, prophylactic low-dose aspirin, β-adrenergic blockers	Unknown[a]
Acute thrombosis	Reduce the risk	Prophylactic low-dose aspirin	33% lower risk in users compared with nonusers (data obtained in men)
Stress	Reduce the risk	Life style modifications	Unknown
Family history	Early detection of risk	Preventive medicine	Unknown

MPA, medroxyprogesterone acetate.
[a]Data from refs. 4 and 445.

implemented to reduce the risk of acute coronary events. More well-designed studies are needed to identify the triggering of acute coronary ischemia in middle-aged and in older women, but the available data indicate the importance of risk factors such as cigarette smoking, stressful and sedentary life style, and estrogen deficiency (447). The Minnesota Heart Survey assessed community trends in the awareness, treatment, and control of hypercholesterolemia during an average of 5 years between 1980 to 1982 and

TABLE 30.5. *Prevalence (%) of common risk factors of coronary artery heart disease in adult women*

	19	25–34	35–44
Age			
Obesity	25	20	27
Cigarette smoking	27	33	34
Total cholesterol[a]	37	18	13
Hypertension[b]		4	11

[a]Defined as ≥170 mg/dL at age 19, ≥220 mg/dL at age 20–25, ≥240 ng/dL at age 30–39, and ≥260 mg/dL at age >40.
[b]Defined as blood pressure ≥160/95 mm Hg.
Data compiled from refs. 3, 4, and 11.

1985 to 1987 (448). In women, mortality from CAHD declined by 12.9%, prevalence of smoking declined by 18%, age-adjusted mean diastolic blood pressure declined by 0.9 mm Hg, mean total plasma cholesterol declined by 5.8 mg/dL, and prevalence of hypercholesterolemia (>240 mg/dL) by 3.5%, from 17.1% to 13.6%. Public awareness, changes in life style such as diet control and routine exercise, and to a lesser extent the use of lipid-lowering medications were felt to account for the 63% of the decline in the mortality from CAHD (448).

Estrogen replacement therapy to postmenopausal women is the single most significant factor in reducing the impact of cardiac ischemia in women (185,253). Estrogens can improve blood flow into the heart, delay and attenuate the development of coronary atherosclerosis, improve the performance of the myocardium, and attenuate myocardial damage following repeat ischemia. Risk-benefit analyses of estrogen replacement therapy to postmenopausal women have been reported in the past (311) and confirmed recently (218,220,449–456). Despite the potential flaws in the underlying studies on which these analyses were based, the conclusions are that the benefits of estrogen replacement far outweigh the risks, including the potential increased risk for breast cancer. Subsequently, the questions to be answered are what women are candidates for the hormone replacement and what treatment modalities should be used.

Whether estrogen replacement therapy in order to reduce the impact of cardiac ischemia should be offered to all postmenopausal women or only to selected high-risk groups is an ongoing debate. Clearly, certain groups of women such as those with premature menopause (see below) or those with a strong family history of heart disease are the primary candidates. Women with other risk factors for cardiac ischemia should be advised to adopt measures to reduce the impact of those risks, as was mentioned above, but can also benefit from estrogen treatment. In contrast, women at risk for developing breast cancer or other estrogen-dependent neoplasia, or women with estrogen-dependent organ/system disease (e.g., liver dysfunction) should be individualized for the hormonal treatment.

The current standard of care dictates using low-dose estrogen replacement, but there are no definitive data on what doses are optimal and what plasma estrogen level/activity is needed to decrease the impact of cardiac ischemia in women. Previous cohort studies suggest that daily doses equivalent to 0.625 mg of oral conjugated estrogen have optimal outcome (218,220), but one should use caution in the interpretation of these results, given the potential methodologic flaws in the studies. The duration of treatment is an equally important subject, as it was suggested that the increase in the incidence of breast cancer begins after about 10 years of estrogen use (218,220). These studies also showed that the beneficial effect of estrogen on heart disease depends on the current use of the hormone and that previous users had a residual effect for about 3 years after cessation (218,220). This conclusion then raises a number of questions, such as at what age after menopause to start estrogen replacement therapy, if treatment should be given continously, etc. A third issue unresolved is the route of administration (e.g., oral vs. transdermal) (457). Oral estrogenic preparations apper to have more beneficial effects on factors that depend on the liver, such as lipid profile (253), but whether the long-term usage of estrogen negates the differences between the various routes of administration remains to be determined. Clearly, more well-designed studies are needed to answer these questions.

A similar debate exists regarding the supplementation of progestins in women with an intact uterus, and it is discussed in other chapters of this book.

Premature Menopause and the Risk for Cardiovascular Disease

One of 100 women between the ages of 15 and 40 will spontaneously develop premature menopause (458), but more will experience medically related menopause as a result of surgical removal of ovaries, irradiation, or chemotherapy (459). Epidemiologic studies suggest that premature menopause increases cardiovascular morbidity and mortality (460), but definitive data are lacking. Women undergoing premature menopause are more likely to seek medical treatment for infertility than for hormone replacement therapy. Most will not be aware of the fact that their risk for developing cardiovascular disease at an early age is high, and a more observant and vigilent approach is usually recommended.

One of the objectives of the management of patients with premature menopause is to prevent the potential ill effects of long-term ovarian hormone deficiency. The present general guidelines for hormone replacement therapy are similar to those in women after natural menopause at ages 50 and above. They are (a) low dose of estrogen that is sufficient to prevent climacteric symptoms, (b) low-dose testosterone to augment the effect of estrogen, and (c) progestin add-on to protect the endometrium from the proliferative effects of estrogen. There are, however, a number of important differences between premature menopause and natural menopause. Patients with premature menopause are deprived of estrogen at a phase of life when the ovaries produce most of the body estrogens. The ensuing plasma and tissue levels of the hormone are significantly higher than those produced by estrogen replacement at the current recommended doses for women after natural menopause. Younger women are usually less obese than older women, and they produce less estrogen in peripheral sites. Also, patients with premature menopause who are treated with hormone replacement therapy usually wish to have regular menstrual cycles, in contrast to women after natural menopause. For these reasons patients with premature menopause may require higher doses of estrogen than are currently prescribed as hormone replacement for older women (459).

An additional issue is the length of treatment. Most patients with premature menopause have climacteric symptoms that may persist for many years, which will motivate them to use hormone replacement therapy. Some women may not regard those symptoms as severe enough to commit themselves to long-term treatment; others may use hormone replacement therapy for a number of months or years and then stop for fear of long-term side effects. No well-controlled prospective data exist with regard to possible ill effects of hormone replacement therapy in patients with premature menopause, including the risk of breast cancer, and patients should be so informed. Some of the protective effects of estrogens on vital organs such as the cardiovascular system (461) and on the bones (462) require exposure to estrogens for many years, even before the age of natural menopause. Bone density in women reaches a peak at ages 35 to 40, and estrogen is the single most important factor for attaining optimal levels (463–465). After menopause, estrogens remain the single most important factor in maintaining bone density, but the effectiveness of estrogen depends on the continuity of treatment, and bone density decreases acutely after cessation of hormone replacement therapy. Whether estrogens have similar effects on the cardiovascular system remains to be seen.

Although estrogen replacement is perhaps the single most important factor in the long-term management of women with premature menopause, other nonestrogen approaches should be recommended, including appropriate life-style changes, nutrition and diet, exercise, vitamins and calcium, and control of known risk factors such as smoking, hypertension, and diabetes.

REFERENCES

1. Anderson RN, Kochanek KD, Murphy SL. *Report of final mortality statistics, 1995. Monthly vital statistics report, vol 45, no. 11, Suppl 2, Table 7.* Hyattsville, MD: National Center for Health Statistics, 1997:23–33.
2. Advance report of final mortality statistics, 1989. *Monthly Vital Stat Rep* 1992; 40(Suppl 2):1–47.
3. NIH. *Chartbook on cardiovascular, lung and blood diseases.* Bethesda, MD: US Department of Health and Human Services, 1992.
4. Manson JE, Tosteson H, Ridker PM, et al. The primary prevention of myocardial infarction. *N Engl J Med* 1992;326:1406–1416.
5. Bush TL. The epidemiology of cardiovascular disease in postmenopausal women. *Ann NY Acad Sci* 1990;592:263–271.
6. Heberden W. Commentaries on the history and cure of diseases. In: Willius FA, Keys TE, eds. *Cardiac classics.* St Louis: CV Mosby, 1941:221–224.
7. Kalin MF, Zumoff B. Sex hormones and coronary disease: a reveiw of the clinical studies. *Steroids* 1990;55:330–352.
8. Ayanian JZ, Epstein AM. Differences in the use of procedures between women and men hospitalized for coronary heart disease. *N Engl J Med* 1991;325:222–225.
9. Steingart RM, Packer M, Hamm P, et al. Sex differences in the management of coronary artery disease. *N Engl J Med* 1991;325:226–230.
10. Maynard C, Litwin PE, Martin JS, Weaver WD. Gender differences in the treatment and outcome of acute myocardial infarction. *Arch Intern Med* 1992;152: 972–976.
11. American Heart Association. *1993 heart and stroke facts.* Dallas: American Heart Association National Center, 1993.
12. Cummings SR, Black DM, Rubin SM. Lifetime risks of hip, Colle's or vertebral fracture and coronary heart disease among white postmenopausal women. *Arch Intern Med* 1989;149:2445–2448.
13. Miller VT. Dyslipoproteinemia in women: special considerations. *Endocrinol Metab Clin North Am* 1990;19:381–398.
14. Kannell WB, Feinleib M. Natural history of angina pectoris in the Framingham study: Prognosis and survival. *Am J Cardiol* 1972;29:154–163.
15. Kannel WB, Abbott RD. Incidence and prognosis of unrecognized myocardial infarction: an update on the Framingham study. *N Engl J Med* 1984;311: 1144–1147.
16. Lerner DJ, Kannel WB. Patterns of coronary heart disease morbidity and mortality in the sexes. A 26 year follow-up of the Framingham population. *Am Heart J* 1986;111:383–390.
17. Sarrel PM, Lindsay D, Rosano GMC, Poole-Wilson PA. Angina and normal coronary arteries in women: Gynecologic findings. *Am J Obstet Gynecol* 1992;167:467–472.
18. Kessler KM. Syndrome X: The epicardial view. *J Am Coll Cardiol* 1992;19: 32–33.
19. Hutchinson SJ, Poole-Wilson PA, Henderson AH. Angina with normal coronary arteries: a review. *Q J Med* 1989;72:677–688.
20. Ockene IS, Shay MJ, Alpert JS, Weiner BH, Dalen JE. Unexplained chest pain in patients with normal coronary arteriograms. *N Engl J Med* 1980;303: 1249–1252.
21. Leppert J, Aberg H, Ringqvist F, Sorensson S. Raynaud's phenomenon in a female population: prevalence and association with other conditions. *Angiology* 1987;38:871–877.
22. Kronenberg F. Hot flashes: Epidemiology and physiology. *Ann NY Acad Sci* 1990;592:52–86.
23. Kahn SS, Nessim S, Gray R, Czer LS, Chaux A, Matloff J. Increased mortality of women in coronary artery bypass surgery: evidence for referral bias. *Ann Intern Med* 1990;112:561–567.
24. Wenger NK. Gender, coronary artery disease, and coronary bypass surgery. *Ann Intern Med* 1990;112:557–558.
25. Loop FD, Golding LR, MacMillan JP, Cosgrove DM, Lytle BW, Sheldon WC. Coronary artery surgery in women compared with men: analyses of risks and long term results. *J Am Coll Cardiol* 1983;1:383–390.
26. Tofler G, Stone P, Muller J, et al. Effect of gender and race on prognosis after myocardial infarction: adverse prognosis for women, particularly black women. *J Am Coll Cardiol* 1987;9:473–482.
27. Moss AJ, Benhorin J. Prognosis and management after a first myocardial infarction. *N Engl J Med* 1990;322:743–751.
28. Greenland P, Reicher-Reiss H, Goldbourt I, Behar S. In-hospital and 1-year mortality in 1524 women after myocardial infarction: comparison with 4315 men. *Circulation* 1991;83:484–491.
29. Chirikos TN, Nickel JL. Work disability from coronary heart disease in women. *Women Health* 1984;9:55–74.
30. Ross R. The pathogenesis of atherosclerosis: an update. *N Engl J Med* 1986; 314:488–500.
31. Ip JH, Fuster V, Badimon L, Badimon JJ, Taubman MB, Chesebro JH. Syndromes of accelerated atherosclerosis: the role of vascular injury and smooth muscle cell proliferation. *J Am Coll Cardiol* 1990;15:1667–1687.
32. Fuster V, Badimon L, Badimon JJ, Chesebro JH. The pathogenesis of coronary artery disease and the acute coronary syndromes (I). *N Engl J Med* 1992;326: 242–250.
33. Stary HC. Evolution and progression of atherosclerotic lesions in coronary arteries of children and young adults. *Arteriosclerosis* 1989;99(Suppl 1):I19–I32.
34. Solberg LA, Strong JP. Risk factors and atherosclerosis lesions: a review of autopsy studies. *Arteriosclerosis* 1983;3:187–198.
35. Berenson GS, Wattiguey WA, Tracy RE, et al. Atherosclerosis of the aorta and coronary arteries and cardiovascular risk factors in persons aged 6 to 30 years and studied at necropsy (The Bogalusa Heart Study). *Am J Cardiol* 1992;70: 851–858.
36. Vlodaver Z, Kahn HA, Neufeld HN. The coronary arteries in early life in three different ethnic groups. *Circulation* 1979;39:541–550.
37. Neufeld HN, Wagenvoort CA, Edwards JE. Coronary arteries in fetuses, infants, juveniles and young adults. *Lab Invest* 1962;11:837–844.
38. Pober JS. Cytokine activation of vascular endothelium: physiology and pathology. *Am J Pathol* 1988;133:426–433.
39. Poston RN, Haskard DO, Coucher JR, Gall NP, Johnson-Tidey RR. Expression of intercellular adhesion molecule-1 in atherosclerosis plaques. *Am J Pathol* 1992;140:665–673.
40. Navab M, Imes SS, Hough GP, et al. Monocyte transmigration induced by modification of low density lipoprotein co-cultures of human aortic wall cell is due to induction of monocyte chemotactic protein synthesis and is abolished by high density lipoprotein. *J Cell Biochem* 1992;16A:A008.
41. Henriksen T, Mahoney EM, Steinberg D. Enhanced macrophage degradation of low density lipoprotein previously incubated with cultured endothelial cells: recognition by receptors for acetylated low density lipoproteins. *Proc Natl Acad Sci USA* 1981;78:6499–6503.
42. Rosenfeld ME, Khoo JC, Miller E, Parthsarathey S, Palinski W, Witztum JL. Macrophage-derived foam cells freshly isolated from rabbit atherosclerotic lesions degrade modified lipoproteins, promote oxidation of low density lipoproteins and contain oxidation specific lipid protein adducts. *J Clin Invest* 1991;87:90–99.
43. Regnstrom J, Nilsson J, Tornvall P, Landon C, Hamsten A. Susceptibility to low density lipoprotein oxidation and coronary atherosclerosis in man. *Lancet* 1992;339:1183–1186.
44. Szczeklik A, Gryglewski RJ, Domagala B, Dworski R, Basista M. Dietary supplementation with vitamin E in hyperlipoproteinemias: effects on plasma lipid peroxides, antioxidant activity, prostacyclin generation and platelet aggregability. *Thromb Haemostas* 1985;54:425–430.
45. Mitchinson MJ, Ball RY. Macrophages and atherogenesis. *Lancet* 1987;1: 146–148.
46. Barrowcliffe TW, Gutteridge JM, Gray E. Oxygen radicals, lipid peroxidation and the coagulation system. *Agents Actions* 1987;22:347–348.
47. Fuster V, Badimon L, Badimon JJ, Chesebro JH. The pathogenesis of coronary artery disease and the acute coronary syndromes (II). *N Engl J Med* 1992;326: 310–318.
48. Editorial: Atherosclerosis goes to the wall. *Lancet* 1992;339:647–648.
49. Davies SW, Marchant B, Lyons JP, et al. Irregular coronary lesion morphology after thrombolysis predicts early clinical instability. *J Am Coll Cardiol* 1991;18: 669–674.
50. Little WC. Angiographic assessment of the culprit coronary artery lesion before acute myocardial infarction. *Am J Cardiol* 1990;66:44G–47G.
51. Moise A, Lesperance J, Theroux P, Taeymans Y, Goulet C, Bourassa MG. Clinical and angiographic predictors of new total coronary occlusion in coronary artery disease: analysis of 313 nonoperated patients. *Am J Cardiol* 1984;54: 1176–1181.
52. Tomanek RJ. Age as a modulator of coronary capillary angiogenesis. *Circulation* 1992;86:320–321.
53. Vane JR, Anggaard EE, Botting RM. Regulatory functions of the vascular endothelium. *N Engl J Med* 1990;323:27–36.
54. Endothelins. *Lancet* 1991;337:79–81.
55. Wright L, Homans DC, Laxson DD, Dai XZ, Bache RJ. Effect of serotonin and thromboxane A_2 on blood flow through moderately well developed coronary collateral vessels. *J Am Coll Cardiol* 1992;19:687–693.
56. Ludmer PL, Selwyn AP, Shook TL, et al. Paradoxical vasoconstriction induced by acetylcholine in atherosclerotic coronary arteries. *N Engl J Med* 1987;315: 1046–1051.

57. Williams JK, Adams MR, Herrington DM, Clarkson TB. Short term administration of estrogen and vascular responses of atherosclerotic coronary arteries. *J Am Coll Cardiol* 1992;20:452–457.
58. Ernst E, Matrai A, Marshall M. Blood rheology in patients with ischemic attacks. *Stroke* 1988;19:634–636.
59. Resch KL, Ernst E, Matrai A, Paulson HF. Fibrinogen and viscosity as risk factors for subsequent cardiovascular events in stroke survivors. *Ann Intern Med* 1992;117:371–375.
60. Vinten-Johansen J, Zhao ZQ, Sato H. Reduction in surgical ischemic gynecological endocrinology reperfusion injury with adenosine and nitric oxide therapy. *Ann Thorac Surg* 1995;60:852–857.
61. Nakanishi K, Vinten-Johansen J, Lefer DJ, et al. Intracoronary L-arginine during reperfusion improves endothelial function and reduces infarct size. *Am J Physiol* 1992;263:H1650–H1658.
62. Lefer DJ, Nakanishi K, Vinten-Johansen J.(1993). Endothelial and myocardial cell protection by a cysteine-containing nitric oxide donor after myocardial ischemia and reperfusion. *J Cardiovasc Pharmacol* 1993;22(Suppl 7):S34–S43.
63. Fung KP, Wu TW, Zeng LH, Wu J. The opposing effects of an inhibitor of nitric oxide synthesis and of a donor of nitric oxide in rabbits undergoing myocardial ischemia reperfusion. *Life Sci* 1994;54:PL491–496.
64. Hattler BG, Gorcsan J 3rd, Shah N, et al. A potential role for nitric oxide in myocardial stunning. *J Cardiac Surg* 1994;9:425–429.
65. Seccombe JF, Pearson PJ, Schaff HV.(1994). Oxygen radical-mediated vascular injury selectively inhibits receptor-dependent release of nitric oxide from canine coronary arteries. *J Thorac Cardiovasc Surg* 1997;107:505–509.
66. Engelman DT, Watanabe M, Engelman RM, et al. Constitutive nitric oxide release is impaired after ischemia and reperfusion. *J Thorac Cardiovasc Surg* 1995;110:1047–1053.
67. Hammon JW Jr, Vinten-Johansen J. Augmentation of microvascular nitric oxide improves myocardial performance following global ischemia. *J Cardiac Surg* 1995;10:423–427.
68. Hiramatsu T, Forbess JM, Miura T, Mayer JE Jr.(1995) Effects of L-arginine and L-nitro-arginine methyl ester on recovery of neonatal lamb hearts after cold ischemia. Evidence for an important role of endothelial production of nitric oxide. *J Thorac Cardiovasc Surg* 1995;109:81–86, discussion 86.
69. Maulik N, Engelman DT, Watanabe M, et al. Nitric oxide signaling in ischemic heart. *Cardiovasc Res* 1995;30,593–601.
70. Seccombe JF, Schaff HV. Coronary artery endothelial function after myocardial ischemia and reperfusion. *Ann Thorac Surg* 1995;60:778–788.
71. Pearson PJ, Lin PJ, Schaff HV. Global myocardial ischemia and reperfusion impair endothelium-dependent relaxations to aggregating platelets in the canine coronary artery. A possible cause of vasospasm after cardiopulmonary bypass. *J Thorac Cardiovasc Surg* 1992;103:1147–1154.
72. Schror K, Woditsch I. Endogenous prostacyclin preserves myocardial function and endothelium-derived nitric oxide formation in myocardial ischemia. *Agents Actions* 1992;(Suppl 37):312–319.
73. Vegh A, Szekeres L, Parratt J. Preconditioning of the ischaemic myocardium; involvement of the L-arginine nitric oxide pathway. *Br J Pharmacol* 1992;107:648–652.
74. Woditsch I, Schror K. Prostacyclin rather than endogenous nitric oxide is a tissue protective factor in myocardial ischemia. *Am J Physiol* 1992;263:H1390–H1396.
75. Hiramatsu T, Forbess J, Miura T, Roth SJ, Cioffi MA, Mayer JE Jr. Effects of endothelin-1 and endothelin-A receptor antagonist on recovery after hypothermic cardioplegic ischemia in neonatal lamb hearts. *Circulation* 1995;92(Suppl II):404–404.
76. Wang QD, Uriuda Y, Pernow J, Hemsen A, Sjoquist PO, Ryden L. Myocardial release of endothelin (ET) and enhanced ET(A) receptor-mediated coronary vasoconstriction after coronary thrombosis and thrombolysis in pigs. *J Cardiovasc Pharmacol* 1995;26:770–776.
77. Wanna FS, Obayashi DY, Young JN, DeCampli WM. Simultaneous manipulation of the nitric oxide and prostanoid pathways reduces myocardial reperfusion injury. *J Thorac Cardiovasc Surg* 1995;110:1054–1062.
78. Pabla R, Buda AJ, Flynn DM, et al. Nitric oxide attenuates neutrophil-mediated myocardial contractile dysfunction after ischemia and reperfusion. *Circ Res* 1996;78:65–72.
79. Lefer DJ. Myocardial protective actions of nitric oxide donors after myocardial ischemia and reperfusion. *New Horizons* 1995;3:105–112.
80. McHugh NA, Cook SM, Schairer JL, Bidgoli MM, Merrill GF. Ischemia- and reperfusion-induced ventricular arrhythmias in dogs: effects of estrogen. *Am J Physiol* 1995;268:H2569–H2573.
81. Delyani JA, Murohara T, Nossuli TO, Lefer AM. Protection from myocardial reperfusion injury by acute administraiton of 17β-estradiol. *J Mol Cell Cardiol* 1996;28:1001–1008.
82. Hale SL, Birnbaum Y, Kloner RA. β-Estradiol, but not α-estradiol, reduces myocardial necrosis in rabbits after ischemia and reperfusion. *Am Heart J* 1996;132:258–262.
83. Kim YD, Lees DE. Estrogen and ischemic heart disease. *Chonnam J Med Sci* 1996;9(1):62–70.
84. Kim YD, Chen B, Beauregard J, et al. 17-Beta-estradiol prevents dysfunction of canine coronary endothelium and myocardium and reperfusion arrhythmias after brief ischemia/reperfusion. *Circulation* 1996;94(11):2901–2908.
85. Levy MN, Utian WH, Yang T, Goldfarb J, Gorodeski GI. Effects of estrogen on cardiac stunning in female rabbits. *Menopause* 1997;4:246(S-2).
86. Andersson LB. Genes and obesity. *Ann Med* 1996;28(1):5–7.
87. Campfield LA, Smith FJ, Burn P. The *OB* protein (leptin) pathway—a link between adipose tissue mass and central neural networks. *Horm Metab Res* 1996;28(12):619–632.
88. Schwartz MW, Peskind E, Raskind M, Boyko EJ, Porte D Jr. Cerebrospinal fluid leptin levels: relationship to plasma levels and to adiposity in humans. *Nature Med* 1996;2(5):589–593.
89. Masuzaki H, Hosoda K, Ogawa Y, et al. Augmented expression of obese *(ob)* gene during the process of obesity in genetically obese-hyperglycemic Wistar fatty *(fa/fa)* rats. *FEBS Lett* 1996;378(3):267–271.
90. Lonnqvist F, Arner P, Nordfors L, Schalling M. Overexpression of the obese *(ob)* gene in adipose tissue of human obese subjects. *Nature Med* 1995;1(9):950–953.
91. Webber LS, Srinivasan SR, Wattigney WA, Berenson GS. Tracking of serum lipids and lipoproteins from childhood to adulthood. The Bogalusa Heart Study. *Am J Epidemiol* 1991;132:884–899.
92. Hubert HB, Feinlab M, McNamara PM, Castelli WP. Obesity as an independent risk factor for cardiovascular disease: A 26 year follow-up of participants in the Framingham heart study. *Circulation* 1983;67:968–977.
93. Harlan WR, Landis JR, Flegal KM, Davis CS, Miller ME. Secular trends in body mass in the U.S., 1960–1980. *Am J Epidemiol* 1988;128:1065–1074.
94. Manson JE, Colditz GA, Stampfer MJ, et al. A prospective study of obesity and risk of coronary heart disease in women. *N Engl J Med* 1990;322:882–889.
95. Wing RR, Mathews KA, Kuller LH, Meilahn EW, Plantinga PL. Weight gain at the time of menopause. *Arch Intern Med* 1991;151:97–102.
96. Ferraro R, Lillioja S, Fontvieille AM, Rising R, Bogardus C, Ravussin E. Lower sedentary metabolic rate in women compared with men. *J Clin Invest* 1992;90:780–784.
97. Tayback M, Kumanyika S, Chee E. Body weight as a risk factor in the elderly. *Arch Intern Med* 1990;150:1065–1072.
98. Martin ML, Jensen MD. Effects of body fat distribution on regional lipolysis in obesity. *J Clin Invest* 1991;88:609–613.
99. Larsson B, Bengtsson C, Bjorntorp P, et al. Is abdominal body fat distribution a major explanation for the sex difference in the incidence of myocardial infarction? *Am J Epidemiol* 1992;135:266–273.
100. Mueller WH, Wear ML, Hanis CL, et al. Which measure of body fat distribution is best for epidemiologic research? *Am J Epidemiol* 1991;133:858–869.
101. Kissebach AH, Peiris AN. Biology of regional body fat distribution: relationship to non-insulin-dependent diabetes mellitus. *Diabetes Metab Rev* 1989;5:83–109.
102. Armellini F, Micciolo R, Ferrari P, et al. Blood pressure, metabolic variables and adipose tissue distribution in pre- and postmenopausal women. *Acta Obstet Gynecol Scand* 1990;69:627–633.
103. Zamboni M, Armellini F, Milani MP, et al. Body fat distribution in pre and post-menopausal women: metabolic and anthropometric variables and their interrelationships. *Int J Obesity* 1992;16:495–504.
104. Jensen DM, Haymond MW, Rizza RA, Cryer PE, Miles JM. Influence of body fat distribution on free fatty acid metabolism in obesity. *J Clin Invest* 1989;83:1168–1173.
105. Report of the National Cholesterol Education Program Expert Panel on detection, evaluation and treatment of high blood cholesterol in adults. *Arch Intern Med* 1988;148:36–49.
106. Jacobs DR, Mebane IL, Bangdiwala SI, Cirqin MH, Tyroler HA. High density lipoprotein cholesterol as a predictor of cardiovascular disease mortality in men and women: The follow-up study of the Lipid Research Clinics Prevalence Study. *Am J Epidemiol* 1990;131:32–47.
107. Chen Z, Peto R, Collins R, MacMahon S, Lu J, Li W. Serum cholesterol concentration and coronary heart disease in population with low cholesterol concentration. *Br Med J* 1991;303:276–282.
108. Perlman JA, Wolf PH, Ray R, Lieberknecht G. Cardiovascular risk factors, premature heart disease and all cause mortality in a cohort of Northern California women. *Am J Obstet Gynecol* 1988;158:1568–1574.
109. Isles CG, Hole DJ, Hawthorne VM, Lever AF. Relation between coronary risk and coronary mortality in women of the Renfrew and Paisley Survey: comparison with men. *Lancet* 1992;339:702–706.
110. Beard CM, Kottke TE, Annegers JF, Ballard DJ. The Rochester Coronary Heart Disease Project: effect of cigarette smoking, hypertension, diabetes and steroidal estrogen use on coronary heart disease among 40 to 59 year-old women, 1960 through 1982. *Mayo Clin Proc* 1989;64:1471–1480.
111. Austin MA. Plasma triglyceride as a risk factor for coronary heart disease. *Am J Epidemiol* 1989;129:249–259.
112. Sharp SD, Williams RR, Hunt SC, Schumacher MC. Coronary risk factors and the severity of angiographic coronary artery disease in members of high risk pedigrees. *Am Heart J* 1992;123:279–285.
113. Ettinger B. Hormone replacement and coronary heart disease. *Obstet Gynecol Clin North Am* 1990;17:741–757.
114. Levy RI, Brensike JF, Epstein SE, et al. The influence of changes in lipid values induced by cholestyramine and diet on progression of coronary artery disease. *Circulation* 1984;69:325–337.
115. Arntzenius AC, Kromhont D, Barth JD, et al. Diet, lipoproteins and the progression of coronary atherosclerosis. *N Engl J Med* 1985;312:805–811.
116. Blankenhorn DH, Nessin SA, Johnson RL, Sanmarco ME, Azen SP, Hemphill CL. Beneficial aspects of combined colestipol-niacin therapy on coronary atherosclerosis and coronary venous bypass grafts. *JAMA* 1987;257:3233–3240.
117. Kannel WB. Nutrition and the occurrence and prevention of cardiovascular disease in the elderly. *Nutr Rev* 1988;46:68–78.
118. Matthews KA, Meilahn E, Kuller LH, Kelsey SF, Cagginla AW, Wing RR.

Menopause and risk factors for coronary heart disease. *N Engl J Med* 1989;321: 641–646.

119. Jensen J, Nilas L, Christiansen C. Influence of menopause on serum lipids and lipoproteins. *Maturitas* 1990;12:321–331.

120. Schuler G, Hambrecht R, Schlierf G, et al. Regular physical exercise and low fat diet. *Circulation* 1992;86:1–11.

121. Ericsson S, Ericsson M, Vitols S, Einarsson K, Berglund L, Angelin B. Influence of age on the metabolism of plasma low density lipoproteins in healthy males. *J Clin Invest* 1991;87:591–596.

122. Wild RA, Painter PC, Coulson PB, Carruth KB, Ranney GB. Lipoprotein lipid concentrations and cardiovascular risk in women with polycystic ovary syndrome. *J Clin Endocrinol Metab* 1985;61:946–951.

123. Wild RA, Alanpovic P, Givens JR, Parker IJ. Lipoprotein abnormalities in hirsute women. *Am J Obstet Gynecol* 1992;167:1813–1818.

124. Working group on hypertension in the elderly. Statement on hypertension in the elderly. *JAMA* 1986;256:70–74.

125. MacMahon S, Peto R, Cutler J, et al. Blood pressure, stroke and coronary heart disease. *Lancet* 1990;335:765–774.

126. Dittrich H, Gilpin E, Nicol P, Cali G, Henning H, Ross J. Acute myocardial infarction in women: influence of gender on mortality and prognostic variables. *Am J Cardiol* 1988;62:1–7.

127. Kannel WB, Wilson PWF, Zhang TJ. The epidemiology of impaired glucose tolerance and hypertension *Am Heart J* 1991;121:1268–1273.

128. Barrett-Connor E, Wingard DL. Sex differential in ischemic heart disease mortality in diabetics. *Am J Epidemiol* 1983;118:489–496.

129. Ford ES, DeStefano F. Risk factors for mortality from all causes and from coronary heart disease among persons with diabetes. *Am J Epidemiol* 1991;133: 1220–1230.

130. Despres J-P, Lamarche B, Mauriege P, et al. Hyperinsulinemia as an independent risk factor for ischemic heart disease. *N Engl J Med* 1996;334:952–957.

131. Reaven GM, Greenfield MS. Diabetic hypertriglyceridemia, evidence for the clinical syndromes. *Diabetes* 1981;30(Suppl):66–75.

132. Jarrett RJ, McCartney P, Keen H. The Bedford Study: ten year mortality rates in newly diagnosed diabetics, borderline diabetics and normoglycaemic controls and risk indices for coronary heart disease in borderline diabetics. *Diabetologia* 1982;22:79–84.

133. Manson JE, Rimm EB, Stampfer MJ, et al. Physical activity and incidence of non-insulin-dependent diabetes mellitus in women. *Lancet* 1991;338:774–778.

134. Bush TL, Comstock CW. Smoking and cardiovascular mortality in women. *Am J Epidemiol* 1983;118:480–488.

135. Rosenberg L, Kaufman DW, Helmrich SP, Miller DR, Stolley PD, Shapiro C. Myocardial infarction and cigarette smoking in women younger than 50 years of age. *JAMA* 1985;253:2965–2969.

136. LaCroix AZ, Lang J, Scherr P, et al. Smoking and mortality among older men and women in three communities. *N Engl J Med* 1991;324:1619–1625.

137. Department of Health and Human Services. *Reducing the health consequences of smoking: 25 years of progress. A report of the Surgeon General (DHHS publication no. CDC 89-8411).* Washington, DC: US Government Printing Office, 1989.

138. Willett WC, Green A, Stampfer MJ, et al. Relative and absolute excess risks of coronary heart disease among women who smoke cigarettes. *N Engl J Med* 1987;317:1303–1309.

139. Craig WY, Palomaki GE, Haddow JE. Cigarette smoking and serum lipid and lipoprotein concentration: an analysis of published data. *Br Med J* 1989;298: 784–788.

140. Palmer JR, Rosenberg L, Shapiro S. "Low yield" cigarettes and the risk of non-fatal myocardial infarction in women. *N Engl J Med* 1989;320:1569–1573.

141. Muscat JE, Harris RE, Haley NJ, Wynder EL. Cigarette smoking and plasma cholesterol. *Am Heart J* 1991;121:141–147.

142. Suarez L, Barrett-Connor E. Interaction between cigarette smoking and diabetes mellitus in the prediction of death attributed to cardiovascular disease. *Am J Epidemiol* 1984;120:670–675.

143. Fowkes FGR, Housley E, Riemersma RA, et al. Smoking, lipids, glucose intolerance and blood pressure as risk factors for peripheral atherosclerosis compared with ischemic heart disease in the Edinburgh Artery Study. *Am J Epidemiol* 1992;135:331–340.

144. Mjos OD. Lipid effects of smoking. *Am Heart J* 1988;115:272–275.

145. Schoenberger JC. Smoking in relation to changes in blood pressure, weight and cholesterol. *Prev Med* 1982;11:441–453.

146. Renaud S, Blache D, Dumont E, Therenon C, Wissendanger T. Platelet function after cigarette smoking in relation to nicotine and carbon monoxide. *Clin Pharmacol Ther* 1984;36:389–395.

147. Davis JW, Davis RF. Acute effects of tocacco cigarette smoking on the platelet aggregate ratio. *Am J Med Sci* 1979;278:139–143.

148. Markowe HLJ, Marmot MG, Shipley MJ, et al. Fibrinogen: a possible link between social class and coronary heart disease. *Br Med J* 1985;291:1312–1314.

149. Facchini FS, Hollenbeck CB, Jeppesen J, Chen YDI, Reaven GM. Insulin resistance and cigarette smoking. *Lancet* 1992;339:1128–1130.

150. Daniel M, Martin AD, Faiman C. Sex hormones and adipose tissue distribution in premenopausal cigarette smokers. *Int J Obesity* 1992;16:245–254.

151. Keil DP, Baron JA, Anderson JJ, Hannan MT, Felson DT. Smoking eliminates the protective effect of oral estrogens on the risk for hip fracture among women. *Ann Intern Med* 1992;116:716–721.

152. Jensen J, Christiansen C, Rodbro P. Cigarette smoking, serum estrogens and

bone loss during hormone replacement therapy early after menopause. *N Engl J Med* 1985;313:973–975.

153. Hartz AJ, Kelber S, Borkowf H, Wild R, Gillis BL, Rimm AA. The association of smoking with clinical indicators of altered sex steroids—a study of 50,145 women. *Public Health Rep* 1987;102:254–259.

154. Lesko SM, Rosenberg L, Kaufman DW, et al. Cigarette smoking and the risk of endometrial cancer. *N Engl J Med* 1985;313:593–596.

155. Baron JA, La Vecchia C, Levi F. The antiestrogenic effect of cigarette smoking in women. *Am J Obstet Gynecol* 1990;162:502–514.

156. Barbieri RL, McShane RM, Ryan KJ. Constituents of cigarette smoke inhibit human granulosa cell aromatase. *Fertil Steril* 1986;46:232–236.

157. Michnovicz JJ, Hershcopf RJ, Naganuma H, Bradlow HL, Fishman J. Increased 2-hydroxylation of estradiol as a possible mechanism for the antiestrogenic effect of cigarette smoking. *N Engl J Med* 1986;315:1305–1309.

158. Rosenberg L, Palmer JR, Shapiro S. Decline in the risk of myocardial infarction among women who stop smoking. *N Engl J Med* 1990;322:213–217.

159. Paffenbarger RS, Hide PHRT, Wing AL, Hsieh CC. Physical activity, all cause mortality and longevity of college alumni. *N Engl J Med* 1986;314:605–613.

160. Berlin JA, Colditz GA. A meta-analysis of physical activity in the prevention of coronary heart disease. *Am J Epidemiol* 1990;132:612–628.

161. Sallis JF, Patterson TL, Buono MJ, Nader PR. Relation of cardiovascular fitness and physical activity to cardiovascular risk factors in children and adults. *Am J Epidemiol* 1988;127:933–941.

162. Jacobs DR, Hahn LP, Folsom AR, Hannan PJ, Sprafka JM, Burke GL. Time trends in leisure-time physical activity in the upper midwest 1957–1987. University of Minnesota Studies. *Epidemiology* 1991;2:8–15.

163. Owens JF, Matthews KA, Wing RR, Kuller LH. Can physical activity mitigate the effects of aging in middle aged women? *Circulation* 1992;85:1265–1270.

164. Voorrips LE, Meijers HH, Sol P, Seidell JC, Van Starern WA. History of body weight and physical activity of elderly women differing in current physical activity. *Int J Obesity* 1992;16:199–205.

165. Considine RV. Invited editorial on acute and chronic effects of exercise on leptin levels in humans *J Appl Physiol* 1997;83(1):3–4.

166. Ross CE, Hayes D. Exercise and psychologic well-being in the community. *Am J Epidemiol* 1988;127:762–771.

168. Powell KE, Thompson PD, Caspersen CJ, Kendrick JS. Physical activity and the incidence of coronary heart disease. *Annu Rev Public Health* 1987;8:253–287.

169. Fraser GE, Strahan TM, Sabate J, Beeson L, Kissinger D. Effects of traditional coronary risk factors on rates of incident coronary events in a low risk population. *Circulation* 1992 86:406–413.

170. Hunt BJ. The relation between abnormal hemostatic function and the progression of coronary disease. *Curr Opin Cardiol* 1990;5:758–765.

170. Scarabin PY, Kopp CB, Bara L, Malmejac A, Guize L, Samama M. Factor VII activation and menopausal status. *Thromb Res* 1990;57:227–234.

171. Herd JA. Cardiovascular response to stress. *Physiol Rev* 1991;71:305–330.

172. Tofler GH, Brezinski D, Schafer AI, et al. Concurrent morning increase in platelet aggregability and the risk of myocardial infarction and sudden cardiac death. *N Engl J Med* 1987;316:1514–1518.

173. Panza JA, Epstein SE, Quyyumi AA. Circadian variation in vascular tone and its relation to sympathetic vasoconstrictor activity. *N Engl J Med* 1991;325: 986–990.

174. Manfredini R, Gallerani M, Portaluppi F, Fersini C. Relationships of the circadian rhythms of thrombotic, ischemic, hemorrhagic, and arrhythmic events to blood pressure rhythms. *Ann NY Acad Sci* 1996;783:141–158.

175. Ballinger SE, Walker WL. *Not THE change of life: Breaking the menopause taboo.* Ringwood, Victoria, Australia: Penguin, 1987.

176. Ballinger S. Stress as a factor in lowered estrogen levels in the early postmenopause. *Ann NY Acad Sci* 1990;592:95–113.

177. Woods NF, Derby GK, Most A. Stressful life events and perimenstrual symptoms. *J Hum Stress* 1982;8:23–31.

178. Hayano J, Sakakibara Y, Yamada M, et al. Decreased magnitude of heart rate spectral components in coronary disease: its relation to angiographic severity. *Circulation* 1990;81:1217–1224.

179. Lipsitz LA, Connelly CM, Kelley-Gagnon M, Kiely DK, Morin RJ. Effects of chronic estrogen replacement therapy on beat-to-beat blood pressure dynamics in healthy postmenopausal women. *Hypertension* 1995;26:711–715.

180. Rosano GM, Patrizi R, Leonardo F, et al. Effect of estrogen replacement therapy on heart rate variability and heart rate in healthy postmenopausal women. *Am J Cardiol* 1997;80(6):815–817.

181. Davy KP, Miniclier NL, Taylor JA, Stevenson ET, Seals DR. Elevated heart rate variability in physically active postmenopausal women: a cardioprotective effect? *Am J Physiol* 1996;271:H455–H460.

182. Kannel WB, Hjortland MC, McNamara PM, Gordon T. Menopause and risk of cardiovascular disease. The Framingham Study. *Ann Intern Med* 1976;85: 447–452.

183. Colditz GA, Willett WC, Stampfer MJ, Rosner B, Speizer FE, Hennekens CH. A prospective study of age at menarche, parity, age at first birth and coronary heart disease in women. *Am J Epidemiol* 1987;126:861–870.

184. LaVecchia C, Decarli A, Franceschi S, Gentile A, Negri E, Parazzini F. Menstrual and reproductive factors and risk of myocardial infarction in women under 55 years of age. *Am J Obstet Gynecol* 1987;157:1108–1112.

185. Stampfer MJ, Colditz GA. Estrogen replacement therapy and coronary heart disease: a quantitative assessment of the epidemiologic evidence. *Prevent Med* 1991;20:47–63.

186. Potocki J. Wplyw leczenia estrogenami na niewydolnose wiencowa u kobiet po menopauzie. *Pol Tyg Lek* 1971;26:1812–1815.
187. Burch JC, Byrd BF Jr, Vaughn WK. The effects of long-term estrogen on hysterectomized women. *Am J Obstet Gynecol* 1974;188:778–782.
188. Talbott E, Kuller LH, Detre K, Perper J. Biologic and psychosocial risk factors of sudden death from coronary disease in white women. *Am J Cardiol* 1977;39:858–864.
189. Jick H, Dinan B, Herman R, Rothman KJ. Myocardial infarction and other vascular diseases in young women: Role of estrogens and other factors. *JAMA* 1978;240:2548–2552.
190. Pfeffer RI, Whipple GH, Kurosaki TT, Chapman JM. Coronary risk and estrogen use in postmenopausal women. *Am J Epidemiol* 1978;107:479–497.
191. MacMahon B. Cardiovascular disease and noncontraceptive oestrogen therapy. In: Oliver MF, ed. *Coronary heart disease in young women.* New York: Churchill Livingstone, 1979:197–207.
192. Hammond CB, Jelovsek FR, Lee LK, Creasman WT, Parker RT. Effects of long-term estrogen replacement therapy. I. Metabolic effects. *Am J Obstet Gynecol* 1979;133:525–536.
193. Nachtigall LE, Nachtigall RH, Nachtigall RD, Beckman EM. Estrogen replacement therapy II: A prospective study in the relationship to carcinoma and cardiovascular and metabolic problems. *Obstet Gynecol* 1979;54:74–79.
194. Adam S, Williams V, Vessey MP. Cardiovascular disease and hormone replacement treatment: A pilot case-control study. *Br Med J* 1981;282:1277–1278.
195. Bain C, Willett WC, Hennekens CH, Rosner B, Belanger C, Speizer FE. Use of postmenopausal hormones and risk of myocardial infarction. *Circulation* 1981;64:42–46.
196. Ross RK, Paganini-Hill A, Mack TM, Arthur M, Henderson BE. Menopausal oestrogen therapy and protection from death from ischaemic heart disease. *Lancet* 1981;1:858–860.
197. Szklo M, Tonascia J, Gordis L, Bloom I. Estrogen use and myocardial infarction risk: A case-control study. *Prev Med* 1984;13:510–516.
198. Lafferty FW, Helmuth DO. Postmenopausal estrogen replacement: The prevention of osteoporosis and systemic effects. *Maturitas* 1985;7:147–159.
199. Bush TL, Barrett-Connor E, Cowan LD, et al. Cardiovascular mortality and noncontraceptive use of estrogen in women: Results from the Lipid Research Clinics Program Follow-up Study. *Circulation* 1987;75:1102–1109.
200. Hunt K, Vessey M, McPherson K, Coleman M. Long-term surveillance of mortality and cancer incidence in women receiving hormone replacement therapy. *Br J Obstet Gynaecol* 1987;94:620–635.
201. Petitti DB, Perlman JA, Sidney S. Noncontraceptive estrogens and mortality: Long-term follow-up of women in the Walnut Creek Study. *Obstet Gynecol* 1987;70:289–293.
202. Criqui MH, Suarez L, Barrett-Connor E, McPhillips J, Wingard DL, Garland C. Postmenopausal estrogen use and mortality. *Am J Epidemiol* 1988;128:606–614.
203. Gruchow HW, Anderson AJ, Barboriak JJ, Sobocinski KA. Postmenopausal use of estrogen and occlusion of coronary arteries. *Am Heart J* 1988;115:954–963.
204. McFarland KF, Boniface ME, Hornung CA, Earnhardt W, Humphries JO. Risk factors and noncontraceptive estrogen use in women with and without coronary disease. *Am Heart J* 1989;117:1209–1214.
205. Croft P, Hannaford PC. Risk factors for acute myocardial infarction in women: Evidence from the Royal College of General Practitioners' oral contraceptive study. *Br Med J* 1989;298:165–168.
206. Avila MH, Walker AM, Jick H. Use of replacement estrogens and the risk of myocardial infarction. *Epidemiology* 1990;1:128–133.
207. Sullivan JM, Zwang RV, Hughes JP, et al. Estrogen replacement and coronary artery disease: Effect on survival in postmenopausal women. *Arch Intern Med* 1990;150:2557–2562.
208. Henderson BE, Paganini-Hill A, Ross RK. Decreased mortality in users of estrogen replacement therapy. *Arch Intern Med* 1991;151:75–78.
209. Stampfer MJ, Colditz GA, Willett WC. Postmenopausal estrogen therapy and cardiovascular disease: Ten year follow-up from the Nurses' Health Study. *N Engl J Med* 1991;325:756–762.
210. Wolf PH, Madans JH, Finucane FF, Higgins M, Kleinman JC. Reduction of cardiovascular disease-related mortality among postmenopausal women who use hormones: evidence from a national cohort. *Am J Obstet Gynecol* 1991;164:489–494.
211. Falkeborn M, Persson I, Adami HO. The risk of acute myocardial infarction after oestrogen and oestrogen-progestogen therapy. *Br J Obstet Gynaecol* 1992;99:821–828.
212. Rosenberg L, Armstrong B, Jick H. Myocardial infarction and estrogen therapy in postmenopausal women. *N Engl J Med* 1976;294:1256–1259.
213. Thompson SG, Meade TW, Greenberg G. The use of hormonal replacement therapy and the risk of stroke and myocardial infarction in women. *J Epidemiol Community Health* 1989;43:173–178.
214. Jick H, Dinan B, Rothman KJ. Noncontraceptive estrogens and nonfatal myocardial infarction. *JAMA* 1978;239:1407–1408.
215. Rosenberg L, Stone D, Shapiro S, Kaufman P, Stolley PD, Miettinen OS. Noncontraceptive estrogens and myocardial infarction in young women. *JAMA* 1980;244:339–342.
216. Wilson PW, Garrison RJ, Castelli WP. Postmenopausal estrogen use, cigarette smoking, and cardiovascular morbidity in women over 50: The Framingham Study. *N Engl J Med* 1985;313:1038–1043.
217. LaVecchia C, Franceschi S, Decarli A, Pampallona S, Tognoni G. Risk factors for myocardial infarction in young women. *Am J Epidemiol* 1987;125:832–843.
218. Grodstein F, Stampfer MJ, Manson JE, et al. Postmenopausal estrogen and progestin use and the risk of cardiovascular disease. *N Engl J Med* 1996;335(7):453–461. (Published erratum appears in *N Engl J Med* 1996;335:1406.)
219. Barrett-Connor E. Postmenopausal estrogen and prevention bias. *Ann Intern Med* 1991;115:455–456.
220. Grodstein F, Stampfer MJ, Colditz GA, et al. Postmenopausal hormone therapy and mortality. *N Engl J Med* 1997;336(25):1769–1775.
221. Grodstein F, Stampfer M. The epidemiology of coronary heart disease and estrogen replacement in postmenopausal women. *Prog Cardiovasc Dis* 1995;38:199–210.
222. Hong MK, Romm PA, Reagan K, Green CE, Rackley CE. Effects of estrogen replacement therapy on serum lipid values and angiographically defined coronary artery disease in postmenopausal women. *Am J Cardiol* 1992;69:176–178.
223. Stumpf WE, Sar M, Aumuller G. The heart: a target organ for estradiol. *Science* 1977;196:319–321.
224. McGill HC, Sheridan PJ. Nuclear uptake of sex steroid hormones in the cardiovascular system of the baboon. *Circ Res* 1981;48:238–244.
225. Horwitz KB, Horwitz LD. Canine vascular tissues are targets for androgens, estrogens, progestins and clucocorticoids. *J Clin Invest* 1982;69:750–758.
226. Lin AL, McGill HC, Shain SA. Hormone receptors of the baboon cardiovascular system. Biochemical characterization of aortic and myocardial cytoplasmic progesterone receptors. *Circ Res* 1982;50:610–616.
227. Sheridan PJ, McGill HC Jr. The nuclear uptake and retention of a synthetic progestin in the cardiovascular system of the baboon. *Endocrinology* 1984;114:2015.
228. Hochner-Celnikier D, Marandici A, Iohan F, Monder C. Estrogen and progesterone receptors in the organs of prenatal cynomolgus monkey and laboratory mouse. *Biol Reprod* 1986;35:633–640.
229. Stumpf WE. Steroid hormones and the cardiovascular system: direct action of estradiol, progesterone, testosterone, gluco- and mineralocorticoids and soltriol (vitamin D) on central nervous regulatory and peripheral tissues. *Experientia* 1990;46:13–25.
230. White MM, Zamudio S, Stevens T, et al. Estrogen, progesterone, and vascular reactivity: potential cellular mechanisms. *Endocr Rev* 1995;16(6):739–751.
231. Baysal K, Losordo DW. Oestrogen receptors and cardiovascular disease. *Clin Exp Pharmacol Physiol* 1996;23,537–548.
232. Kim-Schulze S, McGowan KA, Hubchak SC, et al. Expression of an estrogen receptor by human coronary artery and umbilical vein endothelial cells. *Circulation* 1996;94:1402–1407.
233. Venkov CD, Rankin AB, Vaughan DE. Identification of authentic estrogen receptor in cultured endothelial cells. *Circulation* 1996;94:727–733.
234. Lin AL, Gonzalez R, Carey KD, Shain SA. Estradiol-17β affects estrogen receptor distribution and elevates progesterone receptor content in baboon aorta. *Arteriosclerosis* 1986;6:495–504.
235. Chilton BS, Kaplan HA, Lennarz WJ. Estrogen regulation of the central enzymes involved in O- and N-linked glycoprotein assembly in the developing and the adult rabbit endocervix. *Endocrinology* 1988;123:1237–1244.
236. Weiner CP. Sex hormonal regulation of nitric oxide during ovulation and pregnancy. In: *Effects of gonadal steroids on vascular function. ASPET Colloquium.* Washington DC, April 17–18, 1996.
237. Ishi K, Kano T, Ando J. Calcium channel, Ca⁺⁺ mobilization, and mechanical reactivity of estrogen- and progesterone-treated rat uterus. *Jpn J Pharmacol* 1986;41:47–54.
238. Collins P, Rosano GM, Jiang C, Lindsay D, Sarrel PM, Poole-Wilson PA. Cardiovascular protection by oestrogen—a calcium antagonist effect? *Lancet* 1993;341:1264–1265.
239. Yamamoto T. Effects of estrogens on Ca channels in myometrial cells isolated from pregnant rats. *Am J Physiol* 1995;268:C64–C69.
240. Lippert TH, Seeger H, Mueck AO, Hanke H, Haasis R. Effect of estradiol, progesterone and progestogens on calcium influx in cell cultures of human vessels. *Menopause* 1996;3:33–37.
241. Morley P, Whitfield JF, Vanderhyden BC, Tsang BK, Schwartz JL. A new, nongenomic estrogen action: the rapid release of intracellular calcium. *Endocrinology* 1992;131:1305–1312.
242. Subbiah MTR, Kessel B, Agrawal M, Rajan R, Abplanalp W, Rymaszewski Z. Antioxidant potential of specific estrogens on lipid peroxidation. *J Clin Endocrinol Metab* 1993;77:1095–1097.
243. Yagi K, Komura S. Inhibitory effect of female hormones on lipid peroxidation. *Biochem Int* 1986;13:1051–1055.
244. Schwartz J, Freeman R, Frishman W. Clinical pharmacology of estrogens: cardiovascular actions and cardioprotective benefits of replacement therapy in postmenopausal women. *J Clin Pharmacol* 1994;35:1–16.
245. Taniguchi S, Yanase T, Kobayashi K, et al. Catechol estrogens are more potent antioxidants than estrogens for the Cu²⁺-catalyzed oxidation of low or high density lipoprotein: antioxidative effects of steroids on lipoproteins. *Endocr J* 1994;41:605–611.
246. Lacort M, Leal AM, Liza M, Martin C, Martinez R, Ruiz-Larrea MB. Protective effect of estrogens and catecholestrogens against peroxidative membrane damage *in vitro. Lipids* 1995;30:141–146.
247. Tang M, Abplanalp W, Ayres S, Subbiah MTR. Superior and distinct antioxidant effects of selected estrogen metabolites on lipid peroxidation. *Metab Clin Exp* 1996;45:411–414.
248. Tranquilli AL, Mazzanti L, Cugini AM, Cester N, Garzetti GG, Romanini C. Transdermal estradiol and medroxyprogesterone acetate in hormone replacement therapy are both antioxidants. *Gynecol Endocrinol* 1995;9:137–141.

249. Takanashi K, Watanabe K, Yoshizawa I. On the inhibitory effect of E_{17} sulfo-conjugated catechol estrogens upon lipid peroxidation of rat liver microsomes. *Biol Pharm Bull* 1995;18:1120–1125.

250. Keany J. Antioxidant effects of estrogen. In: *Effects of gonadal steroids on vascular function. ASPET Colloquium.* Washington, DC, April 17–18, 1996.

251. Gorodeski GI. Mechanisms of action for estrogen in cardioprotection. In: Wren BG, ed. *Proceedings of the Eighth International Menopause Congress, Sidney: Progress in the Management of Menopause.* Carnforth, UK: Parthenon, 1997: 402–418.

252. Barrett-Connor E, Bush TL. Estrogen and coronary heart disease in women. *JAMA* 1991;265:1861–1867.

253. Walsh BW, Schiff I, Rosner B, Greenberg L, Ravinkar V, Sacks FM. Effects of postmenopausal estrogen replacement on the concentrations and metabolism of plasma lipoproteins. *N Engl J Med* 1991;325:1196–1204.

254. Sacks FM, McPherson R, Walsh BW. Effect of postmenopausal estrogen replacement on plasma Lp(a) lipoprotein concentrations. *Arch Intern Med* 1994; 154:1106–1110.

255. Bruckert E, Turpin G. Estrogens and progestins in postmenopausal women, influence on lipid parameters and cardiovascular risk. *Horm Res* 1995;43:100–103.

256. Haines CJ, Chung TK, Masarei JR, Tomlinson B, Lau JT. The effect of percutaneous oestrogen replacement therapy on Lp(a) and other lipoproteins. *Maturitas* 1995;22(3):219–225.

257. Haines CJ, Chung TK, Masarei JR, Tomlinson B, Lau JT. An examination of the effect of combined cyclical hormone replacement therapy on lipoprotein(a) and other lipoproteins. *Atherosclerosis* 1996;119:215–222.

258. Kim CJ, Min YK, Ryu WS, Kwak JW, Ryoo UH. Effect of hormone replacement therapy on lipoprotein(a) and lipid levels in postmenopausal women. Influence of various progestogens and duration of therapy. *Arch Intern Med* 1996;156(15): 1693–1700.

259. Orth-Gomer K, Mittleman MA, Schenck-Gustafsson K, et al. Lipoprotein(a) as a determinant of coronary heart disease in young women. *Circulation* 1997; 95(2):329–334.

260. Ohta T, Hattori S, Murakami M, Nishiyama S, Matsuda I. Age and sex related differences in lipoproteins containing apoprotein A-I. *Arteriosclerosis* 1989;9:90–95.

261. Yui Y, Aoyama T, Morishita H, Takahashi M, Takatsu Y, Kawai C. Serum prostacyclin stabilizing factor is identical to apolipoprotein A-1 (Apo-A-1). *J Clin Invest* 1988;82:803–807.

262. Barbaras R, Puchois P, Fruchart JC, Ailhand G. Cholesterol efflux from cultured adipose cells is mediated by LpAI particles but not by LpAI:AII particles. *Biochem Biophys Res Commun* 1987;142:63–69.

263. Soma MR, Osnago-Gadda I, Paoletti R, et al. The lowering of lipoprotein(a) induced by estrogen plus progesterone replacement therapy in postmenopausal women. *Arch Intern Med* 1993;153:1462–1468.

264. Sacks FM, McPherson R, Walsh BW. Effect of postmenopausal estrogen replacement on plasma Lpa lipoprotein concentrations. *Arch Intern Med* 1994; 154:1106–1110.

265. Shewmon DA, Stock JL, Rosen CJ, et al. Tamoxifen and estrogen lower circulating lipoprotein(a) concentrations in healthy postmenopausal women. *Arterioscler Thromb* 1994;14:1586–1593.

266. Kim CJ, Jang HC, Cho DH, Min YK. Effects of hormone replacement therapy on lipoprotein(a) and lipids in postmenopausal women. *Arterioscler Thromb* 1994;14:275–281.

267. The Writing Group for the PEPI Trial. Effects of estrogen or estrogen/progestin regimens on heart disease risk factors in postmenopausal women: The Postmenopausal Estrogen/Progestin Interventions PEPI Trial. *JAMA* 1995;273: 199–208.

268. Haffner SM, Mykkanen L, Stern MP. Leptin concentrations in women in the San Antonio Heart Study: effect of menopausal status and postmenopausal hormone replacement therapy. *Am J Epidemiol* 1997;146(7):581–585.

269. Cho MM, Mack WJ, Hodis HN. Stanczyk effect of long-term estradiol treatment on circulating leptin levels in postmenopausal women. *J Soc Gynecol Invest* 1998;5(1 Suppl):9a.

270. Rich-Edwards JW, Manson JE, Hennekens CH, Buring JE. The primary prevention of coronary heart disease in women. *N Engl J Med* 1995;332:1758–1766.

271. Scandinavian Simvastatin Survival Study Group. Randomized trial of cholesterol lowering in 4444 patients with coronary heart disease: the Scandinavian Simvastatin Survival Study. *Lancet* 1994;344:1383–1389.

272. Sacks FM, Pfeffer MA, Moye LA, et al, for the Cholesterol and Recurrent Events Trial Investigators. The effect of pravastatin on coronary events after myocardial infarction in patients with average cholesterol levels. *N Engl J Med* 1996;335:1001–1009.

273. Gordon DJ, Probstfield JL, Garrison RJ, et al. High-density lipoprotein cholesterol and cardiovascular disease: four prospective American studies. *Circulation* 1989;79:8–15.

274. Walsh JME, Grady D. Treatment of hyperlipidemia in women. *JAMA* 1995;274: 1152–1158.

275. Kovanen PT, Brown MS, Goldstein JL. Increased binding of low density lipoprotein to liver membranes from rats treated with 17β ethinyl estradiol. *J Biol Chem* 1979;254:11367–11373.

276. Tikkanen MJ, Nikkila EA, Kuusi T, Sipinen S. High density lipoprotein-2 and hepatic lipase: reciprocal changes produced by estrogen and norgestrel. *J Clin Endocrinol Metab* 1982;54:1113–1117.

277. Everson GT, McKinley G, Kern F. Mechanisms of gallstone formation in women. *J Clin Invest* 1991;87:237–246.

278. Wagner JD, Clarkson TB, St Clair RW, Schwenke DC, Shirely CA, Adams MR. Estrogen and progesterone replacement therapy reduces low density lipoprotein accumulation in the coronary arteries of surgically postmenopausal cynomolgus monkeys. *J Clin Invest* 1991;88:1995–2002.

279. Meade TW, Haines AP, Imeson JD, Stirling Y, Thompson SG. Menopausal status and haemostatic variables. *Lancet* 1983;1:22–24.

280. Wilhelmsen L, Svardsudd K, Korsan-Bengtsen K, Larsson B, Welin L, Tibblin G. Fibrinogen as a risk factor for stroke and myocardial infarction. *N Engl J Med* 1984;311:501–505.

281. Meade TW, Mellows S, Brozovic M, et al. Haemostatic function and ischaemic heart disease: principle results of the Northwick Park Heart Study. *Lancet* 1986; 2:533–537.

282. Folsom AR, Wu KK, Davis CE, Conlan MG, Sorlie PD, Szklo M. Population correlates of plasma fibrinogen and factor VII, putative cardiac risk factors. *Atherosclerosis* 1991;91:191–205.

283. Yarnell JWG, Baker IA, Sweetnam PM, et al. Fibrinogen, viscosity, and white blood cell count are major risk factors for ischemic heart disease: the Caerphilly and Speedwell Collaborative Heart Disease Studies. *Circulation* 1991;83:836–844.

284. Kannel WB, D'Agostino RB, Belanger AJ. Update on fibrinogen as a cardiovascular risk factor. *Ann Epidemiol* 1992;2:457–466.

285. Ernst E, Resch KL. Fibrinogen as a cardiovascular risk factor: a meta analysis and review of the literature. *Ann Intern Med* 1993;118:956–963.

286. Lee AJ, Lowe GOD, Smith WCS, Turnstall-Pedoe H. Plasma fibrinogen in women: relationships with oral contraception, the menopause and hormone replacement therapy. *Br J Haematol* 1993;83:616–621.

287. Heinrich J, Balleisen L, Schulte H, Assmann G, van de Loo J. Fibrinogen and factor VII in the prediction of coronary risk: Results from the PROCAM study in healthy men. *Arterioscler Thromb* 1994;14:54–59.

288. Scarabin P-Y, Plu-Bureau G, Bara L, Bonithon-Kopp C, Guize L, Samama MM. Haemostatic variables and menopausal status: influence of hormone replacement therapy. *Thromb Haemostas* 1993;70:584–587.

289. Scarabin P-Y, Vissac A-M, Kirzin J-M, et al. Population correlates of coagulation factor VII: importance of age, sex, and menopausal status as determinants of activated factor VII. *Arterioscler Thromb Vasc Biol* 1996;16:1170–1176.

290. Nabulsi AA, Folsom AR, White A, et al, for the Atherosclerosis Risk in Communities Study Investigators. Association of hormone-replacement therapy with various cardiovascular risk factors in postmenopausal women. *N Engl J Med* 1993;328:1069–1075.

291. Meilahn EN, Kuller LH, Matthews KA, Kiss JE. Hemostatic factors according to menopausal status and use of hormone replacement therapy. *Ann Epidemiol* 1992;2:445–455.

292. Kroon U-B. Silfverstolpe G, Tengborn L. The effects of transdermal estradiol and oral conjugated estrogens on haemostasis variables. *Thromb Haemost* 1994; 71:420–423.

293. Sporrong T, Mattsson L-A, Samsioe G, Stigendal L, Hellgren M. Haemostatic changes during continuous oestradiol-progestogen treatment of opstmenopausal women. *Br J Obstet Gynaecol* 1990;97:939–944.

294. Gebara OCE, Mittleman MA, Sutherland P, et al. Association between increased estrogen status and increased fibrinolytic potential in the Framingham Offspring Study. *Circulation* 1995;91:1952–1958.

295. Shahar E, Folsom AR, Salomaa VV, et al, for the Atherosclerosis Risk in Communities ARIC Study Investigators. Relation of hormone-replacement therapy to measures of plasma fibrinlytic activity. *Circulation* 1996;93:1970–1975.

296. Koh KK, Minimoyer R, Bui MN, et al. Effects of hormone-replacement therapy on fibrinolysis in postmenopausal women. *N Engl J Med* 1997;336:683–901.

297. Johnson M, Ramey E, Ramwell PW. Androgen-mediated sensitivity in platelet aggregation. *Am J Physiol* 1977;232:H381–H385.

298. Aune B, Oian P, Omsjo I, Osterud B. Hormone replacement therapy reduces the reactivity of monocytes and platelets in whole blood—a beneficial effect on atherogenesis and thrombus formation? *Am J Obstet Gynecol* 1995;173: 1816–1820.

299. Bar J, Tepper R, Fuchs J, Pardo Y, Goldberger S, Ovadia J. The effect of estrogen replacement therapy on platelet aggregation and adenosine triphosphate release in postmenopausal women. *Obstet Gynecol* 1993;81:261–264.

300. Chang W-C, Nakao J, Orimo H, Murota S-L. Stimulation of prostaglandin cyclooxygenase and prostacyclin synthetase activities by estradiol in rat aortic smooth muscle cells. *Biochim Biophys Acta* 1980;620:472–482.

301. Seillan C, Ody C, Russo-Marie F, Duval D. Differential effects of sex steroids on prostaglandin secretion by male and female cultured piglet endothelial cells. *Prostaglandins* 1983;26:3–12.

302. Witter FR, DiBlasi MC. Effect of steroid hormones on arachidonic acid metabolites of endothelial cells. *Obstet Gynecol* 1984;63:747–751.

303. David M, Griesmacher A, Muller MM. 17-Alpha-ethinylestradiol decreses production and release of prostacyclin in cultured human umbilical vein endothelial cells. *Prostaglandins* 1989;38:431–438.

304. Fogelberg M, Vesterqvist O, Diczfalusy U, Henriksson P. Experimental atherosclerosis: effects of oestrogen and atherosclerosis on thromboxane and prostacyclin formation. *Eur J Clin Invest* 1990;20:105–110.

305. Redmond EM, Cherian MN, Wetzel RC. 17β-Estradiol inhibits flow- and acute hypoxia-induced prostacyclin release from perfused endocardial endothelial cells. *Circulation* 1994;90:2519–2524.

306. Altura BM, Altura BT. Influence of sex hormones, oral contraceptives and pregnancy on vascular muscle and its reactivity. In: Carrier O, Shibata S, eds. *Factors influencing vascular reactivity.* Tokyo: Igaku-Shoin, 1977:221–254.

307. Gisclard V, Flavahan NA, Vanhoutte PM. Alpha adrenergic responses of blood vessels of rabbits after ovariectomy and administration of 17 beta estradiol. *J Pharmacol Exp Ther* 1988;240:466–470.

308. Colucci WS, Giambrone MA, McLaughlin MK, Halpern NW, Alexander RW. Increased vascular catecholamine sensitivity and alpha adrenergic receptor affinity in female and estrogen treated male rats. *Circ Res* 1982;50:805–811.

309. Barone S, Panek D, Bennett L, Stitzel RE, Head RJ. The influence of oestrogen and oestrogen metabolites on the sensitivity of the isolated rabbit aorta to catecholamines. *Arch Pharmacol* 1987;335:513–520.

310. Ganger KF, Vyas S, Whitehead M, Crook D, Meire H, Campbell S. Pulsatility index in internal carotid artery in relation to transdermal oestradiol and time since menopause. *Lancet* 1991;338:839–842.

311. Lobo RA. Cardiovascular implications of estrogen replacement therapy. *Obstet Gynecol* 1990;75(Suppl):18S–25S.

312. Proudler AJ, Ahmed AI, Crook D, Fogelman I, Rymer JM, Stevenson JC. Hormone replacement therapy and serum angiotensin-converting-enzyme activity in postmenopausal women. *Lancet* 1995;346:89–90.

313. Barrett-Connor E, Laakso M. Ischemic heart disease risk in postmenopausal women: Effects of estrogen use on glucose and insulin levels. *Arteriosclerosis* 1990;10:531–534.

314. Abraham GE, Maroulis GB. Affect of exogenous estrogen on serum pregnenolone, cortisol and androgens in postmenopausal women. *Obstet Gynecol* 1975;45:271–274.

315. Magness RR, Rosenfeld CR. Local and systemic estradiol-17β: effects on uterine and systemic vasodilation. *Am J Physiol* 1989;256:E536–E542.

316. Magness RR, Oarker CR, Rosenfeld CR. Systemic and uterine responses to chronic infusion of estradiol-17β. *Am J Physiol* 1993;265:E690–E698.

317. Killam AO, Rosefeld CR, Battaglia FC, Makowski EL, Meschia G. Effect of estrogens on the uterine blood flow of oophorectomized ewes. *Am J Obstet Gynecol* 1973;115:1045–1052.

318. Gorodeski GI, Sheean LA, Utian WH. Sex hormone modulation of flow velocity in the parametrial artery of the pregnant rat. *Am J Physiol* 1995;268:R614–R624.

319. Gisclard V, Miller VM, Vanhoutte PM. Effect of 17β-estradiol on endothelium-dependent responses in the rabbit. *J Pharmacol Exp Ther* 1988;244:19–22.

320. Lieberman EH, Gerhard MD, Uchata A, et al. Estrogen improves endothelium-dependent flow-mediated vasodilation in postmenopausal women. *Ann Intern Med* 1994;121:936–941.

321. Gilligan DM, Badar DM, Panza JA, Quyyumi AA, Cannon RO. Effects of estrogen replacement therapy on peripheral vasomotor function in postmenopausal women. *Am J Cardiol* 1995;75:264–268.

322. Gorodeski GI, Yang T, Levy MN, Goldfarb J, Utian WH. Effects of estrogen *in vivo* on coronary vascular resistance in perfused rabbit hearts. *Am J Physiol* 1995;269:R1333–R1338.

323. Fischer GM, Cherian K, Swain ML. Increased synthesis of aortic collagen and elastin in experimental atherosclerosis: inhibition by contraceptive steroids. *Atherosclerosis* 1981;39:463–476.

324. Fischer GM, Swain ML. Effects of estradiol and progesterone on the increased synthesis of collagen in atherosclerotic rabbit aortas. *Atherosclerosis.* 1985;54:177–185.

325. Morales DE, McGowan KA, Grant DS, et al. Estrogen promotes angiogenic activity in human umbilical vein endothelial cells *in vitro* and in a murine model. *Circulation* 1995;91:755–763.

326. Caulin-Glaser T, Watson CA, Bender JR. Effects of 17β-estradiol on cytokine-induced endothelial cell adhesion molecule expression. *J Clin Invest* 1996;98:36–42.

327. Kolodgic FD, Jacob A, Wilson PS, et al. Estradiol attenuates directed migration of vascular smooth muscle cells *in vitro. Am J Pathol* 1996;148:969–976.

328. Schnaper HW, McGowan KA, Kim-Schulze S, Cid MC. Oestrogen and endothelial cell angiogenic activity. *Clin Exp Pharmacol Physiol* 1996;23:247–250.

329. Suzuki A, Mizuno K, Ino Y, et al. Effects of 17 beta-estradiol and progesterone on growth-factor-induced proliferation and migration in human female aortic smooth muscle cells *in vitro. Cardiovasc Res* 1996;32:516–523.

330. Morey AK, Pedram A, Razandi M, et al. Estrogen and progesterone inhibit vascular smooth muscle proliferation. *Endocrinology* 1997;138:3330–3339.

331. Gilligan DM, Quyyumi AA, Cannon RO. Effects of physiological levels of estrogen on coronary vasomotor function in postmenopausal women. *Circulation* 1994;89:2545–2551.

332. Riedel M., Oeltermann A, Mugge A, Creutzig A, Rafflenbeul W, Lichtlen P. Vascular responses to 17 beta-oestradiol in postmenopausal women. *Eur J Clin Invest* 1995;25(1):44–47.

333. Rajkumar C, Kingwell BA, Cameron JD, et al. Hormonal therapy increases arterial compliance in postmenopausal women. *J Am Coll Cardiol* 1997;30(2):350–356.

334. Williams JK, Adams MR, Klopfenstein HS. Estrogen modulates responses of atherosclerotic coronary arteries. *Circulation* 1990;81:1680–1687.

335. Williams JK, Adams MR, Herrington DM, Clarkson TB. Short-term administration of estrogen and vascular responses of atherosclerotic coronary arteries. *J Am Coll Cardiol* 1992;20:452–457.

336. Reis SE, Gloth ST, Blumenthal RS, et al. Ethinyl estradiol acutely attenuates abnormal coronary vasomotor responses to acetylcholine in postmenopausal women. *Circulation* 1994;89:52–60.

337. Ignarro LJ, Buga GM, Wood KS, Byrns RE, Chaudhuri G. Endothelium-derived relaxing factor produced and released from artery and vein is nitric oxide. *Proc Natl Acad Sci USA* 1987;84:9265–9269.

338. Wellman GC, Brayden JE, Nelson MT. A proposed mechanism for the cardio-protective effect of oestrogen in women: enhanced endothelial nitric oxide release decreases coronary artery reactivity. *Clin Exp Pharmacol Physiol* 1996;23:260–266.

339. Hayashi T, Fukuto JM, Ignarro LJ, Chaudhuri G. Basal release of nitric oxide from aortic rings is greater in female rabbits than in male rabbits: Implication for atherosclerosis. *Proc Natl Acad Sci USA* 1992;89:11259–11263.

340. Farhat MY, Lavigne MC, Ramwell PW. The vascular protective effects of estrogen. *FASEB J* 1996;10:615–624.

341. Miller VM, Barber DA, Fenton AM, Wang X, Sieck GC. Gender differences in response to endothelin-1 in coronary arteries: transcription, receptors and calcium regulation. *Clin Exp Pharmacol Physiol* 1996;23:256–259.

342. Osborne JA, Siegman MJ, Sedar AW, Moores AU, Lefer AM. Lack of endothelium dependent relaxation in coronary resistance arteries of cholesterol-fed rabbits. *Am J Physiol* 1989;256;6591–6597.

343. Mugge A, Riedel M, Barton M, Kuhn M, Lichtlen PR. Endothelium independent relaxation of human coronary arteries by 17β-oestradiol *in vitro. Cardiovasc Res* 1993;27:1939–1942.

344. Chester AH, Jiang C, Borland JA, Yacoub MH, Collins P. Oestrogen relaxes human epicardial coronary arteries through non-endothelium-dependent mechanisms. *Coronary Art Dis* 1997;6:417–422.

345. Vedernikov YP, Liao QP, Jain V, Saade GR, Chwalisz K, Garfield RE. Effect of chronic treatment with 17beta-estradiol and progesterone on endothelium-dependent and endothelium-independent relaxation in isolated aortic rings from ovariectomized rats. *Am J Obstet Gynecol* 1997;176:603–608.

346. Fregly MJ, Thrasher TN. Response of heart rate to acute administration of iso-proterenol in rats treated chronically with norethynodrel, ethinyl estradiol, and both combined. *Endocrinology* 1977;100:148–154.

347. Levin RM, Shofer FS, Wein AJ. Estrogen-induced alterations in the autonomic responces of the rabbit urinary bladder. *J Pharmacol Exp Ther* 1980;215:614–618.

348. Egozi Y, Kloog Y. Muscarinic receptors in the preoptic area are sensitive to 17 beta-estradiol during the critical period. *Neuroendocrinology* 1985;40:385–392.

349. Han SZ, Karaki H, Ouchi Y, Akishita M, Orimo H. 17β-Estradiol inhibits Ca^{2+} influx and Ca^{2+} release induced by thromboxane A_2 in porcine coronary artery. *Circulation* 1995;91:2619–2626.

350. Kessler KM. Syndrome X: the epicardial view. *J Am Coll Cardiol* 1992;19:32–33.

351. Sarrel PM, Lindsay D, Rosano GMC, Poole-Wilson PA. Angina and normal coronary arteries in women: gynecologic findings. *Am J Obstet Gynecol* 1992;167:467–472.

352. Hough JL, Zilversmith DB. Effect of 17 beta estradiol on aortic cholesterol content and metabolism in cholesterol-fed rabbits. *Arteriosclerosis* 1986;6:57–63.

353. Adams MR, Kaplan JR, Manuck SB, et al. Inhibition of coronary artery atherosclerosis by 17 beta estradiol in ovariectomized monkeys. *Arteriosclerosis* 1990;10:1051–1057.

354. Cheng LP, Kuwahara M, Jacobsson J, Foegh ML. Inhibition of myointimal hyperplasia and macrophage infiltration by estradiol in aorta allografts. *Transplantation* 1991;52:967–972.

355. Wagner JD, Clarkson TB, St Clair RW, Schwenke DC, Shively CA, Adams MR. Estrogen and progesterone replacement therapy reduces low density lipoprotein accumulation in the coronary arteries of surgically postmenopausal cynomolgus monkeys. *J Clin Invest* 1991;88:1995–2002.

356. Foegh ML, Asotra S, Howell MH, Ramwell PW. Estradiol inhibition of arterial neointimal hyperplasia after balloon injury. *J Vasc Surg* 1994;19:722–726.

357. Wagner JD, Schwenke DC, Zhang L, Applebaum Bowden D, Bagdade JD, Adams MR. Effects of short-term hormone replacement therapies on low-density lipoprotein metabolism in cynomolgus monkeys. *Arterioscler Thromb Vasc Biol* 1997;17:1128–1134.

358. Sack MN, Rader DJ, Cannon RO. Oestrogen and inhibition of oxidation of low-density lipoproteins in postmenopausal women. *Lancet* 1994;343:269–270.

359. Cho M, Ziats N, Goldfarb J, Utian WH, Gorodeski GI. *Estrogen increases transendothelial cation selectivity: A novel vasculoprotective mechanism.* Paper presented at the seventh annual meeting of the North American Menopause Society, Chicago, September 26–28, 1996.

360. Gallagher LJ, Sloane BF. Effect of estrogen on lysosomal enzyme activities in rat heart. *Proc Soc Exp Biol Med* 1984;177:428–433.

361. Carrington LJ, Bailey CJ. Effects of natural and synthetic estrogens and progestins on glycogen deposition in female mice. *Horm Res* 1985;21:199–203.

362. Payne RM, Friedman DL, Grant JW, Perryman MB, Strauss AW. Creatine kinase isoenzymes are highly regulated during pregnancy in rat uterus and placenta. *Am J Physiol* 1993;265:E624–E235.

363. Weiner CP, Lizasoain J, Baylis SA, Knowles RG, Charles JG, Moncada S. Induction of calcium-dependent nitric oxide synthases by sex hormones. *Proc Natl Acad Sci USA* 1994;91(11):5212–5216.

364. Shiverick KT, Hutchins K, Kikta DC, Squires N, Fregly MJ. Effects of chronic administration of mestranol on alpha and beta adrenergic responsiveness in female rats. *J Pharmacol Exp Ther* 1983;226:362–367.

365. Pines A, Fisman EZ, Levo Y, et al. The effects of hormone replacement therapy in nomal postmenopausal women: Measurements of Doppler-derived parameters of aortic flow. *Am J Obstet Gynecol* 1991;164:806–812.

366. Davis LE, Magness RR, Rosenfeld CR. Role of angiotensin II and α-adrenergic receptors during estrogen-induced vasodilation in ewes. *Am J Physiol* 1992;263:E837–E843.

367. Pines A, Fisman EZ, Shemesh J, et al. Menopause-related changes in left ventricular function in healthy women. *Cardiology* 1992;80:413–416.

368. Blumenthal RS, Brinker JA, Resar JR. Long-term estrogen therapy abolishes acute estrogen-induced coronary flow augmentation in postmenopausal women. *Am Heart J* 1997;133(3):323–328.

369. Herrington DM, Braden GA, Downes TR, Williams JK. Estrogen modulates coronary vasomotor responses in postmenopausal women with early atherosclerosis. *Circulation* 1992;abstract 2461.

370. Rosano GMC, Clarke D, Sarrel PM, Collins P. Estradiol 17 beta improves myocardial ischemia in postmenopausal women with coronary heart disease. *Circulation* 1992;86(Suppl I):abstract 2137.

371. Sbarouni E, Kyriakides ZS, Antoniadis A, Kremastinos DT. Acute hemodynamic effects of estrogen administration in postmenopausal women. *Am J Cardiol* 1997;80(4):532–535.

372. Snabes MC, Herd A, Schuyler N, Dunn K, Spence DW, Young RL. In normal postmenopausal women physiologic estrogen replacement therapy fails to improve exercise tolerance: A randomized, double-blind, placebo-controlled, crossover trial. *Am J Obstet Gynecol* 1996;175:110–114.

373. Lee M, Giardina EG, Homma S, DiTullio MR, Sciacca RR. Lack of effect of estrogen on rest and treadmill exercise in postmenopausal women without known cardiac disease. *Am J Cardiol* 1997;80(6):793–797.

374. Pines A, Fisman EZ, Shapira I, et al. Exercise echocardiography in postmenopausal hormone users with mild systemic hypertension. *Am J Cardiol* 1996;78(12):1385–1389.

375. Malhotra A, Buttride P, Scheuer J. Effect of sex hormones on development of physiological and pathological cardiac hypertrophy in male and female rats. *Am J Physiol* 1990;259:H866–H871.

376. Schaible TF, Malhotra A, Ciambrone G, Scheuer J. The effects of gonadectomy on left ventricular function and cardiac contractile proteins in male and female rats. *Circ Res* 1984;58:38–49.

377. Scheuer J, Malhotra A, Schaible TF, Capasso J. Effects of gonadectomy and hormonal replacement on rat hearts. *Circ Res* 1987;61:12–19.

378. Michel T, Smith TW. Nitric oxide synthases and cardiovascular signaling. *Am J Cardiol* 1993;72:33C–38C.

379. Johansson SR, Hjalmarson A. Age and sex differences in cardiovascular reactivity to adrenergic agonists, mental stress and isometric excercise in normal subjects. *Scand J Clin Lab Invest* 1988;48:183–191.

380. Williams JK, Kim YD, Adams MR, Chen M-F, Myers AK, Ramwell PW. Effects of estrogen on cardiovascular responses of premenopausal monkeys. *J Pharmacol Exp Ther* 1994;271:671–676.

381. Colucci WS, Gimbrone MA, Alexander RW. Regulation of myocardial and vascular α-adrenergic receptor affinity. *Circ Res* 1984;55:78–88.

382. Schwarz P, Diem R, Dun NJ, Forstermann U. Endogenous and exogenous nitric oxide inhibits norepinephrine release from rat heart sympathetic nerves. *Circ Res* 1995;77:841–848.

383. Eckstein N, Nadler E, Barnea O, Shavit G, Ayalon D. Acute effects of 17β-estradiol on the rat heart. *Am J Obstet Gynecol* 1994;171:844–848.

384. Takesawa H, Hayashi H, Sano H, Saito H, Ebihara S. Circadian and estrous cycle-dependent variations in blood pressure and heart rate in female rats. *Am J Physiol* 1994;267:R1250–R1256.

385. Klangkalya B, Chan A. The effects of ovarian hormones on beta-adrenergic and muscarinic receptors in rat heart. *Life Sci* 1988;42:2307–2314.

386. Mitlak BH, Cohen FJ. In search of optimal long-term female hormone replacement: the potential of selective estrogen receptor modulators. *Horm Res* 1997;48:155–163.

387. Fuchs-Young R, Glasebrook AL, Short LL, et al. Raloxifene is a tissue-selective agonist/antagonist that functions through the estrogen receptor. *Ann NY Acad Sci* 1995;761:355–360.

388. Frolik CA, Bryant HU, Black EC, Magee DE, Chandrasekhar S. Time-dependent changes in biochemical bone markers and serum cholesterol in ovariectomized rats: effects of raloxifene HCl, tamoxifen, estrogen and alendronate. *Bone* 1996;18(6):621–627.

389. Dodge JA, Lugar CW, Cho S, et al. Evaluation of the major metabolites of raloxifene as modulators of tissue selectivity. *J Steroid Biochem Mol Biol* 1997;61:97–106.

390. Evista. Indianapolis: Eli Lilly and Company.

391. Jennings RB, Steenbergen C Jr, Reimer KA. Myocardial ischemia and reperfusion. *Monogr Pathol* 1995;37:47–80.

392. Martin LG, Brenner GM, Jarolim KL, Banschbach MW, Coons DL, Wolfe AK. Effects of sex steroids on myocardial anoxic resistance. *Proc Soc Exp Biol Med* 1993;202:288–294.

393. Ames BN, Shigenaga MK, Hagen TM. Oxidants, antioxidants, and the degenerative diseases of aging. *Proc Natl Acad Sci USA* 1993;90:7915–7922.

394. Kendall MJ, Rajman I, Maxweil SRJ. Cardioprotective therapeutics drugs used in hypertension, hyperlipidaemia, thromboemolism, arrhythmias, the postmenopausal state and as antioxidants. *Postgrad Med J* 1994;70:329–343.

395. Sato I, Morita I, Kaji K, Ikeda M, Nagao M, Murota S-I. Reduction of nitric oxide producing activity associated with *in vitro* aging in cultured human umbilical vein. *Biochem Biophys Res Commun* 1993;195:1070–1076.

396. Brunet J, Boily MJ, Cordeau S, Des Rosiers C. Effects of N-acetylcysteine in the rat heart reperfused after low-flow ischemia: evidence for a direct scavenging of hydroxyl radicals and a nitric oxide-dependent increase in coronary flow. *Free Radical Biol Med* 1995;19:627–638.

397. Coughlan MG, Kenny D, Kampine JP, Bosnjak ZJ, Warltier DC. Differential sensitivity of proximal and distal coronary arteries to a nitric oxide donor following reperfusion injury or inhibition of nitric oxide synthesis. *Cardiovasc Res* 1993;27:1444–1448.

398. Patel VC, Yellon DM, Singh KJ, Neild GH, Woolfson RG. Inhibition of nitric oxide limits infarct size in the *in situ* rabbit heart. *Biochem Biophys Res Commun* 1993;194:234–238.

399. Pernow J, Uriuda Y, Wang QD, Li XS, Nordlander R, Rydeen L. The protective effect of L-arginine on myocardial injury and endothelial function following ischaemia and reperfusion in the pig. *Eur Heart J* 1994;15:1712–1719.

400. Amrani M, Chester AH, Jayakumar J, Schyns CJ, Yacoub MH. L-Arginine reverses low coronary reflow and enhances postischaemic recovery of cardiac mechanical function. *Cardiovasc Res* 1995;30:200–204.

401. Depre C, Vanoverschelde JL, Goudemant JF, Mottet I, Hue L. Protection against ischemic injury by nonvasoactive concentrations of nitric oxide synthase inhibitors in the perfused rabbit heart. *Circulation* 1995;92:1911–1918.

402. Engelman DT, Watanabe M, Maulik N, et al. L-Arginine reduces endothelial inflammation and myocardial stunning during ischemia/reperfusion. *Ann Thorac Surg* 1995;60:1275–1281.

403. Naseem SA, Kontos MC, Rao PS, Jesse RL, Hess ML, Kukreja RC. Sustained inhibition of nitric oxide by N^G-nitro-L-arginine improves myocardial function following ischemia/reperfusion in isolated perfused rat heart. *J Mol Cell Cardiol* 1995;27,419–426.

404. Hoshida S, Yamashita N, Igarashi J, et al. Nitric oxide synthase protects the heart against ischemia-reperfusion injury in rabbits. *J Pharmacol Exp Ther* 1995;274:413–418.

405. Sato H, Zhao ZQ, McGee DS, Williams MW, Hammon JW Jr, Vinten-Johansen J. Supplemental L-arginine during cardioplegic arrest and reperfusion avoids regional postischemic injury. *J Thorac Cardiovasc Surg* 1995;110,302–314.

406. Schulz R, Wambolt R. Inhibition of nitric oxide synthesis protects the isolated working rabbit heart from ischaemia-reperfusion injury. *Cardiovasc Res* 1995;30:432–439.

407. Takeuchi K, McGowan FX, Danh HC, Glynn P, Simplaceanu E, del Nido PJ. Direct detrimental effects of L-arginine upon ischemia-reperfusion injury to myocardium. *J Mol Cell Cardiol* 1995;27:1405–1414.

408. Weselcouch EO, Baird AJ, Sleph P, Grover GJ. Inhibition of nitric oxide synthesis does not affect ischemic preconditioning in isolated perfused rat hearts. *Am J Physiol* 1995;268:H242–H249.

409. Williams MW, Taft CS, Ramnauth S, Zhao ZQ, Vinten-Johansen J. Endogenous nitric oxide (NO) protects against ischaemia-reperfusion injury in the rabbit. *Cardiovasc Res* 1995;30:79–86.

410. Sugioka K, Shimosegawa Y, Nakano M. Estrogens as natural antioxidants of membrane phospholipid peroxidation. *FEBS Lett* 1987;210:37–39.

411. Sack MN, Rader DJ, Cannon RO III. Estrogen and inhibition of oxidation of low density lipoproteins in postmenopausal women. *Lancet* 1994;343:269–270.

412. Rifici VA, Khachadurian AK. The inhibition of low-density lipoprotein oxidation by 17-beta estradiol. *Metab Clin Exp* 1992;41:1110–1114.

413. Padwick ML, Pryse-Davis J, Whitehead MI. A simple method for determining the optimal dosage of progestin in postmenopausal women receiving estrogens. *N Engl J Med* 1986;315:930.

414. Henderson BF, Pike MC, Ross RR, Mack TM, Lobo RA. Re-evaluating the role of progestogen therapy after the menopause. *Fertil Steril* 1988;49(Suppl):9S–15S.

415. La Rosa JC. The varying effects of progestins on lipid levels and cardiovascular disease. *Am J Obstet Gynecol* 1988;158:1621–1629.

416. Sherwin BB, Gelfand MM. A prospective one year study of estrogen and progestin in postmenopausal women: Effects on clinical symptoms and lipoprotein lipids. *Obstet Gynecol* 1989;73:759–766.

417. Knopp RH. Effects of sex steroid hormones on lipoprotein levels in pre and postmenopausal women. *Can J Cardiol* 1990;6(Suppl):31B–35B.

418. Cano A, Fernandes H, Serrano S, Mahiques P. Effect of continuous oestradiol-medroxyprogesterone administration on plasma lipids and lipoproteins. *Maturitas* 1991;13:35–42.

419. Crook D, Stevenson JC. Progestogens, lipid metabolism and hormone replacement therapy. *Br J Obstet Gynaecol* 1991;98:749–750.

420. Lobo RA, Pickar JH, Wild RA, Walsh B, Hirvonen E, for the Menopause Study Group. Metabolic impact of adding medroxyprogesterone acetate to conjugated estrogen therapy in postmenopausal women. *Obstet Gynecol* 1994;84:987–995.

421. Yancey MK, Hannan CJ, Plymate SR, Stone IK, Friedl KE, Wright JR. Serum lipids and lipoproteins in continuous or cyclic medroxyprogesterone acetate treatment in postmenopausal women treated with conjugated estrogens. *Fertil Steril* 1990;54:778–782.

422. Haarbo J, Hassager C, Jensen SB, Riis BJ, Christiansen C. Serum lipids, lipoproteins and apolipoproteins during postmenopausal estrogen replacement therapy combined with either 19-nortestosterone derivatives or 17-hydroxy progesterone derivatives. *Am J Med* 1991;90:584–589.

423. Adams MR, Register TC, Golden DL, Wagner JD, Williams K. Medroxyprogesterone acetate antagonizes inhibitory effects of conjugated equine estrogens on coronary artery atherosclerosis. *Arterioscler Thromb Vasc Biol* 1997;17(1):217–221.

424. Sarrel PM. How progestins compromise the cardiovascular effects of estrogens. *Menopause* 1995;2:187–190.

425. Miyagawa K, Rosch J, Stanczyk F, Hermsmeyer K. Medroxyprogesterone interferes with ovarian steroid protection against coronary vasospasm. *Nature Med* 1997;3:324–327.

426. Levy MN, Yang T, Utian WH, Goldfarb J, Gorodeski GI. Progesterone attenuates the estrogen-induced increase in coronary flow. *FASEB J* 1996;A50.

427. Makila UM, Wahlberg L, Vlinikkal L, Ylikorkala O. Regulation of prostacyclin and thromboxane production by human umbilical vessels: The effect of estradiol and progesterone in a superfusion model. *Prostaglandins Leukotrienes Med* 1982;8:115–124.

428. Kuhl H. Effects of progestogens on haemostasis. *Maturitas* 1996;24:1–19.

429. Sita A. Miller SB. Estradiol, progesterone and cardiovascular response to stress. *Psychoneuroendocrinology* 1996;21:339–346.

430. Pecins-Thompson M, Keller-Wood M. Effects of progesterone on blood pressure, plasma volume, and responses to hypotension. *Am J Physiol* 1997;272: R377–R385.

431. Lee WS, Harder JA, Yoshizumi M, Lee ME, Haber E. Progesterone inhibits arterial smooth muscle cell proliferation. *Nature Med* 1997;3:1005–1008.

432. Stuenkel CA. *Women and heart disease.* Paper presented at annual meeting of the Medical Section of the American Council on Life Insurance, 1994:203–215.

433. Ready AE, Drinkwater DT, Ducas J, Fitzpatrick DW, Brereton DG, Oades SC. Walking program reduces elevated cholesterol in women in postmenopause. *Can J Cardiol* 1995;11(10):905–912.

434. Binder EF, Birge SJ, Kohrt WM. Effects of endurance exercise and hormone replacement therapy on serum lipids in older women. *J Am Geriatr Soc* 1996; 44(3):231–236.

435. Bush TL. Evidence for primary and secondary prevention of coronary artery disease in women taking oestrogen replacement therapy. *Eur Heart J* 1996; 17(Suppl D):9–14.

436. Playford DA, Watts GF. Management of lipid disorders in the elderly. *Rev Drugs Aging* 1997;10(6):444–462.

436. Kushi LH, Folsom AR, Prineas RJ, Mink PJ, Wu Y, Bostick RM. Dietary antioxidant vitamins and death from coronary heart disease in postmenopausal women. *N Engl J Med* 1996;334(18):1156–1162.

438. Sullivan JM. Practical aspects of preventing and managing athersclerotic disease in post-menopausal women. *Eur Heart J* 1996;17(Suppl D):32–37.

439. Goldstein MR. Evidence supporting cholesterol-lowering therapy for postmenopausal women with heart disease. *JAMA* 1997;278(8):633–634.

440. Grundy SM. Primary prevention of coronary heart disease: role of cholesterol control in the United States. *J Intern Med* 1997;241(4):295–306.

441. Kushi LH, Fee RM, Folsom AR, Mink PJ, Anderson KE, Sellers TA. Physical activity and mortality in postmenopausal women. *JAMA* 1997;277(16):1287–1292.

442. Mosca L, Manson JE, Sutherland SE, Langer RD, Manolio T, Barrett-Connor E. Cardiovascular disease in women: a statement for healthcare professionals from the American Heart Association. *Circulation* 1997;96(7):2468–2482.

443. Nicklas BJ, Katzel LI, Bunyard LB, Dennis KE, Goldberg AP. Effects of an American Heart Association diet and weight loss on lipoprotein lipids in obese, postmenopausal women. *Am J Clin Nutr* 1997;66(4):853–859.

444. Schrott HG, Bittner V, Vittinghoff E, Herrington DM, Hulley S. Adherence to National Cholesterol Education Program Treatment goals in postmenopausal women with heart disease. The Heart and Estrogen/Progestin Replacement Study (HERS). *JAMA* 1997;277(16):1281–1286.

445. Muller JE, Tofler GH. Circadian variation and cardiovascular disease. *N Engl J Med* 1991;325:1038–1039.

446. Herd JA. Cardiovascular response to stress. *Physiol Rev* 1991;71:305–330.

447. Ornish D, Brown SE, Scherwitz LW, et al. Can lifestyle changes reverse coronary heart disease? The Lifestyle Heart Trial. *Lancet* 1990;336:129–133.

448. Burke GL, Sprafka M, Folsom AR, Hahn LP, Luepker RV, Blackburn H. Trends in serum cholesterol levels from 1980 to 1987: The Minnesota Heart Survey. *N Engl J Med* 1991;324:941–446.

449. Chae CU, Ridker PM, Manson JE. Postmenopausal hormone replacement therapy and cardiovascular disease. *Thromb Haemostas* 1997;78(1):770–780.

450. Ettinger B, Friedman GD, Bush T, Quesenbury CP Jr. Reduced mortality associated with long-term postmenopausal estrogen therapy. *Obstet Gynecol* 1996; 87(1):6–12.

451. Folsom AR, Mink PJ, Sellers TA, Hong CP, Zheng W, Potter JD. Hormonal replacement therapy and morbidity and mortality in a prospective study of postmenopausal women. *Am J Public Health* 1995;85(8 Pt 1):1128–1132.

452. Radford NB. Southwestern Internal Medicine Conference: postmenopausal estrogen supplementation: a cardiologist's perspective. *Am J Med Sci* 1994; 308(1):63–73.

453. Nathan L, Chaudhuri G. Estrogens and atherosclerosis. *Annu Rev Pharmacol Toxicol* 1997;37:477–515.

454. Moerman CJ, Witteman JC, Collette HJ, et al. Hormone replacement therapy: a useful tool in the prevention of coronary artery disease in postmenopausal women? *Eur Heart J* 1996;17(5):658–666.

455. Guetta V, Cannon RO. Cardiovascular effects of estrogen and lipid-lowering therapies in postmenopausal women. *Circulation* 1996;93:1928–1937.

456. Rossouw JE. Estrogens for the prevention of coronary heart disease: putting the brakes on the bandwagon. *Circulation* 1996;94:2982–2985.

457. Steingold KA, Matt DW, DeZiegler D, et al. Comparison of transdermal to oral estradiol administration on hormonal and hepatic parameters in women with premature ovarian failure. *J Clin Endocrinol Metab* 1991;73(2):275–280.

458. Coulam CB, Adamson SC, Annegers JF. Incidence of premature ovarian failure. *Obstet Gynecol* 1986;67(4):604–606.

459. Gorodeski GI. Premature menopause. Menopause management 1997;6:10–17.

460. Eaker ED, Castelli WP. Coronary heart disease and its risk factors among women in the Framingham Study. In: Eaker E, Packard B, Wagner NK, Clarkson TB, Tyroler HA, eds. *Coronary heart disease in women.* New York: Haymarket Doyma, 1987:122–132.

461. Gorodeski GI. Impact of the menopause on the epidemiology and risk factors of coronary artery heart disease in women. *Exp Gerontol* 1994;29:357–375.

462. Ohta H, Sugimoto I, Masuda A, et al. Decreased bone mineral density associated with early menopause progresses for at least ten years: cross-sectional comparisons between early and normal menopausal women. *Bone* 1996;18(3): 227–231.

463. Bagur AC, Mautalen CA. Risk for developing osteoporosis in untreated premature menopause. *Calcif Tissue Int* 1992;51(1):4–7.

464. Pouilles JM, Tremollieres F, Bonneu M. Influence of early age at menopause on vertebral bone mass. *J Bone Miner Res* 1994;9(3):311–315.

465. Hashimoto K, Nozaki M, Inoue Y, et al. The chronological change of vertebral bone loss following oophorectomy using dual energy x-ray absorptiometry: the correlation with specific markers of bone metabolism. *Maturitas* 1995;22(3): 185–191.

Treatment of the Postmenopausal Woman: Basic and Clinical Aspects, Second Edition, edited by Rogerio A. Lobo, Lippincott Williams & Wilkins, Philadelphia © 1999.

CHAPTER 31

Role of Hormone Replacement in Cardiovascular Disease

Meir J. Stampfer and Francine Grodstein

Cardiovascular diseases remain the leading cause of death in women. In particular, rates of coronary heart disease, although relatively low among premenopausal women, rise sharply with age. Moreover, the ratio of rates between men and women grows smaller with increasing age (1). This observation led to speculation that functioning ovaries in premenopausal women were protective. The increased risk of coronary heart disease (CHD) among young women with bilateral oophorectomy (2) further supports the view that estrogens play an important role in reducing the risk of CHD in premenopausal women and that estrogen replacement therapy (ERT) after menopause might decrease the risk.

Attention has also been given to the relation between estrogen and other cardiovascular diseases. Studies have examined the possibility of protecting menopausal women against stroke through the use of ERT; CHD and stroke share many risk factors, and furthermore, some evidence suggests that, as with CHD, surgical removal of the ovaries increases the frequency of cerebrovascular disease (3). Finally, growing evidence indicates that postmenopausal hormone therapy may increase the risk of thromboembolic disease.

This chapter summarizes the epidemiologic investigations regarding the association between postmenopausal estrogen use and cardiovascular diseases (CVDs). For CHD, substantial evidence has accumulated from hospital- and community-based case-control studies, cross-sec-

tional studies, prospective cohort studies, and a small clinical trial. Less consistent information is available on the relationship between stroke and ERT, and only a few studies have addressed thromboembolism. In this chapter, we present the epidemiologic studies; the biologic evidence for these associations is presented in detail in the following chapters.

CORONARY HEART DISEASE

Many different study designs have been used to examine the association between hormone use and heart disease: hospital- and community-based case-control studies, cross-sectional studies, and prospective studies. In the hospital-based case-control design, prior estrogen use among patients hospitalized for CVD is compared to that of patients hospitalized for other reasons. It is essential to choose controls from among patients diagnosed with diseases unrelated to estrogen use. This can be difficult because many diseases are associated in some way with estrogens. For example, in several investigations, many of the controls were subjects admitted for treatment of fracture. These studies were conducted before it was widely appreciated that estrogens reduce the incidence of osteoporosis and fracture. Such controls would be less likely to have taken estrogen than comparably aged women in the population, and their inclusion in a study would tend to reduce the magnitude of the apparent inverse association between estrogens and risk of CVD. Generally, one might expect that hospital-based case-control studies would underestimate the protective effect of estrogen on CVD, and in fact, only the hospital-based case-control studies do not find consistent protection against heart disease for hormone users.

Six hospital-based case-control studies (4–9) have examined the relation between estrogen use and subse-

M. J. Stampfer: Departments of Nutrition and Epidemiology, Harvard School of Public Health, and Channing Laboratory, Department of Medicine, Brigham and Women's Hospital, Harvard Medical School, Boston, Massachusetts 02115.

F. Grodstein: Channing Laboratory, Department of Medicine, Brigham and Women's Hospital, Harvard Medical School, Boston, Massachusetts 02115.

quent risk of heart disease. The relative risks observed in these studies range from 4.2 to 0.5, with most showing no association. Of the two investigations that found strong positive associations, one (5) was based on only 14 cases of coronary disease, had very low participation (10% of those initially eligible), and was restricted to women under the age of 46, and the other (9) used controls in whom 40% had orthopedic disorders.

Relative risks (RR) from the population-based case-control studies of myocardial infarction (MI) and estrogen use range from 0.3 to 1.2 (10–20). Only one study reported a relative risk that was not below 1 (17); although one other study, which combined stroke and MI cases (16), found essentially null results, and a recent study also reported little relation between current hormone use and MI (20). Heckbert et al. (19) closely examined the effect of duration of hormone use on risk of heart disease in a study using 850 cases and 1,974 controls from the Group Health Cooperative in Seattle; they found increasing protection with increasing duration of current use, with a relative risk of 0.91 for less than 1.8 years of use and 0.55 for users of 8.2 years or more.

In the cross-sectional studies, the degree of coronary artery occlusion is assessed among users and nonusers of postmenopausal estrogens in women presenting for coronary arteriography (21–25). It is likely that this design could overestimate the benefit of estrogen use on the risk of CHD because estrogen users have greater contact with the health care system and may be more likely to have angiography than nonusers with the same equivocal symptoms. Hence, it is possible that the estrogen-using group in these investigations is artificially enriched with women who have nonsignificant disease. Nonetheless, the magnitude of such an effect could explain only a small fraction of the apparent benefit of estrogen observed by these studies. And, when one study (22) examined symptoms in users and nonusers in order to address this issue, no difference was found between the two groups, suggesting the absence of any important bias.

The results of the four cross-sectional studies (21–23, 25) examining women with severe occlusion (defined as 70% or more in two, and as an average of or greater than 50% in two) compared to those with no stenosis were nearly identical; each observed a statistically significant decrease of about 60% in the risk of severe coronary disease among women using estrogens compared with nonusers. In a fifth study, the outcome was defined as coronary artery disease or greater than 24% stenosis (24), and the investigators also found a significant decrease of disease in estrogen users, with an 87% reduction in prevalence.

Controlling for total cholesterol and triglyceride levels in the Gruchow et al. study (22) did not change the results at all. However, when high-density lipoprotein (HDL)-cholesterol was included as a confounder in the regression model, the observed association was substantially reduced. This effect is consistent with the view that elevations in HDLs (and a decrease in low-density lipoproteins, LDLs) most likely mediate at least part of the apparent benefit of estrogen. Usually, it is inappropriate to adjust for these variables because they are in the causal pathway for estrogens, and controlling for them is, effectively, controlling for the endpoint. When one does include HDL levels in the model, it is equivalent to asking what the result of estrogen use is on coronary risk above and beyond its effect on HDL levels.

Prospective studies have important advantages over case-control studies, chiefly in avoiding the problems of recall bias and control selection. Most of the studies followed women with and without estrogen exposure and thus had an internal control group; this design is preferable because the exposed and unexposed individuals are generally comparable. However, in a few studies, all subjects were taking estrogens. At the end of the follow-up period, their mortality experience was compared with national statistics. In most instances, patients given estrogen tend to be healthier than the general population, in part by virtue of their connection with the medical care system. As a result, studies that compare estrogen users to a general population probably overestimate the benefit of ERT. One potential limitation of most prospective studies is that hormone use is often assessed only at baseline. With long follow-up in such studies, there can be substantial misclassification of estrogen use because many women will stop or start taking hormones after the baseline assessment; this would lead to an underestimate of the benefit of estrogen.

All the prospective studies (26–52) have observed a protective effect of estrogens on coronary heart disease and mortality, although the results from the Framingham Study (34,35) are equivocal. As expected, those using national statistics for comparison (27,28,43,44) found some of the strongest benefits, with relative risks from approximately 0.3 to 0.4.

The Nurses' Health Study (33) is the largest prospective cohort to investigate hormone use and heart disease. The study was established in 1976 when 121,700 married female registered nurses aged 30 to 55 years completed a mailed questionnaire. Information on coronary risk factors and hormone usage was updated by means of follow-up questionnaires sent every 2 years. Reports of coronary disease are confirmed by medical record review, and data on hormones and other possible risk factors are likely to be reliable because all subjects are registered nurses with a demonstrated interest in medical research. In the analysis of hormones and heart disease, a total of 59,337 postmenopausal women without prior coronary heart disease were followed for up to 16 years; 584 nonfatal MIs and 186 confirmed coronary deaths were documented.

Most of the benefit was observed for current estrogen users, who had a 40% lower risk of heart disease compared to nonusers (RR = 0.60, 95% CI 0.43–0.83) after adjustment for a wide array of CHD risk factors. There was little effect of duration of current use; the protection was similar for short-term (RR = 0.53 for less than 2 years) and long-term users (RR = 0.70 for 10 years or more). However, the relationship was attenuated among past hormone users (RR = 0.85, 95% CI 0.71–1.01); in particular, the inverse association appeared to diminish 3 years or more after the cessation of estrogen use (RR = 0.69 for women who had stopped estrogen use less than 3 years in the past; RR = 0.81 after 3 to 5 years). The multivariate-adjusted relative risk of coronary disease for current users of 0.625 mg of conjugated estrogen was 0.53 (95% CI 0.36–0.78) compared to never users, and only modest protection (not statistically significant) was observed with the 1.25-mg dose (RR = 0.82, 95% CI 0.51–1.33). The inverse association was consistently observed regardless of age; for women under age 50, the relative risk for coronary disease among current estrogen users was 0.18 (95% CI 0.05–0.60), for those 50 to 59 years 0.71 (95% CI 0.52–0.96), and for women 60 to 71 years, 0.66 (0.44–1.01).

The Nurses' Health Study cohort includes predominantly young postmenopausal women, and data for women of older ages are sparse. Ettinger et al. (51) studied 454 women with an average age of 77 years at the end of follow-up and reported a relative risk of 0.40 (95% CI 0.16–1.02) for coronary death among hormone users. In the Leisure World cohort (39,40), estrogen status and other cardiovascular risk factors were ascertained in 8,807 women aged 40 through 101 living in a retirement community in 1981 (median age 73); 203 deaths from MI were identified over 7½ years of follow-up. The rate of fatal myocardial infarction was substantially reduced among estrogen users (RR = 0.60, $p < 0.001$). Current estrogen users, defined by the single baseline questionnaire, were afforded the greatest protection (RR = 0.51).

Results from all the studies of coronary disease were combined in a metaanalysis (Stampfer M. Progress in Cardiovascular Diseases. *Prev Med* 1991;20:47.) (Fig. 31.1). The relative risks for all studies of heart disease ranged from 0.17 to 4.2, with a summary relative risk of 0.65 (95% CI 0.61–0.69). However, evidence from many of these studies indicates that current estrogen users enjoy greater protection against heart disease than past users. Thus, combining investigations of current, past, and ever use in a summary estimate such as this is misleading because the results will be directly affected by the proportion of past and current use in the studies included. Summary estimates based on analyses of current use, where such data were provided, were recalculated; as expected, the estimates were lower than those derived by combining studies of any estrogen use. For the population-based case-control studies, the pooled relative risk for current estrogen use was 0.69 (95% CI 0.50–0.95); for the cross-sectional studies, it was 0.39 (95% CI 0.31–0.48); and for the internally controlled prospective studies, the summary estimate was 0.60

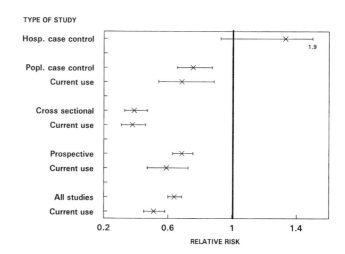

FIG. 31.1. Cardiovascular disease and postmenopausal hormones: meta-analysis of ever and current use.

(95% CI 0.50–0.72). The pooled relative risk for current estrogen use, combining all three study designs, was 0.53 (95% CI 0.47–0.60); we believe that this figure represents the best estimate for the impact of estrogen on CHD risk.

CEREBROVASCULAR DISEASE

Fewer investigations of stroke than of heart disease have been conducted. Three population-based case-control studies of stroke and estrogen use find relative risks ranging from 0.15 to 1.22 (53–56). One of these studies comes from a retirement community (55) and compares 216 women with fatal or nonfatal first stroke identified by hospital discharge diagnostic indices and medical center death records to 1,056 age-matched controls residing in the community during the same time period. The relative risk overall was 0.97, although there was some variation in risks when the data were examined by type of stroke (from 2.79 for transient ischemic attack to 0.49 for embolic infarction). However, the numbers in each of these groups tended to be small, and none of the relative risks attained statistical significance. Stroke was not associated with the duration of estrogen use (mean of 307 days in controls and 225 days in cases) or with past versus current use, but long-term and current users were a minority of the population.

In the most recent study, based on 1,422 cases from the Danish National Patient Register and 3,171 controls (56), the association between nonfatal stroke and hormone use was examined by the type of stroke. Current unopposed estrogen use was not related to thromboembolic infarction (RR = 1.16, 95% CI 0.86–1.58), although there were decreased risks of subarachnoid and intracerebral hemorrhages (RR = 0.52, 95% CI 0.23–1.22 and RR = 0.15, 95% CI 0.02–1.09, respectively); however, the numbers of cases of hemorrhagic stroke were relatively small, and the relative risk estimates were not statistically significant. For current use of combined estrogen and progestin, no association was found for thromboembolic infarction (RR = 1.17), subarachnoid hemorrhage (RR = 1.22), or for intracerebral hemorrhage (RR = 1.17).

Ten prospective studies have examined the influence of estrogen use on risk of stroke (32–34,37,40,43,50,52, 57–60). Five of these studies with internal controls (37,40,52,57,58,60) found estrogen use to be beneficial, with relative risks ranging from 0.23 to 0.79; statistically significant results were attained in only two of the studies (40,60). Three large investigations (33,50,61) found no effect of estrogen on the risk of cerebrovascular disease incidence, and the Framingham Study (34) observed significantly elevated rates of stroke among estrogen users, in particular, atherothrombotic brain infarctions, though the number of cases was small.

One of the largest investigations examining stroke risk was the Nurses' Health Study (33), with 552 cases of fatal and nonfatal first stroke. Estrogen therapy showed no effect on the incidence of stroke, with a relative risk of 1.03 among current estrogen users and 0.99 for past users. Similarly, no association was observed specifically for subarachnoid hemorrhage (RR = 0.90), although there appeared to be a slight increase in the risk of ischemic stroke (RR = 1.40). In addition, there was a trend of increasing risk of stroke with increasing dose of estrogen used (RR = 0.64 for 0.3 mg, RR = 1.24 for 0.625 mg, and RR = 1.44 for 1.25 mg). Interestingly, in a recent analysis of mortality (62), in the Nurses Health Study, there was an apparent overall decrease in stroke death for current hormone users (RR = 0.68, 95% CI 0.39–1.16, based on 28 cases who were current hormone users), consistent with the results of two other studies that specifically focus of deaths from stroke (40,52,58).

In the Leisure World study (40), the endpoint was stroke mortality. Of 8,807 women followed, 92 died from stroke. The relative risk of stroke death was 0.63 for estrogen users compared to nonusers, although this was not statistically significant. The greatest degree of protection was found among current users and those who used estrogen 1 year in the past, where there was 70% (RR = 0.3, p < 0.05) lower mortality from stroke among users compared to nonusers. In contrast, those who had taken estrogen 2 to 14 years ago had an approximately 40% reduction in stroke mortality, whereas those using it 15 years or more in the past had a 30% decrease. The authors note that the observed protection among current users is probably an underestimate of the true benefit of estrogen use because just 60% of these women continued therapy throughout the follow-up period.

THROMBOEMBOLISM

Five studies have reported on the relation between postmenopausal hormones and thromboembolism. Two case-control studies found an increased risk of venous thrombosis for estrogen users (63,64). In one investigation (63), of 103 cases and 178 control patients, Daly et al. found an increased risk of venous thromboembolism for current users of postmenopausal hormones (RR = 3.5, 95% CI 1.8–7.0), although no relation was found with past hormone use.

In the most recent of these studies (65), Gutthann et al. compared 292 women hospitalized for pulmonary embolism or deep vein thrombosis and 10,000 controls from the General Practice Research Database in the United Kingdom; they reported an increased risk of thromboembolism for current hormone users (RR = 2.1, 95% CI 1.4–3.2), with little association for past users (RR = 1.4, 95% CI 0.6–3.6). The dose of estrogen and type of regimen (estrogen alone or combined with a progestin) had little effect on the results.

In the only prospective study (66), there was an increased risk of pulmonary embolism for current hormone users (RR = 2.1, 95% CI 1.2–3.8), which was substantially attenuated after cessation (RR = 1.3, 95% CI 0.7–2.4 for past use). In addition, in a preliminary report from the HERS trial (67), a randomized clinical trial of combined estrogen and progestin therapy, investigators observed an increase in venous thromboembolism in the treatment compared to the placebo group, although no quantitative data were presented.

ASSOCIATION OF HORMONES WITH LOWER RISK OF CORONARY HEART DISEASE: CAUSE AND EFFECT OR SELECTION?

The findings from these studies that estrogen users are at generally lower risk from cardiovascular disease does not necessarily imply cause and effect. Women and their physicians decide on estrogen therapy. Often the health status of the woman will have an important influence on this decision and on the results of studies that examine these women. Thus, some have argued that estrogen use is merely a marker rather than a cause of good health.

Most of the studies reviewed here have provided some information bearing on this critical point. One way to judge the evidence for this position is to examine results of studies in which all the women were judged eligible by their physicians to receive estrogens. Only two small studies of CHD meet that criterion (30,31); the summary relative risk from those two was 0.22 (95% CI 0.06–0.88). These findings do not support the hypothesis that selection of healthy women for estrogen use can explain the lower rate of CHD among estrogen users.

With a similar intent, the Nurses' Health Study (33) tried to evaluate whether increased medical care of women using postmenopausal hormones might be responsible for the benefit observed. In an analysis limited to women who reported regular physician visits (50% of the cohort), results were similar to those found in the larger population of all subjects: the relative risk for major coronary heart disease was 0.52 (95% CI 0.37–0.74) for current hormone use.

Another approach is to examine the risk profile of estrogen users and nonusers to determine if there is a consistent pattern of higher risk among the nonusers and to assess whether the differences, if any, are sufficient to explain the large decrease in risk among estrogen users. Barrett-Connor (68) observed that, in a cohort of postmenopausal women, those taking estrogens reported more intensive health-care behavior, including frequent screening tests such as blood cholesterol measurement and mammograms. An examination of determinants of estrogen therapy in 9,704 women participating in a large, multicenter study of osteoporotic fractures (61) found that hormone users tended to be better educated, less obese, and to drink alcohol and participate in sports more often than nonusers. Similarly, in a prospective study of randomly selected premenopausal women, Matthews et al. (69) observed a better cardiovascular risk factor profile before hormone use among the women who subsequently took hormones at menopause than among women who did not.

However, many of the large studies reviewed here are based on homogeneous groups chosen because of their common profession or community. In the Nurses' Health Study, all women are registered nurses with access to health care and knowledge, and the distribution of established coronary risk factors was similar among current and never users of estrogens (33). The same findings were observed in the Lipid Research Clinics Follow-up Study (36) (Table 31.1). In both of these investigations, multivariate control for risk factors had only modest impact on the relative risk estimates. In the Leisure World Study (40) of women in a retirement community, the age-adjusted relative risk of all-cause mortality was 0.80 (95% CI 0.70–0.87) for estrogen users compared to nonusers; after

further adjustment for high blood pressure, history of angina, MI, or stroke, alcohol use, smoking, body mass index, and age at menopause, the relative risk was virtually the same (RR = 0.79, 95% CI 0.71–0.88), implying an equivalent risk status for users and nonusers. In addition, to further examine this issue, the Nurses' Health Study conducted an analysis limited to a subgroup of low-risk women (i.e., those with no diagnosis of hypertension, diabetes, or high serum cholesterol who were nonsmokers and had a Quetelet's index below 32 kg/m^2). Even with such restrictions, the relative risk for coronary disease was almost 40% lower for current hormone users. In summary, to explain the benefit as a result of confounding by health status, one would have to presume unknown risk factors that are extremely strong predictors of CHD and very closely associated with estrogen use.

Compliance with use of estrogen has also been considered as a marker for low risk of heart disease (68), suggesting to some that the behavioral characteristics of hormone users are more important to their decreased risk of CHD than the estrogen that they are taking. This argument is based on findings from clinical trials, where subjects who were compliant placebo takers had a better outcome than noncompliant subjects on placebo (70). However, it is unclear to what extent these findings from drug therapy trials can be extended to the interpretation of observational studies, where the subjects themselves have chosen to use medication. It is possible, for example, that clinical trial participants with symptoms of preclinical disease may selectively stop taking their randomly assigned regimen, perhaps explaining part of the apparent benefit of compliance. Furthermore, although few studies have specifically examined this issue, there does not consistently appear to be a greater protection against heart disease in long-term estrogen users compared to short-term users, indicating

TABLE 31.1. *Risk factor profiles of estrogen users and nonusers*

	Study of Osteoporotic Fractures (61)(%)				Lipid Research Clinics Programs (36)(%)				Nurses' Health Study (33)(%)	
	Current	Past	Never		Current	Past	Never		Current/past	Never
<High school education	15.8	18.2	27.0	Current heavy smoker	5.5	8.9	9.4	<High school education	16	25
Ever smoker	43.2	43.5	37.0	Hypertension	35.6	35.9	32.9	Smoker	33	31
Physical activity in past week	75.5	73.5	63.0	Diabetes	3.8	5.6	5.8	Regular exercise	12	10
Drink alcohol	76.1	74.8	66.4	High serum cholesterol	43.9	41.9	35.6	Alcohol	82	79
BMI ≥27.3 kg/m^2	28.6	36.2	41.1	Parental MI 60 before age	21.8	26.7	29.6	Mean BMI (kg/m^2)	24.7	25.7
Waist/hip ratio >0.84	28.1	29.8	33.5	Mean alcohol intake (g/day)	6.4	5.5	4.7	Mean age	53.8	52.6
				Mean BMI (kg/m^2)	25.1	25.9	26.3	Mean systolic blood pressure	129.0	127.7
								Mean diastolic blood pressure	79.9	79.5
								Mean cholesterol	234.8	235.2

that the characteristic of long-term compliance cannot explain the apparent benefit of estrogen.

ESTROGEN COMBINED WITH PROGESTIN AND CARDIOVASCULAR DISEASES

Progestin use was quite uncommon during the period that most of the epidemiologic studies were conducted. Hence, most of the data are related directly to use of estrogens alone. Currently, progestins are prescribed along with estrogens in women with a uterus to reduce or eliminate the excess risk of endometrial cancer from unopposed estrogen. However, progestin alone tends to raise LDL and lower HDL and may thus detract from the beneficial effect of estrogens on the lipid profile. In the PEPI trial (71), women were assigned to placebo, conjugated estrogen alone, estrogen combined with cyclic medroxyprogesterone acetate (MPA), estrogen combined with continuous MPA, or estrogen with micronized progesterone. Significant decreases in LDL and increases in HDL were found for women assigned to any hormone regimen compared to those taking placebo. In addition, the extent of LDL decrease was similar for all hormone regimens (by 0.37 to 0.46 mmol/L); however, for HDL, the elevation among users of estrogen with MPA (by 0.03 to 0.04 mmol/L) was less than that for users of estrogen alone (increase of 0.14 mmol/L) or estrogen with micronized progesterone (0.11 mmol/L). Furthermore, although estrogen therapy improves blood flow, limited studies suggest that this benefit may be diminished with the addition of progestin (72,73).

Nonetheless, the epidemiologic studies of heart disease strongly suggest that there is a similar decrease in the risk for users of estrogen alone and combined with a progestin. In a case-control study with 502 cases of myocardial infarction and 1,193 controls, Psaty et al. (18) reported relative risks of 0.68 (95% CI 0.38–1.22) for current users of conjugated estrogen with MPA and 0.69 (95% CI 0.47–1.02) for users of conjugated estrogen alone. In a follow-up study of the population of Uppsala, Sweden, Falkeborn et al. (49) also found that MI was reduced by 47% (RR = 0.53, 95% CI 0.30–0.87) in women taking estrogen (estradiol valerate or conjugated estrogen) with a progestin (levonorgestrel, MPA, and norethisterone acetate) and 31% (RR = 0.69, 95% CI 0.54–0.86) in those taking estrogen alone. In the Nurses' Health Study (33), the risk of CHD was diminished for women using estrogen with progestin (primarily MPA, RR = 0.39, 95% CI 0.19–0.78) or estrogen alone (RR = 0.60, 95% CI 0.43–0.83), after adjusting for an array of coronary risk factors. In one case-control study of women in Massachusetts (17), the relative risk of MI for ever use of combined therapy was 1.2 (95% CI 0.6–2.4), although the confidence interval is quite wide, and the investigators also found no protection against MI for women using estrogen alone (RR = 0.9, 95% CI 0.7–1.2). In a meta-analysis of all the studies of estrogen and progestin, the summary relative risk was 0.61 (95% CI 0.45–0.82).

Only three studies (56,33,60) have examined the relationship of stroke to combined hormone therapy. Pedersen et al. (56) found no association between current use of combined therapy and subarachnoid hemorrhage (RR = 1.22), intracerebral hemorrhage (RR = 1.17), thromboembolic infarction (RR = 1.17), or transient ischemic attack (RR = 1.25). In the Nurses' Health Study (33), there was also no relation between current use of estrogen and progestin and stroke risk (RR = 1.09, 95% CI 0.66–1.80). However, in the Swedish cohort, Falkeborn et al. (60) did report a reduced risk of stroke for users of estrogen and progestin (RR = 0.61, 95% CI 0.40–0.88).

SUMMARY

The preponderance of evidence from the epidemiologic studies strongly supports the view that postmenopausal hormone therapy can substantially reduce the risk for coronary heart disease, although there appears to be an increased risk of venous thromboembolism, and the data on stroke are inconclusive. The results from general population studies may be influenced in part by inherent characteristics of hormone users and nonusers, but much of the epidemiologic data are derived from studies in more homogeneous populations where health status and health-seeking behavior are not largely related to estrogen use. Clinical trials of estrogen for primary prevention are currently under way; however, it will be at least a decade before their outcome is known. Findings from observational studies, in conjunction with the abundant biologic evidence described elsewhere in this book, lend substantial foundation for a causal relation between estrogen and heart disease.

ACKNOWLEDGMENT

The authors' work has been supported by research grants HL 34594, CA 40356, and CA 50385 from the National Institutes of Health; Dr. Grodstein is partially supported by grant AG 13482.

REFERENCES

1. US Department of Health and Human Services, Public Health Service, Centers for Disease Control, National Center for Health Statistics. *Vital Statistics of the United States 1986. Vol II: Mortality, Part A.* Hyattsville, MD: National Center for Health Statistics, 1988.
2. Stampfer MJ, Colditz GA, Willett WC. Menopause and heart disease: a review. *Ann NY Acad Sci* 1990;592:193–203.
3. Upmark E. Life and death without ovaries. *Acta Med Scand* 1962;172:129–135.
4. Rosenberg L, Armstrong B, Jick H. Myocardial infarction and estrogen therapy in postmenopausal women. *N Engl J Med* 1976;294:1256–1259.
5. Jick H, Dinan B, Rothman KJ. Noncontraceptive estrogens and nonfatal myocardial infarction. *JAMA* 1978;239:1407–1408.
6. Rosenberg L, Stone D, Shapiro S, Kaufman P, Stolley PD, Miettinen OS. Noncontraceptive estrogens and myocardial infarction in young women. *JAMA* 1980; 244:339–342.
7. Szklo M, Tonascia J, Gordis L, Bloom I. Estrogen use and myocardial infarction risk: a case-control study. *Prev Med* 1984;13:510–516.
8. Jick H, Kinan B, Herman R, Rothman KJ. Myocardial infarction and other vascular diseases in young women: role of estrogen and other factors. *JAMA* 1978; 240:2548–2552.

9. La Vecchia C, Franceschi S, Decarli A, Pampallona S, Tognoni G. Risk factors for myocardial infarction in young women. *Am J Epidemiol* 1987;125:832–843.

10. Talbott E, Kuller LH, Detre K, Perper J. Biologic and psychosocial risk factors of sudden death from coronary disease in white women. *Am J Cardiol* 1977;39:858–864.

11. Pfeffer RI, Whipple GH, Kurosaki TT, Chapman JM. Coronary risk and estrogen use in postmenopausal women. *Am J Epidemiol* 1978;107:479–487.

12. Ross RK, Paganini-Hill A, Mack TM, Arthur M, Henderson BE. Menopausal oestrogen therapy and protection from death from ischemic heart disease. *Lancet* 1981;1:858–860.

13. Bain C, Willett WC, Hennekens CH, Rosner B, Belanger C, Speizer FE. Use of postmenopausal hormones and risk of myocardial infarction. *Circulation* 1981;64:42–46.

14. Adam S, Williams V, Vessey MP. Cardiovascular disease and hormone replacement treatment; a pilot case-control study. *Br Med J* 1981;282:1277–1278.

15. Beard CM, Kottke TE, Annegers JF, Ballard DJ. The Rochester Coronary Heart Disease Project: effect of cigarette smoking, hypertension, diabetes, and steroidal estrogen use on coronary heart disease among 40–59 year-old women. *Mayo Clin Proc* 1989;64.

16. Thompson SG, Meade TW, Greenberg G. The use of hormonal replacement therapy and the risk of stroke and myocardial infarction in women. *J Epidemiol Commun Health* 1989;43:173–178.

17. Rosenberg L, Palmer JR, Shapiro S. A case-control study of myocardial infarction in relation to use of estrogen supplements. *Am J Epidemiol* 1993;137:54–63.

18. Psaty BM, Heckbert SR, Atkins D, et al. The risk of myocardial infarction associated with the combined use of estrogens and progestins in postmenopausal women. *Arch Intern Med* 1994;154:1333–1339.

19. Heckbert SR, Weiss NS, Koepsell TD, et al. Duration of estrogen replacement therapy in relation to the risk of incident myocardial infarction in postmenopausal women. *Arch Intern Med* 1997;157:1330–1336.

20. Sidney S, Petitti DB, Quesenberry CP. Myocardial infarction and the use of estrogen and estrogen-progestogen in postmenopausal women. *Ann Intern Med* 127;127:501–508.

21. Sullivan JM, Zwagg RV, Lemp GF, et al. Postmenopausal estrogen use and coronary atherosclerosis. *Ann Intern Med* 1988;108:358–363.

22. Gruchow HW, Anderson AJ, Barboriak JJ, Sobocinski KA. Postmenopausal use of estrogen and occlusion of coronary arteries. *Am Heart J* 1988;115:954–963.

23. McFarland KF, Boniface ME, Hornung CA, Earnhardt W, Humphries JO. Risk factors and noncontraceptive estrogen use in women with and without coronary disease. *Am Heart J* 1989;117:1209–1214.

24. Hong MK, Romm PA, Reagan K, Green CE, Rackley CE. Effects of estrogen replacement therapy on serum lipid values and angiographically defined coronary artery disease in postmenopausal women. *Am J Cardiol* 1992;69:176–178.

25. Solymoss BC, Michel M, Wesolowska E, Gilfix BM, Lesperance J, Campeau L. Relation of coronary artery disease in women <60 years of age to the combined elevation of serum lipoprotein(a) and total cholesterol to high-density cholesterol ratio. *Am J Cardiol* 1993;72:1215–1219.

26. Potocki J. Wplyw leczenia estrogenami na niewydolnose wiencowa u kobiet po menopauzie. *Pol Tyg Lek* 1971;117:1209–1214.

27. Burch JC, Byrd BF, Vaughn WK. The effects of long-term estrogen on hysterectomized women. *Am J Obstet Gynecol* 1974;188:778–782.

28. McMahon B. Cardiovascular disease and noncontraceptive oestrogen therapy. In: Oliver MF, ed. *Coronary heart disease in young women.* New York: Churchill Livingstone, 1978:197–207.

29. Hammond CB, Jelovsek FR, Lee LK, Creasman WT, Parker RT. Effects of long-term estrogen replacement therapy. I. Metabolic effects. *Am J Obstet Gynecol* 1979;133:525–536.

30. Nachtigall LE, Nachtigall RH, Nachtigall RD, Beckman EM. Estrogen replacement therapy II: a prospective study in the relationship to carcinoma and cardiovascular and metabolic problems. *Obstet Gynecol* 1979;54:74–79.

31. Lafferty FW, Helmuth DO. Postmenopausal estrogen replacement: the prevention of osteoporosis and systemic effects. *Maturitas* 1985;7:147–159.

32. Stampfer MJ, Colditz GA, Willett WC, et al. Postmenopausal estrogen therapy and cardiovascular disease: ten-year follow-up from the Nurses' Health Study. *N Engl J Med* 1991;325:756–762.

33. Grodstein F, Stampfer MJ, Manson JE, et al. Postmenopausal estrogen and progestin use and the risk of cardiovascular disease. *N Engl J Med* 1996;335:453–461.

34. Wilson PW, Garrison RJ, Castelli WP. Postmenopausal estrogen use, cigarette smoking, and cardiovascular morbidity in women over 50: the Framingham Study. *N Engl J Med* 1985;313:1038–1043.

35. Eaker ED, Castelli WP. Coronary heart disease and its risk factors among women in the Framingham Study. In: Eaker E, Packard B, Wenger NK, Clarkson TB, Tyroler HA, eds. *Coronary heart disease in women.* New York: Haymarket Doyma, 1987:122–132.

36. Bush TL, Barrett-Connor E, Cowan LD, et al. Cardiovascular mortality and noncontraceptive use of estrogen in women: results from the Lipid Research Clinics Program Follow-up Study. *Circulation* 1987;75:1102–1109.

37. Petitti DB, Perlman JA, Sidney S. Noncontraceptive estrogens and mortality: long-term follow-up of women in the Walnut Creek Study. *Obstet Gynecol* 1987;70:289–293.

38. Criqui MH, Suarez L, Barrett-Connor E, McPhillips J, Wingard DL, Garland C. Postmenopausal estrogen use and mortality. *Am J Epidemiol* 1988;159:606–614.

39. Henderson BE, Paganini-Hill A, Ross RK. Estrogen replacement therapy and protection from acute myocardial infarction. *Am J Obstet Gynecol* 1988;159:312–317.

40. Henderson BE, Paganini-Hill A, Ross RK. Decreased mortality in users of estrogen replacement therapy. *Arch Intern Med* 1991;151:75–78.

41. Croft P, Hannaford PC. Risk factors for acute myocardial infarction in women: evidence from the Royal College of General Practitioners' oral contraceptive study. *Br Med J* 1989;298:165–169.

42. Bush TL, Cowan LD, Barrett-Connor E, et al. Estrogen use and all-cause mortality: preliminary results from the Lipid Research Clinics Program Follow-up Study. *JAMA* 1983;249:903–906.

43. Hunt K, Vessey M, McPherson K. Mortality in a cohort of long-term users of hormone replacement therapy: an updated analysis. *Br J Obstet Gynaecol* 1990;97:1080–1086.

44. Hunt K, Vessey M, McPherson K, Coleman M. Long-term surveillance of mortality and cancer incidence in women receiving hormone replacement therapy. *Br J Obstet Gynaecol* 1987;94:620–635.

45. Wolf PH, Madans JH, Finucane FF, Higgins M, Kleinman JC. Reduction of cardiovascular disease-related mortality among postmenopausal women who use hormones: evidence from a national cohort. *Am J Obstet Gynecol* 1991;164:489–494.

46. Persson I, Adami HO, Reinhold B, Brith KU, Hoover R. Survival in women receiving hormone replacement therapy. A record-linkage study of a large population-based cohort. *J Clin Epidemiol* 1990;43:677–685.

47. Avila MH, Walker AM, Jick H. Use of replacement estrogens and the risk of myocardial infarction. *Epidemiology* 1990;1:128–133.

48. Sullivan JM, Zwaag RV, Hughes JP, et al. Estrogen replacement and coronary artery disease. *Arch Intern Med* 1990;150:2557–2562.

49. Falkeborn M, Persson I, Adami HO, et al. The risk of acute myocardial infarction after oestrogen and oestrogen-progestogen replacement. *Br J Obstet Gynaecol* 1992;99:821–828.

50. Folsom AR, Mink PJ, Sellers TA, Hong C, Zheng W, Potter JD. Hormonal replacement therapy and morbidity and mortality in a prospective study of postmenopausal women. *Am J Public Health* 1995;85:1128–1132.

51. Ettinger B, Friedman GD, Bush T, Quesenberry CP. Reduced mortality associated with long-term postmenopausal estrogen therapy. *Obstet Gynecol* 1996;87:6–12.

52. Cauley JA, Seeley DG, Browner WS, et al. Estrogen replacement therapy and mortality among older women. *Arch Intern Med* 1997;157:2181–2187.

53. Rosenberg SH, Fausone V, Clark R. The role of estrogens as a risk for stroke in postmenopausal women. *West J Med* 1980;133:292–296.

54. Pfeffer RI, Van den Noort S. Estrogen use and stroke risk in postmenopausal women. *Am J Epidemiol* 1976;103:445–456.

55. Pfeffer RI. Estrogen use, hypertension and stroke in postmenopausal women. *J Chron Dis* 1978;31:389–398.

56. Pedersen AT, Lidegaard O, Kreiner S, Ottesen B. Hormone replacement therapy and risk of non-fatal stroke. *Lancet* 1997;350:1277–1283.

57. Group A-CC-oS. Persantine aspirin trial in cerebral ischemia, Part III: Risk factors for stroke. *Stroke* 1986;17:12–18.

58. Paganini-Hill A, Ross RK, Henderson BE. Postmenopausal oestrogen treatment and stroke: a prospective study. *Br Med J* 1988;297:519–522.

59. Boysen G, Nyobe J, Appleyard M, et al. Stroke incidence and risk factors for stroke in Copenhagen, Denmark. *Stroke* 1988;19:1345–1353.

60. Falkeborn M, Persson I, Terent A, Adami HO, Lithell H, Bergstrom R. Hormone replacement therapy and the risk of stroke. *Arch Intern Med* 1993;153:1201–1209.

61. Cauley JA, Cummings SR, Black DM, Mascioli SR, Seeley DG. Prevalence and determinants of estrogen replacement therapy in elderly women. *Am J Obstet Gynecol* 1990;163:1438–1444.

62. Grodstein F, Stampfer MJ, Colditz GA, et al. Postmenopausal hormone therapy and mortality. *N Engl J Med* 1997;336:1769–1775.

63. Daly E, Vessey MP, Hawkins MM, Carson JL, Gough P, Marsh S. Risk of venous thromboembolism in users of hormone replacement therapy. *Lancet* 1996;348:977–988.

64. Jick H, Derby LE, Myers MW, Vasilakis C, Newton KM. Risk of hospital admission for idiopathic venous thromboembolism among users of postmenopausal estrogens. *Lancet* 1996;348:981–983.

65. Gutthann S, Rodriguez L, Castellsague J, Ollart A. Hormone replacement therapy and risk of venous thromboembolism: population based case-control study. *Br Med J* 1997;314:796–800.

66. Grodstein F, Stampfer MJ, Goldhaber SZ, et al. Prospective study of exogenous hormones and risk of pulmonary embolism in women. *Lancet* 1996;348:983–987.

67. Grady D, Hulley SB, Furberg C. Venous thromboembolic events associated with hormone replacement therapy (letter). *JAMA* 1997;278:477.

68. Barrett-Connor E. Postmenopausal estrogen and prevention bias. *Ann Intern Med* 1991;115:455–456.

69. Matthews KA, Kuller LH, Wing RR, Meilahn EN, Plantinga P. Prior to estrogen replacement therapy, are users healthier than nonusers? *Am J Epidemiol* 1996;143:971–978.

70. Coronary Drug Project Research Group. Influence of adherence to treatment and response of cholesterol on mortality in the coronary drug project. *N Engl J Med* 1980;303:1038–1041.

71. Postmenopausal Estrogen/Progestin Interventions Trial Writing Group. Effects of estrogen/progestin regimens on heart disease risk factors in postmenopausal women. *JAMA* 1995;273:199–208.

72. Sarrel PM, Lindsay D, Rosano GMC, Poole-Wilson PA. Angina and normal coronary arteries in women: gynecologic findings. *Am J Obstet Gynecol* 1992;167:467–472.

73. Sullivan JM, Shala BA, Miller LA, Lerner JL, McBrayer JD. Progestin enhances vasoconstrictor responses in postmenopausal women receiving estrogen replacement therapy. *Menopause* 1995;2:193–199.

Treatment of the Postmenopausal Woman: Basic and Clinical Aspects, Second Edition, edited by Rogerio A. Lobo, Lippincott Williams & Wilkins, Philadelphia © 1999.

CHAPTER 32

Lipids and Lipoproteins and Effects of Hormone Replacement

Ronald M. Krauss

Levels of plasma lipids and lipoproteins are strong predictors of the development of atherosclerotic cardiovascular disease in postmenopausal women (1). In women, as in men, numerous factors contribute to variations in plasma lipoproteins that may affect cardiovascular disease risk. These include age, dietary components, adiposity, genetic traits, and hormonal changes. Each of these factors may operate to varying degrees in determining changes in plasma lipoprotein profiles accompanying menopause. Cross-sectional (2,3) and longitudinal studies (3–5) have suggested increases in levels of cholesterol, low-density lipoproteins (LDLs), and triglyceride-rich lipoproteins associated with menopause. Levels of high-density lipoproteins (HDLs), which are higher in women than men and are thought to contribute to relative protection of premenopausal women from cardiovascular disease, remain relatively constant in the years following menopause (6), although small, and perhaps transient, reductions in the HDL_2 subfraction have been reported in relation to reduced estradiol level following menopause (4,5). Despite these associations, it has been difficult to determine the role of endogenous hormones in influencing the plasma lipoproteins of postmenopausal women. In principle, the effects of hormone replacement should act to reverse any alterations in lipoprotein metabolism that are caused by postmenopausal hormone changes. However, although there may be beneficial effects on lipoproteins, hormone treatment does not restore a premenopausal lipoprotein profile. Furthermore, it is not clear to what extent exogenous hormone-induced lipoprotein changes contribute to the reduced incidence of cardiovascular disease with hormone replacement therapy (HRT).

R. M. Krauss: Department of Molecular Medicine, Lawrence Berkeley Laboratory, University of California, Berkeley, California 94720.

MAJOR LIPOPROTEINS AND METABOLIC PATHWAYS

Atherogenic Lipoproteins

Endogenously synthesized triglycerides are secreted, along with cholesterol and phospholipids, in the form of very-low-density lipoproteins (VLDLs, density <1.006 g/mL). The VLDLs comprise an array of particles, each of which contains one molecule of a high-molecular-weight structural protein, Apo-B100, and varying amounts of lipids and smaller proteins, Apo-Es and Apo-Cs. The triglycerides in VLDLs are hydrolyzed in peripheral tissues by the action of lipoprotein lipase, releasing VLDL surface lipids, Apo-Es, and Apo-Cs, which may be transferred to HDLs. Triglyceride-depleted VLDL remnants are returned to the liver and taken up by receptor-mediated processes, which are incompletely understood. There is evidence that LDL receptors, LDL receptor-like proteins, and perhaps other uptake mechanisms are involved (Fig. 32.1).

Similar pathways operate in the metabolism of exogenously derived fat, which is transported in plasma in intestinally derived chylomicron particles (not shown in Fig. 32.1). Chylomicrons have a structure similar to that of VLDLs but are generally much larger and contain a smaller-molecular-weight form of Apo-B, designated Apo-B48.

Larger VLDL and chylomicron remnants are generally cleared from plasma over the course of several hours. However, smaller VLDL particles may be metabolized more slowly and accumulate in plasma as cholesteryl ester–rich remnants. Prolonged residence of these particles in plasma may result in further cholesterol enrichment by transfer of cholesteryl ester from HDLs through the action of cholesteryl ester transfer protein. This process, in conjunction with progressive loss of triglyc-

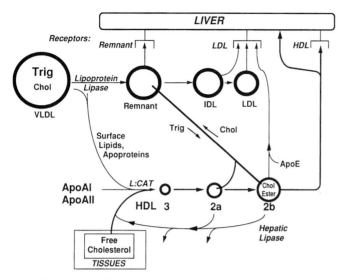

FIG. 32.1. Major lipoproteins and metabolic pathways.

eride and smaller protein constituents from VLDL remnants, results in the formation of intermediate-density lipoproteins (IDLs, density 1.006 to 1.019 g/mL) and ultimately in the production of LDLs (density 1.019 to 1.063 g/mL). The LDL particles retain Apo-B100 and cholesteryl esters as the principal protein and lipid components, respectively, and are responsible for the bulk of cholesterol transport in plasma. As is the case for VLDLs, both IDLs and LDLs are heterogeneous, comprising multiple subpopulations differing in size, density, and composition. The metabolic and possible pathologic features of certain subclasses, particularly small, dense LDLs, have been reviewed elsewhere (7,8).

The major fractions of both IDLs and LDLs are cleared from plasma by hepatic LDL receptors, which recognize both Apo-E and Apo-B100 as ligands. This process is much slower than that for remnant clearance and results in LDL plasma residence times of several days. Alterations in composition of LDLs, and perhaps IDLs and remnants, may occur, likely related in part to prolongation of their circulation in plasma and to interaction with tissues. Transport of these lipoproteins into the subendothelial space of arteries, and their retention by arterial proteoglycans, can lead to oxidative changes and other modifications. Oxidized lipoprotein lipids can trigger release of cytokines from arterial macrophages. These inflammatory agents have a wide range of effects, including cellular proliferation and recruitment of more macrophages. Unregulated uptake of modified lipoproteins by macrophages can in turn lead to cholesterol engorgement of these cells and the development of an early atherosclerotic plaque, designated a fatty streak. Excess arterial lipoprotein influx and the disruption of cholesterol-enriched cells produce extracellular cholesterol deposition in the form of a lipid "core" that is covered by a raised fibrous cap. An increase in size of the

lipid core, together with a weakening of the fibrous cap, and perhaps vasoconstriction as a result of altered endothelial function, can lead to rupture of the atherosclerotic lesion and to further inflammatory and procoagulant changes with resultant thrombus formation and vessel occlusion.

Recently, another type of lipoprotein particle, Lp(a), has been recognized as a factor of potential importance in the development of atherosclerosis (10). The Lp(a) contains Apo-B100 complexed with another large protein, Apo(a), which is highly homologous to plasminogen. Plasma concentrations of Lp(a) vary over a wide range in the general population and appear to be under strong genetic influence. The Lp(a) levels have been highly correlated with coronary disease risk in epidemiologic studies, and Apo(a) has been demonstrated in arterial lesions by immunochemical techniques. Although the mechanisms for the involvement of Lp(a) in atherosclerosis are not known, interactions of Apo(a) with the arterial endothelium, and perhaps also with the fibrinolytic system, may be of importance.

High-Density Lipoproteins

High-density lipoproteins comprise a complex array of particles with differing lipid and protein composition and metabolic behavior (11). Most HDL particles contain the protein Apo-AI, derived from both liver and intestine, and certain subpopulations also contain varying amounts of Apo-AII as well as Apo-Cs and Apo-Es. The bulk of HDLs are thought to arise from lipid-poor precursor particles secreted by both the liver and intestine, which acquire additional lipids and undergo a variety of transformations during their circulation in the blood. The HDL lipids are derived both from the metabolism of Apo-B-containing lipoproteins, as described earlier, and from the direct uptake of cellular lipids, in particular, unesterified cholesterol. The enzyme lecithin cholesterol acyltransferase (LCAT), activated by Apo-AI, converts unesterified to esterified cholesterol and participates in the transformation of nascent HDLs in a stepwise manner to a series of progressively larger particles with increasing cholesterol and apoprotein content. The smaller and denser HDL subclasses are designated HDL₃, whereas the larger and more buoyant are designated HDL₂. Within both HDL₃ and HDL₂, there are multiple discrete subspecies with differing content of Apo-AI and Apo-AII as well as other constituents. Of particular note is the largest major HDL subspecies, HDL₂ᵦ, which contains four molecules of Apo-AI without Apo-AII. Levels of HDL₂ᵦ are higher in women than in men and, in both sexes, correlate with plasma concentrations of HDL-cholesterol.

The HDL components leave the plasma by a variety of pathways. As described earlier, cholesteryl ester transfer protein may mediate cholesterol movement from HDLs to Apo-B-containing lipoproteins, particularly lipolytic remnants, in exchange for triglycerides. The acceptor particles may then be taken up by LDL or remnant receptors. Subpopulations of HDLs containing Apo-E also may be cleared directly by such receptors. Alternatively, HDLs may deliver cholesterol directly to tissues, either by selective uptake of HDL lipids or removal of intact HDL particles. Recently a receptor, designated SR-B1, which is highly expressed in the liver as well as in adrenal and gonadal tissue, has been found to mediate tissue uptake of HDL cholesterol (12).

Another mechanism implicated in regulating plasma HDL levels is the activity of hepatic lipase, an enzyme that catalyzes the hydrolysis of HDL phospholipids and triglycerides and potentiates hepatic HDL lipid uptake. Variations of hepatic lipase activity measured in postheparin plasma have been strongly inversely correlated with levels of HDL-cholesterol. It has also been proposed that triglyceride-enriched HDLs resulting from accelerated cholesterol/triglyceride exchange are catabolized and perhaps more rapidly cleared as a result of hepatic lipase activity.

The potential ability of HDLs to mediate delivery of cholesterol from peripheral tissues to the liver has led to the hypothesis that HDLs have an antiatherogenic effect by promoting "reverse cholesterol transport." However, a number of other factors may underlie the inverse relationship of HDL-cholesterol to risk of atherosclerotic cardiovascular disease (13). For example, levels of HDL-cholesterol are determined in part by the efficacy of clearance of triglyceride-rich lipoproteins and their remnants. Thus, high HDL levels may reflect lower levels or shorter plasma residence time of potentially atherogenic remnant particles. In addition, there has been recent evidence that HDLs may reduce the accumulation of lipid peroxides in LDLs. A direct effect of increased Apo-AI production in atherosclerosis prevention has been demonstrated in transgenic mice overexpressing the human Apo-AI gene (14). This suggests that, whatever the mechanism, genetic and other factors regulating Apo-AI synthesis may have important antiatherogenic effects.

EFFECTS OF ESTROGENS ON PLASMA LIPOPROTEIN METABOLISM

Estrogen treatment has been shown to increase the rates of both hepatic triglyceride production and VLDL-Apo-B100 secretion (Fig. 32.2). Walsh et al. (15) have reported that oral micronized estradiol at a dose of 2 mg/day increased the production of Apo-B in large VLDL particles (of Svedberg flotation rate, S_f, 60 to 400) to a much greater extent than in smaller VLDL particles (S_f 20 to 60). Most of the additional large VLDLs were cleared directly from plasma, with a smaller portion converted to smaller VLDLs and LDLs. In addition, there was an increased fractional catabolic rate of LDLs. The latter finding is consistent with evidence from animal

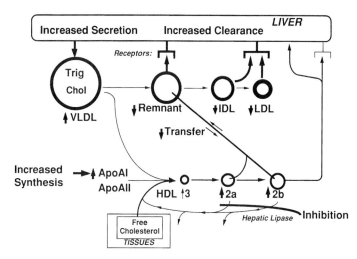

FIG. 32.2. Effects of estrogens on plasma lipoprotein metabolism.

studies that estrogens increase the number of hepatic LDL receptors. The net influence of estrogens on Apo-B-containing lipoproteins thus depends on the balance between increased production of large, triglyceride-rich VLDLs and increased clearance of these particles as well as cholesterol-rich remnants and LDLs.

There is little information on the metabolic mechanisms by which estrogens influence HDL levels. In nonhuman primates, estrogen treatment has been found to increase both Apo-AI and Apo-AII production rates (16). High-dose ethinyl estradiol treatment of premenopausal women was shown to increase production rates of HDL Apo-AI in particular (17). On the other hand, estrogen treatment results in significant suppression of hepatic lipase activity (17,18), and in a study in postmenopausal women, reduced HDL fractional clearance has been reported. Either increased Apo-AI production or reduced hepatic lipase activity might be expected to induce a preferential increase in HDL₂ subclasses. Recently, estrogen has been shown to induce dramatic suppression of the SR-B1 (HDL) receptor in the liver, an effect that may also contribute to accumulation of cholesterol-rich HDL particles in plasma (19).

PROGESTIN EFFECTS ON LIPOPROTEIN METABOLISM

The common practice of using progestins to counteract estrogen-induced endometrial hyperplasia raises the question of what effects this may have on lipoprotein metabolism. Natural progesterone, although not extensively studied, has not been found to cause significant changes in levels of plasma lipoproteins (20–23). On the other hand, synthetic progestins, particularly those with evidence of androgenic activity (e.g., norethindrone, levonorgestrel), may have significant metabolic effects. The best-documented effect of androgenic progestins on lipoprotein metabolism is increased hepatic lipase activity, which in turn has been strongly correlated with reduced levels of HDL-cholesterol, particularly in the HDL$_2$ subclasses (18). Androgenic progestins are also known to reduce triglyceride levels (19), although the mechanism of this effect is not understood. Some effects of these agents may also be mediated by insulin resistance, which has been associated with a dyslipidemia characterized by increased levels of VLDLs and reduced levels of HDL-cholesterol (24).

EFFECTS OF HORMONE REPLACEMENT THERAPY ON PLASMA LIPID AND LIPOPROTEIN CHOLESTEROL LEVELS

A large number of cross-sectional and longitudinal studies have assessed the influence of postmenopausal HRT on plasma lipoprotein concentrations (reviewed in 25,26). The findings of these studies reflect a number of sources of variation, including study designs, size and characteristics of study populations, hormone formulations, treatment regimens, duration of use, and laboratory methodology. The Postmenopausal Estrogen/Progestin Intervention (PEPI) Trial has provided the most definitive information to date on the effects of unopposed estrogen and various combination HRT regimens on plasma lipoproteins and other risk factors for coronary heart disease (27). In this 3-year double-blind study, 875 healthy postmenopausal women aged 45 to 64 were randomly assigned to placebo or treatment with conjugated equine estrogens (CEE), 0.625 mg/day, alone or in combination with cyclic medroxyprogesterone acetate (MPA), 10 mg/day for 12 days/month, continuous MPA 2.5 mg/day, or cyclic micronized progesterone 200 mg/day for 12 days/month. The major findings from this and earlier studies may be summarized as follows:

Estrogen Therapy

Plasma Triglyceride and VLDL Levels Increase in a Dose-Dependent Manner

In the Lipid Research Clinics of North America Study (LRC), a comparison of 370 nonmenstruating 45- to 64-year-old women not using estrogens with 239 women using equine estrogens at various doses demonstrated a 26% higher median triglyceride level in the estrogen users (28). A summary analysis by Bush and Miller (29) of 10 randomized and crossover studies employing conjugated estrogens, adjusted for variables including sample size (ranging from 6 to 265) and duration of treatment (ranging from 1 to 12 months), revealed an overall increase in triglycerides of 20%, with levels increasing as a function of estrogen dose. A similar mean increase (24%) was observed by Walsh et al. (15) in a double-blind placebo-controlled crossover study of 31 postmenopausal

women treated with CEE for 3 months at a dose of 0.625 mg/day, and the mean increase at 1.25 mg/day was substantially greater (38%). These findings are consistent with those of the PEPI Trial, in which CEE, 0.625 mg/day, resulted in a 25% increase in plasma triglyceride among adherent subjects (30). It should be noted that these studies were carried out in normolipidemic women. Women with primary hypertriglyceridemia may develop severe hyperlipemia on estrogen replacement therapy (31), and in such patients, estrogens should be used with caution and only after therapeutic reduction of triglyceride levels to less than 500 mg/dL.

Plasma Total and LDL-Cholesterol Levels Decrease

In the LRC study, median LDL-cholesterol was 11% lower in CEE users than in nonusers (28). Three other large cross-sectional studies revealed similar reductions in LDL-cholesterol (32–34) with dose-response effects between 0.625 mg/day and 0.9 to 1.25 mg/day reported in two of the studies (32,34). In the study by Walsh et al. (15), the reductions were somewhat greater: 15% at the lower dose and 19% at the higher dose, with a nonsignificant dosage effect. The LDL-cholesterol reduction with CEE, 0.625 mg/day in the PEPI Trial, was 10% (27), with a somewhat greater effect when the analyses were restricted to adherent subjects (30).

Plasma HDL-Cholesterol Levels Increase, Principally HDL$_2$

Median HDL-cholesterol was found to be 10% higher in users of conjugated estrogens in the LRC Study (28), with similar increases observed in three other cross-sectional studies (32–34), two of which detected an apparent effect of dose (32,34). In the 10 prospective trials summarized by Bush and Miller (29), the average adjusted increase was also 10%, without an apparent dose effect. The PEPI Trial observed an HDL-cholesterol increase of 9% with CEE 0.625 mg/day (27), and a 13% increase among adherent subjects (30). In the studies of Sherwin and Gelfand (35) and Walsh et al. (15), increases in HDL-cholesterol were 14% and 16% at 0.625 mg CEE/day and 19% and 18% at 1.25 mg/day, suggestive of a small but not significant dose dependence. As in a number of other studies (36,37), the increase was restricted to the HDL2 subclasses. Thus, as is the case with LDL-cholesterol, there may be saturation of the effects of CEE at 0.625 mg/day, although there is clearly much interindividual variation in response.

The Lipid and Lipoprotein Effects of Estrogens Are Greater with Oral Than with Systemic Administration

A number of studies have indicated that systemic estrogen therapy, administered as percutaneous estradiol patches or creams, have little or no impact on plasma lipid and lipoprotein cholesterol levels (38–44). Other studies, however, have detected moderate increases in levels of HDLs (37,45–47) and reductions in LDLs (23,47,48). Although there are a number of differences in experimental methodology among these studies, it has been pointed out that some differences in the findings may be related to the relatively greater plasma levels of systematically administered estrogens that are required to achieve intrahepatic hormone levels comparable to those achieved via the portal circulation after oral administration (15).

Combination Hormone Replacement Therapy

The effects of estrogen/progestin combinations on plasma lipid and lipoprotein cholesterol levels in postmenopausal women have been examined in a large number of studies employing various hormonal replacement regimens, as reviewed elsewhere (25,26). The following represents general observations that may be drawn from an overview of these as well as more recent studies, including the PEPI Trial (27,30).

1. The metabolic effects of added progestin are related to the dose and relative androgenic potency of the hormone preparation and the concomitant dose of estrogen. On a weight basis, the C_{21} hydroxyprogesterone derivatives (e.g., medroxyprogesterone and medrogestone) are less metabolically active than the 19-nortestosterone derivatives (e.g., norethindrone) and levonorgestrel (20,49,50). Progesterone appears to be relatively inert in its effects on lipoprotein metabolism (20).
2. Addition of progestin has small and variable effects on levels of plasma triglyceride and VLDL levels compared with those produced by estrogen alone. In the PEPI Trial, among adherent subjects, triglycerides increased 15% to 20% in each opposed CEE arm versus 25% with CEE alone, although this difference was not statistically significant (30). Estrogen-induced increases in triglyceride level tend to be blunted to a greater extent by the more androgenic progestins (51). This may be related to the finding that a combination of estradiol and (d,l)-norgestrel results in increased fractional VLDL Apo-B clearance without an increase in VLDL Apo-B production rate (51).
3. Estrogen-induced reductions in LDL cholesterol are affected minimally, if at all, by addition of conventional doses of progestins. A number of studies have shown similar reductions of LDL-cholesterol with or without the concomitant administration of progestins (25,27,48,51). Although this would appear to suggest minimal interference of progestogens with the beneficial effects of estrogen on LDL metabolism, it has been reported that an oral estradiol-norgestrel combi-

nation decreased the LDL Apo-B production rate without affecting the fractional LDL Apo-B clearance (52). This finding stands in contrast to the recent report that estrogen therapy alone reduces LDL levels primarily by increasing the fractional LDL Apo-B catabolic rate (15). Thus, estrogens and estrogen-progestin combinations might alter LDL levels by different mechanisms, and this could conceivably have consequences for the prediction of effects on coronary disease risk.
4. Most progestins attenuate estrogen-induced increases in HDL-cholesterol (principally HDL_2). Although this effect has been reported to be more pronounced with high doses of 19-nortestosterone derivatives or levonorgestrel than with 21-hydroxyprogesterone derivatives, substantial reversal of estrogen-induced increases in HDL and HDL_2 cholesterol have been observed with endometrial-suppressive doses of cyclic medroxyprogesterone (10 mg), norethindrone (1 mg), and (d,l)-norgestrel (0.15 mg) (22,47). In PEPI, HDL-cholesterol increased by only 2% with either CEE/MPA regimen (27) and by 7% with the CEE/micronized progesterone combination. Among adherent subjects, these increases were significantly less than with unopposed CEE (30).
5. Observational studies of lipid and lipoprotein levels in older users of combination hormone replacement therapy have not demonstrated the effects on HDL levels observed in short-term clinical trials. A cross-sectional study in a retirement community in California showed no differences in plasma triglyceride, LDL-cholesterol, or HDL-cholesterol levels in users of estrogen-only versus combination hormone replacement therapy (33). Similar results have been observed recently in studies carried out in a second California retirement community (34). In the latter study, there were also no detectable differences in lipids and lipoproteins with doses of medroxyprogesterone ranging from 2.5 to 10 mg/day, administered from 5 to 25 days/month in combination with estrogen. In both studies, differences in lipid and lipoprotein levels between nonusers of hormones and estrogen-only users were comparable to those reviewed earlier. Multiple explanations might be offered for these results, ranging from subject selection to poor progestin compliance, but it should also be noted that longer-term prospective treatment trials (e.g., >3 years) have not been performed in older women, and it is possible that progestin-induced alterations of lipoproteins (notably HDLs) become attenuated over time.

Selective Estrogen Receptor Modulators

Recently, effects on lipoproteins and other cardiovascular risk markers have been described for raloxifene, a selective estrogen receptor modulator that has estrogen-agonistic effects on bone and estrogen-antagonistic effects on breast and uterus (53).

At two doses of raloxifene, LDL-cholesterol was reduced by 12%, similar to the effects of estrogen and HRT. In contrast to HRT, however, there were no significant increases in triglyceride or HDL-cholesterol, although HDL_2 was increased by 11%.

Similar lipoprotein effects have been observed in cholesterol-fed nonhuman primates, in which raloxifene, unlike CEE, had no benefit on atherosclerosis severity (54). As discussed further below, these results are consistent with evidence from humans that estrogen-related increases in HDL may be a marker for cardioprotection, although hormonal effects on mechanisms unrelated to lipoproteins are also of considerable importance.

EFFECTS OF HORMONE REPLACEMENT THERAPY ON OTHER LIPOPROTEIN PARAMETERS THAT MAY AFFECT CARDIOVASCULAR DISEASE RISK

Several recent studies have found reductions in levels of Lp(a) with HRT (55,56). In PEPI, these ranged from 17% to 23% in comparison with placebo and did not differ significantly among treatment arms (56). Raloxifene has also been reported to lower Lp(a), but to a significantly smaller extent (53). Thus, although there is no evidence to date as to the benefits of Lp(a) reduction on cardiovascular disease risk, HRT is one of the few therapies capable of lowering elevated Lp(a) levels.

Changes in composition and metabolism of atherogenic lipoproteins may have an impact on cardiovascular risk that is not reflected in standard measurements of their plasma levels. Estrogens have been shown to increase triglyceride content of LDLs as well as other lipoprotein classes (28,37), but these changes have not been directly related to altered cardiovascular disease risk. Reductions in levels of plasma Apo-B100 have been reported with estrogen replacement (57) and with combined estrogen-progestin therapy (58), but these reductions are not as great as for LDL-cholesterol (37,58). This is a result of preferential reduction in levels of large, buoyant LDL subspecies with a higher ratio of cholesterol to Apo-B LDL than is found in smaller denser LDL (59,60). Recent metabolic studies have indicated that estrogen induces increased turnover of both large and small LDL and that the preferential reduction in plasma levels of large LDL results from a reduced rate of production of these particles (60). Although smaller LDL particles signify increased risk for coronary heart disease (61), the clinical implications of the differing effects of estrogen on metabolism of larger and smaller LDL particles are not known. Estrogens have also been found to increase plasma clearance of potentially atherogenic remnants formed during the course of postprandial triglyceride-rich lipoprotein metabolism (62), an effect consistent with the earlier demonstration of an increase in fractional catabolic rate of smaller VLDL particles (15). Finally, though estrogens have been found to reduce susceptibility of LDLs (63–65) and HDL (65) to oxidative modification, it has not been established to what extent this may contribute to protection from LDL oxidation and atherosclerosis *in vivo*.

RELATION OF HORMONE REPLACEMENT THERAPY EFFECTS ON PLASMA LIPOPROTEINS TO CARDIOVASCULAR DISEASE RISK

Observational epidemiologic evidence has indicated that the substantial reduction in risk of coronary artery disease associated with estrogen therapy is related in part to changes in plasma lipoproteins (66), although it is estimated that these changes account for less than half of the apparent benefit. Among standard lipoprotein measures, the strongest correlate of reduced risk is the estrogen-related increase in HDL-cholesterol (66). Notably, unlike estrogen-induced reductions in LDL, this increase does not represent an effect of estrogen "replacement" but a pharmacologic increase related to oral estrogen administration that results in HDL levels higher than those found in premenopause. It is likely that other changes in plasma lipoprotein metabolism induced by HRT could also contribute to reduced cardiovascular disease risk, for example, reductions in Lp(a), increased clearance of atherogenic lipoprotein subfractions, and reduced lipoprotein oxidation.

An increasing body of evidence, however, has suggested that a major portion of the apparent benefit of estrogen therapy on cardiovascular disease risk may result from effects that are not related to changes in plasma lipoprotein risk measurements. This hypothesis is supported by studies in cholesterol-fed nonhuman primates in which reduction in extent of atherosclerosis, reduction induced by estrogen (67), and lack of reduction with estrogen plus medroxyprogesterone (68) have been found to be largely independent of changes in plasma lipoproteins. A number of mechanisms have been invoked to account for nonlipoprotein effects of HRT on the cardiovascular system including changes in vascular reactivity, lipoprotein retention, and coagulation factors. Ongoing clinical trials and metabolic studies in humans and animals should provide additional information that will help to define the clinically significant lipoprotein effects of various hormonal replacement regimens.

ACKNOWLEDGMENT

This work was supported by the National Institutes of Health grants HL 18574 and HL 33577 from the National Heart, Lung, and Blood Institute, a grant from the National Dairy Promotion and Research Board and administered in cooperation with the National Dairy Council, and was conducted at the Lawrence Berkeley National Laboratory through the U.S. Department of Energy under Contract No. DE-AC03-76SF00098.

REFERENCES

1. Kannel WB. Metabolic risk factors for coronary artery disease in women: perspective from the Framingham study. *Am Heart J* 1987;114:413–419.
2. Hjortland MC, McNamara PM, Kannel WB. Some atherogenic concomitants of menopause: the Framingham study. *Am J Epidemiol* 1976;103:304–311.
3. Jensen J, Nilas L, Christiansen C. Influence of menopause on serum lipids and lipoproteins. *Maturitas* 1990;12:321–331.
4. Matthews KA, Meilahn E, Kuller LH, et al. Menopause and risk factors for coronary heart disease. *N Engl J Med* 1989;321:641–646.
5. Kuller LH, Gutai JP, Meilahn E, et al. Relationship of endogenous sex steroid hormones to lipids and apoproteins in postmenopausal women. *Arteriosclerosis* 1990;10:1058–1066.
6. Rifkind BM, Tamir I, Heiss G, et al. Distribution of high density and other lipoproteins in selected LRC Prevalence Study populations. *Lipids* 1979;14:105–112.
7. Krauss RM. Relationship of intermediate and low-density lipoprotein subspecies to risk of coronary artery disease. *Am Heart J* 1987;113:578–582.
8. Krauss RM. Low-density lipoprotein subclasses and risk of coronary artery disease. *Curr Opin Lipidol* 1991;2:248–252.
9. Witztum JL. The role of oxidized LDL in atherosclerosis. *Adv Exp Med Biol* 1991;285:353–365.
10. Scanu AM, Scandiani L. Lipoprotein(a): structure, biology, and clinical relevance. *Adv Intern Med* 1991;36:249–270.
11. Krauss RM. Regulation of high density lipoprotein levels. *Med Clin North Am* 1982;66:403–430.
12. Acton S, Rigotti A, Landschulz KT, Xu SZ, Hobbs HH, Krieger M. Identification of scavenger receptor SR-BI as a high density lipoprotein receptor. *Science* 1996;271:518–520.
13. Rubin EM, Krauss RM, Spangler EA, et al. Inhibition of early atherogenesis in transgenic mice by human apolipoprotein AI. *Nature* 1991;353:265–267.
14. Tribble DL, Krauss RM. HDL and coronary artery disease. *Adv Intern Med* 1993;38:1–29.
15. Walsh BW, Schiff I, Rosner B, et al. Effects of postmenopausal estrogen replacement on the concentrations and metabolism of plasma lipoproteins. *N Engl J Med* 1991;325:1196–1204.
16. Kushwaha RS, Foster DM, Murthy VN, et al. Metabolic regulation of apoproteins of high-density lipoproteins by estrogen and progesterone in the baboon (*Papio* sp). *Metabolism* 1990;39:544–552.
17. Schaefer EJ, Foster DM, Zech LA, et al. The effects of estrogen administration on plasma lipoprotein metabolism in premenopausal females. *J Clin Endocrinol Metab* 1983;57:262–267.
18. Tikkanen MJ, Nikkila EA, Kuusi T, et al. High density lipoprotein-2 and hepatic lipase: reciprocal changes produced by estrogen and Norgestrel. *J Clin Endocrinol Metab* 1982;54:1113–1117.
19. Landschulz KT, Pathak RK, Rigotti A, et al. Regulation of scavenger receptor, class B, type I, a high density lipoprotein receptor, in liver and steroidogenic tissues of the rat. *J Clin Invest* 1996;98:984–995.
20. Krauss RM. Effects of progestational agents on serum lipids and lipoproteins. *J Reprod Med* 1982;27:503–510.
21. Fahraeus L, Larsson CU, Wallentin L. L-Norgestrel and progesterone have different influences on plasma lipoproteins. *Eur J Clin Invest* 1983;13:447–453.
22. Ottosson UB, Johansson BG, Von Schoultz B. Subfractions of high-density lipoprotein cholesterol during estrogen replacement therapy: a comparison between progestogens and Natural progesterone. *Am J Obstet Gynecol* 1985;151:746–750.
23. Jensen J, Riis BJ, Strom V, et al. Long-term effects of percutaneous estrogens and oral progesterone on serum lipoproteins in postmenopausal women. *Am J Obstet Gynecol* 1987;156:66–71.
24. Laws A, Reaven GM. Evidence for an independent relationship between insulin resistance and fasting plasma HDL-cholesterol, triglyceride and insulin concentrations. *J Intern Med* 1992;231:25–30.
25. Rijpkema AHM, Van der Sanden AA, Ruijs AHC. Effects of post-menopausal oestrogen-progestogen replacement therapy on serum lipids and lipoproteins: a review. *Maturitas* 1990;12:259–285.
26. Sacks FM, Walsh BW. The effects of reproductive hormones on serum lipoproteins: unresolved issues in biology and clinical practice. *Ann NY Acad Sci* 1990;592:272–285.
27. The Writing Group for the PEPI Trial. Effects of estrogen or estrogen/progestin regimens on heart disease risk factors in postmenopausal women: The Postmenopausal Estrogen/Progestin Interventions (PEPI) Trial. *JAMA* 1995;273:199–208.
28. Wahl P, Walden C, Knopp R, et al. Effect of estrogen/progestin potency on lipid/lipoprotein cholesterol. *N Engl J Med* 1983;308:862–867.
29. Bush TL, Miller VT. Effects of pharmacologic agents used during menopause:

impact on lipids and lipoproteins. In: Mishell DR, ed. *Menopause: physiology and pharmacology.* Chicago: Year Book Medical Publishers, 1987:187–208.
30. Barrett-Connor E, Slone S, Greendale G, et al. The Postmenopausal Estrogen/Progestin Interventions Study: primary outcomes in adherent women. *Maturitas* 1997;27(3):261–274.
31. Glueck CJ, Scheel D, Fishback J, et al. Estrogen-induced pancreatitis in patients with previously covert familial type V hyperlipoproteinemia. *Metabolism* 1972;21:657–666.
32. Krauss RM, Perlman JA, Ray R, et al. Effects of estrogen dose and smoking on lipid and lipoprotein levels in postmenopausal women. *Am J Obstet Gynecol* 1988;158:1606–1611.
33. Barrett-Connor CE, Wingard DL, Criqui MH. Postmenopausal estrogen use and heart disease risk factors in the 1980s. Rancho Bernardo, Calif, revisited. *JAMA* 1989;261:2095–2100.
34. Paganini-Hill A, Dworsky R, Krauss RM. Hormone replacement therapy, hormone levels, and lipoprotein cholesterol concentrations in elderly women. *Am J Obstet Gynecol* 1996;174:897–902.
35. Sherwin BB, Gelfand MM. A prospective one-year study of estrogen and progestin in postmenopausal women: effects on clinical symptoms and lipoprotein lipids. *Obstet Gynecol* 1989;73:759–766.
36. Krauss RM, Lindgren FT, Wingerd J, et al. Effects of estrogens and progestins on high density lipoproteins. *Lipids* 1979;14:113–118.
37. Moorjani S, Dupont A, Labrie F, et al. Changes in plasma lipoprotein and apolipoprotein composition in relation to oral versus percutaneous administration of estrogen alone or in cyclic association with utrogestan in menopausal women. *J Clin Endocrinol Metab* 1991;73:373–379.
38. Fahraeus L, Larsson-Cohn U, Wallentin L. Lipoprotein during oral and cutaneous administration of estradiol-17β to menopausal women. *Acta Endocrinol (Kbh)* 1982;101:597–602.
39. Elkik F, Gompel A, Mercier-Bodard C. Effects of percutaneous estradiol and conjugated estrogens on the level of plasma proteins and triglycerides in postmenopausal women. *Am J Obstet Gynecol* 1982;143:888–892.
40. Basdevant A, De Lignieres B, Guy-Grand B. Differential lipemic and hormonal responses to oral and parenteral 17 beta-estradiol in postmenopausal women. *Am J Obstet Gynecol* 1983;147:77–81.
41. Mandel FP, Geola FL, Meldrum DR. Biological effects of various doses of vaginally administered conjugated equine estrogens in postmenopausal women. *J Clin Endocrinol Metab* 1983;57:133–139.
42. Farish ECD, Fletcher DM, Hart F, et al. The effects of hormone implants on serum lipoproteins and steroid hormones in bilaterally oophorectomised women. *Acta Endocrinol (Kbh)* 1984;106:116–120.
43. Chetkowski RJ, Meldrum DR, Steingold KA, et al. Biologic effects of transdermal estradiol. *N Engl J Med* 1986;314:1615–1620.
44. De Lignieres B, Basdevant A, Thomas G, et al. Biological effects of estradiol-17 beta in postmenopausal women: oral versus percutaneous administration. *J Clin Endocrinol Metab* 1986;62:536–541.
45. Lobo RA, March CM, Goebelsmann U, et al. Subdermal estradiol pellets following hysterectomy and oophorectomy. Effect upon serum estrone, estradiol, luteinizing hormone, follicle-stimulating hormone, corticosteroid binding globulin binding capacity, testosterone-estradiol binding globulin binding capacity, lipids, and hot flushes. *Am J Obstet Gynecol* 1980;138:714–719.
46. Stanczyk FZ, Shoupe D, Nunez V, et al. A randomized comparison of nonoral estradiol delivery in postmenopausal women. *Am J Obstet Gynecol* 1988;159:1540–1546.
47. Sharf M, Oettinger M, Lanir A, et al. Lipid and lipoprotein levels following pure estradiol implantation in postmenopausal women. *Gynecol Obstet Invest* 1985;19:207–212.
48. Crook D, Cust MP, Gangar KF, et al. Comparison of transdermal and oral estrogen-progestin replacement therapy: effects on serum lipids and lipoproteins. *Am J Obstet Gynecol* 1992;166:950–955.
49. Dorflinger LJ. Relative potency of progestins used in oral contraceptives. *Contraception* 1985;31:557–570.
50. Sonnendecker E, Polakow ES, Benadé A, et al. Serum lipoprotein effects of conjugated estrogen and a sequential conjugated estrogen-medrogestone regimen in hysterectomized postmenopausal women. *Am J Obstet Gynecol* 1989;1:1128–1134.
51. Miller VT, Muesing RA, LaRosa JC, et al. Effects of conjugated equine estrogen with and without three different progestogens on lipoproteins, high-density lipoprotein subfractions, and apolipoprotein A-I. *Obstet Gynecol* 1991;77:235–240.
52. Wolfe BM, Huff MW. Effects of combined estrogen and progestin administration on plasma lipoprotein metabolism in postmenopausal women. *J Clin Invest* 1989;83:40–45.
53. Walsh BW, Kuller LH, Wild RA, et al. Effects of raloxifene on serum lipids and coagulation factors in healthy postmenopausal women. *JAMA* 1998;279:1445–1451.
54. Clarkson TB, Anthony MS, Jerome CP. Lack of effect of raloxifene on coronary artery atherosclerosis of postmenopausal monkeys. *J Clin Endocrinol Metab* 1998;83:721–726.
55. Soma M, Fumagalli R, Paoletti R, et al. Plasma Lp(a) concentration after oestrogen and progestogen in postmenopausal women. *Lancet* 1991;337:612.
56. Espeland MA, Marcovina SM, Miller V, et al. Effect of postmenopausal hormone therapy on lipoprotein(a) concentration. *Circulation* 1998;97:979–986.
57. Applebaum-Bowden D, McLean P, Steinmetz A, et al. Lipoprotein, apolipoprotein, and lipolytic enzyme changes following estrogen administration in postmenopausal women. *J Lipid Res* 1989;30:1895–1906.

58. Haarbo J, Hassager C, Jensen SB, et al. Serum lipids, lipoproteins, and apolipoproteins during postmenopausal estrogen replacement therapy combined with either 19-nortestosterone derivatives or 17-hydroxyprogesterone derivatives. *Am J Med* 1991;90:584–589.

59. Campos H, Sacks FM, Walsh BW, et al. Differential effects of estrogen on low-density lipoprotein subclasses in healthy postmenopausal women. *Metabolism* 1993;42:1153–1158.

60. Campos H, Walsh BW, Judge H, Sacks FM. Effect of estrogen on very low density lipoprotein and low density lipoprotein subclass Metabolism in postmenopausal women. *J Clin Endocrinol Metab* 1997;82:3955–3963.

61. Gardner CD, Fortmann SP, Krauss RM. Association of small low-density lipoprotein particles with the incidence of coronary artery disease in men and women. *JAMA* 1996;276:875–881.

62. Westerveld HT, Kock LA, van Rijn HJ, et al. 17 Beta-estradiol improves postprandial lipid metabolism in postmenopausal women. *J Clin Endocrinol Metab* 1995;80:249–253.

63. Maziagere C, Auclair M, Ronveaux MF, et al. Estrogens inhibit copper and cell-mediated modification of low density lipoprotein. *Atherosclerosis* 1991;89:175–182.

64. Sack MN, Rader DJ, Cannon RO III. Oestrogen and inhibition of oxidation of low-density lipoproteins in postmenopausal women. *Lancet* 1994;343:269–270.

65. Wakatsuki A, Ikenoue N, Sagara Y. Effects of estrogen on susceptibility to oxidation of low-density and high-density lipoprotein in postmenopausal women. *Maturitas* 1998;28:229–234.

66. Bush TL, Barrett-Connor E, Cowan LD, et al. Cardiovascular mortality and noncontraceptive use of estrogen in women: results from the lipid research clinics program follow-up study. *Circulation* 1987;75:1102–1109.

67. Wagner JD, Clarkson TB, St Clair RW, et al. Estrogen and progesterone replacement therapy reduces low density lipoprotein accumulation in the coronary arteries of surgically postmenopausal cynomolgus monkeys. *J Clin Invest* 1991;88:1995–2002.

68. Adams MR, Register TC, Golden DL, et al. Medroxyprogesterone acetate antagonizes inhibitory effects of conjugated equine estrogens on coronary artery atherosclerosis. *Arterioscler Thromb Vasc Biol* 1997;17:217–221.

Treatment of the Postmenopausal Woman: Basic and Clinical Aspects, Second Edition, edited by Rogerio A. Lobo, Lippincott Williams & Wilkins, Philadelphia © 1999.

CHAPTER 33

Arterial Changes: Estrogen Deficiency and Effects of Hormone Replacement

Michael R. Adams, Scott A. Washburn, Janice D. Wagner, J. Koudy Williams, and Thomas B. Clarkson

In human populations where coronary heart disease is a major public health problem, its incidence is much lower in premenopausal women than in men of similar age. This sex difference in coronary heart disease risk is paralleled by a difference in extent and severity of coronary artery atherosclerosis (1). It is widely believed that ovarian estrogen is responsible for this relative sparing of the coronary arteries in women; however, it remains uncertain whether coronary heart disease risk, or atherosclerosis, in human beings is influenced by conditions that influence endogenous estrogen concentrations (e.g., menopause, pregnancy) (2). Yet compelling evidence suggests that estrogen replacement therapy results in a marked reduction in the risk of coronary heart disease in postmenopausal women (3). The mechanisms by which this effect is mediated are poorly understood. Among multiple possibilities are inhibitory effects on atherosclerosis progression, inhibitory effects on coronary thrombosis, and beneficial effects on vasomotor function of coronary arteries.

In this chapter we have summarized the epidemiologic, clinical, and experimental evidence regarding the effects of estrogen deficiency and estrogen replacement therapy on atherosclerosis progression and arterial vasomotor function.

AUTOPSY AND ANGIOGRAPHIC STUDIES IN HUMAN BEINGS

The results of several large, long-term epidemiologic studies have led scientists to conclude that post-

M. R. Adams, S. A. Washburn, J. D. Wagner, J. K. Williams, T. B. Clarkson: Department of Pathology/Comparative Medicine, The Bowman Gray School of Medicine, Wake Forest University, Winston-Salem, North Carolina 27157.

menopausal women who undergo hormone replacement therapy (HRT) reduce their risk of myocardial infarction by 50% (4). Unfortunately, few studies in human beings have addressed the assumed protective effect of postmenopausal HRT on the extent of coronary artery atherosclerosis in women.

To date, three autopsy studies have specifically related age at surgical menopause to degree of coronary artery atherosclerosis (5–7). All three reveal a trend toward worsened coronary artery atherosclerosis in women who underwent surgical menopause compared with estrogenic or "hyperestrogenic" women. Unfortunately, only the study comparing women who had undergone bilateral oophorectomy with women who were labeled as "hyperestrogenic" as a result of having developed breast carcinoma demonstrated a statistically significant difference in atherosclerosis extent (1,3).

Two case-control studies and one cross-sectional study related the degree of coronary artery lumen stenosis at coronary angiography to postmenopausal estrogen replacement (8–10). A 56% to 63% reduction in risk for developing severe coronary artery stenosis in women who took postmenopausal estrogen replacement was indicated.

Sullivan et al. (11) assessed the 10-year survival rate of 2,268 menopausal women who had varying degrees of angiographically defined coronary artery atherosclerosis with respect to whether they used estrogen replacement. In women without demonstrable coronary artery atherosclerosis at the initial angiogram, no statistically significant difference was found in the 10-year survival rate of women who never used (85%, *n* = 306) versus ever used (95.6%, *n* = 64) postmenopausal estrogens. However, in women with more than 70% lumen stenosis at the initial angiogram, the 10-year survival rate of "never users" dropped to 60% ($n = 789$) and was significantly less than the 97% 10-year survival rate among "ever users" ($n = 53$; $p = 0.027$).

ANIMAL MODEL STUDIES

Effects of Estrogen on Coronary Artery Atherosclerosis: Overview

This discussion emphasizes coronary arteries because (a) the gender difference in atherosclerosis extent is confined to coronary arteries (1); (b) experimental evidence indicates that effects of sex hormones are confined to coronary arteries and, perhaps, femoral arteries (1,12,13); and (c) effects on coronary arteries are of greatest relevance to coronary heart disease—the major clinical sequela of atherosclerosis in human beings. Effects on aortic atherosclerosis, for example, may be of limited relevance and, in fact, can lead to inappropriate conclusions regarding coronary heart disease.

Some of the initial evidence that estrogen inhibits the progression of coronary artery atherosclerosis came from a series of studies done in the 1950s at the Michael Reese Research Institute. Among the important findings from these studies was the resistance of hens to develop coronary artery atherosclerosis relative to roosters (14). Furthermore, ligation of the hen oviduct, which results in a marked elevation in plasma cholesterol concentration, had no effect on the relative resistance of the hen to atherosclerosis, whereas ovariectomy resulted in a marked exacerbation of atherosclerosis (6). In addition, exogenous estradiol in physiologic doses was found to inhibit progression of atherosclerosis (15) and to promote its regression (16) in this species. Subsequent studies using white Carneau pigeons resulted in similar conclusions regarding inhibitory effects of physiologic doses of estrogen on coronary atherosclerosis (17).

The subject of sex hormones and atherosclerosis received relatively little attention until 1977, when McGill et al. (18) studied the effects of exogenous estrogens on atherosclerosis extent in ovariectomized baboons. These investigators determined that ovariectomy was not associated with increased extent or severity of diet-induced atherosclerosis, nor did they find any significant effects of treatment with either physiologic or pharmacologic estrogen replacement therapy. It is important to note that, unlike many other primate species (including humans), the baboon is relatively resistant to diet-induced hyperlipidemia and atherosclerosis. Furthermore, no sex difference is seen in the extent of diet-induced coronary artery atherosclerosis in baboons.

Cynomolgus Macaque Model

In our laboratory, we have used the cynomolgus macaque to study the effects of reproductive steroids on coronary artery atherosclerosis. This nonhuman primate species has been used in atherosclerosis research for approximately 30 years, principally because of its susceptibility to diet-induced atherosclerotic involvement of main branch coronary arteries. We chose it for our research because, in addition to its susceptibility to atherosclerosis, its reproductive physiology is similar to that of human beings; the female has a 28-day menstrual cycle and circulating sex hormone patterns that are similar to those of women (19). Also, a natural menopause occurs in aged monkeys.

In an initial study of the relationship between endogenous sex steroids and atherosclerosis, we studied cynomolgus macaques fed a moderately atherogenic diet for 30 months containing 40% of calories as fat and 0.4 mg of cholesterol per calorie. There were four experimental groups: males ($n = 15$); intact, nonpregnant females ($n = 23$); surgically postmenopausal (i.e., ovariectomized) females ($n = 21$); and pregnant females ($n = 27$). Total plasma cholesterol and plasma high-density lipoprotein (HDL) cholesterol concentrations and blood pressure were determined periodically. After 30 months, all animals were necropsied and the extent of atherosclerosis (lesion cross-sectional area) was determined morphometrically.

As in a previous study (20), males were found to have more extensive coronary artery atherosclerosis than were intact nonpregnant females (21). Males also had significantly lower plasma HDL cholesterol concentrations and higher systolic blood pressure. Ovariectomy, which results in estrogen deficiency, also resulted in a more atherogenic plasma lipoprotein pattern (decreased plasma HDL cholesterol, an increased total plasma cholesterol concentrations), and a twofold increase in coronary artery atherosclerosis extent (22). The hyperestrogenic state of pregnancy was associated with a marked reduction in extent of coronary artery atherosclerosis (23). In this group of animals, both total plasma cholesterol and HDL cholesterol concentrations were markedly decreased during pregnancy. These findings are summarized in Fig. 33.1.

The results of this study provide indirect evidence regarding the effects of endogenous sex hormones on atherosclerosis extent. Males and ovariectomized females did not differ in regard to coronary artery atherosclerosis extent and also had consistently low plasma estradiol concentrations in the range of 20 pg/mL. Atherosclerosis extent was reduced by approximately one half in intact, nonpregnant females, who had much greater plasma estradiol concentrations, fluctuating in the normal range of 60 to 300 pg/mL depending on time of the menstrual cycle. Relative to these intact females, atherosclerosis extent was reduced by approximately 50% in pregnant females, a group that also showed sustained dramatic elevations in plasma estradiol concentrations in the range of 300 to 1000 pg/mL.

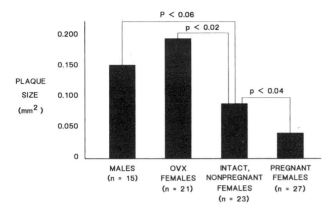

FIG. 33.1. Coronary artery plaque extent (mm²) in four groups of cynomolgus macaques. Although ovariectomized (OVX) females had a far more atherogenic profile, their extent of coronary artery atherosclerosis did not differ from that seen in males. (Adapted from: Kaplan JR, Adams MR, Clarkson TB, et al. Psychosocial influences on female protection among cynomolgus macaques. *Atherosclerosis* 1984;53:283–295; Adams MR, Clarkson TB, Kaplan JR, et al. Ovariectomy, social status, and coronary artery atherosclerosis in cynomolgus monkeys. *Arteriosclerosis* 1985;5: 192–200; and Adams MR, Kaplan JR, Clarkson TB, et al. Pregnancy-associated inhibition of coronary artery atherosclerosis in monkeys: evidence of a relationship with endogenous estrogen. *Arteriosclerosis* 1987;7:378–384.)

Experimental Effects of Hormone Therapy

Direct evidence for an inhibitory effect of endogenous estrogen on progression of coronary artery atherosclerosis is provided by the results of two subsequent studies (24,25). In the first study, ovariectomized monkeys fed an atherogenic diet were assigned randomly to one of three treatment groups: (a) no hormone replacement ($n = 17$), (b) continually administered 17β-estradiol plus cyclically administered progesterone ($n = 20$); and (c) continuously administered 17β-estradiol ($n = 18$). Physiologic patterns of plasma estradiol and progesterone concentrations were maintained by administering the hormones in sustained-release subcutaneous Silastic implants. The experiment lasted 30 months. At necropsy, coronary artery atherosclerosis was inhibited similarly (reduced by approximately one-half) in animals in both hormone replacement groups (Fig. 33.2). Antiatherogenic effects of hormone replacement were independent of variation in total plasma cholesterol, lipoprotein cholesterol, apoprotein A1 and B concentrations, average low-density lipoprotein (LDL) particle size, and HDL subfractional heterogeneity.

Similarly, effects of hormone replacement on atherosclerosis could not be accounted for by other risk variables (e.g., blood pressure or carbohydrate tolerance). This finding suggests that an inhibitory influence of estrogen on atherogenesis and coronary heart disease must be mediated either through other risk factors not measured in this study (or not yet described), or through

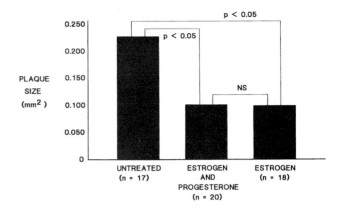

FIG. 33.2. Effect of hormone replacement therapy on coronary artery atherosclerosis extent (mm²) in ovariectomized cynomolgus macaques fed a moderately atherogenic diet. Both hormone therapy groups had half the plaque extent of the untreated group. (Adapted from: Adams MR, Kaplan JR, Manuck SB, et al. Inhibition of coronary artery atherosclerosis by 17-beta estradiol in ovariectomized monkeys. Lack of an effect of added progesterone. *Arteriosclerosis* 1990;10: 1051–1057.)

a direct influence on cellular or biochemical events occurring in the arterial intima.

In a second study (25), ovariectomized monkeys were fed an atherogenic diet and assigned randomly to one of four treatment groups: no treatment ($n = 21$), conjugated equine estrogens (human equivalent of 0.625 mg/day) ($n = 25$), medroxyprogesterone acetate ([MPA]; human equivalent of 2.5 mg/day) ($n = 19$), and conjugated equine estrogens and MPA ($n = 26$). Treatment continued for 30 months. Effects of these treatments on atherosclerosis extent are summarized in Fig. 33.3. Treatment with

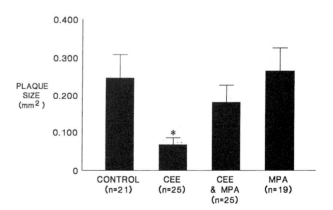

FIG. 33.3. Effects of oral conjugated equine estrogens (CEE), medroxyprogesterone acetate (MPA), and CEE plus MPA on coronary artery atherosclerosis in ovariectomized cynomolgus monkeys. CEE reduced atherosclerosis extent by 70% (*$p = 0.05$). Coadministration of MPA antagonized this effect. (Adapted from: Adams MR, Register TC, Golden DL, et al. Medroxyprogesterone acetate antagonizes inhibitory effects of conjugated equine estrogens on coronary artery atherosclerosis. *Arterioscler Thromb Vasc Biol* 1997;17:217–221.)

conjugated equine estrogens alone resulted in a 70% decrease (p <0.01) in atherosclerosis extent, whereas treatment with MPA alone or MPA in combination with estrogen resulted in atherosclerosis extent that did not differ from that of untreated controls, and it was increased 170% and 290%, respectively, relative to animals treated with estrogen alone (p <0.01) (Fig. 33.3). As in the first study, these effects were largely independent of variation in plasma lipoproteins.

The results of these two studies agree incompletely with the epidemiologic data. The results of the first study are consistent with the protective effect of estrogen monotherapy or combined estrogen and sequential progestin on coronary heart disease (CHD) risk seen in a number of studies (26,27). However, the effects seen in the second study (combined continuous estrogen and MPA) are inconsistent (i.e., atherosclerosis extent is not reduced). One possible explanation for this conflict is that the epidemiologic data for combined HRT represent predominantly data for continuously administered estrogen and sequentially administered (i.e., 7 to 14 days per month) progestin. No data are available that have adequate statistical power to assess the effects of combined continuous therapy, a practice which has become increasingly prevalent in recent years. Our data suggest that this form of therapy may result in increased CHD risk relative to users of estrogen alone or estrogen and sequentially administered progestin.

Our findings also suggest that the inhibitory influences of hormone replacement on atherosclerosis and coronary heart disease are probably mediated through nonlipoprotein risk factors; other risk factors not assessed in our studies; or through direct effects on cellular or biochemical events occurring in the arterial intima. Subsequent studies in our laboratory have addressed the effects of sex hormones on arterial lipoprotein metabolism.

Estrogen Deficiency and Arterial Lipoprotein Metabolism

Rabbit Model

Although the effects of estrogens and progestins on atherosclerosis may be mediated, in part, by beneficial effects on whole-body lipoprotein metabolism (i.e., by reducing lipoprotein levels), evidence also exists that estrogens can directly influence arterial lipoprotein metabolism as well as other cellular and molecular processes associated with early atherogenesis.

One possible mechanism for the protective effect of estrogens is through arterial cholesterol accumulation. Kushwaha and Hazzard (28) found that exogenous estrogen (estradiol cypionate) dramatically reduced (a) dietary hypercholesterolemia, especially in the very low-density lipoprotein (VLDL), (b); intermediate-density lipoprotein (IDL) fractions; and (c) atherosclerosis in rabbits.

However, in some animals fed different amounts of cholesterol to induce similar levels of hypercholesterolemia, estrogen-treated rabbits still had significantly less aortic cholesterol and phospholipid content. A similar finding was made by Haarbo et al. (29), who studied orally administered 17β-estradiol alone or with the contraceptive progestins norethisterone and levonorgestrel in ovariectomized cholesterol-fed rabbits. All hormone replacement therapies significantly reduced total cholesterol, VLDL and IDL cholesterol concentrations, and total aortic cholesterol content. However, as with the study by Kushwaha and Hazzard (28), the reduction in aortic cholesterol accumulation was again found to be independent of serum cholesterol as well as VLDL cholesterol concentration.

Another mechanism for the protective effect of estrogens may be via reduced arterial cholesterol ester influx and hydrolysis. Hough and Zilversmit (30) investigated the effects of estrogen treatment (17β-estradiol cypionate) in cholesterol-fed rabbits on net arterial influx and hydrolysis of plasma cholesteryl ester entering the artery. Although no significant effects were seen on plasma cholesterol concentrations or lipoprotein patterns, estrogen treatment decreased lesion development significantly. Net cholesteryl ester influx, which was positively correlated with the extent of atherosclerosis, was also decreased in estrogen-treated animals. In addition, the percentage of newly entering cholesteryl ester hydrolyzed by the artery was found to be reduced significantly by estrogen treatment independent of the extent of atherosclerosis.

Nonhuman Primate Model

Studies in the rabbit have suggested that estrogen treatment may be decrease arterial lesion formation by directly inhibiting the accumulation or hydrolysis of cholesterol in the arterial wall. To determine the effects of hormone treatment on lipoprotein metabolism in the cynomolgus macaque, we studied LDL coupled to radiolabeled tyramine cellobiose (TC) (31). The labeled TC-LDL, originally described by Pittman et al. (32), allows quantification of the accumulation of products of LDL degradation and undegraded LDL in tissue or arterial samples. When lipoproteins coupled to iodinated tyramine cellobiose are degraded by the cell, the labeled tyramine cellobiose remains trapped in the lysosomes, representing the accumulation of products of LDL degradation and undegraded LDL over time (33,34).

In our laboratory, we studied ovariectomized monkeys fed a moderately atherogenic diet for only 18 weeks to study the effects of hormone treatment on early events in atherogenesis. Estrogen and cyclic progesterone were administered via Silastic implants to one group ($n = 9$), resulting in physiologic hormone concentrations, whereas controls ($n = 8$) had low to undetectable hormone levels. Radiolabeled LDL was injected 24 hours before necropsy

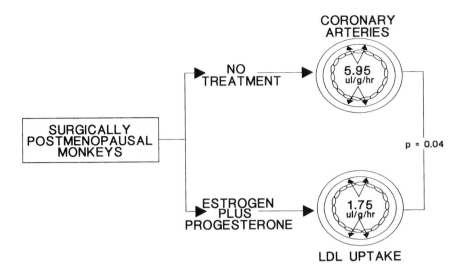

FIG. 33.4. Effect of hormone replacement therapy on arterial uptake of low-density lipoprotein in surgically postmenopausal female cynomolgus macaques fed a moderately atherogenic diet. (Adapted from: Wagner JD, Clarkson TB, St Clair RW, et al. Estrogen and progesterone replacement therapy reduces LDL accumulation in the coronary arteries of surgically postmenopausal cynomolgus monkeys. *J Clin Invest* 1991;88:1995–2002.)

and the whole-body and arterial metabolism was measured. Hormone replacement therapy resulted in significantly reduced accumulation of LDL and products of LDL accumulation in coronary arteries (Fig. 33.4) (31) as well as other arterial sites (34). This occurred despite no significant difference in plasma lipid and lipoprotein concentrations. Furthermore, the reduction in LDL metabolism occurred before any changes in intimal thickening or other indices of endothelial injury had taken place (e.g., increased endothelial cell turnover or numbers of adherent leukocytes to the endothelium).

Studies using both rabbit and monkey models, thus, suggest that estrogen treatment inhibits atherosclerosis independently of changes in plasma lipids and lipoproteins. This effect may be occurring through a number of mechanisms. The study by Hough and Zilversmit (30) and our studies in monkeys (31,34) suggest that estrogen may be acting intracellularly by inhibiting the hydrolysis of cholesterol and degradation of LDL, respectively.

Effects of Estrogen Deficiency on Vasomotor Function in Atherosclerotic Primates

Endothelium and Vasomotor Function

Coronary heart disease develops when blood flow through coronary arteries is no longer sufficient to meet the metabolic demands on the heart. Development of occlusive atherosclerotic plaque or an occlusive mural thrombus can reduce blood flow through coronary arteries, resulting in myocardial ischemia or infarction (35). However, dynamic changes in vascular smooth muscle tone (resulting in vasospasm) also play an important role in narrowing the lumen of atherosclerotic coronary arteries (36). These factors are not entirely independent, and it is likely that interactions between blood elements, the vascular endothelium, various components of the plaque, and the vascular smooth muscle cells are important in the pathogenesis of coronary heart disease.

It has become evident that the endothelium plays a key role in modulating vascular smooth muscle cell reactivity (37,38). Endothelial cells release dilator and constrictor substances, which diffuse to underlying smooth muscle cells and modulate the vascular response of arteries to a wide variety of neurohumoral stimuli (39). Atherosclerosis impairs dilation and augments constriction to platelet products (40) and white blood cell products (41) in arteries of male cynomolgus monkeys. Thus, a consequence of atherosclerosis is a shift in regulatory responses that promote vasoconstriction to cells and cell products (platelets and white blood cells) that are associated with atherosclerotic lesions.

Role of Estrogen

Estrogen and progesterone receptors have been found in arterial endothelial and smooth muscle cells of several species, including human beings (42–44). One study showed that estrogen treatment of baboons results in a redistribution of arterial intercellular estrogen receptors and an increase in the cellular concentration of progesterone receptors (44). These findings imply a role for sex steroids in the regulation of arterial cell function. Other animal studies have shown that estrogen treatment results in reduced lipoprotein-induced arterial smooth muscle cell proliferation (45), inhibited myointimal proliferation associated with mechanical endothelial injury (46–48), reduced arterial cholesterol ester influx and hydrolysis (30), inhibition of platelet aggregation (49), decreased collagen and elastin production (50,51), and increased prostacyclin production by arterial smooth muscle cells (52). Hence, estrogen may inhibit atherogenesis by inhibiting foam cell formation, platelet aggregation, smooth muscle cell proliferation, and the accumulation of collagen and elastin.

Increasing evidence suggests that risk factors for coronary heart disease in women differ from those in men.

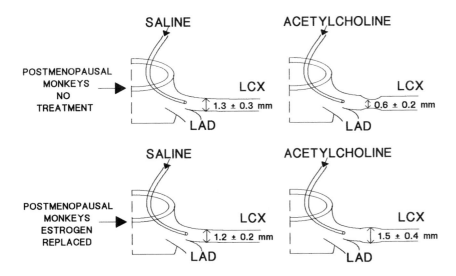

FIG. 33.5. Schematic illustration of effect of estrogen replacement therapy on coronary arteries of surgically postmenopausal cynomolgus macaques. Estrogen therapy prevented the paradoxical arterial dilation to acetylcholine. LAD, left anterior descending artery; LCX, left circumflex artery. (Adapted from: Williams JK, Adams MR, Klopfenstein HS. Estrogen modulates responses of atherosclerotic coronary arteries. *Circulation* 1990;81:1680–1687.)

Although it has been established that patients with atherosclerosis are susceptible to development of coronary vasospasm, particularly at sites of coronary artery stenosis (35,36), such studies have been done only in men or in populations where possible sex differences were not considered. It is known that estrogen replacement therapy in postmenopausal women decreases their risk of CHD, possibly by inhibiting atherogenesis in coronary arteries (53); however, it is likely that estrogen provides major benefits in preventing the clinical expression of CHD unrelated to the extent of coronary artery atherosclerosis. Estrogen modulates vascular responses of arteries at several arterial sites, such as the uterine artery in guinea pigs (54) and the iliac artery in rabbits (55). Preliminary reports by Jiang et al. (56–58) provide evidence that estradiol promotes endothelium-independent dilation of

arteries; it has calcium antagonistic properties; and it attenuates constriction of coronary arteries in rabbits.

The studies mentioned used nonatherosclerotic arteries to examine the effect of estrogen on endothelium-dependent and endothelium-independent vascular responses. Results of our studies using surgically postmenopausal female monkeys with atherosclerosis have shown that subcutaneous administration of estradiol "protects" against impaired endothelium-mediated dilation of atherosclerotic coronary arteries (Fig. 33.5) (59). In addition, the effects of estrogen on vascular responses of atherosclerotic coronary arteries may be rapid. Results of a study by our group (60) indicated that intravenous administration of ethinyl estradiol improved impaired vascular responses of coronary arteries within 20 minutes of administration (Fig. 33.6).

SUMMARY AND CONCLUSIONS

We have reviewed the current evidence concerning the roles of estrogen deficiency and estrogen replacement therapy in atherogenesis, especially in the coronary arteries, and in arterial vasomotor abnormalities. Although it has long been known that women have a lower incidence of coronary heart disease, previous clinical and epidemiologic studies did not investigate possible sex differences in the risk of cardiovascular disease, particularly coronary artery atherosclerosis.

Early experimental models of estrogen-deficient animals with coronary artery atherosclerosis used chickens and pigeons. However, because of greater similarities to human beings these nonhuman primate models have replaced these earlier models. Our studies have focused on the female cynomolgus macaque, especially surgically postmenopausal (i.e., estrogen-deficient) animals fed an atherogenic diet. We found that male and ovariectomized female cynomolgus macaques did not differ with respect to coronary artery atherosclerosis, whereas premenopausal

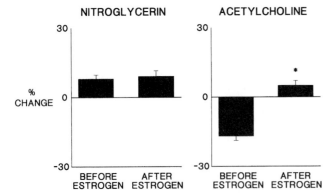

FIG. 33.6. Percentage of change in vascular responses of surgically postmenopausal cynomolgus macaques to nitroglycerin and acetylcholine, both before and after intravenous injection of ethinyl estradiol. *$p < 0.05$ versus before estrogen treatment. (Adapted from: Williams JK, Adams MR, Herrington DM, et al. Effects of short-term estrogen treatment on vascular responses of coronary arteries. *J Am Coll Cardiol* 1992;20:452–457.)

females had half the coronary artery atherosclerosis of their counterparts. In two studies of HRT of ovariectomized cynomolgus macaques, we discovered that estrogen replacement therapy, either parenteral estradiol or oral conjugated equine estrogens, resulted in 50% to 70% reductions in the extent of coronary artery atherosclerosis. However, although combined hormone replacement with continuously administered parenteral estradiol and sequentially administered progesterone resulted in a 50% reduction in atherosclerosis extent, treatment with combined continuous orally administered conjugated equine estrogens and MPA resulted in atherosclerosis extent that did not differ from untreated controls. These results indicate that effects of progestins, when given with estrogen, on coronary arteries may depend on type, dose, route of administration, or pattern (continuous vs. sequential) of administration and that some forms of progestin cotherapy may antagonize favorable effects of estrogen.

Subsequent experiments looked at the effects of estrogen treatment on early atherogenesis and found that estrogen inhibited atherosclerosis independent of changes in plasma lipids and lipoproteins. Results of recent studies focusing on estrogen's effects on coronary artery vasodilation have indicated that estrogen seems to improve endothelium-mediated vascular responses, although the mechanisms by which it does so require further study.

ACKNOWLEDGMENTS

This work was supported in part by grants HL-38964 and HL-45666 and by contract No. HV-53029, National Heart, Lung and Blood Institute, National Institutes of Health, Bethesda, Maryland.

REFERENCES

1. McGill HC Jr., Stern MP. Sex and atherosclerosis. *Atherosclerosis Rev* 1979; 4:157–242.
2. Adams MR, Kaplan JR, Clarkson TB, et al. Effects of psychosocial stress, menopause and pregnancy on coronary artery atherosclerosis. In: Eaker ED, Packard B, Wenger NK, et al., eds. *Coronary heart disease in women.* New York: Haymarket Doyma, 1987:151–157.
3. Bush TL. The epidemiology of cardiovascular disease in postmenopausal women. *Ann NY Acad Sci* 1990;592:263–271.
4. Barrett-Connor E, Bush TL. Estrogen and coronary heart disease in women. *JAMA* 1991;265:1861–1867.
5. Wuest JH, Dry TJ, Edwards JE. The degree of coronary atherosclerosis in bilaterally oophorectomized women. *Circulation* 1953;7:801–809.
6. Rivin AU, Dimitroff SP. The incidence and severity of atherosclerosis in estrogen-treated males, and in females with a hypoestrogenic or a hyperestrogenic state. *Circulation* 1954;9:533–539.
7. Novak ER, Williams TJ. Autopsy comparison of cardiovascular changes in castrated and normal women. *Am J Obstet Gynecol* 1966;80:863–872.
8. Sullivan JM, Vander Zwaag R, Lemp GF, et al. Postmenopausal estrogen use and coronary atherosclerosis. *Ann Intern Med* 1988;108:358–363.
9. McFarland KF, Boniface ME, Hornung CA, et al. Risk factors and noncontraceptive estrogen use in women with and without coronary disease. *Am Heart J* 1989; 117:1209–1214.
10. Gruchow HW, Anderson AJ, Barboriak JJ, et al. Postmenopausal use of estrogen and occlusion of coronary arteries. *Am Heart J* 1988;115:954–963.
11. Sullivan JM, Vander Zwaag R, Hughes JP, et al. Estrogen replacement and coronary artery disease. Effect on survival in postmenopausal women. *Arch Intern Med* 1990;150:2557–2562.
12. Adams MR, Clarkson TB, Koritnik DR, et al. Contraceptive steroids and coronary artery atherosclerosis in cynomolgus macaques. *Fertil Steril* 1987;47:1010–1018.
13. Clarkson TB, Shively CA, Morgan TM, et al. Oral contraceptives and coronary artery atherosclerosis of cynomolgus monkeys. *Obstet Gynecol* 1990;75:217–222.
14. Stamler J, Pick R, Katz LN. Inhibition of cholesterol-induced coronary atherogenesis in the egg-producing hen. *Circulation* 1954;10:251–254.
15. Pick R, Stamler J, Rodbard S, et al. The inhibition of coronary atherosclerosis by estrogens in cholesterol-fed chicks. *Circulation* 1952;6:276–280.
16. Pick R, Stamler J, Rodbard S, et al. Estrogen-induced regression of coronary atherosclerosis in cholesterol-fed chicks. *Circulation* 1952;6:858–861.
17. Prichard RW, Clarkson TB, Lofland HB. Estrogen in pigeon atherosclerosis. Estradiol valerate effects at several dose levels on cholesterol-fed male white Carneau pigeons. *Arch Pathol* 1966;82:15–17.
18. McGill HC Jr, Axelrod LR, McMahan CA, et al. Estrogens and experimental atherosclerosis in the baboon (Papio cynocephalus). *Circulation* 1977;56:657–662.
19. Hamm TE Jr, Kaplan JR, Koritnik DR. Psychosocial influences on ovarian endocrine and ovulatory function in cynomolgus monkeys (Macaca fascicularis). *Physiol Behav* 1985;35:935–940.
20. Hamm TE Jr, Kaplan JR, Clarkson TB, et al. Effects of gender and social behavior on the development of coronary artery atherosclerosis in cynomolgus monkeys. *Atherosclerosis* 1983;48:221–233.
21. Kaplan JR, Adams MR, Clarkson TB, et al. Psychosocial influences on female protection among cynomolgus macaques. *Atherosclerosis* 1984;53:283–295.
22. Adams MR, Clarkson TB, Kaplan JR, et al. Ovariectomy, social status, and coronary artery atherosclerosis in cynomolgus monkeys. *Arteriosclerosis* 1985;5:192–200.
23. Adams MR, Kaplan JR, Clarkson TB, et al. Pregnancy-associated inhibition of coronary artery atherosclerosis in monkeys: evidence of a relationship with endogenous estrogen. *Arteriosclerosis* 1987;7:378–384.
24. Adams MR, Kaplan JR, Manuck SB, et al. Inhibition of coronary artery atherosclerosis by 17-beta estradiol in ovariectomized monkeys. Lack of an effect of added progesterone. *Arteriosclerosis* 1990;10:1051–1057.
25. Adams MR, Register TC, Golden DL, et al. Medroxyprogesterone acetate antagonizes inhibitory effects of conjugated equine estrogens on coronary artery atherosclerosis. *Arterioscler Thromb Vasc Biol* 1997;17:217–221.
26. Psaty B, Heckbert S, Atkins, D, et al. The risk of myocardial infarction associated with the combined use of estrogens and progestins in postmenopausal women. *Arch Intern Med* 1994;133–1339.
27. Grodstein F, Stampfer MJ, Manson JE, et al. Postmenopausal estrogen and progestin use and the risk of cardiovascular disease. *N Engl J Med* 1996;335: 453–461.
28. Kushwaha RS, Hazzard WR. Exogenous estrogens attenuate dietary hypercholesterolemia and atherosclerosis in the rabbit. *Metabolism* 1981;30:359–366.
29. Haarbo J, Leth-Espensen P, Stender S, et al. Estrogen monotherapy and combined estrogen–progestogen replacement therapy attenuate aortic accumulation of cholesterol in ovariectomized cholesterol-fed rabbits. *J Clin Invest* 1991;87:1274–1279.
30. Hough JL, Zilversmit DB. Effect of 17-beta estradiol on aortic cholesterol content and metabolism in cholesterol-fed rabbits. *Atherosclerosis* 1986;6:57–63.
31. Wagner JD, Clarkson TB, St Clair RW, et al. Estrogen and progesterone replacement therapy reduces LDL accumulation in the coronary arteries of surgically postmenopausal cynomolgus monkeys. *J Clin Invest* 1991;88:1995–2002.
32. Pittman RC, Carew TE, Glass CK, et al. A radioiodinated, intracellularly trapped ligand for determining the sites of plasma protein degradation in vivo. *Biochem J* 1983;212:791–800.
33. Carew TC, Pittman RC, Marchand ER, et al. Measurement in vivo of irreversible degradation of low density lipoprotein in the rabbit aorta. Predominance of intimal degradation. *Arteriosclerosis* 1984;4:214–224.
34. Wagner JD, St Clair RW, Schwenke DC, et al. Regional differences in arterial low density lipoprotein metabolism in surgically postmenopausal cynomolgus monkeys: effects of estrogen and progesterone replacement therapy. *Arterioscler Thromb Vasc Biol* 1992;12:716–723.
35. Maseri A, Severi S, De Nes M, et al. "Variant" angina: one aspect of a continuous spectrum of vasospastic myocardial ischemia. Pathogenetic mechanisms, estimated incidence and clinical and coronary arteriographic findings in 138 patients. *Am J Cardiol* 1978;42:1019–1035.
36. Ludmer PL, Selwyn AP, Shook TL, et al. Paradoxical vasoconstriction induced by acetylcholine in atherosclerotic coronary arteries. *N Engl J Med* 1986;315: 1046–1051.
37. Furchgott RF, Zawadski JV. The obligatory role of endothelial cells in the relaxation of arterial smooth muscle by acetylcholine. *Nature* 1980;288:373–376.
38. Vanhoutte PM. Endothelium and responsiveness of vascular smooth muscle. *J Hyperten* 1987;5(Suppl 5):S115–S120.
39. Vanhoutte PM. Endothelium-dependent contractions in arteries and veins. *Blood Vessels* 1987;24:141–144.
40. Lopez JA, Armstrong ML, Piegors DJ, et al. Effect of early and advanced atherosclerosis on vascular responses to serotonin, thromboxane A2, and ADP. *Circulation* 1989;79:698–705.
41. Lopez JA, Armstrong ML, Harrison PG, et al. Vascular responses to leukocyte products in atherosclerotic primates. *Circ Res* 1989;65:1078–1086.
42. Ingegno MD, Money SR, Thelmo W, et al. Progesterone receptors in the human heart and great vessels. *Lab Invest* 1988;59:353–356.
43. Lin AL, McGill HC Jr, Shain SA. Hormone receptors of the baboon cardiovascular system. *Circ Res* 1982;50:610–616.
44. Lin AL, Gonzalez R Jr, Carey KD, et al. Estradiol-17 beta affects estrogen receptor distribution and elevates progesterone receptor content in baboon aorta. *Arteriosclerosis* 1986;6:495–504.
45. Fischer-Dzoga K, Wissler RW, Vesselinovitch D. The effect of estradiol on the pro-

liferation of rabbit aortic medial tissue culture cells induced by hyperlipemic serum. *Exp Mol Pathol* 1983;39:355–363.

46. Rhee CY, Spaet TH, Gaynor E, et al. Suppression of surgically induced vascular intimal hypertrophy by estrogen. *Circulation* 1974;49(Suppl III):III-92.

47. Rhee CY, Drouet RO, Spaet TH, et al. Growth inhibition of cultured vascular smooth muscle cells by estradiol. *Fed Proc* 1978;37:474.

48. Weigensberg BI, Lough H, More MH, et al. Effects of estradiol on myointimal thickening from catheter injury and on organizing white mural nonocclusive thrombi. *Atherosclerosis* 1984;52:253–265.

49. Johnson M, Ramey E, Ramwell PW. Androgen-mediated sensitivity in platelet aggregation. *Am J Physiol* 1977;232:H381–H385.

50. Fischer GM. In vivo effects of estradiol on collagen and elastin dynamics in rat aorta. *Endocrinology* 1972;91:1227–1232.

51. Beldekas JC, Smith B, Geistenfeld LC. Effects of 17-beta estradiol on the biosynthesis of collagen in cultured bovine aortic smooth muscle cells. *Biochemistry* 1981;20:2161–2167.

52. Chang W-C, Nakao J, Orimo H, et al. Stimulation of prostacyclin activity by estradiol in rat aorta smooth muscle cell in culture. *Biochim Biophys Acta* 1980;619: 107–118.

53. Godsland IF, Wynn V, Crook D, et al. Sex, plasma lipoproteins, and atherosclero-sis: prevailing assumptions and outstanding questions. *Am Heart J* 1987;114: 1467–1503.

54. Bell C, Coffey C. Factors influencing estrogen-induced sensitization to acetylcholine of guinea-pig uterine artery. *J Reprod Fertil* 1982;66:133–137.

55. Gisclard V, Miller VM, Vanhoutte PM. Effect of 17 beta-estradiol on endothelium-dependent responses in the rabbit. *J Pharmacol Exp Ther* 1988;244:19–22.

56. Jiang C, Sarrel PM, Lindsay DC, et al. 17-Beta estradiol inhibits contraction in isolated rabbit coronary artery by an EDRF-independent mechanism. *Circulation* 1990;82(Suppl III):III-489.

57. Jiang C, Sarrel PM, Lindsay DC, et al. 17 Beta-estradiol has calcium antagonistic properties in the rabbit coronary artery in vitro. *Circulation* 1991;84(Suppl II):II-272.

58. Jiang C, Sarrel PM, Collins P. Attenuation of endothelin-1 induced rabbit coronary artery contraction by 17 beta-estradiol. *Circulation* 1991;84(Suppl II):II-272.

59. Williams JK, Adams MR, Klopfenstein HS. Estrogen modulates responses of atherosclerotic coronary arteries. *Circulation* 1990;81:1680–1687.

60. Williams JK, Adams MR, Herrington DM, et al. Effects of short-term estrogen treatment on vascular responses of coronary arteries. *J Am Coll Cardiol* 1992; 20:452–457.

Treatment of the Postmenopausal Woman: Basic and Clinical Aspects, Second Edition, edited by Rogerio A. Lobo, Lippincott Williams & Wilkins, Philadelphia © 1999.

CHAPTER 34

Estrogen—Blood Flow and Vasomotion

Peter Collins

Many epidemiologic studies suggest that estrogen replacement can protect the vascular system in postmenopausal women. To date, no randomized trials have confirmed this benefit. However, a body of research has now confirmed that estrogen, probably via its nuclear receptor, can increase the production of nitric oxide (NO) from the vascular endothelium by stimulating the enzyme NO synthase. This effect is important because the postmenopausal state is associated with a decrease in endothelial function. By enhancing this pathway, blood flow autoregulation can be normalized and may result in vascular protection. Other direct and indirect mechanisms may exist whereby estrogen can affect vascular reactivity and, therefore, blood flow control. This chapter primarily presents evidence that estrogen can affect blood flow by both endothelium and non-endothelium dependent mechanisms, and briefly discusses their possible relevance in some pathophysiologic settings in humans.

CORONARY CIRCULATION—INDIRECT, ENDOTHELIUM-DEPENDENT EFFECTS

In ovariectomized cynomolgus monkeys, long-term (2 years) (1) estrogen replacement therapy reverses acetylcholine-induced constriction in atherosclerotic coronary arteries; a similar effect is produced with a 20-minute intravenous infusion of ethinyl estradiol (2). These animal data have been reproduced in postmenopausal women with coronary atherosclerosis. Estrogen attenuates (3) or abolishes (4,5) acetylcholine-induced vasoconstriction when administered acutely (15 to 20 minutes after bolus or continuous intracoronary infusion) in postmenopausal women, resulting in increased coronary diameter and

blood flow. This response of the coronary arteries to acetylcholine after exposure to 17β-estradiol appears to be gender dependent (5). A 20-minute exposure to 17β-estradiol modulated acetylcholine-induced responses of female but not male atherosclerotic coronary arteries *in vivo* (5). Prolonged, physiologic estrogen replacement has also been shown to influence endothelium-dependent and endothelium-independent coronary responsiveness to acetylcholine (6). Estrogen replacement therapy was associated with both an attenuation or reversal of the coronary vasoconstrictor response and a potentiation of the blood flow response to acetylcholine in postmenopausal women. This suggests normalization of an endothelium-dependent mechanism in diseased coronary vessels, which is in agreement with the effect of acutely administered estrogen. Evidence that this effect is caused by NO has been provided by Guetta et al. (7). Physiologic concentrations of estrogen were infused into the coronary arteries of estrogen-deficient women, most of whom had coronary atherosclerosis. Estradiol increased acetylcholine-stimulated blood flow; however, this was abolished after an infusion of the NO synthase inhibitor N^G-monomethyl-L-arginine (L-NMMA).

Estrogen can induce calcium-dependent nitric oxide synthase (8). Basal release of NO was greater in endothelium-intact aortic rings from female rabbits when compared with those from male rabbits (9). A study in humans has shown variation in expired NO production with cyclical hormone changes in premenopausal women, with NO levels peaking at the middle of the menstrual cycle (10), which suggests an influence of gonadal hormones on its synthesis and release in humans. Using serum nitrite or nitrate levels in postmenopausal women taking hormone therapy (transdermal estradiol and sequential norethesterone acetate) for 6, 12, and 18 months, it was demonstrated that both estrogen and combined therapy significantly increased serum nitrite and nitrate levels. These results suggest that hormone therapy

P. Collins: Department of Cardiac Medicine, National Heart & Lung Institute, Imperial College School of Medicine, and Royal Brompton Hospital, London SW3 6LY, United Kingdom.

increases NO levels in postmenopausal women. Use of acetylcholine-induced forearm blood flow responses and L-NMMA suggested that estrogen can enhance the release of basal NO in the forearm vasculature of perimenopausal women (11).

The effect of estrogen on endothelial NO production may be dependent on the classical estrogen receptor. The receptor has been demonstrated in normal coronary arteries, however, variable expression is seen in atherosclerotic coronary arteries from premenopausal women (12). Recent studies using specific monoclonal antibodies and nuclear probes have confirmed the presence of a classical estrogen receptor in cultured human umbilical, aortic, and coronary artery endothelial cells (13,14). A novel estrogen receptor has been cloned in rat prostate, which is termed "estrogen-receptor-beta," (ER-β) (15). This receptor was also found in the ovary and had high affinity to 17β-estradiol. At present no such receptor has been identified in human tissue, but this finding raises the possibility of cardiac or vascular-specific estrogen receptors may be involved in the modulation of vascular responses to estrogen (16).

CORONARY CIRCULATION—DIRECT VASCULAR SMOOTH MUSCLE EFFECTS

Estrogen induces dilation of conductance and resistance in coronary arteries, albeit at supraphysiologic concentrations (> 0.1 μmol/L), in dogs when administered acutely into the coronary circulation (17). By removing the endothelium and using inhibitors of both adenosine triphosphate-sensitive potassium channels and calcium channels, this effect was shown to be endothelium independent. This effect is mediated by effects on adenosine triphosphate-sensitive potassium or calcium channels, and the estrogen receptor is not involved in this acute response. *In vitro* experiments have confirmed that estrogen can affect calcium channels (18,19), large conductance chloride channels (20), and large-conductance calcium and voltage-activated potassium channels (BK_{Ca}) (21). All these mechanisms may contribute to the direct vascular smooth muscle relaxing effect of estrogen.

PERIPHERAL CIRCULATION ENDOTHELIUM-DEPENDENT EFFECTS

The role of endogenous ovarian hormones in modulating peripheral vasoreactivity has been studied in premenopausal women (22). Endothelium-dependent vasodilation, induced by hyperemia, varied significantly with the phase of the menstrual cycle: flow-mediated increases in brachial artery diameter were less during the menstrual phase of the cycle (when serum estradiol levels were low) than in the follicular or luteal phase of the cycle (when serum estradiol levels were elevated). These data suggest that endogenous estradiol may be involved in mediating variations in the endothelium-dependent brachial artery with the menstrual cycle. This emphasizes an effect of ovarian hormones at physiologic plasma levels and confirms similar findings with estrogen treatment.

In postmenopausal women forearm vasodilation induced by acetylcholine is potentiated by the acute local administration of intravenous estradiol (23), suggesting that endothelium-dependent responses in the peripheral circulation may be modulated by steroid hormones in vivo in humans. Estrogen increases flow-mediated vasodilation in the brachial artery of postmenopausal women (24).

A few studies have also shown a beneficial effect of estrogen therapy in male to female transsexuals (25). Vascular function was assessed using brachial artery reactivity. It was shown that high doses of a variety of different estrogens over long periods of time (at least 5 months [25] or 6 months to 21 years [26]) increased flow-mediated dilation of the brachial artery in transsexuals compared with age-matched healthy male controls.

PERIPHERAL CIRCULATION— ENDOTHELIUM-DEPENDENT EFFECTS— THE INFLUENCE OF PROGESTINS

The question of what happens when estrogen is combined with a progestin is an important one because of reports in animal models that certain progestins can reverse the beneficial effects of estrogen on blood flow responses and atheroma development, but others do not. Some studies have shown a detrimental effect of medroxyprogesterone acetate on the beneficial effects of estrogens with regard to atheroma development (27,28) and coronary vascular reactivity (29,30). Other studies have shown that progesterone does not appear to have this inhibitory effect on either atheroma development (31,32) or coronary vascular reactivity in animal models (30,33) or on vascular reactivity (34) and exercise-induced myocardial ischemia in humans (35).

In a recent chronic study, estradiol added to micronized progesterone in postmenopausal women did not attenuate the favorable effect of estradiol on endothelium-dependent vasodilation (34). Similarly, women treated with gonadotrophin-releasing hormone agonists who were given "add-back" continuous oral estradiol and norethisterone acetate showed an improvement of flow-mediated brachial artery reactivity compared with those women who did not receive hormone therapy (36). In a less well-controlled study, the combination of oral estrogen and sequential norethisterone did not appear to enhance endothelium-dependent vasomotor function (37). More studies using different progestins, routes of administration, and doses are required before any general conclusions can be made about combined hormone therapy and its effects on the vascular system.

PERIPHERAL CIRCULATION— PROBABLE DIRECT VASCULAR SMOOTH MUSCLE EFFECTS

In the estrogen depleted state, local and systemic administration of 17β-estradiol has actions on both reproductive and non-reproductive vascular beds (38). The effect of estrogen administration on systemic hemodynamics has been studied in postmenopausal women. Forty minutes after the administration of sublingual 17β-estradiol to postmenopausal volunteers, forearm blood flow was increased and forearm vascular resistance was reduced compared with placebo, with no difference in mean arterial blood pressure noted (39). Relatively high plasma levels of 17β-estradiol (≈ 3,000 pmol/L) were achieved in these women (midcycle level ≈ 1,800 pmol/L); however, the plasma levels are approximately 50% of those found in pregnant women. Similar changes in blood flow have been demonstrated in the blood supply to the leg (40).

Aortic peak flow velocity gradually decreases with time since the onset of the menopause (41), and a significant increase is seen in aortic flow velocity and acceleration after 10 weeks of sequential conjugated equine estrogens medroxyprogesterone acetate (42).

Decreases in arterial waveform pulsatility index in the uterine and carotid arteries have been observed in postmenopausal women after chronic estrogen therapy (43). An increased pulsatility index is closely correlated with the time elapsed after the menopause, and this increase is thought to indicate a reduction in arterial compliance, which, therefore, could reflect a decrease in blood flow. Estrogen therapy reverses increased pulsatility index, suggesting an improvement in arterial compliance.

Another indirect influence on blood flow may involve the parasympathetic and sympathetic nervous systems. The balance of these two systems in the estrogen-deficient postmenopausal woman is in favor of sympathetic overactivity, which could result in impairment of blood flow control. Postmenopausal women have increased basal levels of plasma noradrenaline compared with premenopausal women (44). These increased pressor and neurohormonal responses in postmenopausal women are partially inhibited by estrogen (44). Greater parasympathetic activity in normal women, when compared with men, has been demonstrated by measurement of heart rate variability (45). Sympathetic activity is increased in healthy estrogen-depleted postmenopausal women. Heart rate variability—an indicator of sympathetic activity—is favorably influenced by estrogen therapy (46).

Estrogen also favorably affects the renin–angiotensin system in postmenopausal women (47), and inhibits the effect of the constrictor responses to endothelin-1 (48). These mechanisms may contribute to an overall vasodilator response to estrogen *in vivo*.

CEREBROVASCULAR CIRCULATION

Estrogen status affects the reactivity of cerebral arteries to vasoactive stimuli. Using hormone manipulation in rabbits, estrogen withdrawal selectively increased serotonin reactivity in rabbit basilar arteries (49). Basilar artery segments from chronically oophorectomized animals treated with estrogen, which were subsequently acutely estrogen withdrawn, showed an extremely heightened sensitivity to the vasoconstrictor response to serotonin. This effect may be similar to that in postmenopausal women on hormone replacement who sustain acute estrogen withdrawal, or that associated with estrogen surges in perimenopausal women.

Vascular reactivity changes in the central retinal and ophthalmic arteries can be correlated with estrogen status in pregnant and postmenopausal women (50). Gender differences related to estrogen are also seen in cerebral blood flow. Until the menopause, cerebral blood flow is greater in women than men of the same age (51); however, after menopause, cerebral blood flow decreases in women and remains the same in age-matched males (52). Estrogen therapy in postmenopausal women reduces resistance in the internal carotid (43,53) and middle cerebral arteries (53). Cerebral blood flow is also increased in pregnancy when estrogen levels are substantially increased (54). Velocity changes in the middle cerebral artery have been studied during controlled ovarian hyperstimulation after pituitary suppression (55). Estrogen levels directly correlated with middle cerebral artery velocity and resistance. It was hypothesized that microcirculatory dilation occurs distal to the middle cerebral artery. Estrogenic effects have been identified in smaller vessels (e.g., the central retinal artery) (50).

POTENTIAL THERAPEUTIC BENEFIT OF THE BLOOD FLOW EFFECTS OF ESTROGEN IN THE CARDIOVASCULAR SYSTEM

Myocardial Ischemia

Estrogen-induced reduction in vascular resistance and increases in coronary flow may have clinical implications with regard to exercise-induced myocardial ischemia, wherein coronary stenoses can become flow limiting. Rosano et al. (56) demonstrated a beneficial effect of acute administration of sublingual 17β-estradiol versus placebo on signs of exercise-induced myocardial ischemia on the electrocardiogram (time to 1 mm ST-segment depression) and exercise tolerance in postmenopausal women. Patients with low plasma 17β-estradiol levels generally had a greater response to 17β-estradiol. Plasma levels achieved in this study were approximately 2,500 pmol/L, which is above the peak level found at midcycle (midcycle level ≈1,800 pmol/L) and about one-third of the level found in pregnancy. This effect may result from a direct relaxing effect on the coronary arteries (57), peripheral vasodilation (39), or a combination of the two. Further confirmation of a beneficial effect of acutely administered conjugated estrogen on myocardial ischemia in postmenopausal women with coronary heart disease has been provided by Alpaslan et al. (58). This group investigated the effect of intravenous estrogen on myocardial function using dobutamine stress echocardiography, and showed an improvement in ischemic endpoints after estrogen, compared with placebo, infusion. An anti-ischemic effect of acute sublingual estrogen in postmenopausal women has been demonstrated at physiologic plasma estrogen levels using coronary sinus pH measurements during atrial pacing-induced myocardial ischemia (59). The question of longer-term treatment has recently been addressed. Treatment for 4 and 8 weeks with transdermal 17β-estradiol improves exercise time to myocardial ischemia in postmenopausal women with documented coronary heart disease (60). In this study, the plasma levels of estrogen were within the expected range for postmenopausal estrogen treatment.

Cardiologic Syndrome X

Angina pectoris is usually caused by obstructive atheromatous coronary artery disease; however, angiographically smooth coronary arteries are found in approximately 20% of patients who undergo coronary angiography (61) and most of these patients are women. The triad of angina pectoris, a positive exercise test, and angiographically smooth coronary arteries is commonly referred to as "syndrome X," a term first used by Kemp et al. in 1973 (62). The pathophysiology of the troublesome chest pain in syndrome X is poorly understood, and many mechanisms are suggested to cause it (63–65). Although syndrome X is likely to be a heterogeneous condition, reduced coronary flow reserve induced by dipyridamole has been reported in many patients with this diagnosis (64,66). Most of the women with syndrome X are postmenopausal (67). A recent study that investigated the clinical and gynecologic features of patients with syndrome X found that ovarian hormone deficiency played a role in unmasking the syndrome in these patients (68). Estrogen therapy may be helpful in the treatment of this condition by decreasing the occurrence of chest pain (69). No effect was seen on exercise tolerance, however, which may be because only a small number of patients with syndrome X suffer true myocardial ischemia.

CONCLUSIONS

A wealth of data now shows that estrogen enhances blood flow and has beneficial effects on blood vessel walls in a variety of vascular beds in humans. Many epidemiologic studies suggest a cardioprotective effect of estrogen in postmenopausal women. Well-designed clinical trials are required to confirm or refute this potential benefit.

REFERENCES

1. Williams JK, Adams MR, Klopfenstein HS. Estrogen modulates responses of atherosclerotic coronary arteries. *Circulation* 1990;81:1680–1687.
2. Williams JK, Adams MR, Herrington DM, Clarkson TB. Short-term administration of estrogen and vascular responses of atherosclerotic coronary arteries. *J Am Coll Cardiol* 1992;20:452–457.
3. Reis SE, Gloth ST, Blumenthal RS, et al. Ethinyl estradiol acutely attenuates abnormal coronary vasomotor responses to acetylcholine in postmenopausal women. *Circulation* 1994;89:52–60.
4. Gilligan DM, Quyyumi AA, Cannon RO III. Effects of physiological levels of estrogen on coronary vasomotor function in postmenopausal women. *Circulation* 1994;89:2545–2551.
5. Collins P, Rosano GMC, Sarrel PM, et al. Estradiol–17β attenuates acetylcholine–induced coronary arterial constriction in women but not men with coronary heart disease. *Circulation* 1995;92:24–30.
6. Herrington DM, Braden GA, Williams JK, Morgan TM. Endothelial-dependent coronary vasomotor responsiveness in postmenopausal women with and without estrogen replacement therapy. *Am J Cardiol* 1994;73:951–952.
7. Guetta V, Quyyumi AA, Prasad A, Panza JA, Waclawiw M, Cannon RO III. The role of nitric oxide in coronary vascular effects of estrogen in postmenopausal women. *Circulation* 1997;96:2795–2801.
8. Weiner CP, Lizasoain I, Baylis SA, Knowles RG, Charles IG, Moncada S. Induction of calcium-dependent nitric oxide synthases by sex hormones. *Proc Natl Acad Sci U S A* 1994;91:5212–5216.
9. Hayashi T, Fukuto JM, Ignarro LJ, Chaudhuri G. Basal release of nitric oxide from aortic rings is greater in female rabbits than in male rabbits: implications for atherosclerosis. *Proc Natl Acad Sci U S A* 1992;89:11259–11263.
10. Kharitonov SA, Logan-Sinclair RB, Busset CM, Shinebourne EA. Peak expiratory nitric oxide differences in men and women: relation to the menstrual cycle. *Br Heart J* 1994;72:243–245.
11. Sudhir K, Jennings GL, Funder JW, Komesaroff PA. Estrogen enhances basal nitric oxide release in the forearm vasculature in perimenopausal women. *Hypertension* 1996;28:330–334.
12. Losordo DW, Kearney M, Kim EA, Jekanowski J, Isner JM. Variable expression of the estrogen receptor in normal and atherosclerotic coronary arteries of premenopausal women. *Circulation* 1994;89:1501–1510.
13. Venkov CD, Rankin AB, Vaughan DE. Identification of authentic estrogen receptor in cultured endothelial cells. A potential mechanism for steroid hormone regulation of endothelial function. *Circulation* 1996;94:727–733.
14. Kim-Schulze S, McGowan KA, Hubchak SC, et al. Expression of an estrogen receptor by human coronary artery and umbilical vein endothelial cells. *Circulation* 1996;94:1402–1407.
15. Kuiper GG, Enmark E, Pelto-Huikko M, Nilsson S, Gustafsson JA. Cloning of a novel receptor expressed in rat prostate and ovary. *Proc Natl Acad Sci U S A* 1996;93:5925–5930.
16. Gustafsson JA. Estrogen receptor beta—getting in on the action? *Nat Med* 1997;3:493–494.
17. Sudhir K, Chou TM, Mullen WL, Hausmann D, Collins P, Yock PG, Chatterjee K. Mechanisms of estrogen-induced vasodilation: in vivo studies in canine coronary conductance and resistance arteries. *J Am Coll Cardiol* 1995;26(3):807–814.
18. Jiang C, Sarrel PM, Lindsay DC, Poole-Wilson PA, Collins P. Endothelium-independent relaxation of rabbit coronary artery by 17-oestradiol in vitro. *Br J Pharmacol* 1991;104:1033–1037.
19. Jiang C, Poole-Wilson PA, Sarrel PM, Mochizuki S, Collins P, MacLeod KT. Effect of 17β-oestradiol on contraction, Ca^{2+} current and intracellular free Ca^{2+} in guinea-pig isolated cardiac myocytes. *Br J Pharmacol* 1992;106:739–745.
20. Hardy SP, Valverde MA. Novel plasma membrane action of estrogen and antiestrogens revealed by their regulation of a large conductance chloride channel. *FASEB J* 1994;8:760–765.
21. White RE, Darkow DJ, Lang JL. Estrogen relaxes coronary arteries by opening BKCa channels through a cGMP-dependent mechanism. *Circ Res* 1995;77:936–942.
22. Hashimoto M, Akishita M, Eto M, et al. Modulation of endothelium-dependent flow-mediated dilatation of the brachial artery by sex and menstrual cycle. *Circulation* 1995;92:3431–3435.
23. Gilligan DM, Badar DM, Panza JA, Quyyumi AA, Cannon RO III. Acute vascular effects of estrogen in postmenopausal women. *Circulation* 1994;90:786–791.
24. Lieberman EH, Gerhard MD, Uehata A, et al. Estrogen improves endothelium-dependent, flow-mediated vasodilation in postmenopausal women. *Ann Intern Med* 1994;121:936–941.
25. New G, Timmins KL, Duffy SJ, Tran BT, O'Brien RC, Harper RW, Meredith IT. Long-term estrogen therapy improves vascular function in male to female transsexuals. *J Am Coll Cardiol* 1997;29:1437–1444.
26. McCrohon JA, Walters WA, Robinson JT, et al. Arterial reactivity is enhanced in genetic males taking high dose estrogens. *J Am Coll Cardiol* 1997;29:1432–1436.
27. Adams MR, Register TC, Golden DL, Wagner JD, Williams JK. Medroxyprogesterone acetate antagonizes inhibitory effects of conjugated equine estrogens on coronary artery atherosclerosis. *Arterioscler Thromb Vasc Biol* 1997;17:217–221.
28. Levine RL, Chen SJ, Durand J, Chen YF, Oparil S. Medroxyprogesterone attenuates estrogen-mediated inhibition of neointima formation after balloon injury of the rat carotid artery. *Circulation* 1996;94:2221–2227.
29. Williams JK, Honore EK, Washburn SA, Clarkson TB. Effects of hormone

replacement therapy on reactivity of atherosclerotic coronary arteries in cynomolgus monkeys. *J Am Coll Cardiol* 1994;24:1757–1761.

30. Miyagawa K, Rosch J, Stanczyk F, Hermsmeyer K. Medroxyprogesterone interferes with ovarian steroid protection against coronary vasospasm. *Nat Med* 1997; 3:324–327.

31. Adams MR, Kaplan JR, Manuck SB, Koritnik DR, Parks JS, Wolfe MS, Clarkson TB. Inhibition of coronary artery atherosclerosis by 17-beta estradiol in ovariectomized monkeys. Lack of an effect on added progesterone. *Arteriosclerosis* 1995;10:1051–1057.

32. Register TC, Adams MR, Golden DL, Clarkson TB. Conjugated equine estrogens alone, but not in combination with medroxyprogesterone acetate, inhibit aortic connective tissue remodeling after plasma lipid lowering in female monkeys. *Arterioscler Thromb Vasc Biol* 1998;18:1164–1171.

33. Jiang C, Sarrel PM, Lindsay DC, Poole-Wilson PA, Collins P. Progesterone induces endothelium-independent relaxation of rabbit coronary artery in vitro. *Eur J Pharmacol* 1992;211:163–167.

34. Gerhard M, Walsh BW, Tawakol A, et al. Estradiol therapy combined with progesterone and endothelium-dependent vasodilation in postmenopausal women. *Circulation* 1998;98:1158–1163.

35. Rosano GM, Chierchia SL, Morgagni GL, Gabriele M, Leonardo F, Sarrel PM, Collins P. Effect of the association of different progestogens to estradiol 17 therapy upon effort-induced myocardial ischemia in female patients with coronary artery disease [Abstract]. *J Am Coll Cardiol* 1997;29:344A.

36. Yim SF, Lau TK, Sahota DS, Chung TKH, Chang AMZ, Haines CJ. Prospective randomized study of the effect of "add-back" hormone replacement on vascular function during treatment with gonadotrophin-releasing hormone agonists. *Circulation* 1998;98:1631–1635.

37. Sorensen KE, Dorup I, Hermann AP, Mosekilde L. Combined hormone replacement therapy does not protect women against the age-related decline in endothelium-dependent vasomotor function. *Circulation* 1998;97:1234–1238.

38. Magness RR, Rosenfeld CR. Local and systemic estradiol-17 beta: effects on uterine and systemic vasodilation. *Am J Physiol* 1989;256:E536–E542.

39. Volterrani M, Rosano GMC, Coats A, Beale C, Collins P. Estrogen acutely increases peripheral blood flow in postmenopausal women. *Am J Med* 1995;99:119–122.

40. Riedel M, Oeltermann A, Mugge A, Creutzig A, Rafflenbeul W, Lichtlen P. Vascular responses to 17 beta-oestradiol in postmenopausal women. *Eur J Clin Invest* 1995;25:44–47.

41. Pines A, Fisman EZ, Drory Y, Levo Y, Shemesh J, Ben-Ari E, Ayalon D. Menopause-induced changes in Doppler-derived parameters of aortic flow in healthy women. *Am J Cardiol* 1992;69:1104–1106.

42. Pines A, Fisman EZ, Levo Y, et al. The effects of hormone replacement therapy in normal postmenopausal women: measurements of Doppler-derived parameters of aortic flow. *Am J Obstet Gynecol* 1991;164:806–812.

43. Ganger KF, Vyas S, Whitehead M, Crook D, Meire H, Campbell S. Pulsatility index in internal carotid artery in relation to transdermal oestradiol and time since menopause. *Lancet* 1991;338:839–842.

44. Lindheim SR, Legro RS, Bernstein L, Stanczyk FZ, Vijod MA, Presser SC, Lobo RA. Behavioral stress responses in premenopausal and postmenopausal women and the effects of estrogen. *Am J Obstet Gynecol* 1992;167:1831–1836.

45. Ryne SM, Goldberger AL, Pincus SM, Mietus J, Lipsitz LA. Gender- and age-related differences in heart rate dynamics: are women more complex than men? *J Am Coll Cardiol* 1994;24:1700–1707.

46. Rosano GM, Patrizi R, Leonardo F, Ponikowski P, Collins P, Sarrel PM, Chierchia SL. Effect of estrogen replacement therapy on heart rate variability and heart rate in healthy postmenopausal women. *Am J Cardiol* 1997;80:815–817.

47. Proudler AJ, Hasib Ahmed AI, Crook D, Fogelman I, Rymer JM, Stevenson JC. Hormone replacement therapy and serum angiotensin-converting-enzyme activity in postmenopausal women. *Lancet* 1995;346:89–90.

48. Jiang C, Sarrel PM, Poole-Wilson PA, Collins P. Acute effect of 17β-estradiol on

rabbit coronary artery contractile responses to endothelin-1. *Am J Physiol* 1992; 263:H271–H275.

49. Shay J, Futo J, Badrov N, Moss J. Estrogen withdrawal selectively increases serotonin reactivity in rabbit basilar artery. *Life Sci* 1994;55:1071–1081.

50. Belfort MA, Saade GR, Snabes M, Dunn R, Moise KJ, Jr., Cruz A, Young R. Hormonal status affects the reactivity of the cerebral vasculature. *Am J Obstet Gynecol* 1995;172:1273–1278.

51. Shaw TG, Mortel KF, Meyer JS, Rogers RL, Hardenberg J, Cutaia MM. Cerebral blood flow changes in benign aging and cerebrovascular disease. *Neurology* 1984; 34:855–862.

52. Rodriguez G, Warkentin S, Risberg J, Rosadini G. Sex differences in regional cerebral blood flow. *J Cereb Blood Flow Metab* 1988;8:783–789.

53. Penotti M, Nencioni T, Gabrielli L, Farina M, Castiglioni E, Polvani F. Blood flow variations in internal carotid and middle cerebral arteries induced by postmenopausal hormone replacement therapy. *Am J Obstet Gynecol* 1993;169: 1226–1232.

54. Ikeda T, Ikenoue T, Mori N, et al. Effect of early pregnancy on maternal regional cerebral blood flow. *Am J Obstet Gynecol* 1993;168:1303–1308.

55. Shamma FN, Fayad P, Brass L, Sarrel P. Middle cerebral artery blood velocity during controlled ovarian hyperstimulation. *Fertil Steril* 1992;57:1022–1025.

56. Rosano GMC, Sarrel PM, Poole-Wilson PA, Collins P. Beneficial effect of oestrogen on exercise-induced myocardial ischaemia in women with coronary artery disease. *Lancet* 1993;342:133–136.

57. Chester AH, Jiang C, Borland JA, Yacoub MH, Collins P. Estrogen relaxes human epicardial coronary arteries through non-endothelium-dependent mechanisms. *Coron Artery Dis* 1995;6:417–422.

58. Alpaslan M, Shimokawa H, Kuroiwa-Matsumoto M, Harasawa Y, Takeshita A. Short-term estrogen administration ameliorates dobutamine-induced myocardial ischemia in postmenopausal women with coronary artery disease. *J Am Coll Cardiol* 1997;30:1466–1471.

59. Rosano GMC, Caixeta AM, Chierchia SL, et al. Acute anti-ischemic effect of estradiol-17β in postmenopausal women with coronary artery disease. *Circulation* 1997;96:2837–2841.

60. Webb CM, Rosano GMC, Collins P. Oestrogen improves exercise-induced myocardial ischaemia in women. *Lancet* 1998;351:1556–1557.

61. Likoff W, Segal BL, Kasparian H. Paradox of normal selective coronary arteriograms in patients considered to have unmistakable coronary heart disease. *N Engl J Med* 1967;276:1063–1066.

62. Kemp HG, Jr., Vokonas PS, Cohn PF, Gorlin R. The anginal syndrome associated with normal coronary arteriograms. Report of a six year experience. *Am J Med* 1973;54:735–742.

63. Maseri A, Crea F, Kaski JC, Crake T. Mechanisms of angina pectoris in syndrome X. *J Am Coll Cardiol* 1991;17:499–506.

64. Cannon RO, Epstein SE. "Microvascular angina" as a cause of chest pain with angiographically normal coronary arteries. *Am J Cardiol* 1988;61:1338–1343.

65. Rosano GMC, Lindsay DC, Poole-Wilson PA. Syndrome X: an hypothesis for cardiac pain without ischaemia. *Cardiologia* 1991;36:885–895.

66. Opherk D, Zebe H, Weihe E, et al. Reduced coronary dilatory capacity and ultrastructural changes of the myocardium in patients with angina pectoris but normal coronary arteriograms. *Circulation* 1981;63:817–825.

67. Kaski JC, Rosano GMC, Collins P, Nihoyannopoulos P, Maseri A, Poole-Wilson PA. Cardiac syndrome X: clinical characteristics and left ventricular function. Long term follow-up study. *J Am Coll Cardiol* 1995;25:807–814.

68. Rosano GMC, Collins P, Kaski JC, Lindsay DC, Sarrel PM, Poole-Wilson PA. Syndrome X in women is associated with estrogen deficiency. *Eur Heart J* 1995;16:610–614.

69. Rosano GMC, Peters NS, Lefroy DC, Lindsay DC, Sarrel PM, Collins P, Poole-Wilson PA. 17-beta-estradiol therapy lessens angina in postmenopausal women with syndrome X. *J Am Coll Cardiol* 1996;28:1500–1505.

Treatment of the Postmenopausal Woman: Basic and Clinical Aspects, Second Edition, edited by Rogerio A. Lobo, Lippincott Williams & Wilkins, Philadelphia © 1999.

CHAPTER 35

Hormone Replacement Therapy and Carbohydrate Metabolism in Cardiovascular Risk

Ian F. Godsland

The classic physiologic and metabolic risk factors for cardiovascular disease include hypertension and hypercholesterolemia. Hypertension and hypercholesterolemia, however, explain only a small percentage of the incidence of cardiovascular disease and they have been primarily researched in men. Therefore, a need is seen to explore additional potential risk factors. In this respect, recently considerable interest has focused on the risk potential of disturbances in carbohydrate metabolism. Specifically, diminished sensitivity to the metabolic actions of insulin—insulin resistance—has been the focus of attention. It should be kept in mind, however, that the classic link between disturbances in carbohydrate metabolism and cardiovascular disease is diabetes, and that diabetes is a particularly powerful risk factor for cardiovascular disease in women (1).

Effects of hormone replacement therapy (HRT) on both insulin resistance and insulin secretion should therefore be considered in evaluating the involvement of carbohydrate metabolism on cardiovascular disease risk in postmenopausal women. As in other areas, consideration of the effects of estrogens on carbohydrate metabolism in postmenopausal women has been confounded by inappropriate reference to the effects of oral contraceptives. As will be described, the effects of physiologic estrogen replacement on carbohydrate metabolism are beneficial, although with combination therapy there may be some variation according to progestogen content.

CARBOHYDRATE METABOLISM AND CARDIOVASCULAR RISK

Resistance to the actions of insulin is accompanied by adverse changes in a remarkable number of measures, each of which has been independently related to the development of cardiovascular disease (2,3). Hyperinsulinema is the typical accompanying characteristic of insulin resistance, at least when there is adequate pancreatic insulin secretion. With insulin resistance, pancreatic insulin output is increased to maintain normal basal glucose levels, with either normal or only slightly impaired glucose tolerance. Thus, glucose homeostasis is maintained at the expense of elevations in insulin concentrations.

Chronically elevated insulin levels can have several adverse effects on the vasculature, including increased smooth muscle cell proliferation and arterial lipid deposition (4). Increased insulin levels can also increase sympathetic tone and blood pressure (5), and the production of the antifibrinolytic factor, plasminogen activator inhibitor-1 (6), all of which have been linked with increased vascular disease risk. Insulin has been found to be an independent predictor of coronary heart disease (CHD) in three substantial epidemiologic studies (7–9). A number of studies have found insulin a negative predictor of CHD, but these studies can be criticized for their small size, select groups, or confounding by comorbidity (10).

In addition to adverse effects on glucose metabolism, with accompanying elevations in insulin, insulin resistance adversely affects a number of insulin-dependent processes, primarily in relation to lipid and lipoprotein metabolism (11). Insulin suppression of adipose tissue lipolysis can be diminished, leading to an increased supply of nonesterified fatty acids to the liver and increased triglycerides synthe-

I. F. Godsland: Wynn Department of Metabolic Medicine, Imperial College School of Medicine, London, NW8 9SQ, United Kingdom.

sis. Increased production of triglyceride-enriched lipoproteins leads to a preponderance of the small, dense subfraction of low-density lipoprotein (LDL), which may be particularly atherogenic. It also leads to a reduction in cholesterol carried in the high-density lipoprotein (HDL) fraction, another adverse characteristic with respect to vascular disease risk. Metabolism of triglyceride-rich lipoproteins can also be disrupted by reductions in the activity of the insulin-dependent enzyme lipoprotein lipase, which can also have adverse consequences for HDL metabolism. A feature of this disturbance is impairment of postprandial clearance of triglyceride-rich lipoproteins, which again may be particularly atherogenic; this impairment has been found to be positively associated with the degree of insulin resistance.

Vasodilation, another action of insulin, is diminished in states of insulin resistance, and it can contribute to the increase in blood pressure that has been linked with insulin resistance (12). Other adverse changes that correlate with insulin resistance include decreased levels of sex hormone binding globulin (13), increased levels of the procoagulant factors fibrinogen, factor VII and factor X (14), increased uric acid concentrations (15), and increased centrally distributed body fat (2). Adverse changes associated with insulin resistance are listed in Table 35.1.

The extensive interrelationships that exist in the development of these coordinated disturbances centering on insulin resistance has led to the important concept of the metabolic syndrome or, specifically, the insulin resistance syndrome (16). Quantification of such a syndrome is problematic (3), but recent studies suggest that it is an exceptionally strong predictor of the development of diabetes (17).

The other major disturbance in carbohydrate metabolism with implications for cardiovascular risk, apart from insulin resistance, is diabetes. Insulin resistance, a feature of established diabetes, is in fact, a powerful predictor of the development of diabetes. However, a necessary prerequisite for the markedly elevated glucose levels that are diagnostic of diabetes is a deficiency in pancreatic insulin

TABLE 35.1. *Metabolic and physiologic disturbances associated with insulin resistance and independently with increased risk of cardiovascular disease*

Hyperinsulinemia
Hypertriglyceridemia
Low high density lipoprotein concentrations
Increased small dense low-density lipoprotein
Decreased sex hormone binding globulin
Increased uric acid concentrations
Increased fibrinogen and factor VII
Decreased fibrinolysis
Decreased postprandial fat elimination
Hypertension
Central obesity

secretion. The elevated glucose levels seen in diabetes can adversely affect the vasculature, either directly by protein glycosylation (18) or indirectly by increasing free-radical damage to the vessel wall (19). In addition to increased glucose levels, the deficiency in insulin secretion induces metabolic disturbances that resemble those seen with insulin resistance, which is particularly the case in non–insulin-dependent or type II diabetes (NIDDM). Diabetic dyslipidemia, composed of increased triglyceride and decreased HDL levels, may be an important factor in the increased vascular risk in this condition. It is noteworthy that these lipid and lipoprotein changes are particularly marked in women with NIDDM (20) who are at particular risk of developing cardiovascular disease.

THE MENOPAUSE AND CARBOHYDRATE METABOLISM

Menopause is not associated with any immediate change in glucose or insulin levels; however, underlying changes may have clinical implications, which may become apparent with increasing time since menopause. Pancreatic insulin secretion falls with the decline in estrogen concentrations, although insulin levels are maintained by an increase in the plasma insulin half-life (21). Insulin resistance may not change immediately following menopause, but a progressive increase is seen in insulin resistance and in insulin concentrations that relate to time since menopause rather than to chronological age (22, 23). Thus, postmenopausal women are generally more insulin resistant than would be expected from the effects of age alone. A progressive decrease is seen in the amount of newly secreted insulin taken up by the liver in postmenopausal women (23).

Postmenopausal women exhibit many of the characteristics associated with the insulin resistance syndrome, including increased triglyceride and decreased HDL cholesterol levels, decreased triglyceride elimination, increased uric acid concentrations, and an increased proportion of centrally distributed fat (24). Although estrogen deficiency is likely to be the principal contributing factor, increasing insulin resistance may also provide an added metabolic burden, and the effects of the two combine to generate a characteristic menopausal metabolic syndrome. The progressive decrease in hepatic insulin uptake with increasing time since menopause is also noteworthy because this has been independently linked with adverse changes in HDL metabolism.

Although, in general, the decline in pancreatic insulin secretion at menopause may be compensated for by an increase in insulin half-life, this decline in secretion could lead in certain susceptible or borderline individuals to the emergence of frank diabetes. The US National Health and Nutrition Examination Survey has established that the incidence of diabetes increases more rapidly in middle-aged women than it does in men (25). Moreover, evidence suggests that if onset of diabetes is related to time since menopause rather than to chronological age a very strong relationship may emerge between menopause and the development of diabetes (26).

ESTROGEN AND CARBOHYDRATE METABOLISM

It is well-established that estrogen replacement can reverse many of the adverse clinical and metabolic effects of the menopause, including effects on carbohydrate metabolism. Some confusion has existed over this because of the adverse effects reported in association with oral contraceptive use. These adverse effects stem from the use of potent alkylated estrogens, including ethinyl estradiol, which has been shown to cause deterioration in glucose tolerance and insulin resistance (27). This is also the case in postmenopausal women taking higher doses (±1.25 mg) of conjugated equine estrogens, but with lower doses (0.625 mg) studies are equally divided between those showing no effect and those showing an improvement in insulin sensitivity. With the native estrogen (estradiol) administered orally or transdermally, most studies consistently show an improvement in insulin sensitivity (27). The simplest interpretation of these findings is that physiologic estrogen replacement in postmenopausal women improves insulin sensitivity, whereas estrogen in excess is associated with an adverse effect. Such an adverse effect could result from secondary effects of high estrogen exposure, increased glucocorticoid activity being the most likely candidate. In support of the proposition that the underlying physiologic effect of estrogens is an improvement in insulin sensitivity, it is noteworthy that both muscle and adipose tissue isolated from animals given estrogens show improved responses to insulin (Fig. 35.1) (28,29).

Resistance to both glucagon action on glucose homeostasis and to stimulation of glucagon release by glucose is an additional effect of estrogens on carbohydrate metabolism that should be considered (30,31). These resistant effects are seen primarily in the fasted state, in which effects on gluconeogenesis are most apparent. Significant reductions in both fasting glucose and fasting insulin levels may be seen, particularly with high potency estrogens. Paradoxically, these changes are then accompanied by increased insulin resistance despite the apparent reduction in insulin resistance suggested by the lower fasting insulin levels.

The effects of estrogens on insulin secretion are most strikingly demonstrated in experiments in which administration of estrogens has been found to markedly diminish the development of diabetes in subtotally pancreatectomized animals (Fig. 35.2) (32). This effect is associated with hypertrophy and hyperplasia of the remaining pancreatic tissue and, in accord with these findings, increased pancreatic insulin output has been demonstrated in perfused pancreas preparations exposed to estrogen (33) and in isolated pancreatic islets from estrogen-treated animals (34). These experimental findings contrast with expectations generated by the effects of oral contraceptive use, namely that estrogen replacement in postmenopausal women might increase the incidence of diabetes. Moreover, in the single clinical study to address this issue, it was found that postmenopausal women who took estrogens were less likely to develop diabetes than those who did not (35).

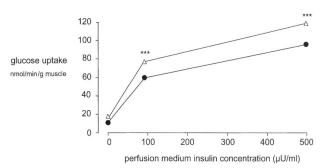

FIG. 35.1. Estrogen-induced improvement in the sensitivity of glucose uptake to insulin in isolated muscle from the rat. Closed circles ●, untreated controls; open triangles △, treated with estradiol benzoate (0.005 mg/d) for 21 days; closed circles, treated with progesterone (5 mg/d) for 21 days. (From Rushakoff R, Kalkhoff R. Effects of pregnancy and sex steroid administration on skeletal muscle metabolism in the rat. *Diabetes* 1981;30:545–550, with permission.)

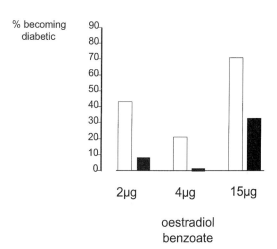

FIG. 35.2. Prevention of diabetes in the partially pancreatectomized rat by daily administration of estradiol benzoate for 6 months at the doses shown. Open bars: untreated controls; filled bars: treated. (Reproduced from Foglia V, Schuster N, Rodriguez R. Sex and diabetes. *Endocrinology* 1947; 41:428–434, with permission.)

COMBINED HORMONE REPLACEMENT THERAPY AND CARBOHYDRATE METABOLISM

The effects of progesterone and progestogens alone have not been studied in postmenopausal women, although a number of studies have been done in premenopausal women using progestogen-only oral contraceptives. Evidence suggests that progesterone alone is probably neutral, although at levels equivalent to those seen in pregnancy some deterioration in carbohydrate metabolism may be seen (27). Most studies of medroxyprogesterone acetate and levonorgestrel use provide evidence for the induction of insulin resistance. With medroxyprogesterone acetate, this can be expected because this steroid has some glucocorticoidlike activity (36). Among the other progestogens that have been employed in HRT, norethindrone acetate has generally been found to be neutral with regard to carbohydrate metabolism, whereas dydrogesterone alone does not appear to have been studied in this respect (27).

Given the variety of regimens used in combined HRT and the relative lack of studies of their effects on carbohydrate metabolism, it is difficult to draw general conclusions. Studies, therefore, are best considered separately according to type of progestogen employed. Increased insulin resistance has been described during the estrogen plus progestogen phase of the treatment cycle with those progestogens—medroxyprogesterone acetate and levonorgestrel—which when given alone are associated with increased insulin resistance (Fig. 35.3) (37–39). With reg-

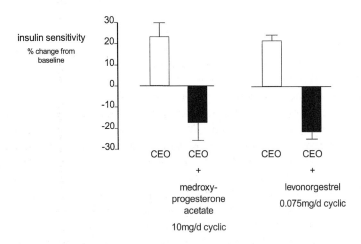

FIG. 35.3. Percentage change in insulin sensitivity, measured by modeling analysis of intravenous glucose tolerance test glucose and insulin concentrations, in 30 women taking conjugated equine estrogens (0.625 mg/day) and cyclical levonorgestrel (0.075 mg/day), tested during the estrogen alone phase (open bar) and the estrogen plus progestogen combined phase (closed bar) of the third treatment cycle. (From Godsland I, Gangar K, Walton C, Cust M, Whitehead M, Wynn V, Stevenson J. Insulin resistance, secretion and elimination in postmenopausal women receiving oral or transdermal hormone replacement therapy. *Metabolism* 1993;42:846–853.)

imens containing these progestogens, evidence points to deterioration in glucose tolerance as the predominant effect of the combination (39–42). One feature that has emerged as a possible contributing factor to these changes is a reduction in the initial insulin output in response to glucose. This was seen in modelling studies of an intravenous glucose tolerance test (IVGTT) in women taking a combination of conjugated equine estrogens and levonorgestrel (39). Interestingly, in the Lobo et al. study of women taking conjugated equine estrogens alone and with varying doses of medroxyprogesterone acetate, oral glucose tolerance test (OGTT) glucose response was significantly increased during at least one of the three cycles studied (cycles 3, 6, and 13) in the combination users, but not in the users of estrogen alone. Also, in accord with a reduction in the initial insulin response to glucose, OGTT insulin response was reduced, primarily during the early part of the OGTT (41)

A combination containing estradiol and norethindrone has been reported to improve glucose tolerance in women with impaired glucose tolerance, but was without effect on either OGTT glucose or insulin levels in diabetic women or women with normal glucose tolerance (43). A similar lack of effect on IVGTT glucose and insulin levels was seen when norethisterone acetate was administered transdermally, in a cyclical regimen with transdermally administered estradiol (39). Neither insulin resistance nor any other measure of insulin metabolism was affected. This was also the case when variables, including insulin resistance, were compared during the estrogen alone phase and during the estrogen plus progestogen phase during the third cycle of treatment. Norethisterone, therefore, appears to be neutral; however, as suggested by the between-phase comparison, it may oppose the favorable effects of estradiol.

Cyclically administered dydrogesterone has been studied at a high dose (20 mg/day) in combination with conjugated equine estrogens (0.625 mg/day) (44). No effect on OGTT glucose or insulin levels was apparent. However, at a lower dose (10 mg/day) with estradiol (2 mg/day), the beneficial effects of estradiol on insulin action and metabolism appeared to be preserved. In 29 women followed for 24 months, fasting glucose levels were unchanged but a steep decline was seen in insulin levels and some increase in fasting C-peptide (45). A similar, albeit nonsignificant trend was apparent with OGTT insulin response. A similar trend toward reduced insulin and increased C-peptide levels has been reported by Gaspard et al. (46).

CONCLUSIONS

Based on the effects of oral contraceptive therapy and contrary to previous expectations, postmenopausal estrogen replacement has the potential for improving carbohydrate metabolism. Changes in carbohydrate metabolism would be expected to contribute to the improvements in the cardiovascular risk profile that have already been established for estrogen replacement. Both reductions in insulin resistance and indirect effects mediated through improvements in the diabetes risk profile could be contributing factors. Reductions in insulin resistance have been most clearly demonstrated in relation to unopposed therapy with the native estrogen, estradiol. Other estrogen regimens may be relatively neutral and this positive effect may be opposed when a progestogen is included in the treatment. However, some progestogens, for example dydrogesterone, may contribute to preserving the improvements seen with estradiol. Improvements in the diabetes risk profile may be less dependent on the type or dose of estrogen used. Experimental support for this effect comes from studies with a variety of different estrogens. Experimental studies of the effects of progestogens on pancreatic insulin release suggest that similar improvements to those with estrogens. It is possible, therefore, that improvements in the diabetes risk profile may be a more general effect of postmenopausal hormone replacement. These possibilities still remain relatively unexplored, but it should be apparent that further investigation would be worthwhile given the potential benefits that could be confirmed.

REFERENCES

1. Barrett-Connor EL, Cohn BA, Wingard DL, Edelstein SL. Why is diabetes mellitus a stronger risk factor for fatal ischemic heart disease in women than in men? The Rancho Bernardo Study. *JAMA* 1991;265:627–631.
2. Després J-P, Marette A. Relation of components of insulin resistance syndrome to coronary disease risk. *Curr Opin Lipidol* 1994;5:274–289.
3. Godsland IF, Stevenson JC. Insulin resistance: syndrome or tendency? *Lancet* 1995;346:100–103.
4. Stout R. Insulin and atheroma: 20-year perspective. *Diabetes Care* 1990;13:631–654.
5. Reaven GM, Lithell H, Landsberg L. Hypertension and associated metabolic abnormalities—the role of insulin resistance and the sympathoadrenal system. *N Engl J Med* 1996;334:374–381.
6. Kooistra T, Bosma P, Töns H, van den Berg A, Meyer P, Princen H. Plasminogen activator inhibitor 1: biosynthesis and mRNA level are increased by insulin in cultured human hepatocytes. *Thromb Haemost* 1989;62:723–728.
7. Eschwege E, Richard J, Thibult N, Ducimetiere P, Warnet J, Claude J, Rosselin G. Coronary heart disease mortality in relation with diabetes, blood glucose and plasma insulin levels: the Paris Prospective Study, ten years later. *Horm Metab Res* 1985;15 (Suppl):41–46.
8. Pyörälä K, Savolainen E, Kaukola S, Haapakoski J. Plasma insulin as coronary heart disease risk factor: relationship to other risk factors and predictive value during 9 1/2 year follow-up of the Helsinki Policemen Study population. *Acta Med Scand* 1985;701 (Suppl):38–52.
9. Després J-P, Lamarche B, Mauriége P, Cantin B, Dagenais GR, Moorjani S, Lupien P-J. Hyperinsulinemia as an independent risk factor for ischemic heart disease. *N Engl J Med* 1996;334:952–957.
10. McKeigue P, Davey G. Associations between insulin levels and cardiovascular disease are confounded by comorbidity. *Diabetes Care* 1995;18:1294–1298.
11. Frayn K. Insulin resistance and lipid metabolism. *Curr Opin Lipidol* 1993;4:197–204.
12. Baron AD. Hemodynamic actions of insulin. *Am J Physiol* 1994;267:E187–E202.
13. Haffner S, Katz M, Dunn J. The relationship of insulin sensitivity and metabolic clearance of insulin to adiposity and sex hormone binding globulin. *Endocr Res* 1990;16:361–376.
14. Godsland IF, Sidhu M, Crook D, Stevenson JC. Coagulation and fibrinolytic factors, insulin resistance and the metabolic syndrome of coronary heart disease risk. *Eur Heart J* 1996;17(Suppl):331.
15. Reaven GM. Role of insulin resistance in human disease (Syndrome X): an expanded definition. *Ann Rev Med* 1993;44:121–131.
16. Reaven G. Banting Lecture 1988. Role of insulin resistance in human disease. *Diabetes* 1988;37:1595–1607.
17. Godsland IF, Leyva F, Bruce R, Walton C, Worthington M, Stevenson JC. The metabolic syndrome predicts development of diabetes in the first follow-up cohort of the RISC Study (RISC-1): an application of factor analysis. *Diabet Med* 1997;14(Suppl 1):S18.
18. Cerami A, Vlassara H, Brownlee M. Role of advanced glycosylation products in complications of diabetes. *Diabetes Care* 1988;11(Suppl 1):73–79.
19. Wolff SP. Diabetes mellitus and free radicals. *Br Med Bull* 1993;49:642–652.
20. Walden C, Knopp R, Wahl P. Sex differences in the effect of diabetes mellitus on lipoprotein triglyceride and cholesterol concentrations. *N Engl J Med* 1984;311:953–959.
21. Walton C, Godsland I, Proudler A, Wynn V, Stevenson J. The effects of the menopause on insulin sensitivity, secretion and elimination in nonobese, healthy women. *Eur J Clin Invest* 1993;23:466–473.
22. Proudler A, Felton C, Stevenson J. Ageing and the response of plasma insulin, glucose and C-peptide concentrations to intravenous glucose in postmenopausal women. *Clin Sci* 1992;83:489–494.
23. Godsland IF, Walton C, Stevenson JC. Impact of menopause on metabolism. In: Diamond MP, Naftolin F, eds. *Metabolism in the female life cycle*. Rome: Ares Serono Symposia, 1993:171–189.
24. Spencer CP, Godsland IF, Stevenson JC. Is there a menopausal metabolic syndrome? *Gynecol Endocrinol* 1997;11:341–355.
25. Harris MI, Hadden WC, Knowler WC, Bennett PH. Prevalence of diabetes and impaired glucose tolerance and plasma glucose levels in U.S. population aged 20-74 years. *Diabetes* 1987;36:523–534.
26. Seige K, Hevelke G. The effect of female gonadal function on the manifestation and frequency of diabetes mellitus. 6th Symposium of the German Endocrinological Society: *Modern Developments in Progestagenic Hormones in Veterinary Medicine*. Kiel: Springer Verlag, 1959:274–279.
27. Godsland IF. The influence of female sex steroids on glucose metabolism and insulin action. *J Intern Med* 1996;240(Suppl 738):1–65.
28. Gilmour K, McKerns K. Insulin and estrogen regulation of lipid synthesis in adipose tissue. *Biochim Biophys Acta* 1966;116:220–228.
29. Rushakoff R, Kalkhoff R. Effects of pregnancy and sex steroid administration on skeletal muscle metabolism in the rat. *Diabetes* 1981;30:545–550.
30. Thomas J. Modification of glucagon-induced hyperglycemia by various steroidal agents. *Metabolism* 1963;12:207–212.
31. Mandour T, Kissebah A, Wynn V. Mechanism of oestrogen and progesterone effects on lipid and carbohydrate metabolism: alteration in the insulin:glucagon molar ratio and hepatic enzyme activity. *Eur J Clin Invest* 1977;7:181–187.
32. Foglia V, Schuster N, Rodriguez R. Sex and diabetes. *Endocrinology* 1947;41:428–434.
33. Sutter-Dub M-T. Preliminary report. Effects of female sex hormones on insulin secretion by the perfused rat pancreas. *J Physiol (Paris)* 1976;72:795–800.
34. Costrini N, Kalkhoff R. Relative effects of pregnancy, estradiol and progesterone on plasma insulin and pancreatic islet insulin secretion. *J Clin Invest* 1971;50:992–999.
35. Manson JE, Rimm EB, Colditz GA, et al. A prospective study of postmenopausal estrogen therapy and subsequent incidence of non-insulin-dependent diabetes mellitus. *Ann Epidemiol* 1992;2:665–673.
36. Siminoski K, Goss P, Drucker DJ. The Cushing Syndrome induced by medroxyprogesterone acetate. *Ann Intern Med* 1989;111:758–760.
37. Elkind-Hirsch K, Sherman L, Malinak R. Hormone replacement therapy alters insulin sensitivity in young women with premature ovarian failure. *J Clin Endocrinol Metab* 1993;76:472–475.
38. Lindheim SR, Presser SC, Ditkoff EC, Vijod MA, Stanczyk FZ, Lobo RA. A possible bimodal effect of estrogen on insulin sensitivity in postmenopausal women and the attenuating effect of added progestin. *Fertil Steril* 1993;60:664–667.
39. Godsland I, Gangar K, Walton C, Cust M, Whitehead M, Wynn V, Stevenson J. Insulin resistance, secretion and elimination in postmenopausal women receiving oral or transdermal hormone replacement therapy. *Metabolism* 1993;42:846–853.
40. Barrett-Connor E, Laakso M. Ischaemic heart disease risk in postmenopausal women: effects of estrogen use on glucose and insulin levels. *Arteriosclerosis* 1990;10:531–534.
41. Lobo RA, Pickar JH, Wild RA, Walsh B, Hirvonen E. Metabolic impact of adding medroxyprogesterone acetate to conjugated estrogen therapy in postmenopausal women. *Obstet Gynecol* 1994;84:987–995.
42. PEPI, The Writing Group for the PEPI Trial. Effects of estrogen or estrogen/progestin regimens on heart disease risk factors in postmenopausal women: the Postmenopausal Estrogen/Progestin Interventions (PEPI) Trial. *JAMA* 1995;273:199–208.
43. Luotola H, Pyörälä T, Loikkanen M. Effects of natural oestrogen/progestogen substitution therapy on carbohydrate and lipid metabolism in post-menopausal women. *Maturitas* 1986;8:245–253.
44. DeCleyn K, Buytaert P, Coppens M. Carbohydrate metabolism during hormonal substitution therapy. *Maturitas* 1989;11:235–242.
45. Crook D, Godsland IF, Hull J, Stevenson JC. Hormone replacement therapy with dydrogesterone progestin and estradiol-17B: effects on serum lipoproteins and on glucose tolerance during 24 month follow-up. *Br J Obstet Gynaecol* 1997;104:298–304.
46. Gaspard UJ, Wery O, Herman P, Scheen AJ, Jaminet CB, Lefebvre PJ. Carbohydrate metabolism in postmenopausal women using oral oestradiol and dydrogesterone. *Int J Gynecol Obstet* 1994;46(Suppl 1):P020.17.

Treatment of the Postmenopausal Woman: Basic and
Clinical Aspects, Second Edition, edited by Rogerio A. Lobo,
Lippincott Williams & Wilkins, Philadelphia © 1999.

CHAPTER 36

Hormone Therapy and Hemostasis

Morris Notelovitz

The pathogenesis of atherogenic disease and the physiology of coagulation are constantly being revised as new information becomes available. As a consequence, we can better understand and anticipate what effects sex steroids do—and do not—have on the vasculature and hemostasis. The subject is of major importance because cardiovascular disease is the primary cause of morbidity and mortality in postmenopausal women, and estrogen therapy is widely touted as the most effective preventive agent (1).

Hormone therapy has been negatively linked to the potential for venous thrombosis via enhanced procoagulant activity (2), and positively linked to reduced risk of atherogenic disease, through normalization of the lipid-lipoprotein moiety (3). Because of better biological markers, it is now apparent that estrogens have little adverse effect on coagulation (4) and that progestins can be beneficial (5). Also, improvement in the lipid profile accounts for only 25% to 50% of the protective effect of estrogen therapy, pointing to other estrogen-influenced mechanisms (3). It is in this context that the contribution of coronary mural thrombosis to atherogenesis and estrogen therapy becomes relevant (6). Finally, as originally postulated by Virchow, blood flow and factors influencing it also have an impact on hemostasis. Sex steroids are known to modulate arterial vasomotion and venous tone (7). This subject is reviewed elsewhere and will not be discussed in detail, but it has an obvious important impact on vascular health. In short, when balancing the benefits and risks of estrogen therapy, clinicians need to consider its effect on the arterial (coronary artery) tree as much as the venous system.

HEMOSTASIS REVISITED

A recent review of hemostasis (8), while endorsing previous in vitro studies, notes variations in the sequential

reactions that lead to blood clot formation in vivo. The process is very complex and has numerous coagulatory and fibrinolytic checks and balances. Figure 36.1 depicts a simplified summary and will serve as a guide to some potential points of clinical relevance when prescribing hormone therapy.

Although the basic process is the same, arterial thrombosis differs from venous thrombosis: the former results in platelet-rich ("white") thrombi, whereas the low blood flow venous thrombosis is fibrin and red cell-rich ("red") and, as a consequence, is more liable to embolism (9). More importantly, thrombus formation is a key event in the origin and progression of atherosclerosis and, as will be discussed, may help to define the clinician's approach to cardiovascular health care in women.

VESSEL WALL

The endothelium, which is a semipermeable barrier between the blood and the deeper layers of the vessel wall, serves two main functions in hemostasis: it helps to regulate vascular tone and it acts as an anticoagulant. The endothelium synthesizes vasodilators such as prostacyclin (PGI_2) and endothelium-derived relaxing factor (nitric oxide [NO]), and vasoconstrictors such as endothelin and platelet-activating factor (PAF) (Fig. 36.1) (10). Prostacyclin and NO act synergistically to prevent platelet activation. Both factors are difficult to assay because they are either only locally active (NO) or are rapidly metabolized (PGI_2). Nevertheless, two studies have shown that nonoral estrogen increases plasma levels of both nitric oxide and prostacyclin (11,12). The serum estradiol level ranged between 80 and 120 pg/dL. A further study involving oral estradiol and norethindrone reported a 21% increased production in prostacyclin but no change in the potent vasoconstrictor, endothelial release (13). The endothelium also inactivates other known vasoactive substances such as serotonin and bradykinin (14). Blood flow—a major determinant of intimal damage—depends on the balance between

M. Notelovitz: Women's Medical & Diagnostic Center, Gainesville, Florida 32605.

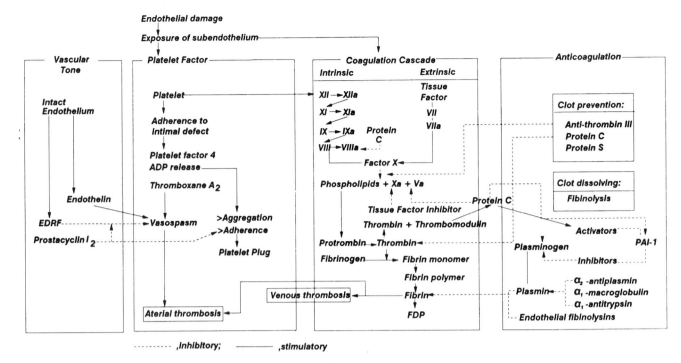

FIG. 36.1. The integrated relationship between four systems (vascular tone, platelet activity, coagulation, and fibrinolysis) is depicted in separate panels showing their interrelationships, both stimulatory (solid lines) and inhibitory (dashed lines). ADP, adenosine diphosphate; EDRF, endothelium derived relaxing factor; FDP, fibrinogen-degradation products; PAI-1, plasminogen activator inhibitor-1.

these various vasoactive substances, many of which are influenced by hormone therapy.

The healthy endothelium prevents thrombosis in at least three ways. It synthesizes thrombomodulin, a protein that is an endothelial receptor for thrombin. The resulting complex activates protein C (see later), the primary inhibitor of factor Va and VIIIa (15); the intact endothelium is a surface anticoagulant. The cells consist of glycoproteins and proteoglycans such as heparin sulfate, the main cofactor to antithrombin III (the most potent endogenous anticoagulant). The glycoproteins emit a negative charge that propels platelets and prevents initiation of the intrinsic arm of the

coagulation cascade (16); tissue plasminogen activator (t-PA) is continuously synthesized and secreted by endothelial cells, and as such regulates the fibrinolytic activity of blood (17). This function may be a major contributor to the prevention of coronary artery disease (CAD). The activity of t-PA is enhanced by progestins (see later discussion).

PLATELET FACTOR

Platelets circulate in blood in an inactive resting form. When they are exposed to the subendothelial layers, platelets develop pseudopodia, attach to the injured sur-

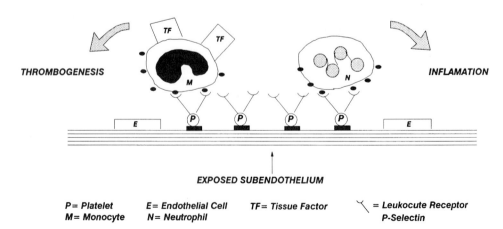

FIG. 36.2. Depiction of the initiation of blood coagulation and formation of the platelet plug within a blood vessel, involving both thrombogenesis and inflammation.

face, and become highly adherent (Fig. 36.2) (8). The binding is determined by various surface receptors that complex with specific ligands such as the von Willebrand factor. The bound platelets degranulate and expose receptors for factor VIII, factor V, and P-selectin (18). Neutrophils and monocytes bind to the P-selectin receptor and participate in the inflammatory response; the monocytes, in addition, secrete tissue factor, the initiator of the extrinsic coagulation cascade (Fig. 36.1). Platelet aggregation is enhanced by modifying and sensitizing their surface receptors to adhesive proteins, such as fibrinogen. The platelet membrane also releases arachidonic acid. Arachidonic acid is metabolized to thromboxane A_2, which in turn promotes further platelet aggregation and local vasoconstriction. The net result is a platelet plug with fibrin formation, the first necessary step to permanent hemostasis and wound healing (9). Aspirin inhibits cyclo-oxygenase activity in both platelets (thereby reducing thromboxane activity), as well as endothelial prostacyclin synthesis. However, the process is more prolonged in platelets (± 2 days) and is short-lived in the endothelium (± 6 hours). It is for this reason that low-dose intermittent aspirin use optimizes its antithrombotic potential (19). Two recent studies have confirmed that hormone replacement therapy (HRT)—involving both combination oral treatment (conjugated equine estrogen with medroxyprogesterone acetate [MPA] and 17β-estradiol and norethindrone acetate—and transdermal estrogen (17β-estradiol plus MPA) decreased platelet aggregation (20) and the cellular reactivity of platelets and monocytes (21). A positive effect of estrogen therapy on platelet activity was the reported decrease in thromboxane metabolism, subsequent to both acutely administered intravenous estradiol and long-term estrogen replacement therapy (ERT) with estradiol pellets (12).

COAGULATION-ANTICOAGULATION

The coagulation system has built-in checks and balances that preclude (in healthy individuals) inappropriate thrombosis, and which conserve the ability to help breach disruptions in the normal vasculature. This is achieved by three mechanisms: the procoagulant factors circulate in an inactive form; activation and, hence, coagulation only occur at the site(s) of trauma. The process is thus localized to a relatively small area of intimal damage; the activated coagulants are inhibited and their activity modulated by naturally occurring anticoagulants. Both coagulants and anticoagulants are present in concentrations far in excess of the physiologic need. As a consequence, when statistically significant alterations in plasma levels of activated zymogens occur in response, for example, to hormone therapy, they usually have little or no clinical impact (22,23).

Factors involved in blood coagulation are summarized in Fig. 36.3. Based on in vitro studies (8), activation of factor X to Xa links the intrinsic and extrinsic pathways

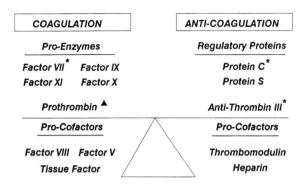

FIG. 36.3. Balance between factors involved in coagulation and anticoagulation. *, systemic tests of possible clinical value; ▲, best prognostic indicator (fragment 1.2).

of the coagulation cascade and leads to the conversion of prothrombin (a vitamin K-dependent hepatic protein) to thrombin, which is the catalyst for the fibrinogen–fibrin reaction (Fig. 36.1). The partial thromboplastin time (PTT) is a dynamic test that assesses the interrelated response of the intrinsic system; the prothrombin time (PT) is a measure of the activity of the extrinsic arm of the coagulation cascade. It has been noted that patients with hereditary factor XII deficiency, for example, have increased PTT but no bleeding diathesis, indicating that this factor is not important for the formation of a blood clot. Thus, the PTT is a test of dubious value (8). Tissue factor (a normal constituent of the surface of nonvascular cells) and stimulated monocytes activate coagulation. The physiologic pathway of blood coagulation appears to bypass the first steps of the intrinsic pathway and is summarized in Fig. 36.4. Coagulation hinges on the formation of a tissue factor-activated VII—a complex that in turn converts factor IX to IXa, and factor X to Xa (24). Activated factors VIIIa and IXa further catalyze the X to Xa conversion. Activated factor Xa, together with activated factor Va, mediates the conversion of prothrombin to thrombin, in the presence of phospholipids and calcium (8). Thrombin, when free in solution, promotes clotting by converting fibrinogen to fibrin, by activating platelets, and, by positive feedback, stimulating the activation of factors XI, VIII, and V (Fig. 36.4). By contrast, thrombin has a local anticoagulant effect (10,25). When thrombin forms a complex with thrombomodulin on the endothelial surface, it inhibits blood clotting by activating protein C (15). The latter is a zymogen formed in the liver and is vitamin K dependent. Protein S, another vitamin K-dependent protein, is a cofactor for protein C (26). Protein C also initiates fibrinolysis by activating plasminogen and neutralizing plasminogen activator inhibitor (9) (PAI-1) (Fig. 36.1). Recently, resistance to activated protein C has been discovered as a hereditary trait in individuals who develop venous thromboembolism without apparent cause. This is now referred to as "factor V Leiden" and is said to occur in approximately 20% of

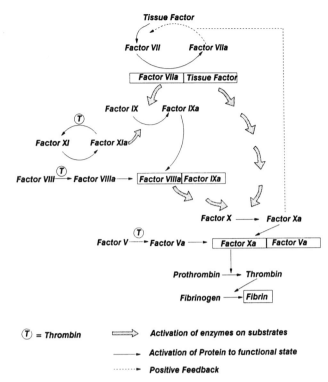

FIG. 36.4. Pathway of coagulation involving factors from tissue and the cascade toward fibrin formation.

patients with venous thromboembolism. In one study, the risk of recurrent venous thromboembolism in carriers of this mutation was increased with a hazard ratio of 2.4 compared with patients without this condition (27).

Antithrombins are inhibitors of thrombin and other coagulation proteases (28). Antithrombin III, which is the most important, probably accounts for at least 50% of the natural fluidity of blood. The action of antithrombin III is catalyzed by heparin and in its complex form neutralizes thrombin instantly (29). Antithrombin III also inhibits other enzymes in the coagulation cascade, such as activated factors Xa, XII, XI, and X (15). However, its main efficacy as a natural anticoagulant is thought by some to be the prevention of factor Xa generation and the activation of prothrombin. A deficiency of antithrombin III is associated with an increased liability of thrombosis (30). The level at which antithrombin III deficiency would cause thrombosis is not known, but it would probably have to be reduced to approximately 50% of its normal activity. This estimate is based on the plasma levels of antithrombin III in families who have congenital antithrombin III deficiency. Not all individuals with antithrombin III deficiency experience thrombosis. As with protein C deficiency, thrombosis usually occurs in conjunction with other events such as trauma and surgery. Reliable assays are now available for the measurements of antithrombin III and protein C levels.

FIBRIN FORMATION AND FIBRINOLYSIS

The introduction of t-PA therapy into clinical practice emphasizes the importance of fibrinolysis in maintaining intimal health and vascular patency. Fibrinogen is a dimer with three polypeptide chains: α, β, and γ. Thrombin acts on the α and β chains and produces two molecules of fibrinopeptide A and two molecules of fibrinopeptide B. This leaves a large residue molecule known as "fibrin monomer," which spontaneously polymerizes into nonstable fibrin polymer. These are cross-linked in the presence of calcium and activated factor XIII to form the stable insoluble clot, fibrin (9). This process is vital to survival and is nature's way of preserving the integrity of the vascular tree subsequent to injury so that healing and normal function of the area concerned can be restored and maintained.

Fibrin formation is regulated by the process of fibrinolysis, which involves the enzymatic degradation of fibrin and fibrinogen by plasmin (9). Plasmin is formed from plasminogen, a β-globulin synthesized by the liver (25). The biologic activity of plasmin and, hence, fibrinolysis is determined by activators and inactivators of plasminogen and plasmin inhibitors (Fig. 36.5). Fibrinolysis is initiated by either factor XIIa or urokinase plasminogen activator (intrinsic pathway) or tissue-type plasminogen activator (t-PA), the extrinsic pathway (31). Tissue plasminogen activator, which is produced by the endothelial cells and released into the circulation, in the presence of fibrin, binds together with plasminogen to generate plasmin, and thus fibrinolysis (17). Fibrin acts both as a substrate and a cofactor to plasminogen activity. Tissue plasminogen activator is inhibited by plasminogen activator inhibitor type 1 (PAI-1) (32). PAI-1 is produced by hepatocytes and endothelial cells. The balance between t-PA and PAI-1 is said to be the major determinant of the spontaneous fibronolytic activity of blood (32). Both fibrinogen and PAI-1 are significantly reduced by combination transdermal estradiol and MPA, and the mean plasma estradiol level was found to be 138 pg/dL (33). In another study, conjugated estrogen (alone and in combination with MPA) significantly reduced plasma PAI-1 antigen levels (34). In this study transdermal estrogen had very little effect on PAI-1.

As noted, plasminogen has to bind to fibrin in order to be activated to plasmin. The binding takes place at the so-called "lysine-binding" sites on the plasminogen molecule. Histidine-rich glycoprotein has an affinity for these sites and can, therefore, control the amount of biologically available free plasminogen (35). Estrogen decreases plasma histidine-rich glycoprotein and may, therefore, enhance fibrinolysis (36). Exogenous progestins and estrogen (37) are associated with increased plasminogen activity (5). Three main plasmin inhibitors exist: α_2-plasmin inhibitor; α_2-macroglobulin, which reacts quickly and as a competitive plasmin inhibitor; and α_2-anti-

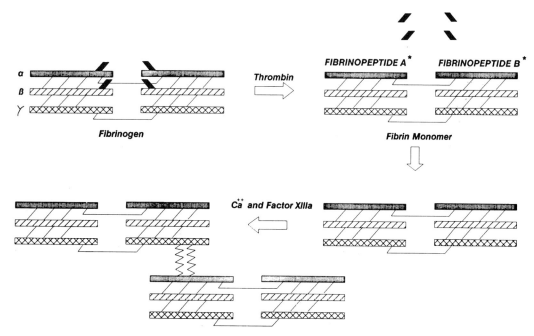

FIG. 36.5. Diagrammatic depiction of how fibrin polymer forms. Asterisks depict potential markers for thrombosis.

trypsin, which reacts more slowly but more firmly. The latter two proteases also inhibit thrombin and so have conflicting functions: they prevent clot formation by antagonizing thrombin and they encourage fibrin and fibrinogen integrity by inhibiting plasmin. Their overall effect on thrombogenesis is not known. Antiplasmin inhibitor (α_2-plasmin inhibitor) is said to inhibit 35% of the plasmin generated from plasminogen (38). It acts in two ways: direct inactivation of plasmin and blockage of plasminogen binding to fibrin. Pharmacologic lowering of α_2-plasmin inhibitor levels can be viewed as a positive side effect, because the net effect will result in increased fibrinolysis.

Cleavage of fibrin and fibrinogen produces a variety of fragments known as "fibrin" or "fibrinogen degradation products" (FDPs). FDPs have potent anticoagulant properties and may interfere with platelet activity as well.

CLINICAL MARKERS OF THROMBOSIS

Given the complexity of hemostasis, it is not surprising that relatively few tests can predict individuals at risk for thrombosis (23,39). Only 15% to 20% of patients with hypercoagulability have an identifiable biochemical abnormality of their plasma proteins (8). Thrombosis is a localized event. Tests based on systemic venous blood samples are insensitive markers of changes occurring on the damaged vascular intima—especially when the latter involves arteries—and tests are performed on venous blood. Also, apart from the physiologic checks and balances of hemostasis, some factors can serve as a systemic procoagulant and a local vessel wall anticoagulant. For

example, thrombin promotes coagulation by catalyzing activation of some zymogens (factors XI, VIII, and V) in the coagulation cascade (8), but it stimulates the intact vascular endothelium to synthesize prostacyclin and NO and also promotes functions of t-PA that together tend to inhibit platelet aggregation and vascular spasm, while enhancing fibrinolysis (10,15,25).

Various studies have identified plasma fibrinogen, factor VIIc (which can be indirectly measured by the prothrombin time), and PAI-1, as markers of arterial thrombosis (39,40). More recently, elevated levels of fragment 1.2, which is derived from the conversion of prothrombin (PT) to thrombin, has been correlated with a thrombotic tendency (41). This test is clinically available and may identify patients at risk for thrombosis. As noted, the PTT is probably of little clinical value, whereas the role of the PT as a measure of anticoagulation is being reevaluated. Native prothrombin antigen has been identified as the sole type of prothrombin in normal blood and can readily be distinguished from abnormal prothrombin, which may be synthesized, for example, in response to treatment with anticoagulants such as warfarin (8). Studies have shown that the adequacy of anticoagulation is better monitored if native prothrombin antigen levels are assayed instead of the PT (42). The effect of exogenous sex steroids on native prothrombin antigen is unknown.

Fibrinopeptides A and B, as well as various FDPs, do change in response to hormone therapy and may be an indirect sign of accelerated coagulation. In this context, the assay of the FDP, D-dimer, may be important. D-dimer, which is an FDP peptide with epitopes that cross-link with those found on activated fibrin, has been used as a marker of ongoing intervascular coagulation, for example, in patients with suspected pulmonary embolism (43).

Reliable assays are available for antithrombin III and proteins C and S. Deficiencies of protein C, protein S, or antithrombin III are associated with thromboembolic disease and are used for screening tests in women with histories of previous thrombotic disease. These protein assays also have to be distinguished from the measurements of activity. Antithrombin III activity must be measured in plasma. Serum antithrombin III only quantifies the amount of antithrombin III left after clotting, and not that consumed during clotting; therefore, it has no clinical relevance to the risk of inappropriate thrombus formation (22). Although activated protein C resistance is said to be present in at least 20% (or more) of patients with venous thrombosis and has been associated with an increased risk of thrombosis in women taking oral contraceptives (see later), routine testing for this factor prior to treating women with HRT is both impractical and costly. Thus, if the prevalence of factor V Leiden is 2% and the positive predictive value of the assay is 44%, the cost of preventing one thromboembolic death is more than $44 million (44).

COAGULATION AND CLINICAL SYNDROMES

The association between accelerated coagulation, venous thrombosis—superficial and deep—and the potential for pulmonary embolism is well recognized and will not be discussed further. Less well recognized is the key role of thrombosis and fibrin formation in the origin and progression of atherosclerosis, and the pathogenesis of acute CAD and associated syndromes. This has recently been reviewed (6). In brief, subsequent to injury of the coronary artery endothelium, macrophages and lipids accumulate at the site of epithelial denudation. The macrophages initiate changes that involve the intima and lead to platelet adhesion and the release of various growth factors. This results in smooth muscle cell proliferation, hypertrophy and migration, and the formation of foam cells, characteristic of the mature atherosclerotic plaque. These lesions appear in most children by the age of puberty (45); however, many regress and it is only in the third decade of life that the lipid-rich plaques are covered by a fibrotic cap with focal areas of microthrombi formation (46). Fibrin and fibrin-related products have been found in the intimal section of these lesions and they are typical of a mature atherosclerotic plaque (47).

Recent angiographic studies have shown that the intimal lesions responsible for subsequent myocardial infarction often have mild (< 50%) to moderate (< 70%) stenosis (48). Thus, recurrent mural thrombi—associated with fissuring and disruption of established plaque—rather than sudden occlusive events may be responsible for much of the unstable angina and eventual myocardial infarctions seen in clinical practice (49). The clinical impact of mural thrombosis is self-evident. The efficacy of thrombolytic therapy when treating patients with acute myocardial infarction is well established. The inhibition or prevention of atherosclerosis by prophylactic antithrombin or fibrinolytic therapy is less clear. Two unrelated (and speculative) observations suggest a potential role for preventive subclinical anticoagulation: pigs with homozygous von Willebrand's disease are resistant to thrombosis and spontaneous atherosclerosis (50). Lower dose aspirin prophylaxis is very effective in preventing coronary thrombosis (51). By inhibiting platelet adhesion at sites of vascular damage, aspirin may prevent microthrombosis and the subsequent evolution of atherosclerosis.

The role of sex steroids in the pathogenesis of the intimal thrombosis and atherogenesis has not been established, but a potential relationship is seen. Apolipoprotein(a), a glycoprotein that is part of the Lp(a) molecule, is structurally similar to plasminogen (52). *In vitro* studies have demonstrated competition between apolipoprotein(a) and plasminogen for the latter's endothelial binding sites (53). By interfering with plasmin generation and clot lysis, endothelial thrombosis results. Lp(a) is also a potent and independent atherogenic moiety. It is absorbed into the arterial intima, where it accumulates in macrophages and is eventually degraded into foam cells, the precursor of arterial plaque (54). Lp(a) also binds to and immobilizes intimal fibrin, promotes plaque formation by the previously discussed thrombin hypothesis. The effect of exogenous estrogen on plasma levels of Lp(a) is variable (55), but some studies have reported a 50% reduction in plasma levels (56). Inconsistency among various studies may be caused by the initial plasma Lp(a) value. Estrogen decreases elevated Lp(a) but has little apparent effect on normal plasma Lp(a) levels. Progestins, and to a lesser extent exogenous estrogen, increase plasma plasminogen antigen and plasminogen activity (5,31). The net potential may be intimal protection via estrogen, because of inhibition of Lp(a) absorption and foam-cell formation, and reduced levels of plasma apolipoprotein(a). This could then free endothelial plasminogen receptors to respond to progestin-stimulated endothelial fibrinolysis if progestins are administered. A recently published study adds some credence to this hypothesis. After 1 year of combination HRT—either estradiol valerate plus MPA or transdermal estrogen plus MPA—significant reductions were noted in plasma levels (compared with baseline) of PAI-1 activity, Lp(a), with corresponding increases in t-PA antigen and the percent of plasminogen (57).

HORMONE REPLACEMENT THERAPY AND VENOUS AND ARTERIAL THROMBOSIS: CLINICAL CONSIDERATIONS

The potential risk of thrombosis in women using estrogen and progestins was based on data of oral contraceptive use prescribed (primarily in the United Kingdom) during the 1960s (2). These data have been extrapolated to postmenopausal hormone therapy, despite the absence—until recently—of a single study demonstrating a significant cause-and-effect relationship between hormone-induced procoagulation and venous or arterial thrombosis. A recent editorial (58) highlighted a basic difference between these earlier studies and currently practiced hormone therapy: the usual dose of estrogen prescribed for menopausal symptom relief and for osteoporosis and cardiovascular protection (conjugated equine estrogen 0.625 mg or its equivalent) is equal to 5 μg of ethinyl estradiol. The earlier oral contraceptives contained between 80 and 100 μg of ethinyl estradiol. The estrogenic enhancement of clotting factors is dose related. For example, low estrogen dose oral contraceptives (30 μg of ethinyl estradiol and 150 mg of norethindrone) were found to increase factors XI and X to a far lesser degree than high-dose preparations (50 μg of mestranol and 1 mg of norethindrone) (59). Use of the low-dose oral contraceptives with the newer progestins (20 μg of ethinyl estradiol and 150 mg of desogesterol) showed similar results with very little change in procoagulation (60). This parallels the reduction in venous thrombosis and thromboembolism following the introduction of low-dose oral contraceptives in Sweden (61). A persistent risk factor is smoking. This effect is also dose related with heavy smokers having a higher relative risk of thrombosis than nonsmokers: 4.3 versus 1.7, respectively (62). The studies cited above are based on oral contraceptive use. A similar relationship with smoking and hormone therapy has not been reported. The adverse effect of smoking may be caused by nicotine-containing tobacco smoke reducing vascular prostacyclin production (63). It is known from epidemiologic studies that estrogen affords protection from cardiovascular disease, even in smokers (see Chapter 20).

Until 1996 epidemiologic studies have not demonstrated a positive association between venous thrombosis and hormonal therapy (4,64). In a 1992 study (65), subjects included women with risks for thrombosis (diabetics, hypertensives) and, once again, the same conclusion was reached. At least two explanations exist for the lowered risk of thrombosis in menopausal women: the menopause is associated with a relative inhibition of blood coagulation, because of higher antithrombin III levels when compared with levels in premenopausal women (66,67); and, as suggested by one study, an enhancement of plasma plasminogen activity is seen (66). Estrogens also increase arterial as well as peripheral blood flow: a deterrent to the stasis of blood associated with venous thrombosis (7,68). Despite this evidence—plus the biologically established nonadverse effect of HRT on hemostasis (see later)—three studies were recently published incriminating HRT with an increased risk of venous thrombosis and thromboembolism (69–71). These studies

provoked a great deal of speculation, but when the findings were confined to their actual clinical impact, the following conclusions were reached: because the incidence of idiopathic venous thromboembolism (VTE) in postmenopausal women is about 1 per 10,000 women, the increased risk of VTE in women on HRT could be 3 per 10,000 treated women per year. In addition, VTE has a mortality risk of less than 1%.

Progestins may have a negative impact on coronary heart disease, depending on the dose and potency of the preparation. Progestins halve the lipid-lowering potential of estrogens; they also may induce peripheral insulin resistance and reduce estrogen-induced vasodilation of coronary arteries. Although progestins have not been shown to be procoagulants (72), they appear to influence the fibrinolytic system favorably, as measured, for example, by plasminogen activity. This is true for studies involving both oral contraceptives (31,73,74) and combination hormone therapy (75). Although the in vivo biologic effect of the increased plasminogen activity is unknown, it may have a preventive or even therapeutic effect on thrombosis. Because of the homology between apolipoprotein(a) and plasminogen (see earlier discussion), it is possible that progestins, by increasing plasminogen activity, can reduce the effect of Lp(a) in inducing atherogenesis (5,57). The effect of progestins on hemostasis was brought into question by the suggestion that the so-called "third generation progestins"—desogestrel and gestodene—were associated with an increased risk of VTE when compared with first (norethindrone) and second (norgestrel group) generation progestin oral contraceptives (76–79). This issue is not relevant to HRT usage because third generation progestins are not prescribed for HRT, but it is important to place these studies in clinical perspective: the probability of death from VTE for women taking third generation oral contraceptives is approximately 20 of 1 million users per year compared with 14 and 5 of 1 million users of second generation oral contraceptives and nonoral contraceptive users, respectively (80). In addition to the low prevalence of VTE in young women, third generation oral contraceptives, in a preliminary interim analysis, are associated with a reduced risk for myocardial infarction compared with second generation oral contraceptives (odds ratio of 0.45) (81).

Extensive literature exists on hormone therapy and its effect on hemostasis (4,82–85). Briefly stated, oral estrogens will induce an increase in the hepatic zymogens—factors VII, X, IX, and II. However, most of the assays measure the inactive proenzyme and the percent increase, although statistically significant in some studies, is invariably well within the physiologic range. It is highly unlikely that these changes have any biologic impact in vivo. Transdermal estrogen has a negligible influence on the hepatic zymogens (86) and is the preferable route of administering estrogen when procoagulant activity is increased, for example, immediately postsurgery. Most importantly, a number of studies have confirmed that, although the effect is variable, ERT does not reduce antithrombin III activity to a clinically meaningful level (86–91). Some studies have shown that conjugated equine estrogens increase plasminogen activity, albeit not to the same degree as with combination hormone therapy. One recent study (91) reported that even markedly reduced doses of ethinyl estradiol (10 μg) increased the factor II-VI-X complex, as well as factor VIIIc—changes that are best avoided, especially in women at high risk for thromboembolic disease. In selected individuals (e.g., those with a previous personal or family history of spontaneous venous thrombosis) testing for factor V Leiden may be appropriate.

The history of hormone therapy and thrombosis needs to be rewritten. The evolving knowledge concerning hemostasis renders much of the published work to date redundant and irrelevant to clinical practice. Even epidemiologic studies showing a positive relationship between thrombosis and plasma fibrinogen (40), for example, must be interpreted and applied with caution. These studies were based on states of endogenous (and pathologic) hyperfibrinoginemia. Elevated levels induced by exogenous hormone therapy are balanced by anticoagulation and enhanced fibrinolysis (75,84,85).

Clinicians are frequently faced with the problem of deciding on the suitability of hormone therapy in women with a history of venous thrombosis. Each patient must be judged individually. In general, if the venous thrombosis was remote (some years previously) and of a nonrecurring nature (e.g., following pelvic surgery), hormone therapy is usually safe. Given the limits of currently available tests and the inability to predict thrombosis accurately, the following tests are recommended—primarily to detect subclinical pathology: plasma fibrinogen; factor VIIa (best tested by measuring the prothrombin time), plasma antithrombin III activity; plasminogen activator inhibitor-1 (PAI-1), protein C; and, possibly, A₂-antiplasmin. If available, the fragment 1.2 test, which is now thought to be the best predictor of thrombosis (41), should be given.

The value of adding androgens when prescribing HRT is gaining increased acceptance. Although definitive studies are lacking, androgens and androgenic progestins are associated with a decrease in PAI-1, a marked decrease in Lp(a), and a general enhancement in fibrinolysis (92).

The type of hormone therapy will be determined by the clinical situation. Preference should be given to the transdermal or subcutaneous (pellets) (93) use of estrogen in those patients at high risk for thrombosis. Believing that progestins enhance fibrinolysis, I would add 1 mg of norethindrone for 2 weeks per month when prescribing cyclic hormone therapy, and 0.35 mg/day of norethindrone when used continuously with the estrogen. As noted, low-dose aspirin (60 to 70 mg every other or third day) should maintain a positive prostacyclin I₂/thromboxane A₂ ratio (94). Smoking should not be allowed. Strenuous exercise induces various degrees of hypercoagulability as well as increased fibrinolysis, which may result from monocyte activation (95) and enhanced thrombin generation (96). However, moderate exercise should be encouraged, because it has an anticoagulant effect and may act synergistically with sex steroids (oral contraceptives) to increase fibrinolytic activity (97).

Coronary artery thrombosis and stroke are listed as absolute contraindications to hormone therapy. This is a wise precaution after a recent event. A number of studies have shown that chronic occlusive coronary artery plaques regress in response to nonsurgical interventions (98,99). Although appropriate prospective studies using hormone therapy have yet to show the same potential, encouraging data associate current hormonal therapy in women with occlusive arterial disease and an improved survival (100). With a better understanding of the pathogenesis of atherogenesis (including the potential role of thrombosis in this process), the safety of estrogen and progestin therapy in menopausal women will become more clearly defined, and the indications for its use widened. At present, the advantages of hormone therapy in preventing CAD and osteoporosis is such that the remote risk of a hormone-induced coagulopathy plays a relatively minor role in the benefit-to-risk equation.

REFERENCES

1. Stampfer MJ, Colditz GA, Willett WC, et al. Postmenopausal estrogen therapy and cardiovascular disease. Ten-year follow-up from the Nurses' Health Study. *N Engl J Med* 1991;325:756–762.
2. Vessey MP, Doll R. Investigation of relation between use of oral contraceptives and thromboembolic disease. *Br Med J* 1968;2:199–205.
3. Barrett-Conner E, Bush TL. Estrogen and coronary heart disease in women. *JAMA* 1991;265:1861–1867.
4. Bush TL, Barret-Connor E. Noncontraceptive estrogen use and cardiovascular disease. *Epidemiol Rev* 1985;7:80–104.
5. Notelovitz M. Progestogens and coagulation. *Int Proc J* 1989;1:229–234.
6. Foster V, Badimon L, Badimon JJ, Cheserro JR. The pathogenesis of coronary artery disease and the acute coronary syndrome. *N Engl J Med* 1992;326:242–250.
7. Gangar KF, Vyas S, Whitehead M, et al. Pulsatility index in internal carotid artery in relation to transdermal estradiol and time since menopause. *Lancet* 1991;338:839–842.
8. Furie B, Furie BC. Molecular and cellular biology of blood coagulation. *N Engl J Med* 1992;326:800–806.
9. Verstraete M, Verhaeghe R. The physiologic mechanism of blood coagulation and fibrinolysis. *Adv Contracept* 1991;(Suppl 3):244–258.
10. Vane JR, Anggard EE, Botting RM. Regularity functions of the vascular endothelium. *N Engl J Med* 1990;323:27–36.
11. Cicinelli E, Ignarro L, Lograno M, Matteo G, Falco N, Schonauer L. Acute effects of transdermal estradiol administration on plasma levels of nitric oxide in postmenopausal women. *Fertil Steril* 1997;67:63–65.
12. Stanczyk F, Rosen G, Ditkoff E, Vijod A, Bernstein L, Lobo R. Influence of estrogen on prostacyclin and thromboxane balance in postmenopausal women. *Men: J of the North Am Men Soc* 1995;2:137–143.
13. Mikkola T, Ranta V, Orpana A, Viinikka L, Ylikorkala O. Hormone replacement therapy modified the capacity of plasma and serum to regulate prostacyclin and endothelin-1 production in human vascular endothelial cells. *Fertil Steril* 1996;66(3):389–393.
14. Golino P, Piscione F, Willerson JT, et al. Divergent effects of serotonin on coronary artery dimensions and blood flow in patients with coronary atherosclerosis and control patients. *N Engl J Med* 1991;324:641–648.
15. Esmon CT. The roles of protein C and thrombomodulin in the regulation of blood coagulation. *J Biol Chem* 1989;264:4743–4746.
16. Marcum JA, Rosenberg RD. Anticoagulantly active heparin-like molecules from vascular tissue. *Biochemistry* 1984;23:1730–1737.

17. Loscalzo J, Braunwald E. Tissue plasminogen activator. *N Engl J Med* 1988;319: 925–931.
18. Larsen E, Celi A, Gilbert GE, et al. PADGEM protein: a receptor that mediates the interaction of activated platelets with neutrophils and monocytes. *Cell* 1989; 59:305–312.
19. Heavey DJ, Barran SE, Hickling NE, Ritter JM. Aspirin causes short-lived inhibition of bradykinin-stimulated prostacyclin in man. *Nature* 1985;318:186–188.
20. Bar J, Tepper R, Fuchs J, Pardo Y, Goldberger S, Ovadia J. The effect of estrogen replacement therapy on platelet aggregation and adenosine triphosphate release in postmenopausal women. *Obstet Gynecol* 1993;81:261–264.
21. Aune B, Ian P, Omsj I, sterud B. Hormone replacement therapy reduces the reactivity of monocytes and platelets in whole blood—a beneficial effect on atherogenesis and thrombus formation? *Am J Obstet Gynecol* 1995;173:1816–1820.
22. Mammen AF. Oral contraceptives and blood coagulation: a critical review. *Am J Obstet Gynecol* 1982;142:781–790.
23. Winkler U. Hormone replacement therapy and hemostasis: principles of a complex interaction. *Maturitas* 1996;24:131–145.
24. Osterud B, Rapaport SI. Activation of factor IX by the reaction product of tissue factor and factor VII: additional pathway for initiating blood coagulation. *Proc Natl Acad Sci U S A* 1977;74:5260–5264.
25. Collen D. On the regulation and control of fibrinolysis. *Thromb Heamost* 1980; 43:77–89.
26. Dahlbäck B. Protein S and C4b-binding protein: components involved in the regulation of the protein C anticoagulant system. *Thromb Haemost* 1991;66:49–61.
27. Simioni P, Prandoni P, Lensing A, et al. The risk of recurrent venous thromboembolism in patients with an ARG^{506} Gln mutation in the gene for factor V (factor V Leiden). *N Engl J Med* 1997;336:399–403.
28. Rosenberg RD. Actions and interactions of anti-thrombin and heparin. *N Engl J Med* 1975;292:146–150.
29. Jordan RE, Fayreau LV, Braswell EH, Rosenberg RD. Heparin with two binding sites for anti-thrombin or platelet factor 4. *J Biol Chem* 1982;257:400–406.
30. Egeberg O. Inherited anti-thrombin deficiency causing thrombophilia. *Thromb Diath Haemorrh* 1965;13:516–530.
31. Jesperson J, Peterson KR, Skouby SO. Effects of newer oral contraceptives on the inhibition of coagulation and fibrinolysis in relation to dosage and type of steroid. *Am J Obstet Gynecol* 1990;163:396–403.
32. Sprengers ED, Kluft C. Plasminogen-activated inhibitors. *Blood* 1987;69: 381–387.
33. Lindoff C, Peterson F, Lecander I, Martinsson G, Åstedt B. Transdermal estrogen replacement therapy: beneficial effects on hemostatic risk factors for cardiovascular disease. *Maturitas* 1996;24:43–50.
34. Koh K, Mincemoyer R, Bui M, et al. Effects of hormone-replacement therapy on fibrinolysis in postmenopausal women. *N Engl J Med* 1997;336:683–690.
35. Lijnen HB, Hoylaerts M, Collen D. Isolation and characterization of a human plasma protein with affinity for the lysine binding sites in plasminogen. Role of the regulation of fibrinolysis and identification of histidine-rich glucoprotein. *J Biol Chem* 1980;255:10214–10222.
36. Haukkamaa M, Morgan WT, Koskelo P. Serum histamine-rich glycoprotein during pregnancy and hormone treatment. *Scand J Clin Lab Invest* 1983;43: 591–595.
37. Conard J, Gompel A, Pelissier C, Mirabel C, Basdevant A. Fibrinogen and plasminogen modifications during oral estradiol replacement therapy. *Fertil Steril* 1997;68:449–453.
38. Aoki N, Saito H, Kamiya T, et al. Congenital deficiency of α^2 plasmin inhibitor associated with severe hemorrhagic tendency. *J Clin Invest* 1979;63:877–884.
39. Kluft C. Disorders of the hemostatic system and the risk of the development of thrombotic and cardiovascular disease: limitation of laboratory diagnosis. *Am J Obstet Gynecol* 1990;163:305–312.
40. Kelleher CC. Clinical aspects of the relationship between oral contraceptives and abnormalities of the hemostatic system: relation to the development of cardiovascular disease. *Am J Obstet Gynecol* 1990;163:392–395.
41. Conway EM, Bauer KA, Barzegar J, Rosenberg RD. Suppression of hemostatic system activation by oral anti-coagulants in the blood of patients with thrombotic diathesis. *J Clin Invest* 1987;80:1533–1544.
42. Hirsh J. Oral anticoagulant drugs. *N Engl J Med* 1991;324:1865–1875.
43. Bounameaux H, Cirafici P, de Moerloose P, et al. Measurement of d-dimer in plasma as diagnostic aid in suspected pulmonary embolism. *Lancet* 1990;1: 196–200.
44. Altés A, Souto J, Mateo J, Borrell M, Fontcuberta J. Activated protein C resistance assay when applied in the general population. *Am J Obstet Gynecol* 1997; 176:358–359.
45. Stary HC. Evolution and progression of atherosclerotic lesions in coronary arteries of children and young adults. *Arteriosclerosis* 1989;99(Suppl 1):I19–I32.
46. Davies MJ, Woolf N, Rowles PM, Pepper J. Morphology of the endometrium over atherosclerotic plaques in human coronary arteries. *Br Heart J* 1988;60: 459–464.
47. Smith EB, Kean A, Grant A. Stirk C. Fate of fibrinogen in human arterial intima. *Arteriosclerosis* 1990;10:263–275.
48. Little WC. Angiographic assessment of the culprit coronary artery lesion before acute myocardial infarction. *Am J Cardiol* 1990;66:44G–47G.
49. Falk E. Unstable angina with fatal outcome: dynamic coronary artery thrombosis leading to infarction and/or sudden death. Autopsy evidence of recurrent mural thrombosis with peripheral embolization culminating in total vascular occlusion. *Circulation* 1985;71:699–708.
50. Foster V, Griggs TR. Porcine von Willebrand disease: implications for the pathophysiology of atherosclerosis and thrombosis. *Prog Hemost Thromb* 1968;8: 159–183.
51. Manson JE, Stampfer MJ, Colditz GA, et al. A prospective study of aspirin use and primary prevention of cardiovascular disease in women. *JAMA* 1991;266: 521–527.
52. Loscalzo J. A unique risk factor for athero-thrombotic disease. *Arteriosclerosis* 1990;10:672–679.
53. Hajjar KA, Gavish D, Breslow JL, Nachman RL. Lipoprotein(a) modulation of endothelial cell surface fibrinolysis and its potential role in atherosclerosis. *Nature* 1989;339:303–305.
54. Smith EB, Cochran S. Factors influencing the accumulation in fibrous plaques of lipid derived from low density lipoprotein. II: Preferential immobilization of lipoprotein(a): LP(a). *Arteriosclerosis* 1990;84:173–181.
55. Lobo RA, Notelovitz M, Bernstein L, et al. Lipoprotein(a) [Lp(a)]: relationship to cardiovascular disease risk factors, exercise and estrogen. *Am J Obstet Gynecol* 1992;166:1182–1190.
56. Henricksen P, Angelin B, Berglund L. Hormonal effects of serum Lp(a) levels: marked reduction during estrogen treatment in males with prostatic cancer [Abstract]. *Arterioscler Thromb Vasc Biol* 1991;11:1423a.
57. Gilabert J, Estellés A, Cano A, et al. The effect of estrogen replacement therapy with or without progestogen on the fibrinolytic system and coagulation inhibitors in postmenopausal status. *Am J Obstet Gynecol* 1995;173:1849–1854.
58. Lobo RA. Estrogen and the risk of coagulopathy. *Am J Med* 1992;92:283–285.
59. Sabra A, Bonner J. Hemostatic system changes induced by 50 μg and 30 μg estrogen/progestogen oral contraceptives. *J Reprod Med* 1983;28(Suppl):85–91.
60. Melis GB, Fruzzetti F, Ricci C, et al. Oral contraceptives and venous thromboembolic disease: the effect of oestrogen dose. *Maturitas* 1988;(Suppl 1): 131–139.
61. Bottiger LE, Boman G, Eklund G, Wetterholm B. Oral contraceptives and thromboembolic disease: effects on lowering oestrogen content. *Lancet* 1980; XX:1097–1101.
62. Craft P, Hannaford PC. Risk factors for acute myocardial infarction in women: evidence from the Royal College of General Practitioners' oral contraception study. *Br Med J* 1989;298:165–168.
63. Nadler JL, Velasco JS, Horton R. Cigarette smoking inhibits prostacyclin formation. *Lancet* 1983;1:1248.
64. The Boston Collaborative Drug Surveillance Program. Surgically confirmed gallbladder disease, venous thromboembolism and breast tumors in relation to postmenopausal estrogen therapy. *N Engl J Med* 1974;290:15–19.
65. Devor M, Barrett-Connor E, Renvall M, et al. Estrogen replacement therapy and the risk of venous thrombosis. *Am J Med* 1992;92:275–282.
66. Notelovitz M, Kitchens CS, Rappaport Y, et al. Menopausal status associated with increased inhibition of blood coagulation. *Am J Obstet Gynecol* 1981;141: 149–152.
67. Meade TW, Dyer S, Howarth DJ, et al. Anti-thrombin III and procoagulant activity: sex differences and effects of the menopause. *Br J Haematol* 1990;74:77–81.
68. Bourne T, Hillard TC, Whitehead MI, et al. Oestrogens, arterial status, and post-menopausal women. *Lancet* 1990;325: 1470–1471.
69. Daly E, Vessey M, Hawkins M, Carson J, Gough P, Marsh S. Risk of venous thromboembolism in users of hormone replacement therapy. *Lancet* 1996;348:977–980.
70. Jick H, Derby L, Myers M, Vasilakis C, Newton K. Risk of hospital admission for idiopathic venous thromboembolism among users of postmenopausal oestrogens. *Lancet* 1996;348:981–983.
71. Grodstein F, Stampfer M, Goldhaber S, et al. Prospective study of exogenous hormones and risk of pulmonary embolism in women. *Lancet* 1996;348:983–987.
72. Aylward M. Coagulation factors in opposed and unopposed oestrogen treatment at the climacteric. *Postgrad Med J* 1978;54(Suppl 2):31–37.
73. Notelovitz M, Kitchens C, Coone R, et al. Low-dose oral contraceptive usage and coagulation. *Am J Obstet Gynecol* 1981;141:71–76.
74. Beller FK, Ebert P. Effects of oral contraceptives on blood coagulation: a review. *Obstet Gynecol Surv* 1985;44:425436.
75. Notelovitz M, Kitchens C, Ware M, et al. Combination estrogen and progestogen replacement therapy does not adversely affect coagulation. *Obstet Gynecol* 1983;62:596–600.
76. World Health Organization Collaborative Study of Cardiovascular Disease and Steroid Hormone Contraception. Venous thromboembolic disease and combined oral contraceptives: results of international multicentre case-control study. *Lancet* 1995;346:1575–1582.
77. World Health Organization Collaborative Study of Cardiovascular Disease and Steroid Hormone Contraception. Effect of different progestogens in low oestrogen oral contraceptives on venous thromboembolic disease. *Lancet* 1995;346: 1582–1588.
78. Jick H, Jick S, Gurewich V, Myers M, Vasilakis C. Risk of idiopathic cardiovascular death and nonfatal venous thromboembolism in women using oral contractive with differing progestogen components. *Lancet* 1995;346:1589–1593.
79. Bloemenkamp K, Rosendaal F, Helmerhorst F, Büller H, Vandenbroucke J. Enhancement by factor V Leiden mutation of risk of deep-vein thrombosis associated with oral contraceptives containing a third-generation progestagen. *Lancet* 1995;346:1593–1596.
80. Spitzer W, Lewis M, Heinemann L, Thorogood M, MacRae K. Third generation oral contraceptives and risk of venous thromboembolic disorders: an international case-control study. *BMJ* 1996;312:83–88.
81. Lewis M, Spitzer W, Heinemann L, MacRae K, Bruppacher R, Thorogood M.

Third generation oral contractive and risk of myocardial infarction: an international case-control study. *BMJ* 1996;312:88–90.

82. Notelovitz M, Ware M. Coagulation risks with postmenopausal oestrogen therapy [Review article]. In: Studd J, ed. *Progress in Obstetrics and Gynecology*, Vol 2. Edinburgh: Churchill-Livingstone, 1983:228–240.

83. Young RL, Goepfert AR, Goldzieher HW. Estrogen replacement therapy is not conducive of venous thromboembolism. *Maturitas* 1991;13:189–192.

84. Kessler C, Szymanski L, Shamsipour Z, Muesing R, Miller V, LaRosa J. Estrogen replacement therapy and coagulation: relationship to lipid and lipoprotein changes. *Obstet Gynecol* 1997;89:326–331.

85. Lobo R, Pickar J, Wild R, Walsh B, Hirvonen E. Metabolic impact of adding medroxyprogesterone acetate to conjugated estrogen therapy in postmenopausal women. *Obstet Gynecol* 1994;84:987–995.

86. Chetkowski RJ, Meldrum DR, Steingold KA, et al. Biologic effects of transdermal estradiol. *N Engl J Med* 1986;314:1615–1620.

87. Steingold KA, Matt DW, de Ziegler D, et al. Comparison of transdermal to oral estradiol administration on hormonal and hepatic parameters in women with premature ovarian failure. *J Clin Endocrinol Metab* 1991;73:275–280.

88. Boschetti C, Cortellaro M, Nencione T, et al. Short- and long-term effects of hormone replacement therapy (transdermal estradiol vs. oral conjugated equine estrogens, combined with medroxyprogesterone acetate) on blood coagulation factors in post-menopausal women. *Thromb Res* 1991;62:1–8.

89. Notelovitz M, Greig HBW. Natural estrogen and anti-thrombin III activity in postmenopausal women. *J Reprod Med* 1976;16:87–90.

90. Notelovitz M, Kitchens CS, Ware MD. Coagulation and fibrinolysis in estrogen-treated surgically menopausal women. *Obstet Gynecol* 1984;63:621–625.

91. Lindberg UB, Crona N, Stigendal L, et al. A comparison between effects of estradiol valerate and low dose ethinyl estradiol on hemostasis parameters. *Thromb Haemost* 1989;61:65–69.

92. Winkler U. Effects of androgens on haemostasis. *Maturitas* 1996;24:147–155.

93. Notelovitz M, Johnston M, Smith S, Kitchen C. Metabolic and hormonal effects of 25 mg and 50 mg 17β-estradiol implants in surgically menopausal women. *Obstet Gynecol* 1987;70:749–754.

94. Clarke RJ, Mayo G, Price P, Fitzgerald GA. Suppression of thromboxane A_2 but not of systemic prostacyclin by controlled-release aspirin. *N Engl J Med* 1991;325:1137–1141.

95. Østerud B, Olsen JO, Wilsgård L. Effect of strenuous exercise on blood monocytes and their relation to coagulation. *Med Sci Sports Exercise* 1989;21:374–378.

96. Bärtsch P, Haeberli A, Straub PW. Blood coagulation after long-distance running: anti-thrombin III prevents fibrin formation. *Thromb Haemost* 1990;6:430–434.

97. Notelovitz M, Zauner C, McKenzie L, et al. The effect of low-dose oral contraceptives on cardiorespiratory function, coagulation, and lipids in exercising young women: a preliminary report. *Am J Obstet Gynecol* 1987;156:591–598.

98. Ornish D, Brown SE, Scherwitz LW, et al. Can lifestyle changes reverse coronary heart disease? *Lancet* 1990;336:129–133.

99. Kane JP, Malloy JM, Ports TA, et al. Regression of coronary atherosclerosis during treatment of familial hypercholesterolemia with combined drug regimens. *JAMA* 1990;264:3007–3012.

100. Sullivan JM, Vanderzwaag R, Lemp G, et al. Estrogen replacement and coronary artery disease. Effect on survival in postmenopausal women. *Ann Intern Med* 1988;108:358–363.

Treatment of the Postmenopausal Woman: Basic and Clinical Aspects, Second Edition, edited by Rogerio A. Lobo, Lippincott Williams & Wilkins, Philadelphia © 1999.

CHAPTER 37

Blood Pressure: Effects of Estrogen and Management of Hypertension in Women

Jay M. Sullivan

Hypertension is a highly prevalent disease in the United States, involving approximately 50 million Americans. It is a major risk factor for coronary heart disease, stroke, and renal failure, and it is one of the major causes of the rising incidence of heart failure in this country (1). The prevalence of hypertension increases with age so that more than half of Americans aged older than 60 years have blood pressures higher than 140 mmHg systolic and 90 mmHg diastolic. Because women constitute the largest proportion of the older population, hypertension is a particular problem for postmenopausal women (2). Rates of control for hypertension are poor in the United States and particularly bad in individuals aged more than 60 years. Recent surveys have shown that no more than 27% of hypertensive Americans are taking sufficient antihypertensive medication to lower their systolic blood pressure to levels beneath 140 mmHg and the diastolic pressure to beneath 90 mmHg (3). The rate of uncontrolled hypertension among Americans aged more than 60 years is greater than 75%. Isolated systolic hypertension (systolic blood pressure > 140 mmHg with diastolic pressure < 90 mmHg) is the most common type of hypertension in individuals in this age group, and it is particularly prevalent in women. Poorly controlled hypertension is a major cause of heart failure, which is the leading cause of hospitalization among older Americans (4).

A serious need exists for better identification and control of hypertension among older Americans, particularly women.

ESTROGEN AND BLOOD PRESSURE

Many physicians are reluctant to prescribe estrogen replacement therapy for women with elevated blood pressure because of their concern that hypertension might worsen. However, a substantial body of evidence exists to support the conclusion that estrogen usually lowers blood pressure. One of the earliest studies to evaluate the relationship between estrogen use and blood pressure was that of Pfeffer et al. (5). This observational study found no difference in blood pressure between those who used estrogen and those who did not, and they also noted a 4.4 mmHg fall in the systolic blood pressure of hypertensive women who received estrogen.

Barrett-Conner et al. (6), in the Leisure World Study, followed 1,057 women aged between 50 and 79 years, noting significantly lower diastolic blood pressure in current estrogen users, although no difference in systolic pressure was found between users versus nonusers. In a prospective, controlled 126-day study of the effect of different forms of hormone replacement therapy on blood pressure in postmenopausal women, Lind et al. (7) found that systolic and diastolic blood pressure fell in approximately 30 of the 41 patients who received treatment. Average systolic and diastolic blood pressures fell significantly, although the decrease was not of great magnitude. The short-term hemodynamic effects of micronized 17β-estradiol was studied in 10 normotensive women who received doses of 2 and 4 mg in a double-blind, placebo-controlled crossover trial (8). A mean reduction of 7 mmHg of systolic blood pressure and 5 mmHg of diastolic blood pressure was observed in the 10 normotensive patients while receiving estradiol. In 10 hypertensive subjects, the average reduction of blood pressure was 11 mmHg (systolic) and 6 mmHg (diastolic). The 4 mg dose of estradiol did not reduce blood pressure more than 2 mg.

J. M. Sullivan: Division of Cardiovascular Diseases, University of Tennessee, Memphis, Tennessee 38163.

Data are beginning to emerge about the effect of trans-dermal estrogen on blood pressure. Mercuro et al. (9) studied 16 hypertensive women randomized to receive 17β-estradiol in a dose of 100 mg/day or placebo. Ambu-latory blood pressure monitoring showed that transder-mal estradiol lowered 24-hour mean systolic blood pres-sure by 9 mmHg and diastolic blood pressure by 5 mmHg ($p < 0.05$) versus placebo. In a study of 90 normotensive women (10), nonrandomly assigned to oral or transder-mal estrogen replacement, 24-hour blood pressure moni-toring found that transdermal estrogen lowered nocturnal and daytime pressures significantly, whereas oral estro-gen had no significant effect. Blood pressure increased in approximately one third of the patients on either form of replacement.

MECHANISMS

A number of studies have evaluated the effect of estro-gen on arterial blood flow and arterial tone. Studies found that estrogen increased uterine blood flow in both animals and humans (11,12). More recent studies have found that brachial blood flow in postmenopausal women was not increased by either intravenous or inter-arterial physiologic doses of 17β-estradiol or by oral conjugated equine estrogens (13,14). However, transder-mal 17β-estradiol has been shown to increase flow-mediated dilation of the brachial artery in postmeno-pausal women, but not men (15).

Estrogen also increases blood flow in the coronary ves-sels. In a study of nonhuman primates, Williams et al. (16) noted that after animals were ovariectomized and fed a high fat diet, they responded to intracoronary acetylcholine with a decrease in coronary artery diameter, indicating vasoconstriction. With estrogen replacement, vasoconstric-tion was less; in some cases, vasodilation occurred. Williams et al. concluded that endothelial function declines during estrogen deprivation and that estrogen replacement reverses this trend. Subsequently, Herrington et al. (17) studied the response to intracoronary acetyl-choline in three postmenopausal women with mild coro-nary disease who were taking hormone replacement and compared their response with that of seven women who did not receive estrogen replacement therapy. Increasing doses of intracoronary acetylcholine caused dose-depen-dent vasoconstriction in women who were not receiving estrogen replacement, whereas dose-dependent relaxation was observed in those who had received estrogen replace-ment. The response of the coronary vessels to intravenous estrogen has also been studied in postmenopausal women. Reis et al. (18) studied 15 postmenopausal women and found that ethinyl estradiol (35 μg) given intravenously lowered coronary vascular resistance by 15% and in-creased coronary blood flow, all within a time frame of 15 minutes. Intravenous estradiol resulted in an increased vasodilatory response to acetylcholine in women with nor-

mal coronary arteries and less vasoconstriction in those women whose coronary arteries were abnormal. These results were confirmed by Gilligan et al. (19), who found that 17β-estradiol increased endothelial-dependent coro-nary vasodilation in postmenopausal women. Collins et al. compared the effect of intracoronary estradiol (2.5 μg 17β-estradiol) in postmenopausal women and comparably aged men (20). Control measurements, made before estradiol administration, showed that intracoronary acetylcholine caused vasoconstriction in both men and women. However, only 20 minutes after receiving intracoronary estradiol, the administration of acetylcholine caused dilation in the coro-nary arteries of women. However, in men, vasoconstriction continued.

The vasodilator effects of estrogens appear to involve several mechanisms. Among the most important is the effect on endothelial function. Estrogen has been found to increase the release of nitric oxide (NO) from the endothelial cells. Results of studies of the effect of estro-gen on the expression of genes that encode for the enzyme NO synthase are contradictory, some showing an increase, whereas others do not (20). Estrogen increases the effect of NO after its release by decreasing the for-mation of oxygen-derived free radicals (21), which com-bine with NO to form a toxic compound. In addition, estrogen has been found to be an antioxidant (22).

Administration of estrogen results in lower circulating levels of endothelin-1 (23). Estrogen also blocks the response of blood vessels to the vasoconstrictor effects of endothelin (24).

In addition, nongenomic membrane effects of estro-gens lead to vasodilation. Estrogen blocks calcium chan-nels (25), which results in lower cytoplasmic calcium concentrations and less forceful interaction between actin and myocin, thus vasodilation. In addition, estrogen opens potassium channels (26), which causes repolariza-tion changes and relaxation of vascular smooth muscle. In studies of estrogen's effect on arachonic acid metabo-lism, it has been observed that estrogen enhances release of prostacyclin, which is a vasodilator, and opposes the action of thromboxane A_2, which is a vasoconstrictor (27).

Although the vasodilator properties of estrogen result in a drop in blood pressure in most women, it must been noted that an occasional women has an idiosyncratic response and manifests an elevation of blood pressure. Therefore, it is important to monitor blood pressure in women who receive estrogen replacement therapy.

ORAL CONTRACEPTIVES AND BLOOD PRESSURE

In contrast to the usual blood pressure lowering effects of estrogens, oral contraceptive agents, which combine estrogens with progestins in higher doses, usu-ally cause an increase in blood pressure. This elevation of pressure is usually not clinically significant because most of the users of oral contraceptives are young and have relatively low blood pressure prior to beginning the use of oral contraceptives. Studies of different populations of women have reported varying occurrence rates of hypertension among oral contraceptive users. The Royal College of General Practitioners reported that 1.5% of women receiving oral contraceptives developed significant hypertension, whereas the incidence was only 0.25% in women who did not use oral contraceptives (28). Over a 5-year period of observation, 5% of the women who used oral contraceptive agents were found to have blood pressures exceeding 140/90 mmHg. However, the frequency with which malignant hypertension was noted was rare. In a prospective study of 83 women, Weir et al. (29) observed an average increase in systolic blood pressure of 9.2 mmHg and of diastolic blood pressure of 5.0 mmHg over a 3-year period of estrogen use. In women who did not take oral contraceptives, no significant change in blood pressure occurred. This study also made the important observation that blood pressure usually returns to pretreatment levels within 3 months of discontinuation of oral contraceptives. The Walnut Creek Contraceptive Drug Study found that systolic blood pressure increased by 5 to 6 mmHg and diastolic pressure increased by 1 to 2 mmHg in women who used oral contraceptives (30). In a study of 16 women who received oral contraceptive agents containing estrogens and progestins, Wineberger et al. (31) observed an increase in blood pressure to hypertensive levels in 11 women with blood pressure rising after 3 to 36 months of use. On discontinuation of oral contraceptive use, blood pressure returned to pretreatment levels in five of the women whereas in six, blood pressure fell, but not to pretreatment levels.

In the Nurses' Health Study, 62,718 women who had never used oral contraceptives were compared with 7,074 who were current users and 42,269 past users (31a). The prevalence of hypertension was 11.8% in nonusers, 12.0% in current users and 16.4% in past users. The higher prevalence in past users was attributed to increased blood pressure monitoring in women receiving oral contraceptives and the practice of discontinuing oral contraceptives when blood pressure becomes elevated.

Studies have not found a significant increase in blood pressure when oral contraceptive agents are used that contained estrogens in doses less that 50 µg (32,33). This observation suggests that the effect is dose related.

Overall, these studies have shown that women who are older than 35 years and who are obese are most likely to develop hypertension while using oral contraceptive agents. In addition, those women who have a positive family history of hypertension are more likely to develop blood pressure elevation with oral contraceptive agent use. Interestingly, hypertension during pregnancy does not predict the development of hypertension with oral

contraceptive agent use (34). The mechanism by which oral contraceptives increase blood pressure remains under debate (35). During the administration of estrogen, levels of angiotensinogen or renin substrate increase because of increased hepatic synthesis. This results in the production of higher levels of angiotensin I and angiotensin II, which in turn causes vasoconstriction and aldosterone secretion. Aldosterone levels are high during estrogen use. However, these changes in the renin-angiotensin-aldosterone axis occur in both women who become hypertensive and those who remain normotensive; therefore, their contribution to the genesis of blood pressure elevations is not clear. It has been proposed that some women fail to suppress renin secretion, whereas renin substrate is elevated and sodium retained (36). However, other studies have questioned this conclusion (37). It has also been proposed that women who have mild impairment of renal function are most susceptible to oral contraceptive-induced hypertension because of a failure of angiotensin II to decrease renal blood flow appropriately.

Data from the Royal College of General Practitioners also implicate progestins in the genesis of hypertension (38). In a recent review, Oelkers (39) proposed that high doses of estrogens such as ethinyl estradiol and mestranol stimulate hepatic production of angiotensinogen, which leads to an increase of angiotension II sufficient to reduce renal blood flow and increase exchangeable sodium and blood pressure in susceptible women. Additionally, he proposes that certain synthetic progestogens are weak estrogen receptor agonists that enhance the effect of estrogens on blood pressure and body sodium.

Few studies have examined the effect of progestins on vascular resistance and reactivity. Limited data indicate that progestins are vasoconstrictors. In studies of uterine blood flow in castrated ewes, Anderson et al. (40) noted that uterine blood flow increased when estradiol was given alone; however, when supplemented with progesterone, the increase in blood flow was blunted. Similarly, Batra et al. (41) found that progesterone reduced the effect of estrogen on blood flow to the uterus, vagina, and urethra in the rabbit. In studies of hind limb vascular reactivity in pregnant ewes, McLaughlin et al. (42) found that progesterone increased the vascular response to phenylephrine but decreased the response to vasoconstrictor response to angiotensin II, suggesting a differential effect on α-adenergic and angiotensin II receptors. In studies of cochlear blood flow in the rat, Laugel et al. (43) also noted that progesterone pretreatment increased the pressor response of angiotensin II. Laugel et al. also found that a combination of progesterone and estrogen increased the blood pressor response to phenylephrine (44).

In human studies, uterine blood flow has been measured by Doppler techniques in postmenopausal women. These studies have found that transdermal estrogen replacement therapy increased blood flow and that vaginal progesterone did not prevent the increase in blood flow induced by estrogen (45). However, another study found that the uterine artery pulsatility index decreases during estrogen replacement therapy but increases when progesterone is added (46). This was confirmed by a study (47) that found less decrease of uterine artery pulsatility index when estrogens were given with progestins in comparison with when estrogen was given alone. Sullivan et al. (14) have also observed that progestin increases forearm vascular resistance, decreases venous compliance, and increases pressor responsiveness to cold in postmenopausal women.

In a series of experiments involving oophorectomized nonhuman primates Adams et al. observed that the addition of medroxyprogesterone acetate attenuates the restoration of endothelial function noted with estrogen replacement in oophorectomized monkeys receiving a high fat diet. In contrast, when natural progesterone was used, the effect of estradiol was unimpaired (48). No studies have reported on the effect of progestins on vascular biology. In contrast, numerous studies have examined the vascular biologic effects of estradiol and have identified two types of estrogen receptors, α and β, in blood vessels. Estrogen

receptors have also been demonstrated in human endothelial and vascular smooth muscle cells (49).

MANAGEMENT OF HYPERTENSION IN WOMEN

Rationale

Neither female gender nor age reduces the cardiovascular risk imposed by untreated hypertension. Systolic blood pressure is a particularly strong predictor of cardiovascular events. For each 10 mmHg rise in systolic pressure, the risk of myocardial infarction or cerebrovascular accident increases by 20% to 30%. A reduction of systolic blood pressure of 10 mmHg reduces the risk of coronary heart disease by 20% to 25%, as does a reduction of 5 mmHg diastolic pressure. Without treatment, a hypertensive woman is approximately 2.5 times more likely to develop coronary artery disease and 3.5 times more likely to have a cerebrovascular accident than a woman whose blood pressure is beneath 140/90. The outcomes of five trials of antihypertensive treatment of older patients are shown in Fig. 37.1 (50).

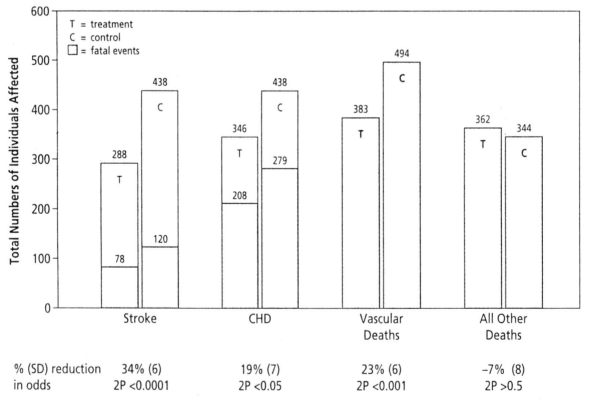

FIG. 37.1. The studies assessed the effects of blood pressure reduction on stroke, coronary heart disease, vascular death, and nonvascular death in 12,483 patients aged more than 60 years (systolic blood pressure difference of 12 to 14 mmHg, diastolic blood pressure difference of 5 to 6 mmHg), follow-up 5 years. SD, standard deviation. (From the sixth report of the Joint National Committee on Prevention, Detection, Evaluation, and Treatment of High Blood Pressure. *Arch Intern Med* 1997;157:2413–2446; with permission.)

TABLE 37.1. *Classification of blood pressure for adults age 18 and older**

Category	Systolic (mmHg)		Diastolic (mmHg)
Optimal†	<120	and	<80
Normal	<130	and	<85
High-normal	130–139	or	85–89
Hypertension‡			
Stage 1	140–159	or	90–99
Stage 2	160–179	or	100–109
Stage 3	≥180	or	≥110

*Not taking antihypertensive drugs and not acutely ill. When systolic and diastolic blood pressures fall into different categories, the higher category should be selected to classify the individual's blood pressure status. For example, 160/92 mmHg should be classified as stage 2 hypertension, and 174/120 mmHg should be classified as stage 3 hypertension. Isolated systolic hypertension is defined as SBP of 140 mmHg or greater and DBP below 90 mmHg and staged appropriately (e.g., 170/82 mmHg is defined as stage 2 isolated systolic hypertension). In addition to classifying stages of hypertension on the basis of average blood pressure levels, clinicians should specify presence or absence of target organ disease and additional risk factors. This specificity is important for risk classification and treatment.

†Optional blood pressure with respect to cardiovascular risk is below 120/80 mmHg. However, unusually low readings should be evaluated for clinical significance.

‡Based on the average of two or more readings taken at each of two or more visits after an initial screening.

(From the sixth report of the joint national committee on prevention, detection, evaluation, and treatment of high blood pressure. *Arch Intern Med* 1997;157:2413–2446; with permission.)

Evaluation

Blood pressure should be measured in the seated position, with the arm and back supported, after a 5-minute wait, with a sphygmomanometer and properly sized cuff. Blood pressure should be measured supine and standing to detect postural hypotension on the first visit. In older patients, consider the possibility of pseudohypertension caused by stiff blood vessels that fail to compress as the sphygmomanometer cuff is inflated (3).

Because older patients can have considerable variability in blood pressure, two or three measurements of blood pressure should be made on two or three separate occasions. These measurement should not be made when the patient has recently eaten or has a full bladder.

The current classification of blood pressure in adults is given in Table 37.1.

In the physical examination, look for vascular changes in the optic retina, evidence of cardiac enlargement, abdominal aorta aneurysm, vascular bruits, diminished peripheral pulses, and evidence of congestive heart failure or prior cerebrovascular accident.

Laboratory studies should consist of complete blood count; urinalysis; blood chemistry for sodium, potassium, creatinine, glucose, total and HDL cholesterol and uric acid; and an electrocardiogram (3).

It is particularly important to note the presence of other cardiovascular risk factors such as family history of cardiovascular disease, obesity, diabetes, hypercholesterolemia, smoking, and physical inactivity. The Sixth Joint National Committee on Prevention, Detection, Evaluation, and Treatment of High Blood Pressure (JNC-IV) report recommends risk stratification and treatment as outlined in Table 37.2.

TABLE 37.2. *Risk stratification and treatment**

Blood pressure stages (mmHg)	Risk group A (No risk factors; no TOD/CCD)†	Risk group B (At least 1 risk factor, not including diabetes; no TOD/CCD)	Risk group C (TOD/CCD and/or diabetes; with or without other risk factors)
High-normal (130–139/85–89)	Lifestyle modification	Lifestyle modification	Drug therapy§
Stage 1 (140–159/90–99)	Lifestyle modification (up to 12 months)	Lifestyle modification‡ (up to 6 months)	Drug therapy
Stages 2 and 3 (≥160/≥100)	Drug therapy	Drug therapy	Drug therapy

For example, a patient with diabetes and a blood pressure of 142/94 mmHg plus left ventricular hypertrophy should be classified as having stage 1 hypertension with target organ disease (left ventricular hypertrophy) and with another major risk factor (diabetes). This patient would be categorized as **Stage 1, Risk Group C,** and recommended for immediate initiation of pharmacologic treatment.

*Lifestyle modification should be adjunctive therapy for all patients recommended for pharmacologic therapy.

†TOD/CCD indicates target organ disease/clinical cardiovascular disease.

‡For patients with multiple risk factors, clinicians should consider drugs as initial therapy plus lifestyle modifications.

§For those with heart failure, renal insufficiency, or diabetes.

(From the sixth report of the Joint national committee on prevention, detection, evaluation, and treatment of high blood pressure. *Arch Intern Med* 1997;157:2413–2446; with permission.)

Secondary causes of hypertension should be suspected in individuals whose blood pressure abruptly rises to levels above 180/110 after the age of 55, if blood pressure cannot be controlled with triple drug therapy taken reliably, if a previously effective program no longer controls blood pressure, or if clinical or laboratory findings suggest a secondary cause of hypertension such as renal failure, hyperaldosteronism, pheochromocytoma, or renal artery stenosis. It should be remembered that bilateral renal artery stenosis is more common in older patients than had been previously suspected (3).

Treatment

Treatment should begin with the setting of a therapeutic goal. In most cases, this should be to lower blood pressure to beneath 140/90 mmHg. In certain older individuals, an intermediate goal might be required first, such as to lower the systolic pressure beneath 160. However, certain high risk groups, such as those with chronic renal failure or diabetes mellitus, should have more aggressive control of blood pressure to levels beneath 135/85 (3).

Treatment should begin with an assessment of the patient's lifestyle to detect areas that might be improved to lower blood pressure. The most effective lifestyle changes for normalizing blood pressure are:

1. Weight loss
2. Sodium restriction
3. Regular aerobic exercise
4. Reduction of alcohol intake to no more than one drink a day for a menopausal woman

In addition, patients should eat a balanced diet, high in fruits and vegetables and low fat dairy products as the DASH Study has shown that this regimen results in effective reduction of blood pressure (51).

In addition, because of its extremely harmful effect on the vasculature, patients should be strongly advised to stop smoking.

In a recent study of the effect of exercise and hormone replacement on blood pressure in 66 healthy, normotensive premenopausal and postmenopausal women, Hunt et al. (52) found that sedentary postmenopausal women had average systolic blood pressure 11 mmHg higher and systemic vascular resistance 50% higher than premenopausal women. Although blood pressure also increased with age in endurance-trained women, systemic vascular resistance increased by only 15% ($p = 0.06$). No significant differences were seen in blood pressure, cardiac output, or vascular resistance in hormone users when compared with nonusers.

The Nurses' Health Study has recently demonstrated a positive correlation between body mass index at age 18 years and at midlife and the occurrence of hypertension (52a). Weight loss lowered the risk of hypertension significantly, whereas weight gain increased the risk. This association was stronger in women aged less than 45 years than in those aged more than 55 years.

If lifestyle changes fail to control blood pressure, it is necessary to begin treatment with an antihypertensive agent. In older patients, it is particularly important to avoid precipitating hypotension and risking cerebrovascular accident or heart attack, the very disorders that an antihypertensive program is designed to avoid. Medication should be started at half the usual the dose and titrated upward very slowly until goal blood pressures are obtained or until drug intolerance is encountered. The

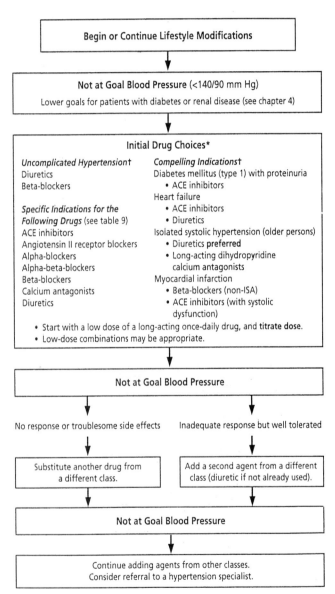

FIG. 37.2. Algorithm for the treatment of hypertension. ACE, angiotensin-converting enzyme; ISA, intrinsic sympathomimetic activity. Based on randomized controlled trials. (From the sixth report of the Joint National Committee on Prevention, Detection, Evaluation, and Treatment of High Blood Pressure. *Arch Intern Med* 1997;157:2413–2446; with permission.)

JNC-VI report recommends beginning therapy with either a diuretic or a β-blocking agent as these are the agents that have been used in earlier randomized, placebo-controlled trials and have been shown to have a statistically significant favorable effect on outcome (3). Although other, more recently developed antihypertensive agents are often as or more effective and frequently better tolerated, these agents have not yet been subjected to outcome studies. Based on the results of the Systolic Hypertension—Europe Trial (53) in which older patients with isolated systolic hypertension were treated with a long-acting dihydropyridine type calcium blocking agent, nitrendipine, JNC-VI also recommends consideration of the use of this type of agent as a second step in older patients in whom systolic blood pressure is not adequately controlled with a diuretic alone. Should these initial steps not work, therapy should be adjusted or increased as outlined in Fig. 37.2.

Compliance

The observation that only approximately 25% of older hypertensive patients are taking sufficient doses of antihypertensive medication with sufficient regularity to control their blood pressure to levels beneath 140/90 is very sobering and points out to physicians the need for persistence and support in the treatment of hypertensive patients. Once blood pressure is controlled, patients should be seen every 4 to 6 months, with those who seem to be missing medications or failing to respond seen more often to encourage proper timing of medications. A careful search for unacceptable side effects should be made in order to advise a patient to change antihypertensive therapy to a more tolerable form.

Several studies have shown that the lower the dose frequency, the better the compliance. Therefore, medications that can be given once a day are preferable. Patients should be instructed about what each medication is, why it is being taken, and what important side effects may occur.

It is particularly important for patients to become partners in their own blood pressure control. One step that encourages this degree of involvement is the use of home blood pressure measurements with regular charting to be discussed with health care providers at each visit.

Finally, it is important to realize that many older patients are living on fixed incomes. Therefore, expensive medications make it necessary for them to cut expenses elsewhere, perhaps reducing their quality of life. It is important to keep the cost of therapy low.

REFERENCES

1. Stamler J, Stamler R, Neaton JD. Blood pressure, systolic and diastolic, and cardiovascular risks: US population data. *Arch Intern Med* 1993;153:598–615.
2. Bush TL. The epidemiology of cardiovascular disease in postmenopausal women. *Ann NY Acad Sci* 1989;592:263–271.
3. The Sixth Report of the Joint National Committee on Prevention, Detection, Evaluation, and Treatment of High Blood Pressure. *Arch Intern Med* 1997;157: 2413–2446.
4. Levy D, Larson MG, Vasen RS, et al. The progression from hypertension to congestive heart failure. *JAMA* 1996;275:1557–1562.
5. Pfeffer RI, Kurosaki TT, Charlton SK. Estrogen use and blood pressure in later life. *Am J Epidemiol* 1979;110:469–478.
6. Barrett-Connor E, Wingard DL, Criqui MH. Postmenopausal estrogen use and heart disease risk factors in the 1980's. Rancho Bernardo, Calif., revisited. *JAMA* 1989;261:2095–2100.
7. Lind T, Cameron EC, Hunter EM, et al. A prospective, controlled trial of six forms of hormone replacement therapy given to postmenopausal women. *Br J Obstet Gynaecol* 1979;86(Suppl 3):1.
8. Luotola H. Blood pressure and hemodynamics in postmenopausal women during estradiol 17-β substitution. *Ann Clin Res* 1983;15(Suppl 38):9.
9. Mercuro G, Zoncu S, Pilia I, Lao A, Melis GN, Cherchi A. Effects of acute administration of transdermal estrogen on postmenopausal women with systemic hypertension. *Am J Cardiol* 1997;80:652-—655.
10. Allad AA, Halligan AW, Abrams K, al-Azzawi F. Differing responses in blood pressure over 24 hours in normotensive women receiving oral or transdermal estrogen replacement therapy. *Obstet Gynecol* 199;89:97–103.
11. Pirhonen JP, Vuento MH, Mäkinen JI, et al. Long-term effects of hormone replacement therapy on the uterus and on uterine circulation. *Am J Obstet Gynecol* 1993;168:620–630.
12. Hillard TC, Bourne TH, Whitehead MI, et al. Differential effects of transdermal estradiol and sequential progestogens on impedance to flow within the uterine arteries of postmenopausal women. *Fertil Steril* 1992:58:959–963.
13. Gilligan DM, Badar DM, Panza JA, Quyyumi AA, Cannon II RO. Acute vascular effects of estrogen in postmenopausal women. *Circulation* 1994;90:786–791.
14. Sullivan JM, Shala BA, Miller LA, Lerner, JL, McBrayer JD. Progestin enhances vasoconstrictor responses in postmenopausal women receiving estrogen replacement therapy. *Menopause: The Journal of the North American Menopause Society* 1995;2:193–199.
15. Kawano H, Motoyama T, Kugiyama K, et al. Gender difference in improvement of endothelium-dependent vasodilation after estrogen supplementation. *J Am Coll Cardiol* 1997;30:914–919.
16. Williams JK, Adams MR, Klopfenstein HS. Estrogen modulates responses of atherosclerotic coronary arteries. *Circulation* 1990;81:1680–1687.
17. Herrington DM, Braden GA, Williams JK, Morgan TM. Endothelial-dependent coronary vasomotor responsiveness in postmenopausal women with and without estrogen replacement therapy. *Am J Cardiol* 1994;73:951–952.
18. Reis SE, Gloth ST, Blumenthal RS, et al. Ethinyl estradiol acutely attenuates abnormal coronary vasomotor responses to acetylcholine in postmenopausal women. *Circulation* 1994;89:52–60.
19. Gilligan DM, Quyyumi AA, Cannon III RO, et al. Effects of physiological levels of estrogen on coronary vasomotor function in postmenopausal women. *Circulation* 1994;89:2545–2551.
20. Collins P, Rosano GMC, Sarrel PM, et al. 17β-Estradiol attenuates acetylcholine-induced coronary arterial constriction in women but not in men with coronary heart disease. *Circulation* 1995:92:24-—30.
21. Arnal JF, Clamens S, Pechet C, et al. Ethinylestradiol does not enhance the expression of nitric oxide synthase in bovine endothelial cells but increases the release of bioactive nitric oxide by inhibiting superoxide anion production. *Proc Natl Acad Sci USA* 1996;93:4108–4113.
22. Liehr JG. Antioxidant and prooxidant properties of estrogen. *J Lab Clin Med* 1996;128:344–345.
23. Polderman KH, Stehouwer CDA, VanKemp GJ, Dekker GA, Verheugt FWA, Gooren LJG. Influence of sex hormones on plasma endothelin levels. *Ann Intern Med* 1993;118:429–432.
24. Jiang C, Sarrel PM, Poole-Wilson PA, Collins P. Acute effect of 17β-estradiol on rabbit coronary artery contractile responses to endothelin-1. *Am J Physiol* 1992: 263:H271–H275.
25. Jiang C, Poole-Wilson PH, Sarrel PM, Mochizuki S, Collins P, MacLeod KT. Effect of 17β-oestradiol on contraction, Ca^{2+} current and intracellular free Ca^{2+} in guinea-pig isolated cardiac myocytes. *Br J Pharmacol* 1992;106:739–745.
26. Harder DR, Coulson PB. Estrogen receptors and effects of estrogen on membrane electrical properties of coronary vascular smooth muscle. *J Cell Physiol* 1979;100:375–382.
27. Fogelberg M, Vesterqvist O, Dicfalusy U, et al. Experimental atherosclerosis: effects of oestrogen and atherosclerosis on thromboxane and prostacyclin formation. *Eur J Clin Invest* 1990;20:105–110.
28. Royal College of General Practitioners. Oral contraceptives and Health. New York: Pitman Publishing, 1974.
29. Weir RJ, Briggs E, Mack A, et al. Blood pressure in women taking oral contraceptives. *Br Med J* 1974;1:533–535.
30. Ramcharan S, Pellegrin FA, Ray RM, et al. The Walnut Creek Contraceptive Drug Study: a prospective study of the side effects of oral contraceptives. *J Reprod Med* 1980;25:345–372.
31. Weinberger MH, Collins RD, Dowdy AJ, et al. Hypertension induced by oral contraceptives containing estrogen and gestagen. *Ann Intern Med* 1969;71:891–902.
31a. Stampfer MJ, Willett WC, Colditz GA, Speizer FE, Hennekens CH. A prospective study of past use of oral contraceptive agents and risk of cardiovascular disease. *N Engl J Med* 1988;319:1313–1317.

32. Briggs M, Briggs M. Oestrogen content of oral contraceptives [Letter]. *Lancet* 1977;2:1233.

33. Woods JW. Oral contraceptives and hypertension. *Hypertension* 1988;(Suppl II): II-11–II-15.

34. Kaplan NM. Hypertension with pregnancy and the pill. In: Kaplan NM, ed. *Clinical hypertension*, 5th ed. Baltimore: Williams & Wilkins, 1990:325–349.

35. Romney B. Oral contraceptive hypertension. *Cardiovascular Review and Reports* 1981;2:75–79.

36. Saruta T, Saade GA, Kaplan NM. A possible mechanism for hypertension induced by oral contraceptives. *Arch Intern Med* 1970;126:621.

37. Beckerhoff R, Luetscher JA, Wilkinson R, et al. PRC, PRA and PRS in hypertension induced by oral contraceptives. *J Clin Endocrinol Metab* 1972;34:1067.

38. Royal College of General Practitioners Study. Effect on hypertension and benign breast disease of progestogen component in combined oral contraceptives. *Lancet* 1977;1:624.

39. Oelkers WK. Effects of estrogens and progestogens on the renin-aldosterone system and blood pressure. *Steroids* 1996;61:166–171.

40. Anderson SG, Hackshaw BT, Still JG, et al. Uterine blood flow and its distribution after chronic estrogen and progesterone administration. *Am J Obstet Gynecol* 1977;127:138–142.

41. Batra S, Bjellin L, et al. Effect of oestrogen and progesterone on the blood flow in the lower urinary tract of the rabbit. *Acta Physiol Scand* 1985;123: 191–194.

42. McLaughlin MK, Quinn P, Farnham JG. Vascular reactivity in the hind limb of the pregnant ewe. *Am J Obstet Gynecol* 1985;152:593–598.

43. Laugel GR, Wright JW, Dengerink HA. Angiotensin II and progesterone effects on laser Doppler measures of cochlear blood flow. *Acta Otolaryngol* 1988;106:34–39.

44. Laugel GR, Dengerink HA, Wright JW. Ovarian steroid and vasoconstrictor effects on cochlear blood flow. *Hear Res* 1987;31(3):245-—251.

45. de Ziegler D, Bessis R, Frydman R. Vascular resistance of uterine arteries: physiological effects of estradiol and progesterone. *Fertil Steril* 1991;55:775-—779.

46. Pirhonen JP, Vuento MH, Makinen JI, et al. Long-term effects of hormone replacement therapy on the uterus and on uterine circulation. *Am J Obstet Gynecol* 1993;168:620–630.

47. Hillard TC, Bourne TH, et al. Differential effects of transdermal estradiol and sequential progestogens on impedance to flow within the uterine arteries of postmenopausal women. *Fertil Steril* 1992;58(5):959–963.

48. Adams MR, Kaplan JR, Manuck SB, et al. Inhibition of coronary artery atherosclerosis by 17-beta estradiol in ovariectomized monkeys: lack of an effect of added progesterone. *Arteriosclerosis* 1990;10:1051–1057.

49. Mendelsohn ME, Kavar RH. Estrogen and the blood vessel wall. *Curr Opin Cardiol* 1994;9:619–626.

50. MacMahon S, Rodgers A. The effects of blood pressure reduction in older patients: an overview of five randomized controlled trials in elderly hypertensives. *Clin Exp Hypertens* 1993;15:967–978.

51. Appel LJ, Moore TJ, Obarzanek E, et al. for the DASH Collaborative Research Group. A clinical trial of the effects of dietary patterns on blood pressure. *N Engl J Med* 1997;336:1117–1124.

52. Hunt BE, Davy KP, Jones PP, DeSouza CA, Van Pelt RE, Tanaka H, Seals DR. Systemic hemodynamic determinants of blood pressure in women: age, physical activity, and hormone replacement. *Am J Physiol* 1997;273:H777–H785.

52a. Huang Z, Willett WC, Manson JE, Rosner B, Stampfer MJ, Speizer FE, Colditz GA. Body weight, weight change, and risk for hypertension in women. *Ann Intern Med* 1998;128:81–88.

53. Staessen JA, Fagard R, Thijs L, et al., for the Systolic Hypertension—Europe (Syst-Eur) Trial Investigators. Morbidity and mortality in the placebo-controlled European Trial on Isolated Systolic Hypertension in the Elderly. *Lancet* 1997;360:757–764.

SECTION VIII

Lifestyle

This section on lifestyle options discusses several variables that are a matter of choice for post-menopausal women. Increasingly and appropriately, postmenopausal women are pursuing a variety of options for treatment of symptoms, but additional lifestyle patterns (exercise and good nutrition) are important for well being and longevity. In this section exercise and nutrition for the post-menopausal woman will be discussed and followed by a review of sexual function and the possible treatment of decreased sexual desire if this is a complaint. The last two chapters in this section deal with compliance and continuance issues of hormonal therapy if this is a woman's choice; also reviewed are alternative therapies and complementary medicine at the end of this section.

Michelle Warren and Cecilia Artacho, who discuss the appropriate prescription for the health of postmenopausal women, author the first chapter. Nancy Phillips and Raymond Rosen next discuss sexual function. Recent data have provided the first real evidence for some benefit with the use of androgen for decreased sexual drive in postmenopausal women and Raymond Rosen provided the questionnaires and instruments for these studies. The recent interest in Viagra for male impotence has led to a wide discussion of the importance of sexual function in older individuals. Largely because of its mechanism of action, Viagra has been shown in recent studies not to be beneficial for sexual function in postmenopausal women; even if it is able to increase vulvovaginal blood flow, they do not relate it to this finding of decreased sexual desire. In the next chapter by Julie Stein and Veron-ica Ravnikar, concerns related to the use of hormonal replacement will be reviewed as well as a dis-cussion of various side effects and strategies for continuance with therapy. All of the long term ben-efits of estrogen (osteoporosis, CVD, Alzheimer's, as well as reduced all cause mortality) are related to continuance of use. On the opposite end of the analysis, risks are also related to long term (exces-sive), use. The major concern is neoplasia that will be discussed in the next section. The last chapter by Adriane Fugh-Berman discusses the important discipline of complementary medicine. A review of the efficacy of the most common herbs and supplements will be provided. While there are clear benefits to some phytoestrogen products, others such as Dong Quai have been shown not to be effec-tive. Risks should be considered as well. A specific discussion of phytoestrogens as an "alternative" may be found in Chapter 53.

Treatment of the Postmenopausal Woman: Basic and Clinical Aspects, Second Edition, edited by Rogerio A. Lobo, Lippincott Williams & Wilkins, Philadelphia © 1999.

CHAPTER 38

Role of Exercise and Nutrition

Michelle P. Warren and Cecilia A. Artacho

ROLE OF EXERCISE AND NUTRITION

The effects of menopause and of the aging process itself cause many physiologic changes, which explain the increased prevalence of chronic diseases observed in postmenopausal women. Exercise and nutrition play important roles in the prevention and treatment of cardiovascular disease, cancer, obesity, diabetes, osteoporosis, and depression, which are some of the major health problems seen in postmenopausal women. Clinicians caring for older women should stress the relevance of these two lifestyle factors to overall health and advise their patients about adequate exercise prescriptions and nutrition.

CARDIOVASCULAR DISEASE— ROLE OF NUTRITION

Cardiovascular disease (CVD) incidence increases with advancing age in women, with a notable increase after menopause, possibly as a result of estrogen deficiency. Coronary heart disease (CHD) is the leading cause of death among postmenopausal women (1,2). It is believed that the atherosclerotic process is attenuated in women until the perimenopause because circulating estrogen prevents the incorporation of low-density lipoprotein cholesterol (LDLc) into atherosclerotic plaques (3). By the year 2015 one-half of all women in the United States will be aged more than 45 years (3), and primary prevention of CVD in this group is becoming increasingly important. Nutrition and exercise both play key roles in the primary prevention of CVD. Smoking, hypertension, hypercholesterolemia, obesity, diabetes mellitus, a sedentary lifestyle, and estrogen deficiency all increase the risk of atherosclerotic plaque formation (4–6). Changes that take place during menopause, including atherogenic changes in serum cho-

lesterol profiles and weight gain, contribute to the increased risk of CHD after menopause (7). Although these CVD risk factors become more pronounced during menopause, they, in turn, are affected by nutrition and decreased physical activity. CVD causes other diseases besides heart disease and stroke that result in significant morbidity in women. As many as 25% of women aged 55 to 74 years suffer from lower extremity atherosclerosis (8). Although hormone replacement therapy (HRT) markedly reduces the incidence of CVD in older women, nutrition, exercise, and smoking cessation also play important roles (4).

Cardiovascular disease risk factors known to become more pronounced during menopause include lipid changes. In a large cohort of premenopausal and postmenopausal French women, menopause was associated with higher levels of serum cholesterol, triglycerides, apolipoprotein (apo) B, and apo A-1, and also with elevated diastolic blood pressure (9). Lipoprotein profiles change with age. LDLc increases in women after age 50 (10). Postmenopausal women not only have higher total LDLc plasma levels, but also the LDL particle itself becomes more dense (11). This smaller, more dense form of LDL is linked to CHD risk (12). The high-density lipoprotein cholesterol (HDLc) plasma level declines with the onset of menopause, and the HDL particle itself is altered. The relative proportions of its two subfractions change and the more dense HDL_3c increases and the less dense HDL_2c decreases (13). The HDL_3b subclass is usually present in individuals with CHD (14). Serum ferritin, total cholesterol, and LDL cholesterol all increase in postmenopausal women, and their parallel rise may be partly responsible for the increased risk of CHD in this population (15).

The Framingham Offspring/Spouse Study, which examined the relationship between diet and plasma total and LDL cholesterol levels in a large sample set of premenopausal and postmenopausal women, showed that cholesterol levels were directly related to consumption of saturated fat and inversely related to total caloric intake, but

M. P. Warren, C. A. Artacho: Department of Obstetrics and Gynecology, Columbia University College of Physicians & Surgeons, New York, New York 10032.

that dietary cholesterol was not a predictor of cholesterol levels (16). Another study of the same cohort showed that plasma triglycerides were inversely related to protein, fiber, and polyunsaturated fat and directly related to saturated fat and oleic acid (17). High triglyceride levels are better predictors of CHD risk in women than in men, and triglycerides are strongly related to HDLc, which is an important predictor of CHD risk in women (18,19). High triglyceride levels are an important risk factor for CHD in women, but the effect of high triglycerides is most pronounced when they are present in conjunction with low HDLc levels. Patients who have both high triglyceride levels and low HDLc levels have an increased incidence of CVD (20). A low HDLc appears to be the strongest predictor of CHD in women (20,21). An association of HDLc with cardiovascular disease in women was also found in the 20-year follow-up of the Donolo-Tel Aviv cohort (21). The importance of HDLc and triglycerides as risk factors for CVD in women was also apparent in the Lipid Research Clinics Follow-up Study (20), which found that HDLc levels of less than 1.3 mmol/L (50 mg/dL) and triglyceride levels of 2.25 to 4.49 mmol/L (200 to 399 mg/dL) were independent predictors of death from CVD. A low HDLc level places women at a greater risk for CHD than a high LDLc level (20). The Framingham, Donolo-Tel Aviv, and Lipid Research Clinics studies all indicate that low HDLc levels in women are stronger predictors of cardiovascular disease mortality than total cholesterol levels (20–22). CHD in women is also more strongly related to the total cholesterol HDLc ratio than to either total cholesterol or to LDLc (23). An age-related increase exists in the ratio of total to HDLc, and when the ratio is greater than 7.5, women have the same CHD risk as men (24).

The entire lipid profile should be assessed yearly, and dietary and exercise interventions should be prescribed to women who are not within the range of optimal cholesterol and lipoprotein profile (Table 38.1). Only one-half of the

TABLE 38.1 *The optimal cholesterol and lipoprotein profile and heart disease risk based on total cholesterol to HDL ratio.*

Optimal Cholesterol/Lipoprotein Profile	
–Total cholesterol	Less than 200 mg/dL (5.2 mmol/L)
–HDL-cholesterol	Greater than 50 mg/dL (1.3 mmol/L)
–LDL-cholesterol	Less than 130 mg/dL (3.4 mmol/L)
–Triglycerides	Less than 250 mg/dL (2.3 mmol/L)
Heart Disease Risk Based on Cholesterol/HDL Ratio	
–Lowest risk	Less than 2.5
–Below average risk	2.5–3.7
–Average risk	3.8–5.6
–High risk	5.7–8.3
–Dangerous	Greater than 8.3

HDL, high-density lipoprotein; LDL, low-density lipoprotein.
(From Byyny RL, Speroff L. *A clinical guide for the care of older women: primary and preventive care,* 2nd ed. Baltimore: Williams & Wilkins, 1996; with permission).

women in the Framingham study met the National Cholesterol Education Program (NECP) guidelines for a desirable blood level of LDLc (< 130 mg/dL) (5). Although women in this cohort were adhering to a moderate cholesterol intake of no more than 300 mg/day, their average fat intake constituted 38% of calories (22). Only one-fifth of the women adhered to the recommended upper limit for fat intake of no more than 30% of calories (22). In light of these findings, it is important for postmenopausal women to receive adequate counseling about ways to reduce their saturated fat, total fat, oleic acid from animal sources, and total caloric intake and to increase their intake of fiber and polyunsatured fat in order to improve their lipoprotein profile and reduce their risk for CVD.

Dietary change resulting in lowered blood cholesterol correlates with a reduction in CHD rates among women in the United States (3.) For each 1% decrease in serum cholesterol, a corresponding 2% to 3% reduction is seen in CVD risk in US adults (25); dietary intervention can lower cholesterol concentrations by approximately 10% (26). One of the important steps in the primary prevention of CHD should be a nutritional intervention aimed at the many women who still consume diets that place them at increased risk for CHD. Women with hypercholesterolemia clearly benefit from a reduction in dietary fat and cholesterol (3). Healthy women with only slightly elevated cholesterol levels may or may not benefit from a dietary intervention, because such a lipid-lowering intervention can also reduce HDLc (3). Because a low HDLc level places women at increased risk of CHD, dietary interventions should be geared toward raising HDL and lowering LDL (3). The American Heart Association (AHA) recommends that total fat intake be reduced to 30% of calories, that saturated fat intake be decreased below 10% of calories, and that dietary cholesterol be lowered to less than 300 mg/day. This AHA Phase I diet (27) should be followed by all nonobese, normocholesterolemic women (28). Women who have a higher CVD risk profile should follow the AHA Phase II or the AHA Phase III diets. Both the AHA step I diet and the AHA step II diet have proved to be equally effective in reducing total serum cholesterol and LDLc in men and women (Fig. 38.1) (29). Reducing fat intake may have additional protective effects. Data from the Iowa Women's health study also indicated that a high fat intake is associated with decreased survival of postmenopausal women with breast cancer (30).

A 5-year randomized trial designed to determine whether increases in LDLc and body weight during menopause can be prevented through changes in diet and physical activity showed that a dietary and behavioral intervention was successful during the first 6 months in a cohort of premenopausal women (7). The risk of CAD can be reduced through dietary intervention, which can improve the lipid profile and lower blood pressure (31). Diet and other nonpharmacologic interventions should be

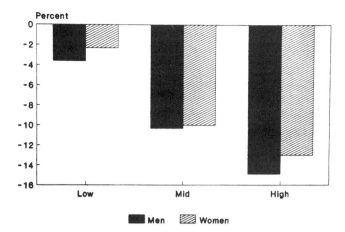

FIG. 38.1. Low-density lipoprotein cholesterol responses in women and men following the American Heart Association step I diet for an 8-week period. Subjects are grouped by tertile based on initial serum cholesterol level. Women had the following serum cholesterol responses: highest titer, initial values 295 (7.6 mmol/L) ± 6 mg/dL, -12.8% ($p < 0.0001$); middle titer, initial values 253 (6.5 mmol/L) ± 2 mg/dL, -9.0% ($p < 0.0001$); lowest titer, initial values 224 (5.8 mmol/L) ± 3 mg/dL, -1.9% ($p = 0.34$). (From Anderson JW. Diet, lipids, and cardiovascular disease in women. *J Am Coll Nutr* 1993; 12:433–437; with permission.)

the first step in management of both hypercholesterolemia and hypertension (32). Lower caloric intake; decreased total, saturated fat and cholesterol intake; weight loss; sodium restriction; and abstinence from alcohol are effective dietary interventions used to lower blood pressure (31,32). In terms of dietary profiles that can affect blood pressure, increased potassium consumption has been shown to significantly lower it (33), and hypertensive patients may benefit from potassium supplements. Complex carbohydrates and soluble fiber have also been shown to lower blood pressure (34). Thus, women should actively attempt to improve unfavorable lipid profiles by restricting caloric intake, losing excess weight, consuming the recommended quantities and types of lipids, consuming sufficient complex carbohydrates and soluble fiber, and exercising.

Oxidative stress, which is defined as an imbalance between pro-oxidative factors and the antioxidative defense mechanisms, has been linked with the development of early stages of arteriosclerosis and cancer (35–38). Epidemiologic studies have shown that diets rich in antioxidants from fruit, vegetables, and vegetable oil sources reduce the relative risk of premature death from CVD and cancer (39). It is believed that an optimal antioxidant status is necessary for optimal health. Threshold antioxidant plasma levels associated with minimal relative risk of premature death by CVD and cancer, in other words, desirable optimal levels, can tentatively be established from available consistent data (36–38,40). At these optimal antioxidant plasma levels, relative risks

seem to disappear (39). Most middle-aged persons can obtain optimal plasma levels by consuming antioxidants at levels close to or only slightly above the current recommended daily allowances (RDAs) (41): 60 to 80 mg vitamin C in nonsmokers, 125 to 130 mg in smokers; 67 mg or more vitamin E in male Americans; 2 to 3 mg β-carotene in nonsmokers, and 9 mg or more in male smokers (39). The risk for CVD and cancer is twice as high at levels 25% to 35% below these levels. Suboptimal levels of a single antioxidant may increase relative risk, and suboptimal levels of several antioxidants further increase relative risk (39). The First US National Health and Nutrition Examination Survey showed that habitual consumption of a vitamin C-containing multivitamin by the general middle-aged US population reduced the mortality rate from CVD by approximately 42% in men and by about 25% in women (42). The effects of vitamin C consumed as a multivitamin did not have a significant effect in terms of lower cancer mortality (42). The US Health Professionals Study and the US Nurses' Health Study, showed that habitual consumption of vitamin E as part of a multivitamin significantly decreased the relative risk of coronary events (43,44). The US Health Professionals Study showed a protective effect against coronary risk for β-carotene supplements in smokers but not in nonsmokers, probably because nonsmokers had above optimal levels of β-carotene even without the use of supplements, but that smokers had low levels and they have an increased requirement (39). Similarly, in US nurses, who had a low intake of preformed vitamin A from food, vitamin A supplementation significantly reduced the relative risk of breast cancer (45).

Randomized antioxidant intervention trials conducted in China and Finland in middle-aged and elderly subjects over a 5 to 6 year period were successful in preventing the earlier stages of CVD and cancer by rectifying previously poor antioxidant levels (46–48). However, antioxidant supplementation did not have an effect on irreversible precancerous lesions, clinically established common cancers, and vascular lesions in chronic smokers (39). It is therefore important for women to start consuming a diet rich in antioxidants as a preventive measure before menopause, when the risk of CVD and cancer begins to escalate with advancing age. Some studies report no association between intake of antioxidant vitamins and relative risk of breast cancer (49), but because of the protective effects of some antioxidants on CVD and possible protective effects against breast cancer and other types of cancers, increasing dietary antioxidant intake seems like a prudent preventive measure. Studies have shown that antioxidant supplementation aimed at preventing or correcting previously poor levels may protect from both CVD and cancer. No evidence indicates that megadoses of antioxidants have an additional protective effect. Practitioners should discourage self-prescribed over-consumption of antioxidant supplements, especially because overdoses of the fat-soluble vitamin A can be extremely toxic. Antioxidants are most effective when overall nutritional status is optimized. Additional large-scale randomized trials of antioxidants in the primary and secondary prevention of CVD should be conducted to prove their effectiveness in reducing CVD risk (50).

Oxidative modification of LDLc may accelerate atherosclerotic plaque formation and dietary antioxidant vitamins may play an important role in preventing CHD. In a large cohort of postmenopausal women, intake of vitamin E from food sources was inversely related to the risk of death from CHD (51). By simply consuming more foods rich in vitamin E, postmenopausal women can lower their risk of CHD. However, intake of two other antioxidant vitamins, vitamins A and C, was not correlated with decreased risk of death from CHD (51). Antioxidant vitamins exert an antioxidant effect on LDL and may also preserve the endogenous antioxidants of LDL (52). Preliminary data indicate that HRT can preserve the LDL particle content of two antioxidants, A-tocopherol and β-carotene, and keep the LDL in a reduced antioxidant state (52).

Nutrition can play a role, not only in the primary prevention of CVD through the effects of the antioxidant vitamins, but also in the treatment of premature arteriosclerotic disease. Mild hyperhomocysteinemia, which is frequently present in patients with premature arteriosclerotic disease, can be corrected by treatment with compounds involved in folic acid metabolism, such as vitamin B6, folic acid, and betaine (53).

Because CVD is one of the main health problems of postmenopausal women, adequate dietary habits should be initiated as early as childhood or adolescence and maintained throughout life, especially during menopause and in the postmenopausal years.

CARDIOVASCULAR DISEASE— ROLE OF EXERCISE

In recent years many studies have shown that increased physical activity plays an independent role in the primary prevention of CHD, the most serious and common form of CVD. Physically active individuals are at lower risk for CHD than those who have a sedentary lifestyle. Physical inactivity is a high risk factor for CVD, but it can also exert its effects by contributing to the physiologic changes associated with atherogenesis, such as hypertension, obesity, diabetes, and hypercholesterolemia. Exercise favorably affects plasma lipids and lipoproteins and, thus, may have protective effects against CVD and CHD mortality (54). Exercise increases the levels of the less dense HDL_2 cholesterol subfraction, which normally decreases during menopause, by causing an increase in lipoprotein lipase, the enzyme that catabolizes triglyceride-rich lipoproteins (28). Higher concentrations of lipoprotein lipase are found in the slow twitch skeletal muscle fibers of endurance athletes (28). Exercise also

lowers triglyceride levels. Population studies such as the Framingham Study have shown that HDLc and triglyceride levels (55) are the best predictors of CHD in women, and dietary or exercise interventions that can alter these lipids can decrease CHD risk.

Thirty of 40 studies conducted between 1985 and 1995 suggest that exercise can reduce cardiovascular risk between 10% and 50% (56). Research on CHD risk and exercise has been conducted mostly in men. Few studies have examined the effects of exercise on CHD in women, and data from available studies are frequently inconsistent, possibly because the number of individuals in the high activity category is too small. Most cross-sectional studies examining the effects of exercise in women show a positive correlation between exercise and HDLc in both premenopausal and postmenopausal women (54). Longitudinal studies on the effects of exercise in women have given inconsistent results because of methodological problems; nevertheless, about half of the studies showed that exercise increases HDLc (54). HDLc can be expected to increase by approximately 10% in both men and women as a result of training (54). Large-scale prospective studies have consistently shown exercise to be effective in reducing heart disease (57–59). A meta-analysis of 27 cohort studies comparing sedentary and physically active individuals indicates an association between lack of physical activity and increased risk of CHD (60). This study also found that the association is stronger when a high activity group is compared with a sedentary group, rather than when the active group only has a moderate activity level, indicating that a dose-response relationship exists between physical activity and protection from CHD (60). Exercise was found to have a protective effect in terms of preventing major cardiovascular events in this study, but not in terms of reducing the severity of such events (60).

Cardiovascular disease risk occurs less in women who exercise than it does in nonexercisers (61). One mechanism that may account for the decreased risk seen in active women is that these women may have more favorable blood pressure-related risk factors than do sedentary women (61). Physically active postmenopausal women in their mid-50s have more favorable systolic blood pressure-related CVD risk factors than do sedentary healthy women in their late-50s (61). The observed decrease in risk may result from the lower levels of abdominal adiposity found in the more active women. The study group was small (active women $n = 18$; less-active controls $n = 34$). Prospective studies need to be conducted with a larger group to establish more definitively the effects of exercise on blood pressure. In light of these findings, however, it would be prudent to advise patients to increase their level of physical activity because of its potential beneficial effects on blood pressure and consequent reduction of CVD risk. Exercise therapy may be particularly appropriate for postmenopausal women, in whom LDLc levels rise sharply with increasing age, because antihypertensive medication, thiazide diuretics, and β-adrenergic blockers all tend to increase blood cholesterol levels (3). Before prescribing antihypertensive medication, a patient's overall CHD risk profile should be evaluated and, in some patients, exercise may be a safer alternative.

Exercise improves cardiovascular fitness, which has been linked to decreased mortality in prospective studies. One study of 3,120 women found that those with the lowest fitness level as measured by maximal treadmill test had a relative risk of death almost fivefold greater than those with the highest fitness level (62). Being in the lowest fitness level was associated with a greater risk of death than the risk from having an elevated systolic blood pressure (> 140 mmHg), a family history of CHD, or obesity. The risk associated with cigarette smoking was approximately equal to the risk associated with being in the lowest fitness category. A blood cholesterol level greater than 260 mg/dL was the only risk factor that was associated with increased risk of death than a low level of fitness (62). A study in an Australian cohort showed that previously sedentary women who improved their fitness level over a 4-year period had significantly improved blood lipid profiles and systolic blood pressure (63). Similar benefits were not reported for the men in this study.

Exercise appears to have many protective effects that can improve the CHD risk profile. In a cross-sectional study of premenopausal and postmenopausal runners and joggers, HDLc was higher in the women who exercised than in the inactive controls (64). The rise in HDLc was the same for premenopausal and postmenopausal women exercisers. In premenopausal women exercise did not affect the HDLc:LDLc ratio, but in postmenopausal women exercise had a favorable effect on the ratio, which increased significantly from 0.57 mg/dL in the inactive women to 0.85 mg/dL in runners (64). Postmenopausal women may exhibit a greater response to exercise (65). In a cross-sectional study of premenopausal and postmenopausal trained runners, the postmenopausal exercise group had a higher HDLc (74 mg/dL vs. 56 mg/dL), a lower LDLc (141 mg/dL vs. 185 mg/dL), and a higher HDLc:LDLc ratio (0.57 mg/dL vs. 0.32 mg/dL) than the sedentary postmenopausal control group (66). In the premenopausal group, only LDL changed significantly with exercise. In these two studies exercise blunted the age-dependent increase in LDLc and prevented the age-dependent decrease in HDLc experienced by menopausal women. Both premenopausal and postmenopausal women who exercise can improve their lipoprotein profile and thereby reduce their risk of developing CHD. In prospective studies, sedentary women had a greater risk of developing hypertension independently of body weight (67). In a large study of perimenopausal women, those who increased their exercise participation over the course of 3 years gained less weight and had a smaller decrease

in HDL$_2$c (68). The activity levels in this study were moderate and seem to indicate that even slight increases in exercise at the time of menopause can help prevent the atherogenic changes in lipid profiles and the weight gain experienced by menopausal women. Thus, moderate exercise seems to lead to improved weight and blood pressure, and to more favorable lipid profiles in both premenopausal and postmenopausal women.

Controversy exists regarding the frequency and intensity of exercise that must be maintained to observe the beneficial rise in HDLc. Few studies have been conducted in postmenopausal women. At least 4 months of fairly strenuous activity, such as running 16 to 24 km per week, may be needed to obtain a significant increase in HDLc (28). More moderate activities, such as walking 48 km per week, require 3 months to observe a significant rise in HDLc (28). Walking can be lower CVD risk because of its effects on cardiorespiratory function and on body fat. Walking 3 or 5 days per week increased peak volume of oxygen utilization (VO$_2$ peak) and decreased body fat, but it did not alter serum lipids of nonobese, normolipidemic postmenopausal women (69). A case-control study of postmenopausal women found that the risk of myocardial infarction in this population is decreased by 50% with energy expenditures corresponding to 30 to 45 minutes of walking three times per week (70). In a large cross-sectional study of female runners participating in the National Runners Health Study, substantial increases in HDLc were observed in women who exercised at levels exceeding current guidelines (71). Official guidelines from the Centers for Disease Control and Prevention (CDC) state that most health benefits from physical activity can be achieved by walking 2 miles (3.2 km) briskly most days, which is the energy equivalent of running 8 to 12 km per week (72). However, the study conducted in runners demonstrated that women obtain additional health benefits from exercise at levels higher than currently recommended, because plasma HDLc concentrations increased for every additional kilometer run per week (Fig. 38.2) (71). A 2-year randomized trial testing the effects of different intensities and formats of exercise on participation rates, fitness and plasma HDLc levels in older men and in postmenopausal women showed that moderate-intensity exercise improved cardiorespiratory fitness levels and improved HDLc levels (Fig. 38.3) (73). Two years were required to observe a change in HDLc. Frequency of participation played an important role in influencing HDLc in this age group (73). This finding differs from previous reports that exercise intensity is the determining factor affecting HDLc levels. In summary, most studies have shown that exercise causes an increase in HDLc, which may be related to the amount, frequency, and intensity of exercise, and that as many as 2 years may be required to produce this increase in HDLc.

The effects of exercise, exercise intensity, and hormone replacement therapy (HRT) on lipid and lipoprotein profiles are controversial. Some studies in women on HRT

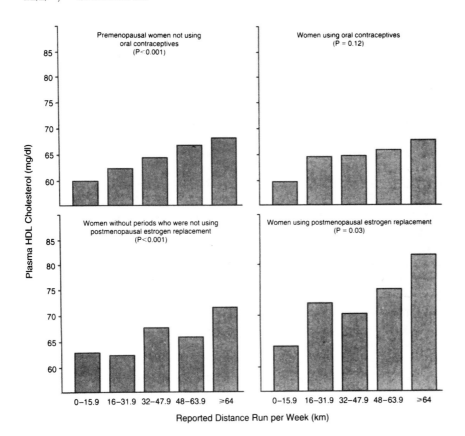

FIG. 38.2. Plasma high-density lipoprotein (HDL) cholesterol concentrations according to weekly distance run. Menstrual periods were reported by 1,390 women; the absence of periods was reported by 447. A total of 236 women reported using oral contraceptives and 176 reported using postmenopausal estrogen-replacement therapy. The *p*-values shown in the figure are for the regression slope of HDL cholesterol plotted against distance run, with adjustment for age, education, progesterone use, and intake of red meat, fish, fruit, and vitamins C and E. (From Williams PT. High-density lipoprotein cholesterol and other risk factors for coronary heart disease in female runners. *N Engl J Med* 1996;334:1325–1327; with permission.)

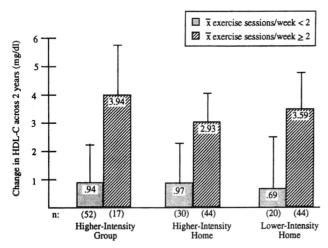

FIG. 38.3. Bar graph shows mean change (with standard error bars) in high-density lipoprotein cholesterol based on the average number of exercise sessions per week completed across 2 years by exercise training condition (higher-intensity, group-based exercise; higher-intensity, home-based exercise; and lower-intensity, home-based exercise). (Adapted King AC, Haskell WL, Young DR, Oka RK, Stefanick ML. Long-term effects of varying intensities and formats of physical activity on participation rates, fitness, and lipoproteins in men and women aged 50 to 65 years. *Circulation* 1995;91:2596–2604; with permission).

indicate that exercisers have higher HDLc levels than nonexercisers (54). In a cross-sectional study of postmenopausal women, regular exercise was associated with significantly greater HDLc concentrations, especially in women using exogenous estrogens (74). In the group of women who were not taking estrogen, the most significant increase in HDLc was observed for the sedentary versus the light activity categories. Increasing activity levels from light to moderate or heavy did not produce an incremental change in HDLc in this study (74). However, other investigators studying the effects of HRT and exercise on lipid metabolism had conflicting results. In a study assessing the independent effects of a moderate exercise program, with and without oral estrogen replacement, on lipids and lipoproteins in a group of postmenopausal women, estrogen therapy alone had the greatest beneficial effect on the lipid and lipoprotein profile (75). Exercise alone also favorably altered lipid and lipoprotein levels, resulting in a significant reduction in cholesterol, triglycerides, and LDLc, and in an increase in the HDL:LDL ratio. The combination of oral estrogen and exercise did not produce additional improvements in lipid metabolism (75). In a controlled, prospective 11-month clinical trial in postmenopausal women who participated in a 2-month, low-intensity exercise regimen followed by a 9-month period of high-intensity exercise for 45 minutes/day, three or more days per week, those in the exercise group had lower total cholesterol and LDLc levels, but HDLc and triglycerides were unaffected by the exercise regimen (76). Those in the exercise plus HRT group had decreased total cholesterol and LDLc and increased HDLc levels. Exercise was found to be protective against the HRT-related increase in triglycerides observed in the HRT group (76).

In postmenopausal women undergoing diagnostic coronary angiography, estrogen replacement therapy (ERT) was associated with an 87% decrease in the incidence of CAD (77). Women on the estrogen replacement therapy (ERT) regimen had significantly higher mean HDLc levels and a lower mean total cholesterol:HDLc ratio (77). Estrogen not only has beneficial effects on lipids, but also has a direct dilatory effect on the coronary arteries, which may be more prominent in women than in men. Women who do not have cardiac disease may not derive as many benefits from ERT as women with cardiac disease. The peripheral vascular effects of estrogen in normal postmenopausal women were investigated in a randomized, crossover trial of oral conjugated estrogen (0.625 mg/day) using exercise echocardiography (78). In normal women ERT did not have significant beneficial effects on treadmill exercise echocardiographic variables at rest or during moderate exercise levels (78).

All women should be encouraged to engage in physical activity starting at a young age so that they can enter menopause with improved CVD risk factors. Exercise is especially important during menopause and in the postmenopausal years as a means of attenuating the development of CVD risk factors that become more pronounced at this time. Evidence suggests that exercise, initiated sufficiently early in a woman's life, also protects against breast cancer, cancers of the reproductive system, nonreproductive system cancers, diabetes, and obesity (79–83.) Exercise is also important for maintaining cardiorespiratory fitness, which decreases as a result of the aging process. Sedentary individuals have a 1% loss of VO_{2max} per year with age, particularly after age 50 (28). Physical activity can slow the natural age-related decline in aerobic power. The age-associated decline in muscle mass, strength, and flexibility can largely be prevented by regular exercise participation. Paradoxically, lowering body fat can adversely affect lipids. Exercise at an intensity that results in reduction in body fat and in a consequent drop in endogenous estrogen can cause atherogenic changes in lipoprotein profiles (3). Fatter postmenopausal women tend to have higher endogenous levels of estrone, because of increased aromatization of androstenedione to estrone. Higher estrone levels are related to higher HDLc and lower LDLc levels in perimenopausal women. Both men and women, but especially women, experience an age-related loss of muscle strength. Before beginning an exercise regimen, all women would probably benefit from a strength training program, especially those women who have been inactive for extended periods.

Few studies have examined whether exercise can effectively prevent CVD. Lack of compliance has been a problem in many studies. Randomized clinical trials should be conducted to prove that exercise reduces cardiovascular risk, and to establish the level of intensity, frequency, and exercise duration that produces maximal protective effects in postmenopausal women. The combined effects of exercise, diet, and HRT on CVD risk remain controversial. The Women's Health Initiative Study will be addressing these issues, but the data from this study will not be available for several years.

OBESITY

Obesity is characterized by excess body fat, or an excess storage of triglycerides in adipose tissue that results from consumption of a high-fat, high-calorie diet and a sedentary lifestyle. Obesity is a condition that has become more prevalent in the United States and one that is often resistant to treatment. Women make up a greater percentage of the obese population than do men (84). The levels of central and total adiposity, which increase with age, contribute to the development of cardiovascular and metabolic disease. The incidence of obesity increases threefold in adult women until age 65 (85). Individuals who are above the 85th percentile of body mass index (BMI), which is the weight in kilograms divided by the height in meters squared, are usually classified as obese. Obesity is a risk factor for diabetes, a low HDLc level, hypertension, degenerative arthritis, lipid disorders, gallbladder disease, renal disease, cirrhosis of the liver, and several forms of cancer (24). Obesity places people at increased risk for CVD, because it is associated with four major risk factors for atherosclerosis: hypertension, diabetes, hypercholesterolemia, and hypertriglyceridemia (24).

The waist:hip ratio is used to estimate the relative proportions of upper body or android obesity and lower body or gynoid obesity. A waist:hip ratio greater than 0.85 is indicative of android obesity and a ratio of less than 0.75 is indicative of gynoid obesity. The waist:hip ratio is the index of obesity most strongly associated with CHD (24). Android obesity is associated with increased risk of CVD. Central body fat is metabolically active: it is sensitive to catecholamines and insensitive to insulin. Gynoid adiposity is a store of fat that does not exhibit significant fatty acid fluxes because, unlike android obesity, it is resistant to catecholamines and sensitive to insulin. Women with gynoid obesity are less likely to develop diabetes mellitus and CHD than are women with android obesity. Body fat in women tends to be distributed superficially on the body frame, whereas men are prone to central-obesity (84). A significant increase in waist:hip ratio, which is indicative of central obesity, is observed in menopausal women, and this increase places women at greater risk for coronary artery disease (84). It is more difficult for the obese woman to lose weight than it is for the obese man; therefore, it is important for women to avoid gaining excessive amounts of weight during middle-age. Men are able to maintain HDLc levels and lose central obesity by diet alone, whereas women must reduce their caloric intake and exercise to obtain the same results (84). Women with a BMI greater than 27 would probably benefit from initiating a dietary and exercise regimen and those with a BMI of 28 or more should definitely be treated (24). Increased mortality is seen at a BMI of 30, which corresponds to roughly 30% excess body weight (24).

Central obesity is associated with an androgenic hormonal status, hypertension, and irregularities in lipid and carbohydrate metabolism in middle-aged women (55), and it places women at an increased risk of CHD (86). Abdominal fat is associated with an atherogenic lipid profile in women that is influenced by insulin and estrogen (87). A direct relationship exists between central adiposity and increased total cholesterol, triglycerides, and LDLc in women and an inverse relationship between central fat and HDLc (88). The waist:hip ratio is the variable that is most strongly and inversely associated with the level of the HDL_2 cholesterol subfraction (89). The HDL_2 cholesterol subfraction is strongly related to protection from CVD. Women with large waist:hip ratios, which are indicative of android obesity, will have low HDL_2 cholesterol levels, and they will therefore be at increased risk of developing CVD. The amount of weight gained during menopause is strongly correlated with the degree to which cardiovascular risk factors such as changes in the lipid profile, blood pressure, and insulin levels become more pronounced (90).

Blood insulin levels are elevated in obesity because excess body fat affects insulin secretion and sensitivity, resulting in insulin resistance. In both men and women, insulin resistance is influenced by total adipose tissue content, daily caloric intake, carbohydrate content of the diet, and daily exercise participation (24). In obese individuals, the observed increase in insulin secretion causes down-regulation of insulin receptors, which in turn leads to insulin resistance. Carbohydrate, fat, and protein metabolism are all adversely affected by insulin resistance and inadequate insulin suppression of fat cells leads to increases in circulating free fatty acids. HDLc levels decrease and LDLc levels increase because of the reduced catabolism of triglycerides caused by the insulin resistance (24). The atherogenic changes in lipid profiles caused by insulin resistance result in increased risk of CVD.

High insulin levels can also contribute to the development of hypertension. Although hyperinsulinemia in obese individuals significantly increases their CVD risk profile, it is responsive to diet and exercise. Hyperinsulinemia is reversible with weight loss. Exercise promotes a more sensitive insulin response (83), and long-term athletic training is associated with a lower risk of developing diabetes (82).

The resting metabolic rate decreases about 2% per decade after age 18, resulting in progressive weight gain over the years if no change occurs in caloric intake or exercise level (24). A study examining the effects of age and sex on energy expenditure independent of differences in body composition found no sex effect and no linear decrease in energy expenditure with increasing age; however, the middle-aged subjects had a lower basal metabolic rate (BMR) than did the younger ones (91). This effect on BMR is independent of body size, body composition, and level of activity (91).

Dietary and exercise interventions to prevent weight gain during menopause may also have a protective effect in terms of breast cancer risk (92). Several studies have shown that a history of weight gain in early adult life is associated with increased breast cancer risk in Western women (92). Obesity also seems to be associated with increased breast cancer risk in Asian women. In a prospective case-control study of 1,086 Singaporean Chinese women, central obesity was associated with the highest risk for breast carcinoma (93). Excessive weight gain in early adult life can lead to the development of hyperinsulinemia in women who are genetically susceptible to insulin resistance (92). The metabolic relationship between weight gain and breast cancer risk in Western women has been supported by evidence of insulin resistance in these women (92). Some studies have found that hyperinsulinemia is related to overall obesity in postmenopausal women; however, in premenopausal women it is related to abdominal adiposity (92). This finding could be the reason why a high BMI is a risk factor for breast cancer in postmenopausal but not in premenopausal women (92). It is believed that over-nutrition and insufficient exercise can promote the development of hyperinsulinemia and increase breast cancer risk in genetically susceptible women, but this hypothesis has not been tested in intervention studies (92).

Overweight and obese postmenopausal women should follow a weight reduction program to reduce their risk for CVD, hypertension, diabetes, and cancer. At the time of menopause, the rise in LDLc, triglycerides and insulin levels is most pronounced in women who put on the most weight (90). The Nurses' Health Study demonstrated the importance of weight reduction in preventing CVD. The study found that women with a BMI of 29 or greater had a threefold increase in risk for CVD (94). In this study, 40% of coronary events were caused by excess body weight. Women who are mildly overweight have a substantial increase in coronary risk, and women who are very overweight have an even higher risk. In the Nurses' Health Study, 70% of coronary events were the result of excess body weight. Physicians should prescribe a diet and actively oversee the management of a realistic weight loss program to which the patient will adhere. In the first month patients should lose 4 to 5 pounds, and in the next 4 to 5 months they should lose 20 to 30 pounds (24). An appropriate rate of weight loss can be achieved when energy expenditure exceeds energy intake by 500 to 1,000 calories (95). As patients lose weight they should decrease their energy intake, because their energy requirements will be lower than they were before. The optimal diet for weight loss should contain 900 to 1,200 calories per day and should be composed of 50% carbohydrates, 15% to 20% protein, and less than 30% fat. This diet will not compromise vitamin and mineral status, but further caloric restriction has an adverse effect on overall nutritional status. Reducing fat intake is the most successful method of weight loss, because fat has twice as many calories per gram than either carbohydrate or protein.

Successful weight loss programs set realistic goals that can be reached by gradual weight loss through diet and exercise, and they teach patients behavior modification strategies. Weight loss and increased physical activity have been shown to reduce LDLc levels and to increase HDLc (96). In overweight and obese women, exercise alone or exercise combined with a low fat diet was found to independently raise HDLc (97,98). Strenuous or prolonged physical activity inhibits appetite for an extended period and increases the resting metabolic rate for 24 to 48 hours. Obese individuals must incorporate increased physical activity into their lifestyles, because exercise is necessary to increase caloric expenditure significantly and to lose weight. It is important for the patient and the physician to design a weight loss program that encourages compliance, because repeated dieting and recidivism have a negative impact on metabolism. With successive diets the body can become more calorically efficient, resulting in difficulty in achieving and maintaining weight loss.

DIABETES

Diabetes mellitus is a chronic metabolic syndrome characterized by glucose intolerance, hyperglycemia, absolute or relative insulin availability, and insulin resistance. The alterations in carbohydrate, protein, and lipid metabolism in diabetics produce atherosclerosis and microvascular complications. Type II, or non–insulin-dependent diabetes mellitus (NIDDM), occurs more frequently with advancing age, and it is one of the major chronic disorders of older women. It is characterized by insulin resistance. A family history of diabetes, obesity, and age are the major risk factors for diabetes (99). An increased prevalence of diabetes is seen in women with advancing age, because women have a high tendency toward weight gain. Diabetes is a more important risk factor for CVD in women than in men, possibly because of its effects on lipoprotein profiles (8). Exercise and weight reduction are effective in the primary prevention of diabetes mellitus in most older women.

Type II diabetics are insulin resistant and thus have hyperinsulinemia. Insulin resistance appears to be caused by decreased insulin receptor numbers and to postreceptor abnormalities, both of which cause alterations in the insulin action system. Genetic predisposition, aging, physical inactivity, and weight gain, especially android

obesity, affect the development of insulin resistance. Hyperinsulinemia in postmenopausal women is related to overall obesity, whereas in premenopausal women hyperinsulinemia is related to abdominal adiposity (92).

Type II diabetics have a high incidence of complications caused by atherosclerosis, such as CHD, cerebrovascular disease, peripheral vascular disease, and premature and severe coronary artery disease (CAD). Type II diabetes also produces multiple lipid disorders, which place patients at increased risk of developing CHD. Elevated LDLc, elevated triglycerides, oxidized LDLc, and decreased HDLc are commonly seen in poorly controlled type II diabetics. Both diet and exercise can prevent many of these complications. Improved diet and exercise are also protective against breast cancer. The incidence of breast cancer is high in societies with a sedentary lifestyle and with diets rich in fat, saturated fat, and refined carbohydrates (100).

Exercise is considered an important intervention, as it increases insulin sensitivity and decreases triglycerides and total cholesterol. Exercise also improves glucose tolerance in both lean and obese type II diabetics under age 55; however, in those older than age 55, this effect is only seen in obese patients (101).

Women who are obese, who have a family history of diabetes, or who have a history of gestational diabetes should periodically monitor their fasting plasma glucose levels, and they should initiate an exercise and weight reduction program for the primary prevention of diabetes mellitus (24). A sedentary individual who initiates an exercise program consisting of walking approximately 5 km per day or swimming, running, or biking 30 to 60 minutes per day is 50% less likely to develop diabetes (24). Long-term athletic training in premenopausal women is associated with a lower risk of developing diabetes (82). Preventing weight gain and possibly losing weight also decrease the likelihood of developing diabetes (82). A group of women aged 34 to 59 years who initiated a once a week exercise program had a 16% decrease in the relative risk of diabetes during an 8-year follow-up (102). Women in this cohort who lost weight and exercised showed a 33% decrease in their relative risk. Primary prevention of type II diabetes mellitus should be initiated at an early age in high-risk women. All women aged more than 30 years who are overweight, hypertensive, or who have a family history of diabetes should exercise at least once a week to lose weight and, thereby, prevent type II diabetes.

Therapy for type II diabetes consists of relieving symptoms and decreasing the risk of vascular complications, which are a frequent problem in these patients. Based on observations in type I diabetics (103,104), it has been hypothesized that lowering glucose levels can reduce microvascular complications in type II diabetics; however, this has not been supported by data in type II diabetics (24). Type II diabetics should attempt to obtain good control of blood glucose through diet and exercise.

Plasma fasting glucose levels should be reduced to less than 140 mg/dL (100 to 140 mg/dL), and postprandial glucose levels should be reduced to less than 200 mg/dL (24). Reductions of this magnitude constitute good control, which could delay and attenuate the onset and progression of vascular complications. Symptomatic patients who have fasting glucose levels greater than 140 mg/dL and postprandial glucose levels greater than 200 mg/dL require oral agents or insulin (24).

Dietary therapy for diabetes focuses on weight loss and reduced consumption of refined carbohydrates (105). Weight gain and overeating should be prevented because they increase insulin resistance (106). Simple carbohydrates such as sucrose should be avoided because they produce sharp increases in blood glucose. Complex carbohydrates such as starch do not cause drastic fluctuations in blood glucose. Women should restrict caloric intake to 34 kcal/kg of ideal body weight (24). Obese patients require a more severe caloric restriction to achieve weight loss. The diet should consist of 60% or less carbohydrates (mostly complex carbohydrates and dietary fiber); approximately 5% refined sugar; 12% to 20% protein; less than 30% total fat, 10% saturated fat, 10% unsaturated fat, 10% monounsaturated fat, and 300 mg or fewer cholesterol/day (105). Dietary fiber has been shown to reduce serum cholesterol and to decrease the postprandial rise in blood glucose (107,108). The American Diabetes Association initially recommended a total of 40 g of crude and soluble fiber intake per day (105), but subsequently found that such a high fiber intake interferes with the absorption of some vitamins and minerals. It now recommends an intake of 20 to 35 g of fiber per day for healthy adults (109). A low protein intake is essential to prevent the renal complications associated with high protein diets. Type II diabetics will benefit from strict adherence to a fixed diet consisting of three meals a day with no snacks, because such a diet will improve plasma glucose levels when insulin levels are limited. Patients should be introduced to the *Exchange Lists for Meal Planning* (105) to ensure proper nutritional balance.

A nutrition assessment and an annual dietary history should be conducted in diabetic patients to determine compliance with the prescribed meal plan (110). Nutritional needs of diabetic patients require particular attention because complications associated with diabetes can affect these requirements (110). Vitamin and mineral requirements in diabetics may exceed the RDAs, and micronutrient imbalances or deficiencies can result (110). Vitamin and mineral deficiencies may play a role in decreased insulin secretion and increased insulin resistance (110). Patients with poor control can lose large amounts of water-soluble vitamins and minerals (110). Careful dietary monitoring and supplementation may be useful in patients at risk of developing deficiencies; however, routine vitamin and mineral supplementation is not indicated in the management of most patients (110).

OSTEOPOROSIS

Osteoporosis is a multifaceted disease in which genetics, endocrine function, exercise, and nutrition play important roles. Risk factors for osteoporosis include menopause, smoking, poor vitamin D and calcium nutrition, lack of weight-bearing exercise, high alcohol intake, and a family history of the disease (111,112). Osteoporosis is a growing health problem. Prevention of osteoporosis is extremely important, because once the disease becomes established treatment options are not highly effective. Preventive strategies are aimed at achieving and maintaining peak bone mass through diet, exercise, HRT, and avoiding behaviors such as smoking that have adverse effects on bone (111).

The contribution of dietary factors, most notably calcium intake, and exercise to peak bone development has recently been under increased scrutiny. Improved diet and exercise during childhood are essential to reach adulthood with optimal bone mass. Bone mass accumulation until the age of 20 is determined largely by hereditary factors (113). Heredity accounts for 50% to 70% of the accumulated bone mass, but the remaining 30% to 50% is probably determined by dietary and other lifestyle factors until early adulthood (113). After age 20, lifestyle factors such as diet and physical activity become increasingly important in promoting an increase in bone mass. Attainment of peak bone mass (PBM) and peak bone density (PBD) during the adolescent and early adult years and reducing bone loss after menopause are factors believed to be most important in preventing osteopenia and osteoporotic fractures during the postmenopausal years.

Proper calcium nutrition increases bone mineral density (BMD) during periods of skeletal growth and prevents loss of bone and osteoporotic fractures in the elderly (114). Calcium supplementation slows the rate of postmenopausal bone loss by 30% to 50% (115). In postmenopausal women loss of bone density in the forearm is significantly attenuated by daily calcium supplementation with 1,000 to 2,000 mg (116–118). Several studies indicate that calcium supplementation does not have a beneficial effect on spinal bone loss in early postmenopausal women (116,119,120). One study in immediately postmenopausal women reports a beneficial effect on cortical bone from calcium supplements (121). Calcium supplementation in women 3 to 6 years postmenopause significantly reduced the rate of total body and femoral neck bone loss (122). In late postmenopausal women with low dietary calcium intakes (< 400 mg/day), a 500 mg/day calcium supplement resulted in improvements in bone density of the spine, proximal femur, and radius as compared with the control group; however, the supplementation did not benefit women with higher initial calcium intakes (120). A 4-year randomized, placebo-controlled trial of 1 g/day calcium supplements in late postmenopausal women found significant reductions in the rate of bone loss from the total body, lumbar spine, and proximal femur (123,124). In the second half of the study, the group receiving calcium supplement showed statistically significant less bone loss in the total body. Based on evidence from this study, it can be concluded that the long-term use of calcium supplements produces small but significant cumulative benefits at baseline calcium intakes of 750 mg, which are typical of postmenopausal women in Western countries (115,124). A 2-year randomized, placebo-controlled study examining the effects of calcium supplementation (1 g/day) and weight-bearing exercise in women who were more than 10 years postmenopausal found that calcium supplementation resulted in cessation of bone loss at the hip and in a significant reduction in the rate of bone loss at the tibia (125). Exercise plus calcium supplementation resulted in less bone loss at the femoral neck than calcium supplementation alone.

Bone loss in elderly women may be attenuated by calcium and vitamin D supplementation (112). In elderly women who are vitamin D deficient, rectification of the deficiency has been associated with a significant decline in hip fractures (126,127). Vitamin D deficiency results in secondary hyperparathyroidism and increased rates of bone catabolism. The effects of the potent vitamin D metabolites such as calcitriol and alphacalcidol on postmenopausal bone density remains controversial (115). HRT or the potent bisphosphonates produce greater increases in BMD than the vitamin D metabolites (115). HRT is routinely used to prevent and treat osteoporosis. Several studies investigating whether calcium supplementation is beneficial to women on HRT seem to indicate that it is, but more study is needed in this area (119,128,129).

Studies examining the effect of calcium supplementation on fracture number in postmenopausal women indicate that calcium supplements may be effective in preventing fractures despite only a modest 1% to 4% difference in BMD between the treated and placebo groups (124,130). A 4-year follow-up study of elderly women found that calcium supplementation is associated with a 45% reduction in the incidence of vertebral fractures in women with a preexisting fracture, but had no effect on women who were fracture free at the beginning of the study (131). The difference in BMD in the two groups in this study was less than 2%. Small effects on BMD may thus result in significant protective effects on fracture risk, especially in high risk women who have already suffered a fracture. Calcium supplements cause decreases in bone turnover rates, which result in the preservation of trabercular connectivity (115). Supplements improve neuromuscular function and, therefore, may prevent falls, ultimately resulting in fewer fractures. Long-term studies are needed to definitively assess whether the small benefit on BMD in postmenopausal women is protective against fractures.

In most studies, calcium supplementation produced small but significant benefits on axial bone density in women more than 5 years after the menopause. Calcium supplementation is probably most effective when given in several doses, because divided doses will prevent saturation of the calcium-active transport system and will result in its increased absorption (115). Calcium-active transport is also stimulated by the major vitamin D metabolite, 1,25-dihydroxyvitamin D. Consuming supplements with meals allows food acids to contribute to the dissolution of insoluble calcium salts and lengthens its transit time in the upper small bowel, also resulting in improved absorption (115). It is important to have calcium available at night, when bone resorption rates are greatest. Ideally, patients should consume small amounts of calcium with meals and at bedtime. Consuming 500 mg of calcium carbonate after breakfast and after dinner, or 1,000 mg of calcium lactate-gluconate at night is probably easier for most patients (115). Postmenopausal women who are not taking HRT should consume 1,500 mg of calcium per day, whereas estrogen-replete women only require 1,000 mg/day (132). All women older than 65 years should consume 1,500 mg/day of calcium (131). Calcium-rich foods such as diary products should constitute the primary source of daily calcium intake, but supplements can be used by patients who cannot consume adequate amounts of calcium through diet alone. Optimal calcium absorption is dependent on proper vitamin D nutrition. Elderly patients are at increased risk of vitamin D deficiency, and their vitamin D status should consequently be monitored. Daily supplementation with 600 to 800 IU of vitamin D in institutionalized elderly patients improves calcium balance and reduces fracture risk (132). A recent study of daily calcium and vitamin D supplementation in men and women aged more than 65 years found that 500 mg of calcium and 700 IU of vitamin D_3 moderately reduced bone loss in the femoral neck, spine, and total body during the 3-year study period (133). The supplementation program also reduced the incidence of nonvertebral fractures.

The type, duration, and frequency of physical activity needed to result in observable beneficial effects on bone remains controversial. In a study of female college athletes, activities that involve high skeletal impacts, such as gymnastics, were found to be especially osteotropic for young women (134). Bone mineral density at the lumbar spine and femoral neck was found to respond dramatically to the mechanical loading exercises typical of gymnastics training, whereas running and swimming did not have pronounced effects on BMD. Muscle strengthening activity did not seem to have a significant effect on BMD in gymnasts (134). A study of mature female athletes had similar findings, namely that women who regularly engage in high impact physical activity in the premenopausal years have higher BMD than nonathletic controls (135). Amenorrhea in premenopausal women, particularly in competitive athletes, can adversely affect bone mass however (136).

Increasing physical activity can slow bone loss in postmenopausal women, even if exercise produces no significant increase in BMD (137). Longitudinal studies examining the effects of walking interventions show that walking, which is frequently prescribed to postmenopausal women, does not prevent bone loss (138–141). Higher intensity exercises may be required to attenuate menopausal bone loss. A randomized, controlled trial of high-intensity strength training exercises 2 days per week conducted in postmenopausal women aged 50 to 70 years showed that the exercises preserved bone density and improved muscle mass, strength, and balance (142). No evidence indicates that exercise alone can replace bone loss during menopause (137). A 12-month study investigating the effects of aerobic training conducted three times a week at 70% to 85% of maximal heart rate (Fig. 38.4) for 30 to 45 minutes and calcium supplementation did not find significant increases in forearm or lumbar BMD, but the training did attenuate lumbar BMD loss in early postmenopausal women (≤ 6 years of the onset of menopause) (143). The exercise program produced significant gain in aerobic power. Prospective studies of strength-training, muscle loading, and aerobic exercise programs in postmenopausal women are difficult to compare because they differ in terms of exercise prescription, length of follow-up, subject age, hormonal status, and method and site of BMD measurement. Nevertheless, the literature seems to indicate that exercise increases forces on bone and may thereby attenuate loss of bone mass (144).

It is important to understand the influence of behavioral and genetic factors on BMD in premenopausal and postmenopausal women to assess adequately the effectiveness of interventions aimed at increasing or maintaining BMD. A study conducted on 25 elderly women, whose mean age was 72 years, and on their premenopausal daughters, whose mean age was 41 years, investigated the associations between lifetime milk consumption, calcium intake from supplements, lifetime weight-bearing exercise, premenopausal and postmenopausal hormone use, and BMD to determine the relative importance of lifestyle factors, such as calcium intake and physical activity, and genetic contributions (145). In the older women, multiple regression analyses showed that total and peripheral BMD were positively related to calcium intake from supplements after age 60, body weight, current ERT, and past oral contraceptive (OC) use. Axial BMD in this group was positively associated with body weight and past OC use. By contrast, in the premenopausal women, total and peripheral BMD were found to be determined by lifetime weight-bearing exercise, and axial BMD was found to be determined by

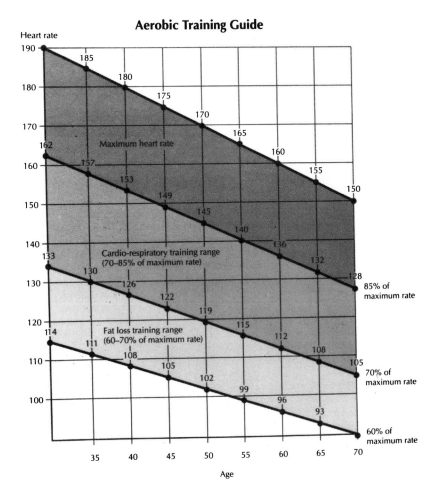

FIG. 38.4. Aerobic training guide. Exercise performed at 70% to 85% of the maximal heart rate was found to be protective against lumbar bone loss in early postmenopausal women and to produce significant gain in aerobic power. (From Byyny RL, Speroff L. *A clinical guide for the care of older women: primary and preventive care*, 2nd ed. Baltimore: Williams & Wilkins, 1996; with permission.)

total lean body mass. Mothers and daughters had similar lifetime milk consumption patterns (145). The results of this study indicate that supplemental calcium intake and exogenous estrogen have a positive effect on bone mass in postmenopausal women and that physical activity is effective in preventing osteoporosis. Behavioral and hormonal factors had a stronger effect on BMD than did familial similarity in the premenopausal and postmenopausal women studied. Women, therefore, are capable of increasing their genetically determined bone mass by engaging in weight-bearing physical activity, following a postmenopausal ERT regimen, and consuming an adequate amount of calcium (145).

The effects of HRT and exercise on bone have been found to be synergistic in many studies; however, some studies have not found a complementary effect. A placebo-controlled, 2-year prospective trial of two estrogen–progestin regimens in healthy postmenopausal women investigating the effects of HRT and exercise on bone density, muscle strength, and lipid metabolism found that exercise exerted a positive effect on BMD in the placebo group; however, in the HRT group no synergistic effect of exercise and estrogen on BMD was observed (146). Exercise cannot substitute for HRT, which clearly has the most significant impact on BMD. Estrogen therapy is effective in the prevention of osteoporosis and in treatment of established osteoporosis (147). A double-blind, placebo-controlled randomized study conducted in 120 postmenopausal women (mean age 56 years) with low forearm bone density examined the effects of an exercise regimen, exercise combined with 1,000 mg of supplemental calcium, and exercise plus estrogen and progesterone (Fig. 38.5) (117). The control group, which consisted of women with normal bone density, had a 2.7% decrease in distal forearm bone density per year. The exercise group showed a similar 2.6% decrease. The exercise–calcium group had significantly reduced bone loss (−0.5% of the baseline value per year). Bone density actually increased by 2.7% over the baseline value per year in the exercise–estrogen group. Similar patterns of bone loss and accrual were observed in the median forearm. In postmenopausal women with low BMD, bone loss can be slowed or prevented by a combined regimen of HRT and exercise or by calcium supplementation plus exercise (117). An exercise–estrogen regimen was more effective in increasing bone mass than calcium plus exercise. The exercise regimen used in this study—a 1-hour low-impact aerobics session per week with 30% of the time devoted to arm exercises, and two 30-minute brisk walks per week—was fairly moderate. A more significant exercise effect might have been observed at a higher training intensity. Nevertheless, the results of this study seem to indicate that both exercise and nutrition play important roles in the prevention and treatment of osteoporosis.

Body weight also contributes to BMD. Obesity and NIDDM are associated with increased bone mineral density. In a study of 559 women, fasting insulin levels were

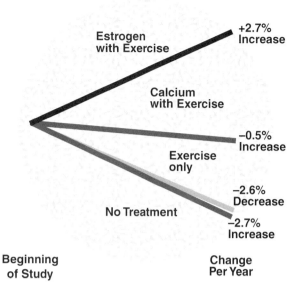

FIG. 38.5. How various treatments affect bone density. Effects of exercise only, calcium with exercise, and estrogen with exercise in postmenopausal women. (Adapted from Prince RL, Smith M, Dick IA, et al. Prevention of postmenopausal osteoporosis. A comparative study of exercise, calcium supplementation, and hormone-replacement therapy. *N Engl J Med* 1991;325:1189–1195; with permission.)

significantly and positively associated with bone density in the radius and in the spine (148). This study indicates that hyperinsulinemia may partly explain the association of diabetes and obesity with BMD in women (148). Weight loss in postmenopausal women can lead to decreased BMD. The number of pregnancies and a BMI of less than 20 kg/m² also had an adverse effect on BMD in a group of Mexican women (149). Increasing age and lack of exercise were found to be significant predictors of bone demineralization in this group.

In summary, women with established osteoporosis can be treated with estrogen, or with estrogen and progestin, calcium, and vitamin D (112). It is probably advisable to prescribe HRT and calcium supplementation to all postmenopausal women to prevent osteoporosis. HRT has the most significant impact on bone. Neither calcium supplementation nor exercise can substitute for HRT at the time of menopause, but their importance should not be overlooked. Estrogen-related bone loss usually takes place 3 to 6 years postmenopause, but loss caused by calcium deficiency results in continued bone loss until the nutritional inadequacy is corrected (150). Many postmenopausal women have low calcium intakes. Absorption efficiency decreases with age, exacerbating the existing nutritional inadequacy. Supplementation is therefore important in this population. Weight-bearing exercise is essential for the proper development and maintenance of the skeleton, and sedentary women can slightly increase their bone mass and prevent further bone loss by becoming more active (137). Exercise programs for older women should aim to improve muscle tone, strength, flexibility, and coordination, which may reduce falls in older women and prevent osteoporotic fractures (112, 137). Many postmenopausal women are inactive. Clinicians should help their patients design an individualized moderate exercise program that is both safe and encourages compliance. The osteogenic effects of such a program may be modest, but the long-term effects on cardiorespiratory fitness, strength, and agility will improve the overall health and quality of life of postmenopausal women well into old age.

TRACE ELEMENTS

Although the role of trace minerals in osteoporosis is still controversial, increasing evidence indicates that trace minerals are important for adequate bone formation and maintenance. Calcium, vitamin D, fluoride, magnesium, and trace elements such as copper, manganese, and zinc are essential for optimal bone matrix development and the maintenance of bone mineral density (151). These trace elements are necessary because they serve as cofactors for certain enzymes.

A study investigating the role of copper, manganese, and zinc in bone metabolism in a rat model, found that female rats placed on diets low in manganese or in copper and manganese for a period of 12 to 24 months had significantly lower BMD than those placed on a trace mineral-sufficient diet (152). The trace element-deficient groups had higher serum calcium concentrations. Serum and femur calcium content were inversely correlated; examination of isolated femurs showed an increase in femur porosity. Based on this observation, the authors concluded that trace mineral deficiency can result in changes in bone crystal composition and alteration of calcium control at the level of the bone (manifested as decreased mineralization or increased bone resorption), intestine, or kidney (152).

Another group investigated the effects of dietary copper or manganese restriction on serum levels of calcium, copper, and manganese and on body mass density of the right femoral shaft in male rats kept on one of four diets for 12 weeks (153). By 8 weeks BMD in the femoral shaft was significantly lower in the rats that were copper and manganese deficient than in the controls; rats placed on diets deficient in only one of the two trace minerals had intermediate BMD (153).

Subcutaneous implants of demineralized bone powder (DBP) and bone powder (BP) were used to determine the effects of long-term dietary deficiencies in manganese and copper on the cellular activity of bone formation and bone resorption *in vivo* (154). This study found that osteoblast activity is compromised more than osteoclast activity, resulting in increased bone resorption. Both bone formation and resorption are impaired by long-term

dietary manganese and copper deficiency (154). manganese deficiency in rats also resulted in lowered proteoglycan content in the organic matrix of bone (151).

Evidence from animal studies for the importance of trace elements in bone formation and maintenance led investigators to study the role of trace elements in humans. A retrospective study in normal and osteoporotic women showed that bone integrity correlates with serum manganese levels (155). The osteoporotic women had low trabecular bone volume, low bone mineral content, low BMD, and significantly lower serum manganese levels than the control group. Cross-sectional studies in a group of postmenopausal women showed a strong correlation between low BMD and low dietary calcium intake and serum copper levels (156). A 2-year prospective, double-blind, placebo-controlled clinical trial evaluating the effect of supplementary calcium with and without a combination of copper, manganese, and zinc found a significant association between BMD and supplementation with calcium and trace minerals (157,158). Dietary calcium, copper, manganese, and zinc supplements could significantly decrease the loss of BMD in postmenopausal women (157,158).

These studies suggest that trace elements are needed for optimal bone development and for maintaining bone density. Postmenopausal women who consume a balanced diet can significantly reduce the incidence of osteoporosis. The amount of calcium used in the clinical trial (1,000 mg/day) and the amount of zinc (15 mg) (157,158) correspond to the current US RDA (41). Currently, no RDA is published for manganese. The amounts of copper used (5 and 2.5 mg) were greater than the current US RDA of 2 mg (41,157,158). Many multivitamin supplements with minerals contain similar amounts of copper, zinc, and manganese. It, therefore, might be prudent for postmenopausal women to take a daily multivitamin with minerals in addition to consuming at least 1,000 mg of calcium through the diet or by the use of supplements.

DEPRESSION

The incidence of psychiatric disorders increases with each decade of life (159), and depression is more prevalent in women than in men. Many women deny they are suffering from depression and often refuse to see psychiatrists. Women have a 20% to 25% lifetime risk of suffering from a major depression (158). Many women and some clinicians share the misconception that women are likely to become depressed or irritable during menopause. Cross-sectional and longitudinal analyses of 2,565 women aged 45 to 55 years participating in the Massachusetts Women's Health Study (MWHS) found no association between menopause status or change in menopause status and depression (160,161). Prior depression was found to be highly predictive of increased depression. A lengthy perimenopausal period was associated with increased depression (161).

Depression typically manifests itself as depressed mood; however, older women more often have other symptoms such as loss of appetite, weight loss, decreased energy levels, decreased motivation, and sleep disturbances (24). Physicians should prescribe a suitable course of antidepressant medication and psychotherapy for treatment of depression, but the potentially adverse impact of a depressive disorder on a woman's nutritional status should be carefully monitored. No hard data exist on the role of nutrition in the management of depression. Nevertheless, the use of nutritional supplements, which provide a good balance of essential nutrients, might prove helpful in the depressed patient who may not have the appetite nor the motivation to consume regular meals.

Health professionals and regular exercisers share the belief that exercise produces psychological benefits (162). The effects of exercise on anxiety, depression, personality, cognition, fatigue, socialization, and work performance have been extensively investigated, but most of the studies were not carefully designed or controlled (162,163). Hughes reviewed randomized, controlled experiments conducted mostly in male populations of all age groups on the psychological effects of habitual aerobic exercise on mood, personality, and cognition (162). He found evidence that exercise improves self-concept; however, he did not find significant evidence to substantiate claims that exercise improves anxiety, depression, body image, personality, or cognition (162). An earlier review of the literature found suggestion that physical fitness results in improved mood, self-concept, and work behavior, and that improvements in physical fitness have an effect on self-concept but not on other personality traits in male and female cohorts of various age groups (163). A popular belief that does not appear to be supported by the scientific literature is the concept of the runner's high, a feeling of euphoria believed to result from release of β-endorphin. A study examined the effect of running on plasma β-endorphin in 6 female and 20 male trained long distance runners (164). Although running did produce increases in plasma β-endorphin that were more pronounced at higher training intensities, the authors caution that the decrease in anxiety reported after running, the other mood changes, and the runner's high, cannot be caused by the small changes that occurred in peripheral plasma β-endorphin concentration (164).

Most studies of the effects of exercise on psychological health have been conducted in men. A clear need exists for well-designed studies in women, especially because preliminary evidence indicates that postmenopausal women will derive benefits from exercise in terms of fitness, psychological well-being, and overall health (165). A randomized, controlled trial studying the impact of a 12-month exercise program on the physical and psychological health in 124 postmenopausal, osteopenic women aged 50 to 70 years, found that exercise produced significant increases in functional fitness, psychological well-being, and self-perceived health (165). The exercise program consisted of weight-bearing exercises, aerobic dancing, and flexibility exercises performed for 60 minutes three times per week. This program was tailored for osteopenic women, who also benefited from decreased back pain and a stabilization of spinal BMD, but similar programs suited to all postmenopausal women should be studied in controlled, randomized trials. All women should be encouraged to exercise because of the potential physical and psychological benefits they can derive from exercise. Even if future studies do not find a scientific basis for a psychological benefit from exercise, the placebo effect can be beneficial and possibly more effective in motivating women to exercise.

PHYTOESTROGENS

Natural estrogenlike substances called phytogens found in plants are attracting increasing attention, particularly with reference to their role in the menopause. Epidemiologic data from Asian countries, where the diet naturally contains large amounts of these products, suggest that they may behave like estrogen by modifying symptoms such as hot flashes and thus attenuating menopausal symptoms. This diet may offer an intriguing alternative treatment in the menopause and may explain why some countries appear to have a lower incidence of menopausal symptoms.

Phytoestrogens are naturally occurring compounds that are structurally or functionally similar to estradiol (E_2). They consist of a number of classes, including isoflavones, lignans, coumestrans, and resorcyclic acid lactones. They are biologically active and this biologic activity has been shown in animals (166). In general the human diet provides precursors for mammalian lignans and isoflavones. Even more intriguing is that the metabolism of the precursors to the phytoestrogens may be highly variable, suggesting that the production of the phytoestrogens can vary from individual to individual.

The major components of isoflavones, genistein and daidzein, are found in chick peas, lentils, soy beans, blue grass, and red clover. Most of the metabolism occurs as a result of fermentation by gut flora, but the liver may also be involved (167). In humans, 30% to 70% of dietary isoflavones are converted into various metabolites (168,169). Four isoflavones—formononetin, biochanin, daidzein, and genistein—appear to have a wide range of biologic effects on human cells, including activating the steroid receptor. Countries where soy and legumes are a major part of the diet can provide 30 to 100 mg of the four isoflavones daily.

In addition to their effect on the menopause, some studies show that the excretion of phytoestrogen is associated with a substantial reduction in breast cancer risk. Thus, the action of these phytoestrogens may be different in some respects from estradiol, which has been associated with a slight increase in breast cancer risk (170). This suggests that the phytoestrogens may act selectively on some estrogen receptors and not on others, in particular on the estrogen receptor β. This receptor is expressed more prominently in the brain, prostrate, and urinary tract and only weakly in the breast cells, where the classic estrogen receptor A is prominent.

SUMMARY AND CONCLUSIONS

Physicians should encourage their patients to initiate or continue a program of regular physical activity and improved nutrition. A better diet and regular exercise can help prevent the development of the chronic diseases of older women. In patients with established disease, exercise and nutrition may delay its progression, help reverse the disease, and improve prognosis. Aerobic exercise has beneficial effects on cardiovascular disease, cancer, obesity, diabetes, and, possibly, on depression; it specifically improves lipid profiles and insulin resistance and lowers body fat. Strength training and flexibility exercises can reduce bone loss and prevent osteoporotic fractures, respectively. Trace minerals may be important in the management of osteoporosis. Phytoestrogens improve menopausal symptoms and reduce breast cancer risk.

Healthy women can safely initiate an exercise program or change their diet with adequate counseling. Exercise and changes in diet, however, may pose serious health risks in women with certain conditions. These patients should be carefully evaluated to determine the safety of a dietary and exercise regimen, and they should be monitored on a regular basis. Exercise frequency and intensity should be prescribed according to the ability and motivation of each patient. Frequent, relatively high intensity exercise might be more beneficial, but such a regimen is less likely to encourage compliance, may result in increased injury rates, and thus may not have lasting effects on overall health. Exercise performed at 70% to 75% of the maximal heart rate at least three times per week for 50 to 60 minutes is protective against cardiovascular disease and osteoporosis (24). A brief period of warm-up and cool-down is important. Jumping, bouncing, and quick bending of the spine should be avoided.

Compelling evidence suggests that improved nutritional and activity profiles can significantly affect the development of chronic diseases that accelerate after menopause. Diet composition should be altered in specific conditions such as CHD and diabetes and appropriate exercise programs prescribed. At risk patients should also be aware of nutritional and exercise interventions that can significantly attenuate the development of such conditions as osteoporosis. Overall, these interventions can be complementary to pharmacologic interventions such as HRT, although present studies indicate that they are not a substitute for them.

REFERENCES

1. Sharp PC, Konen JC. Women's cardiovascular health. *Prim Care* 1997;24:1–14.
2. Wenger NK, Speroff L, Packard B. Cardiovascular health and disease in women. *N Engl J Med* 1993;329:247–256.
3. Meilahn EN, Becker RC, Corrao JM. Primary prevention of coronary heart disease in women. *Cardiology* 1995;86:286–298.
4. Sullivan JM. Practical aspects of preventing and managing atherosclerotic disease in postmenopausal women. *Eur Heart J* 1996;17(Suppl D):32–37.
5. National Cholesterol Education Program, National Heart La. Summary of the Second Report of the National Cholesterol Education Program (NCEP) Expert Panel on Detection, Evaluation and Treatment of High Blood Cholesterol in Adults (Adult Treatment Panel II). *JAMA* 1993;269:3015–3023.
6. Eaker ED, Packard B, Thom TJ. Epidemiology and risk factors for coronary heart disease in women. *Cardiovasc Clin* 1989;19:129–145.
7. Simkin-Silverman L, Wing RR, Hansen DH, et al. Prevention of cardiovascular risk factor elevations in healthy premenopausal women. *Prev Med* 1995;24: 509–517.
8. Gerhard M, Baum P, Raby KE. Peripheral arterial-vascular disease in women: prevalence, prognosis and treatment. *Cardiology* 1995;86:349–355.
9. Dallongeville J, Marecaux N, Isorez D, Zylbergberg G, Fruchart JC, Amouyel P. Multiple coronary heart disease risk factors are associated with menopause and influenced by substitutive hormonal therapy in a cohort of French Women. *Atherosclerosis* 1995;118:123–133.
10. Heiss G, Tamir I, Davis CE, et al. Lipoprotein-cholesterol distributions in selected North American populations: the Lipid Research Clinics Prevalence Study. *Circulation* 1980;61:302.
11. Campos H, McNamara JR, Wilson PWF, Ordovas JM, Schaefer EJ. Differences in low density lipoprotein subfractions and apolipoproteins in premenopausal and postmenopausal women. *J Clin Endocrinol Metab* 1988;67:30–35.
12. Campos H, Genest JJ, Blijlevens E, et al. Low-density lipoprotein particle size and coronary artery disease. *Arterioscler Thromb Vasc Biol* 1992;12:187–195.
13. Mathews KA, Meilahn E, Kuller LH, Kelsey SF, Caggiula AW, Wing RR. Menopause and risk factors for coronary heart disease. *N Engl J Med* 1989;321: 641–646.
14. Cheung MC, Brown BG, Wolf AC, Albers JJ. Altered particle size distribution of apolipoprotein AI-containing lipoproteins in subjects with coronary artery disease. *J Lipid Res* 1991;32:383–394.
15. Berge LN, Bonaa KH, Nordoy A. Serum ferritin, sex hormones, and cardiovascular risk factors in healthy women. *Arterioscl Thromb* 1994;14:857–861.
16. Mullen BE, Franz MM, Quatromoni PA, et al. Diet and plasma lipids in women. I. Macronutrients and plasma total low-density lipoprotein cholesterol in women: the Framingham nutrition studies. *J Clin Epidemiol* 1996;49:657–663.
17. Sonnenberg LM, Quatromi PA, Gagnon DR, et al. Diet and plasma lipids in women. II. Macronutrients and plasma triglycerides, high-density lipoprotein, and the ratio of total to high-density lipoprotein cholesterol in women: the Framingham nutrition studies. *J Clin Epidemiol* 1996;49:665–672.
18. Stensvold I, Tverdal A, Urdal P, Graff-Lissner L. Non-fasting serum triglyceride concentration and mortality from coronary heart disease and any cause in middle aged Norwegian women. *Br Med J* 1993;307:1318–1322.
19. Jacobs DRJ, Mebane IL, Bangdiawala SI, Criqui MH, Tyroler HA. High density lipoprotein cholesterol as a predictor of cardiovascular disease mortality in men and women: the follow-up study of the Lipid Research Clinic Prevalence Study. *Am J Epidemiol* 1990;131:32–47.
20. Bass KM, Newschaffer CJ, Klaq MJ, Bush TL. Plasma lipoprotein levels as predictors of cardiovascular death in women. *Arch Intern Med* 1993;153: 2209–2216.
21. Brunner D, Weisbort J, Meshulam N, et al. Relation of serum total cholesterol and high-density lipoprotein cholesterol percentage to the incidence of definite coronary events: twenty-year follow-up of the Donolo-Tel Aviv Prospective Coronary Artery Disease Study. *Am J Cardiol* 1987;59:1271–1276.
22. Posner BM, Cupples AD, Gagnon D, Wilson PWF, Chetwynd K, Felix D. The rationale and potential efficacy of preventive nutrition in heart disease: the Framingham Offspring-Spouse Study. *Arch Intern Med* 1993;153:1549–1556.
23. Hong MK, Romm PA, Reagan K, Green CE, Rackley CE. Usefulness of total cholesterol to high-density lipoprotein cholesterol ratio in predicting angiographic coronary artery disease in women. *Am J Cardiol* 1991;68:1646–1650.
24. Byyny RL, Speroff L. *A clinical guide for the care of older women: primary and preventive care*, 2nd ed. Baltimore: Williams & Wilkins, 1996.
25. National Heart La. Declining serum cholesterol levels among U.S. adults. *JAMA* 1993;269:23.
26. Wilson PWF, Christiansen JC, Anderson KM, Kannel WB. Impact of national guidelines for cholesterol risk factor screening: the Framingham Offspring Study. *JAMA* 1989;262:41–44.
27. National Cholesterol Education Program, National Heart La. Report of the National Cholesterol Education Program Expert Panel on detection, evaluation and treatment of high blood cholesterol in adults. *Arch Intern Med* 1988;148: 36–39.

28. Notelovitz M. Nutrition and the coagulation effects of estrogen replacement on cardiovascular health. *Obst Gynecol Clin North Am* 1987;14:121–141.
29. Anderson JW. Diet, lipids, and cardiovascular disease in women. *J Am Coll Nutr* 1993;12:433–437.
30. Zhang S, Folsom AR, Sellers TA, Kushi LH, Potter JD. Better breast cancer survival for postmenopausal women who are less overweight and eat less fat. The Iowa Women's Health Study. *Cancer* 1995;76:275–283.
31. Preuss HG. Nutrition and disorders of women: cardiovascular disorders. *J Am Coll Nutr* 1993;12:417–425.
32. Wild RA, Taylor LE, Knehans A. The gynecologist and the prevention of cardiovascular disease. *Am J Obstet Gynecol* 1995;172:1–13.
33. Siani A, Stazzullo P, Russo L, et al. Controlled trial of long term oral potassium supplements in patients with mild hypertension. *Br Med J* 1987;294:1453–1456.
34. Ryttig K. Treatment of mild to moderate hypertension with dietary fibre. *Lancet* 1987;1:622–623.
35. Ames BN, Shigenaga MK. Antioxidants are a major contributor to cancer and ageing. In: Halliwell B, Arumona OI, eds. *DNA and free radicals*. Chichester: Horwood, 1993:1–15.
36. Gey KF. Ten-year retrospective study on the antioxidant hypothesis of arteriosclerosis: threshold plasma levels of antioxidant micronutrients related to minimum cardiovascular risk. *J Nutr Biochem* 1995;6:206–236.
37. Gey KF. Optimum plasma levels of antioxidant micronutrients. Ten years of antioxidant hypothesis on arteriosclerosis. *Bibl Nutr Dieta* 1994;51:84–99.
38. Gey KF. Prospects for the development of free radical disease, regarding cancer and cardiovascular disease. *Br Med Bull* 1993;49:679–699.
39. Gey KF. Cardiovascular disease and vitamins. Concurrent correction of 'suboptimal' plasma antioxidant levels may, as important part of 'optimal' nutrition help to prevent early stages of cardiovascular disease and cancer, respectively. *Bibl Nutr Dieta* 1995;52:75–91.
40. Gey KF. Vitamin E and other essential antioxidants regarding coronary heart disease: risk assessment studies. Epidemiological basis of the antioxidant hypothesis of cardiovascular disease. In: Packer L, Fuchs J, eds. *Vitamin E: biochemistry and clinical applications*. New York: Dekker, 1993:589–633.
41. Food and Nutrition Board, National Research Council. *Recommended dietary allowances*. Washington, DC: National Academy Press, 1989.
42. Enstrom JE, Kanim LE, Klein MA. Vitamin C intake and mortality among a sample of the United States population. *Epidemiology* 1992;3:194–202.
43. Rimm EB, Stampfer MJ, Ascherio A, Giovannucci E, Colditz GA, Willett WC. Vitamin E consumption and risk of coronary heart disease in men. *N Engl J Med* 1993;328:1450–1456.
44. Stampfer MJ, Hennekens CH, Manson JAE, Colditz GA, Rosner B, Willett WC. Vitamin E consumption and the risk of coronary heart disease in women. *N Engl J Med* 1993;328:1444–1449.
45. Hunter DJ, Manson JE, Colditz GA, et al. A prospective study of the intake of vitamins C, E, and A and the risk of breast cancer. *N Engl J Med* 1993;329:234–240.
46. Blot WJ, Li JY, Taylor PR, et al. Nutrition intervention trials in Linxian, China: supplementation with specific vitamin/mineral combinations, cancer incidence and disease-specific mortality in the general population. *J Natl Cancer Inst* 1993;85:1483–1492.
47. Blot WJ, Li JY, Taylor RR, Guo W, Dawsey SM, Li B. The Linxian trials: mortality rates by vitamin-mineral intervention group. *Am J Clin Nutr* 1995;62:1424S–1426S.
48. Heinonen OP, Albanes D. The effect of vitamin E and beta-carotene on the incidence of lung cancer and other cancers in male smokers. *N Engl J Med* 1994;330:1029–1035.
49. Kushi LH, Fee RM, Sellers TA, Zheng W, Folsom AR. Intake of vitamins A, C, and E and postmenopausal breast cancer. The Iowa Women's Health Study. *Am J Epidemiol* 1996;144:165–174.
50. Manson JE, Gaziano JM, Jonas MA, Hennekens CH. Antioxidants and cardiovascular disease: a review. *J Am Coll Nutr* 1993;12:426–432.
51. Kushi LH, Folsom AR, Prineas RJ, Mink PJ, Wu Y, Bostick RM. Dietary antioxidant vitamins and death from coronary heart disease in postmenopausal women. *N Engl J Med* 1996;334:1156–1162.
52. Clemente C, Caruso MG, Berloco P, Buonsante A, Giannandrea B, Di Leo A. Alpha-tocopherol and beta-carotene serum levels in women treated with transdermal estradiol and oral medroxyprogesterone acetate. *Horm Metab Res* 1996;28:558–561.
53. Franken DG, Boers GH, Blom HJ, Trijbels FJ, Kloppenborg PW. Treatment of mild hyperhomocysteinemia in vascular disease patients. *Arterioscl Thromb* 1994;14:465–470.
54. Krummel D, Etherton TD, Peterson S, Kris-Etherton PM. Effects of exercise on plasma lipids and lipoproteins of women. *Proc Soc Exp Biol Med* 1993;204:123–137.
55. Lapidus L, Bengtsson C, Lindquist O, Sigurdsson J, Rybo E. Triglycerides—main lipid risk factor for cardiovascular disease in women. *Acta Med Scand* 1985;217:481–489.
56. Powell KE, Thompson PD, Caspersen CJ, Kendrick JS. Physical activity and the incidence of coronary heart disease. *Annu Rev Pub Health* 1987;8:253–287.
57. Slattery ML, Jacobs DRJ, Nichaman MZ. Leisure time physical activity and coronary heart disease death: the US railroad study. *Circulation* 1989;79:304–311.
58. Leon AS, Connet J, Jacobs DR, Raumaraa R. Leisure-time physical activity levels and risk of coronary heart disease and death: the Multiple Risk Factor Intervention Trial. *JAMA* 1987;258:2388–2395.
59. Paffenbarger RSJ, Hyde RT, Wing AL, Hsieh CC. Physical activity, all-cause mortality and longevity of college alumanganesei. *N Engl J Med* 1986;314:605–613.
60. Berlin JA, Colditz GA. A meta-analysis of physical activity in the prevention of coronary heart disease. *Am J Epidemiol* 1990;132:612–628.
61. Stevenson ET, Davy KP, Jones PP, Desouza CA, Seals DR. Blood pressure risk factors in healthy postmenopausal women: physical activity and hormone replacement. *J Appl Phsiol* 1997;82:652–660.
62. Blair SN, Kohl HW, Paffenberger RS, Clark DG, Cooper KH, Gibbons LW. Physical fitness and all-cause mortality. A prospective study of healthy men and women. *JAMA* 1989;262:2395–2401.
63. Sedgwick AW, Thomas DW, Davies M. Relationships between changes in aerobic fitness and changes in blood pressure and plasma lipids in men and women: The 'Adelaide 1000' 4-year follow-up. *J Clin Epidemiol* 1993;461:141–151.
64. Hartung GH, Moore CE, Mitchell R, Kappus CM. Relationship of menopausal status and exercise level to HDL cholesterol in women. *Exp Aging Res* 1984;10:13–18.
65. Douglas PS, Clarkson TB, Flowers NC, et al. Exercise and atherosclerotic heart disease in women. *Med Sci Sports Exerc* 1992;24(6):S266–S276.
66. Rainville S, Vaccaro P. The effects of menopause and training on serum lipids. *Int J Sports Med* 1984;5:137–141.
67. Blair SN, Goodyear NN, Gibbons LW, et al. Physical fitness and incidence of hypertension in healthy normotensive men and women. *JAMA* 1984;252:487–490.
68. Owens JF, Matthews KA, Wing RR, Kuller LH. Can physical activity mitigate the effects of aging in middle-aged women? *Circulation* 1992;85:1265–1270.
69. Ready AE, Naimark B, Ducas J, et al. Influence of walking volume on health benefits in women post-menopause. *Med Sci Sports Exerc* 1996;28:1097–1105.
70. Lemaitre RN, Heckbert SR, Psaty BM, Siscovik DS. Leisure-time physical activity and the risk of nonfatal myocardial infarction in postmenopausal women. *Arch Intern Med* 1995;155:2302–2308.
71. Williams PT. High-density lipoprotein cholesterol and other risk factors for coronary heart disease in female runners. *N Engl J Med* 1996;334:1325–1327.
72. Pate RR, Pratt M, Blair SN, et al. Physical activity and public health: a recommendation form the Centers for Disease Control and Prevention and the American College of Sports Medicine. *JAMA* 1995;273:402–407.
73. King AC, Haskell WL, Young DR, Oka RK, Stefanick ML. Long-term effects of varying intensities and formats of physical activity on participation rates, fitness, and lipoproteins in men and women aged 50 to 65 years. *Circulation* 1995;91:2596–2604.
74. Reaven PD, McPhillips JB, Barret-Connor EL, Criqui MH. Leisure time exercise an lipid and lipoprotein levels in an older population. *J Am Geriatr Soc* 1990;38:847–854.
75. Lindheim SR, Notelovitz M, Feldman EB, Larsen S, Khan FY, Lobo RA. The independent effects of exercise and estrogen on lipids and lipoproteins in postmenopausal women. *Obstet Gynecol* 1994;83:167–172.
76. Binder EF, Birge SJ, Kohrt WM. Effects of endurance exercise and hormone replacement therapy on serum lipids in older women. *J Am Geriatr Soc* 1996;44:231–236.
77. Hong MK, Romm PA, Reagan K, Green CE, Rackley CE. Effects of estrogen replacement therapy on serum lipid values and angiographically defined coronary artery disease in postmenopausal women. *Am J Cardiol* 1992;69:176–178.
78. Lee M, Giardina EG, Homma S, DiTullio MR, Sciacca RR. Lack of effect of estrogen on rest and treadmill exercise in postmenopausal women without known cardiac disease. *Am J Cardiol* 1997;80:793–797.
79. Frisch RE, Wyshak G, Albright NL, Albright TE, Schiff I, Witschi J. Former athletes have a lower lifetime occurrence of breast cancer and cancers of the reproductive system. *Adv Exp Med Biol* 1992;322:29–39.
80. Frisch RE, Wyshak G, Witschi J, Albright NL, Albright TE, Schiff I. Lower lifetime occurrence of breast cancer and cancers of the reproductive system among former college athletes. *Int J Fertil* 1987;32:217–225.
81. Frisch RE, Wyshak G, Albright NL, Albright TE, Schiff I. Lower prevalence of non-reproductive system cancers among female former college athletes. *Med Sci Sports Exerc* 1989;21:250–253.
82. Frisch RE, Wyshak G, Albright TE, Schiff I. Lower prevalence of diabetes in female former college athletes compared with nonathletes. *Diabetes* 1986;35:1101–1105.
83. Frisch RE, Snow RC, Johnson LA, et al. Insulin response of women athletes in relation to body fat quantified by magnetic resonance imaging. *Gynecol Obstet Invest* 1995;40:195–199.
84. Legato MJ. Gender-specific aspects of obesity. *Int J Fertil Womens Med* 1997;42:184–197.
85. Barret-Connor E. Obesity, atherosclerosis, and coronary artery disease. *Ann Intern Med* 1995;103:1010
86. Wing RR, Matthews KA, Kuller LH, Meilahn EN, Platinga P. Waist-to-hip ratio in middle-aged women. Associations with behavior and psychosocial factors and with changes in cardiovascular risk factors. *Arterioscler Thromb Vasc Biol* 1992;11:1250–1257.
87. Soler JT, Folsom AR, Kaye SA, Prineas RJ. Associations of abdominal adiposity, fasting insulin, sex hormone binding globulin and estrogen with lipids and lipoproteins in postmenopausal women. *Atherosclerosis* 1989;79:21–27.
88. Haarbo J, Hassager C, Riis BJ, Christiansen C. Relation of body fat distribution to serum lipids and lipoproteins in elderly women. *Atherosclerosis* 1989;80:57–62.
89. Ostlund REJ, Staten M, Kohrt W, Schultz J, Malley M. The ratio of waist-to-hip

circumference, plasma insulin level, and glucose intolerance as independent predictors of the HDL2 cholesterol level in older adults. *N Engl J Med* 1990;322:229–234.

90. Wing RR, Mathews KA, Kuller LH, Meilahn EN, Plantinga PL. Weight gain at the time of menopause. *Arch Intern Med* 1991;151:97–102.

91. Klausen B, Toubro S, Astrup A. Age and sex effects on energy expenditure. *Am J Clin Nutr* 1997;65:895–907.

92. Stoll BA. Timing of weight gain in relation to breast cancer risk. *Ann Oncol* 1995;6:245–248.

93. Ng EH, Gao F, Ji CY, Ho GH, Soo KC. Risk factors for breast carcinoma in Singaporean Chinese women: the role of central obesity. *Cancer* 1997;80:725–731.

94. Manson JE, Colditz GA, Stampfer MJ, et al. A prospective study of obesity and risk of coronary heart disease in women. *N Engl J Med* 1990;322:882–889.

95. Garrow JS. Treatment of obesity. *Lancet* 1992;340:409–413.

96. Weisweiler P. Plasma lipoproteins and lipase and lecithin: cholesterol acyltransferase activities in obese subjects before and after weight reduction. *J Clin Endcrinol Metab* 1987;65:969–973.

97. Nieman DC, Haig JL, Fairchild KS, DeGuia ED, Dizon GP, Register UD. Reducing-diet and exercise-training effects on serum lipids and lipoproteins in mildly obese women. *Am J Clin Nutr* 1990;52:640–645.

98. Wood PD, Stefanick ML, Williams PT, Haskell WL. The effects on plasma lipoproteins of a prudent weight-reducing diet, with or without exercise, in overweight men and women. *N Engl J Med* 1991;325:461–466.

99. Shimokata H, Muller DC, Fleg JL, Sorkin J, Ziemba AW, Andres R. Age as independent determinant of glucose tolerance. *Diabetes* 1991;40:44–51.

100. Kaaks R. Nutrition, hormones and breast cancer: is insulin the missing link? *Cancer Causes Control* 1996;7:605–625.

101. Zierath JR, Wallberg-Henriksson H. Exercise training in obese diabetic patients. Special considerations. *Sports Med* 1992;14:171–189.

102. Manson JE, Rimm EB, Stampfer MF, et al. Physical activity and incidence of non-insulin-dependent diabetes mellitus. *Lancet* 1991;338:774–778.

103. The Diabetes Control and Complications Trial Research Group (DCCT). The effect of intensified treatment of diabetes on the development and progression of long-term complications in insulin-dependent diabetes mellitus. *N Engl J Med* 1993;329:977

104. Reichard P, Britz A, Carlsson P, et al. Metabolic control and complications over 3 years in patients with insulin dependent diabetes (IDDM): the Stockholm Diabetes Intervention Study. *J Intern Med* 1990;228:511–517.

105. American Diabetes Association. Nutritional recommendations and principles for individuals with diabetes mellitus: 1986. *Diabetes* Care 1987;10:126–132.

106. Kitamura S. Diet therapy and food exchange lists for diabetic patients. *Diabetes Res Clin Pract* 1994;24:S233–S240.

107. Anderson JW, Ward K. Long term effects of high carbohydrate high fiber diets on glucose and lipid metabolism: a preliminary report on patients with diabetes. *Diabetes Care* 1978;1:77–82.

108. Simpson HCR, Simpson RW, Lousley S, et al. A high carbohydrate leguminous fiber diet improves all aspects of diabetic control. *Lancet* 1981;1:1–5.

109. American Dietetic Association. Position of the American Dietetic Association: health implications of dietary fiber—technical support paper. *J Am Dietetic Assoc* 1988;88:217–221.

110. Mooradian AD, Failla M, Hoogwerf B, Marynuik M, Wylie-Rosett J. Selected vitamins and minerals in diabetes. *Diabetes Care* 1994;17:464–479.

111. Bellantoni MF. Osteoporosis prevention and treatment. *Am Fam Physician* 1996;54:986–992.

112. Wark JD. Osteoporotic fractures: background and prevention strategies. *Maturitas* 1996;23:193–207.

113. Anderson JB, Metz JA. Contributions of dietary calcium and physical activity to primary prevention of osteoporosis in females. *J Am Coll Nutr* 1993;12:378–383.

114. Murray TM. Prevention and management of osteoporosis: consensus statements from the Scientific Advisory Board of the Osteoporosis Society of Canada. 4. Calcium nutrition and osteoporosis. *Can Med Assoc J* 1996;155:935–939.

115. Reid IR. Therapy of osteoporosis: calcium, vitamin D and exercise. *Am J Med Sci* 1996;312:278–286.

116. Riis B, Thomsen SK, Christiansen C. Does calcium supplementation prevent postmenopausal bone loss? *N Engl J Med* 1987;316:173–177.

117. Prince RL, Smith M, Dick IA, et al. Prevention of postmenopausal osteoporosis. A comparative study of exercise, calcium supplementation, and hormone-replacement therapy. *N Engl J Med* 1991;325:1189–1195.

118. Smith EL, Gilligan C, Smith PE, Sempos CT. Calcium supplementation and bone loss in middle-aged women. *Am J Clin Nutr* 1989;50:833–842.

119. Ettinger B, Genant HK, Cann CE. Postmenopausal bone loss is prevented by treatment with low-dosage estrogen with calcium. *Ann Intern Med* 1987;106:40–45.

120. DawsonHughes B, Dallal GE, Krall EA, Sadowski L, Shayoun N, Tannenbaum S. A controlled trial of the effect of calcium supplementation on bone density in postmenopausal women. *N Engl J Med* 1990;323:878–883.

121. Elders PJ, Netelenbos JC, Lips P, et al. Calcium supplementation reduces vertebral bone loss in perimenopausal women: a controlled trial in 248 women between 46 and 55 years of age. *J Clin Endocrinol Metab* 1991;73:533–540.

122. Aloia JF, Vaswani A, Yeh JK, Ross PL, Flaster E, Dilamanian A. Calcium supplementation with and without hormone replacement therapy to prevent postmenopausal bone loss. *Ann Intern Med* 1994;120:97–103.

123. Reid IR, Ames RW, Evans MC, Gamble GD, Sharpe SJ. Effect of calcium supplementation on bone loss in postmenopausal women. *N Engl J Med* 1993;328:460–464.

124. Reid IR, Ames RW, Evans MC, Gamble GD, Sharpe SJ. Long-term effects of calcium supplementation on bone loss in postmenopausal women—a randomized controlled trial. *Am J Med* 1995;98:331–335.

125. Prince R, Devine A, Dick I, et al. The effects of calcium supplementation (milk powder or tablets) and exercise on bone density in postmenopausal women. *J Bone Miner Res* 1995;10:1068–1075.

126. Chapuy MC, Arlot ME, Delmas PD, Meunier PJ. Effect of calcium and cholecalciferol treatment for three years on hip fractures in elderly women. *BMJ* 1994;308:1081–1082.

127. Heikinheimo RJ, Inkovaara JA, Harju EJ, et al. Annual injection of vitamin D and fractures of aged bones. *Calcif Tissue Int* 1992;51:105–110.

128. Haines CJ, Chung TKH, Leung PC, Hsu SY, Leung DHY. Calcium supplementation and bone mineral density in postmenopausal women using estrogen replacement therapy. *Bone* 1995;16:529–531.

129. Davis JW, Ross PD, Johnson NE, Wasnich RD. Estrogen and calcium supplement use among Japanese-American women: effects on bone loss when used singly and in combination. *Bone* 1995;17:369–373.

130. Chevalley T, Rizzoli R, Nydegger V, et al. Effects of calcium supplements on femoral bone mineral density and vertebral fracture rate in vitamin-D-replete elderly patients. *Osteoporos Int* 1994;4:245–252.

131. Recker RR, Kimmel DB, Hinders S, Davies KM. Anti-fracture efficacy of calcium in elderly women. *J Bone Miner Res* 1994;9(Suppl 1):S154

132. Anonymous. Optimal calcium intake: NIH Consensus Statement 1994 June 6–8. *Nutrition* 1995;12:1–31.

133. Dawson-Hughes B, Harris S, Krall EA, Dallal GE. Effect of calcium and vitamin D supplementation on bone density in men and women 65 years of age and older. *N Engl J Med* 1997;337:670–676.

134. Taaffe DR, Robinson TL, Snow CM, Marcus R. High-impact exercise promotes bone gain in well-trained female athletes. *J Bone Miner Res* 1997;12:255–260.

135. Dook JE, James C, Henderson NK, Price RI. Exercise and bone mineral density in mature female athletes. *Med Sci Sports Exerc* 1997;29:291–296.

136. Constantini NW, Warren MP. Physical activity, fitness, and reproductive health in women: clinical observations. In: Bouchard C, Shephard RJ, Stephens T, eds. *Physical activity, fitness, and health: International Proceedings and Consensus Statement*. Champaign: Human Kinetics, 1994:955–966.

137. Anonymous. American College of Sports Medicine position stand on osteoporosis and exercise. *Med Sci Sports Exerc* 1995;27:i–vii.

138. Cavanaugh DJ, Cann CE. Brisk walking does not stop bone loss in postmenopausal women. *Bone* 1988;9:201–204.

139. Nelson ME, Fisher EC, Dilmanian FA, Dallal GE, Evans WJ. A 1-year walking program and increased calcium in postmenopausal women: effects on bone. *Am J Clin Nutr* 1991;53:1304–1311.

140. Sandler RB, Cauley JA, Hom DL, Sashin D, Kriska AM. The effects of walking on cross-sectional dimensions of the radius in postmenopausal women. *Calcif Tissue Int* 1987;41:65–69.

141. White MK, Martin RB, Yeater RA, Butcher RL, Radin EL. The effects of exercise on the bones of postmenopausal women. *Int Orthop* 1984;7:209–214.

142. Nelson ME, Fiatarone MA, Morganti CM, Trice I, Greenberg RA, Evans WJ. Effects of high-intensity strength training on multiple risk factors for osteoporotic fractures. A randomized controlled trial. *JAMA* 1994;272:1909–1914.

143. Martin D, Notelovitz M. Effects of aerobic training on bone mineral density of postmenopausal women. *J Bone Miner Res* 1993;8:931–936.

144. Snow CM, Shaw JM, Matkin CC. Physical activity and risk for osteoporosis. In: Marcus R, Feldman D, Kelsey J, eds. *Osteoporosis*. New York: Academic Press, 1996:511–528.

145. Ulrich CM, Georgiou CC, Snow-Harter CM, Gillis DE. Bone mineral density in mother-daughter pairs: relations to lifetime exercise, lifetime milk consumption, and calcium supplements. *Am J Clin Nutr* 1996;63:72–79.

146. Heikkinen J, Kyllonen E, Kurttila-Matero E, Wilen-Rosenqvist G, Lankinen KS, Rita H, et al. HRT and exercise: effects on bone density, muscle strength and lipid metabolism. A placebo controlled 2-year prospective trial on two estrogen-progestin regimens in healthy postmenopausal women. *Maturitas* 1997;26:139–149.

147. Lindsay R. Hormone replacement therapy for prevention and treatment of osteoporosis. *Am J Med* 1993;95:37S–39S.

148. Barret-Connor E, Kritz-Silverstein D. Does hyperinsulinemia preserve bone? *Diabetes Care* 1996;19:1388–1392.

149. Parra-Cabrera S, Hernandez-Avila M, Tamayo-y-Orozco J, Lopez-Carrillo L, Meneses-Gonzalez F. Exercise and reproductive factors as predictors of bone density among osteoporotic women in Mexico City. *Calcif Tissue Int* 1996;59:89–94.

150. Heaney RP. Nutrition and risk for osteoporosis. In: Marcus R, Feldman D, Kelsey J, eds. *Osteoporosis*. New York: Academic Press, 1996:483–509.

151. Saltman PD, Strause LG. The role of trace minerals in osteoporosis. *J Am Coll Nutr* 1993;12:384–389.

152. Strause L, Saltman P. The role of manganese in bone metabolism. Washington, DC: American Chemical Society, 1987:45–55.

153. Andon M, Luhrsen K, Kanerva R, Chatzidakis C. Effects of dietary copper and manganese restriction on serum mineral concentrations and femoral shaft bone density in rats. *J Am Coll Nutr* 1992;11:600

154. Strause L, Saltman P, Glowacki J. The effect of deficiencies of manganese and copper on resorption of bone particles in rats. *Clacif Tissue Int* 1987;41:145–150.

155. Reginster JY, Strause LG, Saltman P, Franchimont P. Trace elements and post-

menopausal osteoporosis: a preliminary study of decreased serum manganese. *Med Sci Res* 1988;16:337–338.

156. Howard G, Andon M, Bracker M, Saltman P, Strause L. Serum trace mineral concentrations, dietary calcium intake and spine bone mineral density in postmenopausal women. *J Trace Elem Med Biol* 1992;5:23–31.

157. Strause L, Saltman P, Smith K, Andon M. Calcium, copper, manganese and zinc supplementation sustains bone density in postmenopausal women. In: Burckhardt P, Heaney RP, eds. *Nutritional aspects of osteoporosis*. New York: Raven Press, 1991:223–232.

158. Strause L, Saltman P, Smith KT, Bracker M, Andon MB. Spinal bone loss in postmenopausal women supplemented with calcium and trace minerals. *J Nutr* 1994;124:1060–1064.

159. Butler RN. The geriatric patient. In: Usdin G, Lewis JM, eds. *Psychiatry in general medical practice*. New York: McGraw-Hill, 1979.

160. McKinlay JB, McKinlay SM, Brambilla D. The relative contributions of endocrine changes and social circumstances to depression in middle-aged women. *J Health Soc Behav* 1987;28:345–363.

161. Avis NE, Brambilla D, McKinlay SM, Vass K. A longitudinal analysis of the association between menopause and depression. Results from the Massachusetts Women's Health Study. *Ann Epidemiol* 1994;4:214–220.

162. Hughes JR. Psychological effects of habitual aerobic exercise: a critical review. *Prev Med* 1984;13:66–78.

163. Folkins CH, Sime WE. Physical fitness training and mental health. *Am Psychol* 1981;36:373–389.

164. Colt EWD, Wardlaw SL, Frantz AG. The effect of running on plasma beta-endorphin. *Life Sci* 1981;28:1637–1640.

165. Bravo G, Gauthier P, Roy PM, et al. Impact of a 12-month exercise program on the physical and psychological health of osteopenic women. *J Am Geriatr Soc* 1996;44:756–762.

166. Kaldas R, Hughes CL, Jr. Reproductive and general metabolic effects of soy extracts in mammals. *Reprod Toxicol* 1989;25:1917–1925.

167. Nilsson A. Demethylation of the plant oestrogen biochanin A in the rat. *Nature* 1961;192:358.

168. Kelly GE, Nelson C, Waring MA, et al. Metabolites of dietary (soya) isoflavones in human urine. *Clinica Chimica* 1993;223:2–22.

169. Joannou GE, Kelly GE, Reeder AY, Waring M, Nelson C. A urinary profile study of dietary phytoestrogens. The identification and mode of metabolism of new sioflavonoids. *J Steroid Biochem Mol Biol* 1995;54:167–184.

170. Ingram D, Sanders K, Kolyabba M, Lopez D. Case control study of phytoestrogens and breast cancer. *Lancet* 1997;350:990–994.

Treatment of the Postmenopausal Woman: Basic and Clinical Aspects, Second Edition, edited by Rogerio A. Lobo, Lippincott Williams & Wilkins, Philadelphia © 1999.

CHAPTER 39

Menopause and Sexuality

Nancy A. Phillips and Raymond C. Rosen

Sexuality is a complex human phenomenon that is influenced by biologic, psychologic, and physiologic forces. Sexuality is additionally a learned behavior, one that undergoes lifelong development and change as it is influenced by personal experience, interest, and cultural attitudes (1). Sexuality, in its expression, is also dependent on interpersonal relationships and, as such, is influenced by the desires, beliefs, and physiology of another person.

Sexuality, therefore, is difficult to define and even more difficult to assess in terms of a single event or influential force. Few contest that puberty marks the initiation of physical sexuality, and as puberty is so clearly a hormonal event, the belief has developed that menopause, also clearly a hormonal event, is the physiological marker of the cessation of sexuality. Unfortunately, societal and medical beliefs have reinforced this view and unfairly apply it to those in this age group.

However, as this segment of the population grows, and as women can expect to live one-third of their lives after menopause, these myths are being challenged and the concept of sexual retirement is strongly disputed.

MENOPAUSE AND SEXUALITY

Several problems exist in collecting information in the field of sexuality and menopause. Importantly, differentiating between specific effects of menopause and more general effects of the physiological process of aging is challenging, if not impossible. Another problem lies in that the population studied is often recruited from menopause clinics and may, therefore, be self-selected to represent a portion of the population with more menopausal or other health problems. Large population-based studies typically rely on patient recall, often requiring retrospective information on activities and feelings from years earlier. Additionally, studies over the last 20 years have been based on a cohort of women whose attitudes toward sexuality may reflect a time of less sexual permissiveness and independence, and may not necessarily represent those of menopausal women of today or of the next 20 years. Finally, studies employ varying definitions of sexuality, often using intercourse, an activity which requires a functional partner, as the defining act, and less attention is paid to other markers of sexuality, such as sexual thoughts, fantasies, desire, and masturbation.

Despite these limitations, however, several studies do suggest a menopausal decline in measures of sexuality (2), especially as measured in terms of desire (3–5) and frequency of intercourse (3 6,7).

Bachmann, for example surveyed 1,000 consecutive gynecologic outpatients and noted a significantly greater number of sexual complaints in patients aged older than 50 years (8). She also found that 45.1% of women younger than age 35 compared with 20.3% of women older than age 50 reported having intercourse more than once a week (4). Cawood and Bancroft (2) interviewed 141 women aged 40 to 60 years and found a significant correlation between loss of interest in sex and onset of menopause, although this correlation was not found for sexual arousal or orgasm during sexual activity. In the largest population-based survey to date, Dennerstein et al. (5) telephone interviewed 2,001 Australian women aged 45 to 55 and found a significant negative relationship between menopause and sexual interest.

Although these studies are generally representative of most findings in this field, contrasting results have been

N.A. Phillips: Department of Obstetrics and Gynecology, University of Otago, Wellington, New Zealand.

R.C. Rosen: Department of Psychiatry, Center for Sexual and Marital Health, UMDNJ—Robert Wood Johnson Medical School, Piscataway, New Jersey 08854.

reported. For example, Cutler et al. (9) interviewed 124 perimenopausal and early menopausal women and found them not to be suffering from deficits in sexual desire, response, or satisfaction. Several other studies have reported that general feeling of physical and psychologic well-being, prior attitudes to sexuality, and current and past sexual relationship, rather than the occurrence of menopause, are the major factors determining post-menopausal sexuality (2,6,10,11).

Finally, it would be remiss not to recognize that a small percentage of women do report increasing sexual interest or enjoyment following menopause (5).

ESTROGEN AND SEXUALITY

The defining event of menopause is the development of a hypoestrogenic state. The profound effects of this lack of estrogen on cardiovascular disease and osteoporosis is well documented. Many studies also suggest substantial effects on mood and overall sense of well-being, factors found to significantly affect attitudes toward sexuality (2).

In addition, the hypoestrogenic state of menopause causes dramatic physical changes, affecting not only the reproductive system, but also skin, muscle, and overall body habitus (Table 39.1). These changes, especially the tendency in many women toward obesity, can lead to alterations in self-image and loss of self-esteem, with subsequent feelings of decreased attractiveness and sexual desirability. These effects can be compounded by a sense of worthlessness because of the loss of reproductive potential.

The frequent occurrence of vasomotor symptoms, present in up to 80% of women, and leading frequently to sleep interruption with resultant insomnia and fatigue, also contribute to decreasing sexuality. In fact, Cawood and Bancroft (2) found tiredness to be the strongest predictor of overall well-being, which in turn affected sexual interest and responsiveness.

TABLE 39. 1. *Physiologic changes of menopause*

Skin: decreased activity in sweat and sebaceous glands, decreased tactile stimulation
Breasts: decreased fat content; decreased breast swelling and nipple erectile response with sexual arousal
Vagina: shortening and loss of elasticity of vaginal barrel, fewer physiologic secretions, rise in vaginal pH from 3.5–4.5 to > 5, thinning of epithelial layers
Internal reproductive organs: ovaries and tubes diminish in size, ovarian follicles undergo atresia, ovarian stroma becomes fibrotic, uterine body weight decreases 30% to 50%, cervix atrophies and decreases mucous production
Bladder: urethra and bladder trigone atrophy

Adapted from Bachmann GA, Leiblum SR, Grill J. Brief inquiry in gynecologic practice. *Obstet Gynecol* 1989;73(3): 425–427.

UROGENITAL ATROPHY

Perhaps a more direct role of menopausal estrogen deficiency and sexuality lies in the loss of estrogen's maintenance of vaginal health. The development of urogenital atrophy contributes to vaginal irritation and burning, pressure, and discharge with an increased susceptibility to infection, the latter owing to an increase of vaginal pH from premenopausal levels of 3.5 to 4.5 to postmenopausal levels greater than 5. Any of these symptoms can cause intercourse or any form of genital stimulation to be aversive, and combined with the increased fragility of the vaginal epithelium, and decreased arousal and lubrication, may result in post coital bleeding or dyspareunia. Not surprisingly, dyspareunia is the most common sexual complaint of menopausal women .

As an unfortunate consequence of these urogenital changes avoidance of sexual activity may occur. Conversely, with continued uncomfortable sexual activity secondary sexual dysfunctions may ensue, whereby the anticipation of pain can further inhibit arousal or lubrication, leading to worsening dyspareunia or even vaginismus. A male partner may also respond to the woman's discomfort with feelings of guilt or fear of hurting her, leading to further avoidance of sexual contact, or occasionally development of male erectile dysfunction (impotence).

The role of systemic or vaginal estrogen in the reversal of urogenital atrophy is perhaps its most significant contribution in the treatment of menopausal sexual complaints of women. Remembering the frequent development of arousal or desire disorders related to urogenital discomfort further underscores the potential benefits of estrogen therapy.

It should be noted that not all women develop significant urogenital atrophy. In fact, some studies have shown a poor correlation between objective criteria for urogenital atrophy and subjective complaints of dyspareunia (3,12,13). Laan and vanLusen (3) evaluated 42 postmenopausal women by means of vaginal plethysmography (an indirect measure of vaginal blood flow, felt to correlate with levels of sexual arousal) during neutral films, self-induced erotic fantasy, and erotic films, and compared them with premenopausal women. Although the postmenopausal women displayed lower vaginal pulse amplitude prior to erotic stimulation, no differences were observed between premenopausal and postmenopausal women during the period of erotic stimulation. In this study none of the women had severe urogenital atrophy or were suffering from an arousal disorder, but these findings suggest that other factors may be contributing to diminished lubrication or arousal, such as a psychological arousal disorder. Other authors have observed differences in vaginal blood flow between premenopausal and postmenopausal women. For example, Hoon (14) found that the menopausal subjects in his study had decreased vaginal pulse amplitude both at baseline and after erotic stimulation, although the posterotic differences between the groups were corrected with estrogen treatment.

These differences in outcome emphasize again the importance of carefully selecting a homogeneous study population. More importantly, they point to the clinical necessity of a careful pretreatment evaluation which includes a multifactorial assessment of sexual functioning, as well as post-treatment reevaluation and adjustment or adjuvant therapy, as needed.

Park et al. (15) proposed another possible mechanism for postmenopausal lubrication and arousal difficulties. He and his colleagues suggest that atherosclerotic changes in the vaginal and clitoral vasculature cause decreased blood flow and eventual fibrosis in the vessels of these organs, resulting in vaginal engorgement and clitoral erectile insufficiency. These authors have demonstrated this phenomenon in a rabbit model, and propose that similar changes in women lead to a decreased ability to lubricate and become sexually aroused, and that this effect is primarily caused by atherosclerosis, not estrogen deficiency. Atherosclerosis is well documented in men as a cause of erectile dysfunction, and this theory is the basis for new investigations of vasodilators in the treatment of female arousal disorders.

SYSTEMIC HORMONE LEVELS AND SEXUALITY

Beyond the end organ effects of estrogen deficiency, researchers have attempted to correlate menopausal sexual activity with circulating gonadal and adrenal hormone levels. These studies have reported inconsistent, and even surprising results. For example, Laan and von-Lunsen (3), in correlating measures of sexuality and hormone levels, found significance in only 5 of 56 observations. Three of these involved prolactin, which was shown to correlate negatively with lubrication, desire and arousal. High estradiol levels were related to lower levels of sexual desire, and high estrone levels to increased sexual satisfaction. Cutler et al. (9) noted that a subset of perimenopausal women with estradiol levels less than 35 pg/mL had reduced coital activity compared with those with higher levels.

Many other studies have failed to find a consistent relationship between these variables. In general, estrogen, progesterone, androstenedione, follicle-stimulating hormone (FSH) and luteinizing hormone (LH) have not been shown to affect coital frequency, sexual arousal or dyspareunia (2,10,16,17).

In other studies, free testosterone levels have been shown to correlate positively with levels of sexual desire (10,11) and dehydroepiandrosterone (DHEA) with a sense of well-being (2).

HORMONE REPLACEMENT THERAPY AND SEXUALITY

How effective is hormone replacement therapy (HRT) in restoring normal sexual function in menopausal women? Although results in this area again have been inconsistent, positive effects have been observed in a number of studies. For example, Nathort-Boos et al. (18) randomly allocated 242 postmenopausal women to either transdermal estradiol or placebo for 12 weeks. The estradiol-treated group reported an improvement in frequency of sexual activity and fantasies, enjoyment of intercourse, and lubrication, and decreased pain compared with the placebo group, although no change was noted in sexual arousal or orgasm. Other placebo-controlled studies have reported similar results (19,20), although this positive response has not been found universally. Meyers et al. (21) reported the opposite finding in their 10-week double-blind study comparing conjugated equine estrogens alone and with testosterone or medroxyprogesterone compared with placebo. These authors found no significant change in sexual behavior or psychophysiologically measured sexual arousal in any group, and these results confirmed an earlier study by Meyers et al. (22).

The apparent discrepancy in these results may be accounted for by potential confounding factors that may have mediated the positive effects of estrogen treatment. First, urogenital atrophy, as previously discussed, is known to have deleterious effects on intercourse directly and sexual desire indirectly, and indirect effects via correction of urogenital atrophy should be considered. Additionally, hot flushes, depression, and overall sense of well-being affect sexuality. Estrogen replacement can cause significant alterations in these symptoms, again secondarily improving sexuality measures. These mediating factors might explain the variable results seen with systemic estrogen replacement.

Overall, most authors agree that estrogen is probably without a direct effect on the motivational aspects of sexual behavior such as libido, arousal, and fantasy, but it might be effective in the alleviation of specific urogenital and vasomotor complaints with increasing sexual drive or responsiveness occurring as a secondary result (16,19).

As most women will have an intact uterus, a progestational agent needs to be added to the regimen. Although few studies have evaluated the specific effect of progesterone on sexuality, it has been suggested that medroxyprogesterone might dampen mood and adversely affect sexuality by decreasing available androgens (23).

ANDROGENS AND SEXUALITY

Evidence has accumulated that supports the role of androgens in female sexuality, beginning with the reported increase in libido found in breast cancer patients treated with high doses of testosterone in the 1950s (24). The role of testosterone in male sexuality has been clearly demonstrated, and its age-related decline parallels a man's declining libido (25).

Premenopausally, the ovary secretes approximately 25% of circulating testosterone, 50% androstenedione, and 20% DHEA, with the adrenal gland contributing the remainder. The levels of these hormones in postmenopausal women are estimated to drop from 15% to 50%, compared with their younger years, because of declining ovarian function and decreased adrenal production. The latter effect is age related, although independent of menopause (7,26). The ovary, however, does continue androgen secretion following menopause and is responsible for approximately 50% of the total circulating testosterone.

Androgen's importance in sexuality has been demonstrated not only in the correlation of baseline levels of androgens with sexual desire (10,12), but also in studies which have confirmed higher rates of sexual desire, arousal, and number of fantasies in women treated with a combination of androgen and estrogen versus placebo or estrogen alone (19,27,28).

Kaplan and Owett (24) describe a "female androgen deficiency syndrome." These authors studied 11 women after chemotherapy with cytotoxic agents or bilateral salpingoophorectomy, each with a plasma testosterone level of 10 ng/dL or less, and compared them with a group of women with similar medical and surgical histories, but with testosterone levels greater than 30 ng/dL. Although sexual complaints were similar in both groups, the testosterone-deficient women had more global inability to experience sexual desire or erotic pleasure, compared with the group with a normal testosterone level. Additionally, all of the testosterone-deficient women who were treated felt relief of their symptoms, whereas evaluation of the women with normal testosterone levels uncovered dyspareunia and depression as a frequent basis for their sexual complaints.

Although this study would have been more valuable had both groups been treated with testosterone, it does underscore an important aspect of the relationship between androgens, especially testosterone, and sexuality; that is, a true deficiency state may be the precursor for successful treatment. In most studies, the beneficial effects of testosterone have been found at higher than physiologic levels and, therefore, may represent a pharmacologic rather than a physiologic property of testosterone. Clinically, this difference may be important both in selecting the patients most likely to benefit from testosterone therapy (i.e., those with lower than normal levels) and in evaluating treatment efficacy, as at normal physiologic levels the testosterone-deficient women may find relief, whereas those with normal baseline levels might need supraphysiologic levels to show a response. Unfortunately, no consensus currently exists concerning normal levels of testosterone.

Significant side effects of testosterone include potential lowering of high-density lipoproteins, cosmetic side effects such as hirsutism and acne, and virilizing effects such as deepening of the voice and clitoromegaly. In actuality, the lipoprotein effects are successfully countered with simultaneous estrogen administration, and other side effects are rare, especially if dosages in excess of 100 mg

of methyltestosterone per month are avoided. Testosterone administration, however, should not be considered for women suffering from hirsuitism or acne, and any new symptoms such as these should prompt careful reevaluation of dosage.

Studies on other available androgens such as DHEA are currently lacking, and no clear recommendations exist to their use.

EFFECTS OF AGING AND SEXUALITY

Concomitant with declining hormone levels are a multitude of social, physical, and psychological challenges. Our society as a whole places great emphasis on youth and physical attractiveness, and as the aging woman feels these to be waning, feelings of diminished self-worth may ensue. Coupled with sadness related to the loss of reproductive ability, these feelings can escalate into depression or anxiety and place stress on interpersonal relationships at a time when children are leaving, parents are ill or have died, retirement issues arise, and frequent financial strains may already be causing significant personal or interpersonal stress.

Not surprisingly, several studies have found affective involvement with the partner (11), quality of the relationship (2), and interpersonal factors (10) among the most important variables in predicting the continued quality of a sexual relationship.

MEDICAL ILLNESS

Medical illnesses and the medications used in their treatment can interfere with the physiologic sexual response via endocrine, neurologic, or vascular mechanisms; they may promote physical discomfort or increase psychologic barriers to sexuality such as a negative body image or fear of self-harm (25).

Minor physical ailments such as decreased flexibility, minor arthritis, and urinary incontinence can add discomfort and embarrassment to sexual encounters.

Cardiovascular disease and hypertension can be associated with diminished sexuality in a variety of ways. Those patients with disease sufficiently severe to restrict activity will be most impaired, but disease at any stage, or the medications required for treatment, can affect sexuality. Studies of return to sexual functioning following myocardial infarction (MI) show decreased frequency of intercourse in 40% to 58% of patients (29). Reasons for decreased activity with cardiovascular disease, especially following MI, include depression, anxiety about recurrence of disease, fear of coital death, or physical symptoms such as dyspnea or angina with sexual activity. These fears, which can be present in the patient, partner, or both, can lead to avoidance of sexual encounters.

Diabetes has been extensively studied in men and has been clearly shown to cause erectile dysfunction. Although similarly convincing evidence is not available in women, decreased desire, orgasmic dysfunctions, and diminished lubrication have been suggested by some studies (29–31).

Hysterectomy for benign disease is a common surgical procedure and one which often raises sexual concerns, as the uterus carries substantial psychological importance to many women as a symbol of femininity. Some studies suggest that hysterectomy itself does not routinely impair sexual function, although significant individual variation does occur (32). Virtanen et al. (33) noted a significant improvement in dyspareunia and sexual desire with no change in orgasmic capacity in a review of 102 patents, whereas a review of the literature by Goldstein et al. (32) found that 33% to 37% of women reported a decrease in sexual responsiveness following hysterectomy. The literature suggests that the indication for hysterectomy may be a major factor in affecting outcome, as those patients who experience relief from pain or severe bleeding are likely to improve sexual functioning, whereas those who are relatively asymptomatic beforehand fare less well (34).

Cancer and its related treatments cause devastating physical and psychological trauma for both the patient and her partner. Breast cancer, which will affect one of eight women, results in physical alteration of an organ that is both visible and highly emphasized as a source of femininity. This frequently results in feelings of diminished sexuality and, of these patients, 21% to 39% are estimated to develop a sexual dysfunction (32). One-third of women have not resumed intercourse 6 months after mastectomy, and in those who have, the female superior position which directly exposes the breast, is often avoided, and frequency of breast stimulation decreases substantially (35). The trend toward less disfiguring surgery and the widespread use of reconstruction may help minimize these feelings.

Gynecologic malignancies also fare poorly in terms of postoperative sexuality. Thranov and Klee (36) surveyed patients at varying intervals following surgery for endometrial, cervical, and ovarian cancer. Little or no sexual desire was found in 74% of these patients. Of the sexually active group, 40% experienced dyspareunia. Other studies have also shown that up to 90% of women with gynecologic malignancies report some form of sexual dysfunction (37).

Medications are another common source of sexual dysfunctions and can affect arousal, orgasm, or both, either via direct effect on physiologic mechanisms of normal sexual functioning or indirect effect through concomitant alterations in mood, mental alertness, or social interaction (Table 38.2) (38,39). Chronic use of nonprescription medications such as antihistamines are a frequently overlooked source of arousal disorders. Alcohol, although it lessens inhibitions and is generally perceived as a sexual stimulant, actually inhibits arousal, even in small amounts. These side effects should be considered both in medication changes and new prescriptions.

TABLE 39.2 *Common drugs that affect sexuality in women*

Decreased Desire
  Antilipid medications (e.g., Atromid, Lopid)
  Antipsychotics (e.g., Prolixin, Thorazine)
  Barbiturates
  Benzodiazepines (e.g., Ativan, Valium, Xanax)
  Beta-blockers (e.g., Inderal)
  Clonidine (Catapres)
  Danazol
  Digoxin
  Fluoxetine (Prozac)
  Gonatropin-releasing hormone Agonists (Lupron, Synarel)
  H_2 blockers and anti-reflux agents (e.g., Tagamet, Zantac, Reglan)
  Indomethacin (Indocin)
  Ketoconazole (Nizoral)
  Lithium
  Phenytoin (Dilantin)
  Spironolactone (Aldactone)
  Tricyclic Antidepressants (e.g., Elavil, Anafranil)
Diminished Arousal
  Alcohol
  Anticholinergics (eg., ProBanthine)
  Antihistamines (eg., Seldane, Benadryl)
  Antihypertensives (eg., Clonidine, Aldomet)
  Benzodiazepines (eg., Valium, Ativan)
  Selective serotonin reuptake inhibitors (SSRIs) (eg., Prozac, Zoloft)
  Monoamine oxidase inhibitors
  Tricyclic antidepressants (eg., Elavil, Anafranil)
Orgasmic Dysfunction
  Aldomet
  Amphethamines and related anorexic drugs
  Antipsychotics (eg., Mellaril, Thorazine)
  Benzodiazepines (eg., Valium, Xanax, Ativan)
  Selective serotonin reuptake inhibitors (SSRIs) (e.g., Prozac, Zoloft)
  Narcotics (eg., Methadone)
  Trazadone
  Tricyclic antidepressants (eg., Elavil, Anafranil)*

*Also associated with painful orgasm
Adapted from Weiner DN, Rosen RC. Medications and their impact. In: Sipski ML, Alexander CJ, eds. *Sexual function in people with disability and chronic illness.* Gaithersberg, MD: Aspen Publishers, 1997;856–118.

MALE FACTORS

Women face yet another sexual obstacle as they age: an available, functional male partner. Demographics certainly do not favor women. Past the age of 60, it has been estimated that 74% of married men and 56% of married women maintained an active sex life, whereas only 31% of unmarried men and 5% of unmarried women were sexually active, and by the age of 80, there are four women for every man (40).

Another obstacle to continued sexuality within the context of a relationship is the high rate of erectile dysfunction in men, especially older men. The Massachusetts Male Aging Study estimated erectile dysfunction to occur in 52% of men between the age of 40 and 70, with the incidence of complete impotence tripling from 5% at age 40 to 15% at age 70 years (41). Older women are less likely to be with younger men, and when the incidence of erectile dysfunction in available men and the declining numbers of male partners are combined, an unfortunate disparity in society occurs for women.

Normal physiologic male aging changes in the sexual response cycle also occur. These include longer time to achieve erection; diminished penile rigidity, which can cause difficulty in penetration; increase in stimulation and time required for orgasm; and an increase in refractory time, sometimes requiring several days. These normal changes should be understood by both the male partner and the woman to aid in successful sexual encounters.

DIAGNOSIS AND TREATMENT OPTIONS

The key to identifying a sexual problem is to inquire about sexuality during a medical history. Once a problem is identified, a detailed description including onset, frequency, duration, and associated symptoms should be sought. Distinguishing whether the problem is situational or global can further help in uncovering causes, as the former is less likely to be purely physiologic. A careful evaluation of menopausal symptoms, medical conditions, medications, habits, and symptoms of underlying disease such as diabetes and cardiovascular or thyroid disease should be sought.

Physical examination should include a thorough pelvic examination with a careful assessment of vaginal health, including evaluation for atrophy, vaginitis, and vulvar dystrophies. The evaluation for atrophy should include assessment of introital size, the presence or absence of rugal folds, vaginal depth, labial fat content, and skin elasticity and turgor (7). Deep dyspareunia should be evaluated as needed.

Once a diagnosis has been made, medical intervention, if possible, should be initiated (Table 38.3). Hormone replacement therapy should be considered in women who are acceptable candidates and who complain of vasomotor or urogenital symptoms. Vaginal estrogen creams or estradiol-containing vaginal rings are options for patients who do not wish to use systemic hormones and for those who may also need a supplement to systemic hormone replacement. The use of lubricants such as KY Jelly (*Johnson & Johnson, New Brunswick, NJ*), or Replens (*Warner Wellcome, Morris Plains, NJ*) are nonhormonal options.

For those women who are suffering from vaginismus or who have a narrowed introitus, vaginal dilators and progressive relaxation techniques should be encouraged.

Desire disorders should prompt an evaluation that includes exploring the presence of depression, fatigue, or relationship problems, including a sexual dysfunction in the partner. Consideration of testosterone supplementation in the form of pills, creams, or subcutaneous implants is appropriate for women who continue to complain of desire disorders despite systemic estrogen replacement. Sex therapy referral should be considered for those women who do not respond and for those for whom depression, relationship conflicts, or no cause for the disorder is uncovered.

Female patients should also be educated to the normal physiologic changes of aging and their effect on the sexual response cycle. Specific examples include the following:

1. Arousal may require more time and stimulation. The increased sensitivity of the vulvar skin and vaginal mucosa can make prolonged stimulation uncomfortable. Warm baths before genital sexual activity, lubricants, use of fantasy, vibrators, or oral stimulation can be useful suggestions for a slow arousal response.
2. Orgasm, which can become harder to achieve as well, consists of less rhythmic muscular contractions. Muscle tension lessens as well, and the overall intensity of orgasm often diminishes, but individual responses are variable. The use of masturbation, vibrators, and, if necessary, sexual counseling is recommended.
3. For those women and their partners who cannot achieve penetration, massage and sexual activity without intercourse as the goal can be mutually satisfying and should be encouraged. In fact, removal of intercourse as the goal for every sexual encounter is useful advice for all couples, regardless of age.

Above all, menopausal women need to be aware that continued sexuality is a realistic and expected part of aging, and health care professionals need to be sensitive and informed about sexuality issues to best serve these patients.

TABLE 39.3 *Counseling and treatment strategies*

Educate and Encourage
  Normal age-related changes in sexual response cycle
  Women: diminished lubrication, need for increased time and stimulation for arousal, decreased orgasmic contractions, decreased breast fullness and nipple erection
  Men: decreased penile rigidity, need for increased time and stimulation for erection and orgasm, longer refractory time
  Potential sexual strategies
  Masturbation
  Use of sexual fantasies, erotic materials, vibrators
  Changes in sexual routine (place, time of day)
  Sensual massage, noncoital sexual activity
Offer Medical Interventions
  Hormone replacement therapy
  Testosterone supplementation
  Vaginal dilators, relaxation techniques
  Changes in medications
Specialized Referrals
  Psychotherapy
  Individual or marital counseling
  Sex therapy
  Medical endocrinologists

REFERENCES

1. Drench ME, Losee RH. Sexuality and sexual capacities of elderly people. *Rehabilitation Nursing* 1996;21(3):118–123.
2. Cawood, EH, Bancroft J. Steroid hormones, the menopause, sexuality and well-being of women. *Psychol Med* 1996;26(5):925–936.
3. Laan E, vanLunsen RH. Hormones and sexuality in postmenopausal women: a psychophysiological study. *J Psychosom Obstet Gyaecol* 1997;18(2):126–133.
4. Bachmann GA. Influence of menopause on sexuality. *Int J Fertil Menopausal Stud* 1995;40(Suppl 1):16–22.
5. Dennerstein L, Smith AMA, Morse CA, Burger HG. Sexuality and the menopause. *J Psychosom Obstet Gynaecol* 1994;15:59–66.
6. Bachmann GA. Sexual dysfunction in postmenopausal women: the role of medical management. *Geriatrics* 1988;43(11):79–83.
7. Davis SR, Burger HG. Clinical review 82: androgens and the postmenopausal woman. *J Clin Endocrinol Metab* 1996;81(8):2759–2763.
8. Bachmann GA, Leiblum SR, Grill J. Brief inquiry in gynecologic practice. *Obstet Gynecol* 1989;73(3):425–427.
9. Cutler WB, Garcia CR, McCoy N. Perimenopausal sexuality. *Arch Sex Behav* 1987;16(3):225–234.
10. Bachmann GA, Leiblum SR. Sexuality in sexagenarian women. *Maturitas* 1991;13:43–50.
11. Huerta R, Mena A, Malacara JM, Diaz de Leon. Symptoms at perimenopausal period; its association toward sexuality, life-style, family function, and FSH levels. *Psychoneuroendocrinology* 1995;20(2):135–148.
12. Leiblum SR, Bachmann GA, Kemmann E, Colburn D, Schwartzman L. Vaginal atrophy in the postmenopausal woman: the importance of sexual activity and hormones. *JAMA* 1983;249:2195–2198.
13. Bachmann GA, Leiblum SR, Kemmann E, Colburn DW, Schwartzman L. Sexual expression and its determination in the postmenopausal woman. *Maturitas* 1984;6:19–29.
14. Hoon PW. Physiologic assessment of sexual response in women: the unfulfilled promise. *Clin Obstet Gynecol* 1984;27(3):767–780.
15. Park K, Goldstein I, Andry C, Siroky MB, Krane RJ, Azadzoi KM. Vasculogenic female sexual dysfunction: the hemodynamic basis for vaginal engorgment insufficiency and clitoral erectile insufficiency *Int J Impot Res* 1997;9(1):27–37.
16. Loewit K. Hormone treatment of sex disorders in menopause-causal therapy or placebo [Abstract]. *Geburtshilfe Frauenheilkd* 1993;53(11):814–818.
17. Tungphaisal S, Chandeying V, Sutthijumroon S, Krisanapan O, Udomratn P. Postmenopausal sexuality in Thai women. *J Obstet Gynaecol* 1991;17(2):143–146.
18. Nathorst-Boos J, Wiklund I, Mattsson LA, et al. Is sexual life influenced by estrogen therapy? A double-blind placebo-controlled study in postmenopausal women. *Acta Obstet Gynecol Scand* 1993;72:656–660.
19. Sherwin BB, Gelfand MM. The role of androgen in the maintenance of sexual functioning in oophorectomized women. *Psychosom Med* 1987;49:397–409.
20. Dennerstein L, Burrows G, Wood C, Hyman G. Hormones and sexuality: effects of estrogen and progestogen. *Obstet Gynecol* 1980;56:316–322.
21. Myers LS, Dixen J, Morrissette D, Carmichael M, Davidson JM. Effects of estrogen, androgen, and progestin on sexual psychophysiology and behavior in postmenopausal women. *J Clin Endocrin Metab* 1989;70(4):1124–1131.
22. Myers LS, Morokoff PJ. Physiologic and subjective sexual arousal in pre- and postmenopausal women taking replacement therapy. *Psycophysiology* 1986;23:283–292.
23. Sherwin BB. The impact of different doses of estrogen and progestin on mood and sexual behavior in postmenopausal women. *J Clin Endocrinol Metab* 1991;72:336–343.
24. Kaplan HS, Owett T. The female androgen deficiency syndrome. *J Sex Marital Ther* 1993;19(1):3–24.
25. Meston, CM. Aging and sexuality. *West J Med* 1997;167(4):285–290.
26. Longcope C. The endocrinology of the menopause. In: Lobo R, ed. *Treatment of the postmenopausal woman*. New York: Raven Press, 1994:47–56.
27. Montgomery JC, Appleby L, Brincat M, Versi E, Tapp A, Fenwick PBC, Studd JWW. Effect of oestrogen and testosterone implants on psychological disorders in the climacteric. *Lancet* 1987;1:297–299.
28. Sherwin BB, Gelfand MM, Brender W. Androgen enhances sexual motivation in females: a prospective cross over study of sex steroid administration in the surgical menopause. *Psychosom Med* 1985;7:339–351.
28a. Sipski ML, Alexander CJ. Impact of disability or chronic illness on sexual function. In: Sipski ML, Alexander CJ, eds. *Sexual Function in People with Disability and Chronic Illness*. Gaithersberg, MD:Aspen Publishers, 1997:3–11
29. Leiblum SR, Rosen RC, eds. *Principals and practice of sex therapy. Update for the 1990s*. New York; Guilford Press, 1989.
30. Roughan PA, Kaiser FE, Morley JE. Sexuality and the older woman. *Clin Geriatr Med* 1993;9:87–106.
31. Spector IP, Leiblum SR, Carey MP, Rosen RC. Diabetes and female sexual function: a critical review. *Ann Behav Med* 1993;15(4):257–264.
32. Goldstein MK, Teng NNH. Gynecologic factors in sexual dysfunction of the older woman. *Clin Geriatr Med* 1991;7(1):41–61.
33. Virtanen H, Makinen J, Tenho T, Kilholma P, Pitkanen Y, Hirvonen T. Effects of abdominal hysterectomy on urinary and sexual symptoms. *Br J Urol* 1993;72:868–872.
34. Sloan D. The emotional and psychosexual aspects of hysterectomy. *Am J Obstet Gynecol* 1978;131(6):598–605.
35. Droegmueller W. Sexuality and sexual dysfunction. In: Visscher H, ed. *Precis V. An update in obstetrics and gynecology*. Washington DC: American College of Obstetrics and Gynecology 1994:97–103.
36. Thranov I, Klee M. Sexuality among gynecologic cancer patients—a cross sectional study. *Gynecol Oncol* 1994;52:14–19.
37. Bachmann GA, Ayers CA. Psychosexual gynecology. *Med Clin North Am* 1995;79(6):1299–1317.
38. Weiner DN, Rosen RC. Medications and their impact. In: Sipski ML, Alexander CJ, eds. *Sexual Function in People with Disability and Chronic Illness*. Gaithersberg, MD: Aspen Publishers, 1997;85–118.
39. *The Medical Letter* 1992;876(34):73–8.
40. Holzapfel S. Aging and sexuality. *Can Fam Physician* 1994;40:748–766.
41. Feldman HA, Goldstein I, Hatzichristou G, Krane RJ, McKinlay JB. Impotence and its medical and psychosocial correlates: results of the Massachusetts male aging study. *J Urol* 1994;151:54–61.

Treatment of the Postmenopausal Woman: Basic and Clinical Aspects, Second Edition, edited by Rogerio A. Lobo, Lippincott Williams & Wilkins, Philadelphia © 1999.

CHAPTER 40

Postmenopausal Compliance with Hormone Therapy

Julie Stein and Veronica Ravnikar

Hormone replacement therapy (HRT) is prescribed primarily to alleviate menopausal symptoms and to prevent future osteoporosis-related fractures and arteriosclerotic heart disease. Newer studies also show a probable beneficial effect of estrogen in preventing colon cancer, tooth loss, Alzheimer's disease, and ocular macular degeneration. Although the optimal preventative health benefits are obtained with long-term use in the postmenopausal woman, a review of studies shows that at least 25% of users discontinue estrogen in the first 9 months (1). Discontinuance is linked in large part to side effects, fear of breast and endometrial cancers, lack of education, and cultural biases. Physicians need to educate patients in an organized but sympathetic manner and ensure that they understand the reasons for beginning HRT, the reasons for maintaining therapy, and the difference between nuisance and serious side effects. This chapter explores issues of compliance with menopausal hormone therapy given for various clinical end points.

To maximize compliance or adherence with HRT, it is crucial to understand why women begin HRT and why physicians prescribe it. The end points of therapy are varied according to the previously described goals. With perimenopausal use, estrogen is helpful in alleviating the symptoms of hot flushes (also called hot flashes), sleep disturbances, and vaginal dryness. With long-term uninterrupted use (10 to 20 years), HRT can decrease the relative risk of osteoporotic fractures and cardiovascular disease by approximately 50%. These two goals are often difficult to reconcile, because women do not understand

the benefit of long-term therapy, they are fearful of medical risks, or they are intolerant of nuisance side effects such as bloating, weight gain, and vaginal bleeding. The American College of Physicians makes a distinction between use of HRT for relief of symptomatic menopause and for prevention of disease to prolong life (2). It suggests that, when treating menopausal symptoms, hormones should be given for a limited time (1 to 5 years). Although this period can serve as a window during which the physician may begin to discuss the benefits and risks of long-term HRT, the decision to prolong treatment should be made separately and with full patient cooperation.

Compliance with HRT is quite poor. In a preliminary 5-year study of the Massachusetts Women's Health Survey by Dr. Sonjay McKinley and supported by the National Institutes of Aging, 2,500 women between the ages of 45 and 55, few continued taking the therapy beyond the first year (3), and few even filled their prescriptions after the first visit.

For the postmenopausal population older than 60 years of age, HRT is known to be beneficial as secondary intervention therapy for osteoporosis treatment end points. It also may be helpful for cardiovascular treatment as a secondary intervention. Definitive studies (e.g., HERS clinical trial) on cardiac benefits are still pending. Adherence in this group has additional barriers. These women made the transition into menopause before HRT was widely prescribed, thereby missing much of the media onslaught. Having enjoyed several years of amenorrhea and long past hot flushes, they are often less tolerant of the side effects that can accompany replacement therapy. Because older women have largely outgrown or become used to the symptoms of menopause, their motivation to begin HRT has less to do with alleviating an immediate discomfort and more to do with halting disease progression.

J. Stein: Department of Obstetrics and Gynecology, University of Michigan, Ann Arbor, Michigan 48109.

V. Ravnikar: Division of Reproductive Endocrine and Infertility, Department of Obstetrics and Gynecology, University of Massachusetts Medical Center, Worcester, Massachusetts 01655.

Similarly, there is often difficulty with adherence issues in the black and Hispanic communities, which in part may be physician influenced. Because the incidence of osteoporosis is one-third to one-half that seen in the white population, doctors may view HRT as less important for these patients. This would, however, be a grave oversight, because cardiovascular disease rates remain significant for blacks and Hispanics and the incidence of osteoporosis in these women could still benefit from reduction. However, poor adherence also depends on the patient. For reasons that may include a distrust of physicians or cultural norms that keep women from seeking medical assistance for menopausal symptoms, these populations are not widely reached. An article from Duke University (4) finds black study participants to be 83% less likely to report estrogen use and 66% less likely than white participants to report current use. Past arguments have attempted to rely on socioeconomic reasons for this disparity, but the Duke study found these differences to be independent of education or income. If we are to understand why women stop or never start taking estrogen, we must first understand their cultural biases.

The remainder of this chapter deals with ways to gather, organize, and present crucial information to improve adherence with HRT. With a standardized approach to determine risk factors for osteoporosis, heart disease, and breast cancer, physicians may be able to select patients who would benefit from HRT and help them contribute to their own preventative health with a sense of reassurance. A glimpse at newer products provides the potential for greater flexibility in prescribing HRT regimens to minimize the number of patients who discontinue therapy because of nuisance side effects.

PATIENT ATTITUDES

The North American Menopause Society (NAMS) evaluated a cohort of women in an attempt to understand the patients' perspective (5). Using a Gallup survey, they interviewed 833 women between the ages of 45 and 60. The subjects were asked where they received information on HRT, and 36% of women polled reported their physicians. Of the remaining subjects, 27% reported gaining their knowledge of HRT through magazines or journals, and 6% obtained information from friends, newspapers, or television. Women who had gone through menopause were more likely to identify their doctors as a primary source of information on HRT.

With respect to the perceived adequacy of education, less than one-half of women surveyed were very satisfied with information provided by their physicians; 1 in 4 was somewhat satisfied; and 16% said they were not satisfied. Women who were current users of HRT, compared with past or never users, were more likely to report being satisfied with information provided by their physicians. It would seem that the onus is on physicians to become better care providers by becoming better information providers.

The NAMS study also looked at concerns leading women to HRT. The most frequently mentioned medical reason is the risk of osteoporosis (33%). Depression and mental attitude and increased risk of heart disease were the next most frequent concerns (28% and 27%, respectively) of women. Of the women who commented on emotional problems of the menopause, only 3% cited a decreased interest in sex as their primary concern. Although women bothered by emotional rather than physical symptoms of menopause were more likely to report having visited their doctors, the most common complaints at physician visits were physical (e.g., night sweats, hot flushes, irregular bleeding). This finding suggests that prescribers are not doing a thorough enough job of investigating emotional complaints because these are less likely to be volunteered by patients and more likely to be wrapped in the guise of somatic complaints. Overall, 60% of women polled said they chose to take HRT for relief of menopausal symptoms.

DECISION-MAKING MODELS

Col et al. (6) proposed a Markov model to examine the risks and benefits of HRT. By use of such a model, physicians can present patients with a statistical value of their risks and estimate changes in life expectancy with therapy. This approach to decision-making, while seemingly impersonal, is helpful in dispensing prescribing biases for the physician and the confusing and often contradictory information for the patient. The model analyzes the impact of HRT on coronary heart disease, breast cancer, hip fracture, and endometrial cancer. Using risk weights for each of these categories, the relative benefits are determined with the help of a partitioning diagram (Fig. 40.1). The model then bases its recommendations for or against HRT on whether the therapy would increase life expectancy by at least 6 months.

Col weighed several risk factors for the probability of coronary artery disease: systolic blood pressure, cholesterol to high-density lipoprotein (HDL) ratio, electrocardiographic evidence of left ventricular hypertrophy, history of diabetes, and cigarette smoking. Those for breast cancer include age of menarche, previous benign breast biopsies, age at first live birth, and number of affected first-degree relatives. Hip fracture risk factors include history of maternal hip fracture, previous hyperthyroidism, current use of sedating medications, and several items that consider risks of falling, such as height, level of activity, and overall performance status. Objective measurements of bone density are not included in this model (Fig. 40.1).

Col's approach is limited in that the numbers are derived from a hypothetical cohort and an estimation of the likelihood of developing certain diseases from regres-

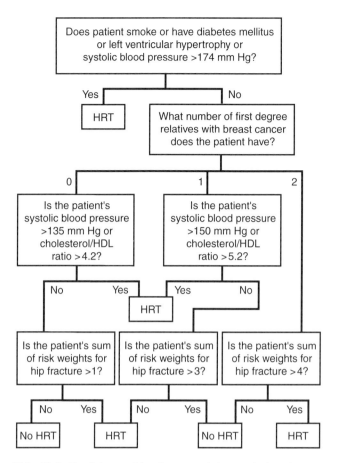

FIG. 40.1. Decision-making framework for analyzing the use of hormone replacement therapy (HRT) in patients at risk for breast cancer, coronary heart disease, hip fracture, or endometrial cancer. (From ref. 6, with permission.)

sion models that link risk factors to disease incidence. Although the model considers family history of breast cancer and osteoporosis, it fails to look at a family history of early heart disease as a potential influencing factor. This method disregards bone densitometry, a useful means of obtaining quantitative information on a woman's risk of osteoporosis. Despite these criticisms, Col provides a reasonable framework in which to organize complicated information for the layperson and the physician. The hope is that simplification of this material will lead to improved comprehension and adherence to therapy.

DISEASE PREVENTION AND TREATMENT

Osteoporosis

For women with diagnosed osteoporosis, HRT becomes a treatment modality instead of a preventative measure. Peak bone mass, achieved in early adulthood, remains stable at the vertebral level (with perhaps a slight decrease at the hip) until the decline of ovarian function (7). During the first 5 to 8 postmenopausal years, there may be a period of accelerated bone loss, with annual rates approaching 3% to 5% and later decreasing to a steady state of about 1% to 2% per year (7). It follows that maintenance of hormone levels should forestall this trend.

Treatments for established osteoporosis have broadened to include bisphosphonates, calcitonin, anabolic steroids, and parathyroid hormone, but HRT remains a viable and most practical option. The Postmenopausal Estrogen/Progestin Interventions (PEPI) trial looked at bone mineral density (BMD) measurements in women on various hormone combinations compared with placebo (8). After 36 months, they found that those in the placebo group had lost an average of 2.8% of spinal BMD, whereas those in any of the active treatment groups had gained approximately 5.1%. With regard to the hip, the placebo group lost an average of 2.2% while those adhering to an active treatment gained 2.3%.

Benefits of hormone replacement on bone loss in some women are seen with estrogen doses as little as 0.3 mg of esterified estrogens per day (9). Using the lowest possible dose that is still effective may increase compliance by decreasing nuisance side effects. Recommendations for the prevention and treatment of osteoporosis made by the American College of Endocrinology are listed in Table 40.1.

Several studies have looked at whether the diagnosis of osteoporosis or screening BMD improves patient continuance with HRT. The European and National Osteoporosis foundations recommend that BMD measurements be obtained if the results would determine treatment modality (7). They also recommend that measurements be repeated at least twice after initiation of treatment at intervals greater than or equal to 1 year. Unfortunately, although screening has been shown to improve HRT new starts, there is little evidence to suggest that it alone improves long-term adherence. A second British source found that, despite a knowledge of

TABLE 40.1. *Recommendations for prevention and treatment of osteoporosis*

Preparation	Osteoporosis indication	Recommended dosing	Available strengths (mg)
Conjugated equine estrogens (Premarin)	Prevention and treatment	0.625 mg/d	0.3, 0.625, 0.9, 1.25, 2.5
Conjugated estrogens	Prevention	0.3	
Estradiol, micronized (Estrace)	Prevention	0.5	0.5, 1,2
17β-Estradiol (Estraderm patch)	Prevention	0.05	0.05, 0.1
Estropipated (Ogen)	Prevention	0.75	0.75, 1.5, 3

Adapted from ref. 3, with permission.

low BMD, nearly 40% of these patients discontinue HRT within 8 months (10).

When screening BMD was combined with support services such as education and counseling, adherence varied from 84% to 92% over 5 years (11). This study was in part predicated on earlier work not specific to osteoporosis or HRT that found improved compliance by patients who were seen promptly and to whom advice was provided in an accessible manner with simple written instructions (12). It appears that optimal adherence to HRT is achieved by providing patients with concrete evidence of osteoporosis in the form of BMD measurements and by providing them with support throughout their therapy: reassurance that their side effects are expected and minimizing their fears through increasing understanding about risks and benefits.

Hypercholesterolemia

For women with elevated serum lipids, the reduction of low-density lipoprotein (LDL) cholesterol and the elevation of HDL may have a significant and beneficial impact on their cardiac risk profile. The cardiovascular benefit from estrogen is not caused by cholesterol entirely. This effect on lipids is, however, a well-known end point and one that may explain about 25% of the cardiac benefit of estrogens. As with BMD measurements, fasting lipid profiles may be used to help patients understand where they fall with respect to disease. Likewise, serial measurements are often helpful in guiding hormone therapy and encouraging patient adherence. Oral estrogen taken at doses of 0.625 mg per day can decrease mean LDL cholesterol by 15% and increase HDL cholesterol by 16% (13). Estrogen may adversely effect serum triglycerides and should be used cautiously in women with hypertriglyceridemia. Transdermal estrogen, although modestly increasing HDL levels, has no significant effect on reductions in very-low-density lipoprotein or LDL (13). Because changes in lipid profiles are not always predictable, at least one repeat assessment is recommended for patients with borderline or increased values to evaluate the need for second-line agents.

Patients must realize that, even though lipid measurements are important, this assessment does not tell the entire story of how estrogen works on the cardiovascular system. Hormone therapy's main effect may be as an antioxidant in decreasing the incorporation of LDL cholesterol into plaques and improving coronary blood flow. Measurement of lipids, however, give the patient a concrete measure of estrogen's effects.

SIDE EFFECTS

Minimizing Nuisance Side Effects

A significant number of women begin HRT enthusiastically but discontinue it because of undesirable side effects such as abnormal bleeding, weight gain, and headaches. With a wide spectrum of formulations, doses, and delivery systems, the options for HRT are greater than ever, providing many alternatives to minimize these symptoms. The physician who is willing to tailor the estrogen and progestin component of a patient's regimen will probably see much improved long-term adherence to therapy.

Abnormal Uterine Bleeding

In nearly every study on adherence and HRT, improved use was observed among women who had undergone surgical menopause. Because postmenopausal bleeding is one of the most common complaints with treatment, it is understandable why hysterectomized women have an easier time maintaining long-term use. Abnormal uterine bleeding is seen frequently in the perimenopausal woman on continuous combined HRT. This method generally employs 0.625 mg of conjugated estrogen and 2.5 mg of medroxyprogesterone acetate (MPA) daily. Because basal levels of exogenous hormone are irregular in perimenopausal patients who retain some ovarian function, endometrial dyssynchrony can occur and result in breakthrough bleeding. In the early postmenopausal years, when HRT is generally sought out by symptomatic patients, a preferred method may be cyclic therapy that tends to create a more predictable monthly bleed. Although the idea of continued menses is not ideal for most women in this age group, it is generally preferable to irregular breakthrough bleeding. This method employs 0.625 mg conjugated estrogen daily and 5 mg of MPA for 14 consecutive days each month. After patients achieve ovarian quiescence, they can be transitioned to continuous combined therapy if amenorrhea is desired.

In the older postmenopausal woman, erratic bleeding is often caused by an atrophic endometrium. These women often find it necessary to increase the dose of estrogen to thicken the uterine lining. Uterine malignancy must first be excluded in all age groups of patients experiencing abnormal bleeding. This can be accomplished easily with in-office endometrial biopsy or vaginal ultrasound.

Weight Gain

HRT users, despite little supportive evidence, frequently attribute weight gain to HRT. Fat stores and distribution probably change in all menopausal women as a result of the natural decrease in metabolic rate that accompanies this phase of life. Patients may, however, experience bloating and breast tenderness as a result of replacement hormones that is sometimes misinterpreted as weight gain. In the normally menstruating woman, these symptoms generally peak in the mid-luteal phase when estradiol increases up to 150 pg/mL (14). Menopausal symptom relief and osteoporosis prevention generally require levels of about 50 to 100 pg/mL of plasma estradiol (14). This can vary from patient to patient, and dose alterations may be required within this range according to patient complaints.

A review of information from the PEPI trials found that hormone replacement may decrease the amount of weight gained in the first postmenopausal decade. This reduction was independent of the hormone regimen selected (15).

With or without HRT, regular aerobic exercise along with a judicious diet is perhaps the most effective means of maintaining weight and can improve cardiovascular conditioning, increase HDL, and increase agility and flexibility to reduce fracture risk.

Headaches

Migraine-like headaches are a common complaint in the perimenopausal woman or the woman beginning HRT. Much of this is caused by decreased or fluctuating levels of circulating estrogen. DeLignieres found concentrations below 40 pg/mL to be associated with an increased incidence of headache (14). When considering estrogen replacement in these women, the newer estrogen patches such as Fempatch (*Parke-Davis, Morris Plains, NJ*) maintain more constant blood levels of hormone than oral or first-generation transdermal estrogens and may be a reasonable first-line therapy. However, standard doses of this patch preparation may be insufficient for osteoporosis and cardiovascular disease treatment and prevention. In women who prefer oral agents, continuous combined regimens are preferable to cyclic therapy to reduce hormone level fluctuations. Anecdotal evidence suggests that micronized progesterone (100 to 200 mg) may be better tolerated by patients who experience headaches related to medroxyprogesterone acetate.

Serious Side Effects

Endometrial Cancer

Unopposed estrogen in the nonhysterectomized woman poses an increased risk of endometrial cancer. Statistics from the PEPI cohort trial reveal the following rates of disease found on endometrial biopsy in women on unopposed estrogen compared with those on placebo: simple (cystic) hyperplasia, 27.7% versus 0.8%; complex (adenomatous) hyperplasia, 22.7% versus 0.8%; and atypical hyperplasia, 11.8% versus 0%. Study participants on estrogen and progestin, regardless of regimen, had rates similar to those given placebo (16). Patient fears of cancer play a significant role in adherence issues. What most physicians know and need to convey to their patients is that the protective effect of progestins, whether used daily or in a cyclic fashion, negates this added risk for endometrial cancer. For women who tolerate progestins poorly, physicians may elect to use it to promote a withdrawal bleed only once every 3 months. Some physicians prescribe unopposed estrogen to a select group of women. This method is advocated only for those who are willing to follow patients closely for signs of bleeding and for routine yearly surveillance in the form of endometrial biopsy.

Venous Thromboembolism

The association between the use of oral contraceptives and the increased risk of venous thromboembolism is well established. Several studies have examined whether this prothrombotic effect is as significant in the doses used in HRT. Although the risk of clot formation does appear to be elevated over that of nonusers, the number of extra cases is no greater than 1 to 2 cases per 10,000 women (17). This risk probably is limited to the first year of therapy and is independent of estrogen dose, route of delivery (oral versus transdermal), or the concurrent use of progestins (17). In counseling patients on HRT, this risk is perhaps significant only for women with preexisting tendencies toward thromboembolism.

Breast Cancer

Perhaps the greatest fear standing in the way of long-term adherence with HRT is the fear of breast cancer. Media coverage of this issue is pervasive and largely conflicting, such that even the most informed patient is left with anxiety-provoking questions. The Nurse's Health Study is the largest cohort study looking at this issue. It followed more than 100,000 women since 1976 (many of whom are now in their 50s and 60s) and determined the relative risk of breast cancer in hormone users with or without progestin to be 1.3 to 1.4 (18). This same study looked at older women (60 to 64 years) on post-menopausal hormone therapy for 5 or more years and found the relative risk of breast cancer to be 1.71. Although many studies echo these findings, it is difficult to prove increased mortality for women on HRT.

Persson et al. looked at breast cancer incidence and mortality in more than 22,000 Swedish women, and although they discovered a 1.4 relative risk in HRT users over that of nonusers, they did not see an associated increase in mortality after 13 years of follow-up (19). This study estimated the risk for liver, biliary tract, and colon cancers to be reduced by about 40% in women on replacement hormones, most notably combined estrogen and progestin.

A large, population-based case-control study in Seattle found no increase in breast cancer among women between the ages of 50 and 64 on estrogen or estrogen-progestin therapy for a period of exposure of up to 20 years (20). It showed that use of combined therapy for 8 or more years was associated with a reduction in breast cancer. The American Cancer Institute looked at more than 400,000 women prospectively and found a 16% decrease in fatal breast cancer among estrogen users (21).

A metanalysis, involving a collaborative analysis of data from 51 epidemiologic studies that enrolled 52,705 women with breast cancer and 108,411 women without breast cancer, showed the following:

1. Current or recent use increased breast cancer risk to 1.35 (95% confidence interval [CI], 1.21–1.49) with a relative risk of duration of use increased by 1.023 for each additional year of use.
2. Once stopped, 5 years of no HRT use brings patient back to baseline.
3. Risk of metastatic disease with long-term use was not increased (contrary to Nurse's Health Study data).
4. Although weight was a factor in increasing breast cancer rates, HRT caused higher levels of breast cancer in thinner women.

A related issue involves the decreased sensitivity and specificity of mammography screening in women on HRT. The unadjusted mammographic sensitivities (95% CI) for never users of estrogen replacement therapy is 94% but is lowered to 69% in current users (22). The specificity for never users is 86%, but for current users it is 82% (22). Imaging difficulties arise because of the increased density of breast tissue under hormonal stimulation. Methods to sidestep this problem include obtaining baseline mammograms before instituting HRT and stopping therapy for a time before annual screening.

Because of breast cancer concerns, there has been a trend over the last few years toward developing a more refined selection process in identifying candidates for HRT. With the assistance of decision-making models such as that proposed by Col (6), we can rule out women who run a higher risk of breast cancer and women whose risk profiles for osteoporosis and cardiac disease are so low that even a slight increase in cancer risk is not worth the potential benefit. The risk of breast cancer with HRT is still essentially unknown, and if elevated, it is only a slight increase with deviation of use.

NEW ESTROGENS AND PROGESTINS

Strategies to improve adherence to HRT are in continued development. Tissue-specific estrogens such as Raloxifene may make replacement issues easier for patients with personal or strong family histories of breast cancer. These designer estrogens, as they are called, have shown promise in lowering serum cholesterol and slowing bone loss. Their effect on cardiovascular disease is unknown.

Progestins are being developed that increase the number of HRT options. Vaginal preparations such as Crinone (*Wyeth-Ayerst, Philadelphia, PA*) are promising. Local application of progestin may provide the benefit of endometrial protection to estrogen users without many of the systemic side effects seen with larger doses of oral progestins. Because Crinone uses a base of bioadhesive

polymer, it acts in a sustained release, allowing for doses as low as 45 mg to be administered every other day (23). Crinone is not yet approved for use in postmenopausal women. Women using such preparations for progesterone replacement need to have their endometrium followed carefully.

CONCLUSIONS

Successful continuation with hormone replacement is simple if treatment helps the patient to feel better and recognize the difference immediately. Adherence to therapy for preventative purposes is a far more complex problem. If the therapy is relatively benign with few side effects, such as an aspirin each day to allay heart attack, compliance largely depends on helping patients to remember their medication.

The issue of hormone replacement is more difficult. With this therapy physicians and patients must put forth effort to minimize nuisance side effects and real medical risks. Responsibility falls on the physician to thoroughly screen patients to determine which of them are appropriate candidates for HRT, to educate patients on the myriad risks and benefits, and to formulate a regimen that best conforms to their needs while minimizing side effects. A women may fair well on one combination of hormones at the beginning of her menopause, but this may not satisfy her needs indefinitely. Recognition of this fact is the first step in understanding that HRT is an evolutionary process, not only for the field of medicine in general, but also for the patient specifically as she proceeds through postmenopausal life.

REFERENCES

1. Coop J, Marsh J. Can we improve compliance with long-term HRT? *Maturitas* 1992;15:151–158.
2. American College of Physicians. Guidelines for counseling postmenopausal women about preventive hormone therapy. *Ann Intern Med* 1992;117:1038–1041.
3. Ravnikar VA. Barriers for taking long-term hormone replacement therapy: why do women not adhere with therapy? Presented at the Novo Nordisk International Health Care Symposium; Barcelona, Spain, 1996.
4. Handa VL, Landerman R, Hanlon JT, et al. Do older women use estrogen replacement? Data from the Duke Established Populations for Epidemiologic Studies of the Elderly (EPESE). *J Am Geriatr Soc* 1996;44:1–6.
5. Utian WH, Schiff I. NAMS-Gallup survey on women's knowledge, information sources, and attitudes menopause and hormone replacement therapy. *Menopause* 1994;1:39–48.
6. Col NF, Eckman MH, Karas RH, et al. Patient specific decisions about hormone replacement therapy in postmenopausal women. *JAMA* 1997;277:1140–1147.
7. Hodgson S, Johnston CC. AACE Clinical practice guidelines for the prevention and treatment of postmenopausal osteoporosis. *Endocr Pract* 1996;2:155–171.
8. Writing group for the Postmenopausal Estrogen/Progestin Interventions (PEPI) trial. Effects of hormone therapy on bone mineral density—results from the PEPI trial. *JAMA* 1996;276:1389–1396.
9. Genant HK, Lucas J, Weiss S, et al. Low dose esterified estrogen therapy. Effects on bone, plasma estradiol levels, endometrim and lipid levels. *Arch Intern Med* 1997;157:2609–2615.
10. Ryan PJ, Harrison R, Blake GM, et al. Compliance with hormone replacement (HRT) after screening for postmenopausal osteoporosis. *Br J Obstet Gynaecol* 1992;99:325–328.
11. European Foundation for Osteoporosis and the National Osteoporosis Foundation. Consensus development statement. *Osteoporos Int* 1997;7:1–6.
12. Carr A. Compliance with medical advice. *Br J Gen Pract* 1990;40:358–360.
13. Walsh BW, Schiff I, Rosner B, et al. Effect of postmenopausal estrogen replace-

ment on the concentrations and metabolism of plasma lipoproteins. *N Engl J Med* 1991;325:1196–1204.

14. DeLignieres B. Hormone replacement therapy: clinical benefits and side-effects [Review]. *Maturitas* 1996;23[Suppl]:S31–S36.

15. Espeland MA, Stefanick ML, Kritz-Silverstein D, et al. Effect of postmenopausal hormone therapy on body weight and waist and hip girths. *J Clin Endocrinol Metab* 1997;82:1549–1556.

16. Writing group for the Postmenopausal Estrogen/Progestin Interventions (PEPI) trial. Effects of hormone therapy on endometrial histology in postmenopausal women: the Postmenopausal Estrogen/Progestin Interventions (PEPI) trial. *JAMA* 1996;275:370–375.

17. Perez Gutthann S, Garcia Rodriguez LA, Castellsague J, et al. Hormone replacement therapy and risk of venous thromboembolism: population-based case-control study *BMJ* 1997;314:796–800.

18. Colditz GA, Hankinson SE, Hunter DJ, et al. The use of estrogens and progestins and the risk of breast cancer in postmenopausal women. *N Engl J Med* 1995;332:1589–1593.

19. Persson I, Yuen J, Bergkvist L, et al. Cancer incidence and mortality in women receiving estrogen and estro-progestin replacement therapy—long-term follow-up of a Swedish cohort. *Int J Cancer* 1996:67:327–332.

20. Stanford JL, Weiss NS, Voight LF, et al. Combined estrogen and progestin hormone replacement therapy in relation to risk of breast cancer in middle-aged women. *JAMA* 1995;274:137–142.

21. Willis DB, Calle EE, Miracle-McMahill HL, et al. Estrogen replacement therapy and risk of fatal breast cancer in a prospective cohort of postmenopausal women in the United States. *Cancer Causes Control* 1996;7:449–457.

22. Johannes CB, Crawford SL, Posner JG, et al. Longitudinal patterns and correlates of hormone replacement therapy use in middle-aged women. *Am J Epidemiol* 1994;140:439–452.

23. Cansanas-Roux F, Nisolle M, Marbaix E, et al. Morphometric, immunohistological and three-dimensional evaluation of the endometrium of menopausal women treated by oestrogen and Crinone, a new slow-release vaginal progesterone. *Hum Reprod* 1996;11:357–363.

Treatment of the Postmenopausal Woman: Basic and Clinical Aspects, Second Edition, edited by Rogerio A. Lobo, Lippincott Williams & Wilkins, Philadelphia © 1999.

CHAPTER 41

Complementary Medicine: Herbs, Phytoestrogens, and Other Treatments

Adriane Fugh-Berman

Complementary medicine goes by many names: alternative, unconventional, natural, integrative, traditional, and nontraditional are just a few variations. By whatever name, complementary practices and therapies are extremely popular. A telephone survey of 2,055 English-speaking adults found that 42.1% had used at least one alternative therapy in 1997 (1), up from 33.8% in 1990 (2). Undoubtedly the use of herbal and other traditional therapies is even higher among non–English-speaking people.

Between 1990 and 1997, women became more common users of alternative therapies (48.9%) than men (37.8%), and expenditures on visits to alternative practitioners increased from an estimated 14.6 to 21.2 billion dollars (1). The percentage of those using alternative therapies who discussed this use with their physician did not change appreciably; it was 38.5% in 1990 and 39.8% in 1997. All physicians should familiarize themselves with complementary therapies enough to be able to counsel patients about them. This chapter reviews studies addressing phytoestrogens, herbs, and other complementary therapies relevant to postmenopausal women.

SOY AND OTHER DIETARY PHYTOESTROGENS

Phytoestrogens, or plant estrogens, may function as naturally occurring selective estrogen receptor modulators (SERMs). Phytoestrogens occupy estrogen receptors but are less than 1% as potent as endogenous estrogens (3). The two major classes of dietary phytoestrogens are isoflavones and lignans. Beans are rich in isoflavones, which include genestein and daidzein. Soybeans are particularly rich in isoflavones and also contain some lignan

A. Fugh-Berman: Department of Health Care Services, George Washington University School of Medicine, Washington, D.C. 20036.

precursors (4). Flaxseed (i.e., linseed) is very high in lignans, which are also found in whole grains, seed, fruits, and berries.

A multi-ethnic study of 50 premenopausal women in the United States measured urinary phytoestrogen levels and found the highest levels of lignans and coumestrol in white women; African-American women and Latinas had the lowest levels of these two phytoestrogens (5). Latinas, however, had the highest levels of genestein, which is found mainly in beans. Other isoflavone levels did not differ significantly by ethnicity. These findings are interesting but are limited by the study's small size.

Hot Flushes

Asian women complain less about hot flushes (also called hot flashes) and other menopausal symptoms than do Western women. Although it is difficult to factor in the effect of cultural differences (e.g., the fact that Asians respect age while Westerners worship youth), it has been suggested that eating soy products serves as a type of hormone replacement therapy (6).

There is evidence that phytoestrogen supplementation can help hot flushes. A double-blind, placebo-controlled study randomized 104 postmenopausal women to 60 g of isolated soy protein or to casein as a control for 12 weeks. Hot flushes were reduced by 45% in the soy group compared with 30% in the placebo group (the difference was statistically significant) (7). Differences between the two groups were evident by the third week. Adverse effects (mainly gastrointestinal complaints) were similar in the two groups.

A 12-week study in 145 Israeli women with menopausal symptoms (114 completed the study) found that the 78 women assigned to a phytoestrogen-rich diet (approximately one-fourth of caloric intake) had fewer hot flushes than the 36 women in the control group (8). Total scores on a menopausal symptom questionnaire were not significantly different between the two groups.

Another study with 58 women enrolled compared daily intake of 45 g of soy flour with the same amount of wheat flour for 12 weeks. The soy-treated group had significantly fewer hot flushes (9).

Effect on Vaginal Epithelial Cells

Four studies have looked at whether supplementing the diet with phytoestrogens resulted in estrogenic changes in vaginal epithelial cells; two had positive results, and two had negative results. A study of 25 women tested 45 g of soy flour daily and found significant improvements in the vaginal maturation index (10).

The Brzezinski study mentioned earlier also found improvements in vaginal cytology (9). However, the Murkies study did not find significant changes in vaginal cytology (10). Another study of 97 women (91 completed the study) found that soy foods supplying a daily intake of 165 mg of isoflavones resulted in an increase in the percentage of vaginal superficial cells in 19% of the soy group compared with 8% of controls; however, the results did not achieve statistical significance (11). This study apparently used an unusual method of collecting vaginal cells that may have underestimated estrogenized cells (12).

Effects on Endogenous Hormones

Studies of the effects of soy on hormone levels in premenopausal women have not been consistent. The best study was a randomized, controlled, cross-over trial enrolling 14 premenopausal women in Minnesota that compared high-isoflavone soy powder (2 mg/kg/day, or approximately 128 mg) with low-isoflavone (1 mg/kg/day, or approximately 64 mg) and isoflavone-free (0.15 mg/kg/day) soy powder (13) and found only small changes in reproductive hormones. This 9-month trial found that the high-isoflavone diet decreased free triiodothyronine (T_3) and dehydroepiandrosterone sulfate (DHEAS) during the early follicular phase and decreased estrone levels during the mid-follicular phase. The low-isoflavone diet decreased luteinizing hormone (LH) and follicle-stimulating hormone (FSH) during the periovulatory phase. There were no other significant changes in sex hormone–binding globulin (SHBG) or hormone levels (including progesterone, testosterone, prolactin, androstenedione, thyroxine [T_4], thyroid-stimulating hormone [TSH], insulin, or cortisol) nor any change in the length of the follicular or luteal phase of the menstrual cycle. Endometrial biopsies showed no changes in histologic dating.

Although this is the most definitive study on this subject, it only examined different doses of isoflavones and did not report baseline levels of hormones. Although isoflavones are assumed to be the only endocrinologically active components of soy, it is possible that other substances in soy besides isoflavones affect hormone levels.

A smaller study of six women between the ages of 22 and 29 years used a higher isoflavone dose and found that daily consumption of 36 ounces of soy milk (containing about 200 mg of isoflavones) for 1 month decreased serum 17β-estradiol levels by 81% at midcycle and 49% in the luteal phase (14). This decrease persisted for two to three cycles. Progesterone levels during the luteal phase decreased by 35%, and DHEAS levels decreased 14% to 30%. Another study of six women with regular menstrual cycles who consumed 60 g of soy protein (containing 45 mg of isoflavones) daily for 1 month found that the soy supplementation increased follicular phase length, decreased midcycle LH and FSH surges, and delayed menstruation (15).

Prevention of Breast Cancer

It is unclear whether phytoestrogen supplementation reduces breast cancer risk. Breast cancer patients excrete lower amounts of phytoestrogens than other women; in areas of the world where breast cancer risk is low, excretion of phytoestrogens is high. Japanese women who eat traditional food have lower breast cancer rates than those who eat a Western diet (16). However, phytoestrogens are not the only factor that separates these two diets; among other things, a traditional diet is lower in meat and fat and higher in vegetables and fiber.

One study of Chinese women in Singapore found that soy product intake was associated with lower rates of breast cancer in premenopausal, but not postmenopausal, women (17). Another study (18) found that phytoestrogen supplementation markedly increased SHBG levels in postmenopausal women.

There is scant evidence that postmenopausal phytoestrogen supplementation benefits breast cancer risk. Although breast cancer rates in Asia are lower at all ages than breast cancer rates in the West, it is unclear to what extent phytoestrogens contribute to this disparity. There is no evidence that merely adding phytoestrogens to a Western diet would decrease these rates. Dosage, formulation, duration, and timing may all have an effect. It has been theorized, for example, that the most important period for phytoestrogen intake is around puberty, when phytoestrogens may affect terminal end bud differentiation. This effect would not be possible to extract from epidemiologic data in which the consumption of soy foods is lifelong. There is no evidence that soy foods increase risk; these foods have been consumed for thousands of years and clearly are not dangerous to consume. Until recently, dietary intake of phytoestrogens was primarily determined by cultural differences in diet. Although purified isoflavone capsules have become readily available to consumers, there are no long-term safety data on these food-free phytoestrogens.

It would be difficult to predict the effect of deliberate high-dose supplementation of phytoestrogens by post-menopausal women who consumed low amounts of phytoestrogens premenopausally. *In vitro*, estradiol and phytoestrogens each stimulate the growth of cultured breast cancer cells (19). When both are added together, little to no growth occurs. Although soy intake can protect against a number of induced cancers in animals (20), this is not always the case. For example, phytoestrogen implants can stimulate growth of estrogen receptor–positive breast cancer implants in immunocompromised mice (21).

Endometrial Cancer

Soy foods do not increase endometrial cancer rates and may be protective. A case-control study of 332 endometrial cancer cases and 511 controls from a multi-ethnic population in Hawaii found that high soy intake appears to protect against endometrial cancer in premenopausal and postmenopausal women (22).

Cardiovascular Disease

Soybeans also may have a beneficial effect on cardiovascular disease. A metanalysis of 38 controlled clinical trials found that high consumption of soy was associated with a 9.3% reduction in total cholesterol, a 12.9% reduction in low-density lipoprotein cholesterol, and a 10.5% reduction in triglycerides. High-density lipoprotein cholesterol was unaffected (23).

One study randomized 189 oophorectomized cynomolgus monkeys fed an atherogenic diet to supplementation with soy, isoflavone-free soy, or conjugated estrogens (in a dose equivalent to 0.625 mg/day) (24). Supplementation with isoflavone-intact soy equaled conjugated estrogens for most lipid and lipoprotein parameters and was superior in increasing apolipoprotein A-1. Soy, unlike the conjugated estrogens, did not increase triglycerides. Soy supplementation also was equivalent to conjugated estrogens in decreasing coronary artery reactivity.

Osteoporosis

In a double-blind trial of 66 postmenopausal, hypercholesterolemic women between the ages of 49 and 73 (25), subjects were randomly assigned to 40 g of protein each day from one of three sources: milk (nonfat dried milk and casein), soy protein with medium isoflavone content (equivalent to 55.6 mg of isoflavones daily), or isolated soy protein with high isoflavone content (equivalent to 90 mg of isoflavones daily). All women also followed a low-fat, low-cholesterol diet. Dual-energy x-ray absorptiometry (DEXA) bone density studies of the lum-

bar spine, proximal femur, and total body were done at the beginning of the study (after a 2-week lead-in) and at the end of the 6-month study.

No differences were seen among the three groups in bone density studies of the hip or total body, but subjects receiving the high isoflavone preparation experienced a significant increase in lumbar bone density and mineral content (2%) compared with the milk protein group.

HERBS

A variety of herbs have been used to treat menopausal symptoms. Ginseng *(Panax ginseng)*, chaste-tree berry *(Vitex agnus-castus)*, Dong quai *(Angelica sinensis)*, black cohosh *(Cimicifuga racemosa)*, and licorice *(Glycyrrhiza glabra)* are a few of the herbs commonly used to treat hot flushes and other symptoms associated with menopause. However, there are few clinical studies on these therapies and little information on the long-term effects of medicinal herbs.

Black Cohosh

Black cohosh is an estrogenic herb that contains alkaloids, including *N*-methylcytisine, the isoflavone formononetin, and terpenoids. Side effects of black cohosh include nausea, vomiting, dizziness, visual disturbances, and bradycardia (26).

One placebo-controlled, double-blind trial showed improvements in the vaginal maturation index in women using black cohosh (27). An unconvincing trial of 110 women with menopausal symptoms (off hormonal treatment for at least 6 months) found that those treated with commercial tablets of black cohosh in a dose equivalent to 40 mg of standardized extract daily had lower LH levels than a control group after 2 months of treatment (28). Follicle-stimulating hormone (FSH) levels were unchanged. However, because baseline levels of hormones were not drawn in this study, preexisting differences in the two groups cannot be excluded.

Several uncontrolled trials published in German showed improvement in depression and measures of well-being among menopausal women. However, the lack of control groups renders these results unreliable, especially considering that mood is highly responsive to placebo.

Black cohosh contains formononetin, a phytoestrogen stronger than those found in beans and whole grains. There is a theoretical concern that long-term use of this herb unopposed by progesterone may lead to endometrial hyperplasia, although such cases has not been reported in the literature.

Dong Quai

Dong quai is a Chinese herb commonly prescribed to menopausal women. A double-blind, placebo-controlled study of 71 symptomatic postmenopausal women with

FSH levels higher than 30 mIU/mL found that 6 months of treatment with dong quai did not affect number of hot flushes, estrogenization of vaginal epithelial cells, or endometrial thickness measured by sonogram (29). Dong quai is most commonly used as part of an individually tailored mixture of Chinese herbs.

Evening Primrose

Oil of evening primrose *(Oenethera biennis)*, a good source of linoleic and γ-linolenic acid, was evaluated in a double-blind controlled trial of 56 women. It was found to be no more effective than placebo for hot flushes (30).

Kava

Widely used in Polynesia, the rhizome of the kava shrub *(Piper methysticum)*, a psychoactive member of the pepper family, is used medicinally for anxiety and insomnia. Active constituents in kava are the kavapyrones (also called kavalactones),

A study of kava for climacteric symptoms in 40 women using doses of 30 to 60 mg/day for 56 to 84 days found significant improvements in the human anti-murine antibody (HAMA) scale and Kupperman index (31). Another trial by the same investigator but using a higher dose (equivalent to 210 kavapyrones/day) in 40 menopausal women also found improvements in symptoms, HAMA, Kupperman index, and Depression Status Inventory (DSI) (32).

Extremely heavy, chronic recreational use of kava results in yellowing of the skin and an ichthyosiform eruption known as kava dermopathy, often accompanied by eye irritation (33).

Ginseng

There are different types of ginseng, the most common of which are Chinese ginseng *(Panax ginseng)*, American ginseng *(Panax quinquefolius)*, and Siberian ginseng *(Eleutherococcus senticosus)*, which is not ginseng at all but is in the same family. Ginseng contains terpenoids, especially a group of compounds called ginsenosides. Ginseng can cause estrogenic effects, although the plant does not actually contain phytoestrogens. Several cases of postmenopausal uterine bleeding after ingesting ginseng have been reported (34,35); another case occurred after use of a face cream that contained ginseng (36). Ginseng may cause hypertension in some individuals. Mastalgia has also been reported in a 70-year-old woman who had consumed a ginseng powder for 3 weeks (37). The same effect, with nipple enlargement and "increased sexual responsiveness" was reported in five cases (38).

Licorice

Licorice contains coumarins, flavonoids, and terpenoids. Glycyrrhizinic acid and its derivatives affect the metabolism of the steroid cortisol, apparently by inhibiting the 11β-hydroxysteroid dehydrogenase system that converts cortisol to cortisone (39). Large chronic doses may result in a pseudoprimary aldosteronism with symptoms that may include edema, hypertension, and hypokalemia (39,40). Cardiac arrhythmias and cardiac arrest, including two deaths, have occurred in users of licorice products. Cardiomyopathy (41), hypokalemic myopathy (42), and pulmonary edema (43) have been reported.

In Chinese medicine, licorice is always used as part of a mixture, and the synergistic effects of mixtures and perhaps dose limitations may prevent problems. All of the reported cases of licorice-induced problems were from licorice-containing candies, gum, laxatives, or chewing tobacco, not from the use of licorice as herbal medicine. (Most "licorice" candies manufactured in the United States are actually flavored with anise; imported candies usually contain real licorice.) However, licorice tinctures, extracts, capsules, and lozenges are available in the United States, and it is useful to know about possible side effects. Hypokalemia due to licorice may be potentiated by the use of diuretics, and the side effects of systemic steroids and licorice probably are additive.

Sage

Sage *(Salvia officinalis)* is reputed to help hot flushes and night sweats. It contains a volatile oil called thujone, other monoterpenes, and tannins. Thujone is toxic, and long-term use can cause seizures or other neurologic symptoms (44).

Vitex

Vitex or chaste-tree berry contains flavonoids and an alkaloid called viticin. There have been no clinical studies on vitex for menopausal symptoms; herbalists believe that it balances hormone levels. Vitex has been reputed to lower libido in women and men—hence its common names of chaste-tree berry and monk's pepper. Chaste-tree berry may have profound hormonal effects. In a double-blind, placebo-controlled trial of 52 women with luteal phase defect due to latent hyperprolactinemia, one 20-mg capsule of vitex daily reduced prolactin levels, normalized the length of luteal phases, and normalized luteal phase progesterone levels (45). Prolactin inhibition of rat pituitary cells has also been demonstrated in an *in vitro* experiment (46). A case of ovarian hyperstimulation in a premenopausal woman apparently caused by ingestion of vitex has been reported (47). It is not clear what effect vitex has on postmenopausal women.

Ginkgo

Ginkgo *(Ginkgo biloba)* is helpful in Alzheimer's disease (48–50). There is less evidence for less severe memory problems. A double-blind study of 31 patients older than 50 with mild to moderate memory impairment found a beneficial effect on some (digit copying, speed of response in a classification task) but not other tests of cognitive function (51).

A metanalysis of 40 controlled trials for cerebral insufficiency (a syndrome not accepted in the United States that includes memory and concentration problems, confusion, fatigue, depression, ringing in the ears, and headache) found that in 26 studies the group receiving ginkgo did significantly better than the control group. In 13 studies, there was a trend toward a benefit or a benefit for some but not all effect measurements. Most of the studies were deemed to be of poor methodologic quality. Of the eight well-performed trials, all showed a significant benefit for the ginkgo group (52).

Ginkgo should not be used by those with bleeding problems or who are on anticoagulants, as ginkgo inhibits platelet function; subdural hematoma and other bleeding complications have been reported, usually in patients on anticoagulant therapies (53).

St. John's Wort

The herb St. John's wort *(Hypericum perforatum)* has gained much popularity in the United States as an antidepressant. There have been many studies performed on this herb in Europe, primarily in Germany. A metanalysis evaluated 23 randomized trials (20 were double-blind studies) of St. John's wort in a total of 1,757 outpatients with mild to moderate depression (54). Improvement in depressive symptoms was observed in all groups. In 15 placebo-controlled trials, St. John's wort was found to be significantly better than placebo. In eight treatment-controlled trials, clinical improvement in those receiving St. John's wort did not differ significantly from those receiving tricyclic antidepressants (the doses of antidepressants were lower than those normally used in the United States). Side effects were reported less often with St. John's wort; 19.8% of those on St. John's wort reported symptoms, compared with 52.8% of those on tricyclic antidepressants. Gastrointestinal effects and fatigue have been reported with St. John's wort; photosensitization may be the most common effect.

Cranberry Juice

The juice of cranberries *(Vaccinia macrocarpon)* has been used as a home remedy for acidifying the urine; it also decreases bacterial adherence (55). In one study (56), 153 elderly women drank 300 mL each day of cranberry juice or of a placebo juice matched for taste, appearance, and vitamin C content. Those who drank the placebo drink had more than twice the incidence of bacteriuria and pyuria as those who drank the cranberry juice. Researchers in Israel tested a number of fruit juices

on the adhesive ability of *Escherichia coli* and found that only juices of cranberry and blueberry (both members of the *Vaccinia* genus) were beneficial (57).

OTHER COMPLEMENTARY TREATMENTS

Exercise

A Swedish survey of regular exercisers found that moderate to severe hot flushes and sweating were half as common in the exercisers compared with women in the general population (58). However, this was not a prospective study, and there may be other differences between gym members and the general population.

Relaxation and Deep Breathing

A randomized, controlled 10-week trial of relaxation response training in 33 women experiencing at least five hot flushes every 24 hours compared the treatment group with a group assigned to reading and an attention control group (59). The women in the relaxation group experienced significant reductions in hot flush intensity, tension-anxiety, and depression. The reading group experienced significant reductions in trait-anxiety and confusion-bewilderment. There were no significant changes in the control group. Deep breathing exercises that reduced respiratory rate and increase tidal volume reduced hot flush frequency by 39% from pretreatment levels (60).

Acupuncture

A study of the effects of acupuncture on hot flushes randomized 24 women to electroacupuncture (i.e., electrical stimulation of acupuncture needles inserted to the proper depth) at standardized points or to shallow acupuncture needle insertion at the same points as a control (61). Women were treated twice weekly for 2 weeks and then weekly for an additional 6 weeks. No significant differences were seen between the two groups; both groups showed a significant decrease in hot flushes and a significant benefit in the Kupperman index.

Biofeedback for Hot Flushes and Incontinence

Biofeedback techniques have been used to control hot flushes with some success. The effect was measured by skin conductance measurements (60).

Many obstetrician-gynecologists recommend Kegel exercises for patients with urinary incontinence. These exercises appear effective; a study of 50 female patients compared surgery with Kegel exercises and found that, although surgery was superior, 42% of the Kegeling patients improved enough that surgery was no longer considered necessary (62). Another study of 36 women with stress incontinence (63) found that 56% of the women who were taught Kegel exercises showed improvement on urinary flow studies and considered their stress incontinence substantially improved or cured.

Because not everyone can learn to Kegel with verbal instruction alone, Kegeling aids, such as biofeedback using various forms of vaginal balloons, may be useful. Women with stress incontinence can reduce the frequency of incontinence episodes by 80% to 90% after bladder-sphincter biofeedback (64–66). A simpler intervention uses weighted vaginal cones; a patient starts by retaining the lightest cone for a set amount of time and then gradually increases the weights (67).

A controlled study of 135 women compared pelvic Kegel exercises and biofeedback with untreated controls and found that urine losses were reduced by 54% in the Kegel group and 61% in the biofeedback group. Controls increased their urine loss by 9% (68,69). Of the 40 patients in the biofeedback group, 23% were completely cured. Of the 43 patients in the Kegel group, 16% were cured; only 3% (1) of 38 women in the control group was cured.

CONCLUSIONS

There is evidence that phytoestrogens may be helpful for menopausal symptoms, but further research needs to be done to delineate the effect of high-phytoestrogen diets on rates of cardiovascular disease, breast cancer, and osteoporosis. Although current evidence on the use of herbs for hot flushes and other menopausal symptoms is not impressive, more studies should be done to delineate benefits and risks. Because several herbs used for menopause have estrogenic effects, effects on endometrial proliferation must be studied. There is substantial evidence showing that St. John's wort is helpful in depression and that ginkgo may be helpful for memory problems. Behavioral techniques may be helpful for some women. A variety of complementary therapies deserve further research.

REFERENCES

1. Eisenberg DM, Davis RB, Ettner SL, et al. Trends in alternative medicine use in the United States, 1990–1997: results of a follow-up national survey. *JAMA* 1998; 280:1569–1575.
2. Eisenberg DM, Kessler RC, Foster C, et al. Unconventional medicine in the United States: prevalence, costs, and patterns of use. *N Engl J Med* 1993;328: 246–252.
3. Kiegler J. Soybeans show promise in cancer prevention. *J Natl Cancer Inst* 1994; 86:1666–1667.
4. Adlercreutz H, Mousavi Y, Clark J, et al. Dietary phytoestrogens and cancer: *in vitro* and *in vivo* studies. *J Steroid Biochem Mol Biol* 1992;41:331–337.
5. Horn-Ross PL, Barnes S, Kirk M, et al. Urinary phytoestrogen levels in young women from a multiethnic population. *Cancer Epidemiol Biomarkers Prev* 1997; 6:339–345.
6. Adlercreutz H, Hamalainen E, Gorbach S, Goldin B. Dietary phytoestrogens and the menopause in Japan. *Lancet* 1992;339:1233.
7. Albertazzi P, Pansini F, Bonaccorsi G, et al. The effect of dietary soy supplementation on hot flushes. *Obstet Gynecol* 1998;91:6–11.
8. Brzezinski A, Adlercreutz H, Shaoul R, et al. Short-term effects of phytoestrogen-rich diet on postmenopausal women. *Menopause* 1997;4:89–94.
9. Murkies AL, Lombard C, Strauss BJG. Dietary flour supplementation decreases postmenopausal hot flushes: effect of soy and wheat. *Maturitas* 1995;21:189–195.
10. Wilcox G, Wahlqvist ML, Burger HG, Medley G. Oestrogenic effects of plant foods in postmenopausal women. *BMJ* 1990;301:905–906.
11. Baird DD, Umbach DM, Lansdell L, et al. Dietary intervention study to assess estrogenicity of dietary soy among postmenopausal women. *J Clin Endocrinol Metab* 1995;:80:685–690.
12. Knight DC, Eden JA. A review of the clinical effect of phytoestrogens. *Obstet Gynecol* 1996;87:897–904.
13. Duncan AM, et al. Soy isoflavones exert modest effects in premenopausal women. *J Clin Endocrinol Metab* 1999;84:192–197.
14. Lu L-JW, Anderson KE, Grady JJ, Nagamani M. Effects of soya consumption for one month on steroid hormones in premenopausal women: implications for breast cancer risk reduction. *Cancer Epidemiol Biomarkers Prev* 1996;5:63–70.
15. Cassidy A, Bingham S, Setchell KDR. Biological effects of a diet of soy protein rich in isoflavones on the menstrual cycle of premenopausal women. *Am J Clin Nutr* 1994;60:333–340.
16. Adlercreutz H, Honjo H, Higashi A, et al. Urinary excretion of lignans and isoflavonoid phytoestrogens in Japanese men and women consuming a traditional Japanese diet. *Am J Clin Nutr* 1991;54:1093–1100.
17. Lee HP, Gourley L, Duffy SW, et al. Dietary effects on breast cancer risk in Singapore. *Lancet* 1991;337:1197–1200.
18. Brzezinski A, Adlercreutz H, Shaoul R, et al. Short-term effects of phytoestrogen-rich diet on postmenopausal women. *Menopause* 1997;4:89–94.
19. Mousavi Y, Adlercreutz H. Enterolactone and estradiol inhibit each other's proliferative effect on MCF-7 breast cancer cells in culture. *J Steroid Biochem Biol* 1992;41:615–619.
20. Hawrylewicz EJ, Zapat JJ, Blair WH. Soy and experimental cancer: animal studies. *J Nutr* 1995;125(Suppl 3):698S–708S.
21. Helferich WG. Paradoxical effects of the soy phytoestrogen genistein on growth of human breast cancer cells *in vitro* and *in vivo*. *Am J Clin Nutr* 1009;68[Suppl]: 1524S(abst).
22. Goodman MT, Wilkems LR, Hankin JH, et al. Association of soy and fiber consumption with the risk of endometrial cancer. *Am J Epidemiol* 1997;146:294–306.
23. Anderson JW, Johnstone BM, Cook-Newell ME. Meta-analysis of the effects of soy protein intake on serum lipids. *N Engl J Med* 1995;33:276–282.
24. Clarkson TB, Anthony MS, Williams JK, et al. The potential for soybean phytoestrogens for postmenopausal hormone replacement therapy. *Proc Soc Exp Biol Med* 1998;217:365–368.
25. Potter SM, Baum JA, Teng H, et al. Soy protein and isoflavones: their effects on blood lipids and bone density in postmenopausal women. *Am J Clin Nutr* 1998; 68[Suppl 6]:1375S–1379S.
26. Newall CA, Anderson LA, Phillipson JD. *Herbal medicines:* a guide for health care professionals. London: Pharmaceutical Press, 1996.
27. Beuscher N. *Cimicifuga racemosa*. *Z Phytoter* 1995;16:301–310. [Translated in *Q Rev Nat Med* 1996;Spring:19–27.]
28. Duker E-M, Kopanski L, Jarry H, Wuttke W. Effects of extracts from Cimicifuga racemosa on gonadotropin release in menopausal women and ovariectomized rats. *Planta Med* 1991;57:420–424.
29. Hirata JD, Ettinger B, Small R, et al. Does dong quai have estrogenic effects in postmenopausal women? A double-blind, placebo-controlled trial. *Fertil Steril* 1997;68:981–986.
30. Chenoy R, Hussain S, Tayob Y, et al. Effect of oral gamolenic acid from evening primrose oil on menopausal flushing. *BMJ* 1994;308:501–503.
31. Warnecke G, Pfaender H, Gerster G, Gracza E. Wirksamkeit von Kava-Kava-Extrakt beim klimakterischen Syndrom. *Z Phytoter* 1990;11:81–86.
32. Warnecke G. Psychosomatic dysfunctions in the female climacteric: clinical effectiveness and tolerance of kava extract [WS 1490]. *Fortschr Med* 1991;109: 119–122.
33. Norton SA, Ruze P. Kava dermapathy. *J Am Acad Dermatol* 1994;31:89–97.
34. Greenspan EM. Ginseng and vaginal bleeding. *JAMA* 1983;249:2018.
35. Punnonen R, Lukola A. Oestrogen-like effect of ginseng. *Br Med J* 1980;281: 1110.
36. Hopkins MO, Androff L, Benninghoff AS. Ginseng face cream and unexplained vaginal bleeding. *Am J Obstet Gynecol* 1988;159:1121–1122.
37. Palmer BV, Montgomery ACV, Monteiro JCMP. Ginseng and mastalgia. *Br Med J* 1978;1:1284.
38. Koriech OM. Ginseng and mastalgia. *Br Med J* 1978;1:1556.
39. Farese RV, Biglieri EG, Shackleton CHL, et al. Licorice-induced hypermineralocorticoidism. *N Engl J Med* 1991;325:1223–1227.
40. Epstein MT, Espiner EA, Donald RA, Hughes H. Effect of eating licorice on the renin-angiotensin aldosterone axis in normal subjects. *Br Med J* 1977;1:488–490.
41. Chandler RF. Glycyrrhiza glabra. In: De Smet PAGM, Keller K, Hansel R, Chandler RF, eds. *Adverse effects of herbal drugs*. Berlin: Springer-Verlag, 1997.
42. Shintani S, Murase H, Tsukagoshi H, Shiigai T. *Glycyrrhizin* (licorice)-induced hypokalemic myopathy. *Eur Neurol* 1992;32:44–51.
43. Chamberlain JJ, Abolnik IZ. Pulmonary edema following a licorice binge. *West J Med* 1997;167:184–185.
44. Wichtl M. *Herbal drugs and phytopharmaceuticals*. Stuttgart: Medpharm Scientific Publishers, 1994.
45. Milewicz A, Gejdel E, Sworen H, et al. *Vitex agnus-castus* extrakt zur Behandlung von Regeltempoanomalien infolge latenter Hyperrolaktinamie. *Arzneimittelforschung* 1993;43:752–756.
46. Sliutz G, Speiser P, Schultz AM, et al. Agnus castus extracts inhibit prolactin secretion of rat pituitary cells. *Horm Metab Res* 1993;25:253–255.

47. Cahill DJ, Fox R, Wardle PG, Harlow CR. Multiple follicular development associated with herbal medicine. *Hum Reprod* 1994;9:1469–1470.
48. Le Bars PL, Katz MM, Berman N, Itil TM, Freedman AM, Schatzberg AF. A placebo-controlled, double-blind, randomized trial of an extract of *Ginkgo biloba* for dementia. *JAMA* 1997;278:1327–1332.
49. Kanowski S, Herrmann WM, Stephan K, et al. Proof of efficacy of *Ginkgo biloba* special extract Egb 761 in outpatient suffering from mild to moderate primary degenerative dementia of the Alzheimer type or multi-infarct dementia. *Pharmacopsychiatry* 1996;29:47–56.
50. Hofferberth B. The efficacy of Egb 761 in patients with senile dementia of the Alzheimer type: a double-blind, placebo-controlled study on different levels of investigation. *Hum Psychopharmacol* 1994;9:215–222.
51. Rai GS, Shovlin C, Wesnes KA. A double-blind, placebo-controlled study of *Ginkgo biloba* extract (Tanakan) in elderly outpatients with mild to moderate memory impairment. *Curr Med Res Opin* 1991;12:350–355.
52. Kleijnen J, Knipschild P. Ginkgo biloba for cerebral insufficiency. *Br J Clin Pharmacol* 1992;34:352–358.
53. *Ginkgo biloba* for dementia. *Med Lett* 1998;40:63–64.
54. Linde K, Ramirez G, Mulrow CD, et al. St John's wort for depression—an overview and meta-analysis of randomized clinical trials. *BMJ* 1996; 313: 253–358.
55. Sobota AE. Inhibition of bacterial adherence by cranberry juice: potential use for the treatment of urinary tract infections. *J Urol* 1984;131:1013–1016.
56. Avorn J, Monane M, Gurwitz JH. Reduction of bacteriuria and pyuria after ingestion of cranberry juice. *JAMA* 1994;271:751–754.
57. Ofek I, Goldhar J, Zafriri D, et al. Anti-*Escherichia coli* adhesion activity of cranberry and blueberry juices. *N Engl J Med* 1991;324:1599.
58. Hammar M, Berg G, Lindgren R. Does physical exercise influence the frequency of postmenopausal hot flushes? *Acta Obstet Gynecol Scand* 1990;69:409–412.
59. Irvin JH, Friedman R, Zuttermeister PC, et al. The effect of relaxation response training on menopausal symptoms. *J Psychosom Obstet Gynecol* 1996;17: 201–207.
60. Freedman RR, Woodward S. Behavioral treatment of menopausal hot flushes: evaluation by ambulatory monitoring. *Am J Obstet Gynecol* 1992;167:436–439.
61. Wyon Y, Lindgren R, Lundeberg T, Hammar M. Effects of acupuncture on climacteric vasomotor symptoms, quality of life, and urinary excretion of neuropeptides among postmenopausal women. *Menopause* 1995;2:3–12.
62. Klarskov P, Belving D, Bischoff N, et al. Pelvic floor exercise versus surgery for female urinary stress incontinence. *Urol Int* 1986;41:129–132.
63. Elia G, Bergman A. Pelvic muscle exercises: when do they work? *Obstet Gynecol* 1993;81:283–286.
64. Burgio KL, Whitehead WE, Engel BT. Urinary incontinence in the elderly. *Ann Intern Med* 1985;104:507.
65. Cardozo LD, Abrams PD, Stanton SL, et al. Idiopathic bladder instability treated by biofeedback. *Br J Urol* 1978;50:521.
66. Shepherd AM, Montgomery E. Treatment of genuine stress incontinence with a new perineometer. *Physiotherapy* 1983;69:113.
67. Brubaker L, Kotarinos R. Kegel or cut? Variations on his theme. *J Reprod Med* 1993;38:672–678.
68. Burns PA, Pranikoff K, Nochajski T, et al. Treatment of stress incontinence with pelvic floor exercises. *J Am Geriatr Soc* 1990;38:341–344.
69. Burns PA, Pranikoff K, Nochajski TH, et al. A comparison of effectiveness of biofeedback and pelvic muscle exercise treatment of stress incontinence in older community-dwelling women. *J Gerontol* 1993;48:M167–M174.

Neoplasia

Whenever we contemplate treatment options, we have to consider risks. Neoplasia is the risk most women worry about. This section details the major reproductive cancers women worry about, namely breast, uterine and ovarian cancers. Not covered here is lung cancer, the leading cause of cancer death in women, and colon cancer. These will be discussed in the following section on "Risk-Benefit Assessment" (Chapter 50).

In the first chapter, Darcy Spicer and Malcolm Pike outline the epidemiology of reproductive cancers. Following this John Park, Malcolm Pike, Jinha Park, and Michael Press provide the basic science background to understand breast proliferation. Some of the intricacies of estrogen action are presented including the influence of ERα, ERß , signal transduction and growth factors. In these two chapters and the next, they note that progesterone enhanced breast proliferation while inhibiting estrogen-induced proliferation in the endometrium. This topic remains controversial. In the chapter by Ron Ross and Leslie Bernstein, they estimate that the risk of estrogen in the development of breast cancer is estimated to be about 1% to 3% per year of use. They concede, however, that there is no definitive answer because the overall risk is not great, and is likely to be about 20% to 30%. They stress confounding variables and that these contribute to the difficulty in getting definitive information. One variable, which has been believed to increase the risk of the association between estrogen and breast cancer, is alcohol consumption. They have not addressed the presumed reduced risk of lower doses because of the paucity of data. Surveillance for neoplasia is key to the health care of postmenopausal women, and Bill Hindle, who runs a large clinic for breast problems, has updated the topic of breast surveillance.

Endometrial cancer is first addressed by John Collins and Jim Schlesselman, who provide valuable information concerning epidemiology and the effects of estrogen and progestogens. Anna Parsons and Jorge Londono discuss surveillance of the endometrium comprehensively. Ultrasound has been an extremely valuable tool for this purpose. Following this, Richard Jaffe discusses ovarian surveillance by ultrasound. The last chapter in this section is a discussion of screening for ovarian cancer by Thomas Randall and Stephen Rubin. They also cover the controversial issue of the BRCA1 and BRCA2 mutations.

An issue which women frequently wish to discuss is whether they may receive hormones if they have been treated for uterine or breast cancer. Some of this discussion will be found in the next section on "Risk-Benefit Assessment" (Chapter 52). For uterine cancer the answer is more straightforward. Women with well-differentiated endometrial cancer who have received complete treatment may receive estrogen under close follow-up. For breast cancer survivors there are no good data. In spite of the theoretical cancer-promoting effect of estrogen, the existing "trials" have not shown a higher rate of recurrence among estrogen users. Although it is much preferred to use non-hormonal treatments for symptomatic complaints these options may not be sufficient for some women. Ingestion of large quantities of plant-based phytoestrogens should be viewed as the same as giving estrogen as phytoestrogens bind to ERß with reasonably good affinity. In women treated with early stage breast cancer who request and wish to use hormones after having tried non-hormonal remedies, a consensus view is that it may be considered. At the recent Boar's Head conference, the following statement was offered:

> In women who have had an established diagnosis of breast cancer, we should seek other established symptomatic or health-promoting interventions before considering the use of estrogens. When estrogen is used as a last resort, it should be used in the lowest dose for the shortest duration of time and only after full discussion of concerns regarding potential risks with respect to breast cancer outcomes. When estrogen is being considered, the role of the informed woman as the final decision-maker should be accepted by the healthcare practitioner.

REFERENCE

Santen R, Pritchard K, Burger H. The consensus Conference on Treatment of Estrogen Deficiency Symptoms in Women Surviving Breast Cancer. Obstet Gynecol Surv [Suppl no. 10] 1998; S1-83.

Treatment of the Postmenopausal Woman: Basic and Clinical Aspects, Second Edition, edited by Rogerio A. Lobo, Lippincott Williams & Wilkins, Philadelphia © 1999.

CHAPTER 42

Epidemiology of Cancer in the Female

Darcy V. Spicer and Malcolm C. Pike

The incidence of the common non–hormone-dependent adult cancers (e.g., colon, lung, stomach) rise continuously and progressively with age, and increasing age is the biggest risk factor for these cancers. For the purpose of understanding the cause of these cancers, it is useful to plot the age-incidence curve on a log-log scale. Such a log-log plot produces a straight line; female colorectal cancer incidence (1) plotted in this way is shown in Fig. 42.1*A*. The data are plotted on arithmetic scales in Fig. 42.1*B*.

Figure 42.2*A* shows the log-log age-incidence curves for breast cancer, endometrial cancer, and ovarian cancer, the three female cancers discussed in this chapter. The incidences of all three cancers continue to increase with age, but in contrast to the common non–hormone-dependent cancers, there is a distinct slowing of the rate of increase around the age of 50 (i.e., around the age at menopause). The important etiologic elements for these cancers appear to be present in premenopausal women and to be sharply reduced after menopause. This is possibly the most important epidemiologic fact known about these cancers. The contrast between the age-incidence curves of these three female cancers and the common non–hormone-dependent cancers is not so clear when the female cancer curves are plotted on arithmetic scales (Fig. 42.2*B*). It is also not clear that the profound change that occurs around age 50 continues from that age on. For purposes of understanding the causes of female cancers, plotting age-incidence curves on a log-log basis is preferred.

The age-incidence curves shown in Figs. 42.1 and 42.2 are from the Birmingham Region Cancer Registry in the United Kingdom for 1968 through 1972; the reason for choosing these figures rather than some U.S. data is that U.S. age-incidence curves are distorted by the high rates

of hysterectomy and oophorectomy in the United States. Because cancer rates are computed on a per-person basis rather than on an organ-at-risk basis, hysterectomy distorts the age-incidence curve for endometrial cancer by artificially lowering the rates from about age 40, and oophorectomy similarly distorts the age-incidence curve for ovarian cancer. Oophorectomy also distorts the age-

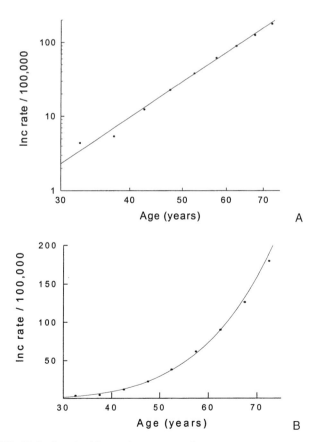

FIG. 42.1. Age-incidence (per 100,000) curves for colorectal cancer in women the Birmingham region of the United Kingdom from 1968 through 1972 (1) are given as a log-log plot **(A)** and an arithmetic-arithmetic plot **(B)**.

D. V. Spicer: Department of Medicine, University of Southern California School of Medicine, Los Angeles, California 90089.

M. C. Pike: Department of Preventative Medicine, University of Southern California School of Medicine, Los Angeles, California 90089.

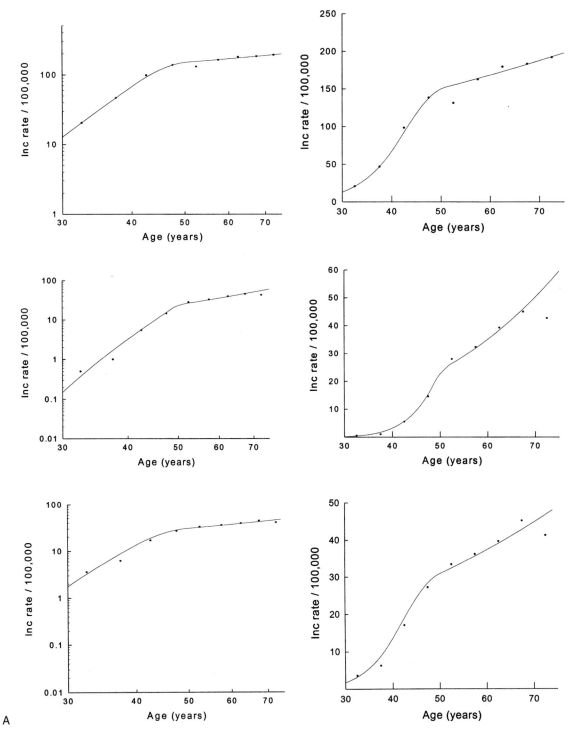

FIG. 42.2. A: Log-log plot of age-incidence (per 100,000) curves for women in the Birmingham region of the United Kingdom from 1968 through 1972 (1) for breast cancer (top), endometrial cancer (middle), and ovarian cancer (bottom). **B:** Arithmetic-arithmetic plot of age-incidence (per 100,000 women) curves for women in the Birmingham region of the United Kingdom from 1968 through 1972 (1) for breast cancer (top), endometrial cancer (middle), and ovarian cancer (bottom).

incidence curve for breast cancer, because early oophorectomy (like early natural menopause) significantly reduces the risk of breast cancer. Moreover, these U.K. figures are only affected to a minor extent by any effect of hormone replacement therapy (HRT) on cancer rates, because HRT was still uncommon in the United Kingdom at that time. The 1970 U.K. breast cancer rates are also not inflated by mammographic screening to any significant extent. Later breast cancer rates in the United Kingdom and in the United States are greatly affected by the mammographic detection of early invasive tumors and carcinoma *in situ* of the breast (which is not recorded by cancer registries as breast cancer), which severely distorts the age-incidence curves at postmenopausal ages.

CELL PROLIFERATION AND CARCINOGENESIS

Studies of chemical carcinogenesis have identified a large group of substances that induce cancer in animal bioassays but are not genotoxic (2–4). Many of these nongenotoxic carcinogens appear to act solely by increasing cell proliferation. Cellular DNA is subject to damage from a variety of sources with great frequency, but such damage is generally rapidly repaired. If, however, DNA replication and cell division occur before repair, the damage may be converted into a stable genetic error (e.g., oncogene activation). An agent that increases (decreases) mitotic activity increases (decreases) the probability of converting DNA damage (exogenously and endogenously induced) into mutations. More profound DNA changes, including nondisjunction, gene conversions, and reduction to homozygosity of tumor suppressor genes, also require cell division and occur with increased (decreased) frequency with increased (decreased) cell division. These carcinogenic effects of mitotic activity depend on the rate and the duration of the mitotic activity.

The natural ovarian hormones, estrogen and progesterone, and the hormones used in HRT and hormonal contraceptives profoundly affect breast and endometrial epithelial cell division rates, and their effects on breast and endometrial cancer rates are in large part explicable in these terms. The situation is not as clear for cancer of the ovary, in which epithelial cell division rates are significantly affected by ovulation. There is, however, evidence that ovarian hormones and gonadotropins affect ovarian epithelial cell division rates, and the epidemiology of ovarian cancer is also in large part explicable in terms of ovarian epithelial cell proliferation effects.

Because the carcinogenic effects of cell division are rate and duration dependent, the effects of endogenous and exogenous hormones need to be discussed in the context of dose and duration and, in particular, considerations of the effects ever-never use of particular exogenous hormones are of little value.

EPITHELIAL CELL PROLIFERATION
Breast

Breast epithelial cell mitotic rates have been studied in normal breast tissue removed at mastectomy, biopsy, reduction mammoplasty, and forensic autopsy (Chapter 43). The epithelial cells of the terminal duct lobular unit (TDLU), from which most breast cancers arise undergo significant changes during the menstrual cycle. TDLU cell proliferation is lowest during the follicular phase and then increases some twofold during the luteal phase. Estradiol (the most important endogenous estrogen) and progesterone are both breast cell mitogens. Estradiol alone induces breast epithelial cell division, and combined estradiol and progesterone further increase cell division, supporting the estrogen-progestin hypothesis of breast cancer. In the postmenopausal period, when estrogen levels are low and progesterone is effectively absent, TDLU cell proliferation is very low.

The estrogen-progestin hypothesis for breast cancer provides a most satisfactory explanation of almost all epidemiologic observations on the disease. However, it does not provide an explanation of the protection afforded by an early first pregnancy, and finding the basis of this protective effect warrants a major research effort, because it holds the promise of a one-time intervention with long-term consequences.

Endometrium

Estrogen stimulates endometrial epithelial cell division but only in the absence of significant progestin. The endometrial cell proliferation hypothesis for endometrial cancer is also known as the unopposed estrogen hypothesis for endometrial cancer. During a normal menstrual cycle, endometrial cell mitotic activity peaks during the early follicular phase (5), when unopposed serum estradiol levels are approximately 50 pg/mL; further increases in unopposed estradiol concentrations do not appear to increase the mitotic rate. After ovulation, the serum progesterone level steadily rises to peak about 7 days later, and endometrial cell proliferation ceases despite continued elevated levels of estradiol. At low serum concentrations of unopposed estradiol (5 pg/mL), such as those occurring in slender postmenopausal women, endometrial cell mitotic activity is very low. There is a clear dose-response relationship between endometrial cell mitotic rate and unopposed estradiol concentrations, somewhere in the range of 5 to 50 pg/mL.

The unopposed estrogen hypothesis provides a most satisfactory explanation of almost all epidemiologic observations on the disease, but it fails to provide a satisfactory explanation of some observations on endometrial cancer risk associated with estrogen-progestin replacement therapy. These observations suggest that it is not just the period of unopposed estrogen that is etiologically important, but also possibly the extent of change brought about in the endometrium by any progestin administered after a period of unopposed estrogen and the subsequent extent of endometrial sloughing.

Ovary

Ovarian (epithelial) cancers are considered by most investigators to arise from the ovarian surface epithelium and from the epithelium of ovarian epithelial inclusions (6). Fathalla (7) proposed that ovarian cancer risk is essentially determined by the increased mitotic activity of the ovarian surface epithelium required to accomplish repair of the surface after each ovulation (i.e., incessant ovulation hypothesis for ovarian cancer). A simple incessant ovulation hypothesis does not, however, provide a satisfactory explanation for the observation that most early-stage ovarian cancers are found within the ovary rather than on its surface (6). To account for this observation, ovarian cancers are thought to arise principally from ovarian epithelial inclusions rather than directly from the ovarian surface epithelium. The incessant ovulation theory can, however, accommodate this by arguing that ovarian epithelium inclusions are formed during the repair of the ovarian surface after ovulation and that the extent of such inclusions strongly correlates with ovulation frequency. There is some evidence for this sequence of events in that the number of inclusions increases with age (8).

The incessant ovulation hypothesis provides a most satisfactory explanation of the reduction in ovarian cancer risk with increasing parity and duration of oral contraceptive use, which are important ovarian cancer risk factors. It cannot explain the continued, although slower, increase in the incidence of ovarian cancer after menopause or the much reduced incidence rates of ovarian cancer found, until recently, in low-risk Asian countries.

Stadel (9) and subsequently Cramer and Welch (10) proposed that elevated gonadotrophin levels increased ovarian cancer risk. The much slower rate of increase in ovarian cancer in the postmenopausal period despite the high levels of gonadotropins postmenopausally appear to argue against this (11), but it may be that gonadotropins need to be released in an episodic fashion (as in the premenopausal but not the postmenopausal period) to have a large effect (12). An indirect effect of gonadotrophin levels is possible by mean of increasing intraovarian estrogen levels (13) exerting paracrine mitogenic effects on the ovarian epithelium (14). The apparent lack of or extremely low level of estrogen receptors in normal ovarian surface epithelium and ovarian epithelial inclusions argues against the latter suggestion, but intraovarian estradiol levels are so high that even very low levels of receptors may be sufficient; it is also possible that the cell of origin of ovarian cancer is not ovarian surface epithe-

lium but müllerian remnants in the ovary, as argued by Dubeau (15).

Estradiol and follicle-stimulating hormone (FSH) have been demonstrated to be mitogenic in two ovarian cancer cell lines (14) and in cell lines established from benign ovarian epithelial tumors (12). These cell lines express gonadotropin receptors and estrogen receptors. These experiments also provide some preliminary evidence that progesterone and possibly luteinizing hormone (LH) may block the estradiol and FSH effects, respectively. The evidence implicating specific gonadotropins and sex steroids (including ovarian androgens) remains unclear (16); more innovative clinical and experimental approaches are needed to elucidate these effects.

EPIDEMIOLOGIC RISK FACTORS

Breast Cancer

The key epidemiologic observations on breast cancer risk (17,18) are discussed in this section, with an explanation of the risk in terms of the estrogen-progestin hypothesis.

Menopause

The age-incidence correlation for breast cancer increases at a much slower rate in the postmenopausal period than in the premenopausal period. In the postmenopausal period, the increase in risk is sharply reduced by the sharp drop in the levels of estradiol and progesterone to which postmenopausal women are exposed.

Menarche

Early menarche increases breast cancer risk. For a given age at menarche, the sooner regular menstruation is established, the greater the breast cancer risk is. Early menarche increases risk by increasing the length of time the breasts are exposed to high levels of estradiol and progesterone. Early onset of regular cycles accentuates this.

Obesity

Postmenopausal obesity increases breast cancer risk, but premenopausal obesity may slightly decrease breast cancer risk. These contrasting effects are readily explained. The low progesterone levels and increased anovulation associated with premenopausal obesity decrease breast exposure to estradiol and progesterone. After menopause, the decreased risk associated with premenopausal obesity is gradually eliminated, and an increased risk is observed at older ages because of the increased levels of bioavailable estradiol associated with postmenopausal obesity.

Hormone Replacement Therapy

The estrogen-progestin hypothesis predicts that menopausal estrogen replacement therapy (ERT) increases breast cancer risk and that the addition of a progestin further increases the risk. ERT has been found to increase risk about 2.1% per year of use (19). There are sparse data on the effects of menopausal estrogen-progestin therapy (EPRT) on breast cancer risk. The available data suggest that the breast cancer risk from EPRT use is greater than that associated with ERT use (19). Further evidence suggesting that EPRT is associated with a greater breast cancer risk than ERT is provided by the finding of a much greater increase in mammographic densities in postmenopausal women taking EPRT than in women taking ERT in the randomized Postmenopausal Estrogen/Progestin Interventions (PEPI) trial (20). These mammography results suggest that the effect of EPRT may be as much as threefold greater than the effect of ERT.

Hormonal Contraceptive Use

Oral contraceptive (OC) use slightly increases breast cancer risk in young women, but the effect does not extend to older ages (21). Direct observational studies of breast cell proliferation in women taking OCs have been made by two groups of investigators (Chapter 43), and these studies suggest that the total breast cell proliferation is similar over an OC cycle and a normal menstrual cycle. These results predict that breast cancer risk should not be substantially affected by OC use. This is effectively what is observed. Issues that need further consideration include the possibility that the effects of early OC use are modified by a subsequent pregnancy.

The epidemiologic finding of no reduction in breast cancer risk with use of Depo-Provera (DMPA) also provides support for the estrogen-progestin hypothesis and adds to the evidence suggesting that the risk from EPRT is greater than that from ERT. DMPA is a 3-month injectable progestin contraceptive that suppresses ovulation and estradiol levels on average by 20% below the normal early follicular phase level (22.23). If progestin was protective or irrelevant to breast cancer risk, use of DMPA should have been associated with a decrease in breast cancer risk; the fact that it was not is evidence of a mitogenic effect of the progestin on breast cells.

Other Risk Factors

Late first full-term pregnancy (FFTP) is associated with increased breast cancer risk. MacMahon et al. (24), in a large international study, found that women younger than 20 years of age with a FFTP have about one-half the risk of nulliparous women but that nulliparous women did not have as high a risk as women whose FFTP was after age 35. Further studies showed that early FFTP is associated with a decreased risk but only after about age 40, and increasing parity causes further small decreases in risk. At younger ages, the risk of developing breast cancer is lower in nulliparous than in parous women. These complex effects of first birth and parity are not immediately explicable in terms of their effects on breast cell proliferation. Animal models suggest that the effects are a combination of increased cell division during pregnancy and the counteracting effect of a long-term decrease in the number of stem cells brought about by breast stem cell differentiation during pregnancy (25). A mathematical model of these ideas provides an excellent quantitative fit to the observed epidemiologic data (26,27).

International Variation

There is a large international variation in breast cancer rates (28). This variation has decreased over time because of large increases in rates during the past 30 years in countries with previously low rates. Breast cancer rates in migrants from low-risk countries tend toward the rates in their adopted country with time (29). Until recently, breast cancer rates in the United States were some fourfold to sixfold greater than the breast cancer rates in Japan. Late menarche (some 2 years later in Japan) and low postmenopausal weight (approximately 17 kg lower in Japan [30]) explain about one half of the difference in rates (26). The remaining difference can be explained by the approximately 25% lower premenopausal ovarian estrogen and progesterone levels of traditional Asian women (31–33).

Endometrial Cancer

The key epidemiologic observations on endometrial cancer risk (34,35) are discussed in this section with an explanation of the risk in terms of the unopposed estrogen hypothesis.

Menopause

The age-incidence correlation of endometrial cancer increases at a much slower rate in the postmenopausal period than in the premenopausal period. In the postmenopausal period, the increase in risk is sharply reduced by the sharp drop in serum estrogen. In postmenopausal women, serum estradiol levels are a small fraction (10% to 20%) of premenopausal levels. This reduction in estrogen exposure is so large that it results in much less exposure of the endometrium to unopposed estrogen, despite the fact that the estrogen is continuous with no premenopausal luteal phase break and with high progesterone levels. The effect is most clear in slender women in whom serum estradiol is particularly low and serum sex hormone–binding globulin (SHBG) levels are high.

The steep rise in endometrial cancer incidence with age in the premenopausal period occurs in all countries, including those where obesity is uncommon. It appears therefore that luteal phase high progesterone levels are not of sufficient duration to negate the increased endometrial cancer risk from the unopposed estrogen stimulation of the earlier part of the cycle.

Menarche

Early menarche increases endometrial cancer risk. Early menarche increases risk by increasing the length of time the endometrium is exposed to high (follicular phase) levels of unopposed estradiol, and luteal phase progesterone does not eliminate this risk.

Obesity

Obesity increases endometrial cancer risk at all ages. The increased anovulation associated with premenopausal obesity increases endometrial exposure to unopposed estrogen at follicular phase levels, which causes near maximal stimulation of the endometrium. In obese postmenopausal women, serum estrogen is greatly increased through increased peripheral conversion of adrenal androgens to estrogens, and serum SHBG is decreased, so that there is a significant increase in unopposed bioavailable (non-SHBG bound) and free estrogen within the dose-response range. Serum estrogen levels increase, and SHBG levels decrease steadily with increasing weight in the postmenopausal period. Increasing weight strongly correlates with increasing endometrial cancer risk in postmenopausal women over the complete weight range.

Parity

Increasing parity decreases endometrial cancer risk. During pregnancy, there is no unopposed estrogen.

Oral Contraceptive Use

OC use decreases endometrial cancer risk by approximately 11.7% per year of use (36). Endometrial cell proliferation is decreased in women using OCs, because OCs contain, in addition to estrogen, a high-dose progestin, and endometrial cells are exposed to unopposed estrogen only during the 7 days in 28 during which the OC is not taken. Endogenous estrogen levels during these 7 days remain quite low. The slope of the age-incidence curve is much reduced during the time of OC use and then increases again after OC use is stopped (37). The protective effect should be lifelong.

Hormone Replacement Therapy

Menopausal unopposed ERT substantially increases endometrial cancer risk. In early studies, some cases of endometrial hyperplasia may have been diagnosed as endometrial cancer, which would have led to inflated estimates of the risk of ERT, but results of a study in which misclassified hyperplasia was not a significant problem showed that the incidence of the disease is increased 2.17-fold with 5 years of ERT use (38). Unopposed ERT, as is commonly prescribed, contains sufficient estrogen to cause endometrial cell proliferation (39) of a sufficient magnitude to account for the observed risk.

To counteract this endometrial cancer risk, progestins were added to ERT for 5 to 15 days per month (i.e., sequential estrogen-progestin replacement therapy [SEPRT]), and subsequently continuous combined replacement therapy (CCRT) regimens were developed in which estrogen and a lower dose of progestin are always taken together. There have been a few studies of the endometrial cancer risks associated with SEPRT, but only one study of the effect of CCRT (38). As expected, CCRT use was not associated with any increased risk of endometrial cancer. For SEPRT-short progestin (SEPRT-SP) with the progestin given for less than 10 days (effectively 7 days) per month, the risk was increased 1.87-fold with 5 years of use, 26% less than the added risk associated with ERT but still a significant increase. For SEPRT-long progestin (SEPRT-LP) with the progestin given for 10 days or more (effectively 10 days) per month, the endometrial cancer risk was increased only 1.07-fold with 5 years of use (not significantly different from no increase and no different from the risk associated with CCRT).

Medroxyprogesterone acetate (MPA) at doses between 5 and 10 mg per day (the usual doses of MPA used as progestin in SEPRT) reduces ERT-induced cell proliferation to effectively zero within 6 days (40). This abolition of cell proliferation and the observation that 7 is the number of days that the level of progesterone is above 5 ng/mL in the normal menstrual cycle (41) persuaded many gynecologists that 7 days of progestin was sufficient to abolish any risk. However, progestin use for 7 days does not completely remove the risk of hyperplasia. Paterson et al. (42) found with ERT given for 21 days per 28-day cycle that the incidence of hyperplasia was 21.0 (per 1,000 woman-months), declining to 4.0 when a progestin was used for the last 5 to 7 days, to 1.3 when used for 10 days, and to 0 when used for 13 days. This effect may be caused by the considerable between-individual variability of uptake and metabolism of MPA (40) and may reflect the fact more than 6 days of progestin treatment are needed to change the morphology of the endometrial cells to a secretory pattern (43), although why this should be important is not clear.

If endometrial cell proliferation in the basalis (stem cell) layer was the key to increased risk from ERT, there would still be an increased risk, even with 10 days of progestin, because there would still be unopposed estrogen for 2 weeks per treatment cycle. If the protection from progestin use is solely caused by the reduction in endometrial cell proliferation, the effects on endometrial cancer can be estimated on the basis of a mathematical model of endometrial cancer (27). In a standard regimen with conjugated estrogen given for 25 days in a 28-day cycle, the total cell proliferation is reduced by about 16% with 7 days of progestin and by 28% with 10 days, based on the time taken by progestin to reduce endometrial cell proliferation to zero. These translate into reductions in the added endometrial cancer risk from ERT of 24% and 40% (the figures given in Pike et al. [38] are incorrect). The figure for 7 days of progestin use agrees completely with the observed reduction in risk. The predicted reduction with SEPRT for 10 days is much less than that observed.

If the protection is caused by the reduction in hyperplasia, the risk of ERT compared with SEPRT may be estimated from the reduction in the incidence of hyperplasia according to the number of days of progestin. Paterson et al. (42) found an 81% reduction in hyperplasia between ERT and SEPRT-SP and a 94% to 100% reduction with SEPRT-LP. We found a much smaller reduction in the risk of endometrial cancer between SEPRT-SP and ERT than these results would suggest.

Flowers et al. (41) found that SEPRT-SP did not cause all the endometrium to desquamate to the basalis layer: "[only] 40% to 50% of the functional layer . . . was lost." If these functionalis cells are susceptible to cancer, and a greater proportion of such cells are lost with longer progestin therapy, this could provide an explanation for the sharp distinction between SEPRT-SP and SEPRT-LP (and between the normal menstrual cycle and SEPRT-LP). It would also be consistent with the observation of pathologists that early stage endometrial tumors often appear to have arisen in the functionalis. This possibility can be studied directly and may lead to a deeper understanding of the origin of endometrial cancer and help to predict the effects of proposed SEPRT regimens in which progestin is added for 13 days every 3 months (44). This latter regimen is important because it would be predicted to have much less of an effect on breast cancer risk than the current SEPRT-LP regimen.

International Variation

International variations in endometrial cancer rates are difficult to interpret because of marked variation between countries and within a country over time in the incidence of and mortality from malignant neoplasms of the uterus (part unspecified). This issue is discussed at length by Mant and Vessey (45). Estimated endometrial cancer rates for women between the ages of 45 and 54 in the United States were some 10-fold greater than the endometrial cancer rates in Japan around 1970, despite the high hysterectomy rates in the United States, and the difference became greater with increasing age. Tradi-

tional Japanese women's late menarche (about 2 years later in Japan than in the United States) and low premenopausal and postmenopausal weight (approximately 17 kg lower in Japan) are major factors explaining these large difference in rates, and by 1970, ERT had become a major factor in the incidence of endometrial cancer in the United States (30).

Ovarian Cancer

The key epidemiologic observations on ovarian cancer risk (45,46) are discussed in this section with an explanation of the risk in terms of the incessant ovulation hypothesis and the possible mitogenic effects of FSH and estradiol and antimitogenic effects of LH and progesterone.

Menopause

The age-incidence correlation for ovarian cancer increases at a much slower rate in the postmenopausal period than in the premenopausal period. In the postmenopausal period, the increase in risk is reduced by the cessation of ovarian surface repair after ovulation and possibly by the sharply reduced intraovarian (paracrine) estradiol levels and the cessation of pulsatile gonadotropin release.

Menarche

Early menarche increases ovarian cancer risk. Early menarche increases risk by increasing the length of time the ovarian epithelium is exposed to repair after ovulation and possibly exposed to high levels of paracrine estradiol and episodic FSH.

Obesity

The results of epidemiologic studies have been inconsistent regarding the effect of weight on ovarian cancer risk; the effect, if any, is likely to be small. Postmenopausal obesity is associated with higher levels of bioavailable serum estrogen levels, but these levels are low compared with intraovarian estrogen levels in premenopausal women. At premenopausal ages, obesity is associated with an increase in anovulation frequency and, according to the incessant ovulation hypothesis, should be associated with an increase in risk. Further epidemiologic data that clearly characterizes premenopausal weight may be useful in this regard.

Parity

Increasing parity decreases ovarian cancer risk. The effect is larger with the first birth than with subsequent births. Pregnancy decreases risk by decreasing the length of time the ovarian epithelium is exposed to repair after ovulation and possibly to much decreased levels of paracrine estradiol and of episodic FSH. The high levels of progesterone during pregnancy may also be protective. The first pregnancy may be more protective, because the nulliparous women group contain a subgroup of women who have difficulty getting pregnant and who for this reason may be at higher ovarian cancer risk, but there are few data relevant to this possibility. Ongoing studies of ovarian cancer risk for infertile women and particularly for women receiving infertility treatments should provide valuable data.

Hormone Replacement Therapy

The results of epidemiologic studies have been inconsistent regarding the effect of HRT on ovarian cancer risk; the effect, if any, is likely to be small. HRT increases serum estrogen levels to approximately those of early follicular phase levels (or slightly lower), but these levels are very low compared with intraovarian estrogen levels in premenopausal women. HRT would therefore not be expected to be associated with an increased risk. HRT does reduce gonadotropin levels and may have been expected to reduce risk slightly, but the dose-response relationship between gonadotropins and ovarian tissue is not understood at this level, and no predictions of the expected effect can be made.

Oral Contraceptive Use

OC use decreases ovarian cancer risk by approximately 7.5% per year of use (27,37). Ovarian cell proliferation is decreased in women using OCs because ovulation does not occur, reducing ovarian surface repair, and paracrine estradiol levels are very low. The age-incidence curve is almost flat during the time OCs are used and then increases again when OC use is stopped (27). The protective effect should be lifelong.

International Variation

There is a large international variation in ovarian cancer rates (45). Until recently, ovarian cancer rates were very much lower in China and Japan than in the United States In 1970, before the widespread use of OCs began to cause a significant drop in ovarian cancer in young women in the United States, the ovarian cancer incidence for women between the ages of 45 and 54 was 4.8-fold higher among U.S. white women than in Japan (or a little bit higher if we adjust for the higher oophorectomy rate in the United States). Japanese women born around 1920 had menarche about 1.7 years later than U.S. women born around that time (30), and they had a mean parity of 3.2 compared with 2.7 for U.S. white women (48,49). They may also have had an average cycle length 2 days longer than U.S. whites (50). These three factors can account for

a 1.7-fold greater rate in U.S. women according to the incessant ovulation hypothesis (26), far from the observed 4.8-fold difference observed. However, studies done in the 1980s of traditional Asian women showed their average serum estradiol level was approximately 75% that of U.S. white women (31–33). If this is mirrored in such lower intraovarian estradiol levels and estradiol was mitogenic to ovarian epithelial cells, this would predict a 3.2-fold increased rate in U.S. women and, taken together with the three factors discussed previously, would predict a 5.4-fold increased risk for U.S. white women. The same would hold if the lower estradiol level was a product of lower FSH and FSH was mitogenic to ovarian epithelium. The difference in ovarian cancer rates between Japanese women and U.S. white women provides evidence against the simple incessant ovulation hypothesis and is accurately predicted by including estradiol or FSH as mitogenic factors.

DISCUSSION

Twelve to 13 days of progestin therapy is required to control endometrial hyperplasia completely (43). Such a regimen may not be required each month. Ettinger et al. (44) showed that a 13-day progestin course given every 3 months leads to a slightly more severe bleeding episode each 3 months than is associated with the progestin given every month, but the incidence of hyperplasia was very low and equal to that seen in women on the monthly progestin regimen. A 13-day progestin course every four to six cycles may be adequate to control endometrial cancer risk. Such intermittent progestin regimens warrant much further serious investigation, because they would greatly reduce the stimulation to the breast associated with current estrogen-progestin regimens. An even more desirable delivery system would allow delivery of progestin continuously, directly and solely to the endometrium. This is possible using a progestin-containing intrauterine device designed for contraceptive use (51). The ideal device would remain in place, delivering an adequate local progestin dose for up to 5 years and would be specifically designed for postmenopausal women.

By reducing the rapid rise in the rates of breast, endometrial, and ovarian cancer rates in the premenopausal period, the rates in older women can be greatly reduced, because cumulative mitogenic exposure is responsible for the high rates of these cancers in older women (27). OCs appear to achieve this reduction for endometrial and ovarian cancer. Current hormonal contraceptives do not achieve this reduction for breast cancer. We have suggested that a hormonal contraceptive comprising a gonadotropin-releasing hormone agonist (GnRHA) plus ultra-low-dose add-back estrogen with intermittent progestin may achieve this for breast cancer and have provided preliminary data in support of this claim (52–54). This GnRHA regimen should also reduce ovarian cancer incidence to the same or greater extent than OC use (54). Its effect on endometrial cancer rates depends on the mechanism of protection provided by a 12-day course of progestin, which remains unclear (38). It may also be possible to achieve this for breast cancer through the use of tamoxifen or another selective estrogen response modulator (SERM) in the premenopausal period, but these agents may cause ovarian stimulation and thereby increase ovarian cancer rates (56).

This is an extraordinarily optimistic time for female cancer prevention. OCs and tamoxifen in postmenopausal women have demonstrated that these cancers can be prevented to a significant extent if stimulation of the relevant tissue can be reduced. Our increasing knowledge of the factors controlling activity in all three of the tissues discussed leads us to confidently predict the effective control of all of these cancers over the next decade.

REFERENCES

1. Waterhouse J, Muir C, Correa P, Powell J, eds. *Cancer incidence in five continents*, vol III. Lyon, France: International Agency for Research on Cancer, 1976.
2. Ames BN, Gold LS. Too many rodent carcinogens: mitogenesis increases mutagenesis. *Science* 1990;249:970–971.
3. Cohen SM, Ellwein LB. Cell proliferation in carcinogenesis. *Science* 1990;249:1007–1011.
4. Preston-Martin S, Pike MC, Ross RK, et al. Increased cell division as a cause of human cancer. *Cancer Res* 1990;50:7415–7421.
5. Ferenczy A, Bertrand G, Gelfand MM. Proliferation kinetics of the human endometrium during the normal menstrual cycle. *Am J Obstet Gynecol* 1979;133:859–867.
6. Scully RE. Pathology of ovarian cancer precursors. *J Cell Biochem* 1995;23[Suppl]:208–218.
7. Fathalla MF. Increased ovulation—a factor in ovarian neoplasia? *Lancet* 1971;716:163–165.
8. Westhoff C, Murphy P, Heller D, Halim A. Is ovarian cancer associated with an increased frequency of germinal inclusion cysts? *Am J Epidemiol* 1993;138:90–93.
9. Stadel BV. The etiology and prevention of ovarian cancer. *Am J Obstet Gynecol* 1975;123:772–773.
10. Cramer DW, Welch WR. Determinants of ovarian cancer risk. II. Inferences regarding pathogenesis. *J Natl Cancer Inst* 1983;71:717–721.
11. Mohle J, Whittemore A, Pike MC, Darby S. Gonadotrophins and ovarian cancer risk. *J Natl Cancer Inst* 1985;75:178–180.
12. Luo MP, Pike MC, Stallcup M, et al. Menstrual cycle hormones regulate growth and signal transduction in benign ovarian epithelial tumors (in press).
13. Casagrande JT, Pike MC, Ross RK, et al. "Incessant ovulation" and ovarian cancer. *Lancet* 1979;2:170–173.
14. Zheng W, Lu J, Luo F, et al. Ovarian epithelial tumor growth promotion by FSH and inhibition of the effect by LH (in press).
15. Dubeau L. The cell of origin of ovarian epithelial tumors and the ovarian surface epithelium dogma: does the emperor have no clothes? *Gynecol Oncol* 1999;72:437–442.
16. Risch HA. Hormonal etiology of epithelial ovarian cancer, with a hypothesis concerning the role of androgens and progesterone. *J Natl Cancer Inst* 1998;90:1774–1786.
17. Key TJA, Pike MC. The role of oestrogens and progestagens in the epidemiology and prevention of breast cancer. *Eur J Cancer Clin Oncol* 1988;24:29–43.
18. Kelsey JL, Horn-Ross PL. Breast Cancer: magnitude of the problem and descriptive epidemiology. *Epidemiol Rev* 1993;15:7–16.
19. Collaborative Group on Hormonal Factors in Breast Cancer. Breast cancer and hormone replacement therapy. *Lancet* 1997;350:1047–1059.
20. Greendale GA, Reboussin BA, Sie A, et al. Effects of estrogen and estrogen-progestin on mammographic parenchymal density. *Ann Intern Med* 1999;130:262–269.
21. Collaborative Group on Hormonal Factors in Breast Cancer. Breast cancer and hormonal contraceptives. *Lancet* 1996;347:1713–1727.
22. Jeppsson S, Johansson EDB, Ljungberg O, Sjoberg N-O. Endometrial histology and circulating levels of medroxyprogesterone acetate (MPA), estradiol, FGSH and LH in women with MPA induced amenorrhoea compared with women with secondary amenorrhoea. *Acta Obstet Gynecol Scand* 1977;56:43–48.
23. Mishell DR. Long-acting contraceptive steroids. In: Mishell DR, Davajan V, Lobo RA, eds. *Infertility, contraception and reproductive endocrinology.* Boston: Blackwell Scientific, 1991:872–911.
24. MacMahon B, Cole P, Lin TM, et al. Age at first birth and breast cancer risk. *Bull World Health Organ* 1970;43:209–221.
25. Russo J, Tay LK, Russo IH. Differentiation of the mammary gland and susceptibility to carcinogenesis—review. *Breast Cancer Res Treat* 1982;2:5–73.
26. Pike MC, Krailo MD, Henderson BE, et al. Hormonal risk factors, breast tissue age and the age-incidence of breast cancer. *Nature* 1983;303:767–770.
27. Pike MC. Age-related factors in cancers of the breast, ovary, and endometrium. *J Chron Dis* 1987;40[Suppl 2]:59–69.
28. Ursin G, Bernstein L, Pike MC. Breast cancer. In: Doll R, Fraumeni J, Muir CS, eds. *Cancer surveys:* trends in cancer incidence and mortality, vol 19/20. Plainview, NY:Cold Spring Harbor Laboratory Press, 1994.
29. Ziegler RG, Hoover RN, Pike MC, et al. Migration patterns and breast cancer risk. *J Natl Cancer Inst* 1993;85:1819–1827.
30. Hoel DG, Wakabayashi T, Pike MC. Secular trends in the distributions of the breast cancer risk factors: menarche, first birth, menopause and weight, in Hiroshima and Nagasaki, Japan. *Am J Epidemiol* 1983;118:78–89.
31. Goldin BR, Adlercreutz H, Gorbach SL, et al. The relationship between estrogen levels and diets of Caucasian American and Oriental immigrant women. *Am J Clin Nutr* 1986;44:945–953.
32. Bernstein L, Yuan J-M, Ross RK, et al. Serum hormone levels in premenopausal Chinese women in Shanghai and white women in Los Angeles: results from two breast cancer case-control studies. *Cancer Causes Control* 1990;1:51–58.
33. Key TJA, Chen J, Wang DY, et al. Sex hormones in women in rural China and in Britain. *Br J Cancer* 1990;62:631–636.
34. Key TJA, Pike MC. The dose-effect relationship between unopposed oestrogens and endometrial mitotic rate: its central role in explaining and predicting endometrial cancer risk. *Br J Cancer* 1988;57:205–212.
35. Grady D, Gebretsadik T, Kerlikowske K, et al. Hormone replacement therapy and endometrial cancer risk: a meta-analysis. *Obstet Gynecol* 1995;85:304–313.
36. Henderson BE, Ross RK, Pike MC. Hormonal chemoprevention of cancer in women. *Science* 1993;259:633–638.
37. Pike MC, Spicer DV. Oral contraceptives and cancer. In: Shoupe D, Haseltine F, eds. *Contraception.* New York: Springer-Verlag, 1993.
38. Pike MC, Peters RK, Cozen W, et al. Estrogen-progestin replacement therapy and endometrial cancer. *J Natl Cancer Inst* 1997;89:1110–1106.
39. Whitehead MI, Townsend PT, Pryse-Davies J, et al. Effects of estrogens and progestins on the biochemistry and morphology of the postmenopausal endometrium. *N Engl J Med* 1981;305:1599–1605.
40. Lane G, Siddle NC, Ryder TA, et al. Is Provera the ideal progestin for addition to postmenopausal estrogen therapy? *Fertil Steril* 1986;45:345–352.
41. Flowers CE, Wilborn WH, Hyde BM. Mechanisms of uterine bleeding in postmenopausal patients receiving estrogen alone or with a progestin. *Obstet Gynecol* 1983;61:135–143.
42. Paterson MEL, Wade-Evans T, Sturdee DW, et al. Endometrial disease after treatment with oestrogens and progestogens in the climacteric. *Br Med J* 1980;22:822–824.
43. Whitehead MI, Townsend PT, Pryse-Davies J, et al. Actions of progestins on the morphology and biochemistry of the endometrium of postmenopausal women receiving low-dose estrogen therapy. *Am J Obstet Gynecol* 1982;142:791–795.
44. Ettinger B, Selby J, Citron JT, et al. Cyclic hormone replacement therapy using quarterly progestin. *Obstet Gynecol* 1994;83:693–700.
45. Mant JWF, Vessey MP. Ovarian and endometrial cancers. In: Doll R, Fraumeni J, Muir CS, eds. *Cancer surveys:* trends in cancer incidence and mortality, vol 19/20. Plainview, NY:Cold Spring Harbor Laboratory Press, 1994.
46. Westhoff C. Ovarian cancer. *Annu Rev Public Health* 1996;17:85–96.
47. Whittemore AS, Harris R, Itnyre J. Characteristics relating to ovarian cancer risk: collaborative analysis of 12 US case-control studies. II. Invasive epithelial ovarian cancers in white women. *Am J Epidemiol* 1992;136:1184–1203.
48. Statistics Bureau, Management and Coordination Agency. *Japan statistical yearbook 1998.* Tokyo: Government of Japan, 1997:Table 2-25.
49. Grove RD, Hetzel AM. Vital statistics rates in the United States, 1940–1960. Washington, DC: U.S. National Center for Health Statistics, U.S. Government Printing Office, 1968:i-ix, 881.
50. Harlow SD, Ephross SA. Epidemiology of menstruation and its relevance to women's health. *Epidemiol Rev* 1995;17:265–285.
51. Pharriss BB. Clinical experience with the intrauterine progesterone contraceptive system. *J Reprod Med* 1978;20:155–165.
52. Spicer DV, Pike MC, Pike A, et al. Pilot trial of a gonadotropin hormone agonist with replacement hormones as a prototype contraceptive to prevent breast cancer. *Contraception* 1993;47:427–444.
53. Spicer DV, Ursin G, Parisky YR, et al. Changes in mammographic densities induced by a hormonal contraceptive designed to reduce breast cancer risk. *J Natl Cancer Inst* 1994;86:431–436.
54. Pike MC, Daniels JR, Spicer DV. A hormonal contraceptive approach to reducing breast and ovarian cancer risk: an update. *Endocr Rel Cancer* 1997;4:125–133.
55. Spicer DV, Shoupe D, Pike MC. GnRH agonists as contraceptive agents: predicted significantly reduced risk of breast cancer. *Contraception* 1991;44:289–310.
56. Spicer DV, Pike MC, Henderson BE. Ovarian cancer and long-term tamoxifen in premenopausal women. *Lancet* 1991;337:1414.

Treatment of the Postmenopausal Woman: Basic and Clinical Aspects, Second Edition, edited by Rogerio A. Lobo, Lippincott Williams & Wilkins, Philadelphia © 1999.

CHAPTER 43

Hormones and Breast Cell Proliferation

John J. Park, Malcolm C. Pike, Jinha M. Park, and Michael F. Press

Breast cancer is the most common malignancy among women in the United States, with approximately 178,700 new cases diagnosed in 1998 (1). It is the second most common cause of cancer-related death. Despite the importance of this disease, relatively little is known about the control mechanisms of cell proliferation in breast epithelium, although proliferative activity is considered to be a critically important determinant of carcinogenesis (2).

Development of malignant phenotypes appear to involve multiple stages, with the accumulation of mutational events occurring within DNA of cells. Cell division increases the risk of genetic errors and serves to propagate the errors to daughter cells. Because single-stranded DNA errors can be repaired, the rate of DNA repair and the rate of cell division are both important in establishing a mutation in the genome. Single-stranded DNA damage may be converted through mitotic activity to gaps or mutations and through nondisjunction into more substantial changes. Activation or alteration of protooncogene expression and the loss or inactivation of tumor suppressor genes, which control normal cellular activity, is considered to be particularly important. Many of the genes that are altered in human cancers are growth factors, growth factor receptors, signal transducers, or transcription factors. The progressive accumulation of genetic alterations is thought to lead to the development of carcinoma *in situ* and, with accumulation of additional genetic alterations, to invasive carcinoma.

PROLIFERATIVE ACTIVITY IN BREAST CANCER DEVELOPMENT

There is considerable evidence that ovarian hormones have an important effect on breast cancer risk (3). Late

J. J. Park, J. M. Park, M. F. Press: Department of Pathology, University of Southern California School of Medicine, Los Angeles, California 90089.

M. C. Pike: Department of Preventive Medicine, University of Southern California School of Medicine, Los Angeles, California 90089.

menarche and early menopause (or ovariectomy) are associated with a lower risk of developing breast cancer (4,5). The protective effect of early menopause (4,6,7) is an important risk factor that illustrates the role of ovarian hormones in the cause of breast cancer. For almost all non–hormone-dependent cancers, when the logarithm of incidence is plotted against the logarithm of age, the result approximates a single straight line (Fig. 43.1A), but for breast cancer and endometrial cancer, it can be approximated by two straight lines, one with a very steep slope before age 50 years and another with a diminished slope thereafter (Fig. 43.1B). The increase in incidence with age is much steeper during the premenopausal period than after the menopause (8). Women who stop menstruating before age 40, naturally or through surgical intervention, have about half the risk of breast cancer of women who continue to menstruate to age 50 (Fig. 43.1C). This strongly suggests that the hormonal pattern of premenopausal women (i.e., cyclic production of relatively large amounts of estradiol and progesterone) causes a greater rate of increase in the risk of breast cancer than the hormonal pattern of postmenopausal women (i.e., constant low estrogen and very low progesterone). However, the protective effect of early menopause gives no information on the relative importance of these two ovarian hormones in determining risk.

Studies of endometrial cancer have led to the "unopposed-estrogen hypothesis" for this cancer (3,9). This hypothesis maintains that estrogen unopposed by a progestin increases the risk of endometrial cancer by stimulating normal endometrial cell division; high-dose progestins block the action of estrogen on the endometrium. This hypothesis provides a very satisfactory explanation of the major risk factors for endometrial cancer: a reduced risk from early menopause, high parity, and combination-type oral contraceptive (COC) use, in contrast with an increased risk from obesity and postmenopausal estrogen replacement therapy (ERT) (10). Endometrial cell division in premenopausal

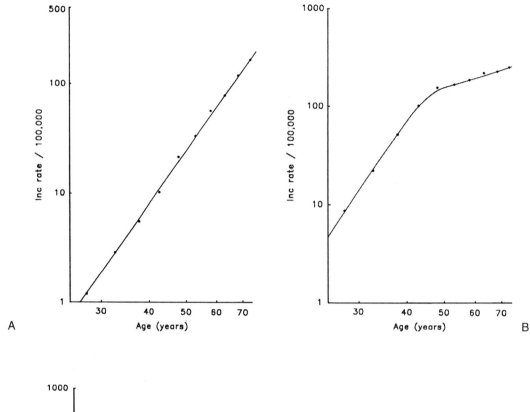

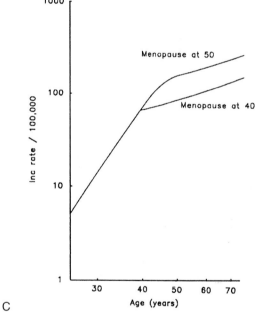

FIG. 43.1. Comparison of the incidence of colon carcinoma and breast carcinoma with increasing age. **A:** Logarithm of the colorectal cancer incidence per 100,000 persons plotted against age at diagnosis. **B:** Logarithm of breast cancer incidence per 100,000 persons plotted against age at diagnosis. **C:** The incidence of breast cancer in women whose menopause occurred by age 40 is compared with the incidence for women whose menopause occurred after age 50.

women is effectively confined to the preovulatory follicular phase and immediate postovulation phase of the menstrual cycle, and maximal cell proliferation is induced by the relatively low unopposed levels early in the follicular phase (10,11). As serum progesterone levels begin to rise in the postovulatory luteal phase, endometrial cell proliferation ceases, despite elevated levels of estradiol. Early menopause reduces endometrial cancer risk by reducing the unopposed-estradiol

concentration and the associated cell division rate from the relatively high level during the premenopausal follicular phase to the low level during the postmenopausal period. This reduction in estradiol concentration is more than sufficient to compensate for the fact that all estrogen exposure in the postmenopausal period is not opposed by a progestin. Parity reduces risk because pregnancy is associated with high progesterone levels. COC use reduces the risk because COCs reduce the period of endometrial exposure to unopposed estrogen from the 14 days of the normal follicular phase to the 7 days per 28-day cycle during which the COC is not used and because endogenous estrogen concentrations are very low during these 7 days. Postmenopausal obesity is associated with significantly increased endogenous estrogen levels, which are also more bioavailable because of the decreased levels of sex hormone–binding globulin (SHBG) and increased peripheral conversion of androgens to estrone in obese women (12–14). Premenopausal obesity is also associated with a greatly increased endometrial cancer risk. Premenopausal obesity is associated with more anovular (no progesterone) cycles, in which the endogenous estrogen level is similar to follicular-phase levels and the endometrium is exposed to unopposed estrogens for a longer period. ERT increases the bioavailable estradiol concentration of a postmenopausal woman to approximately two thirds of the level found in the early follicular phase (10), greatly increasing the endometrial cell division rate.

The success of the unopposed-estrogen hypothesis in explaining the epidemiology of endometrial cancer has stimulated an effort to develop an hypothesis along similar lines for breast cancer. However, it appears clear that an "unopposed-estrogen" hypothesis is not tenable for breast cancer. Although postmenopausal obesity is associated with a small increase in breast cancer risk, premenopausal obesity is actually associated with a decrease in risk. Moreover, COCs with an estrogen-progestin mix in each pill do not protect against breast cancer, and even high-dose ERT (conjugated equine estrogen [1.25 mg daily]) produces at most only a modest increase in breast cancer risk (15,16). In contrast to the situation with endometrial cancer, there is evidence that use of a progestin as part of the ERT for postmenopausal women is associated with an increased, not a decreased, risk of breast cancer (17). COC use by women of reproductive age may actually slightly increase breast cancer risk (18–20), in stark contrast to the clear protective effect against endometrial cancer. In light of these disparate results, characterization of control mechanisms for proliferative activity in normal breast epithelial cells would clearly be useful in understanding breast carcinogenesis.

STEROID HORMONE MECHANISM OF ACTION

Steroid hormones play important roles in promoting proliferation and cell differentiation in normal breast epithelium and breast cancer cells. Because only cells with steroid hormone receptors respond to the steroids, these biologic effects are thought to be mediated through transcriptional activation of specific sets of genes recognized by particular receptor proteins.

The estrogen receptors (ERs) and progesterone receptors (PRs) appear to have little in common functionally, but they share a remarkable amount of structural similarities. Two forms of PR have been described, PR-A and PR-B, which are identical except that PR-A has a truncation of the first 164 amino acids from the amino terminus. This truncated region is thought to play a role in the functional differences between the two PR isoforms. Until recently, only one type of estrogen receptor (ER-α) was thought to exist. However, with the cloning of a second estrogen receptor (ER-β), it is clear that ER-α is not the only mechanism by which estrogens have their influence on target, estrogen-responsive cell types. The following discussion refers to ER-α, and ER-β is described later in this chapter. Through the use of *in vitro* mutagenesis assays, deletion mutation studies and domain-swapping experiments, four major regions have been demonstrated for the ER and the PR. These domains are, in order from the carboxyl-terminal end, a hormone-binding domain (HBD), a hinge region, a DNA-binding domain (DBD), and a variable or regulatory domain (AF-1) (Fig. 43.2) (21–25).

Substantial progress has been made in the past decade in understanding the mechanisms of action for ERs and PRs, members of the steroid-thyroid-retinoid nuclear receptor superfamily (26,27). The HBDs of ERs and PRs are critical for hormone recognition and receptor regulation. In the absence of ligand, this region appears to be inhibitory, preventing the receptor (ER or PR) from binding to its DNA response element in the promoter region of a target gene. This inhibition is caused by the interaction between the HBD and a heat shock protein-90 (HSP-90), which leads to the formation of a transcriptionally inactivated complex of proteins consisting of monomeric receptor, HSP-90, p59, and possibly HSP-70 (28,29). It is believed that the formation of

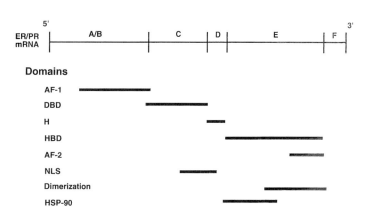

FIG. 43.2. Functional domains of the steroid hormone receptors. AF-1, ligand-independent transactivation domain; DBD, DNA-binding domain; H, hinge region; HBD, hormone-binding domain; AF-2, ligand-dependent transactivation domain; NLS, nuclear localization domain; HSP-90, heat shock protein-90 binding region.

this complex prevents the receptor from binding DNA, possibly by disrupting key areas of the DBD. Receptors lacking the HBD no longer have this regulatory element and results in an altered receptor that is constituitively active (30).

Binding of ligand to receptor is thought to result in an allosteric change that allows the receptor-hormone complex to bind to its DNA response element. In the presence of a hormone agonist, the receptor undergoes a conformational change resulting in the dissociation of the monomeric receptor from the heat shock complex. This change in conformation results in the spontaneous dimerization of receptors, followed by DNA binding through their specific hormone response elements (HREs) and activation of a second, ligand-dependent transcriptional activation domain (AF-2) contained within the HBD (31,32). This ligand-mediated process is highly regulated and hormone specific. Only an agonist can induce the proper allosteric effects to enable DNA binding and transcriptional activation. Antagonists that bind to the HBD have been shown to elicit DNA binding but cannot induce the correct conformational changes necessary for *trans*-activation (33). Because of all of these important functions, it is easy to understand why this domain is highly conserved within each class of steroid receptors.

The other highly conserved domain is the DBD, which lies immediately downstream of the highly variable, ligand-independent transcriptional activation domain (AF-1). This region enables each receptor to recognize and bind its own special hormone response element after ligand binding and dimerization have occurred. In addition to this DNA binding function, this domain has also been demonstrated to be important in dimerization, nuclear localization of receptor, and HSP-90 binding (34).

The amino acids between the HBDs and DBDs have been referred to as the hinge region, because it is thought to be important in establishing the allosteric association of the hormone-binding and the regulatory domains. This region also contains sequences that are critical in directing the receptor protein to the nucleus after it is synthesized in the cytoplasm (35,36). These "nuclear-localization signals" are sufficient to direct these proteins to the nucleus. In addition to the primary nuclear localization signals in the hinge region, a second signal is present in the HBD that specifies nuclear localization in the presence of hormone (37).

The nuclear localization of the steroid-unoccupied form of ER and PR requires continuous metabolic activity. Various inhibitors of energy synthesis in cultured cells expressing ERs or PRs demonstrate that the nuclear residency of the receptor reflects a dynamic state. In the presence of energy inhibitors, receptor diffuses from the nucleus to the cytoplasm. When the inhibitors are removed and glucose is returned to the culture medium, ERs and PRs are transported back to the nucleus (37). The steroid-occupied and steroid-unoccupied forms of

receptor reside in the nucleus, not the cytoplasm, of the intact cell. ERs and PRs can be thought of primarily as regulators of transcriptional activity, and their location in the nucleus is most appropriate for this function. Although the DNA sequences of estrogen- and progesterone-response elements in promoter regions have been characterized, only a limited number of specific ER/PR-inducible genes are identified. The genes responsible for the proliferative activity of hormone-responsive cells are unknown.

There are two subtypes of ER, designated ER-α and ER-β. ER-α has been localized to the long arm of chromosome 6 (band q24-27) (38) and is the "classic" ER. It is a relatively large gene, spanning at least 140 kilobases, and contains eight exons that encode the ER-α protein product. These exons are 684, 191, 117, 336, 139, 134, 184, and 4537 base pairs long (Fig. 43.3), have been well characterized, and have various functions. The transactivational amino-terminal hypervariable region (AF-1) is predominantly coded for by exon 1. Exons 2 and 3 each code for one zinc finger of the DNA binding domain. The hinge region is coded for by exon 4. The large hydrophobic hormone-binding domain (HBD/AF-2) is encoded by five different exons, including part of exon 4; exons 5, 6, and 7; and part of exon 8 (39). Combined, these four domains make up the 595–amino acid ER-α (Fig. 43.3*A*).

ER-β, which was initially cloned from a rat prostate cDNA library (40) and subsequently from humans (41) and mice (42), maps to chromosome 14 (band q22-24) (43). The ER-β gene spans a region of 30 to 40 kilobases, and like ER-α, it is composed of eight exons that code for a 530–amino acid protein product (Fig. 43.3*B*). These exons have been shown by various groups to share significant homology to their ER-α counterparts, especially in the areas of the DBD (97%) and the HBD (59.1%) (40–44). It was this high degree of sequence conservation between the two subtypes that initially alerted researchers that ER-β was actually a second type of ER. Subsequent studies have shown that ER-β is a novel ER subtype, suggesting that ER-α is not the only mechanism by which estrogens have their influence on target, estrogen-responsive cell types. Because of the heterogeneous tissue distribution patterns of the two ERs (43), it is suspected that there may exist heretofore unrecognized mechanisms of estrogen signaling in tissues that exclusively express just the ER-α or ER-β subtype or express both (45).

Unlike the ERs, there is only one type of PR, although multiple isoforms have been shown to exist. The two major isoforms are PR-A (94 kd) and PR-B (114 kd), both of which are encoded by the same gene, which is located on the long arm of chromosome 11 (band q22-23) and spans more than 90 kilobases (46). It was once thought that the two isoforms arose from the same mRNA transcript through different in-frame translational initiation sites, but the two isoforms are the products of two different transcripts generated by alternative estrogen-

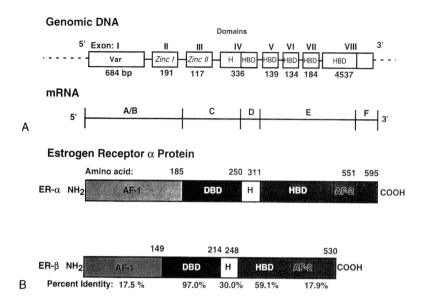

Genomic DNA

mRNA

Estrogen Receptor α Protein

A
B

FIG. 43.3. Schematic illustration of the estrogen receptor (ER) genome and messenger RNA with protein structure. **A:** ER-α genomic DNA. Exons I through VIII, depicted as boxes separated by variable intronic sequences, are shown with their respective sizes. The mRNA structure of the ER-α transcript and its protein product are also shown. ER-β is the product of a different gene and is located on a separate chromosome than ER-α. Var, amino terminal hypervariable domain; Zinc, zinc finger DNA-binding domains; H, hinge region; DBD, DNA-binding domain; HBD, hormone-binding domain; AF-1, ligand-independent transactivation domain; AF-2, ligand-dependent transactivation domain. **B:** The protein structure of ER-β is shown with the percent identity between the functional domains of the two ER subtypes. The genomic structure and mRNA transcript for ER-β have not been included.

responsive promoters (47). These promoters, however, lack the consensus palindromic estrogen responsive element (GGTCAnnnTGACC) typical for other estrogen-responsive genes (48,49), suggesting that alternative estrogen-responsive regulatory elements may exist, such as the imperfect palindromic elements that mediate estrogen's induction of transforming growth factor-α (50). The PR is encoded by eight exons of 2380, 152, 117, 306,

145, 131, 158, and 153 base pairs (46). These exons code for functional domains similar to those of their ER counterparts, demonstrating the high degree of functional and structural conservation among the different steroid receptors (the androgen receptor also shares this basic structural identity) (Fig. 43.4*A, B*). A third isoform of PR (60-kd PR-C) has been described (51), but it remains to be seen if this form plays a major functional role in progestin-mediated signaling. PR-C is smaller than the other two PR isoforms as it is truncated in its amino terminus.

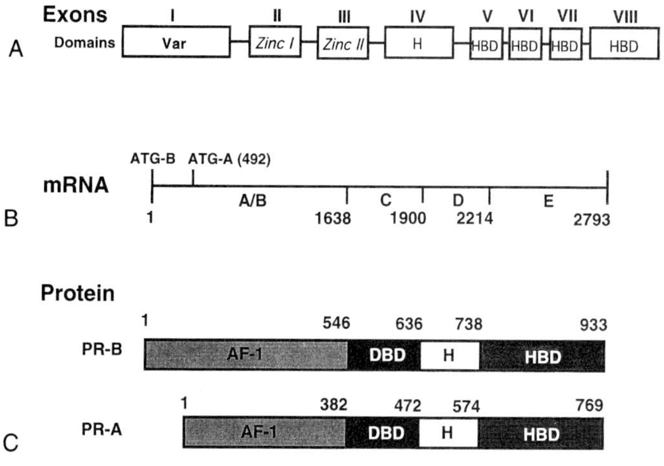

ESTROGEN RECEPTOR AND PROGESTERONE RECEPTOR CONTENT OF NORMAL BREAST TISSUE

Normal Menstrual Cycles

Because ER-β was discovered only recently, little is known about its expression in normal breast tissue. The following discussion applies only to ER-α. Because the actions of steroid hormones influencing the normal breast are considered to be mediated directly or indirectly by their respective receptors, determining the expression pattern of these receptors is important for an understanding of hormonal effects on the breast. However, there is limited information available on the pattern of ER and PR expression in the normal breast during the menstrual cycle and during oral contraceptive pill use. Conventional biochemical assays are not well suited for characterization of ERs and PRs in normal breast tissue because of the low content of epithelial cells. The homogenization of normal breast tissue required for biochemical assays is likely to result in false-negative results because of the low cellularity. Immunohistochemical localization with monoclonal ER and PR antibodies is, however, well suited to address this issue.

FIG. 43.4. Schematic illustration of the progesterone receptor (PR) genome and messenger RNA with protein structure. **A:** PR genomic DNA includes exons and functional domains. **B:** The mRNA structure of PR has two distinct ATG sites. PR-B is encoded by a full-length transcript and initiates from the first of the two ATG initiation sites, whereas PR-A initiates from a downstream in-frame ATG site. Whether the two isoforms of PR are translated from the same transcript or from two distinct transcripts is not clear. **C:** Protein structures of PR-B and PR-A. AF-1, ligand-independent transactivation domain; DMB, DNA-binding domain; H, hinge region; HBD, hormone-binding domain.

TABLE 43.1. *Estrogen receptor status in normal breast tissue during different phases of the menstrual cycle*

Study	Measure	Week of menstrual cycle[a]			
		Week 1	Week 2	Week 3	Week 4
Ricketts et al., 1991 (54)[b]	ER-positive cases	25.0% (60)		11.5% (52)	
Williams et al., 1991 (55)[c]	ER-positive cells	4.3% (17)	4.3% (14)	3.7% (8)	2.2% (6)
Battersby et al., 1992 (57)[d]	ER-positive cases	58% (14)	64% (27)	30% (20)	35% (24)
Weighted average[e]		100%	103%	53%	52%

[a]Values given are averages when appropriate; values based on the number of observations are given in parentheses.

[b]Measurements appear to have been made in small ducts and lobules. Normal tissue was obtained by fine-needle aspiration. Data are given as the percent of cases with >50% of cells ER position Nulliparous versus parous: 7/35, 20%; 15/75, 20%. Age: 25, 2/12, 17%; 26–35, 7/35, 20%; 36–45, 8/52, 15%.

[c]Measurements were made in lobules. No significant effects of age or parity were observed.

[d]Only TDLU cells were considered. Data are given as the percent of cases with 5% of cells ER positive. Nulliparous versus Parous: 20/47, 43%; 22/41, 54%. Age: 25, 15/33, 45%; >25, 27/55, 49%.

[e]Standardized to 100% at week 1.

Data on the study of Jacquemier et al. (53) are not presented in the tables because, for premenopausal women, the researchers did not distinguish between women cycling naturally from women using oral contraceptives.

ERs and PRs are heterogeneous in the normal breast with regard to frequency and intensity of immunostaining (52–57). ERs and PRs are found almost exclusively in nuclei of ductal and lobular epithelial cells, not in myoepithelial or stromal cells. Studies examining ER and PR expression in normal premenopausal breast tissue have reported higher percentages of epithelial cells expressing PRs than expressing ERs (Tables 43.1 and 43.2). However, a double-labeling study using antibodies directed against ERs and PRs with antigen retrieval in paraffin-embedded tissues demonstrated that the two receptors are coexpressed in approximately 96% of cells that are steroid receptor positive (58). The researchers stated that they found antigen retrieval of paraffin-embedded tissue sections "to be more sensitive for ER detection" than ER immunostaining of frozen tissue sections. This is contrary to the experience of most investigators. The very terminology of antigen "retrieval" indicates recovery of antigens observed in frozen tissues but lost with paraffin-embedded tissues.

TABLE 43.2. *Progesterone receptor status in normal breast tissue during different phases of the menstrual cycle*

Study	Measure	Week of menstrual cycle[a]			
		Week 1	Week 2	Week 3	Week 4
Ricketts et al., 1991 (54)[b]	ER-positive cases	25.0%		11.5%	
Ricketts et al., 1991 (54)[b]	PR-positive cases	23.9% (46)		31.7% (41)	
Williams et al., 1991 (55)[c]	PR-positive cells	11.5% (14)	10.2% (13)	16.8% (9)	9.0% (6)
Battersby et al., 1992 (57)[d]	PR-positive cases	70% (13)	82% (21)	72% (17)	73% (18)
Weighted average[e]		100%	103%	124%	114%

[a]Values given are averages when appropriate; values based on the number of observations are given in parentheses.

[b]Measurements appear to have been made in small ducts and lobules. Normal tissue was obtained by fine-needle aspiration. Data are given as the percent of cases with >50% of cells PR positive Nulliparous versus parous: 6/26, 23%; 18/64, 28%. Age: 25, 2/6, 33%; 26–35, 5/26, 19%; 36–45, 12/45, 27%. High body mass, pregnancy before age 20, and family history of breast cancer were associated with PR-positive cases.

[c]Measurements made in lobules. No significant effects of age or parity were observed.

[d]Only TDLU cells were considered. Data are given as the percent of cases with 5% of cells PR positive. Nulliparous versus parous: 29/37, 78%; 22/33, 67%. Age: 25, 20/25, 80%; >25, 31/45, 69%.

[e]Standardized to 100% at week 1.

Data on the study of Jacquemier et al. (53) are not presented in the tables because, for premenopausal women, the researchers did not distinguish between women cycling naturally from women using oral contraceptives.

TABLE 43.3. *Estrogen receptor status in normal breast tissue during different weeks of combination-type oral contraceptive (COC) pill use*

Study	Measure	Week of COC use[a]			
		Week 1 (off COC)	Week 2	Week 3	Week 4
Williams et al., 1991 (55)[b]	ER-positive cells	2.9% (8)	0.1% (5)	0.4% (8)	1.3% (7)
	Proportion of natural cycle value	67%	2%	11%	59%
Battersby et al., 1992 (57)[c]	ER-positive cases	40% (13)	34% (19)	20% (16)	16% (20)
	Proportion of natural cycle value	69%	53%	67%	46%

[a]Values given are averages when appropriate; values are based on the number of observations given in parentheses.

[b]Measurements were made in lobules. No significant effects of age or parity were observed.

[c]Only TDLU cells were considered. Data are given as the percent of cases with 5% of cells ER positive. No significant effect of age was found. Expression was lower in parous women in the first few years post-partum than in nulliparous women and higher than in nulliparous thereafter.

ERs and PRs usually have been characterized in the lobules of the breast and, in the study of Battersby et al. (57), only in the terminal duct lobular units (TDLUs) (Tables 43.1 through 43.4). The nuclei of lobular cells showing receptor immunostaining are scored as positive without making a distinction with regard to lobular cell type (i.e., lobular ductules versus intralobular ducts). ER is higher in the follicular phase of the cycle (Table 43.1). Overall, ER levels in the luteal phase are less than 60% of the levels in the follicular phase. In contrast, PR has been found to be relatively stable during the menstrual cycle (Table 43.2). These studies show little or no effect of age or parity on ERs or PRs.

The percentage of epithelial cells expressing ERs or PRs is low compared with observations made in breast cancers (59–61). Studies reporting the actual percentage of positive cells find an average of less than 5% to 12% of epithelial cells expressing ERs and less than 20% expressing PRs in normal breast (Tables 43.1 and 43.2) (55,58). Other studies suggest that the actual percentage of positive cells may be higher, although numbers of positive epithelial cells are not reported (Tables 43.1 and

43.2) (54,57,58). Battersby et al. (57) reported the percentage of women whose breast biopsy contained at least 5% ER-positive cells.

Expression of ERs varies depending on the phase of the menstrual cycle. About 60% of women biopsied during the follicular phase have been found to have had at least 5% ER-immunostained cells, but when the biopsy is performed during the luteal phase, this decreases to 30% to 35% (Table 43.1) (57). The other report with a much higher percentage of ER-positive cells is a study of fine-needle aspirates from breasts of normal women (54). In this study, more than 50% of epithelial cells are reported to be ER positive in 25% (follicular phase) and 12% (luteal phase) of women (Table 43.1). The results obtained by these investigators (54) are incompatible with the results reported by the other groups shown in Table 43.1.

PR expression in normal women appears to be only slightly affected by phase of the cycle (Table 43.2) (53,54,56). Battersby et al. (57) found PRs in 5% or more of breast epithelial cells in approximately 75% of women biopsied for benign breast lesions. Ricketts et al. (54) reported that fine-needle aspirates contained immunos-

TABLE 43.4. *Progesterone receptor status in normal breast tissue during different weeks of combination-type oral contraceptive (COC) pill use*

Study	Measure	Week of COC use[a]			
		Week 1 (off COC)	Week 2	Week 3	Week 4
Williams et al., 1991 (55)[b]	PR-positive cells	8.6% (6)	13.4% (4)	10.5% (7)	11.0% (6)
	Proportion of natural cycle value	75%	131%	62%	122%
Battersby et al., 1992 (57)[c]	PR-positive cases	58% (12)	59% (17)	77% (13)	84% (19)
	Proportion of natural cycle value	83%	72%	107%	115%

[a]Values given are averages when appropriate; values are based on the number of observations given in parentheses.

[b]Measurements were made in lobules. No significant effects of age or parity were observed.

[c]Only TDLU cells were considered. Data are given as the percent of cases with 5% of cells PR positive. Expression was higher in older women. Expression was lower in parous women in the first few years post-partum than in nulliparous women and higher than in nulliparous thereafter.

taining for PRs in more than 50% of cells from approximately 28% of normal women (24% in the follicular and 32% in the luteal phase) (54). The results obtained by this group are incompatible with the results of the other groups (Table 43.2).

Oral Contraceptive–Regulated Cycles

Observations have been made in women using oral contraceptives in two studies (Tables 43.3 and 43.4). The findings for ERs are discrepant. One study finds the number of ER-positive cells to be lowest in the second and third weeks of COC cycles (i.e., in the first 2 weeks of COC use). In contrast, Battersby et al. (57) found fewer women with at least 5% ER-positive cells in the third and fourth weeks of the cycle than in the first and second weeks. Their results show a decline in the percentage of ER-positive cells during the third and fourth weeks of the COC cycle is most consistent with the trend observed during natural cycles (i.e., a reduction in ER during the progestin-dominant portion of the cycle). PR content remains level throughout the COC cycle or is slightly increased in weeks 3 and 4 of COC use (Table 43.4), in agreement with the relatively minor fluctuations in PR concentration during natural cycles.

Postmenopausal Period

A study examining ER and PR expression in normal postmenopausal breast tissue has reported higher percentages of epithelial cells expressing ERs than expressing PRs (53), which is the opposite of observations made in the premenopausal breast (Tables 43.1 and 43.2). Twenty-six percent of epithelial cells in postmenopausal breast were immunostained for ERs and 2% for PRs, in contrast to the approximately 5% and 10% to 15%

observed in premenopausal breast tissue for ERs and PRs, respectively.

Other than the nuclear distribution of receptor, observations of ERs and PRs in the breast contrast strikingly with observations made in the endometrium. Uterine ERs and PRs are found in endometrial epithelial cells, stromal cells, and myometrial smooth muscle cells (62–65). Breast ERs and PRs are identified only in epithelial cells. Cyclic variation of ERs and PRs is substantial in the endometrium but not in the breast. In endometrial epithelial cells, ERs and PRs are expressed at maximal levels during the follicular phase of the cycle and are difficult to identify in glandular epithelium during the middle and late luteal phases. During the follicular phase, more than 90% of endometrial epithelial cells express ERs and PRs. Although the number of ERs in the breast appears to be greater during the follicular than the luteal phase, 10% or fewer cells express the receptor. It is also remarkable that lower ER expression is found in breast cells during that portion of the menstrual cycle associated with the most active breast cell proliferative activity (i.e., luteal phase), while the reverse is found for ER expression and proliferative activity in the endometrium.

PROLIFERATIVE ACTIVITY OF NORMAL BREAST TISSUE

Normal Menstrual Cycles

The relation of steroid hormone receptor levels to breast cell proliferation is controversial (66–69). Breast epithelial cell division has been studied in benign surgical specimens and in normal tissue from reduction mammoplasties and autopsies. In sharp contrast to the endometrium, ^{3}H-thymidine labeling index (TLI) studies of the breast (55,70–74) show most proliferative activity is during the luteal phase of the cycle with peak activity

TABLE 43.5. *Thymidine labeling index in normal breast epithelium during different weeks of the menstrual cycle*

Study	Week of menstrual cycle[a]			
	Week 1	Week 2	Week 3	Week 4
Meyer, 1977 (71)[b]	0.17% (21)		0.79 (19)	
Anderson, et al., 1989 (74)[c]	0.51% (20)	0.37% (53)	0.78% (53)	1.25% (48)
Williams et al., 1991 (55)[d]	1.8% (33)	1.5% (37)	3.4% (31)	3.6% (26)
Weighted average[e]	100%	82%	191%	257%

[a]Values given are averages when appropriate; values are based on the number of observations given in parentheses.

[b]TDLU cells. No data were available on parity. Labeling decreases with age: <20, 2.1%; 20–34, 1.9%; 35+, 1.6%.

[c]TDLU cells. Measurements shown are unweighted averages of parous and nulliparous women. Results were adjusted for breast age. No effect of parity was observed. Labeling decreases with age: <20, 1.5%; 20–34, 0.9%; 35+ 0.6%.

[d]Measurements were made in lobules. No effect of parity was observed. Labeling decreases with age.

[e]Standardized to 100% at week 1.

TABLE 43.6. *Mitotic rate per lobule in normal breast epithelium during different weeks of the menstrual cycle*

Study	Week of menstrual cycle[a]			
	Week 1	Week 2	Week 3	Week 4
Anderson, 1982 (76)	0.10%	0.07%	0.11%	0.40%
	(24)	(25)	(21)	(29)
Longacre & Bartow, 1986 (77)	0.25%	0.25%	0.25%	0.60%
	(19)	(20)	(12)	(24)
Weighted average[b]	100%	82%	106%	318%

[a]Values given are averages when appropriate; values are based on the number of observations given in parentheses.

[b]Standardized to 100% at week 1.

between postovulation days 9 and 12 (72–76). The percentage of cells incorporating thymidine is 2 to 2.5 times higher in the luteal phase than in the follicular phase (Table 43.5), whereas epithelial mitotic counts appear to be approximately three times higher in the late luteal phase than in the follicular phase (Table 43.6) (76,77). A decline in TLI and mitotic activity with age has been consistently observed. Anderson et al. (74) found that the TLI of women under age 20 years was 2.5 times greater than that of women 35 years of age or older. The results are inconsistent with regard to parity. Anderson et al. (74) found that nulliparous women have a much greater TLI in the late luteal phase than parous women, but this was not found by Williams et al. (55).

Oral Contraceptive–Regulated Cycles

Proliferative activity of normal breast tissue through the oral contraceptive-regulated cycle is lowest in week 1, when COCs are not taken (Table 43.7). The data are inconsistent about whether proliferative activity is constant or is rising as COC use continues through weeks 2 to 4. Anderson et al. (74) found a steadily increasing TLI with week of COC use, but Williams et al. (55) reported no change over the 3 weeks of COC uses. Two of the studies demonstrate increased proliferative activity in COC-regulated cycles compared with normal menstrual cycles (71,74). In the third study (55), the total TLI over the 28-day COC cycle was almost identical to that found over the normal menstrual cycle. A slight increase in proliferative activity in the normal breast is consistent with a slightly increased risk of developing breast cancer in young women who have used COCs (18–20).

These observations suggest that estrogen alone (in the follicular phase) induces some cell division but that estrogen and progesterone together (in the luteal phase) induce much more cell division. However, progesterone has not been found to augment the mitogenic effect of estrogen in human breast tissue samples transplanted to athymic nude mice (69,78,79). *In vitro* studies of cultured normal human mammary epithelial cells obtained from surgically excised tissue are inconclusive (80). In other studies, some synthetic progestins have been shown to inhibit the *in vitro* mitogenic effect of estrogen (81). However, in

TABLE 43.7. *Thymidine labeling index (TLI) of normal breast tissue during different weeks of combination-type oral contraceptive use*

Study	Measure	Week of COC use[a]			
		Week 1 (off COC)	Week 2	Week 3	Week 4
Meyer, 1977 (71)[b]	TLI	0.81%		2.12%	
		(2)	(7)		
	Proportion of natural cycle value	476%		268%	
Anderson et al., 1989 (74)[c]	TLI	0.63%	0.56%	0.98%	1.96%
		(32)	(38)	(40)	(50)
	Proportion of natural cycle value	124%	151%	126%	157%
Williams et al., 1991 55[d]	TLI	1.5%	2.8%	2.9%	3.0%
		(12)	(16)	(11)	(10)
	Proportion of natural cycle value	83%	187%	85%	83%

[a]Values given are averages when appropriate; values are based on the number of observations given in parentheses.

[b]TDLU cells. No data on parity were available. The decline with age was not significant.

[c]TDLU cells. Refer to Table 43.2. Measurements shown are unweighted averages of parous and nulliparous women. Results are adjusted for breast age. Labeling was much greater in nulliparous than parous women in week 4.

[d]Measurements were made in lobules. No statement was made on the effect of parity. Labeling decreases with age.

a study by Cline et al. (82) using postmenopausal cynomolgus macaques, conjugated equine estrogens alone and in combination with medroxyprogesterone acetate was administered for 30 months at low doses "equivalent" to the doses used in hormone replacement therapy. They found that combined therapy induced greater breast cell proliferation than estrogen alone, suggesting that progesterone does augment the mitogenic effect of estrogen in normal breast cell proliferation. An alternative possibility to estrogen-progestin induction of mitotic activity is that only estrogens stimulate proliferative activity with a dose-response relationship between cell division and plasma estrogen concentration in the range of estrogen concentrations occurring during the normal menstrual cycle and with a 4- to 5-day lag time between changes in estrogen concentration and the induced changes in cell division. If there is an increase in mitotic activity during the later weeks of the COC cycle, this may be caused by a lag in breast cell response or to an increase in serum concentrations of synthetic steroid in certain women over the 21-day cycle of pill taking (83). Other interpretations are possible; estrogen may be solely responsible for interlobular ductal cell division, and the addition of progesterone may be responsible for the greatly increased terminal duct lobular unit cell division in the luteal phase. At menarche, ductal growth is stimulated by estrogen; the addition of progestin is required for lobular development (84). Full proliferative development of the terminal region of the mammary tree occurs during pregnancy when estrogen and progesterone are present. However, these anatomic distinctions in ductal epithelium are not addressed in the studies of ER, PR, and thymidine labeling in which intralobular ducts and lobular ductular epithelium are characterized together.

In the luteal phase of the menstrual cycle, terminal ducts per lobule are greatly increased with an increase in the number of cells per TDLU (77). In the late luteal and early follicular phase, there is a great loss of TDLU cells (75). Another important observation concerning breast cell proliferation is the tremendous interpersonal variation. This variability is evident in studies of specimens obtained on the same day of the normal menstrual cycle and on the same day of a COC cycle. No studies relate the observed cell division rates with serum hormone concentrations that are known to show large between-person variability. Hormonal effects on the TDLU are important, because most breast carcinomas arise in the TDLU (84).

PROLIFERATION OF BREAST CANCER CELLS

ERs and PRs are important cellular proteins of demonstrated clinical importance in breast carcinomas. Because normal breast tissue responds to steroid hormonal stimulation, cancer cells derived from breast epithelium can be expected to retain some of the regulatory pathways of the normal tissue and therefore be influenced by the hormonal environment. The ER and PR content of breast cancers is important in predicting response to endocrine therapy, presumably because of the influence on mitotic activity. Women whose breast cancers are ER positive and PR positive and who develop recurrent disease are likely to respond to endocrine therapy (60% respond) with regression or growth arrest of the tumor, whereas women with ER-negative, PR-negative breast cancers seldom respond (<10%) (85–92).

Estrogen-responsive breast cancer cell lines, particularly MCF-7 cells, have been extensively used to examine hormonal influences on breast cancer cell growth (93–96). Phenol red, the pH indicator in tissue culture media, acts as a weak estrogen (97). Early studies of estrogen effects on breast cancer cells are flawed by the inclusion of phenol red in the medium. The direct stimulatory effects of estrogen on cell growth are clearly evident in MCF-7 cells grown under the appropriate culture conditions (phenol red–free medium and low concentrations of steroid-stripped serum) (98,99). However, estrogen-induced cellular proliferation varies among different hormone-responsive cell lines and among various subclones of the cell lines (67).

Loss of estrogenic stimulation can have potent antiproliferative effects, as observed clinically in some patients with ER-rich metastatic breast cancer who are treated by estrogen ablation or by antiestrogens. A similar effect can be achieved in animal models of breast cancer. Withdrawal of estrogen from MCF-7 human breast cancer xenografts in nude mice causes a greater than 70% regression of the tumor as a result of apoptotic cell death and reduced proliferative activity (100).

Treatment of MCF-7 and ZR-75 human breast cancer cells with estradiol causes a dose-dependent reduction in ER messenger RNA and protein (101,102). Downregulation of ER by estradiol is inhibited by a 100-fold excess of tamoxifen (101). Although estradiol-induced growth is accompanied by a reduction in ER levels of MCF-7 and ZR-75 cells, this is not true of the ER-positive breast cancer cell line MDA-MB-134. In this cell line, estrogen stimulates growth, but the ER levels are undiminished (103). In cell lines with low levels of ERs, such as T47D, estradiol can stimulate increased expression of the ERs (101). The ER response of different cell lines to estrogen appears to be variable.

Tamoxifen has biphasic, dose-dependent, estrogenic-antiestrogenic effects on breast cancer cell lines. At low concentrations, it is estrogenic and results in PR induction, and high concentrations inhibit cell growth and suppress PRs (94). Moreover, tamoxifen, like estrogen, can activate the transcription of genes that are regulated by an AP1 element (104), which may explain why long-term tamoxifen use increases the occurrence of uterine abnormalities (105).

Several studies have demonstrated the growth-inhibitory effect of progestins behaving similarly to tamoxifen by inducing cells to accumulate in the G_1 phase of the cell cycle (81,106–109). In MCF-7 and ZR-75 cells, estradiol induces PR synthesis, and treatment with progestin causes a reduction in PR levels and suppression of proliferative activity. The synthetic progestin R5020 inhibits estrogen-induced growth of an estrogen-responsive clone of T47D cells and R27 (an antiestrogen resistant variant of MCF-7 cells) (110). The antiestrogen activity of progesterone may be mediated through reduced replenishment of ERs and through the synthesis of 17β-hydroxysteroid dehydrogenase, which accelerates the metabolism of the potent estradiol to the weaker estrone (81).

Conversely, several studies report growth stimulatory effects of progestins in animal models (111–113) and in human mammary cancer cells (80,107,114–116). This proliferative effect has been attributed to the absence of phenol red from the culture media, with subsequent loss of progestin antagonism of estrogen-induced proliferation. When the same cell lines are grown in the presence of estrogen, the stimulatory effects of progestins are masked, and the inhibitory effects predominate (115,117).

The antiprogestin RU486 exerts antiproliferative activity against cultured breast cancer cells (118,119). RU486 acts as an antiprogestin and as an antiestrogen (116).

Although estrogens and progestins appear to play important roles in breast cell proliferation, many other hormones and growth factors are also potentially important in regulating proliferative activity in breast cells (Table 43.8). Insulin and estrogen exert synergistic effects on breast cancer cell proliferation (120,121). It has been suggested that estrogen directly stimulates cellular proliferation through induction of the *FOS* protooncogene. However, estrogen alone fails to induce genes from the *JUN* family that are essential for successful transcriptional activity. Insulin and insulin-like growth factors are efficient inducers of *JUN* and can act synergistically with estrogen to stimulate cellular proliferation. MCF-7 human breast cancer cells also respond to epidermal growth factor and insulin-like growth factor-1 by increasing cell proliferation.

CONCLUSIONS

Much remains to be learned about breast cell proliferation. The cellular distribution and level of expression of steroid hormone receptors in the breast are different than in the endometrium. The breast responds differently to steroid hormonal stimulation than the endometrium. Proliferative activity in the breast occurs throughout the menstrual cycle and peaks in the luteal phase, whereas proliferative activity in the endometrium occurs predominantly in the follicular phase. The effects of estrogens and progestins on the breast epithelium remain poorly understood. Proliferative activity plays a significant effect in the risk of developing breast cancer. Understanding the regulation of breast cell proliferation could be critically important to our understanding of breast cancer.

ACKNOWLEDGEMENTS

The work described in this chapter was supported in part by grants CA48780, CA14089, and CA50589 from the National Cancer Institute.

TABLE 43.8. *Hormones and growth factors potentially involved in breast development and differentiation*

Transforming growth factor-α
Transforming growth factor-β
Platelet-derived growth factor
Insulin-like growth factor 2
Insulin-like growth factor 1
Epidermal growth factor
Fibroblast growth factor
Growth hormone
Thyroid hormone
Glucocorticoids
Gonadotropins
Somatostatin
Heregulin
Progestin
Estrogen
Prolactin
Insulin

REFERENCES

1. Landis S, Murray T, Bolden S, Wingo P. Cancer statistics, 1998. *CA Cancer J Clin* 1998;48:6–30.
2. Cohen SM, Ellwein LB. Cell proliferation in carcinogenesis. *Science* 1990;249:1007–1011.
3. Henderson BE, Ross RK, Pike MC, Casagrande JT. Endogenous hormones as a major factor in human cancer. *Cancer Res* 1982;42:3232–3239.
4. Kelsey JL, Gammon MD, John EM. Reproductive factors and breast cancer. *Epidemiol Rev* 1993;15:36–47.
5. Moore DH, Moore DH, Moore CT. Breast carcinoma etiological factors. *Adv Cancer Res* 1983;40:189–253.
6. Trichopolous D, MacMahon B, Cole P. The menopause and breast cancer risk. *J Natl Cancer Inst* 1972;48:605–613.
7. MacMahon B, Cole P, Brown J. Etiology of human breast cancer: a review. *J Natl Cancer Inst* 1973;50:21–42.
8. Pike MC. Age-related factors in cancers of the breast, ovary, and endometrium. *J Chron Dis* 1987;40[Suppl II]:59S–69S.
9. Siiteri PK. Steroid hormones and endometrial cancer. *Cancer Res* 1978;38:4360.
10. Ferenczy A, Bertrand G, Gelfand MM. Proliferation kinetics of human endometrium during the normal menstrual cycle. *Am J Obstet Gynecol* 1979;133:859–867.
11. Key TJA, Pike MC. The dose-effect relationship between "unopposed" oestrogens and endometrial mitotic rate: its central role in explaining and predicting endometrial cancer risk. *Br J Cancer* 1988;57:205–212.
12. Longcope C. Metabolic clearance and blood production rates of estrogens in postmenopausal women. *Am J Obstet Gynecol* 1971;111:778–781.
13. MacDonald PC, Edman CD, Hemsell DL, Porter JC, Siiteri PK. Effect of obesity on conversion of plasma androstenedione to estrone in postmenopausal women with and without endometrial cancer. *Am J Obstet Gynecol* 1978;130:448–455.
14. Folsom AR, Kaye SA, Prineas RJ, Potter JD, Gapstur SM, Wallance RB. Increased incidence of carcinoma of the breast associated with abdominal adiposity in postmenopausal women. *Am J Epidemiol* 1990;131:794–803.
15. Key TJA, Pike MC. The role of oestrogens and progestagens in the epidemiology and prevention of breast cancer. *Eur J Cancer Clin Oncol* 1988;24:29–34.

16. Colditz GA, Hankinson SE, Hunter DJ, et al. The use of estrogens and progestins and the risk of breast cancer in postmenopausal women. *N Engl J Med* 1995;332: 1589–1593.
17. Bergkvist L, Adami H-O, Persson I, Hoover R, Schairer C. The risk of breast cancer after estrogen and estrogen-progestin replacement. *N Engl J Med* 1989; 321:293–297.
18. Collaborative Group on Hormonal Factors in Breast Cancer. Breast cancer and hormonal contraceptives. *Lancet* 1996;347:1713–1727.
19. Collaborative Group on Hormonal Factors in Breast Cancer. Breast cancer and hormonal contraceptives: further results. *Contraception* 1996;54(Suppl 3): 1S–106S.
20. Pike MC, Bernstein L, Spicer DV. Exogenous hormones and breast cancer risk. In: Niederhuber JE, ed. *Current therapy in oncology*. St. Louis: Mosby–Year Book, 1993.
21. Green S, Walter P, Kumar V, Krust ABJ-M, Argos P, Chambon P. Human oestrogen receptor cDNA: sequence, expression and homology to v-erb-A. *Nature* 1986;320:134–139.
22. Greene GL, Gilna P, Waterfield M, et al. Sequence and expression of human estrogen receptor complementary DNA. *Science* 1986;231:1150–1154.
23. Misrahi M, Atger M, d'Auriol L, et al. Complete amino acid sequence of the human progesterone receptor deduced from cloned cDNA. *Biochem Biophys Res Commun* 1987;143:740–748.
24. Kumar V, Green S, Staub A, Chambon P. Localisation of the oestradiol-binding and putative DNA-binding domains of the human oestrogen receptor. *EMBO J* 1986;5:2231–2236.
25. Green S, Chambon P. Oestradiol induction of a glucocorticoid-responsive gene by a chimaeric receptor. *Nature* 1987;325:75–78.
26. Evans RM. The steroid and thyroid hormone receptor superfamily. *Science* 1988; 240:889–895.
27. Tsai MJ, O'Malley BW. Molecular mechanisms of action of steroid/thyroid receptor superfamily. *Annu Rev Biochem* 1994;63:451–486.
28. Rehberger P, Rexin M, Gehring U. Heterotetrameric structure of the human progesterone receptor. *Proc Natl Acad Sci USA* 1992;89:8001–8005.
29. Segnitz B, Ghering U. Subunit structure of the nonactivated human estrogen receptor. *Proc Natl Acad Sci USA* 1995;92:2179–2183.
30. Tora L, Mullick A, Metzger D, Ponglikitmongkol M, Park I, Chambon P. The cloned human oestrogen receptor contains a mutation which alters its hormone binding properties. *EMBO J* 1989;8:1981–1986.
31. Giangrande P, Pollio G, McDonnell D. Mapping and characterization of the functional domains responsible for the differential activity of the A and B isoforms of the human progesterone receptor. *J Biol Chem* 1997;272:: 32889–32900.
32. Wahli W, Martinez E. Superfamily of steroid nuclear receptors: positive and negative regulators of gene expression. *FASEB J* 1991;5:2243–2249.
33. Xu J, Nawaz Z, Tsai S, Tsai M-J, O'Malley B. The extreme C terminus of progesterone contains a transcriptional repressor domain that functions through a putative corepressor. *Proc Natl Acad Sci USA* 1996;93:12195–12199.
34. Levenson A, Jordan C. Transfection of human estrogen receptor (ER) cDNA into ER-negative mammalian cell lines. *J Steroid Biochem Mol Biol* 1994;54: 229–239.
35. Fuller PJ. The steroid receptor superfamily: mechanisms of diversity. *FASEB J* 1991;5:3092–3099.
36. Picard D, Kumar V, Chambon P, Yamamoto K. Signal transduction by steroid hormones: nuclear localization is differentially regulated in estrogen and glucocorticoid receptors. *Cell Regul* 1990;1:291–299.
37. Guiochon-Mantel A, Lescop P, Chgristin-Maitre S, Losfelt H, Perrot-Applanat M, Milgrom E. Nucleocytoplasmic shuttling of the progesterone receptor. *EMBO J* 1991;10:3851–3859.
38. Kumar V, Green S, Stack G, Berry M, Jin JR, Chambon P. Functional domains of the human estrogen receptor. *Cell* 1987;51:941–951.
39. Ponglikitmongkol M, Green S, Chambon P. Genomic organization of the human oestrogen receptor gene. *EMBO J* 1988;7:3385–3388.
40. Kuiper GG, Enmark E, Pelto-Huikko M, Nilsson S, Gustafsson J. Cloning of a novel estrogen receptor expressed in rat prostate and ovary. *Proc Natl Acad Sci USA* 1996;93:5925–5930.
41. Mosselman S, Polman J, Dijkema R. ER-β: identification and characterization of a novel human estrogen receptor. *FEBS Lett* 1996;392:49–53.
42. Tremblay GB, Tremblay A, Copeland NG, Gilbert DJ, Jenkins NA, Labrie F, Giguere V. Cloning, chromosomal localization, and functional analysis of the murine estrogen receptor β. *Mol Endocrinol* 1997;11:353–365.
43. Enmark E, Pelto-Huikko M, Grandien K, et al. Human estrogen receptor β gene structure, chromosomal localization, and expression pattern. *Clin Endocrinol Metab* 1997;82:4258–4265.
44. Ogawa S, Inoue S, Watanabe T, et al. The complete primary structure of human estrogen receptor β (hERβ) and its heterodimerization with ER α *in vivo* and *in vitro*. *Biochem Biophys Res Commun* 1998;243:122–126.
45. Kuiper GG, Gustafsson J. The novel estrogen receptor-β subtype: potential role in the cell- and promoter-specific actions of estrogens and anti-estrogens. *FEBS Lett* 1997;410:87–90.
46. Misrahi M, Venenci PY, Saugier-Veber P, Sar S, Dessen P, Milgrom E. Structure of the human progesterone receptor gene. *Biochem et Biophys Acta* 1993;1216: 289–292.
47. Kastner P, Krust A, Turcotte B, Stropp U, Tora L, Gronemeyer H, Chambon P. Two distinct estrogen-regulated promoters generate transcripts encoding the two
48. functionally different human progesterone receptor forms A and B. *EMBO J* 1990;9:1603–1614.
48. Klein-Hitpass L, Ryffel G, Heitlinger E, Cato A. A 13 bp palindrome is a functional estrogen response element and interacts specifically with estrogen receptor. *Nucleic Acids Res* 1987;16:647–663.
49. Klock G, Strahle U, Schutz G. Oestrogen and glucocorticoid responsive elements are closely related but distinct. *Nature* 1987;329:734–736.
50. El-Ashry D, Chrysogelos S, Lippman M, Kern F. Estrogen induction of TGF-α is mediated by an estrogen response element composed of two imperfect palindromes. *J Steroid Biochem Mol Biol* 1996;59:261–269.
51. Wei LL, Norris BM, Baker CJ. An N-terminally truncated third progesterone receptor protein, PRc, forms heterodimers with PRB but interferes in PRB-DNA binding. *J Steroid Biochem Mol Biol* 1997;62:287–297.
52. Petersen OW, Hoyer PE, van Deurs B. Frequency and distribution of estrogen receptor-positive cells in normal, nonlactating human breast tissue. *Cancer Res* 1987;47:5748–5751.
53. Jacquemier JD, Hassoun J, Torrente M, Martin PM. Distribution of estrogen and progesterone receptors in healthy tissue adjacent to breast lesions at various stages: immunohistochemical study of 107 cases. *Breast Cancer Res Treat* 1990; 15:109–117.
54. Ricketts D, Turnbull L, Ryall G, et al. Estrogen and progesterone receptors in the normal female breast. *Cancer Res* 1991;51:1817–1822.
55. Williams G, Anderson E, Howell A, et al. Oral contraceptive (OCP) use increases proliferation and decreases oestrogen receptor content of epithelial cells in the normal human breast. *Int J Cancer* 1991;48:206–210.
56. Markopoulos C, Berger U, Wilson P, Gazet J-C, Coombes RC. Oestrogen receptor content of normal breast cells and breast carcinomas throughout the menstrual cycle. *BMJ* 1988;296:1349–1351.
57. Battersby S, Robertson BJ, Anderson TJ, King RJB, McPherson K. Influence of menstrual cycle, parity and oral contraceptive use on steroid hormone receptors in normal breast. *Br J Cancer* 1992;65:601–607.
58. Clarke R, Howell A, Potten C, Anderson E. Dissociation between steroid receptor expression and cell proliferation in the human breast. *Cancer Res* 1997;57: 4987–4991.
59. Pertschuk LP. *Immunocytochemistry for steroid receptors*. Boca Raton, FL: CRC Press, 1990.
60. Ballare C, Bravo A, Laucella S, et al. DNA synthesis in estrogen receptor-positive human breast cancer takes place preferentially in estrogen receptor-negative cells. *Cancer* 1989;64:842–848.
61. Fanelli M, Vargas-Roig L, Gago F, Teilo O, Lucero De Angelis R, Ciocca D. Estrogen receptors, progesterone receptors, and cell proliferation in human breast cancer. *Breast Cancer Res Treat* 1996;37:217–228.
62. Press MF, Greene GL. An immunocytochemical method for demonstrating estrogen receptor in human uterus using monoclonal antibodies to human estrophilin. *Lab Invest* 1984;50:480–486.
63. Press MF, Nousek-Goebl NA, King WJ, Herbst AL, Greene GL. Immunohistochemical assessment of estrogen receptor distribution in the human endometrium throughout the menstrual cycle. *Lab Invest* 1984;51:495–504.
64. Press MF, Udove JA, Greene GL. Progesterone receptor distribution in the human endometrium: analysis using monoclonal antibodies to human progestin receptor. *Am J Pathol* 1988;131:112–124.
65. Lessey BA, Killam AP, Metzger DA, Haney AF, Greene GL, McCarty KS Jr. Immunohistochemical analysis of human uterine estrogen and progesterone receptors throughout the menstrual cycle. *J Clin Endocrinol Metab* 1988;67: 334–340.
66. McCarty KS Jr. Proliferative stimuli in the normal breast: estrogens or progestins? *Hum Pathol* 1989;20:1137.
67. King RJB. A discussion of the roles of estrogen and progestin in human mammary carcinogenesis. *J Steroid Biochem Mol Biol* 1991;39:811–818.
68. Pike M, Urskin G, Spicer D. Experiments on proliferation of normal human breast tissue in nude mice do not show that progesterone does not stimulate breast cells. *Endocrinology* 1996;137:1505–1506.
69. Laidlaw I, Clarke R, Howell A, Owen A, Potten C, Anderson E. The proliferation of normal human breast tissue implanted into athymic nude mice is stimulated by estrogen but not progesterone. *Endocrinology* 1995;136:164–171.
70. Masters JRW, Drife JO, Scarisbrick JJ. Cyclic variations of DNA synthesis in human breast epithelium. *J Natl Cancer Inst* 1977;58:1263–1265.
71. Meyer JS. Cell proliferation in normal human breast ducts, fibroadenomas, and other duct hyperplasias, measured by nuclear labeling with tritiated thymidine. *Hum Pathol* 1977;8:67–81.
72. Going JJ, Anderson TJ, Battersby S, MacIntyre CC. Proliferative and secretory activity in human breast during natural and artificial menstrual cycles. *Am J Pathol* 1988;130:193–204.
73. Potten CS, Watson RJ, Williams GT, et al. The effect of age and menstrual cycle upon proliferative activity of the normal human breast. *Br J Cancer* 1988;58: 163–170.
74. Anderson TJ, Battersby S, King RJB, McPherson K, Going JJ. Oral contraceptive use influences resting breast proliferation. *Hum Pathol* 1989;20:1139–1144.
75. Ferguson DJP, Anderson TJ. Morphologic evaluation of cell turnover in relation to the menstrual cycle in the "resting" human breast. *Br J Cancer* 1981;44: 177–181.
76. Anderson FJ, Ferguson DJP, Raab GM. Cell turnover in the "resting" human breast: influence of parity, contraceptive pill, age and laterality. *Br J Cancer* 1982;46:376–382.

77. Longacre TA, Bartow SA. A correlative morphologic study of human breast and endometrium in the menstrual cycle. *Am J Surg Pathol* 1986;10:382–393.

78. McManus MJ, Welsch CW. The effects of estrogen, progesterone, thyroxine, and human placental lactogen on DNA synthesis of human breast ductal epithelium maintained in athymic nude mice. *Cancer* 1984;54:1920–1927.

79. Clarke R, Howell A, Anderson E. Estrogen sensitivity of normal human breast tissue *in vivo* and implanted into athymic nude mice: analysis of the relationship between estrogen-induced proliferation and progesterone receptor expression. *Breast Cancer Res Treat* 1997;45:121–133.

80. Longman SM, Buehring GC. Oral contraceptives and breast cancer: *in vitro* effect of contraceptive steroids on human mammary cell growth. *Cancer* 1987;59:281–287.

81. Mauvais-Jarvis P, Kuttenn F, Gompel A. Anti-estrogen action of progesterone in breast tissue. *Breast Cancer Res Treat* 1986;8:179–187.

82. Cline JM, Soderqvist G, von Schoultz E, Skoog L, von Schoultz B. Effect of hormone replacement therapy on the mammary gland of surgically postmenopausal cynomolgus macaques. *Am J Obstet Gynecol* 1996;174:93–100.

83. Stanczyk JZ, Brenner PF, Mishell DR, Ortiz A, Gentzchein EKE, Goebelsmann U. A radioimmunoassay for norethindrone (NET): measurement of serum NET concentrations following ingestion of NET-containing oral contraceptive steroids. *Contraception* 1978;18:615–633.

84. Russo J, Gusterson BA, Rogers AE, Russo IH, Sellings SR, van Zwieten MJ. Comparative study of human and rat mammary tumorigenesis. *Lab Invest* 1990;62:244–278.

85. McCarty KS Jr, Miller LS, Cox EB, Konrath J, McCarty KS Sr. Estrogen receptor analyses: correlation of biochemical and immunohistohemical methods using monoclonal antireceptor antibodies. *Arch Pathol Lab Med* 1985;109:716–721.

86. Pertschuk LP, Eisenberg KB, Carter AC, Feldman JG. Immunohistologic localization of estrogen receptors in breast cancer with monoclonal antibodies: correlation with biochemistry and clinical endocrine response. *Cancer* 1985;55:1513–1518.

87. McClelland RA, Berger U, Miller LS, Powles TJ, Coombes RC. Immunocytochemical assay for estrogen receptor in patients with breast cancer: relationship to a biochemical assay and to outcome of therapy. *J Clin Oncol* 1986;4:1171–1176.

88. Jonat W, Maass HM, Stegner HE. Immunohistochemical measurement of estrogen receptors in breast cancer tissue. *Cancer Res* 1986;46[Suppl 8]:4296s–4298s.

89. Betta PG, Cosimi MF, Spinoglio G, Bobutti F. Determinazione immunocitochemica con anticorpo monoclonale dei recettori per estrogeni nel carcinoma della mammella in fase avanzata e correlazione con la risposta alla terapia antiestrogenica. *Pathologica* 1987;79:135.

90. De Lena M, Marzullo F, Simone G, et al. Correlation between ERICA and DCC assay in hormone receptor assessment of human breast cancer. *Oncology* 1988;45:308–312.

91. Pertschuk LP, Kim DS, Nayer K, et al. Immunocytochemical estrogen and progestin receptor assays in breast cancer with monoclonal antibodies. *Cancer* 1990;66:1663–1670.

92. Joseph H, Guy JM, Przywara L, Coombes RC, Kiang DP, Pertschuk LP. The usefulness of Abbott ER-ICA in predicting response to hormonal therapy in advanced breast cancer. *J Tumor Marker Oncol* 1987;2:83.

93. Lippman M, Bolan G, Huff K. The effects of estrogens and antiestrogens on hormone responsive human breast cancer in long term tissue culture. *Cancer Res* 1976;36:4595–4601.

94. Horwitz KB, Koseki Y, McGuire WL. Estrogen control of progesterone receptor in human breast cancer; role of estradiol and antiestrogen. *Endocrinology* 1978;103:1742–1751.

95. Edwards DP, Murthy SR, McGuire WL. Effects of estrogen and antiestrogen on DNA polymerase in human breast cancer. *Cancer Res* 1980;1:1722–1726.

96. Aitken SC, Lippman ME. Effects of estrogens and antiestrogens on growth regulatory enzymes in human breast cancer cells in tissue culture. *Cancer Res* 1985;45:1611–1620.

97. Berthois Y, Katzenellenbogen JA, Katzenellenbogen BS. Phenol red in tissue culture media is a weak estrogen: implications concerning the study of estrogen-responsive cells in culture. *Proc Natl Acad Sci USA* 1986;83:2496–2500.

98. Katzenellenbogen BS, Kendra KL, Norman MJ, Berthois Y. Proliferation, hormonal responsiveness, and estrogen receptor content of MCF-7 human breast cancer cells grown in the short-term and long-term absence of estrogens. *Cancer Res* 1987;47:4355–4360.

99. Bezwoda WR, Meyer K. Effect of alpha-interferon, 17 beta-estradiol and tamox-

ifen on estrogen receptor concentration and cell cycle kinetics of MCF-7 cells. *Cancer Res* 1990;50:5387–5391.

100. Kyprianou N, English HF, Davidson NE, Isaacs JT. Programmed cell death during regression of the MCF-7 human breast cancer following estrogen ablation. *Cancer Res* 1991;51:162–166.

101. Read LD, Greene GL, Katzenellenbogen BS. Regulation of estrogen receptor messenger ribonucleic acid and protein levels in human breast cancer cell lines by sex steroid hormones, their antagonists, and growth factors. *Mol Endocrinol* 1989;2:295–304.

102. Poulin R, Simard J, Labrie C, et al. Down-regulation of estrogen receptors by androgens in the ZR-75-1 human breast cancer cell line. *Endocrinology* 1989;125:392–399.

103. Reiner GC, Katzenellenbogen BS. Characterization of estrogen and progesterone receptors and the dissociated regulation of growth and progesterone receptor stimulation by estrogen in MDA-MB-134 human breast cancer cells. *Cancer Res* 1986;46:1124–1131.

104. Webb P, Lopez G, Uht R, Kusher P. Tamoxifen activation of the estrogen receptor/AP-1 pathway: potential origin for the cell-specific estrogen-like effects of antiestrogens. *Mol Endocrinol* 1995;9:443–456.

105. Kedar R, Bourne T, Powles T, et al. Effects of tamoxifen on uterus and ovaries of postmenopausal women in a randomised breast cancer prevention trial. *Lancet* 1994;343:1318–1321.

106. Allegra JC, Kiefer SM. Mechanisms of action of progestational agents. *Semin Oncol* 1985;12[Suppl 1]:3–5.

107. Braunsberg H, Coldham NG, Leake RE, Cowan SK, Wong W. Actions of a progestagen on human breast cancer cells: mechanisms of growth stimulation and inhibition. *Eur J Cancer Clin Oncol* 1987;23:563–571.

108. Sutherland RL, Hall RE, Pang GYN, Musgrove EA, Clarke CL. Effect of medroxyprogesterone acetate on proliferation and cell cycle kinetics of human mammary carcinoma cells. *Cancer Res* 1988;48:5084–5091.

109. Gill PG, Tilley WD, De Young NJ, Lensink IL, Dixon PD, Horsfall DJ. Inhibition of T-47-D human breast cancer cell growth by the synthetic progestin R5020: effects of serum, estradiol, insulin and EGF. *Breast Cancer Res Treat* 1991;20:53–62.

110. Vignon F, Bardon S, Chalbos D, Rochefort H. Antiestrogenic effect of R5020, a synthetic progestin in human breast cancer cells in culture. *J Clin Endocrinol Metab* 1983;56:1124–1130.

111. Kiss R, Paridaens RJ, Heuson JC, Danguy AJ. Effect of progesterone on cell proliferation in the MXT mouse hormone-sensitive mammary neoplasm. *J Natl Cancer Inst* 1986;77:173–177.

112. Manni A, Badger B, Wright C, Ahmed SR, Dehmers LM. Effects of progestins on growth of experimental breast cancer in culture: interaction with estradiol and prolactin and involvement of the polyamine pathway. *Cancer Res* 1987;47:3066–3071.

113. Robinson SP, Jordan VC. Reversal of the antitumor effects of tamoxifen by progesterone in the 7,12-dimethylbenzanthracene induced rat mammary carcinoma model. *Cancer Res* 1987;47:5386–5390.

114. Braunsberg H, Coldham NG, Wong W. Hormonal therapies for breast cancer: can progestogens stimulate growth? *Cancer Lett* 1986;30:213–218.

115. Hissom JR, Moore MR. Progestin effects on growth in the human breast cancer cell line T47D; possible therapeutic implications. *Biochem Biophys Res Commun* 1987;145:706–711.

116. Hissom JR, Bowden RT, Moore MR. Effects of progestins, estrogens and antihormones on growth and lactate dehydrogenase in the human cell line T47D. *Endocrinology* 1989;125:418–423.

117. Clarke CL, Sutherland RL. Progestin regulation of cellular proliferation. *Endocr Rev* 1990;11:266–301.

118. Bardon S, Vignon F, Chalbos D, Rochefort H. RU486, a progestin and glucocorticoid antagonist, inhibits the growth of breast cancer cells via the progesterone receptor. *J Clin Endocrinol Metab* 1985;50:692–697.

119. Gill PG, Vignon F, Bardon S, Derocq D, Rochefort H. Difference between R5020 and the antiprogestin RU486 in antiproliferative effects on human breast cancer cells. *Breast Cancer Res Treat* 1987;10:37–45.

120. Van der Burg B, Rutteman GR, Blankenstein MA, de Laat SW, van Zoelen EJJ. Mitogenic stimulation of human breast cancer cells in a growth factor-defined medium: synergistic action of insulin and estrogen. *J Cell Physiol* 1988;134:101–108.

121. Sutherland RL, Lee CSL, Feldman RS, Musgrove EA. Regulation of breast cancer cell cycle progression by growth factors, steroids and steroid antagonists. *J Steroid Biochem Mol Biol* 1992;41:315–321.

Treatment of the Postmenopausal Woman: Basic and Clinical Aspects, Second Edition, edited by Rogerio A. Lobo, Lippincott Williams & Wilkins, Philadelphia © 1999.

CHAPTER 44

Influence of Sex Hormones on Breast Cancer Risk and Mortality

Ronald K. Ross and Leslie Bernstein

Breast cancer is a disease whose development is highly dependent on the hormones associated with ovarian function (1). Although the risk of breast cancer in U.S. women increases throughout life, it is in effect a disease of the reproductive period. Breast cancer incidence begins to increase in women in their early 20s; thereafter, the rate of increase is very rapid until around age 50, at which time ovarian hormone production ceases, and the rate of increase in breast cancer incidence slows dramatically (2). Although breast cancer incidence rates continue to increase throughout the remainder of life, the rate of increase in postmenopausal U.S. women is only about 10% to 15% that of the premenopausal period (Fig. 44.1) (3).

Many hormones are involved in ovarian function, but there is little doubt that the estrogens are largely responsible for the close association of ovarian activity and breast cancer. We reviewed the extensive epidemiologic and experimental evidence linking estrogens and breast cancer (1). Among the most important risk factors for breast cancer are age at menarche and age at menopause. Breast cancer risk is reduced by approximately 10% for each year that menarche is delayed and is increased by a comparable amount for each year the menopause is delayed, whether menopause occurs naturally or through surgical intervention.

Postmenopausal obesity is also an important breast cancer risk factor. Evidence is strong that this effect is caused by the close association between obesity and estrogen production postmenopausally (4). The principal

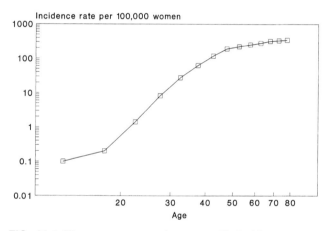

FIG. 44.1. The average annual age-specific incidence rates for female breast cancer in Los Angeles County between 1972 and 1987 is depicted on log scales.

source of estrogens after cessation of ovarian function is fat cells, which contain an enzyme (aromatase) that converts the adrenal androgen androstenedione to estrone. Estrone can be converted to the more biologically potent estrogen, estradiol. It is the influence of obesity on breast cancer risk postmenopausally that is thought to account for the continued slow rise in breast cancer incidence after age 50, despite the cessation of or marked reduction in ovarian function experienced by most women by this age. In Japan, where the prevalence of postmenopausal obesity is low, breast cancer incidence remains relatively constant after age 50 (5).

Estrogens are established carcinogens in experimental settings, increasing the incidence of mammary tumors in various animal models, even in the absence of any additional chemical carcinogen (6). Evidence strongly suggests that populations at higher risk of breast cancer, such

R. K Ross, L. Bernstein: Department of Preventive Medicine, University of Southern California School of Medicine, Los Angeles, California 90089.

as U.S. white women or first-degree relatives of breast cancer patients, have higher circulating or excretion levels of estrogen than women at lower risk, such as Asian women living in Japan or China (7) or women without a family history of breast cancer (8), respectively.

Although the epidemiologic and experimental evidence is not nearly as substantial as for the estrogens, progestogens may also play a role in human breast cancer development (9). The most important data supporting this possible link have come from studies of the relation between mitotic activity in breast epithelium and the menstrual cycle (10). Mitotic activity peaks during the luteal phase of the cycle between days 20 and 25, at the time of maximum progesterone stimulation. This is important, because mitotic activity is a cause of human cancer (11).

Epidemiologic data also seem to support a role of progestogens in human breast carcinogenesis. For example, even though age at menarche and age at menopause are important breast cancer risk factors, the cumulative number of ovulatory cycles rather than the total number of years of menstrual activity appears to be the more critical factor (12). Women who establish regular ovulatory cycles quickly have a substantially higher breast cancer risk than women who start menstruating at the same age but take longer intervals to begin having regular ovulatory cycles (13). A small part of the low risk of breast cancer among Japanese women may result from the longer average cycle length (and therefore fewer ovulatory cycles) of Japanese women during their reproductive years (1).

In this setting of strong evidence that estrogens and probably progestogens influence a woman's risk of developing breast cancer, the relation between hormone replacement therapy (HRT), in the form of unopposed estrogen or estrogen in combination with progestogen, becomes of great public health interest and importance. Before reviewing the considerable epidemiologic literature on this correlation and discussing some of the complex methodologic issues that must be addressed in studying this possible association, it is useful to consider our current understanding of the relation between exogenous estrogens and progestogens administered for reasons other than replacement therapy and breast cancer risk.

ORAL CONTRACEPTIVES

Numerous epidemiologic studies have examined the association between oral contraceptives and the risk of breast cancer. Results have been published from more than 50 epidemiologic studies without uncovering evidence of any strong overall correlation (14). The most detailed analyses of the world's extensive literature on the relation between oral contraceptive use and breast cancer was conducted and reported by the Collaborative Group on Hormonal Factors in Breast Cancer (14,15). The Collaborative Group arranged for individual data on oral contraceptive use from more than 53,000 women with breast cancer and more than 100,000 control women from 54 studies around the world to be sent to a centralized unit for collation, checking, and analysis. (This represents about 90% of all epidemiologic data on this question until that time.) There was one main conclusion from this massive effort. Women who are taking oral contraceptives have a modest increase in breast cancer incidence (relative risk [RR] = 1.24, 95% CI = 1.15, 1.33), which gradually dissipates after cessation of use (1 to 4 years after stopping, RR = 1.16; 5–9 years after stopping, RR = 1.07; 10+ years after stopping, RR = 1.01). Women who used oral contraceptives at a young age (before age 20) had higher risks than women who used them at older ages for comparable duration of use. Breast cancers diagnosed in women taking oral contraceptives were, on average, diagnosed at a less advanced stage clinically than in women who had never used oral contraceptives.

We have argued for several years that the periods of greatest concern regarding oral contraceptive use and their possible impact on breast cancer risk are the postmenarcheal and the perimenopausal periods. These are both periods of reproductive life when anovulatory menstrual cycles are common. Such cycles are characterized by lower integrated levels during a monthly period of progesterone and of estrogen than are normal ovulatory cycles. During these periods of life, the hormonal exposure to breast tissue resulting from oral contraceptive use is likely to be greater, on average, than that experienced by the same woman when not using oral contraceptives.

Metanalyses (a statistical technique for combining risk estimates from multiple studies into a single risk estimate) of oral contraceptive use early in reproductive life support a small but important increase in risk of about 3.1% for each year of pill use, relative to a woman of comparable age not taking the pill (3). However, in a large British study, which examined women younger than 36 at breast cancer diagnosis and controls matched on exact age, a highly significant trend in risk of breast cancer was associated with increasing total duration of oral contraceptive use, regardless of whether that use occurred before or after a woman's first term pregnancy (i.e., regardless of whether the oral contraceptive use was very early or later in reproductive life) (16). The women using oral contraceptives with relatively low estrogen content (less than 50 µg/pill) appeared to have a lower risk of breast cancer than women using oral contraceptives with higher estrogen content per pill (17).

Fewer studies have examined breast cancer risk associated with oral contraceptive use around the time of menopause. However, five studies found an elevation in risk with such use, albeit with a wide range of reported relative risk estimates (18–22).

Even though metanalyses of oral contraceptive use in the early reproductive years and summary analyses of oral contraceptive use in the late reproductive years suggest that use during both periods conveys at least a small increment in risk of breast cancer, the largest U.S. study, the Contraceptive and Steroid Hormone (CASH) study, a collaborative case-control study involving eight areas of the United States, found no increased risk of breast cancer for any duration of oral contraceptive use category overall, early in reproductive life or before a term pregnancy (23).

The combined evidence suggests at most a very modest association between breast cancer risk and use of the older, higher steroid dosage contraceptive formulations, even in subgroups of the population for whom larger effects could be predicted. With newer, lower-dose formulations, there is reason for some optimism about a modest reduction in breast cancer risk in oral contraceptive users. Some published data indicate that women who carry mutations of the *BRCA1* and *BRCA2* breast cancer susceptibility genes may be at particularly high risk of breast cancer if they have used oral contraceptives (24). This finding, if confirmed, has substantial public health implications.

OTHER EXOGENOUS HORMONE USE

Depo-medroxyprogesterone acetate (DMPA) is a long-acting, injectable contraceptive that is widely used outside the United States. An advisory committee of the U.S. Food and Drug Administration has recommended approving DMPA for general use. Such approval was delayed for an extended period because of concerns about its carcinogenicity. DMPA has been shown to induce malignant breast nodules in female beagle dogs (25) and endometrial carcinomas in rhesus monkeys (26).

If estrogens alone are a cause of breast cancer, DMPA should decrease breast cancer risk, because its primary mode of action is to inhibit ovulation, reducing endogenous estrogen levels without providing any exogenous estrogen supplement as occurs with oral contraceptives (9). A case-control study conducted in Costa Rica reported an overall statistically significant increased risk of breast cancer associated with use of DMPA (users had a 2.6-fold increase in risk relative to nonusers), and it appeared that risk increased with increasing duration of use (27). A case-control study in New Zealand found no overall increase in breast cancer risk in women 25 to 54 years of age using DMPA but did find a twofold increase in risk among the subgroup of women 25 to 34 years of age (28). However, the largest study, an international World Health Organization-sponsored study, found no consistent association between DMPA use and breast cancer risk overall or among specific age groups (29). Although there remains a need for additional data to determine whether DMPA increases breast cancer risk overall or in specific subgroups, existing evidence is convincing that DMPA does not reduce risk.

TABLE 44.1. *Effect of tamoxifen treatment on the risk of primary contralateral breast cancer in women with postmenopausal breast cancer: results from five randomized controlled clinical trials*

Study	Rate of contralateral breast cancer per 100 women followed per year	
	Tamoxifen group	Control group
NATO (36)	0.43 (564)[a]	0.38 (567)
Ribeiro and Swindell (37)	0.34 (282)	0.37 (306)
Fisher et al. (38)	0.51 (1318)	1.18 (1326)
Fornander et al. (39)	>0.43 (931)	>0.78 (915)
Stewart and Knight (40)	0.27 (282)	0.38 (531)

NATO, Nolvadex and Adjuvant Trial Organization.
[a]Numbers in parentheses are numbers of patients randomized.
Adapted from ref. 32.

Tamoxifen is a synthetic, nonsteroidal antiestrogen in breast tissue that has proven effective in the treatment of breast cancer (30). Tamoxifen blocks estrogen receptors at the level of the tumor by competitively inhibiting estradiol binding. In 1986, Cuzick et al. suggested that use of tamoxifen be extended to healthy postmenopausal women at high risk of breast cancer for the purpose of primary prevention of this disease. The most compelling argument to extend the use of tamoxifen to such women was the substantially lower risk of contralateral primary breast cancer observed among women receiving adjuvant tamoxifen therapy for breast cancer. Spicer et al. (32) summarized these data in tamoxifen-treated versus control patients from five randomized trials, which overall showed a 38% reduction in risk of contralateral breast cancer (Table 44.1). This sharp reduction in risk occurred even though tamoxifen was used in these trials for only relatively short periods. Based on this observation and in conjunction with the extensive epidemiologic and experimental evidence summarized previously supporting a major role for estrogens in breast cancer development, large national clinical trials for the hormonal chemoprevention of breast cancer in healthy women using tamoxifen were undertaken in the United States, United Kingdom, and Italy. Results from these three trials were reported. The U.S. trial that targeted women at high risk of breast cancer based on a risk equivalent to that of a 60-year-old women found a 49% reduction in breast cancer incidence among women randomized to the treatment arm of 20 mg of tamoxifen daily, compared with women randomized to placebo (33). Preliminary results from the United Kingdom and Italian studies that targeted women at average risk and hysterectomized women, respectively, found no substantial risk modifications, and these trials continue (34,35).

HORMONE REPLACEMENT THERAPY

HRT in the form of unopposed estrogen therapy became widely popular in the United States in the 1960s and early 1970s (41). By 1974, there were nearly 30 million prescriptions of estrogen replacement therapy (ERT) being filled annually in the United States, and the most popular brand, the conjugated equine estrogen Premarin, had become the fourth most frequently prescribed drug in the country. Usage decreased dramatically in the mid-1970s, after the initial reports showing that ERT caused endometrial cancer (42,43). As subsequent studies demonstrated the enormous benefits to be derived from such treatment in the form of reduced mortality from cardiovascular disease (44), possibly from cerebrovascular disease (45), and from reduced morbidity from osteoporotic fractures (46), the prevalence of use began to increase again (Fig. 44.2). Overall use has now surpassed that of the peak period of the 1970s. As evidence began to accumulate that the addition of a progestogen to ERT would reduce risk of endometrial cancer relative to use of unopposed estrogen, progestogen prescriptions for menopausal women have also increased rapidly. By the mid-1980s, nearly 30% of all noncontraceptive estrogen prescriptions were already combined with a progestogen prescription (Fig. 44.2) (47).

In the past two decades, there have been more than 50 publications on the relation between various forms of HRT and breast cancer. These, or some subset of these, have been summarized in various ways, but the conclusions from these summarized results have been generally comparable. None of these studies, when considered individually or jointly, has demonstrated any dramatic increase in breast cancer associated with use of ERT, even after an extended duration of treatment. However, even a small increase in breast cancer risk is important to document, given the underlying morbidity and mortality associated with breast cancer and the psychosocial implications of a breast cancer diagnosis in an individual patient.

Persson et al. (48) summarized the literature on this issue by looking simultaneously at the point estimates of risk for ERT users overall and for "long-term" users versus nonusers from each of the individual studies examining this association. Among the 19 studies included in this analysis, five found small but statistically significant increases in breast cancer risk among ERT users compared with nonusers, whereas the others found no significant overall change in risk. Although the definition of long-term use has varied across studies, results were somewhat more consistent when Persson et al. (48) examined the effects of long-term use on risk, with most studies finding at least a modest (typically less than twofold) increased risk of breast cancer among those who have used ERT for extended periods.

Metanalytic statistical techniques were developed to increase the power of clinical trials by combining results across multiple studies. When applied to observational epidemiologic studies, metanalysis allows investigators to combine risk estimates from multiple studies into a single summary risk estimate. Although this summary risk estimate can be weighted by the size and exposure prevalence of the various study populations contributing to it, this summary risk cannot be weighted by any other methodologic strengths or weaknesses of the individual studies. When metanalysis is applied to observational studies (as opposed to clinical trials), the results should be interpreted especially cautiously. Several metanalyses have been conducted on the relation between ERT and breast cancer. One was conducted by investigators at the Centers for Disease Control in Atlanta, Georgia (44). This particular analysis concluded that, across all studies, there was some evidence of a duration-related increase in breast cancer risk associated with ERT use but that this effect was of relatively small magnitude, with about a 10% increase in risk for each 5 years of therapy relative to nonusers. Another metanalysis concluded that this duration effect, if it exists at all, is even smaller (50).

Pike et al. (3) conducted a third metanalysis that was limited to the 10 population-based epidemiologic studies of ERT and breast cancer published at that time (Table 44.2). They omitted the results of the many hospital-based studies (in which controls are hospitalized patients with other diseases), concluding that the magnitude for potential bias was too great in this type of study, especially when small relative risks are being investigated. Nine of the 10 studies included in this analysis showed a positive association between use of ERT and breast cancer risk, with the results from five of these achieving statistical significance. Across all studies, breast cancer risk increased 3.1% for each year of estrogen therapy. Only the seven U.S. studies permitted a quantitative analysis of the effects of conjugated equine estrogen. When only these studies were considered, the increment in risk associated with each year of estrogen therapy decreased to 2.2%, but the results remained highly statistically significant (Table 44.2).

Pike et al. tried to determine whether such an increment in risk is reasonable based on the effects of conju-

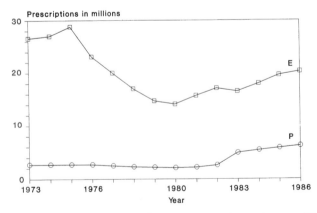

FIG. 44.2. The number of noncontraceptive estrogen (E) and progestogen (P) prescriptions written between 1973 and 1986.

TABLE 44.2. *Population-based studies of the effect of menopausal estrogen replacement therapy on breast cancer risk*

Study (type of study)	Cases/controls	Percentage of controls ever exposed	Percent change in breast cancer risk/year of HRT use (95% confidence limits)	
Ross et al. (51) (case-control)	131/262	48	+10.3	(0.9, 20.4)
Hoover et al. (52) (case-control)	345/611	29	+6.7	(1.4, 12.3)
Hiatt et al. (53) (case-control)	119/119	90	+5.7	(−0.4, 12.3)
Brinton et al. (54) (case-control)	1960/2258	52	+1.9	(0.4, 3.4)
Nomura et al. (55) (case-control)	341/341	56	+0.7	(−3.9, 5.5)
Wingo et al. (56) (case-control)	1369/1645	32	+0.1	(−0.5, 0.7)
Ewertz (57) (case-control)	596/568	28	+9.3	(3.3, 15.7)
Rohan and McMichael (58) (case-control)	281/288	24	-2.3	(−20.6, 20.3)
Bergkvist et al. (59) (case-control)	219/653	100	+8.5	(0.4, 17.3)
Colditz et al. (60) (cohort)	722/—	47	+2.0	(−0.3, 4.3)
Weighted average	All studies: studies permitting analysis for CEE at 0.625 mg/day		+3.1 +2.2	(1.2, 5.1) (0.4, 3.9)

CEE, conjugated equine estrogen; HRT, hormone replacement therapy.
Adapted from ref. 3.

gated equine estrogen administration on circulating levels of estradiol, the most biologically potent endogenous human estrogen fraction. In postmenopausal U.S. women, the mean serum level of non–sex hormone—binding globulin (non-SHBG)–bound estradiol (i.e., bioavailable estradiol) is approximately 12 pg/mL in the absence of any exogenous estrogen therapy (61). After age 50, breast cancer incidence rates increase about 2.1% per year (62). Use of conjugated equine estrogen approximately doubles the serum level of non-SHBG-bound estradiol (63). Pike et al. argued that an incremental increase of roughly 2% per year in breast cancer risk (i.e., a doubling of the usual increase) from the use of conjugated equine estrogen is therefore reasonable (3).

The Collaborative Group on Hormonal Factors in Breast Cancer used a variation of the metanalysis approach, and their results provide the most detailed summary data available on this association (64). This large group of investigators was able to collect raw individual data from 51 of the studies conducted on this association, which they believe constituted over 90% of all data available. The combined analysis included 52,705 women with breast cancer and 108,411 control women. Only the group of 54,000 women whose age at menopause based on loss of ovarian function could be determined (women, for example, who had had a hysterectomy without oophorectomy were excluded) were included in the final analysis. One-third of these women had used HRT, and one-third of these had used HRT for 5 years or longer. The summary findings were of interest. The risk of breast cancer increased approximately 2.3% for each year of use of HRT, so that women who used HRT for an average of 11 years (the average use in women who used HRT for more than five years) had a 35% increase in risk relative to women who never used replacement therapy. These

combined data were sufficiently powerful that potential risk modifiers could be examined in some detail. The only strong risk modifier was body weight (body mass index), such that thin women (<60 kg) showed a 65% increase in risk with 5 years of use of HRT, compared with 32% for women weighing between 60 and 69 kg and just 5% for women weighing 70 kg or more. A reasonable explanation for the reduced influence of HRT on breast cancer risk in heavier women is the higher endogenous estrogen levels in such women.

Other breast cancer risk factors that had previously been suggested as risk modifiers in small single studies, including a history of benign breast disease, type of menopause, and a family history of breast cancer had no substantial risk modification in these extensive combined data. The latter factor is of special interest, because there is some evidence that oral contraceptive use may enhance penetrance in women carrying a mutation of the *BRCA1* or *BRCA2* breast cancer susceptibility genes (24). The data from the combined analysis do not totally address this issue, because women with a mutation in either of these genes comprise only a small subset of the women reporting a family history of breast cancer; moreover, it is likely that usage patterns of HRT differ in complex ways from the general population among women with a family history of breast cancer.

Other issues of widespread interest related to the association between HRT and breast cancer were addressed in some detail in this combined analysis. One group of investigators have argued that the effect of HRT on breast cancer risk is limited to women who are current users (65), but most individual studies have had insufficient sample sizes to evaluate the effects of current use independent of the highly correlated variable of duration of use. In the combined analyses, current use was associated with a 2.6% increase in breast cancer per year of use, whereas women who had stopped use 1 to 5 years earlier showed a 1.8% increase in risk per year of use. Women who had stopped use many years previously still had a 0.7% increase in risk, although this risk was not statistically significant from that of nonusers (64). Nonetheless, these results suggest that, even though risk dissipates relative to nonusers of HRT as time elapses since last use, risk may never reach that of a lifetime nonuser.

In the combined collaborative analysis, no details were reported on types of HRT and dosage patterns as they relate to risk, but it was stated that little difference in risk was detected by type of estrogen preparation or usual daily pill dose. It is reasonable to expect that, if ERT increases breast cancer risk, this effect would be related to usual pill dose. However, there is good reason to believe that any dose-response effect may not be strictly linear. Pike et al. (3) observed that an increase in conjugated equine estrogen dose is associated with an increase in serum estrogens and with an increase in SHBG, so that the biologically effective increase in dose may be less than the apparent increase. For example, a doubling of conjugated equine estrogen dose from 0.625 to 1.25 mg results in less than a 10% increase in the circulating non-SHBG-bound estradiol level (3).

Few data exist on the relation between combination HRT and breast cancer. The best known data on this issue come from a large cohort of Swedish women known through prescription records to have taken some form of HRT. Bergkvist et al. (59) reported that the subgroup of these women who had used combination therapy for more than 6 years had a 4.4-fold increase in risk relative to women with no history of use of HRT. However, there was no evidence of any increase in risk with shorter-term use and the 4.4-fold increase was based on only 10 patients and did not reach statistical significance. Because of the limited data on the overall association between combination therapy and breast cancer, there are no adequate published data on the effects of different formulations, schedules, and doses on risk of breast cancer.

In the Collaborative Group combined analysis, about 12% of all HRT use was a combination of estrogen and progestogen (64). Although the results indicated some difference in risk levels between estrogen-only use compared with combined HRT use for comparable duration categories (typically higher risk with combination therapy), these differences were not marked. Nonetheless, even relatively small differences in risk would have important biologic and public health implications. Even in this large, combined dataset, the numbers of combined HRT users were sufficiently few, especially in the long-duration categories, that it could not be determined with confidence whether any observed differences from ERT risk levels were real. Additional detailed, large-scale studies of combination therapy and breast cancer must be a continued high priority.

Limited data are available on the relation between HRT and breast cancer mortality. In the Swedish cohort study of Bergkvist et al., women who were current HRT users when they developed breast cancer had a 5-year relative survival of 84%, compared with 74% for women who had discontinued such therapy before diagnosis (66). Although these investigators provided no specific data on breast cancer mortality rates in current estrogen users compared with past users, these survival data suggest that the mortality experience from breast cancer among women using replacement therapy in this cohort is more favorable than the morbidity experience (59). Several other groups have observed a reduction in mortality from breast cancer among ERT users overall (44,67), although no one has reported yet on the breast cancer mortality experience among women who have used replacement therapy for extended periods. One possible explanation for this apparent anomaly between incidence and mortality effects, consistent with what has been proposed to explain a similar phenomenon occurring with endometrial cancer (68), is that HRT users are diagnosed with breast (or endometrial) cancer at an earlier stage, on average, because as a group such women are under closer medical surveillance than nonusers.

Another important observation from the combined analysis described earlier was the clear relation between HRT use and extent of disease at diagnosis. Breast cancers among women who used HRT were significantly more likely to be localized to the breast than were breast cancers among women who had never used HRT (64). Nonetheless, even among women whose tumors were not localized, risk increased significantly with increasing duration of HRT use. Although the most obvious explanation for an excess risk of localized versus more advanced tumors in women using HRT is that women who use HRT are under increased medical surveillance (i.e., physician examination or mammography on a more regular basis) than women who do not take HRT; alternative explanations are possible. It is feasible that replacement therapy leads to a detection bias, although no data exist to suggest that screening by mammography or by other means picks up breast tumors that would otherwise not come to medical attention. It is also plausible that the biologic behavior or in the response to therapy of breast cancers diagnosed in women taking HRT is fundamentally different from that of unexposed women.

It is surprising that, given all the intense interest in the association between use of HRT and breast cancer and despite the evidence supporting the possibility of a cause and effect association, it has been exceedingly difficult to prove that a real association exists. At least part of the reason for this may include several complex methodologic issues, which must be addressed to adequately study this possible association. The most important of these are related to statistical power, the strong likelihood of confounding variables, and the selection of an appropriate comparison group.

Although it is sensible to expect to find an association between HRT and breast cancer, based on empiric data and on hormonally based statistical models of breast cancer incidence (1), the anticipated increment in risk is small. Metanalyses suggest that the increment may be on the order of 5% to 15% for each 5 years of treatment with the most commonly prescribed formulations. Such small effects are at the limits of detectability of epidemiologic studies, because it is extremely difficult to cull these small effects from confounding by other breast cancer risk factors. Moreover, the detection of such small effects with statistical precision requires thousands of study subjects, if the prevalence of long-term exposure is small in the population. Few individual epidemiologic studies of this association have had sufficient statistical power to detect such small risk levels overall, much less to examine possible interactions with other risk factors.

Breast cancer risk factors can serve as risk modifiers of the association between HRT and breast cancer and as potentially powerful confounders. A confounding variable is one that is related to the exposure of interest (i.e., HRT) and to the disease in question (i.e., breast cancer), which can explain some or all of any observed association between them. A list of some of the likely possible confounders in studies of the relation between HRT and breast cancer is provided in Table 44.3. With the exception of factors related to social class, the expected effect of inadequate adjustment for these confounding variables is to *underestimate* the true strength of the correlation. Among all the possible confounding variables listed in the table, age at menopause may be the most important, partly because it is so difficult to accurately assess (especially in women using replacement therapy, because one of the side effects is menstrual bleeding). Women with breast cancer would be expected, on average, to have a later average age at menopause than healthy control women, because age at menopause is an established

TABLE 44.3. *Possible confounding variables in studies of hormone replacement therapy and breast cancer*

Variable	Expected effect of "adjustment" on relative risk
Age	Increase, decrease[a]
Weight	Increase
Age at menopause	Increase
Type of menopause	Increase
Family history of breast cancer	Increase
Benign breast disease history	Increase
Social class	Decrease

Breast cancer rates increase for women between 20 and 50 years of age but decreases after ovarian hormone production ceases.

[a]From ref. 69, with permission.

breast cancer risk factor (1). Late menopause is also associated with lower use of HRT in most populations, and failure to adjust for this variable overestimates the prevalence of such use in controls (relative to cases) and lead to an underestimation of the actual relative risk; proper adjustment correctly increases the relative risk, but this can only occur if the variable has been measured accurately.

Most studies that have explored the relation between HRT and breast cancer have been case-control studies. Among the most critical determinants about whether a case-control study can provide an accurate assessment of an exposure-outcome association is the appropriateness of the control selection algorithm in terms of providing an unbiased estimate of the prevalence of the exposure of interest in the healthy "source" population. Among recent case-control studies, there have been a wide variety of strategies used for selecting controls, and even small biases (in providing an accurate measure of the exposure prevalence) can cause a small association to be observed when there is none or no association to be observed when a small one exists. Generally, case-control studies that have used hospitalized patients as controls have found lower risk levels than those that have drawn their controls from the healthy population (1). The reasons for the relatively clear distinction in the net results between these two general design strategies is unknown, but it emphasizes the importance of selecting an appropriate comparison population.

Although it is generally agreed among the scientific and clinical community who are seriously engaged in HRT research or therapeutic implementations that, on a population basis, the benefits of such therapy (especially in terms of cardioprevention and protection from bone loss) outweigh the risks (especially in terms of endometrial cancer and breast cancer), there are subgroups of women (e.g., thin women, women with a family history of breast cancer) for whom the balance of the risk-benefit equation, although still positive, may be less favorable. The group that has received the greatest attention in terms of the risk-benefit equation is women with a personal history of breast cancer. Traditionally, HRT use has been widely regarded as absolutely contraindicated in such women. There are several related reasons for this. The primary reason for this clinical dogma is that breast cancer is estrogen responsive and a late metastasizing disease. Estrogen even in low doses may shorten the time to recurrence. Individuals with prior breast cancer are at increased risk for a second primary breast cancer, and because HRT is associated with a small increase in breast cancer in the population as a whole, it is possible that this risk may be enhanced in women with a personal history of breast cancer.

Standard practice is to discontinue HRT in women when they develop breast cancer, but little information is available about whether HRT increases the risk of breast cancer recurrence. There are indirect data that can help provide a perspective on this issue. Obesity is associated with increased circulating estrogen levels in postmenopausal women. Studies suggest a strong adverse effect of obesity on the risk of recurrence in postmenopausal women (70,71). However, obesity also appears to increase risk of recurrence in premenopausal women in whom estrogen levels are unaffected by weight (72). This observation raises some doubts about whether this adverse effect is mediated by estrogens, although many patients who are premenopausal at diagnosis become anovulatory temporarily after treatment or permanently during follow-up.

Pike and Spicer argued, based on the effects of obesity on recurrence in postmenopausal women, the impact of weight on circulating estrogen levels, and the circulating levels of estrogen in women using HRT, that the effect of HRT on recurrence in women with a history of breast cancer could be profound (on the order of doubling the expected rate in women with early-stage disease) (32). An equally strong piece of evidence that HRT may adversely affect recurrence rates is the observation that oophorectomy in premenopausal women with breast cancer reduces recurrence by 30% and death by 28% (73). Spicer and Pike have made the only serious attempt to establish a risk-benefit equation for HRT use in women with a history of breast cancer by weighing hypothetical risks of recurrence against the benefits to be derived from cardiovascular disease and hip fracture mortality (32). In women with breast cancer, the risk-benefit equation is greatly altered compared with healthy women. In women with a personal history of breast cancer, even low-risk patients with good prognoses, breast cancer remains the greatest single contributor to mortality for many years after diagnosis. In patients with node-negative disease and primary tumors less than 1 cm in diameter, for example, the mortality rate from breast cancer averages approximately 1% per year for the first 10 years after diagnosis and roughly 0.7% per year for the next 10 (32). Because the estimated annual mortality benefit from HRT use up to age 70 never exceeds 0.07%, this benefit would be completely negated by as little as a 10% increase in recurrence as a result of HRT use. This increase in recurrence is much less than predicted by the effects of obesity (32).

CONCLUSIONS

Although there have been few studies with adequate statistical power or that have been otherwise totally sound methodologically, the balance of evidence suggests that a small duration-related increase in breast cancer risk associated with ERT. Future studies will continue to have difficulty in establishing this relation beyond any reasonable doubt, because the alteration in risk is at the limits of detectability of epidemiologic research. There is,

nonetheless, a real need to understand better any modifying effect of other breast cancer risk factors (e.g., family history of breast cancer) on the ERT and breast cancer association. There also is a great need to better understand the apparent disparity between the effects of replacement therapy on breast cancer mortality compared with that on breast cancer incidence. Little is known about the effects on breast cancer risk of adding a progestogen to replacement therapy, and studies of this effect should receive high priority for future research.

Even if HRT causes breast cancer, it is critical that this effect be weighed against the enormous health benefits to be derived from HRT (45). Noncontraceptive estrogens offer substantial protection against osteoporosis and associated fractures (46), but most importantly, ERT greatly reduces risk of dying from ischemic heart disease (44). According to some sophisticated calculations, using the best available epidemiologic data, approximately six deaths from heart disease probably are prevented for each incident case of breast cancer induced by such therapy (45). Whether this balance point in the risk-benefit equation is altered by the addition of a progestogen to replacement therapy still must be determined.

REFERENCES

1. Henderson BE, Ross RK, Bernstein L. Estrogens as a cause of human cancer: the Richard and Hinda Rosenthal Foundation Award Lecture. *Cancer Res* 1988;48:246–253.
2. Pike MC. Age-related factors in cancers of the breast, ovary, and endometrium. *J Chron Dis* 1987;40(Suppl 2):59s–69s.
3. Pike MC, Bernstein L, Spicer DV. Exogenous hormones and breast cancer risk. In: Niederhuber JE, ed. *Current therapy in oncology.* Philadelphia: Decker 1993;292–303.
4. MacDonald PC, Edman CD, Hemsell DL, et al. Effect of obesity on conversion of plasma androstenedione to estrone in postmenopausal women with and without endometrial cancer. *Am J Obstet Gynecol* 1978;130:448–455.
5. Waterhouse J, Muir C, Correa P, Powell J, eds. *Cancer incidence in five continents,* vol 3. IARC publication no. 15. Lyon: International Agency for Research on Cancer, 1973.
6. Bittner JJ. The causes and control of mammary cancer in mice. *Harvey Lect* 1948;42:221–246.
7. Bernstein L, Yuan J-M, Ross RK, et al. Serum hormone levels in premenopausal Chinese women in Shanghai and white women in Los Angeles: results from two breast cancer case-control studies. *Cancer Causes Control* 1990;1:51–58.
8. Henderson BE, Gerkins V, Rosario I, et al. Elevated serum levels of estrogen and prolactin in daughters of patients with breast cancer. *N Engl J Med* 1975;293:790–795.
9. Henderson BE, Ross RK, Lobo RA, Pike MC, Mack TM. Re-evaluating the role of progestogen therapy after the menopause. *Fertil Steril* 1989;49s:9–15.
10. Ferguson DJP, Anderson TJ. Morphological evaluation of cell turnover in the "resting" human breast. *Br J Cancer* 1981;44:177–181.
11. Preston-Martin S, Pike MC, Ross RK, Jones PA, Henderson BE. Increased cell division as a cause of human cancer. *Cancer Res* 1990;50:7415–7421.
12. Henderson BE, Ross RK, Judd HL, et al. Do regular ovulatory cycles increase breast cancer risk? *Cancer* 1985;56:1206–1208.
13. Henderson BE, Pike MC, Casagrande JT. Breast cancer and the oestrogen window hypothesis. *Lancet* 1981;2:363–364.
14. Collaborative Group on Hormonal Factors in Breast Cancer. Breast cancer and hormonal contraceptives. *Lancet* 1996;347:1713–1727.
15. Collaborative Group on Hormonal Factors in Breast Cancer. Breast cancer and hormonal contraceptives: further results. *Contraception* 1996;54(Suppl 3):1S–106S.
16. UK National Case-Control Study Group. Oral contraceptive use and breast cancer risk in young women. *Lancet* 1989;1:973–982.
17. UK National Case-Control Study Group. Oral contraceptive use and breast cancer risk in young women: subgroup analyses. *Lancet* 1990;1:1507–1509.
18. Vessey MP, Doll R, Jones K, et al. An epidemiological study of oral contraceptives and breast cancer. *Br Med J* 1979;1:1757–1760.
19. Jick H, Walker AM, Watkins RM, et al. Oral contraceptives and breast cancer. *Am J Epidemiol* 1980;112:577–585.

20. Royal College of General Practitioners. Breast cancer and oral contraceptives: findings in Royal College of General Practitioners' study. *Br Med J* 1981;282: 2089–2093.
21. Brinton LA, Hoover R, Szklo M, et al. Oral contraceptives and breast cancer. *Int J Epidemiol* 1982;11:316–322.
22. Lipnick RJ, Buring JE, Hennekens CH, et al. Oral contraceptives and breast cancer: a prospective cohort study. *JAMA* 1986;255:58–61.
23. Centers for Disease Control. Long-term oral contraceptive use and the risk of breast cancer. *JAMA* 1983;249:1591–1595.
24. Ursin G, Henderson B, Haile RW, Zhou N, Diep A, Bernstein L. Oral contraceptive use is more common in women with BRCA1/BRCA2 mutations than in other women with breast cancer. *Cancer Res* 1997;57:3678–3681.
25. Finkel MC, Berlinger VR. The extrapolation of experimental findings (animal to man): the dilemma of systematically administered contraceptives. *Bull Soc Pharmacol Environ Pathol* 1973;4:13–18.
26. Geil RC, Lamar K. FDA studies of oestrogen, progestogen and oestrogen-progestogen combinations. *J Toxicol Environ Health* 1977;3:179–193.
27. Lee NC, Rosero-Bixby L, Oberle MW, Grimaldo C, Whatley AS, Rovira EZ. A case-control study of breast cancer and hormonal contraception in Costa Rica. *J Natl Cancer Inst* 1987;79:1247–1254.
28. Paul C, Skegg DCG, Spears GFS. Depo medroxyprogesterone (Depo-Provera) and risk of breast cancer. *BMJ* 1989;299:759–762.
29. WHO Collaborative Study of Neoplasia and Contraceptives. Breast cancer and depomedroxyprogesterone acetate: a multinational study. *Lancet* 1991;2: 833–838.
30. Early Breast Cancer Trialists' Collaborative Group. Effects of adjuvant tamoxifen and of cytotoxic therapy on mortality in early breast cancer: an overview of 61 randomized trials among 28,896 women. *N Engl J Med* 1988;319:1681–1692.
31. Cuzick J, Wang DY, Bulbrook RD. The prevention of breast cancer. *Lancet* 1986; 2:83–86.
32. Spicer D, Pike MC, Henderson BE. The question of estrogen replacement therapy in patients with a prior diagnosis of breast cancer. *Oncology* 1990;4:49–62.
33. Fisher B, Costantino JP, Wickerham DL, et al. Tamoxifen for prevention of breast cancer: report of the National Surgical Adjuvant Breast and Bowel Project P-1 Study. *J Natl Cancer Inst* 1998;90:1371–1388.
34. Powles T, Eeles R, Ashley S, et al. Interim analysis of the incidence of breast cancer in the Royal Marsden Hospital tamoxifen randomised chemoprevention trial. *Lancet* 1998;352:98–101.
35. Veronesi U, Maisonneuve P, Costa A, et al. Prevention of breast cancer with tamoxifen: preliminary findings from the Italian randomised trial among hysterectomised women—Italian Tamoxifen Prevention Study. *Lancet* 1998;352: 93–97.
36. Nalvadex and Adjuvant Trial Organization (NATO). Controlled trial of tamoxifen as a single adjuvant agent in the management of early breast cancer. *Br J Cancer* 1988;57:608–611.
37. Ribeiro G, Swindell R. The Christie Hospital adjuvant tamoxifen trial: status at 10 years. *Br J Cancer* 1988;57:601–603.
38. Fisher B, Constantino J, Redmond C, et al. A randomized clinical trial evaluating tamoxifen in the treatment of patients with node-negative breast cancer who have estrogen-receptor-positive tumors. *N Engl J Med* 1989;320:479–484.
39. Fornander T, Rutqvist LE, Cedermark B, et al. Adjuvant tamoxifen in early breast cancer: occurrence of new primary cancers. *Lancet* 1989;1:117–120.
40. Stewart HJ, Knight GM. Tamoxifen and the uterus and endometrium [Letter]. *Lancet* 1989;1:375–376.
41. Kennedy DL, Baum C, Forbes MF. Noncontraceptive estrogens and progestins: use patterns over time. *Obstet Gynecol* 1985;65:441–446.
42. Mack TM, Pike MC, Henderson BE, et al. Estrogens and endometrial cancer in a retirement community. *N Engl J Med* 1976;194:1262–1267.
43. Ziel WD, Finkle WD. Increased risk of endometrial carcinoma among users of conjugated estrogens. *N Engl J Med* 1975;293:1167–1170.
44. Henderson BE, Paganini-Hill A, Ross RK. Decreased mortality in users of estrogen replacement therapy. *Arch Intern Med* 1991;151:75–78.
45. Ross RK, Pike MC, Henderson BE, et al. Stroke prevention and oestrogen replacement therapy [Letter]. *Lancet* 1989;1:505.
46. Paganini-Hill A, Ross RK, Gerkins VR, et al. Menopausal estrogen therapy and hip fractures. *Ann Intern Med* 1981;95:28–31.
47. Hemminki E, Kennedy DL, Baum C, McKinlay SM. Prescribing of non-contra-

ceptive estrogens and progestogens in the United States, 1974–1986. *Am J Public Health* 1988;78:1479–1481.
48. Persson I, Adami HO, Bergkvist L. Hormone replacement therapy and the risk of cancer in the breast and reproductive organs: a review of epidemiological data. In: Drife JO, Studd JWW, eds. *HRT and osteoporosis*. London: Springer-Verlag, 1990:165–175.
49. Steinberg K, Thacker SB, Smith SJ, et al. A meta-analysis of the effect of estrogen replacement therapy on the risk of breast cancer. *JAMA* 1991;265: 1985–1990.
50. Dupont WD, Page DL. Menopausal estrogen replacement therapy and breast cancer. *Arch Intern Med* 1991;151:67–72.
51. Ross RK, Paganini-Hill A, Gerkins VR, et al. A case-control study of menopausal estrogen therapy and breast cancer. *JAMA* 1980;243:1635–1638.
52. Hoover R, Glass A, Finkle WD, Azevedo D, Milne K. Conjugated estrogens and breast cancer risk in women. *J Natl Cancer Inst* 1981;67:815–820.
53. Hiatt RA, Bawol R, Friedman GD, Hoover R. Exogenous estrogen and breast cancer after bilateral oophorectomy. *Cancer* 1994;54:139–144.
54. Brinton LA, Hoover R, Fraumeni JF. Menopausal oestrogens and breast cancer risk: an expanded case-control study. *Br J Cancer* 1986;54:825–832.
55. Nomura AMY, Kolonel LN, Hirohata T, Lee J. The association of replacement estrogens with breast cancer. *Int J Cancer* 1986;37:49–53.
56. Wingo PA, Layde PM, Lee NC, et al. The risk of breast cancer in postmenopausal women who have used estrogen replacement therapy. *JAMA* 1987;257:209–215.
57. Ewertz M. Influences of non-contraceptive exogenous and endogenous sex hormones on breast cancer risk in Denmark. *Int J Cancer* 1988;42:832–838.
58. Rohan TE, McMichael AJ. Non-contraceptive exogenous oestrogen therapy and breast cancer. *Med J Aust* 1988;148:217–221.
59. Bergkvist L, Adami O, Persson I, Hoover P, Schairer C. The risk of breast cancer after estrogen and estrogen-progestin replacement. *N Engl J Med* 1989;321: 293–297.
60. Colditz GA, Stampfer MJ, Willett WC, et al. Prospective study of estrogen replacement therapy and risk of breast cancer in postmenopausal women. *JAMA* 1990;264:2648–2653.
61. Shimizu H, Ross RK, Bernstein L, Pike MC, Henderson BE. Serum estrogen levels in postmenopausal women: comparison of US whites and Japanese in Japan. *Br J Cancer* 1990;62:451–454.
62. Cutler SY, Young JL. *Third National Cancer Survey: incidence data*, vol 41. Washington DC: National Cancer Institute Monograph; 1975.
63. Key TJA, Pike MC. The dose-effect relationship between "unopposed" estrogens and endometrial mitotic rate: its central role in explaining and predicting endometrial cancer risk. *Br J Cancer* 1988;57:205–212.
64. Collaborative Group on Hormonal Factors in Breast Cancer. Breast cancer and hormone replacement therapy: collaborative reanalyses of data from 51 epidemiological studies of 52,705 women with breast cancer and 108,411 women without breast cancer. *Lancet* 1997;350:1047–1059.
65. Golditz GA, Hankinson SE, Hunter DJ, et al. The use of estrogens and progestins and the risk of breast cancer in postmenopausal women. *N Engl J Med* 1995;332: 1589–1593.
66. Bergkvist L, Adami HO, Persson I, et al. Prognosis after breast cancer diagnosis in women exposed to estrogen and estrogen-progestogen replacement therapy. *Am J Epidemiol* 1989;130:221–228.
67. Pike MC, Bernstein L, Ross RK, Henderson BE. Estrogen replacement therapy and risk of breast cancer in postmenopausal women [Letter]. *JAMA* 1991;265: 1824.
68. Chu J, Schweid A, Weiss NS. Survival among women with endometrial cancer: a comparison of estrogen users and non-users. *Am J Obstet Gynecol* 1982;143: 569–573.
69. Ross RK, Bernstein LB. Why can't we prove that hormone replacement therapy causes breast cancer? Methodological and biological challenges. In: Mann RD, ed. *Hormone replacement therapy and breast cancer risk*. London: Parthenon Publishing, 1992:241–251.
70. Donegan WL, Hartz AJ, Rimm AJ. The association of body weight with recurrent cancer of the breast. *Cancer* 1978;41:1590–1594.
71. Boyd N, Campbell J, Germanson T, Thomson D, Sutherland D, Meakin J. Body weight and prognosis in breast cancer. *J Natl Cancer Inst* 1981;67:785–789.
72. Greenberg ER, Vessey MP, McPherson K, Doll R, Yeates D. Body size and survival in premenopausal breast cancer. *Br J Cancer* 1985;51:691–697.

Treatment of the Postmenopausal Woman: Basic and Clinical Aspects, Second Edition, edited by Rogerio A. Lobo, Lippincott Williams & Wilkins, Philadelphia © 1999.

CHAPTER 45

Postmenopausal Breast Surveillance

William H. Hindle

At menopause, with its subsequent estrogen deficiency, the breasts begin to atrophy; the glandular tissue continues to diminish and be progressively replaced by fat; benign breast diseases, including neoplasms, subside; and tenderness and palpable nodularity clear. Estrogen replacement therapy (ERT) can reverse or delay these breast-aging changes in some cases. However, the incidence of cancer continues to rise with advancing age.

Annual screening mammography is the most important tool in the surveillance of the breasts of postmenopausal women. To detect small cancers, which have an excellent prognosis when treated, physicians who care for postmenopausal women should obtain annual mammograms (bilateral craniocaudal and mediolateral oblique views) for and perform complete annual breast examinations on all their patients.

Breast cancer is the most common cancer of postmenopausal women. The incidence of breast cancer is more than twice the combined incidence of cervical, endometrial, and ovarian cancer in this age group (1). The incidence rate of breast cancer continues to increase every year as a woman grows older (Fig. 45.1) (2,3). The cumulative lifetime risk of breast cancer is 1 in 8 for women born in the United States (1). The age-specific incidence rates (4) and the aging of the population combine to make breast cancer an ever-increasing health care dilemma.

Benign breast disease, including cysts, fibroadenomas, fibrocystic changes, and mastalgia, markedly decrease with menopause and its subsequent estrogen deficiency. Elicited milky nipple discharge subsides after menopause, However, spontaneous watery, serous, or bloody nipple discharge from a single duct must be investigated. These may be signs of underlying carcinoma, although

W. H. Hindle: Department of Obstetrics and Gynecology, University of Southern California School of Medicine, Women's and Children's Hospital, LAC-USC Medical Center, Los Angeles, California 90033.

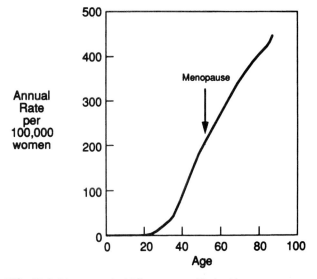

FIG. 45.1. Linear scale U.S. age-specific incidence rates per 100,000 white women for breast cancer based on the Surveillance, Epidemiology, and End Results (SEER) program data, 1978–1984. (From ref. 31, with permission.)

such nipple discharges are most commonly related to intraductal papillomas. Ductography (galactography) is useful in defining the extent of the intraductal lesion and whether it is single or multiple. Multiple papilloma formation is more commonly associated with papillary carcinoma. Cytology of bloody nipple discharge can be useful but only if malignant cells are identified. Nipple discharge cytology is not cost effective, does not alter the clinical management, and does not circumvent the need for definitive surgery. Surgical excision should be limited to the involved collecting duct draining a single glandular lobe into a single opening (i.e., galactophore) on the nipple. However, all of the ductal system showing intraductal abnormalities should be excised. This can usually be performed through a limited circumareolar incision and microdochectomy. Only permanent section histologic evaluation of the excised duct can establish the definitive diagnosis. If ductography is not available, the oncologic surgeon can pass a fine probe down the single duct that produces the discharge.

Mammary ectasia (i.e., periductal mastitis), which is most common during the perimenopausal ages, usually presents as dark greenish discharge, often from multiple duct openings on the nipple. Treatment is usually not necessary for this self-limited, benign condition. Hemostix or similar dipsticks are useful to determine if dark nipple discharge contains hemoglobin. If so, it must be investigated.

Monthly breast self-examination (BSE) should be encouraged for postmenopausal women. Because the aging breast usually becomes smaller, less tender, less nodular, and less thickened, BSE is potentially more accurate in detecting palpable breast masses.

Significant changes from prior BSE and new differences between the right and left breast, such as dimpling of the skin or inversion of the nipple, which can be secondary signs of underlying breast cancer, must be evaluated. If a new mass is identified, it must be definitely diagnosed. Contrary to the case for younger women, a high percentage of palpable dominant breast masses in postmenopausal women are cancers.

Methodical bilateral clinical breast examination (CBE) should be performed at least once each year and include both axillae and the supraclavicular and subareolar areas. The vertical strip method recommended by the American Cancer Society is the most effective technique for detecting palpable breast masses (5). Unfortunately, palpable breast cancers have usually already reached stage II or are even more advanced and carry an unfavorable prognosis. It is critical that CBE findings be recorded in the medical record, particularly any abnormal findings. A pictorial diagram is useful to record the exact location of any abnormality, especially a suspected or suspicious mass. A specific follow-up plan should be recorded.

All palpable dominant masses and suspicious mammographic lesions in postmenopausal women must be specifically diagnosed in a timely manner to definitively exclude cancer. Palpable masses can be evaluated by fine-needle aspiration (FNA), with cysts being evacuated and aspirates of solid masses sent for cytology. Because FNA may produce hematoma formation, which can mammographically mimic a suspicious lesion in the breast, mammography should be done before or 2 weeks after FNA (6). However, if the mammogram is taken shortly thereafter and the mammographer is aware that an FNA has been performed (including the exact location in the breast), clinical management is rarely altered (7).

FNA is performed with a 22-gauge, 1-inch needle with a transparent plastic hub and a 10-cc syringe. Most physicians prefer a pistol-type syringe holder or a three-finger control syringe. The FNA technique is illustrated in Fig. 45.2. The dominant breast mass must be completely immobilized, preferably over a rib, with the fingers of the

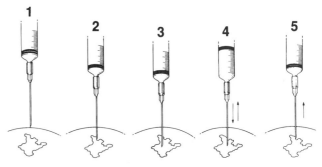

FIG. 45.2. Five-step technique of fine-needle aspiration for cytology of a palpable dominant breast mass.

nonaspirating hand. The skin is cleaned with an alcohol wipe, and the needle tip is sharply thrust downward in jackhammer-like motions back and forth about 20 times within the mass while negative pressure is maintained in the syringe. At all times during the aspiration (negative pressure), the needle tip is kept within the mass. Local anesthesia usually is not necessary because the procedure is no more painful than a venipuncture and takes about the same amount of time to perform.

An alternate method for FNA is the needle-alone technique, which requires more thrusts (preferably 30 or more) as the cellular material is accumulated in the barrel of the needle by capillary action, not by negative pressure in the syringe. With this technique, usually less cellular material is obtained. However, the learning curve is shorter, less blood is obtained, and tactical sensation (and control) is increased.

A cyst should be completely drained and followed to be certain there is no residual mass and that the cyst does not reform. Cytology of cyst fluid is rarely rewarding and is indicated only for frankly bloody fluid. Routine cytology of cyst fluid is not cost effective and rarely alters clinical management.

Cellular material that collects in the bore of the needle during the FNA of a solid mass should be quickly ejected onto a properly identified slide, smeared, and fixed. The slide can then be stained at leisure, usually with Papanicolaou or hematoxylin and eosin stain. An alternate method of slide preparation is air drying and then staining, usually with some version of Wright-Giemsa. With an adequate cell sample, as many as 90% of solid breast masses can be specifically diagnosed by FNA cytology (8). If a specific cytologic diagnosis is not made by FNA, a definitive histologic diagnosis should be obtained by tissue core-needle biopsy or open surgical biopsy. Open surgical excision biopsies are usually done under local anesthesia in an outpatient setting. Evaluation of multiple permanent histologic sections is required for definitive diagnosis. Excision biopsies should be done following the National Surgical Adjuvant Breast Project (NSABP) guidelines for lumpectomy with clear margins (9).

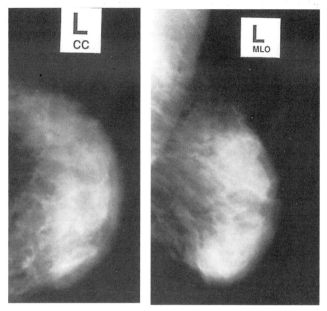

FIG. 45.3. Typical normal mammogram (left craniocaudal and mediolateral oblique views) of a premenopausal woman.

Nonpalpable masses can be evaluated by stereotactic mammography-guided FNA or tissue core-needle biopsy (10). However, if a specific diagnosis is not obtained, mammographic needle localization of the nonpalpable mass and lumpectomy with clear surgical margins are required. These procedures are usually performed simultaneously on an outpatient basis using local anesthesia. Specimen radiography before the operation is completed is essential to be certain the nonpalpable mammographic lesion has been excised. If not, repeat excision is required. The weight and dimensions of the lumpectomy specimen should be recorded. Multiple histologic sections should be evaluated to establish a definitive diagno-

sis and that all the surgical margins are clear. The maximum diameter of the malignant lesion should be measured and recorded.

Screening mammography is the only proven method of meaningfully decreasing the overall mortality from breast cancer (11,12). Clinically significant mammographic findings that should be specifically reported are a spiculated mass, a circumscribed mass, microcalcifications, an asymmetric density, and skin changes (i.e., thickening and retraction). The mammographic impression can be negative (i.e., normal or no abnormalities noted), benign finding, probably benign finding, suspicious abnormality, or highly suggestive of malignancy. Most mammographers add a qualifier about their level of confidence in the mammographic impression and add their recommendation. The mammogram report should follow the breast imaging reporting and data system (BIRADS) format and terminology, including the complete assessment category (1 to 5) (13).

Even complete mammographic evaluation and workup does not give a definitive clinical diagnosis, although experienced mammographers develop a high clinical correlation. Definite cytology by FNA or histology by open biopsy is necessary for the final specific definitive diagnosis of a breast lesion. A "negative" mammogram does not exclude cancer and gives no useful clinical information other than the fact that the mammographer does not perceive a significant abnormality on viewing the films. A negative mammogram does not ensure disease-free status.

Even though the overall accuracy of mammography is about 90% (14–16) and the progressive fatty replacement of glandular tissue in the aging breast increases the accuracy of mammography (14,15), CBE must continue to be performed in the postmenopausal group. Typical changes in premenopausal and postmenopausal mammograms are illustrated in Figs. 45.3 and 45.4.

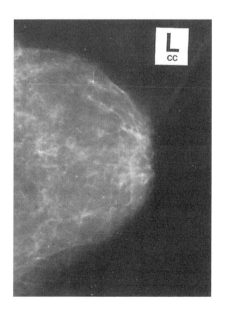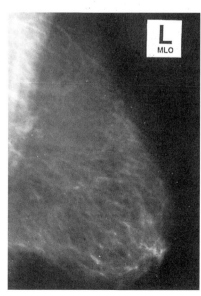

FIG. 45.4. Typical normal mammogram (left craniocaudal and mediolateral oblique views) of a postmenopausal woman.

Screening mammography is useful throughout a woman's life, and there is no upper-age limit (17). However, after age 85, estimated life expectancy and quality of life issues may outweigh the benefits, particularly when viewed on a population-wide basis and with consideration of health care costs. Each elderly woman should be evaluated individually, her family consulted, and her informed consent obtained.

Breast infections occur in postmenopausal women but are unusual. Diffuse mastitis must be differentiated from inflammatory carcinoma. If the mastitis does not respond to antibiotic therapy, a skin biopsy should be done to look for possible carcinoma involvement of the dermal lymphatics. Subareolar fistulas continue to occur in postmenopausal women. Excision often is necessary to eradicate these chronic or recurrent infections.

Before initially prescribing ERT for a patient, the physician should obtain a mammogram unless one has been performed within the preceding year. Annual mammograms should be obtained thereafter. CBE should also be done before ERT and every year thereafter. Monthly BSE should be encouraged. Breast cysts or fibroadenomas may become symptomatic, palpable, or enlarged when a women begins ERT. Such symptoms and palpable masses must be definitively diagnosed to exclude cancer. The diagnostic triad of CBE, mammography, and FNA (Fig. 45.5) should give a specific diagnosis. However, if uncertainty remains in the mind of the patient or her physician, a definitive histologic diagnosis should be obtained by tissue core-needle biopsy or open surgical biopsy.

Women who have been treated for breast cancer should be followed in the same manner as other postmenopausal women with annual mammography and CBE. They should have an annual chest film and blood obtained for alkaline phosphatase. Further studies such as bone, liver, or brain scans should be done to evaluate symptoms that suggest recurrent disease.

Women on tamoxifen should be monitored for evidence of osteoporosis (by evaluation of bone mineral content) or cardiovascular disease (by measurements of blood pressure, serum cholesterol or lipid profile, and weight). However, osteoporosis and cardiovascular disease are not thought to be adversely affected by tamoxifen therapy. Studies on the long-term effects of tamoxifen indicate, however, that there is an increased incidence of endometrial carcinoma (18,19), warranting close monitoring of each woman with a uterus. Data suggest decreased osteoporosis (20–22) and unchanged or decreased cardiovascular disease with tamoxifen (23–25).

The National Surgical Adjuvant Breast Project (NSABP) clinical trials are evaluating tamoxifen therapy as a prevention strategy for invasive breast cancer in high-risk women (NSABP P-1), as adjuvant therapy after lumpectomy for ductal carcinoma *in situ* (DCIS), for prevention of ipsilateral or contralateral invasive cancer (NSABP B-24), and as adjuvant therapy after lumpectomy for occult invasive carcinoma with and without adjuvant radiation therapy (NSABP B-21).

Compliance with surveillance decreases as women become elderly (26). A personal physician's recommendations and advice are the strongest motivators for compliance (27). A careful follow-up system with automatic reminders assists the physician in maintaining compliance. Twelve major medical organizations recommend screening mammography for women every year after 50 years of age (28.29). Annual mammography and CBE are required for postmenopausal women to have the best chance for early diagnosis of breast cancer (14,30).

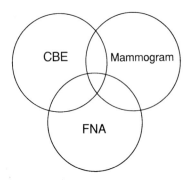

FIG. 45.5. The diagnostic triad of clinical breast examination (CBE), mammography, and fine-needle aspiration (FNA) for a persistent dominant breast mass. Congruence of all three techniques provides a definitive specific diagnosis.

REFERENCES

1. Landis SH, Murray T, Bolden S, Wingo PA. Cancer statistics, 1998. *CA Cancer J Clin* 1998;48:6–29.
2. Boring MS, Squires T, Tong T. Cancer statistics, 1991. *Cancer* 1991;1:19–39.
3. National Cancer Institute. Division of Cancer Prevention and Control: 1987 annual cancer statistics review, including cancer trends: 1950–1985, publication no. 88-2789. Bethesda, MD: National Institutes of Health, 1988:III-36.
4. Miller BA, Feuer EJ, Hankey BF. The increasing incidence of breast cancer since 1982: relevance of early detection. *Cancer Causes Control* 1991;2:67–74.
5. Saunders KJ, Pilgrim CA, Pennypacker HS. Increased proficiency of search in breast self-examination. *Cancer* 1986;58:2531–2537.
6. Sickles EA, Klein DL, Goodson WH 3rd, Hunt TK. Mammography after fine-needle aspiration of palpable breast masses. *Am J Surg* 1983;145:395–397.
7. Hindle, WH, Chen EC. Accuracy of mammographic appearance after breast fine-needle aspiration. *Am J Obstet Gynecol* 1997;176:1286-92.
8. Kline TS, Kline IK. Breast: guides to clinical aspiration biopsy. New York: Igaku-Shoin Medical Publishers, 1989:1–19.
9. Margolese R, Poisson R, Shibata H, Pilch Y, Lerner H, Fisher B. The technique of segmental mastectomy (lumpectomy) and axillary dissection: a syllabus from the National Surgical Adjuvant Breast Project Workshops. *Surgery* 1987;102:828–834.
10. Duffy SW, Tabar L, Fagerberg G, et al. Breast screening, prognostic factors and survival: results from the Swedish two county study. *Br J Cancer* 1991;64:1133–1138.
11. Costanza ME. Breast cancer screening in older women: synopsis of a forum. *Cancer* 1992;69:1925–1931.
12. Tabar L, Fagerberg G, Duffy SW, Day NE. The Swedish two county trial of mammographic screening for breast cancer: recent results and calculation of benefit. *J Epidemiol Commun Health* 1998;43:107–114.
13. BIRADS American College of Radiology (ACR). *Breast imaging reporting and data system (BI-RADS)*, 2nd ed. Reston, VA: American College of Radiology, 1995.
14. Edeiken S. Mammography in the symptomatic woman. *Cancer* 1989;63:1412–1414.
15. Bender HG, Schnurch HG, Beck L, et al. Breast cancer detection: age-related significance of findings on physical exam and mammography. *Gynecol Oncol* 1988;31:166–175.

16. Feig SA. Should breast self-examination be included in a mammographic screening program? *Recent Results Cancer Res* 1990;119:151–164.
17. Mandelblatt JS, Wheat ME, Monane M, Moshief RD, Hollenberg JP, Tang J. Breast cancer screening for elderly women with and without comorbid conditions. *Ann Intern Med* 1992;116:722–730.
18. Fornander T, Cedemark B, Mattsson A, et al. Adjuvant tamoxifen in early breast cancer: occurrence of new primary cancers. *Lancet* 1989;1:117–120.
19. Killackey MA, Hakes TB, Pierce VK. Endometrial adenocarcinoma in breast cancer patients receiving antiestrogens. *Cancer Treat Rep* 1985;69:237–238.
20. Love RR, Mazess RB, Barden HS, et al. Effects of tamoxifen on bone mineral density in postmenopausal women with breast cancer. *N Engl J Med* 1992;326:852–856.
21. Fornander T, Rutquist LE, Sjoberg HE, et al. Long-term adjuvant tamoxifen in early breast cancer: effect on bone mineral density in postmenopausal women. *J Clin Oncol* 1990;8:1019–1024.
22. Love RR, Mazess RB, Tormey DC, et al. Bone mineral density in women with breast cancer treated with adjuvant tamoxifen for at least two years. *Breast Cancer Res Treat* 1988;12:297–302.
23. Love RR, Wiebe DA, Newcomb PA, et al. Effects of tamoxifen on cardiovascular risk factors in postmenopausal women. *Ann Intern Med* 1991;115:860–864.
24. Bagdade JD, Rayn G, Wolter JM. Effects of tamoxifen treatment on plasma lipids and lipoprotein composition. *J Clin Endocrinol Metab* 1990;70:1132–1135.
25. Love RR, Newcomb PA, Wiebe DA, et al. Effects of tamoxifen therapy on lipid and lipoprotein levels in postmenopausal patients with node-negative breast cancer. *J Natl Cancer Inst* 1990;82:1327–1332.
26. Weinberger M, Saunders AF, Samsa GP, et al. Breast cancer screening in older women: practice and barriers reported by primary care physicians. *J Am Geriatr Soc* 1991;39:22–29.
27. Glockner SM, Holden MG, Hilton SVW, Norcross WA. Women's attitudes toward screening mammography. *Am J Prev Med* 1992;8:69–77.
28. American College of Obstetricians and Gynecologists. Report of task force on routine cancer screening. ACOG committee opinion 68. Washington DC: American College of Obstetricians and Gynecologists, 1989.
29. Medical News and Perspectives. Breast cancer screening guidelines agreed on by AMA, other medically related organizations. *JAMA* 1989;262:1155.
30. Council on Scientific Affairs. Mammographic screening in asymptomatic women aged 40 years and older. *JAMA* 1989;261:2535–2542.
31. Ernster VL, et al. U.S. cancer incidence rates by sex, race, and age: graphics of SEER Program data 1978 to 1984. Atlanta: American Cancer Society, 1988.

Treatment of the Postmenopausal Woman: Basic and Clinical Aspects, Second Edition, edited by Rogerio A. Lobo, Lippincott Williams & Wilkins, Philadelphia © 1999.

CHAPTER 46

Hormone Replacement Therapy and Endometrial Cancer

John A. Collins and James J. Schlesselman

Endometrial cancer is the most common gynecologic malignancy. The incidence rises substantially after menopause and peaks between the ages of 70 and 80 years (1,2). Endometrial cancer originates within the glandular epithelium of the endometrium and comprises two main types: endometrioid and serous. The serous or papillary serous types are found typically in older women who have not received estrogens, whereas the more common endometrioid type is associated with exposure to endogenous estrogen (3). Whether exogenous estrogen also increases the risk of endometrial cancer is an important issue in clinical decisions about hormonal treatment of menopausal symptoms.

Estrogenic compounds became available during the late 1930s, and they were used initially to treat menopausal symptoms and endometriosis (4,5). In each of these conditions, there was concern about the dangers of continuous stimulation of the endometrium (4,6). Studies in postmenopausal women suggested only small increased risks of endometrial cancer in estrogen users until 1975, when two epidemiologic studies reported materially higher risks (7–11). Epidemiologic studies since then have consistently reported a significantly increased risk with unopposed estrogen use.

Prescriptions for hormone replacement therapy (HRT) and patients' use of this treatment have fluctuated according to perceptions of the benefits and risks. From 1975 to 1980, prescriptions in the United States declined from 28 million per annum to 14 million (12) and thereafter returned to pre-1975 levels (13–15). In surveys, the prevalence of current use of HRT ranges from 15% to 25% among women between the ages of 50 and 54 years (16–18). This low level of use mainly reflects the fear of bleeding and breast cancer, whereas fear of endometrial cancer is a less important factor (17,19,20). Only one-fourth of HRT prescriptions included a progestin (13,15), although most postmenopausal U.S. women have not had a hysterectomy. Even in the late 1990s, many HRT users remain at increased risk of endometrial hyperplasia and endometrial cancer. As a consequence, increased endometrial cancer risk continues to be a clinical concern more than 20 years after the first published evidence of an association with estrogen use.

This chapter on HRT and invasive endometrial cancer begins with a brief account of the incidence and mortality of endometrial cancer in the United States. It then covers the biologic plausibility for effects of exogenous hormones on endometrial cancer risk, presents summary estimates of the effect of hormone replacement use on endometrial cancer incidence and mortality, and provides a clinical perspective on the results of epidemiologic studies.

EPIDEMIOLOGIC BACKGROUND

Age-Specific Rates of Uterine Cancer Occurrence

Figure 46.1 shows for the United States the age-specific incidence rates of invasive cancer of the corpus uteri (21). *Incidence rate* refers to the number of newly diagnosed cases of primary cancer during the 5-year period 1991–1995 expressed per 100,000 women per year. If *r* denotes the incidence rate at a given age, such as age 50 or 65, then 5 times *r* would be the risk of developing cancer over the succeeding 5-year period, from age 50 to 54 or from age 65 to 69.

J.A. Collins: Department of Obstetrics and Gynecology, McMaster University, Hamilton, Ontario, Canada, L8N 3Z5.

J.J. Schlesselman: Department of Epidemiology and Public Health, University of Miami School of Medicine, Miami, Florida 33136.

There is a clear rise in the incidence of endometrial cancer with increasing age, corresponding to the pattern seen with other cancers. Figure 46.1 shows that, as of 1991 through 1995, invasive uterine cancer was diagnosed in American women between the ages of 20 and 24 at the rate of 2 cases per million women per year. For women between the ages of 50 and 54, the corresponding rate of diagnosis was 44 cases per 100,000 per year, and for women between the ages of 70 and 74, the rate was 107 per 100,000 per year, a 500-fold increase over the incidence rate for women between the ages of 20 and 24.

Between 1973 and 1995, uterine cancer incidence for U.S. women of all races declined by 26%, although the last 4 years, from 1991 to 1995, saw a small increase of 2% in total incidence (21).

Although Fig. 46.1 shows the incidence rates of cancer of the uterine corpus, including corpus sites not otherwise specified (NOS), epidemiologic studies of HRT have focused on *endometrial* cancer. The reported rates for uterine cancer approximate those for endometrial cancer, because most uterine corpus cancers are endometrial carcinomas: adenocarcinomas, adenoacanthomas, adenosquamous carcinomas, and other histologic subtypes. In the United States, about 90% of whites and 80% of blacks diagnosed with uterine corpus cancer have endometrial cancer (22). Other corpus cancers include leiomyosarcomas and malignant lesions of mixed origin, such as carcinosarcoma and müllerian mixed tumors.

Adjustment of Rates for Population at Risk

Another qualification when interpreting the incidence rates in Fig. 46.1 is that their "denominators" are based on the estimated total number of women in the population, rather than the number of women actually at risk of

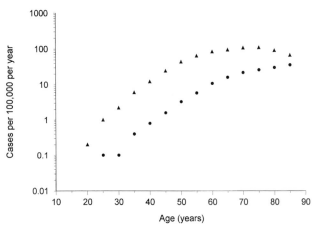

FIG. 46.1. Age-specific rates of invasive cancer of the uterine corpus for U.S. women of all races, 1991–1995. Uterus, corpus uteri plus not otherwise specified; ▲, incidence; ●, mortality.

gynecologic cancer. In particular, the rates do not account for hysterectomies, which effectively eliminate the risk of uterine corpus cancer. If adjustment for hysterectomies were made, the incidence rates in Fig. 46.1 would be substantially higher at older ages. For example, by 40 years of age, 11% of American women have had a hysterectomy, and by age 70, the corresponding figure is 33% (22). If the rates of uterine cancer in U.S. women shown in Fig. 46.1 were expressed as rates per 100,000 nonhysterectomized women, the incidence rates would be about 3% higher for women age 30, about 12% higher for women age 40, and about 49% higher for women age 70. Unquestionably, this correction varies by age, race, and country. Because reported incidence data do not adjust for hysterectomy, we accept that such incidence rates are *underestimates* of gynecologic cancer risk, particularly at older ages.

Age-Adjusted Rates of Uterine Cancer Occurrence

One means of summarizing the overall frequency of cancer occurrence is the age-adjusted incidence rate. This computation is based on a weighted average of the age-specific incidence rates, in which the weights correspond to the proportion of the population within each age range. For the period of 1991 through 1995, the age-adjusted incidence rate for U.S. women of all races was 13.1 cases of uterine cancer per 100,000 women younger than 65 years and 98.5 cases per 100,000 women who ere 65 or older (21). The age-adjusted incidence rate for all U.S. women was 21.6 cases per 100,000, which is 25% higher than the average reported from around the world, 17.8 per 100,000.

International Variation in Cancer Risk

International variation in cancer risk can be represented by age-adjusted incidence rates, as in the example just cited, or by cumulative risk. The *cumulative risk* of cancer is the probability (risk) that cancer is diagnosed at some time within a specified range of age throughout the entire span of time under consideration or until cancer becomes clinically evident at some point within it. The computation assumes that no premature deaths occur over the period in question. It therefore allows comparisons of cancer incidence across populations that are subject to markedly different risks of mortality. For example, if a woman who is free of cancer dies at age 40 from infectious disease or at age 50 from cardiovascular disease, she is obviously not at risk of developing cancer at older ages, the time at which the incidence rate is greatest.

The cumulative risk of cancer of the uterine corpus (plus NOS) is highest among women in Canada (2.1% cumulative risk), Czechoslovakia (2.2%), and whites in the United States (2.7%). The cumulative risk is lowest among Asian women—less than 0.5% for India, China, Thailand, and all but one cancer registry in Japan (21,22).

Risk Factors for Endometrial Cancer

Much of the epidemiologic data concerns the endometrioid type of endometrial cancer, which is more common than the serous or papillary serous varieties (3,23). Aside from the association with age and the international variation described previously, the well-established risk factors for endometrial cancer have in common a degree of exposure to unopposed endogenous or exogenous estrogen as an underlying factor. These risk factors include early age at menarche, late age at menopause, obesity, chronic anovulation, and nulliparity (2,24).

Mortality and Survival Rates for Uterine Cancer

An estimated 36,100 new cases of endometrial cancer occurred in the United States in 1998, along with approximately 6,300 deaths (25). The extent of mortality associated with a given cancer can be represented by the *case-fatality rate,* the number of deaths per annum divided by the number of newly diagnosed cases. Using the estimates for 1998, the case-fatality rate for endometrial cancer was 6,300/36,100 (17.5%).

For individual patients, the likelihood of cure or survival is more relevant and important than case-fatality rates derived from population or registry statistics. Cure is difficult to ascertain, but survival rates can be determined from follow-up of patients. For endometrial cancer, survival through 5 years is accepted for clinical purposes as an approximation of the probability of cure. Rates based on follow-up of patients through 1995 indicate that 5-year *relative survival* is 88% for women younger than 65 years of age (21). In other words, women diagnosed with endometrial cancer have survival over the next 5 years diminished by only 12% compared with 5-year survival for women of similar age. Five-year relative survival is 81% for women 65 years of age or older (21).

BIOLOGIC PLAUSIBILITY FOR EFFECTS OF EXOGENOUS HORMONES

Endometrial cancers are hormonally dependent neoplasms, many of which are considered to be a consequence of excess estrogenic stimulation in the presence of inadequate exposure to progestin (3,26). Consistent with this mechanism are studies showing that estrogen increases cellular proliferation and induces the synthesis of estradiol receptors in the endometrium (27). Progestins diminish both of these effects (27,28) and increase the conversion of estradiol to estrone, which has a lower affinity for estrogen receptors (29). Progestins also pre-

vent or reverse endometrial hyperplasia associated with use of unopposed estrogen (30–32).

The exact mechanisms by which estrogen and progestin affect the development of endometrial cancer are unknown. It makes sense to consider the role of these hormones within the context of the current theoretical framework of carcinogenesis, which visualizes a multistep process involving a series of mutations affecting a single cell and its progeny (33–35). When the resulting genetic damage to a cell impairs its control of cell division, the affected cell has the potential to develop into cancer. The initial damage can arise from spontaneous mutation, irradiation, viral infection, or chemical exposure. For example, mutations of the *p53* tumor suppressor gene are found in 23% of endometrial carcinomas (36). Estrogen is unlikely to cause such genetic damage, because it does not have the molecular instability that characterizes carcinogenic aromatic hydrocarbons (37). More plausible is the likelihood that estrogen stimulates endometrial cell division while the genetically damaged cells are still in a precancerous state (38). More rapid cell division presumably could increase the odds that the precancerous cells will undergo sufficient divisions to become an autonomous cancer.

Another role for estrogen late in the preclinical stage of cancer development is also plausible, possibly through continuing stimulation of endometrial cell division or by means of effects on tissue resistance, immune defenses, or angiogenesis (24,39). Among these possibilities, an effect on angiogenesis seems plausible, because a developing tumor requires an adequate blood supply. Estrogen induces vasodilation, which with the movement of endothelial cells, appears to facilitate angiogenesis (40). Estradiol enhances the rapid growth of spiral arterioles during the proliferative phase of the menstrual cycle (41). It also increases arteriolar dilatation through mechanisms including stimulation of nitric oxide synthesis and prostacyclin activity and by attenuating the vasoconstrictor activity of endothelin on vascular smooth muscle (42,43).

In theory, estrogen may have early precancer effects and later preclinical effects on endometrial cancer development. An early precancer effect from estrogen-induced division of genetically damaged cells would increase cancer incidence only after a relatively long period of exposure (i.e., long latent phase), and the increased cancer incidence would not decline immediately after cessation of exposure (i.e., residual effect). Later estrogen influences at the preclinical stage of cancer development would be associated with an early rise in cancer incidence (i.e., short latent phase) and a rapid decline after cessation of use (i.e., negligible residual effect). The data summarized in the next section reveal a short latent phase and a long residual effect, consistent with a combination of both mechanisms. Not to be overlooked is the alternate premise that estrogen-induced bleeding prompts diagnostic tests that disclose the presence of cancer before it would otherwise have become symptomatic.

ESTIMATED EFFECT OF HORMONE REPLACEMENT THERAPY ON ENDOMETRIAL CANCER

Use of Hormone Replacement Therapy

The evidence associating endometrial cancer with HRT is based mainly on studies in which unopposed estrogen was the dominant therapy (i.e., estrogen replacement therapy [ERT]). Use of HRT including progestin is referred to here as HRT, and this exposure is addressed separately.

Ever use of ERT was reported in 30 case-control studies (35 estimates) and 7 cohort studies (7 estimates) (7,8,10,11,44–76). The studies included 8,410 cancer patients, 2,766 of whom (33%) had used unopposed estrogen (i.e., ERT). The typical risk was increased 2.8-fold (95% CI, 2.4–3.2) in the case-control studies, 2.7-fold (2.3–3.3) in the cohort studies, and 2.8-fold (2.6–3.0) if all of the estimates are taken into account.

Closer surveillance of ERT users may lead to the discovery of latent endometrial cancer in ERT users. Such latent cancer would be missed in controls if they were not similarly evaluated and thereby result in a spuriously increased risk associated with estrogen use. Seven of the studies referred to had controls who were undergoing gynecologic procedures, ensuring comparable diagnostic assessment of the endometrium for cases and controls (8,10,47,50,53,54,66). Of these, three studies involving 1,158 cancer patients, of whom 407 were ERT users, provided separate estimates based on gynecologic and other controls. The typical risk of endometrial cancer for ERT users compared with nonusers was increased 2.0-fold (95% CI, 1.5–2.6) when the controls were gynecologic patients and 2.5-fold (1.9–3.4) when the controls were other hospital or community subjects (53,54,66). Differential diagnostic assessment of cases and controls does not explain the association between ERT and endometrial cancer.

Duration of Estrogen Replacement Therapy

Estimates of risk based on duration of ERT use are more relevant than estimates based on ever use, because individuals are exposed for various periods. Figure 46.2 shows 106 estimates of the relative risk of endometrial cancer by duration of HRT using unopposed estrogen. The estimates are drawn from 27 case-control and 6 cohort studies (10,11,44,46,47,50–55,57–62,64–69,73, 74,77–84). Most of the estimates were adjusted for age, and many were also adjusted for other possible confounding variables, such as obesity, diabetes, and smoking. Increasing duration of use is associated with a significant trend of increasing risk. The estimated relative

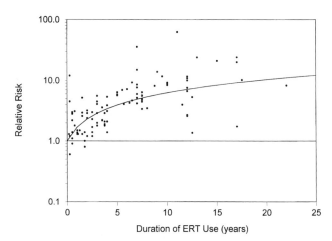

FIG. 46.2. Relative risk of endometrial cancer by duration of unopposed estrogen use (ERT).

risks are 1.7, 3.4, 5.4, and 7.1 at 1, 4, 8, and 12 years, respectively (trend: $p < 0.0001$). The relative risk associated with use for less than 5 years is 2.0 (95% CI, 1.8–2.2); the corresponding estimate for use of 5 or more years is 6.7 (95% CI, 5.9–7.6).

Discontinued Use of Estrogen Replacement Therapy

Figure 46.3 shows 40 estimates of endometrial cancer risk after discontinuing ERT. The data are from 13 case-control studies and one cohort study (46,47,54,56,59,60, 62,64,66,68,74,77,83,84). The elevated risk of endometrial cancer associated with ERT use diminishes on stopping but remains significantly higher compared with nonusers for many years after cessation of use. The estimated relative risk in former users compared with nonusers is 3.7 at 1 year after discontinuation and remains as high as 1.9 at 12 years after discontinued treatment. The relative risk associated with use discontinued for less than 5 years is 3.5 (95% CI, 3.0–4.0) and 2.5 (95% CI, 1.9–3.2) for use discontinued for 5 or more years.

Type of Estrogen Replacement and Estrogen Dose

Conjugated equine estrogens comprise the most frequently prescribed form of ERT in North America. Separate estimates of endometrial cancer risk were available for conjugated estrogens and other types of estrogen from eleven studies (46,50,52,54,57,60,61,64,73,75,85). The estimated relative risk of endometrial cancer compared with nonusers is 2.6 (95% CI, 2.0–3.4) for users of ERT consisting of other estrogens and 3.0 (95% CI, 2.5–3.7) for users of ERT consisting of conjugated estrogens, a difference that is not statistically significant ($p = 0.65$).

Estimates of the relative risk of endometrial cancer compared with nonusers according to estrogen dosage

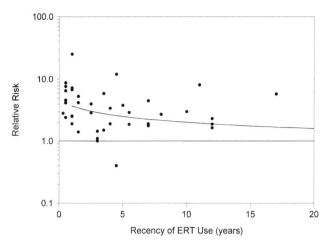

FIG. 46.3. Relative risk of endometrial cancer by recency of unopposed estrogen use (ERT).

were drawn from 16 studies (44,46,47,50,54,56,60–62, 65,66,68,73,74,79,83). Increasing estrogen content is associated with a trend of increasing risk: the estimated relative risks are 3.2, 4.0 and 5.0 for preparations containing less than 0.625 mg of conjugated equine estrogens, 0.625 mg, or more than 0.625 mg, respectively (trend: $p = 0.05$) (Figs. 46.2 and 46.3).

Use of Progestins in Hormone Replacement Therapy

Progestins are included in only a minority of hormone prescriptions for menopause in North America (13), and consequently, the small number of estimates of endometrial cancer risk associated with combined estrogen-progestin therapy are based on relatively few cases. Figure 46.4 shows 21 estimates of endometrial cancer risk by duration of combined estrogen-progestin therapy. The estimates are drawn from five case-control studies and

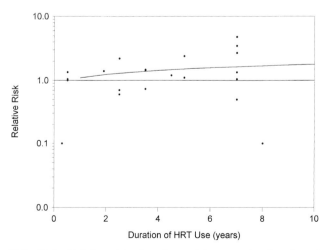

FIG. 46.4. Relative risk of endometrial cancer by duration of estrogen and progestin use (HRT).

one cohort study (45,46,67,75,77,84). For use less than 5 years, endometrial cancer risk is 1.2-fold higher than for nonusers (95% CI, 1.0–1.5), a result compatible with only a small increased risk. With use for 5 years or more, endometrial cancer risk was 2.9-fold higher than in nonusers (95% CI, 1.5–5.4).

An important consideration is the duration of progestin exposure in each cycle of HRT use. With use of progestin for less than 10 days, the relative risk of endometrial cancer relative to nonusers is 2.0 (95% CI, 1.6–2.6) compared with a relative risk of 1.1 (95% CI, 0.9–1.3) when progestin was used for 10 days or more in each cycle ($p = 0.04$). Estimates of relative risk associated with daily continuous use of combined estrogen and progestin were reported in only one study: the relative risk of endometrial cancer with continuous HRT was 1.1 for use less than 2 years and 1.3 for use longer than 5 years (84).

Although the data on HRT use with progestins are based on only 424 exposed cases, the evidence consistently indicates that use of progestins lessens the adverse effect of unopposed estrogen on the overall risk of endometrial cancer. As with prevention of endometrial hyperplasia, the key element appears to be a sufficient duration of progestin exposure (84,86,87).

Tumor Characteristics

Estrogen use tends to be identified with favorable categories of the known prognostic factors, such as earlier stage and lower grade of the tumor (44,47,55,60,61). It remains unclear, however, whether this association arises from earlier detection of tumors because of increased surveillance among users or because tumors arising with estrogen use are truly less aggressive.

With respect to stage, the relative risk associated with ERT use was 3.3 (95% CI, 2.7–4.0) for stage I disease, compared with 1.6 (95% CI, 1.2–2.2) for more advanced stages (trend: $p = 0.016$), based on eight reported estimates (44,47,50,52,55,57,61,88). With respect to grade, the ERT-associated relative risk was 3.6 (95% CI, 3.0–4.4) for grade 1 tumors and 2.3 (95% CI, 2.0–2.7) for higher histologic grades ($p = 0.016$), based on 10 studies (44,47,50,52,55,57,60,61,88,89). Although grade 1 tumors are well differentiated and more likely to occur with less advanced clinical stage, most estimates for grade were not adjusted for stage.

Before myometrial invasion was incorporated into clinical staging, it was measured by different methods and not reported uniformly (3). We therefore consider the following categories to be minimal invasion: no myometrial invasion, superficial myometrial invasion, and penetration to less than one-half depth. Based on nine studies (44,47,55,60,61,68,84,88,89), the average relative risk associated with ERT was 4.1 (95% CI, 3.3–5.1) for minimal invasion compared with 2.5 (95% CI, 2.0–3.1) for deeper degrees of myometrial invasion (trend: $p = 0.02$).

Two studies described the association between estrogen-progestin HRT and tumor characteristics. In the first of these, with use of estrogen plus cyclic or continuous progestin for 3 or more years, the relative risk of endometrial cancer was 1.7, 1.9, and 1.4 for grade 1, 2, and 3 lesions, respectively (89). The relative risk was 2.1 (95% CI, 1.2–3.7) for tumor confined to the endometrium and 1.3 (95% CI, 0.8–2.2) for myometrial invasion (89). In the second of these studies, with continuous use of estrogen combined with progestin, the relative risk was 1.3 (95% CI, 0.7–2.2) for endometrial cancer confined to the endometrium and 1.2 (95% CI, 0.8–1.6) for invasion up to the first half of the myometrium (84). Although estrogen use is associated with favorable endometrial cancer prognostic factors, no such trend is seen with use of estrogen-progestin combinations. The lower risk of endometrial cancer with HRT compared with ERT, which was discussed in the forgoing section, may reflect a reduced risk of tumors with more favorable characteristics.

Endometrial Cancer Survival

Because estrogen use appears to be associated with endometrial cancers that have less tendency to metastasize, it should also be associated with better survival. This expectation is confirmed by the results of six follow-up studies reporting 2,442 cancer patients, 851 of whom (35%) were users of ERT (55,74,90–93). In the two studies that made use of survival analysis techniques to adjust for age, stage, grade, and myometrial invasion, the risk of death from any cause was 2.4-fold higher in nonusers than estrogen users (95% CI, 1.4–4.0). Considering deaths from endometrial cancer only, the relative likelihood was 4.8-fold higher in nonusers than in estrogen users (95% CI, 2.2–10.3) (91,92).

INTERPRETATION OF THE HRT ASSOCIATION WITH ENDOMETRIAL CANCER

The increased risk of endometrial cancer associated with the use of ERT is consistent among the reported studies and does not result from known sources of bias and confounding, for which adjustments have been made. Risk increases with longer duration of ERT and with higher ERT dosage, and there is a residual increased risk from prior use. In view of the biologic rationale reviewed earlier, these findings indicate that the increased risk of endometrial cancer associated with use of ERT is a biologic effect of replacement therapy.

The risk of endometrial cancer rises soon after ERT use begins, showing no intervening latent period, and a residual elevated risk remains after discontinuing therapy. The residual effect of ERT on endometrial cancer incidence could be caused by tumors arising from cells affected near the beginning of cancer development, which would take years to reach clinical detection, in some cases long after therapy had been discontinued. The lack of a latent period implies that preclinical tumors may respond promptly to estrogen exposure and become clinically recognizable. Such response could be caused by estrogen-induced cell division or angiogenesis. The epidemiologic studies are consistent with an estrogen effect on cancer progression at two stages of tumor development: an early effect on cells that have undergone genetic damage and a later effect on existing preclinical cancers.

The absence of a latent period is also consistent with a nonbiologic effect of HRT arising from increased diagnostic surveillance. Hormone-induced bleeding in estrogen users (32,94,95) may prompt diagnostic tests and reveal the presence of latent cancers that remain undetected in nonuser controls. Closer surveillance is not a sufficient explanation for the association between estrogen and endometrial cancer, but the association remains even when the control groups also have complete endometrial assessment (53,54,66), and no appreciable risk occurs with short-term use of estrogen-progestin combined HRT, which is also associated with hormone-induced bleeding and increased medical attention (32). Nevertheless, it must be acknowledged that eliminating potential diagnostic bias does reduce the magnitude of the relative risk, suggesting that earlier diagnosis of latent tumors in HRT users may account for a small portion of the increased risk of endometrial cancer.

The link between ERT and more favorable tumor characteristics could be explained by the tendency toward earlier diagnosis among estrogen users compared with nonusers. Women with endometrial cancer who have used estrogen have a shorter interval between symptoms and diagnosis than nonusers (60), which is consistent with the association between estrogen use and earlier stage, lower grade, less myometrial invasion, and younger age at diagnosis (92,93).

The better survival associated with estrogen use could arise from earlier diagnosis in estrogen users, better health in estrogen users who develop cancer, or less aggressive tumors associated with estrogen use (74,90, 91). Earlier diagnosis does occur for estrogen users, but the better survival associated with estrogen use remains after adjustment for less advanced disease. On average, those who are able to pay for optional prescriptions such as estrogen would be expected to enjoy better health, and among patients with endometrial cancer, deaths from any cause were less likely for estrogen users. Because deaths from endometrial cancer were also less likely in these patients, it remains possible that the tumors associated with estrogen use are less aggressive, perhaps because hormone-dependent mechanisms of tumor growth are only possible in cancer cells that have not undergone advanced disruption of cell regulation mechanisms (Fig. 46.4).

TABLE 46.1. *Cumulative number of uterine cancer cases arising between 50 and 74 years of age in 100,000 U.S. women (all races) using replacement therapies*

Cases	Duration of replacement therapy (years)			
	0	4	8	12
Estrogen only				
Total cases	2061	4202	6330	8008
Additional cases		2141	4269	5947
Estrogen with progestin				
Total cases	2061	2445	2761	2972
Additional cases		383	700	911

NET EFFECT OF ESTROGEN REPLACEMENT AND HORMONE REPLACEMENT THERAPIES ON UTERINE CANCER

To determine the absolute risk of uterine cancer associated with the relative risks described previously, Table 46.1 shows estimates of the cumulative incidence of uterine corpus cancer by duration of use of ERT and HRT. The first column in Table 46.1 shows that, in a cohort of 100,000 U.S. women who never use ERT or HRT, 2,061 are expected to develop invasive cancer of the uterine corpus at some time between the ages of 50 and 74 years. Columns 2 through 4 show the corresponding estimated numbers of cancer cases in cohorts of 100,000 women using ERT (upper panel) or HRT (lower panel). For example, among 100,000 U.S. women who use ERT for 4 years beginning at the age of 50, a total of 4,202 cases of invasive cancer of the uterine corpus, or an *additional* 2,141 cases, are estimated to occur from age 50 through 74 years. For women using ERT for 8 years or 12 years, the additional number of invasive cancers among 100,000 users would be 4,269 and 5,847, respectively.

The lower panel of Table 46.1 refers to women who use HRT (i.e., estrogen and progestin). For example (column 2), among 100,000 U.S. women who begin 4 years of HRT use at age 50, 2,445 are expected to develop invasive cancer of the uterine corpus at some time between the ages of 50 and 74 years. This represents an *additional* 383 cases per 100,000 users. For women using HRT for 8 years or 12 years, the additional number of invasive cancers per 100,000 users is 700 and 911, respectively.

The calculations in Table 46.1 are based on our estimates of the age-specific incidence rate of uterine cancer in women using ERT or HRT (I_{users}), calculated as a function of women's age, duration of replacement-therapy use, and recency of use by means of the following equation:

$$I_{users} = I_{age} \times RR_{dur} \times RR_{rec}$$

I_{age} denotes the age-specific rate of invasive cancer of the uterine corpus (plus NOS) in nonusers of replacement therapy. The values were assumed to equal the incidence rates reported for the time period 1991–1995 in U.S. women (21). RR_{dur} and RR_{rec} denote our estimates of rel-

ative risk by duration and recentness of use of ERT or HRT. The calculation of cumulative incidence in Table 46.1 was based on standard life-table methods (96) applied to the values of I_{users} on the assumption that any duration-related effect of replacement therapy appears immediately (i.e., there is no latent effect) and that use of replacement therapy begins at age 50 and continues without interruption for 4, 8, or 12 years.

Figure 46.5 is a graphic representation of cumulative incidence of uterine cancer by women's age and duration of replacement therapy; the values at age 75 were summarized in Table 46.1. Use of unopposed estrogens is expected to lead to a large number of uterine cancers, because a high multiple of risk from ERT is applied to a high baseline incidence rate and because the effect of ERT is not immediately eliminated on discontinuing therapy. It is critical to ensure that such therapy includes progestin for each woman who has a uterus (15). Prevention is important because the diagnosis of cancer leads to signif-

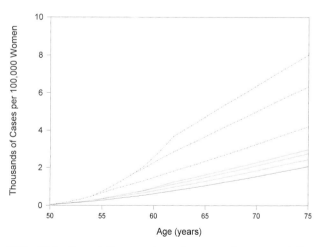

FIG. 46.5. Cumulative number of cases of cancer of the uterine corpus for U.S. women of all races, 1991–1995. Effects of unopposed estrogen (ERT) and estrogen with progestin (HRT) are demonstrated. Solid line indicates no HRT use. Dotted lines indicate HRT use; the lower, middle, and upper lines represent use for 4, 8, and 12 years, respectively. Broken lines indicate ERT use; the lower, middle, and upper lines represent use for 4, 8, and 12 years, respectively.

icant morbidity, cost, and attendant anxiety. Although use of progestin does not eliminate entirely the estrogen-associated risk, the number of additional cases of invasive uterine cancer in women using HRT is substantially reduced. For women beginning HRT at age 50 and continuing for 12 years, the risk of uterine cancer through age 74 is reduced from 6% to 1% with the use of progestin. For women on therapy for 8 years, the corresponding reduction in risk is from 4.3% (ERT) to 0.7% (HRT).

CONCLUSIONS

Epidemiologic studies consistently show that a woman with a uterus who is on estrogen replacement therapy is at increased risk of developing endometrial cancer. The risk of endometrial cancer in women using replacement therapy consists of a baseline risk shared with nonusers and a further risk due to hormonal effects on transformed cells and preclinical cancers. Progestins ameliorate but do not completely abolish the estrogen-related components of the HRT-associated risk. Survival of patients with endometrial cancer is better for those who have used estrogen, but this does not reassure potential hormone users, who prefer to avoid endometrial cancer entirely.

HRT offers relief of menopausal symptoms and is potentially associated with other important benefits, including a reduced likelihood of osteoporotic fractures and myocardial infarction (81,97–99). Although use of progestins diminishes the beneficial effects of estrogen on lipid markers of cardiovascular disease, there is no clear evidence that progestins reduce the important cardiovascular outcomes (100). Our estimates indicate that 6% of a cohort of 50-year-old American women who use unopposed estrogen for 12 years would develop endometrial cancer before reaching 75 years of age and that the use of progestins would reduce this figure to 1%. The cardiovascular benefits of unopposed estrogen compared with the combination with progestin would have to be well proven to warrant a policy of prescribing unopposed estrogen for a long period.

REFERENCES

1. Wynder EL, Escher GC, Mantel N. An epidemiologic investigation of cancer of the endometrium. *Cancer* 1966;10:489–520.
2. Sulak PJ. Endometrial cancer and hormone replacement therapy. *Endocrinol Metab Clin North Am* 1997;26:399–411.
3. Kurman RJ, Zaino RJ, Norris HJ. Endometrial carcinoma. In: Kurman RJ, ed. *Blaustein's pathology of the female genital tract*, 4th ed. New York: Springer-Verlag, 1994:439–486.
4. Henry JS. The avoidance of untoward effects of estrogenic therapy in the menopause. *Can Med Assoc J* 1945;53:31–37.
5. Hurxthal LM, Smith AT. Treatment of endometriosis and other gynecologic conditions with large doses of estrogens. *N Engl J Med* 1952;247:339–343.
6. Scott RB, Wharton LR. The effects of excessive amounts of diethylstilbestrol on experimental endometriosis in monkeys. *Am J Obstet Gynecol* 1955;69:573–587.
7. Jensen EI, Ostergaard E. Clinical studies concerning the relationship of estrogens to the development of cancer of the corpus uteri. *Am J Obstet Gynecol* 1954;67:1094–1102.
8. Dunn LJ, Bradbury JT. Endocrine factors in endometrial carcinoma. *Am J Obstet Gynecol* 1967;97:465–471.
9. Quint BC. Changing patterns in endometrial adenocarcinoma. *Am J Obstet Gynecol* 1975;122:498–501.
10. Smith DC, Prentice R, Thompson DJ, Herrmann WL. Association of exogenous estrogen and endometrial carcinoma. *N Engl J Med* 1975;293:1164–1166.
11. Ziel HK, Finkle WD. Increased risk of endometrial carcinoma among users of conjugated estrogens. *N Engl J Med* 1975;293:1167–1170.
12. Kennedy DL, Baum C, Forbes MB. Noncontraceptive estrogens and progestins: use patterns over time. *Obstet Gynecol* 1985;65:441–446.
13. Wysowski DK, Golden L, Burke L. Use of menopausal estrogens and medroxyprogesterone in the United States, 1982–1992. *Obstet Gynecol* 1995;85:6–10.
14. Ross RK, Paganini-Hill A, Roy S, Chao A, Henderson BE. Past and present preferred prescribing practices of hormone replacement therapy among Los Angeles gynecologists: possible implications for public health. *Am J Public Health* 1988;78:516–519.
15. Harris RB, Laws A, Reddy VM, King A, Haskell WL. Are women using postmenopausal estrogens? A community survey. *Am J Public Health* 1990;80:1266–1268.
16. Thompson W. Estrogen replacement therapy in practice: trends and issues. *Am J Obstet Gynecol* 1995;173:990–993.
17. Oddens BJ, Boulet MJ. Hormone replacement therapy among Danish women aged 45–65 years: prevalence, determinants, and compliance. *Obstet Gynecol* 1997;90:269–277.
18. Lancaster T, Daly E, Yudkin P, et al. Hormone replacement therapy: characteristics of users and non-users in a British general practice cohort identified through computerised prescribing records. *J Epidemiol Commun Health* 1995;49:389–394.
19. Kadri AZ. Hormone-replacement therapy—a survey of perimenopausal women in a community setting. *Br J Gen Pract* 1991;41:109–112.
20. Mattsson LA, Milsom I, Stadberg E. Management of hormone replacement therapy: the Swedish experience. *Eur J Obstet Gynecol Reprod Biol* 1996;64:S3–S5.
21. Ries LAG, Kosary CL, Hankey BF, Miller BA, Edwards BK. *SEER cancer statistics review, 1973–1995*. Bethesda, MD: National Cancer Institute, 1998.
22. Schlesselman JJ, Collins JA. Influence of steroids on the incidence and severity of gynecologic cancer. In: Fraser IS, Jansen R, Lobo RA, Whitehead M, eds. *Estrogens and progestogens in clinical practice*. New York: Churchill-Livingstone, 1999:831–864.
23. Sherman ME, Sturgeon S, Brinton LA, et al. Risk factors and hormone levels in patients with serous and endometrioid uterine carcinomas. *Mod Pathol* 1997;10:963–968.
24. Kelsey JL, Whittemore AS. Epidemiology and primary prevention of cancers of the breast, endometrium, and ovary: a brief overview. *Ann Epidemiol* 1994;4:89–95.
25. Landis SH, Murray T, Bolden S, Wingo PA. Cancer Statistics, 1998. *CA Cancer J Clin* 1998;48:6–29.
26. King R, Whitehead M, Campbell S, Minardi J. Effect of estrogen and progestin treatments on endometria from postmenopausal women. *Cancer Res* 1979;39:1094–1101.
27. Whitehead M, Townsend P, Pryse-Davies J, Ryder T, King R. Effects of estrogens and progestins on the biochemistry and morphology of the postmenopausal endometrium. *N Engl J Med* 1981;305:1599–1605.
28. Henderson BE, Ross RK, Bernstein L. Estrogens as a cause of human cancer: the Richard and Hinda Rosenthal Foundation award lecture. *Cancer Res* 1988;48:246–251.
29. Wu ML, Einstein M, Geissler WM, Chan HK, Elliston KO, Andersson S. Expression cloning and characterization of human 17-beta-hydroxysteroid dehydrogenase type 2, a microsomal enzyme possessing 20-alpha-hydroxysteroid dehydrogenase activity. *J Biol Chem* 1993;268:12964.
30. PEPI Trial Writing Group. Effects of hormone replacement therapy on endometrial histology in postmenopausal women. *JAMA* 1996;275:370–375.
31. Woodruff JD, Pickar JH. Incidence of endometrial hyperplasia in postmenopausal women taking conjugated estrogens (Premarin) with medroxyprogesterone acetate or conjugated estrogens alone. *Am J Obstet Gynecol* 1994;170:1213–1223.
32. Speroff L, Rowan J, Symons J, Genant H, Wilborn W. The comparative effect on bone density, endometrium, and lipids of continuous hormones as replacement therapy (CHART study): a randomized controlled study. *JAMA* 1996;276:1397–1403.
33. Cavenee WK, White RL. The genetic basis of cancer. *Sci Am* 1995;272:72–79.
34. Clarkson BD. Consistent genetic abnormalities in human cancers as targets for selective therapies. *Mt Sinai J Med* 1992;59:400–404.
35. Rabbitts TH. Translocations, master genes, and differences between the origins of acute and chronic leukemias. *Cell* 1991;67:641–644.
36. Enomoto T, Fujita M, Inoue M, et al. Alterations of the p53 tumor suppressor gene and its association with activation of the c-K-ras-2 protooncogene in premalignant and malignant lesions of the human uterine endometrium. *Cancer Res* 1993;53:1883–1888.
37. Hoffmann D, Hecht S, Schmeltz I, Wynder E. Polynuclear aromatic hydrocarbons: occurrence, formation, and carcinogenicity. In: Asher IM, Zervos C, eds. *Structural correlates of carcinogenesis and mutagenesis: a guide to testing priorities?* Washington, DC: Office of Science, Food and Drug Administration, 1978:120–127.
38. Christopherson WM, Gray LA. Premalignant lesions of the endometrium: endometrial hyperplasia and adenocarcinoma in situ. In: Coppleson M, Monaghan JM, Morrow CP, Tattersall MHN, eds. *Gynecologic oncology*, 2nd ed. New York: Churchill Livingstone, 1992:731–745.

39. Grossman C. Regulation of the immune system by sex steroids. *Endocr Rev* 1984;5:435–455.

40. Folkman J. Clinical applications of research on angiogenesis. *N Engl J Med* 1995;333:1757–1763.

41. Giudice LC, Ferenczy A. The endometrial cycle. In: Adashi EY, Rock JA, Rosenwaks Z, eds. *Reproductive endocrinology, surgery and technology.* Philadelphia: Lippincott-Raven, 1996:271–300.

42. White MM, Zamudio S, Stevens T, et al. Estrogen, progesterone, and vascular reactivity: potential cellular mechanisms. *Endocr Rev* 1995;16:739–751.

43. Chester AH, Jiang C, Borland JA, Yacoub MH, Collins P. Oestrogen relaxes human epicardial coronary arteries through non–endothelium-dependent mechanisms. *Coron Artery Dis* 1995;6:417–422.

44. Antunes C, Stolley P, Rosenshein N, et al. Endometrial cancer and estrogen use: report of a large case-control study. *N Engl J Med* 1979;300:9–13.

45. Beresford SAA, Weiss NS, Voigt LF, McKnight B. Risk of endometrial cancer in relation to use of oestrogen combined with cyclic progestagen therapy in postmenopausal women. *Lancet* 1997;349:458–461.

46. Brinton LA, Hoover RN, Endometrial Cancer Collaborative Group. Estrogen replacement therapy and endometrial cancer risk: unresolved issues. *Obstet Gynecol* 1993;81:2:265–271.

47. Buring JE, Bain CJ, Ehrmann RL. Conjugated estrogen use and risk of endometrial cancer. *Am J Epidemiol* 1986;124:434–441.

48. Ewertz M, Schou G, Boice JD. The joint effect of risk factors on endometrial cancer. *Eur J Cancer Clin Oncol* 1988;24:189–194.

49. Franks AL, Kendrick J, Tyler C, The Cancer and Steroid Hormone Study Group. Postmenopausal smoking, estrogen replacement therapy, and the risk of endometrial cancer. *Am J Obstet Gynecol* 1987;156:20–23.

50. Gray LA, Christopherson WM, Hoover RN. Estrogens and Endometrial carcinoma. *Obstet Gynecol* 1977;49:385–391.

51. Henderson BE, Casagrande JT, Pike MC, Mack T, Rosario I, Duke A. The epidemiology of endometrial cancer in young women. *Br J Cancer* 1983;47:749–756.

52. Hoogerland DL, Buchler DA, Crowley JJ, Carr WA. Estrogen use—risk of endometrial carcinoma. *Gynecol Oncol* 1978;6:451–458.

53. Horwitz R, Feinstein AR. Alternative analytic methods for case-control studies of estrogens and endometrial cancer. *N Engl J Med* 1978;299:1089–1094.

54. Hulka B, Fowler W, Kaufman D, et al. Estrogen and endometrial cancer: cases and two control groups from North Carolina. *Am J Obstet Gynecol* 1980;137:92–101.

55. Jelovsek F, Hammond C, Woodard B, et al. Risk of exogenous estrogen therapy and endometrial cancer. *Am J Obstet Gynecol* 1980;137:85–91.

56. Jick SS, Walker AM, Jick H. Estrogens, progesterone, and endometrial cancer. *Epidemiology* 1993;4:20–24.

57. Kelsey JL, Livolsi VA, Holford TR, et al. A case-control study of cancer of the endometrium. *Am J Epidemiol* 1982;116:333–342.

58. La Vecchia C, Franceschi S, Decarli A, Gallus G, Tognoni G. Risk factors for endometrial cancer at different ages. *J Natl Cancer Inst* 1984;73:667–671.

59. Levi F, La Vecchia C, Gulie C, Franceschi S, Negri E. Oestrogen replacement treatment and the risk of endometrial cancer: an assessment of the role of co-variates. *Eur J Cancer* 1993;29A:1445–1449.

60. Mack TM, Pike MC, Henderson BE, et al. Estrogens and endometrial cancer in a retirement community. *N Engl J Med* 1976;294:1262–1267.

61. McDonald TW, Annegers JF, O'Fallon WM, Dockerty MB, Malkasian GD, Kurland LT. Exogenous estrogen and endometrial carcinoma: case-control and incidence study. *Am J Obstet Gynecol* 1977;127:572–579.

62. Rubin GL, Peterson HB, Lee NC, Maes EF, Wingo PA, Becker S. Estrogen replacement therapy and the risk of endometrial cancer: remaining controversies. *Am J Obstet Gynecol* 1990;162:148–154.

63. Salmi T. Endometrial carcinoma risk factors, with special reference to the use of oestrogens. *Acta Endocrinol* 1980;233:37–43.

64. Shapiro S, Kelly J, Rosenberg L, et al. Risk of localized and widespread endometrial cancer in relation to recent and discontinued use of conjugated estrogens. *N Engl J Med* 1985;313:969–972.

65. Spengler R, Clarke E, Woolever C, Newman A, Osborn R. Exogenous estrogens and endometrial cancer: a case-control study and assessment of potential biases. *Am J Epidemiol* 1981;114:497–506.

66. Stavraky K, Collins JA, Donner A, Wells G. A comparison of estrogen use by women with endometrial cancer, gynecologic disorders, and other illnesses. *Am J Obstet Gynecol* 1981;141:547–555.

67. Voigt LF, Weiss NS, Chu J, Daling JR, McKnight B, Van Belle G. Progestagen supplementation of exogenous oestrogens and risk of endometrial cancer. *Lancet* 1991;338:274–277.

68. Weiss NS, Szekely DR, English DR, Schweid AI. Endometrial cancer in relation to patterns of menopausal estrogen use. *JAMA* 1979;242:261–264.

69. Wigle DT, Grace M, Smith ESO. Estrogen use and cancer of the uterine corpus in Alberta. *Can Med Assoc J* 1978;118:1276–1278.

70. Folsom AR, Mink PJ, Sellers TA, Hong C-P, Zheng W, Potter JD. Hormonal replacement therapy and morbidity and mortality in a prospective study of postmenopausal women. *Am J Public Health* 1995;85:1128–1132.

71. Gambrell RD, Massey F, Castaneda TA, Ugenas A, Ricci C, Wright J. Use of the progestogen challenge test to reduce the risk of endometrial cancer. *Obstet Gynecol* 1980;55:732–738.

72. Hoover R, Fraumeni JF, Everson R, Myers MH. Cancer of the uterine corpus after hormonal treatment for breast cancer. *Lancet* 1976;1:885–887.

73. Jick H, Watkins RN, Hunter JR, et al. Replacement estrogens and endometrial cancer. *N Engl J Med* 1979;300:218–222.

74. Paganini-Hill A, Ross RK, Henderson BE. Endometrial cancer and patterns of use of oestrogen replacement therapy: a cohort study. *Br J Cancer* 1989;59:445–447.

75. Persson I, Adami H-O, Bergkvist L, et al. Risk of endometrial cancer after treatment with oestrogens alone or in conjunction with progestogens: results of a prospective study. *BMJ* 1989;298:147–151.

76. Petitti D, Perlman J, Sidney S. Noncontraceptive estrogens and mortality: long-term follow-up of women in the Walnut Creek study. *Obstet Gynecol* 1987;70:289–293.

77. Jick SS. Combined estrogen and progesterone use and endometrial cancer. *Epidemiology* 1993;4:384–384.

78. Ettinger B, Golditch IM, Friedman G. Gynecologic consequences of long-term, unopposed estrogen replacement therapy. *Maturitas* 1988;10:271–282.

79. Hammond CB, Jelovsek FR, Lee KL, Creasman WT, Parker RT. Effects of long-term estrogen replacement therapy: II. Neoplasia. *Am J Obstet Gynecol* 1979;133:537–547.

80. Hunt K, Vessey M, McPherson K, Coleman M. Long-term surveillance of mortality and cancer incidence in women receiving hormone replacement therapy. *Br J Obstet Gynaecol* 1987;94:620–635.

81. Lafferty FW, Helmuth DO. Post-menopausal estrogen replacement: the prevention of osteoporosis and systemic benefits. *Maturitas* 1985;7:147–159.

82. Vakil D, Morgan R, Halliday M. Exogenous estrogens and development of breast and endometrial cancer. *Cancer Detect Prev* 1983;6:415–424.

83. Cushing KL, Weiss NS, Voigt LF, McKnight B, Beresford SAA. Risk of endometrial cancer in relation to use of low-dose, unopposed estrogens. *Obstet Gynecol* 1998;91:35–39.

84. Pike MC, Peters RK, Cozen W, et al. Estrogen-Progestin Replacement Therapy and Endometrial Cancer. *J Natl Cancer Inst* 1997;89:1110–1116.

85. Shapiro S, Kaufman D, Slone D, et al. Recent and past use of conjugated estrogens in relation to adenocarcinoma of the endometrium. *N Engl J Med* 1980;303:485–489.

86. Whitehead M. Prevention of endometrial abnormalities. *Acta Obstet Gynecol Scand Suppl* 1986;134:81–91.

87. Varma T. Effect of long-term therapy with estrogen and progesterone on the endometrium of post-menopausal women. *Acta Obstet Gynecol Scand* 1985;64:41–46.

88. Hulka B, Kaufman D, Fowler W Jr, Grimson R, Greenberg B. Predominance of early endometrial cancers after long-term estrogen use. *JAMA* 1980;244:2419–2422.

89. Shapiro JA, Weiss NS, Beresford SAA, Voigt LF. Menopausal hormone use and endometrial cancer by tumor grade and invasion. *Epidemiology* 1998;9:99–101.

90. Chu J, Schweid A, Weiss N. Survival among women with endometrial cancer: a comparison of estrogen users and nonusers. *Am J Obstet Gynecol* 1982;143:569–573.

91. Collins JA, Allen L, Donner A, Adams O. Oestrogen use and survival in endometrial cancer. *Lancet* 1980:961–963.

92. Schwartzbaum JA, Hulka BS, Fowler WC, Kaufman DG, Hoberman D. The influence of exogenous estrogen use on survival after diagnosis of endometrial cancer. *Am J Epidemiol* 1987;126:851–860.

93. Elwood JM, Boyes D. Clinical and pathological features and survival of endometrial cancer patients in relation to prior use of estrogens. *Gynecol Oncol* 1980;10:173–187.

94. Archer DF, Pickar JH, Bottiglioni F. Bleeding patterns in postmenopausal women taking continuous combined or sequential regimens of conjugated estrogens with medroxyprogesterone acetate. *Obstet Gynecol* 1994;83:686–692.

95. Clisham PR, de Ziegler D, Lozano K, Judd HL. Comparison of continuous versus sequential estrogen and progestin therapy in postmenopausal women. *Obstet Gynecol* 1991;77:241–246.

96. Cutler S, Ederer F. Maximum utilization of the life table method in analyzing survival. *J Chron Dis* 1958;8:699–712.

97. Naessen T, Persson I, Adami H-O, Bergstrom R, Bergkvist L. Hormone replacement therapy and the risk of first hip fracture: a prospective, population-based cohort study. *Ann Intern Med* 1990;113:95–103.

98. Falkeborn M, Persson I, Hans-Olov A, et al. The risk of acute myocardial infarction after oestrogen and oestrogen-progestogen replacement. *Br J Obstet Gynaecol* 1992;99:821–828.

99. Stampfer MJ, Willett W, Colditz GA, Rosner B, Speizer F, Hennekens C. A prospective study of postmenopausal estrogen therapy and coronary heart disease. *N Engl J Med* 1985;313:1044–1049.

100. Grady D, Rubin SM, Petitti DB, et al. Hormone therapy to prevent disease and prolong life in postmenopausal women. *Ann Intern Med* 1992;117:12:1016–1037.

Treatment of the Postmenopausal Woman: Basic and Clinical Aspects, Second Edition, edited by Rogerio A. Lobo, Lippincott Williams & Wilkins, Philadelphia © 1999.

CHAPTER 47

Detection and Surveillance of Endometrial Hyperplasia and Carcinoma

Anna K. Parsons and Jorge L. Londono

Endometrial cancer is the most commonly diagnosed gynecologic cancer in the United States, and 75% of cases occur in the postmenopausal years. It has well-defined risk factors, most of which have excessive endogenous or exogenous estrogen exposure in common (1–4). It accounts for 6% of all cancers diagnosed in women, behind those of the breast (30%), lung and bronchus (13%), and colon and rectum (11%). It is the seventh most frequent neoplastic cause of death, accounting for 2% of deaths from cancer in women. The American Cancer Society estimates that 36,100 women were diagnosed in 1998 and that 6,300 women died of this type of cancer, which seems to represent a plateau in incidence and a slight increase in death rate in this decade. There is a lower incidence among Hispanic and black women than white women. The 5-year survival rates are 81% for Hispanic women (5), 86% for white women (6), but only 55% for black women (much lower than the 74% rate with breast cancer) because of detection of more virulent cancers at a later stage (7). Most endometrial cancers announce themselves by bleeding at an early stage (8).

General screening for endometrial cancer is neither endorsed by the American College of Obstetricians and Gynecologists (ACOG) (9) nor the American Cancer Society (ACS). Even so, the ACS Task Force on Gynecologic Cancer recommended on October 3, 1993, that screening office sampling should be considered for women with a history of infertility, obesity, anovulation, abnormal uterine bleeding at menopause, unopposed estrogen therapy, or tamoxifen therapy. They mention that 30% of the virulent tumors that develop are found in low-risk women (10). The ACOG recommends uterine evaluation only for women with abnormal bleeding.

POSTMENOPAUSAL BLEEDING: EFFECTS OF HORMONE REPLACEMENT THERAPY

Unexpected vaginal bleeding in the postmenopausal woman has been considered an absolute indication for prompt endometrial sampling, an interesting situation now that most bleeding is iatrogenic. Fewer than 2 of 10 women with abnormal postmenopausal bleeding are found to have endometrial cancer (11,12), and there is a much lower incidence in populations treated with standard regimens of estrogen and progestin hormone replacement therapy (HRT) (13–18).

Ettinger et al. found that, when used in general practice, cyclic and continuous combined regimens induced a significant incidence of bleeding requiring evaluation for up to 2 years after beginning treatment of women who continued treatment (19). No atypical hyperplasia or cancer occurred in either group (Fig. 47.1) (1). A Swedish randomized, double-blind study of 568 postmenopausal women on estrone and continuous 2.5-, 5.0, or 10-mg doses of medroxyprogesterone acetate (MPA) reported amenorrhea in 77%, 80%, and 81%, respectively, by 6 months (20). However after 2 years, there was still bleeding in 10% of women remaining in each group, none of whom had any endometrial abnormality found on biopsy.

Archer et al. reported that about 45% of 678 highly selected, low-risk, white postmenopausal women on a continuous combined regimen of 0.625 mg of conjugated equine estrogen (CEE) and 2.5 or 5.0 mg of MPA bled in the last 7 months of a year's observation, with the rate decreasing to 25% during the final 3 months. As expected, 95% of 699 similar women taking 0.625 mg CEE daily and 5 or 10 mg of MPA 14 days per month had cyclic bleeding at the end of a year (21).

A.K. Parsons, J.L. Londono: Department of Obstetrics and Gynecology, University of South Florida, Tampa, Florida 33606.

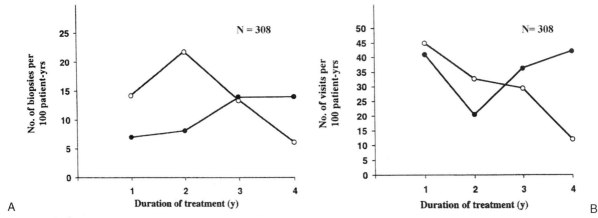

FIG. 47.1. A: Endometrial biopsies per 100 patient-years for unexpected bleeding in first-time users of continuous combined (○) or cyclic (●) hormone replacement therapy (HRT). **B:** Clinic visits per 100 patient-years for unexpected vaginal bleeding in 308 women using continuous combined (○) or cyclic (●) HRT. Ettinger et al. (19) reviewed clinical records in an unscreened health maintenance organization clinic population of 284 women starting continuous combined HRT and 306 women starting cyclic HRT. Until the third year after initiation of treatment, most biopsies were performed in women treated with continuous regimens. One of three women starting either regimen went to the clinic for unexpected bleeding, and in one-half of those visits, a biopsy was done during the first 2 years of treatment.

Although these women were screened with endometrial biopsy on admission to this study, we also evaluated the subset of 26 women who completed this protocol at our center with sonohysterography. We found that 11% of them had an intrauterine lesion that may have influenced the bleeding pattern throughout treatment; one woman on a continuous combined regimen and one on unopposed estrogen had a benign polyp; one woman on a cyclic regimen had a 1-cm intracavitary myoma (unpublished data). All three had a pattern of unremitting or increasing and unexpected bleeding throughout the 13 cycles of treatment. All three were initially asymptomatic, with atrophic biopsy results and baseline endometrial measurements of 5 to 10 mm. After 13 cycles of treatment, the total measurements of endometrial thickness were 10, 15, and 38 mm. After subtracting the measurement of the polyp or myoma obtained with saline infusion, the sums of the two endometrial layers were 5 mm (continuous combined), 8 mm (cyclic) and 10 mm (estrogen only), respectively. Both polyps were benign when sampled during the study and when all (including the myoma) were removed at the end of the study by ultrasound-directed biopsy in the office.

Endometrial biopsy results from a single pathologist obtained while screening 801 low-risk, untreated women for this same study included a 0.6% incidence of cancer or atypical hyperplasia (5 women), atrophy in 47% (373 women), proliferation in 16.7% (133 women), secretory changes in 6.8% (54 women), and typical hyperplasia in 5.2% (41 women) (22). Of the 195 biopsies, 24.5% produced insufficient tissue, and polyp tissue (associated with the described backgrounds) was retrieved in 1% (not including our patients with polyps).

The similarly low yield of endometrial cancer (1.3 per 1,000) and atypical hyperplasia (5.2 per 1,000) in this and another asymptomatic population of 2,964 healthy women (23) of normal weight supports previous evidence that a pretreatment screening biopsy for all such women is excessive. Koss found a prevalence of endometrial cancer of 6.96 cases per 1,000 in a more heterogeneous group of 2,586 New Yorkers (24).

The sonographic demonstration of benign intracavitary lesions in 11% of our small sample of women that were undetected by blind biopsy corroborate other reports that these lesions may contribute significantly to persistent abnormal bleeding in some women when given HRT. Focal endometrial lesions were found on hysteroscopy in 43% of 157 selected women who commenced abnormal bleeding on HRT in one report (13), and in 27% of 106 in another (25), twice as many as were found in asymptomatic women.

Benign uterine bleeding is a frequent reason for abandoning HRT (26) and is a nuisance and source of worry for patients, requiring a large expenditure of time and resources for evaluation. A minimally invasive, efficient, and widely available method is needed to promptly identify which bleeding patients require surgery for cure and which may benefit from hormonal manipulation or observation. Our job is exclude cancer and to find the cause of bleeding and stop it.

New treatments involving stimulation and modulation of estrogen receptors are being developed for HRT and for prevention and treatment of breast cancer. A clear understanding of their long- and short-term effects on the uterus is needed.

METHODS OF DETECTION

Blind Sampling Techniques

Blind methods of obtaining biopsy specimens from the uterine cavity are less informative than those directed by inspection, although they may be reasonably sensitive for cancer. *Cervical dilatation and curettage* (D&C) of the uterine cavity under general or regional anesthesia missed focal pathology because of incomplete sampling of the uterine cavity in classic studies (27–29). Diagnostic D&C has been largely replaced by *office biopsy*, with considerable reductions in expense and anesthetic risk (30). However, results of trials involving presurgical sampling have shown a range of efficacy for accurate diagnosis by office sampling devices. The 3.1-mm piston vacuum Pipelle was found to sample less than 15% of the endometrial surface, mostly in the midline (31), when compared with the 4-mm Vabra trap suction device, which sampled about 41% of the surface, equivalent to a D&C.

Accurate results depend on the location, size, and nature of the lesion. Small, focal endometrial lesions off the midline, polyps, and myomas are most likely to escape office biopsy (32). Van Den Bosch et al. (33) diagnosed all cancers and diffuse hyperplasias with the Pipelle but missed 93% of polyps and myomas and 36% of cases of hyperplasia, producing an overall sensitivity for disease detection of 44% for 138 bleeding untreated women. Two biopsies were prevented by cervical stenosis. In this group, compared with surgical inspection, vaginal ultrasound also detected all cancers, and using a normal upper threshold of 4 mm, ultrasound had a sensitivity of 82%. Four cases of focal hyperplasia and one 3-mm submucosal myoma were missed by ultrasound at this thickness.

In a randomized trial comparing the Pipelle with the hollow metal Novak curet (34), insufficient tissue was retrieved in 12.8% of 149 procedures with the Pipelle and in 9.6% of the 126 procedures with the Novak. However, 48 (96%) Pipelle samples of 50 were representative of the tissue found at hysterectomy. Cancer was detected using a Pipelle in 39 (97%) of 40 known cases by Stovall (35), and a similar experiment by Ferry et al. yielded positive results in only 67% of 37 cancerous uteri (36). These failures occurred in cases of well-differentiated, small, focal, superficial tumors. There was 90% agreement between a Pipelle biopsy and D&C in 159 cases of bleeding in another series (37), but 7 cases of hyperplasia were not detected, although the 3 cases of cancer were. In the 40 postmenopausal women in this group, vaginal ultrasound (with a threshold of 5 mm for the upper limit of normal endometrial thickness) accurately detected 100% of endometrial abnormalities.

Although in most series the majority of neoplastic lesions have been detected by office biopsy, underestimation of the tumor grade by blind biopsy is common (38).

Larson et al. used a 3.1-mm-diameter piston-type aspiration device (Z-sampler) to biopsy 131 women in the office and D&C in 52 to diagnose cancer. The grade at hysterectomy varied from the preoperative cancer grade in 42% of the former and in 23% of the latter group. About one-half of both of the inaccurate subsets, or 26% overall, were undergraded (39). Dunton et al. found cancer at hysterectomy in one-half of a group of 23 uteri in which atypical hyperplasia was diagnosed by blind sampling methods (40).

The use of *cytologic sampling* with flushing and aspiration or brushing of the cavity requires an experienced, specially trained cytologist for interpretation (41) and has proven to be no more accurate than blind biopsy for benign or malignant lesions. In one large study, the sensitivity for detecting endometrial cancer was only 90%, mainly because of missed focal lesions (42). The sensitivity for detection of all endometrial hyperplasia was only 58%, but all those with atypia were identified.

Techniques for Inspecting the Endometrial Cavity

The ability to fully image or visualize the endometrial cavity allows accurate disease detection, precise location of lesions, and ascertainment of a normal cavity, which obviates the requirement for further investigation. Bleeding from atrophic endometrium is not synonymous with bleeding from a normal cavity, and although the histology of a biopsy may be reassuring, the patient who is still bleeding has not been helped. The strength of hysteroscopy and vaginal sonography (including saline infusion sonohysterography [SIS]) is their ability to detect focal lesions.

Hysteroscopy was the first widely used method for direct evaluation of the uterine cavity (43,44) and is the current method of choice for intracavitary surgery: myomectomy, polypectomy, septum resection, or directed biopsy of focal lesions. Hysteroscopy has enabled accurate diagnosis of benign focal causes of bleeding that are obscure when D&C curettings are the reference for disease, making it clear that about one-third to one-half postmenopausal women with bleeding have a polyp, myoma, or benign, abnormal, focal proliferation. The incidence of benign lesions (i.e., polyps, myomas, and typical hyperplasia) was similar among 157 bleeding women taking HRT (48%) and 146 postmenopausal women with spontaneous bleeding (35%), but four cancers were found in the untreated women (45). Two other cancers and four polyps in seven bleeding women taking tamoxifen were also detected. Only 62% of the lesions could be biopsied, and all patients with polyps and resectable myomas and the 5.7% of women in whom office hysteroscopy could not be done then underwent operative hysteroscopy for directed biopsy or treatment.

Hysteroscopy with directed biopsy is an improvement on blind sampling for gaining diagnostic information about the bleeding uterus (46,47). Gimpelson reported agreement between an initial office hysteroscopy and subsequent D&C in 80% of 276 cases, with superior clinical information supplied by diagnostic hysteroscopy for 16% and by D&C for 4% (48). The reported sensitivity of the technique declines from between 92% and 100% for cancer to 70% for identification of hyperplasia (49), and general curettage is customary after operative hysteroscopy.

Office hysteroscopy is a useful but invasive and expensive method of evaluating abnormal bleeding, and focal lesions must often then be removed by a second operative procedure. However, if roughly one-half of postmenopausal bleeding is from normal cavities, the anesthetic risk and cost in time and resources makes it difficult to justify operative hysteroscopy under anesthesia for routine initial diagnosis of postmenopausal bleeding. As with any endoscopic procedure, hysteroscopy requires a fair amount of expertise to maximize benefit and minimize risk for complication. In general, hysteroscopy is most effectively reserved for directed biopsy or surgical therapy after sonographic diagnosis of focal lesions or for persistent, undiagnosed bleeding.

Vaginal Ultrasound

There is enough experience with the use of transvaginal ultrasound (TVU) imaging of the endometrium to recommend it as the first-line method of investigation of postmenopausal bleeding when it is available. For more than 15 years, numerous independent investigators, in comparing the transvaginal endometrial image with biopsy, D&C, hysteroscopy, and hysterectomy, have arrived at the same conclusions:

1. TVU of the uterus, with a consistent and systematic imaging protocol, provides accurate measurement of endometrial thickness of the entire cavity (50).
2. In a well-imaged uterus, when the sum of both endometrial layers is no more than 5 mm at any point in the longitudinal view, the risk of endometrial cancer as a cause of bleeding is about 1% for untreated women and about 0.1% for women on standard HRT regimens (51).
3. SIS, a minor variation of TVU, defines the anatomy of the endometrial cavity as accurately as diagnostic hysteroscopy and is indicated for the evaluation of abnormal bleeding or when the endometrial image is unclear or abnormal (52).

Endometrial Thickness as a Practical Bioassay of Estrogen Effect

Interpretation of any TVU image depends on the context of the woman's history and treatment, informed by an understanding of uterine structure and physiology. When the endometrial functionalis layer is absent or completely suppressed, only the basalis layer remains. The normal postmenopausal fixed endometrium is atrophic and is histologically described as less than 1 mm thick, with sparse, tiny glands and dense stroma and with the occasional dilated gland (Fig. 47.2A) (53,54). It consists of a 1-mm layer of basalis and epithelium over the myometrium (Fig. 47.2) (55), allowing thickening or distortion to be readily appreciated. In adequately imaged uteri, it is possible to measure endometrial thickness to within 1 mm (56).

A similar sonographic effect of absence or suppression of functionalis development is found at any age in irradiated uteri (57,58); after castration or premature ovarian failure (59); with prolonged use of oral or injectable contraceptives containing MPA, norethindrone, or norgestrel (Fig. 47.3) (60); and after gonadotropin-releasing hormone–induced pituitary suppression. The entire functionalis layer is also removed at menses or after progesterone-induced withdrawal, a time when the sonographic thickness of the normal postmenstrual endometrium is also 4 mm or less throughout the cavity. Cyclic HRT recreates the appearance of the normal endometrial cycle, and continuous combined HRT with adequate progestin suppresses the functionalis layer (Fig. 47.4) (4).

Endometrial thickness in the normal uterus is a reliable bioassay of the presence or absence of an estrogen effect. It is equivalent to the classic bioassay of estrogen status, the progesterone challenge, in which an endometrial thickness of 5 mm or less predicts no or scanty withdrawal, but a thickness of 6 mm or more ensures a withdrawal bleed (61,62). Sonographic endometrial thickness (considered with the ovarian morphology) discriminates between euestrogenic and hypoestrogenic amenorrhea in young women better than spot estradiol levels.

This is true in postmenopausal women as well, with an interesting addition. There is a clear correlation between endogenous postmenopausal estrogen levels, body mass index (BMI), and endometrial thickness. Andolf et al. (Table 47.1) (63) observed that a persistent endometrial thickness of 5 mm or more found in 11 of 279 asymptomatic untreated women within 7 years of menopause correlated with a significantly elevated BMI (5). Likewise, Douchi et al. (64) studied a group of 212 untreated postmenopausal Japanese women, one-third of whom had bleeding. A strong correlation between BMI and endometrial thickness was demonstrated at all sizes, but no association was demonstrated between endometrial thickness and age or years since menopause in this mixed group, probably because a high percentage of them had lesions. Endometrial or uterine abnormalities, many of which are estrogen dependent, also increase endometrial thickness, but the 4-mm threshold for normalcy retains its usefulness because neither functionalis proliferation nor lesions are desirable in postmenopausal women.

In a larger Italian population of 930 untreated bleeding women with an 11.5% prevalence of endometrial cancer

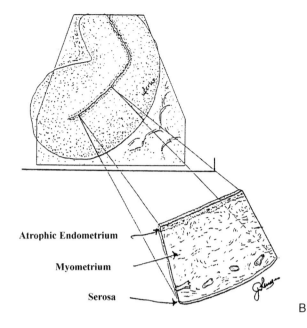

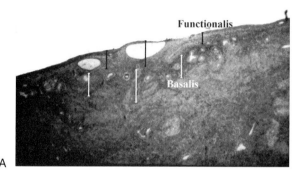

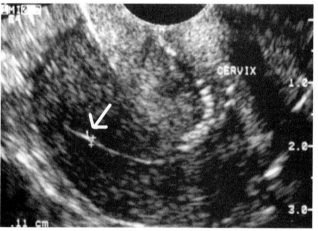

FIG. 47.2. **A:** A photomicrograph of atrophic endometrium shows two residual, dilated glands in the functionalis layer, below which is the very thin, unchanging basalis layer with randomly oriented glands (*arrows*). **B:** A sketch of the layers of the senescent uterus. (Courtesy of Jorge Lense, M.D.) **C:** In a comparable sonographic sagittal image of the uterus, the two basalis layers are condensed with the specular reflection of the intracavitary interface into a thin, echogenic line (*arrow*) that is of uniform thickness (1.1 mm) from the internal os to the fundus. The fundus is sharply anteflexed on the cervix, and the cervical canal has been enhanced as a thicker, white line after the use of a Papanicolaou (Pap) screening smear cytobrush (CERVIX).

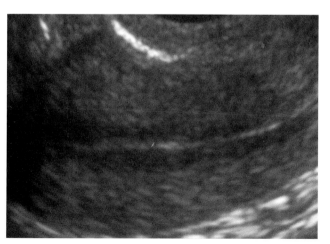

FIG. 47.3. Suppressed endometrium, without the functionalis, appears as a uniform echogenic line surrounded by the hypoechogenic inner myometrium in this uterus of a 19-year-old woman taking an oral contraceptive with 35 μg of ethinyl estradiol and 0.4 mg of norethindrone acetate. Compare with Fig. 47.2C.

and a 50% prevalence of atrophy, logistic regression analysis identified a strong correlation among endometrial cancer and the independent variables of increasing BMI and age, even at an endometrial thickness of less than 4 mm (65). These observations are congruent with the well-established association of obesity, relatively high endogenous estrone due to peripheral conversion of androgens, and increased risk for endometrial cancer. The Italian investigators were able to refine the estimates of individual risk for endometrial cancer compared with endometrial atrophy at various measured thicknesses (i.e., posttest risk) for this population. They showed a dramatic decline in risk for the women found to have endometrial thicknesses of 4 mm or less (only 2 of 298 women had cancer on biopsy) (Fig. 47.5) (6).

Meuwissen et al. monitored proliferation in postmenopausal uteri by measuring endometrial growth rates of initially normal endometrium (≤4 mm) in response to various forms of unopposed estrogen therapy, recording a mean rate in of 0.2 mm/week (66). Only 2 of 159 estro-

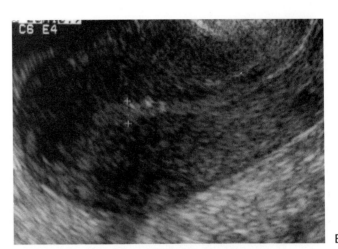

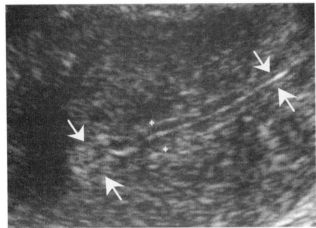

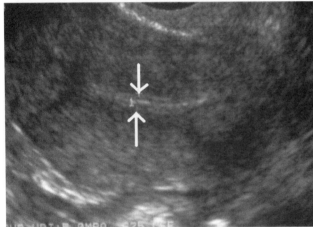

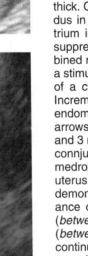

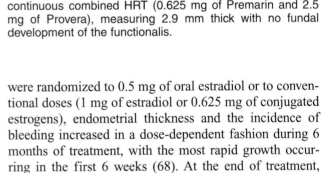

FIG. 47.4. When the functionalis is stimulated, the endometrial thickness is perceptibly greater in the fundus than in the rest of the uterus, even though it may be less than 5 mm thick. Compare the gradual increase in thickness at the fundus in **A** and **B** with the uniform thickness of the endometrium in Figs. 47.3 and 47.4C, in which there is adequate suppression of functionalis growth on a continuous combined regimen. **A:** Vaginal ultrasound scan of the uterus with a stimulated endometrium in a 72-year-old woman on day 10 of a cyclic hormone replacement therapy (HRT) regimen. Incremental estrogen exposure creates the typical layered endometrial pattern of proliferative functionalis (between arrows), in this case measuring 4.5 mm thick in the fundus and 3 mm in the lower segment. (Day 1–25, 0.625 mg/day of connjugated equine estrogen; day 12–25, add 10 mg/day of medroxyprogesterone acetate). **B:** Vaginal ultrasound of the uterus in the same woman on day 25 of the artificial cycle, demonstrating the typical white, solid sonographic appearance of a 4.2-mm secretory functionalis endometrial layer (*between arrows*). **C:** Sonogram of the endometrium (*between arrows*) in a different 65-year-old woman taking continuous combined HRT (0.625 mg of Premarin and 2.5 mg of Provera), measuring 2.9 mm thick with no fundal development of the functionalis.

gen-treated endometria were less than 6 mm thick. After chronic estrogen exposure, a single progestin challenge did not produce complete regression in many cases, but the decline in thickness was directly related to the intensity and duration of the withdrawal bleeding (67).

The effects of even low doses of unopposed estrogen are sonographically apparent. When Californian women

TABLE 47.1. *Hormone levels and body mass index in asymptomatic postmenopausal women*

Endometrial thickness	≥5 mm	≤5 mm	P
Estrone (pmol/L)	219 ± 20	175 ± 35	0.01
Estradiol (pmol/L)	38 ± 17	13 ± 2.7	0.05
Progesterone (nmol/L)	1.0 ± 0.2	0.87 ± 0.05	
Body mass index (Kg/m²)	29.1 ± 1.2	25.6 ± 0.3	0.02

From Andolf et al, *Obstet Gynecol* 82:937,1993.

were randomized to 0.5 mg of oral estradiol or to conventional doses (1 mg of estradiol or 0.625 mg of conjugated estrogens), endometrial thickness and the incidence of bleeding increased in a dose-dependent fashion during 6 months of treatment, with the most rapid growth occurring in the first 6 weeks (68). At the end of treatment, about 15% of women on 0.5 mg of oral estradiol and about 40% of those on standard doses had an endometrial thickness of 10 mm or more. As in Meuwissen's patients, a few women had surprisingly little endometrial response.

Regardless of the few women with significant endometrial synechiae and unusual uterine metabolism, the physician must assume that all women can have a proliferative endometrial response to estrogen. Unless the physician plans to intervene with intermittent progestins and evaluate complete removal of the functionalis periodically, TVU is not an appropriate method with which to monitor the endometrium in women taking unopposed estrogens, because the tissue virtually always grows

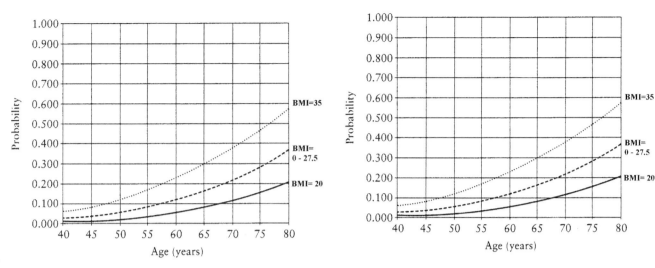

FIG. 47.5. The risk of cancer increased with age and obesity in bleeding postmenopausal Italian women studied in a multicenter trial, but the risk declined by more than 90% when the endometrium was thin. **A:** Pretest probability of endometrial cancer according to age and body mass index (BMI). **B:** Posttest probability of endometrial cancer according to age and BMI for women with endometrial thickness of 4 mm or less. (From ref. 65, with permission.)

thicker than 5 mm. Ultrasound cannot distinguish between benign and neoplastic proliferation. Regular endometrial biopsy is necessary to determine when the line between proliferation and hyperplasia is crossed, as it is within 12 months in as many as one third of women so treated (69).

Cyclic or sequential HRT regimens should grow and deplete the functionalis layer with each artificial cycle in a manner similar to a spontaneous cycle. There is no need to change the criteria for deciding which patient is best served by sampling if sonographic endometrial measurement is timed for the post withdrawal phase. No large studies have completely characterized the endometrial effects of cyclic regimens, but loss of functionalis with an adequate withdrawal should occur as it does at spontaneous menses. Gull et al., studying asymptomatic women, reported endometrial thickness during cycle days 1 through 7 to be 4.3 ± 1.0 mm (SEM) in 4 women, during days 8 through 14 to be 6.8 ± 1.2 mm in 13; during cycle days 15 through 21 to be 6.0 ± 0.3 mm in 11; and during cycle days 22 through 28 to be 6.2 ± 0.6 mm in 14. These rather meager data, expressed as means without ranges, suggest that postwithdrawal measurements during week 1 represent the cycle nadir.

Goldstein was mindful of sonography's inability to reflect the histology of functionalis, but he knew that the postmenstrual endometrium is the histologic equivalent of the thin residual basalis layers he had previously characterized in postmenopausal women as 5 mm or less (70). He therefore imaged 21 perimenopausal women with irregular bleeding on days 4 to 6 after the onset of spontaneous bleeding (71). The nine women with appropriate postmenstrual endometrium all had symmetric bilayer

measurements of 4 mm or less. Eight polyps, three submucosal myomas, and one 8-mm hyperplasia demonstrated inappropriately thickened bilayer measurements or abnormal asymmetric cavities. Diagnosis of the various masses was obviously not cycle dependent, but ascertainment of the normal cavities and of the failure of the hyperplasia to regress was possible only after menses. He and his colleagues went on to test this hypothesis in a series of 433 perimenopausal women with menorrhagia or menometrorrhagia. Seventy-nine percent (341) demonstrated appropriate symmetric endometrium thickness of 5 mm or less, ending the investigation. Eighteen percent harbored focal masses such as polyps (n = 58) or myomas (n = 22), which were addressed by operative hysteroscopy. Ten had global thickening sampled immediately by Pipelle, which demonstrated abnormal proliferation in one-half and hyperplasia in one-half. Two failures went on to hysteroscopy. Although it was not stated whether symptoms resolved with SIS-directed management, the effectiveness of timed evaluation was well demonstrated.

A continuous combined HRT regimen maintained the endometrial thickness at 4 mm or less in 91% of a small group. Biopsy results were consistent with suppression of functionalis or atrophy in 32 of 33 women; the one proliferative endometrium was more than 4 mm thick (72). Varner et al. published similar findings for 13 of 14 women on continuous HRT in 1991; in this group, only a bleeding woman with an 8-mm endometrium demonstrated proliferation. Cyclic regimens also produced a range of thickness, from 4 to 8 mm, when scanned randomly, and the tissue demonstrated inactive, proliferative, or secretory histology. Sixty women with endometrial measurements of 5 mm or less had suppressed, insufficient, or atrophic histology, and two bleeding women with 5-mm-thick endometria had cancer and hyperplasia, respectively.

Sonographic evaluation of women on continuous combined regimens is simplified: a smooth-surfaced symmetric endometrium of 5 mm or thicker suggests inappropriate proliferation. Persistent proliferation is not desirable in a postmenopausal uterus, although this histology may be technically normal and expected because of treatment. Persistent bleeding in such a uterus suggests that the estrogen dose should be decreased or the progestin should be increased to counteract the effects of endogenous estrogen (73) and that symptoms and endometrial response should be monitored.

Bleeding from the Apparently Normal Cavity

By imaging the uterus instead of imagining it, we have the opportunity to better understand mechanisms of abnormal bleeding. Most postmenopausal bleeding episodes occur seemingly inexplicably in women with atrophic or inactive histology demonstrated on biopsy or D&C. Complete evaluation of the bladder, urethra, distal sigmoid, adnexa, cervix, and uterus with ultrasound, a Papanicolaou (Pap) smear, inspection of the vaginal vault, and rectal examination with testing for fecal occult blood in a single visit is an effective workup. If these tests results are negative, the physician is left with the possibilities of endogenous or exogenous dysfunctional hormone effects, endometritis (as reported in women with new spotting on oral contraceptives [74]), or after exclusion of other possibilities, "atrophic" bleeding.

In 12 consecutive women in our practice with new bleeding on continuous combined HRT and normal, smooth cavities on SIS, seven Pipelle endometrial biopsies revealed various degrees of proliferation (with dual-layered endometria ranging from 3.5 to 5.4 mm thick), with no growth in aerobic and anaerobic cultures of endometrial tissue. The other five biopsies (from endometria ranging from 2 to 4 mm) grew *Enterococcus* (associated only with bacterial vaginosis in this patient), *Escherichia coli*, *Peptostreptococcus*, *Propionibacterium*, and *Streptococcus viridans*, respectively, when cultured. These last five biopsies did not demonstrate proliferation. Although all 12 patients presented with mild cramping and bleeding, the five women also were found to have specific bilateral adnexal tenderness during the ultrasound-guided pelvic examination. Three also had sonographic findings in the sigmoid colon of thickened muscularis traversed by focally painful diverticula that were adherent to the left adnexa (Fig. 47.6) (7). Endometritis was not demonstrated in the scanty samples of endometrium recovered, because there was no functionalis in which to identify plasma cells (75). The fourth patient weighed nearly 400 pounds and had difficulty

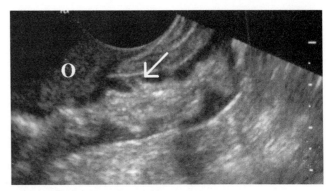

FIG. 47.6. Sonographic evidence for descending infection from transmural tubal contamination producing postmenopausal bleeding. A postmenopausal woman had left lower quadrant pain and new onset of light uterine bleeding from an unstimulated, sonographically normal-appearing uterine cavity (not shown). Early colonic diverticula appear as fine tracks of mucosa traversing the hypertrophic and edematous muscularis layers of the sigmoid (*arrow*). Gentle pressure with the ultrasound probe produces focal pain at the site and fails to disengage the colon from the contiguous and apparently adherent ovary *(O)*. Endometrial biopsy produced scant superficial epithelium, but when cultured, it grew *Peptostreptococcus*.

with perineal hygiene because of obesity and bladder incontinence. The fifth patient had a husband with recurrent infectious complications of benign prostatic hypertrophy and demonstrated a small, painful hydrosalpinx that regressed after treatment with doxycycline (unpublished data).

It appears that the first group of women had sufficient endogenous estrogens to render the progestin dose inadequate to prevent proliferation and ceased to bleed on a higher dose of progestin. The latter group apparently bled from endometritis. Without changing their continuous combined HRT, all of the latter five women responded to appropriate oral antibiotics with resumption of amenorrhea and resolution of pelvic discomfort.

In women within a few years of menopause, recurrent ovarian activity can prompt an isolated episode of bleeding from a normal cavity. The rare ovulation in a postmenopausal woman has been documented in excised ovaries, but simple follicular growth and regression is apparently not unusual. This may be the case when a woman reports breast tenderness or other estrogenic symptoms occurred before bleeding occurs. Yearly ultrasound screening of postmenopausal women for the past 10 years has yielded one corpus luteum associated with bleeding in a 59-year-old woman who was 6 years postmenopausal and 12 occasions of identification of a simple ovarian cyst that disappeared after a subsequent bleed (unpublished data).

Ovarian tumors (particularly mucinous) may increase sex steroid production in postmenopausal women (76), as do steroid-producing tumors such as granulosa cell neoplasms. This is an unusual cause of bleeding but readily identified on the ultrasound-assisted pelvic examination.

Evidence for the Use of Vaginal Ultrasound to Detect Cancer

During the last 10 years, reports of the use of TVU to evaluate postmenopausal bleeding have varied in their estimation of the upper limit of normal total endometrial thickness in untreated women, from 4 mm (77) to 5 mm (78,79) to 6 mm (80,81) to 7 mm (82,83). Those who had neither small cancers nor atypical hyperplasia in their populations initially adopted a higher upper limit of normal. Most reported the sum total of both opposed walls (47,70,78); others reported one half or the "single wall thickness" of the total measurement obtained. However, all agreed that 30% to 50% of biopsies could be avoided by using the thresholds derived from their populations and that endometria measuring less than 5 mm thick were unlikely to harbor cancer.

Although sonographic measurement of the endometrial function is accurate, assessment of its histology with ultrasound is not. The utility of the 4- or 5-mm threshold is to exclude the presence of inappropriate proliferative tissue in the endometrial cavity of the postmenopausal woman. Sonographic monitoring of women on unopposed estrogen or random scanning of women on cyclic HRT is nonspecific and unhelpful (84–86), because most have endometria of thicker than 5 mm.

Granberg et al. published their preliminary experience with 205 bleeding postmenopausal women in 1991 (87). Each of the 150 women with endometrium measuring 5 mm or less in total thickness was found to have atrophic or no endometrim on D&C. One colon cancer, five bladder tumors, and 18 adnexal lesions, including seven tumors, were simultaneously diagnosed by ultrasound. Seven specimens from endometria measuring between 6 and 15 mm were also atrophic, a finding that led them to confirm their findings using hysteroscopy. In a study of 51 women, they demonstrated that a discrepancy between atrophic histology and sonographically thick endometrium indicated the presence of a benign polyp or myoma.

This group had meanwhile begun a landmark multicenter study in 1989 at eight centers in four countries to test the validity of the use of simple endometrial thickness to predict any pathology. A variety of machines were used, scanning at between 5 and 7.5 MHz. Only very experienced imagers were involved, and they used well-defined maneuvers. The results of this Nordic trial, published in 1995, established the reliability of their technique and a standard for data analysis (88). They constructed a receiver-operator curve to determine the best measurement to discriminate between normal and abnormal endometrium (Fig. 47.7) (8) based on the data derived from 1,168 bleeding postmenopausal women

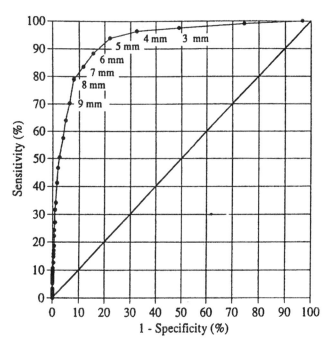

FIG. 47.7. A receiver-operator characteristics curve illustrates the performance of vaginal ultrasound at various endometrial thicknesses (marked on the curve) when used by experts in the detection of endometrial abnormalities (e.g., hyperplasia, polyps, cancer) in a population of postmenopausal women with bleeding. One-third took hormone replacement therapy. Optimal sensitivity compared with specificity is obtained with a threshold for normal defined as 4 mm. (From ref. 88, with permission.)

who were scanned within 3 days of a D&C. Using an endometrial threshold of 4 mm, the probability of any abnormality in the curettage specimen was about 3.6%, with a 95% confidence limit of 5.5%. Any finding other than atrophy, insufficient tissue, or "hormonal effect" was considered abnormal. One-third of the population took estriol as a very-low-potency vaginal cream or cyclic HRT. The prevalence of cancer was 9.7%. At 4 mm or less, the sensitivity for abnormality was 96%, specificity was 68%, and accuracy was 78%, with a negative predictive value of 97% and positive predictive value of 61%. The corresponding ratios when 5 mm was used as the upper limit of normal were 94%, 78%, 84%, 96%, and 69%.

In the 518 uteri with endometrium that was 4 mm or less, there were no endometrial cancers or atypical hyperplasia. There were 491 atrophic uteri (43%), 2 cervical cancers (0.17%), 6 cases of simple hyperplasia (0.5%), and 6 polyps retrieved (0.5%), and 13 cases of hormonal effect (1.09%) were indecipherable.

Although using D&C as a less than perfect gold standard, these data confirmed the high negative predictive value for disease using a 4-mm threshold in postmenopausal uteri in the hands of highly experienced imagers. They also reinforced the point that TVU should

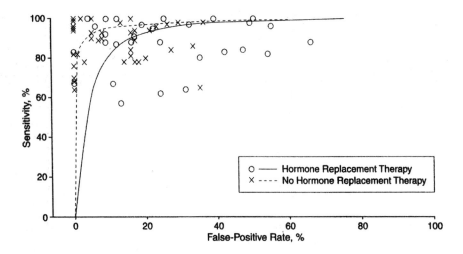

FIG. 47.8. Summary receiver-operator characteristics curve illustrates the acceptable performance of vaginal ultrasound in detecting endometrial abnormalities using 5 mm as a cutoff. This summarizes data from 35 studies, stratified by hormone use, in a metanalysis. (Fig. 47.8 and Table 47.2 are from Smith-Bindman et al. [ref. 51] EVUS to exclude endometrial cancer and other endometrial abnormalities. *JAMA* 1998; 280:1510–1517. Copyright 1998, American Medical Association.)

be accompanied by a vaginal inspection and cervical cytology in the evaluation of postmenopausal bleeding.

The Italian multicenter trial evaluating postmenopausal bleeding involved participation of a representative mix of imaging centers, imager experience, and equipment rather than research-oriented sites with long experience in postmenopausal gynecologic imaging. Among the 10 university centers and eight general hospitals, results were comparable, although with twice as many indecipherable images as occurred in the "expert" Nordic study: 4.7%. These women took no hormones; there was a prevalence of endometrial cancer of 11.4% and prevalence of atrophy of 49%. The comparison procedure was D&C. The test performance was somewhat lower than in the hands of experts but was still excellent, with a sensitivity for detection of cancer of 98% and a negative predictive value of 99.3% for endometrium of 4 mm.

The reproducibility of these data has been further confirmed by a metanalysis of 35 studies (89) involving prospective ultrasound examination followed by endometrial sampling in 5,892 women, a fraction of the studies that have been reported. Overall, 94% of these subjects were bleeding; 40% had cancer, hyperplasia, or polyps, and there was a 13% prevalence of cancer. Using a 5-mm threshold, 96% of women with cancer had abnormal TVU results (95% CI, 94–98%); 92% with hyperplasia or polyps were abnormal (95% CI, 90–93%), and sensitivity was quite consistent between studies. Twenty-three percent of women on HRT had a stimulated but normal endometrium measuring more than 5 mm, and 8% of untreated women did. Specificity varied considerably between studies that included women on hormones, depending on when in the cycle they were scanned.

As expected, more women with disease were detected as the threshold for normal was lowered to 4 mm, and there were more false-positive results. Because hormone therapy can stimulate the endometrium, "endovaginal ultrasound (EVUS) or TVU was more accurate in women

who were not using hormone replacement therapy . . . [but] the sensitivity did not vary significantly with hormone use, being 96% for cancer detection." The receiver-operator curves reflected the decline in specificity in hormonally treated women (Fig. 47.8) (9), but it is clear that the threshold should not be increased, as has been suggested, to accommodate a population more likely to have stimulated functionalis, because the consequences of false-negative results are more detrimental than those of false-positive results. The endometrium can be manipulated hormonally and the test timed to minimize false-positive results.

The researchers observe that "this meta-analysis suggests that the sensitivity of [TVU] is at least as good as office-based endometrial biopsy techniques (to exclude endometrial abnormality). Endovaginal ultrasound has similar sensitivity as endometrial biopsy and can be used when endometrial biopsy is not available, nondiagnostic or unsuccessful." A normal TVU result diminished the pretest risk of cancer by 90%; in the untreated woman, it declined from 10% to 1%, and in a woman on HRT, it declined from 1% to 0.1% (Table 47.2). These data agree

TABLE 47.2.

HRT	Pretest probability, %	Posttest probability of endometrial disease after an EVUS, %	
		Normal result	Abnormal result
No	1	0.1	11
Yes		0.1	4
No	5	0.3	39
Yes		0.6	17
No	10	0.6	57
Yes		1.3	31
No	20	1.3	75
Yes		2.9	50
No	50	5.1	92
Yes		11.0	80

with those of the Italian trial, which were not included in this analysis.

Ultrasound does not replace biopsy unless the threshold and regularity criteria are clearly met. The role of ultrasound is to determine at the initial presentation who is likely to benefit from biopsy and to determine who can be observed or treated medically. A poor image provides no data, and another test must be done. This is particularly critical because a poorly imaged endometrium is more likely to harbor severe disease and to be misinterpreted by the inexperienced examiner.

Saline Infusion Sonohysterography

SIS consists of infusion of sterile saline into the uterine cavity through a 2-mm (5.3-French) flexible catheter during systematic uterine scanning. SIS enhances the uterine image by providing the exquisite intrauterine surface detail afforded by amniotic fluid in pregnancy.

When expanded by saline, the normal postmenopausal lumen appears quite smooth, and the endometrium around it is symmetric and no more than 3 mm in *single-layer* thickness (Fig. 47.9) (10). SIS can accomplish the following:

1. Clarify difficult uterine anatomy and enhance definition of the entire uterine cavity and endometrial surface and thickness
2. Define the anatomy of endometrium that appears abnormal or ill defined by TVU or any other imaging method
3. Accurately identify the location, size, and attachment of focal abnormalities

The clinical role of SIS for the postmenopausal woman is to distinguish between bleeding that can be treated medically and lesions that require surgery. Polyps, intracavitary myomas, and synechiae are benign causes of bleeding that are not always identifiable on TVU. In an abnormal uterus, the physician can immediately make the distinction between focal and global endometrial abnormalities to refine the approach to biopsy, surgery, or hormonal treatment. It has also been used in randomized comparisons of conventional estrogen replacement therapy (ERT), HRT, and the selective estrogen receptor modulator (SERM), raloxifene, a relative of tamoxifen. The effort was made to characterize the uterus before and during treatment to observe, measure, and compare treatment effects in normal and abnormal uteri before widespread use of the drug was underway (90).

During the past 15 years, the idea of clear fluid enhancement of the uterine cavity occurred independently to many investigators around the world (91–97), with even earlier reports of its use with abdominal ultrasound continuing to come to light (98). Widrich et al. were the first to report independent comparison with office hysteroscopy (99) in 130 bleeding women for the detection of intraluminal abnormalities. They found it had a sensitivity of 96% and specificity of 88% for histologic diagnosis of lesions, and it identified hyperplasia more accurately than hysteroscopy. Numerous other comparisons between surgical examination and SIS have demonstrated that the procedure can define virtually all irregularities of the endometrial surface (Table 47.3) (11), and even in inexperienced hands, it has a negative predictive value of 100% (100). It cannot, however, reliably differentiate disorderly proliferation, hyperplasia, and neoplasia (Fig. 47.10) (12), and histologic diagnosis remains in the domain of the pathologist. As with TVU, timing the saline infusion to follow complete endometrial sloughing minimizes diagnostic confusion in cycling women.

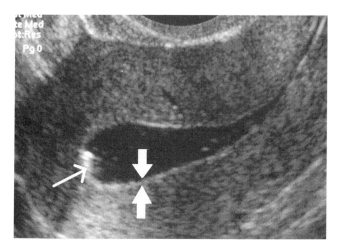

FIG. 47.9. Sonogram of a postmenopausal uterus during saline infusion sonohysterography shows a normal atrophic endometrial cavity. It is seen in a mid-sagittal view, with the fundus on the left. The bright echo (*thin arrow*) is a minor typical midfundal artifact caused by the catheter. The isolated posterior basalis layer (*between thick arrows*) is less than 3 mm thick.

TABLE 47.3. *Comparison of SIS to surgical inspection for intracavitary abnormality*

Author	Year	N	Sens.	Spec.	PPV	NPV
Syrop	1993	14	100%	100%	100%	100%
Bonilla-Musoles	1992	76	96%	97%	96%	98%
Parsons	1993	59	100%	94%	96%	100%
Widrich	1995	130	96%	88%		
Gaucherand	1995	104	94%	98%		
Hill	1996	50	98%	100%	100%	98%
Wolman	1996	47	*86%	100%		
Keltz	1997	34	100%	100%	100%	100%
Tepper	1997	68	100%	95%	95%	100%
Bernard	1997	109	99%	76%		
Schwarzler	1998	104	*87%	91%	92%	86%
Williams	1998	39	100%	85%	75%	100%

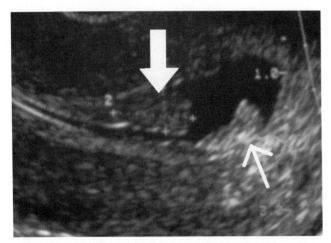

FIG. 47.10. Saline infusion sonohysterography in a retroverted uterus in a postmenopausal woman with spontaneous bleeding at age 58. The fundus is on the left, and there is a supracervical posterior polyp (*wide arrow*) and an anterior fundal area of hyperplasia (*thin arrow*). Biopsies of these lesions were immediately performed under ultrasound guidance for removal and diagnosis. Cyclic hormone replacement therapy was instituted for three cycles, followed by a continuous combined regimen, on which she is amenorrheic and has a normal cavity.

In a blinded comparison of sonography, SIS, and diagnostic hysteroscopy in 104 women, SIS could not be done in 6 because of stenosis, myomas, or cervical polyps. However, it improved sonographic detection of focal masses, equal to that of diagnostic hysteroscopy, and better regarding detection and description of submucosal myomas (101). The use of a flexible, 2-mm, straight catheter minimizes obfuscatory artifacts; in this and another series that demonstrated rather low sensitivity, 8- or 9-French bladder catheters were used, often with the balloons inflated in the cavity (102) (Table 47.3).

O'Connell et al. (103) compared the findings from Pipelle biopsy, SIS, and hysteroscopy or D&C in 1,000 postmenopausal bleeding women in a military clinic. Seventy-two percent were treated with cyclic or continuous HRT, and scanning was not timed to cycles. Eight were treated with tamoxifen, and the investigators found these cases very hard to interpret. Untreated women were significantly more likely to have neoplastic lesions. Sonohysterography alone correlated with hysteroscopy in 92% of cases, with 88% sensitivity and 96% specificity. Two small cornual polyps were missed, and three false-positive results included an intramural myoma mistaken as a submucosal myoma and two echogenic areas in the endometrium mistaken as very small polyps. The researchers observed that these mistakes all occurred within the first 30 women in whom they did SIS but concluded that the combination of SIS and endometrial biopsy was most reliable for accurate diagnosis, yielding a 95% correlation with surgical findings, 94% sensitivity, and 96% specificity. Endometrial biopsy alone yielded a 64% correlation with hysteroscopic or hysterectomy findings and 23% sensitivity but 100% specificity, whereas the use of the endometrial thickness alone also gave a 64% correlation.

SIS, like hysteroscopy, identifies all causes of bleeding better than Pipelle endometrial biopsy and is more sensitive for abnormality than TVU. Dubinsky et al. reported sonographic identification of 43 (54%) focal lesions in 79 of consecutive bleeding postmenopausal women in whom aspiration endometrial biopsies were negative. TVS identified endometrium thicker than 5 mm and SIS demonstrated intracavitary masses in 43; these patients were found at hysteroscopy curettage or hysterectomy to have 3 endometrial cancers, 18 myomas, 14 polyps, 4 focal hyperplasias, and 2 normal cavities (two false-positive results) (104). Almost one-fourth of the lesions were multiple.

Considering the high ratio of information gained to money and time spent, safety, patient acceptance, and ease of performance in almost any clinical setting, SIS is superior to diagnostic hysteroscopy (105–107). The information supplied regarding the causes of abnormal bleeding frequently reduced the extent of surgery required or obviate it completely (108). Because of the minimal investment in materials, training, and time required, SIS can and should be available wherever TVU is performed. Suspected pelvic infection or pregnancy are the only gynecologic contraindications to performing SIS.

Imaging Technique

The expected image of the normal untreated postmenopausal uterus, viewed in midsagittal section at an angle of insonation to the uterine axis of between 60 and 90 degrees, is a regular "stripe" with a width of 4 mm or less. The term *stripe* seems descriptive, but because it inaccurately suggests a two-dimensional object, it is probably better to call this structure the *endometrium.* Normally, it is a constant surface layer of a three-dimensional cavity. Asymmetry in this layer in a postmenopausal woman is the anatomic hallmark of abnormality at any thickness (13,109–111). In the absence of intracavitary fluid, it is a symmetric, single stratum that represents the sonographic condensation of the two basalis layers and the specular reflection produced by apposition of their intracavitary surfaces. When unstimulated, the thickness is uniform throughout (Figs. 47.2C and 47.4C). If functionalis development is stimulated, it is thicker at the fundus (Fig. 47.4). The term *endometrial thickness,* unless otherwise specified, refers to the sum of both layers measured together.

A three-dimensional assessment of endometrial symmetry and thickness is obtained rapidly by orienting the transducer to image the midsagittal plane of the uterus and scanning from cornu to cornu and then turning it 90 degrees to image the transverse uterus and scanning from external cervical os to the fundal serosa. The midsagittal uterine view is identified by imaging the entire length of the cervical canal, which leads to the cavity at the internal os (Fig. 47.11) (14).

Focal intracavitary lesions are measured separately from the endometrium for more accurate description when SIS is used. The sum of each endometrial wall, when measured separately during SIS, tends to be slightly (up to 1 mm on average) greater than when measured together without cavitary expansion. For comparative and threshold purposes, the dual-layer endometrial thickness without fluid is the key measurement.

In the absence of myometrial abnormality, the basalis-myometrium interface is further defined by the "dark halo" of the hypoechoic subendometrial inner circular layer, or junctional zone. This smooth inner layer of compact smooth muscle, first described by Fleischer et al., is a landmark that defines the regularity of the basalis layers (Figs. 47.2C and 47.3) (112).

Abnormal processes disrupt or distort the basalis-myometrium interface (i.e., when glands invade myometrium or vice versa). Processes emanating from the endometrium include the diffuse basalis-blurring

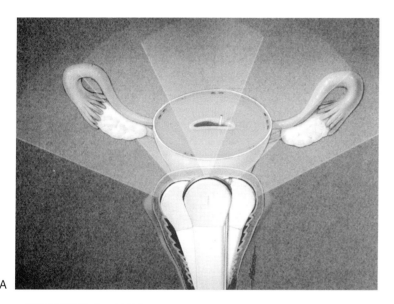
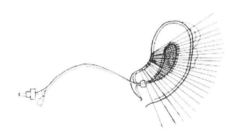
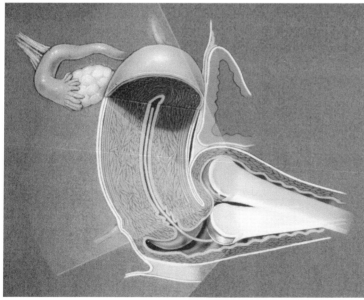
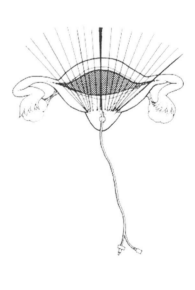

FIG. 47.11. Basic maneuvers for sonographic uterine evaluation. **A:** The sagittal maneuver is used to scan the entire cavity and fundus from cornu to cornu after obtaining a well-oriented sagittal view. **B:** In the transverse maneuver, the transducer is turned 90 degrees from the sagittal view, and the uterus is scanned from cervix to fundus. These maneuvers are done for the baseline transvaginal ultrasound scan and repeated during saline infusion sonohysterography after catheter placement to inspect every millimeter of the endometrial cavity systematically.

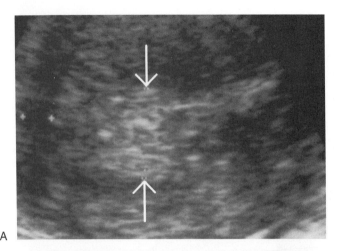

A

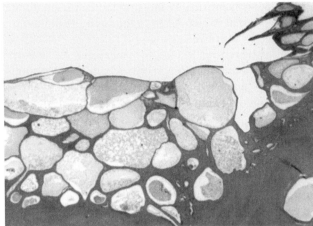

B

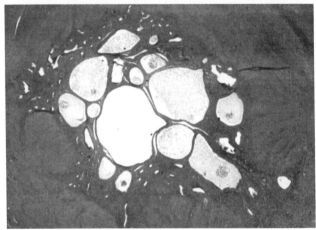

C

FIG. 47.12. Glands are the largest structures in the endometrium. When they are dilated and fill most of the endometrial volume (i.e., in secretory, hyperplastic, or neoplastic endometrium), the sonographic appearance is that of hyperechoic, thickened endometrium. These images illustrate cystic atrophy in an obese 68-year-old woman who underwent hysterectomy for an ovarian cystadenoma. Cystic atrophy is a benign condition in which glands are dilated without proliferation. **A:** Transvaginal ultrasound of the uterus shows a thickened, irregular endometrium. The endometrium appears to invade the myometrium, and echogenic foci are seen in the myometrium remote from the endometrium, both caused by extensive adenomyosis. **B:** Photomicrograph of the endometrium shows cystic atrophy. **C:** Similar histology is identified in a focus of adenomyosis.

effect of adenomyosis (Fig. 47.12) (15) and focal disruption by invasive endometrial cancer (Fig. 47.13) (16). Lesions that push from the myometrium through the basalis layer into the cavity include stalked intracavitary myomas and submucosal myomas, which are covered with a layer of endometrium and distort the shape of the endometrial cavity (Fig. 47.14) (17) but may not be visible by hysteroscopy. Uterine sarcomas and metastases are rare, and as a heterogeneous group, they are characterized by behavior rather than appearance: rapid growth and relentless bleeding when they invade the endometrium. Endometrial polyps do not interrupt the basalis layer and are confined and conform to the shape of the endometrial cavity (Fig. 47.15*A*) (18). Polyps are defined histologically by a thick muscular blood vessel arising from the basalis layer, and this is virtually always visible using amplitude ("power") color Doppler ultrasound set for slow flows (Fig. 47.15*B*).

The SIS technique consists of the insertion of a 5-French flexible catheter through a speculum and into a cleansed cervix (Fig. 47.16) (19,113). The tip of the catheter is placed at the fundus, the speculum is removed, and a sheathed, lubricated vaginal transducer is inserted into the vagina. It is placed in the anterior fornix

(above the plane of the catheter) in an anteverted uterus and into the posterior fornix (below the plane of the catheter) in a retroverted uterus. In cases of a dilated internal cervical os, a very large uterine cavity, or intracavitary synechiae or when tubal patency is being tested, a 2-mL balloon catheter (H/S catheter, *Ackrad Labs, Inc., Cranston, NJ*) is placed instead, with the balloon lodged in the cervix to avoid obscuring the cavity. Intravenous, injectable-grade sterile saline (or 1% lidocaine if biopsy is anticipated [114]) in a 10- to 20-mL syringe are attached to the catheter and slowly infused during the standard sagittal and transverse scanning maneuvers described in Fig. 47.11 until a three-dimensional evaluation of the cavitary contours is obtained. Including the essential baseline TVU, cervical preparation, and catheter insertion, this procedure takes 15 minutes, except in rare cases of cervical obstruction. Most cervical "stenosis" is caused by uterine flexion and is easily overcome by deflexion of the fundus through manual abdominal pressure, manipulation of the speculum, or as a last resort, application of a cervical tenaculum for traction. Optimal performance requires the use of comfortable patient support and lighting for gynecologic examination.

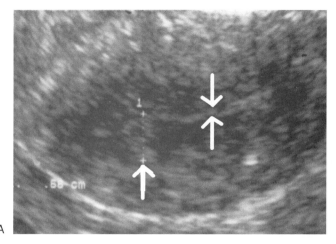

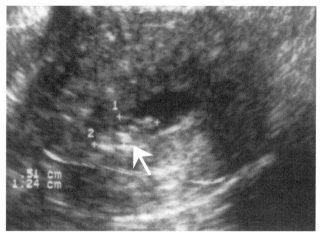

A B

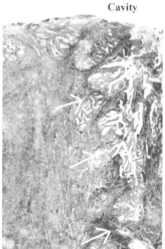

Cavity

C

FIG. 47.13. The uterus of a 73-year-old woman with a single episode of moderate vaginal bleeding and a Pap smear finding of a few cells of adenocarcinoma. The Pipelle biopsy and the dilatation and curettage results were negative, and both procedures produced scant normal epithelial cells. **A:** Transvaginal ultrasound demonstrated a single area of irregularity extending into the myometrium in the right cornu (*single arrow*) in an otherwise atrophic, 3.5-mm endometrium (*double arrows*). **B:** Saline infusion sonohysterography demonstrated a small, fine, filmy irregularity (*arrow*) in the right cornu in an otherwise normal cavity. **C:** Opening of the uterus at hysterectomy did not reveal any surface intracavitary abnormality, but step sectioning of the entire cavity uncovered the tiny (2 × 6 mm) focus of invasive adenocarcinoma (*outlined by arrows*) in the right cornu that had proliferated into the myometrium rather than the cavity.

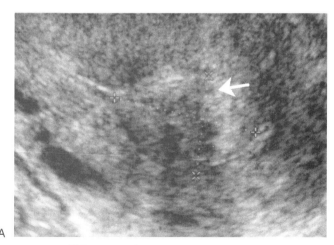

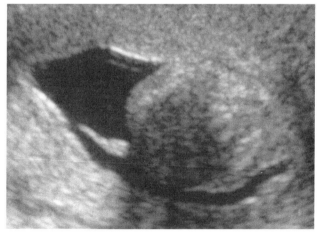

A B

FIG. 47.14. **A:** Transvaginal ultrasound of a uterus that bled on various regimens of hormone replacement therapy. A myoma obscured the endometrium. **B:** Saline infusion sonohysterography demonstrated the myoma to be submucosal in an atrophic cavity. The shape of the cavity conforms to that of the myoma. A strand of blood clot is at the supracervical edge of the myoma.

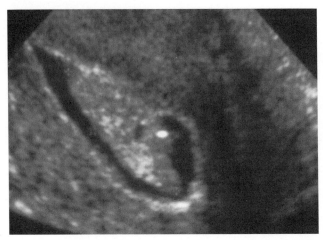
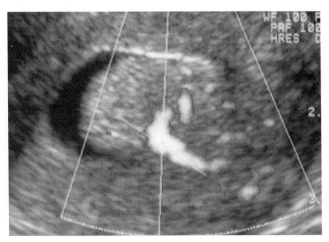

A

B

FIG. 47.15. A: A benign endometrial polyp was demonstrated by saline infusion sonohysterography in an atrophic cavity. The woman had undergone a biopsy and two dilatation and curettage procedures, which produced atrophic tissue without remission of symptoms. The polyp conforms to the shape of the endometrial cavity. B: In another patient with a polyp, the single feeding vessel is demonstrated with power or amplitude Doppler. The smooth border of the polyp, typical vessel, and otherwise atrophic cavity (not well seen here) suggest a benign polyp. The calibration scale on the right is marked in 5-mm increments.

Cancer is suspected in the woman with bleeding and thickened or highly irregular endometrial contours. Reporting of sonographic evaluation of endometrial lesions should specify the presence and depth of myometrial invasion, involvement of the lower segment or cervix, presence of ascites, and adnexal involvement, all of which affect prognosis.

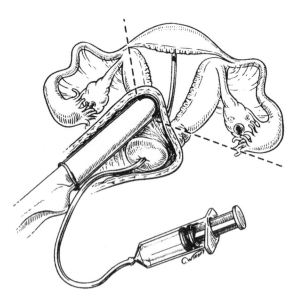

FIG. 47.16. Position of the 2-mm catheter placed for saline infusion sonohysterography. The tip is advanced gently to the fundus, and sterile, intravenous, injectable-quality saline is infused during sonographic inspection of the cavity. (From ref. 113, with permission.)

The use of low-pressure saline infusion without cervical occlusion is unlikely to produce significant retrograde flow of fragments of endometrium into the peritoneal cavity to any greater extent than does spontaneous bleeding, endometrial washing, D&C or hysteroscopy, or hysterosalpingography with an occluded cervix (115).

Several techniques can ensure optimal imaging of the endometrium:

1. The method of measurement should be consistent. The transducer should be in contact with the fundus through the vaginal wall for optimal resolution. Endometrium is conventionally measured as the sum of both walls, from one basalis boundary with the myometrium to that of the opposite wall. We perform SIS in all women with bleeding, obscure, or irregular endometria. The addition of 5 minutes, a $7.00 disposable catheter, and a 20-mL syringe of sterile saline to the basic TVU does not add sufficient cost to justify missing the few small polyps or areas of irregular proliferation or (rarely) tiny cancers that may be present under these circumstances. Biopsy is reserved for irregular thickening, global thickening over 5 mm (both layers) despite hormonal adjustment, or persistent bleeding.

2. The axis of the uterus should be as perpendicular to the axis of insonation as possible. Scanning down the barrel of the uterus produces an ill-defined image. The image may be improved by emptying the bladder completely, using manual pressure on the abdomen to push a midposition uterus into retroversion, using saline infusion to delineate the cavity (with a cervi-

cal balloon in some cases), or using an abdominal or side-firing rectal transducer.

3. A three-dimensional mental evaluation of the cavity is essential, using the sagittal planes from cornu to cornu and then turning 90 degrees to "bread loaf" the uterus from the external cervical os to the fundal serosa, evaluating the endometrial cavity for symmetry and shape in every frame (Fig. 47.11).

4. If a well-defined three-dimensional image of the endometrial cavity is not obtained, the examiner can make no judgment about the endometrium, and another test must be used.

Accuracy of Measurements

The primary limitations on the use of ultrasound as a method of evaluation of the uterus are the ability of the imager to obtain interpretable images and the ability to interpret them in the context of the patient's history and treatment. Reproducibility of measurements of endometrial thickness is excellent for normal endometria of all thicknesses in young women and in normal postmenopausal women (at less than 5 mm), but clinical judgment should be exercised when measurements are near the chosen threshold. We have found that uterine compression with the transducer or contractions can change the repeated endometrial measurement at one site by up to 1 mm. The ability of a single observer to make consecutive reproducible measurements to within ±1 mm 95% of the time was confirmed by Delisle et al. (116), with 94% interobserver agreement regarding whether the endometrium was less than or more than 5 mm in young women undergoing ovulation induction. Wolman et al. (117), studying women with postmenopausal bleeding, found that interobserver variation was negligible at measurements of 4 mm or less (0.1 mean difference ±0.2 mm), but that at 5 to 10 mm, the mean difference was 0.3 mm, with a range of up to 4 mm. Above 10 mm, the mean difference between examiners was 1 mm, but with a range of up to 6.7 mm.

In another exercise, an experienced examiner's measurements of endometrium in bleeding postmenopausal women were compared with those of five gynecologists with experience in sonography but not specifically experiences in postmenopausal endometrial evaluation (118). These imagers were each instructed in the technique in three patients, and then each evaluated 20 women independently while the experienced examiner scanned all 100. In 71% of cases, an inexperienced and experienced examiner agreed within 1 mm, but in the balance of studies, there was a discrepancy of 2 to 18 mm, with a mean difference of 1.5 mm. When compared individually with the experienced imager, the other five observers demonstrated a range of standard deviations from very narrow to rather broad, indicating variable innate ability. However, in these 100 women, no serious pathology was

missed by any examiner using a 4-mm threshold for normal. The widest discrepancies were in uteri with abnormalities such as myomas and cancer. The experienced examiner found the endometrium to be obscure in 5% (two of whom had cancer), and the others had obscure (nondiagnostic) images in 10%. In a separate group of 25 women, who were examined just before hysterectomy, the experienced examiner's measurements invariably exceeded the gross ruler measurements made on the two layers together in the fixed specimen. Although dehydration and exsanguination of the uterus undoubtedly condenses the tissue somewhat, it is clear that the sonographic image of the endometrium is slightly broadened or splayed compared with histologic measurements.

A comparison of three large multicenter studies conducted under different circumstances and their results revealed a range of image adequacy that depends on experience. A multicenter study in which all imaging was performed by highly experienced sonologists using a strict protocol reported a rate of 2.8% of unsatisfactory images. There was a high frequency of serious abnormality (by endometrial curettage) when the image was unclear, including one each of stage IV cervical cancer, endometrial cancer, and atypical hyperplasia. There also were 5 polyps, 1 hematometra, 19 atrophic cavities, and 2 cases of "exogenous hormonal effects." In another study in which "routine" scanning was done by available sonographers with nonspecific training and variable experience (119), the rate of uninterpretable scans was about 9% and involved significantly more serious abnormalities and myomas than other scans. A third multicenter study was carefully designed to involve academic and community hospital centers with a variety of gynecologic sonographic experience, and the scanning physicians used a common, prospectively designed protocol. In this case, the rate of uninterpertable images was 4.7%, midway between the study conducted under rigorous conditions and the one conducted as an afterthought to a randomized estrogen treatment protocol.

There is an irreducible number of unclear scans even in the best of hands. It is also apparent that obscure endometrium cannot be construed as normal, especially because less experienced imagers are more likely to be unable to recognize abnormal endometrial contours. These cases generally benefit from the immediate performance of SIS. The remaining (<0.5%) unclear cavities are caused by severe synechiae that prevent uterine expansion or intractable cervical stenosis that precludes SIS (unpublished data).

Ultrasound-Directed Office Biopsy

We sought to combine ultrasound-guided diagnosis and therapy for small focal lesions such as polyps and subcentimeter intracavitary myomas (120). Using TVU and SIS and adding transabdominal ultrasound for guidance in one-half of the procedures, focal lesions were identified, measured, and removed entirely or at least biopsied in 54 of 56 women with abnormal bleeding (44 of them postmenopausal). A 23-cm pediatric broncho-scopic malleable alligator grasper (Storz 50372) with a 2.5 mm diameter could be inserted in all except two women. Removal of the complete lesion at the first visit was possible in 44%, and adequate tissue for diagnosis was obtained immediately in 96% of 54. Findings included 50 simple or hyperplastic polyps, 1 placental polyp, 1 atypical focal hyperplasia, and 2 myomas. A total of 82 procedures were done in 54 women; some were repeated to remove enough tissue to allow symptom remission. Symptoms did not recur in 88%; one hystero-scopic polypectomy and four hysterectomies for atypical hyperplasia (1), adnexal masses (2), and continued bleed-ing from a large submucosal myoma after polypectomy were required for five women.

EFFECTS OF SELECTIVE ESTROGEN RECEPTOR MODULATORS ON ENDOMETRIUM

SERMs are nonsteroidal estrogen receptor ligands that, when complexed with estrogen receptors α or β and an adaptor protein, promote transcription of key proteins that alter the cell's phenotype and products. Their tissue-specific effects produce a range of estrogen or antiestro-genic responses that vary with the compound, the avail-able adapter proteins in the organ, and the hormonal milieu (121,122), a process that is under intense scrutiny for natural steroids and SERMs.

The use of tamoxifen in premenopausal women indi-rectly promotes estradiol and progesterone production by hypothalamic stimulation of follicle-stimulating hormone with consequent enhancement of follicular growth, ovu-lation, and luteal phase progesterone. For this reason,

tamoxifen, like a related SERM, clomiphene, is also used for ovulation induction in infertile women (123). This enhancement of ovulatory cycles may promote endome-triosis and myoma growth but does not elevate endome-trial cancer risk in premenopausal women. The National Surgical Adjuvant Breast Project report (124) of the pro-phylactic use of 20 mg of tamoxifen per day for up to 5 years (mean, 24 months) in healthy women described an insignificantly increased risk ratio for endometrial cancer of 1.21 in women younger than 50 on tamoxifen com-pared with those on placebo (95% CI, 0.41–3.60).

For women 50 years of age or older, the risk of endometrial cancer was increased fourfold over that of women taking placebo (risk ratio = 4.01; 95% CI, 1.70–10.90). This is approximately the middle of the range of the estimates of the increased risk reported with unopposed estrogen in case-control studies (125). The accelerated incidence of cancers occurred within a year of beginning treatment with tamoxifen, suggesting there were preexisting lesions in some women. In women older than 50 years of age taking placebo (n = 4,194), the aver-age annual incidence of endometrial cancer was 0.76 women per thousand; in those on tamoxifen (4,097), it was 3.05 cases per 1,000 women. This concurs with pre-vious reports of healthy women in prophylactic trials. Kedar et al. (126) reported that only 61% of tamoxifen-treated women had atrophic endometria on hysteroscopic biopsy (although tamoxifen levels were undetectable in six of them) compared with 90% of 50 untreated controls. No controls had hyperplasia (using ultrasound and office biopsy), but 10 (16%) treated women had hyperplasia, and all cases were judged to be atypical.

In a percentage of hypoestrogenic postmenopausal women, tamoxifen acts as a weak estrogen to produce significant uterine stimulation and endometrial prolifera-tion (Fig. 47.17) (20). The degree of individual response is at this time unpredictable, and ACOG has recom-

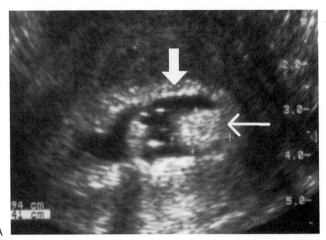
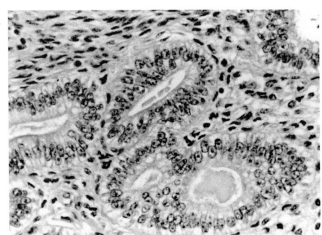

FIG. 47.17. A: Sonogram of a uterus with a thickened, hyperplastic endometrium (*thick arrow*) and irregular surface surrounding a polyp (*thin arrow*). **B:** Typical endometrial hyperplasia.

mended endometrial biopsy only if bleeding occurs (127). Screening of asymptomatic women by hysteroscopy, sonography, or biopsy is not encouraged, but it may be done at the discretion of the physician.

The lack of pretreatment evaluation and controls has caused much confusion regarding the real effects of tamoxifen, which seem to be primarily those of a weak unopposed estrogen. The polyps arising in tamoxifen-treated women have the same genetic abnormalities as other estrogen-promoted benign tumors (i.e., spontaneous polyps and myomas [128]). Estrogen-like proliferative responses (including cancer in up to 3%) have been reported in 15% to 70% of women in uncontrolled series of asymptomatic women taking tamoxifen. Tepper et al. found that two-thirds of 68 women had normal cavities by hysteroscopy and SIS and that, of the remaining 22, 19 were found to have had polyps or hyperplasia, 1 had a myoma, 2 had septa, and 1 had inactive endometrium (129).

Cohen et al., comparing 175 asymptomatic women with breast cancer on tamoxifen with 27 untreated breast cancer patients as controls (130), found 80% of cavities in both groups to be normal, with approximately the same incidence in polyps (8%) and hyperplasia (12%) but with more of the tamoxifen-treated polyps associated with endometrial hyperplasia. In another controlled series, 72% of 51 tamoxifen-treated, asymptomatic women had abnormal endometrial stimulation, compared with 13% of 52 controls with breast cancer (131). These investigators found that the tamoxifen group had significantly thicker endometria and larger uterine volumes than the controls. Thirty-six percent had polyps (including 1% involving cancer and 2% with hyperplasia), compared with 10% of controls. Uziely found 15% of 95 asymptomatic tamoxifen-treated patients to have abnormalities, including three with cancer and three with hyperplasia (132).

There has been further confusion regarding tamoxifen's endometrial effects because of a nonprogressive minimally or nonproliferative effect of basalis glandular distention, similar to but more exaggerated than typical cystic atrophy, which can be mistaken for functionalis proliferation in about one-half of asymptomatic women with abnormal ultrasound images (133). When Achiron et al. (134) used sonohysterography to evaluate the cavities of 20 women with tamoxifen-associated cystic, thickened endometria, 8 had endometrial polyps, and 12 had irregular, cystic endometrial-myometrial junctions without endometrial proliferation on biopsy.

It appears from our experience that more than one-half of the women on tamoxifen do have inactive endometrium with massively dilated but essentially atrophic glands that protrude into the myometrium at the basalis layer (Fig. 47.18) (21), but as Goldstein showed, the essentially smooth cavity and lack of development of the functionalis is revealed by SIS (135). This peculiar but innocuous condition has been called *pseudopolypoid glandulocystic endometrial atrophy* (136), and the hysteroscopic effect of the endometrium has been likened to the bouncy surface of a waterbed by Dr. Patrick Neven (personal communication). Schwarz et al. (137) used SIS to demonstrate the cavities in 44 asymptomatic tamoxifen-treated breast cancer patients. 68% had endometria that appeared to be thicker than 5 mm and that 11% had obscure endometria. One-third of these 79% had atrophic endometria with typical tamoxifen-induced subendometrial cysts; the others had a variety of abnormal proliferative lesions that required biopsy.

Berliere et al. helped put the findings in the tamoxifen database in perspective (138). In a 3-year prospective study of postmenopausal patients prescribed tamoxifen, 264 women were studied with ultrasound and hysteroscopy before treatment and yearly during treatment. Seventeen percent had asymptomatic polyps or hyperplasia before starting tamoxifen, two of them with atypia. The lesions were removed. After 3 years of treatment, 9 of the original 46 women with lesions reformed lesions, 3 of them with atypical hyperplasia, and 51 (23%) originally normal patients developed new polyps or hyperplasia, with only one being atypical, a significant difference in incidence of atypia ($p = 0.0009$). Although a similar proportion (about 20%) developed lesions in both groups, one-third of the women with original lesions developed precancerous changes, compared with 1.8% in women with lesions induced by tamoxifen.

These data suggest that pretreatment or early endometrial evaluation can substantially diminish the opportunity for tamoxifen to exacerbate existing estrogen-sensitive lesions and identifies a select group of high-risk women for yearly scrutiny. Conventional HRT does not mandate pretreatment screening of asymptomatic women, because the therapy prevents hyperplasia. However, early or pretreatment evaluation of women on tamoxifen is desirable, because the treatment itself can be expected to induce some degree of uncontrollable proliferation in about one-half of the women treated and can exacerbate preexisting lesions (103).

Between 25% and 50% of asymptomatic women taking tamoxifen seem to maintain unstimulated endometria after years of treatment (139,140). Our experience also suggests that those in whom tamoxifen has a stimulatory effect are revealed within the first year of treatment by some form of endometrial proliferation. The severity of proliferative lesions increases in these women as treatment progresses, but significant new proliferation does not seem to occur in women without any by 1 year. Our practice has been to scan and perform SIS for all women on tamoxifen at the time of initial referral to characterize their response. Our annual examination of all postmenopausal women includes an ultrasound-assisted pelvic examination, and SIS is added only for bleeding or in women with irregular, unclear, or thickened endome-

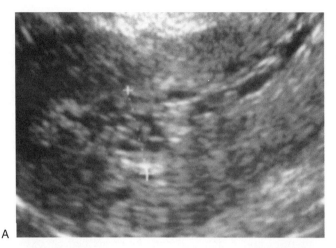
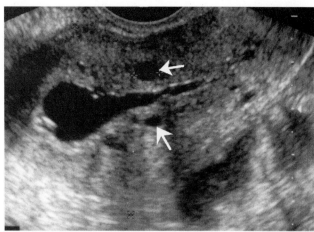
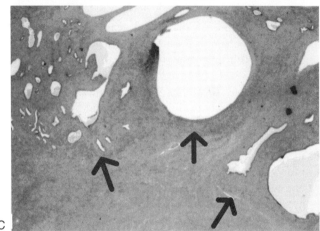

FIG. 47.18. Macrocystic distention of endometrial basalis glands produced by tamoxifen. **A:** Transvaginal ultrasound of a uterus exposed to tamoxifen for 10 years demonstrates a visibly cystic endometrium measuring 7 mm thick. The 67-year-old woman had no bleeding, and biopsy revealed an inactive endometrium. **B:** Saline infusion sonohysterography demonstrates a regular cavity, except for the protrusion of two small cysts and an ill-defined endometrium, enhanced at some points by through-transmission of the ultrasound through the cysts that border it and protrude into the myometrium (*arrows*). On yearly scans, this pattern had not changed for 5 years. **C:** The hysterectomy specimen from the same patient had been removed at the time of oophorectomy for an ovarian fibroma. The lumen is at the top of the slide. The macrocystic basalis glands produce a highly irregular interface with the myometrium (*arrows*) as they protrude into it. There is also some cystic atrophy of the smaller glands in the otherwise inactive basalis. These changes produce the appearance of an ill-defined endometrium with visible hypoechoic cysts where the dilated glands are large enough to be resolved on ultrasound (about 1 mm) and hyperechoic areas where they are smaller.

trium over 4 mm. In the past 9 years, we have followed 56 postmenopausal women referred while taking tamoxifen, 9 of whom presented with polyps or progressive proliferation, hyperplasia, or cancer. Two of the remaining 42 have developed fibrous benign polyps in otherwise atrophic endometria. MPA proved ineffective in suppressing polyp growth; growth was instead promoted, as others have reported (141). The rest (40) have maintained sonographically unstimulated endometria without uterine enlargement. Although most have developed typical dilated endometrial basalis layer glands, none of these has bled.

Raloxifene Hydrochloride

To avoid the ambiguities that have plagued the use of tamoxifen, a stringent ultrasound and biopsy protocol was used to study the uterine effects of raloxifene. This benzothiophene SERM is used to prevent osteoporosis, but it also lowered serum low-density lipoprotein levels and diminished the incidence of new breast cancers by over 50% compared with placebo in a normal early postmenopausal population. It also demonstrated a primarily antiestrogenic effect on the uterus in biopsy-based studies (142,143).

A randomized, placebo-controlled, double-blind protocol was used to compare the uterine effects of two doses of raloxifene with those of 0.625 mg of CEE. This trial involved 415 postmenopausal women with an endometrial thickness of no more than 5 mm and a single-wall thickness of no more than 3 mm determined using SIS. They were randomized to placebo, 60 or 150 mg of raloxifene, or estrogen. The endometrium was evaluated with a Pipelle biopsy. TVU and SIS were done during screening and after 6 months and 1 year of treatment. The TVU for endometrial thickness was done every 3 months during treatment, with SIS performed at 6 months. The endometrial status of enrolled women was clearly free of focal abnormalities (except submucosal myomas) at baseline and did not change in thickness throughout treatment with either dose of raloxifene or placebo. Endometrial thickness did increase by a mean of 5.5 mm in women treated with estrogen (144), 23% of whom developed hyperplasia, and 39% of whom had proliferation. Three women in the 60-mg raloxifene group, each with a BMI greater than 29, developed proliferative changes; none did in the 150 mg group. In the placebo group, 2% each developed hyperplasia and proliferation. There were no subendometrial cysts seen in women treated with raloxifene.

Other Selective Estrogen Receptor Modulators

Various tamoxifen-related compounds are or will be available for the treatment of advanced breast cancer. There is a paucity of data about these compounds; no uterine safety studies have been published. Toremifene appears to produce vaginal bleeding at a rate similar to tamoxifen. Idoxifene reportedly produces stromal changes and apparent sonographic thickening without proliferation, which requires further evaluation. Because scanty tissue is retrieved on biopsy from these women, the intense echogenic thickening may represent some form of cystic atrophy. They do not appear to develop macrocysts, however. (Art Fleischer, M.D., personal communication).

USE OF DOPPLER FOR DISCRIMINATION OF ENDOMETRIAL CANCER

Duplex Doppler sonography provides simultaneous vessel imaging and flow studies. Color flow imaging translates red blood cell movement to a velocity-defined color spectrum, and amplitude Doppler imaging evaluates the density of moving red blood cells without regard to their direction. The latter technique vividly depicts small tortuous vessels with slow flow and is highly effective for demonstration of uterine vascular anatomy. Accurate identification of the direction of a vessel allows calculation of systolic and diastolic flow velocity. The waveform produced by Doppler shifts caused by changes in velocity through the cardiac cycle is characterized by a mathematical index of the actual Doppler shifts at systole

and diastole. The most common of these indices are the pulsatility index (PI) and the resistance index (RI), which are calculated as follows:

$$PI = \frac{(A - B)}{Mean}$$

$$RI = \frac{(A - B)}{A}$$

In these equations, A is the maximum or peak systolic frequency shift (highest point on the waveform), and B is the minimum or end diastolic frequency shift. *Mean* refers to the calculated mean frequency shift over the entire cardiac cycle. The lower these numbers are, the less variation there is in flow rates over the cardiac cycle, and the less impedance there is to blood flow distal to the point of observation. Reproducibility and interpretation of the results of flow velocity require an understanding and appropriate use of angle settings and transducer frequency. Descriptions of waveforms by these indices merely describe flow characteristics of individual vessels without regard to actual velocity and are independent of insonation angle or transducer frequency.

Unimpeded forward diastolic flow is typical of a low-resistance vascular bed. Angiogenesis of relatively acontractile vessels in a tumor bed (35,36,145,146), in trophoblast (37,38), or in the functional ovarian corpus luteum (39) produces a low-impedance wave form with a low PI and RI in afferent vessels.

The addition of estrogen decreases impedance in the uterine vessels of estrogen-deficient women at any age (147,148). The PI and RI of the dominant ovarian artery decrease dramatically during peak estrogen and progesterone output in the ovulatory cycle (149). However, neither the nondominant ovary nor the uterine vessels reflect such dramatic cyclic changes in impedance, although flow velocities may change (150).

The small decline in the impedance of postmenopausal uterine vasculature produced by low-dose exogenous estrogen (151) appears to be a systemic response. Pines et al. demonstrated a small increase in stroke volume and aortic flow acceleration in estrogen-treated postmenopausal women, and a small but significant decrease in carotid artery PI has been reported in another well-designed study (152). Others have documented ultrasound and Doppler-derived evidence of diminished systemic vascular resistance after exposure to high estrogen levels during ovulation induction and early pregnancy (153,154).

An early impression that the impedance of uterine arteries and (subendometrial) radial arteries was significantly lowered in postmenopausal women with endometrial cancer (155,156) has been modified. Further experience, the confounding effects of estrogen and tamoxifen, and improvements in Doppler ultrasound technology that allow detection of ever smaller normal vessels indicate that Doppler data are probably not sufficient for diagnosis or prognosis. Although uteri with cancer do have significantly more visible subendometrial and endometrial vessels than those without, there is substantial overlap between the two groups. Sladkevicius et al. showed the endometrial thickness in postmenopausal bleeders, even scanned randomly during cyclic HRT, to be a much better discriminator between benign and malignant processes than any Doppler characteristic of the uterine, radial, or endometrial vessels (157).

PREDICTION OF TUMOR INVASION WITH TRANSVAGINAL ULTRASOUND

More than 70% of patients present with disease confined to the corpus, and reliable preoperative evaluation can help tailor treatment to minimize trauma and expense. Stage Ia or Ib cancers are effectively treated by vaginal hysterectomy in selected patients (158,159); total abdominal hysterectomy and bilateral salpingo-oophorectomy with lymphadenectomy is required for higher-stage disease; and radical hysterectomy is recommended with cervical involvement.

Hata et al. tested whether tumor vascularity measured as the RI and the peak systolic velocity of intratumoral vessels correlated with grade, local invasion, and likelihood of nodal involvement in 36 tumors with the same result: endometrial thickness produced the only significant (positive) correlation with grade and stage of disease (160). This agrees with the older observation that increasing surgical tumor size is highly prognostic of nodal involvement (161) but not more recent observations that higher numbers of microvessels in the tumor confer a poorer prognosis (162). As power- or amplitude-dependent Doppler becomes more widely used, it may discriminate these tumors with the aid of other techniques, including contrast agents and Doppler pulse inversion.

Because prognosis depends on the extent of tumor invasion and cervical involvement at the time of diagnosis, non-Doppler ultrasound and magnetic resonance imaging (MRI) have been tested for their ability to predict these features. In a number of small series, they are comparable in their ability to do so and suffer from similar problems. Uterine polyps, myomas, and adenomyosis can be confounding, as can cervical polyps, using either modality. The most commonly cited cause of error is overestimation of invasion by a superficial polypoid intracavitary cancer, caused by stretching and thinning of the adjacent myometrium. Saline infusion during scanning can satisfactorily delineate the borders and site of attachment of such lesions, differentiating an expanding intracavitary mass from myometrial invasion.

Ten years ago, abdominal ultrasound provided an accuracy of 80% for myometrial depth of invasion and 93% for cervical involvement in 93 women (163). In a total of 486 cases in 11 studies (164–173), the accuracy for vaginal sonographic determination of depth of invasion is

about 87%, ranging from 78% to 90%, with slightly more mistakes (overestimates and underestimates) in larger uteri with high-grade, ill-defined tumors or other benign pathology. Preoperative vaginal ultrasound made the gross distinction between more than and less than 50% myometrial invasion in 90% of 20 cases, essentially the same as was found with open inspection of the uterus (174).

Accuracy for sonographic determination of cervical involvement ranges from 33% to 94%. MRI, described in five reports of a total of 210 patients (175), gave an accuracy for level of invasion of 71% to 89% and for cervical invasion of 98% (one study). A series of 27 accurately diagnosed cases suggests that parasagittal MRI with contrast demonstrates cervical involvement (176) most precisely.

Three-dimensional ultrasound may refine the accuracy of cancer diagnosis (177) and invasion, and it may shorten scanning time, but this has yet to be proven (178).

COST EFFECTIVENESS OF STRATEGIES TO EVALUATE POSTMENOPAUSAL BLEEDING

In 1983, Feldman et al. compared office biopsy, D&C, hysterectomy and observation in various combinations for their cost effectiveness and effect on life expectancy at different risk levels (179). They concluded that an initial endometrial biopsy was the most effective strategy by far, but that the overall cost per life-year saved rose enormously for women with a low risk of cancer. They speculated that a method for predicting individual risk, such as sonographic endometrial thickness, would prevent a costly series of evaluations (including more invasive testing when insufficient endometrium was retrieved) by clearly identifying a low-risk group of women with less than 1% risk of cancer.

Weber et al. compared the costs of two diagnostic algorithms (180). The first used standard vaginal ultrasound as the initial test for bleeding, followed by office biopsy for all abnormal results. The second used endometrial biopsy as the initial test, with ultrasound for those that are nondiagnostic. Hysteroscopy or D&C was the next test for the estimated 10% of abnormal cases expected from ultrasound screening. Hysteroscopy or D&C was likewise done for the estimated 10% of nondiagnostic endometrial biopsies in the second diagnostic pathway. Using cost estimates from their institution, they concluded that the initial use of ultrasound to estimate cancer risk was always less costly, albeit by $14 to $20 per patient, because their ultrasound costs were less than their biopsy costs. By their literature-based estimate, about 50% of women undergoing ultrasound would require biopsy.

These investigators then suggested the obvious next step: although ultrasound thickness is effective in assessing risk for cancer, it is less sensitive than hysteroscopy

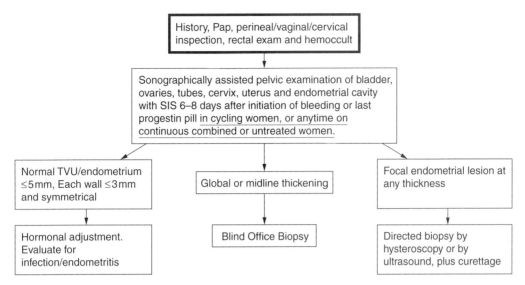

FIG. 47.19. Algorithm for the evaluation of postmenopausal bleeding. Pap, Papanicolaou screening, TVU, transvaginal ultrasound; SIS, saline infusion sonohysterography.

for other benign causes of bleeding, and endometrial biopsy is much less sensitive. The inclusion of SIS, which their group previously showed was an equivalent to hysteroscopy for diagnosis of intracavitary lesions, shortens the diagnostic process by increasing sensitivity and decreases cost by reserving surgery for therapy rather than diagnosis. Their primary reservation regarding recommending its routine use was the "lack of availability" of the technique—a limitation of practitioners, not the procedure.

CONCLUSIONS

Postmenopausal bleeding has increased with the use of HRT. The cost in lost time from work and investigative procedures incurred because of iatrogenic bleeding with HRT can be minimized by prompt characterization of the uterus and endometrial thickness using ultrasound with saline infusion at the initial visit. The time-honored concept that endometrial atrophy is the cause of most postmenopausal bleeding, based on blind curettings, has given way to an appreciation for the ubiquity of polyps and submucosal and intracavitary myomas in the postmenopausal population.

Sonographic identification of unstimulated endometrium is highly accurate in excluding neoplasia as a cause of bleeding. Saline infusion discriminates between focal and global intracavitary and extracavitary lesions for a more specific identification of all causes of uterine bleeding. The technology is safe, inexpensive, and widely available. Polyps, myomas, hyperplasia, and cancers produce demonstrable irregularities in the luminal contour of the endometrial surface and increase the thickness of the endometrial layer. The timing of evaluation in the postbleed window is essential for rational management of bleeding during artificial cycles. Continuous combined regimens with adequate antiproliferative effects can be expected to maintain the total combined layers of endometrium at 5 mm or less, with a smooth normal cavity.

Tamoxifen is a weak estrogen and unpredictably promotes proliferation in the postmenopausal uterus during a 5-year course of treatment. It therefore seems no more acceptable to wait until the tamoxifen-treated woman bleeds for uterine surveillance than it is when giving unopposed estrogen. The increased risk of ovarian and endometrial cancer of patients with breast cancer also suggests that an annual ultrasound-assisted pelvic examination has added value for these patients. However, the development and broader use of SERMs that decrease bone resorption, diminish the incidence of breast cancer in healthy women, and lower cholesterol without uterine stimulation can prevent bleeding and diminish the widespread need for repetitive uterine evaluation.

The primary limitation on the optimal use of ultrasound is the imager's technical ability, understanding of pelvic anatomy and physiology, and use of a systematic, rigorous imaging protocol. Based on the principal that all endometrial functionalis should be eliminated after progesterone withdrawal, leaving a basalis-lined cavity of recognizably normal contour, an algorithm for evaluation of postmenopausal bleeding is provided in Fig. 47.19.

REFERENCES

1. Lochen ML, Lund E. Childbearing and mortality from cancer of the corpus uteri. *Acta Obstet Gynecol Scand* 1997;76:373–377.
2. Parazzini F, La Vecchia C, Bocciolone L, Franceschi S. The epidemiology of endometrial cancer. *Gynecol Oncol* 1991;41:1–16.

3. American College of Obstetricians and Gynecologists. ACOG technical bulletin no. 162. Washington, DC: American College of Obstetricians and Gynecologists, December 1991.
4. Persson I, Yuen J, Bergkvist L, Schairer C. Cancer incidence and mortality in women receiving estrogen and estrogen-progestin replacement therapy—long term follow-up of a Swedish cohort. Int J Cancer 1996;29:67:327–332.
5. Schiff M, Key CR, Gilliland FD, Becker TM. Ethnic differences in uterine corpus cancer incidence and mortality in New Mexico's American Indians, Hispanics and non-Hispanic whites, Int J Epidemiol 1997;26:249–255.
6. Landis SH, Murray T, Bolden S, Wingo P. Cancer statistics. CA Cancer J Clin 1998;48:6–30.
7. Parker SL, Davis KJ, Wingo PA, Ries LAG, Heath CW. Cancer statistics by race and ethnicity. CA Cancer J Clin 1998;48:31–48.
8. Shipley CF, Nelson GH. Seeking early medical attention after vaginal bleeding will not ensure mild disease in postmenopausal endometrial carcinoma. Am J Obstet Gynecol 1993;168:555–556.
9. ACOG Committee on Gynecologic Practice, ACOG Committee Opinion. Routine cancer screening, technical bulletin no. 185. Washington, DC: American College of Obstetricians and Gynecologists, 1997.
10. Mettlin C, Jones G, Averette H, Gusberg SB, Murphy GP. Defining and updating the American Cancer Society Guidelines for the cancer related check-up: prostate and endometrial cancers. CA Cancer J Clin 1993;43:42–46.
11. MacKenzie IZ, Bibby JG. Critical assessment of dilatation and curettage in 1,209 women. Lancet 1978;2:566–568.
12. Hoist J, Koseila O. Endometrial findings following curettage in 2,018 women according to age and indications. Ann Chir Gynaecol 1983;72:274–277.
13. Nagele F, O'Connor H, Baskett TF, Davies A, Mohammed H, Magos AL. Hysteroscopy in women with abnormal uterine bleeding on HRT: a comparison with postmenopausal bleeding. Fertil Steril 1996;65:1145–1150.
14. Grady D, Rubin SM, Petitti DB, et al. Hormone therapy to prevent disease and prolong life in postmenopausal women. Ann Intern Med 1992;117:1016–1037.
15. Rubin GL, Peterson HB, Lee NC, Maes EF, Wingo PA, Becker S. Estrogen replacement therapy in the risk of endometrial cancer: remaining controversies. Am J Obstet Gynecol 1990;162:148–154.
16. Voight LF, Weiss NS, Chu J, Daling J, McKnight B, van Delle G. Progestogen supplementation of exogenous estrogens and risk of endometrial cancer. Lancet 1991;338:274–277.
17. Woodruff JD, Pickar JH and The Menopause Study Group, Incidence of endometrial hyperplasia in postmenopausal women taking conjugated estrogens (Premarin) with medroxyprogesterone acetate or conjugated estrogens alone. Am J Obstet Gynecol 1994;170:1213–1223.
18. Ettinger B, Selby JV, Citron JT, Ettinger VM, Zhang D. Gynecologic complications of cyclic estrogen progestin therapy. Maturitas 1993;17:197–204.
19. Ettinger B, Li D, Klein R. Unexpected vaginal bleeding and associated gynecologic care in postmenopausal women using hormone replacement therapy: comparison of cyclic versus continuous combined schedules Fertil Steril 1998;69:865–869.
20. Nand SL, Wester MA, Baber R, O'Connor V. Bleeding pattern and endometrial changes during continuous combined hormone replacement therapy: the Ogen/Provera Study Group. Obstet Gynecol 1998;91:678–684.
21. Archer DF, Pickar JH, Bottiglioni F, et al. Bleeding patterns in postmenopausal women taking continuous combined or sequential regimens of conjugated estrogens with medroxyprogesterone acetate. Obstet Gynecol 1994;83:686–692.
22. Archer DF, McIntyre-Seltman K, Wilborn WW, et al. Am J Obstet Gynecol 1991;165:317–322.
23. Korhonen MO, Sumons JP, Hyde BM, et al. Histologic classification and pathologic findings for endometrial biopsy specimens obtained from 2964 perimenopausal nd postmenopausal women undergoing screening for continuous hormones as replacement therapy. Am J Obstet Gynecol 1997;176:377–380.
24. Koss LG, Schreiber K, Oberlander SG, Moussouris HF, Lesser M. Detection of endometrial carcinoma and hyperplasia in asymptomatic women. Obstet Gynecol 1984;64:1–11.
25. Akkad AA, Habiba MA, Ismail N, et al. Abnormal uterine bleeding on hormone replacement: The importance of intrauterine structural abnormalities. Obstet Gynecol 1995;86:330–334.
26. Hahn RG. Compliance considerations with estrogen replacement: withdrawal bleeding and other factors. Am J Gynecol 1989;161:1854–1858.
27. Stock R, Kanbour A. Prehysterectomy curettage. Obstet Gynecol 1975;45:537–541.
28. Word B, Gravlee L, Wideman G. The fallacy of simple uterine curettage. Obstet Gynecol 1958;12:642–647.
29. Stovall TG, Solomon S, Ling F. Endometrial sampling prior to hysterectomy. Obstet Gynecol 1989;73:405–409.
30. Feldman S, Berkowitz RS, Tosteson ANA. Cost-effectiveness of strategies to evaluate postmenopausal bleeding. Obstet Gynecol 1993;81:968–975.
31. Rodriguez GC, Yaqub N, King ME. A comparison of the Pipelle device and the Vabra aspirator as measured by endometrial denudation in hysterectomy specimens: the Pipelle device samples significantly less of the endometrial surface than the Vabra aspirator. Am J Obstet Gynecol 1993;168:55–59.
32. Dijkhuizen PFJB, Brolmann HAM, Potters A, Bongers MY, Heintz APM. The accuracy of transvaginal ultrasonography in the diagnosis of endometrial abnormalities. Obstet Gynecol 1996;87:345–349.
33. Van den Bosch T, Vandendael A, Van Schoubroeck D, Wranz PA, Lombard DJ. Combining vaginal ultrasonography and office endometrial sampling in the diagnosis of endometrial disease in postmenopausal women. Obstet Gynecol 1995;85:349–352.
34. Stovall TG, Ling FW, Morgan PL. A prospective randomized comparison of the Pipelle endometrial sampling device with the Novak curette. Am J Obstet Gynecol 1991;165:1287–1290.
35. Stovall TG, Photopulos GJ, Poston WM, Ling FW, Sandles LG. Pipelle endometrial sampling in patients with known endometrial carcinoma. Obstet Gynecol 1991;77:954–956.
36. Ferry J, Farnsworth A, Webster M, Wren B. The efficacy of the Pipelle endometrial biopsy in detecting endometrial carcinoma. Aust N Z J Obstet Gynaecol 1993;33:76–78.
37. Goldchmit R, Katz Z, Blickstein I, Caspi B, Dgani R. The accuracy of endometrial Pipelle sampling with and without sonographic measurement of endometrial thickness. Obstet Gynecol 1993;82:727–730.
38. Creasman WT. New gynecologic cancer staging. Obstet Gynecol 1990;75:287–288.
39. Larson DM, Johnson KK, Broste SK, Krawisc BR, Kresl JJ. Comparison of D&C and office endometrial biopsy in predicting final histopathologic grade in endometrial cancer. Obstet Gynecol 1995;86:38–42.
40. Dunton CG, Baak JPA, Palazzo JP, van Diest PJ, McHugh M, Widra EA. Use of computerized morphometric analyses of endometrial hyperplasias in the prediction of coexistent cancer. Am J Obstet Gynecol 1996;174;1518–1521.
41. Mencaglia L, Valle RF, Perino A, Gilardo G. Endometrial cancer and its precursors: early detection and treatment. Int J Gynecol Obstet 1990;31:107–116.
42. LaPolla JP, Nicosia S, Mccurdy C, et al. Experience with the EndoPap device for the cytologic detection of uterine cancer and its precursors: a comparison of the EndoPap with fractional curettage and hysterectomy. Am J Obstet Gynecol 1990;163:1055–1060.
43. Valle RF. Hysteroscopic evaluation of patients with abnormal uterine bleeding. Surg Gynecol Obstet 1981;153:521.
44. Englund S, Ingelman-Sundberg A, Weston B. Hysteroscopy in diagnosis and treatment of uterine bleeding. Gynaecologia 1957;143:217.
45. Nagele F, O'Connor H, Baskett TF, Davies A. Hysteroscopy in women with abnormal uterine bleeding on hormone replacement therapy: a comparison with postmenopausal bleeding. Fertil Steril 1996;65:1145–1150.
46. Valle RF. Hysteroscopic evaluation of patients with abnormal uterine bleeding. Surg Gynecol Obstet 1981;153:521.
47. Karlsson B, Granberg S, Hellberg P, Wikland M. Comparative study of transvaginal sonography and hysteroscopy for the detection of pathologic endometrial lesions in women with postmenopausal bleeding. J Ultrasound Med 1994;13:757–762.
48. Gimpelson R, Rappold H. A comparative study between panoramic hysteroscopy with directed biopsies and dilation and curettage: a review of 276 cases. Am J Obstet Gynecol 1988;158:489–492.
49. Mencaglia L, Perino A, Hamou J. Hysteroscopy in perimenopausal and postmenopausal women with abnormal uterine bleeding. J Reprod Med 1987;32:577–582.
50. Karlsson B, Granberg S, Ridell B, Wikland M. Endometrial thickness as measured by transvaginal sonography: interobserver variation. Ultrasound Obstet Gynecol 1994;4:320–5.
51. Smith-Bindman R, Kerlikowske K, Feldstein VA, et al. Endovaginal ultrasound to exclude endometrial cancer and other endometrial abnormalities. JAMA 1998;280:1510–1517.
52. Parsons A, Lense J. Sonohysterography for endometrial abnormalities: preliminary results. J Clin Ultrasound 1993;21:87–95.
53. Gompel C, Silverberg SG. The corpus uteri. In: Pathology in gynecology and obstetrics, 4th ed. Philadelphia: JB Lippincott, 1994:186.
54. Demopoulos RI, Mittal KR. Anatomy, histology and physiology. In: Altchek A, Deligdisch L, eds. The uterus. New York: Springer-Verlag, 1991:2.
55. Dallenbach-Hellweg G. Histopathology of the endometrium. New York: Springer-Verlag, 1987.
56. Delisle M, Villeneuve M, Boulvain M. Measurement of endometrial thickness with transvaginal ultrasonography: is it reproducible? J Ultrasound Med 1998:17:481–4.
57. MacBride JM. The normal post-menopausal endometrium. Br J Obstet Gynecol 1954;61:691–697.
58. Kraus FT. Irradiation changes in the uterus. In: Hertig AT, Norris HG, Abell MR, eds. The uterus. Baltimore: Williams & Wilkins, 1973:457–488.
59. Board JA, Redwine FO, Moncure CW, Frable WJ, Taylor JR. Identification of differing etiologies of clinically diagnosed premature menopause. Am J Obstet Gynecol 1979;134:936–944.
60. Evrard JR, Buxton BH Jr, Erickson D. Amenorrhea following oral contraception. Am J Obstet Gynecol 1976;124:88–91.
61. Shulman A, Shulman N, Weissenglass L, Bahary C. Ultrasonic assessment of the endometrium as a predictor of oestrogen status in amenorrhoeic patients. Hum Reprod 1989;4:61–69.
62. Nakamura S, Douchi T, Oki T, Ijuin H, Ymamoto S, Nagata Y. Relationship between sonographic endometrial thickness and progestin-induced withdrawal bleeding. Obstet Gynecol 1996;87:722–725.
63. Andolf E, Kahlander K, Aspenberg P. Ultrasonic thickness of the endometrium correlated to body weight in asymptomatic postmenopausal women. Obstet Gynecol 1993;82:936–940.
64. Douchi T, Yoshinaga M, Katanozaka M, et al. Relationship between body mass

index and transvaginal ultrasonographic endometrial thickness in postmenopausal women. *Acta Obstet Gynecol Scand* 1998;77:905–908.

65. Ferrazzi E, Torri V, Trio D, et al. sonographic endometrial thickness: a useful test to predict atrophy in patients with postmenopausal bleeding: an Italian multicenter study. *Ultrasound Obstet Gynecol* 1996;7:315–321.

66. Meuwissen JHJM, van Langen H, Moret E, Navarro-Morquecho I. Monitoring of oestrogen replacement therapy by vaginosonography of the endometrium. *Maturitas* 1992;15:33–37.

67. Meuwissen JHJM, van Langen H, Navarro I. Ultrasound determination of the effect of progestogens on the endometrium in postmenopausal women receiving hormone replacement therapy. *Maturitas* 1994;18:77–85.

68. Ettinger B, Bainton L, Upmalis DH, et al. Comparison of endometrial growth produced by unopposed conjugated estrogens or by micronized estradiol in postmenopausal women. *Am J Obstet Gynecol* 1997;176:112–117.

69. Woodruff JD, Pickar JH. Incidence of endometrial hyperplasia in postmenopausal women taking conjugated estrogens and medroxyprogesterone acetate or conjugated estrogens alone. *Am J Obstet Gynecol* 1994;170:1213–1223.

70. Goldstein SR, Nachtigall M, Snyder JR, Nachtigall L. Endometrial assessment by vaginal ultrasonography before endometrial sampling in patients with postmenopausal bleeding. *Am J Obstet Gynecol* 1990;163:119–123.

71. Goldstein SR. Use of ultrasonohysterography for triage of perimenopausal patients with unexplained uterine bleeding. *Am J Obstet Gynecol* 1994;170:565–570.

72. Affinito P, Palomba S, Pellicano M, Sorrentino C, Di Carlo C, et al. Ultrasonographic measurement of endometrial thickness during hormonal replacement therapy in postmenopausal women. *Ultrasound Obstet Gynecol* 1998;11:343–346.

73. Magos AL, Brincat M, Studd WW, et al. Amenorrhea and endometrial atrophy with continuous oral estrogen and progestogen therapy in postmenopausal women. *Obstet Gynecol* 65:496–499.

74. Krettek JE, Arkin SI, Chaisilwattana P, Monif GRG. *Chlamydia trachomatis* in patients who used oral contraceptives and had intermenstrual spotting. *Obstet Gynecol* 1993;81:728–731.

75. Vasudeva K, Thrasher TV, Richart RM. Chronic endometritis: a clinical and electron microscopic study. *Am J Obstet Gynecol* 1972;112:749–758.

76. Heinonen PK, Koivula T, Pystynen P. Elevated progesterone levels in serum and ovarian venous blood in patients with ovarian tumors. *Acta Obstet Gynecol Scand* 1985;64:649–652.

77. Varner RE, Sparks JM, Cameron CD, Roberts LL, Soong SJ. Transvaginal sonography of the endometrium in postmenopausal women. *Obstet Gynecol* 1991;78:195–199.

78. Nasri MN, Shepherd JH, Setchell MM, Lowe DG, Chard T. The role of vaginal scan in measurements of endometrial thickness in postmenopausal women. *Br J Obstet Gynaecol* 1991;98:470–475.

79. Karlsson BS, Granberg S, Wikland M, et al. Endovaginal scanning of the endometrium compared with cytology and histology in women with postmenopausal bleeding. *Gynecol Oncol* 1993;50:173–178.

80. Fleischer AC, Kalemeris GC, Mackin JE, Entman SS, James AE. Sonographic depiction of normal and abnormal endometrium with histopathologic correlation. *J Ultrasound Med* 1986;5:445–453.

81. Dijkhuizen FPHLJ, Brolmann HAM, Potters AE, Bongers MY, Heintz APM. The accuracy of transvaginal ultrasonography in the diagnosis of endometrial abnormalities. *Obstet Gynecol* 1996;87:345–349.

82. Osmers R, Volksen M, Schauer A. Vaginosonography for early detection of endometrial carcinoma? *Lancet* 1990;335:1569–1571.

83. Smith P, Bakos O, Heimer G, Ulmsten U. Transvaginal ultrasound for identifying endometrial abnormality. *Acta Obstet Gynecol Scand* 1991;70:591–694.

84. Langer RD, Pierce JJ, O'Hanlan KA, et al. Transvaginal ultrasonography compared with endometrial biopsy for the detection of endometrial disease. *N Engl J Med* 1997;337:1792–1798.

85. Holbert T. Transvaginal ultrasonographic measurement of endometrial thickness in postmenopausal women receiving estrogen replacement therapy. *Am J Obstet Gynecol* 1997;176:1334–1339.

86. Parsons A. Evaluation of postmenopausal endometrium. *Ultrasound Obstet Gynecol* 1998;12:295–300.

87. Granberg S, Wikland M, Karlsson B, Norstrom A, Friberg LG. Endometrial thickness as measured by endovaginal ultrasonography for identifying endometrial abnormality. *Am J Obstet Gynecol* 1991;164:47–52.

88. Karlsson B, Granberg S, Wikland M, et al. Transvaginal ultrasonography of the endometrium in women with postmenopausal bleeding—a Nordic multicenter study. *Am J Obstet Gynecol* 1995;172:1488–1494.

89. Smith-Bindman R, Kerlikowske K, Feldstein VA, et al. Endovaginal ultrasound to exclude endometrial cancer and other abnormalities. *JAMA* 1998;280:1510–1517.

90. Goldstein R, Srikanth R, Parsons A, et al. Effects of raloxifene on the endometrium in healthy postmenopausal women. *Ultrasound Obstet Gynecol* 1998;12[Suppl 1]:59(abst).

91. Nannini R, Chelo E, Branconi F, Tantini C, Scarselli GF. Dynamic echohysteroscopy: a new diagnostic technique in the study of female infertility. *Acta Eur Fertil* 1981;12:165–171.

92. Randolph JR, Ying YK, Maier DB, et al. Comparison of real-time ultrasonography, hysterosalpingography, and laparoscopy/hysteroscopy in the evaluation of uterine abnormalities and tubal patency. *Fertil Steril* 1986;46:828–832.

93. Van Roessel J, Wamsteker K, Exalto N. Sonographic investigation of the uterus during artificial uterine cavity distension. *J Clin Ultrasound* 1987;15:439–450.

94. Deichert U, Schlief R, Van De Sandt M, Juhnke I. Transvaginal hysterosalpingo-contrast sonography compared with conventional tubal diagnostics. *Hum Reprod* 1989;4:418–424.

95. Mitri FF, Andronikou AD, Perpinyal S, Hofmeyr GJ, Sonnendecker EWW. A clinical comparison of sonographic hydrotubation and hysterosalpingography. *Br J Obstet Gynecol* 1991;98:1031–1036.

96. Bonilla-Musoles F, Simon C, Serra V, Sampaio M, Pellier A. An assessment of hysterosalpingosonography (HSSG) as a diagnostic tool for uterine cavity defects and tubal patency. *J Clin Ultrasound* 1992;20:175–181.

97. Syrop CG, Sahakian V. Transvaginal sonographic detection of endometrial polyps with fluid contrast augmentation. *Obstet Gynecol* 1992;79:1041–1043.

98. Beyth Y, Beller U, Yarkoni S. A simple technique for visualization of the uterine cavity and its pathology during ultrasound scanning. *Isr J Med Sci* 1982;18:817.

99. Widrich T, Bradley LD, Mitchinson AR, Collin RL. Comparison of saline infusion sonography with office hysteroscopy for the evaluation of the endometrium. *Am J Obstet Gynecol* 1996;174;1327–1334.

100. Williams CD, Marshburn PB. A prospective study of transvaginal hydrosonography in the evaluation of abnormal uterine bleeding. *Am J Obstet Gynecol* 1998;179:292–298.

101. Schwarzler P, Concin H, Bosch H, et al. An evaluation of sonohysterography and diagnostic hysteroscopy for the assessment of intrauterine pathology. *Ultrasound Obstet Gynecol* 1998;11:337–342.

102. Wolman I, Jaffa AJ, Hartoov J, Bar-Am A, David MP. Sensitivity and specificity of sonohysterography for the evaluation of the uterine cavity in perimenopausal patients. *J Ultrasound Med* 1996;15:285–288.

103. O'Connell LP, Fries MH, Zeringue E, Grehm W. Triage of abnormal postmenopausal bleeding: a comparison of endometrial biopsy and transvaginal sonohysterography versus fractional curettage with hysteroscopy. *Am J Obstet Gynecol* 1998;178:956–961.

104. Dubinsky TJ, Parvey R, Gormaz G, Curtis M, Maklad N. Transvaginal hysterosonography: comparison with biopsy in the evaluation of postmenopausal bleeding. *J Ultrasound Med* 1995;14:887–893.

105. Schwayder JM. Hysterosonography as an alternative to office hysteroscopy. *J Am Assoc Gynecol Laparosc* 1995;2[Suppl 4]:S77.

106. Laughead MK, Stones LM. Clinical utility of saline solution infusion sonohysterography in a primary care obstetric-gynecologic practice. *Am J Obstet Gynecol* 1997;176:1313–1318.

107. Bernard JP, Iecuru F, Darles C, Robin F, deBievre P, Taurelle R. Saline contrast sonohysterography as a first-line investigation for women with uterine bleeding. *Ultrasound Obstet Gynecol* 1997;10:121–125.

108. Lev-Toaff AS, Toaff ME, Liu JB, Merton DA, Goldberg BB. Value of sonohysterography in the diagnosis and management of abnormal uterine bleeding. *Radiology* 1996;201:179–184.

109. Cecchini S, Ciatto S, Bonardi R, Grazzini G, Mazzota A. Endometrial ultrasonography—an alternative to invasive assessment in women with postmenopausal vaginal bleeding. *Tumori* 1996;82:38–39.

110. Weber G, Merz E, Bahlmann F, Rosch B. Evaluation of different transvaginal sonographic diagnostic parameters in women with postmenopausal bleeding. *Ultrasound Obstet Gynecol* 1998;12:265–270.

111. Weigel M, Friese K, Strittmatter H-J, Melchert F. Measuring the thickness—is that all we have to do for sonographic assessment of endometrium in postmenopausal women? *Ultrasound Obstet Gynecol* 1995;6:97–102.

112. Fleischer AC, Kalemeris GC, Entman SS. Sonographic depiction of the endometrium during normal cycles. *Ultrasound Med Biol* 1986;12:271–277.

113. Parsons AK, Lense J. sonohysterography for endometrial abnormalities: preliminary results. *J Clin Ultrasound* 1993;21:87–95.

114. Cicinelli E, Didonna T, Ambrosi G, Schonauer LM, et al. Topical anaesthesia for diagnostic hysteroscopy and endometrial biopsy in postmenopausal women: a randomised placebo-controlled double-blind study. *Br J Obstet Gynaecol* 1997;104:316–319.

115. DeVore GR, Schwartz TE, Morris J. Hysterography: a five-year follow-up in patients with endometrial carcinoma. *Obstet Gynecol* 1982;60:369–372.

116. Delisle M-F, Villeneuve M, Boulvain M. Measurement of endometrial thickness with transvaginal ultrasonography: is it reproducible? *J Ultrasound Med* 1998;17:481–484.

117. Wolman I, Amster R, Hartoov J, et al. Reproducibility of transvaginal ultrasonographic measurements of endometrial thickness in patients with postmenopausal bleeding. *Gynecol Obstet Invest* 1998;46:191–194.

118. Karlsson B, Granberg S, Ridell B, Wikland M. Endometrial thickness as measured by transvaginal sonography: interobserver variation. *Ultrasound Obstet Gynecol* 194;4:320–325.

119. Langer RD, Pierce JJ, O, Hanlan KA, et al. Transvaginal ultrasonography compared with endometrial biopsy for the detection of endometrial disease. *N Engl J Med* 1997;337:1792–1798.

120. Londono J, Jevars G, Parsons A. Ultrasound-directed endometrial biopsy in the office. *Ultrasound Obstet Gynecol* 1998;12[Suppl 1]:56(abst).

121. Brzozowski AM, Pike AC, Dauter Z, et al. Molecular basis of agonism and antagonism in the oestrogen receptor. *Nature* 1997;389:753–758.

122. Horwitz KB, Jackson TA, Bain DL, et al. Nuclear receptor coactivators and corepressors. *Mol Endocrinol* 1996;10:1167–1177.

123. Messinis IE, Nillius SJ. Comparison between tamoxifen and clomiphene for induction of ovulation. *Acta Obstet Gynecol Scand* 1982;61:377–379.

124. Fisher B, Constantino JP, Wickerham DK, et al. Tamoxifen for prevention of breast cancer: report of the National Surgical Adjuvant Breast and Bowel Project P-1 study. *J Natl Cancer Inst* 1998;90:1371–1388.

125. DiSaia PJ, Creasman WT, eds. *Clinical gynecologic oncology,* 5th ed. St. Louis: Mosby, 1997:116.
126. Kedar RP, Bourne TH, Powles TJ, et al. Effects of tamoxifen on uterus and ovaries of postmenopausal women in a randomised breast cancer prevention trial. *Lancet* 1994;343:1318–1321.
127. American College of Obstetricians and Gynecologists. ACOG Committee opinion: tamoxifen and endometrial cancer, publication no. 169. Washington, DC: American College of Obstetricians and Gynecologists, 1996.
128. Dal Cin P, Timmerman D, Van den Berghe I, et al. Genomic changes in endometrial polyps associated with tamoxifen show no evidence for its action as an external carcinogen. *Cancer Res* 1998;58:2278–2281.
129. Tepper R, Beyth Y, Altaras MM, et al. Value of sonohysterography in asymptomatic postmenopausal tamoxifen-treated patients. *Gynecol Oncol* 1997;64: 386–391.
130. Cohen I, Rosen DJ, Shapira J, Cordoba M, et al. Endometrial changes with tamoxifen: comparison between tamoxifen-treated and nontreated asymptomatic postmenopausal breast cancer patients. *Gynecol Oncol* 1994;52:185–190.
131. Lahti E, Blanco G, Kauppila A, et al. Endometrial changes in postmenopausal breast cancer patients receiving tamoxifen. *Obstet Gynecol* 1993;81:660–664.
132. Uziely B, Lewin E, Brufman G, et al. The effect of tamoxifen on the endometrium. *Breast Cancer Res Treat* 1993;26:101.
133. Dijkhuizen FP, Brolmann HA, Oddens BJ, Roumen RM, et al. Transvaginal ultrasonography and endometrial changes in postmenopausal breast cancer patients receiving tamoxifen. *Maturitas* 1996;45–50.
134. Achiron R, Lipitz S, Sivan E, Goldberg G, Mashiach S. Sonohysterography for ultrasonographic evaluation of tamoxifen-associated cysts thickened endometrium. *J Ultrasound Med* 1995:685–688.
135. Goldstein SR. Unusual sonographic appearance of the uterus in patients receiving tamoxifen. *Am J Obstet Gynecol* 1994;170:447–451.
136. Neven P, Van Belle Y, De Muylder X, Campo R, Vanderick G. The hysteroscopic assessment of women taking tamoxifen. *Acta Obstet Gynecol Scand* 1997; 76[167 Suppl 1]:13.
137. Schwartz LB, Snyder J, Horan C, Porges RF, Nachtigall LE, Goldsten SR. The use of transvaginal ultrasound and saline infusion sonohysterography for the evaluation of asymptomatic postmenopausal breast cancer patients on tamoxifen. *Ultrasound Obstet Gynecol* 1998:11:48–53.
138. Berliere M, Charles A, Galant C, Donnez J. Uterine side effects of tamoxifen: a need for systematic preteatment screening. *Obstet Gynecol* 1998;91:40–44.
139. Cohen I, Tepper R, Rosen DJ, et al. Continuous tamoxifen treatment in asymptomatic postmenopausal breast cancer patients does not cause aggravation of endometrial pathologies. *Gynecol Oncol* 1994;55:138–143.
140. Lahti E, Vuopala S, Kauppila A, et al. Maturation of vaginal and endometrial epithelium in postmenopausal breast cancer patients. *Gynecol Oncol* 1994;55:114–119.
141. Berezowsky J, Chalvardjian A, Murry M. Iatrogenic endometrial megapolyps in women with breast carcinoma. *Obstet Gynecol* 1994;84:727–730.
142. Boss SM, Huster WJ, Neild JA, et al. Effects of raloxifene hydrochloride on the endometrium of postmenopausal women. *Am J Obstet Gynecol* 1997;177: 1458–1464.
143. Delmas PD, Bjarnason NH, Mitlak BH, et al. Effects of raloxifene on bone mineral density, serum cholesterol concentrations, and uterine endometrium in postmenopausal women. *N Engl J Med* 1997;337:1641–1647.
144. Goldstein S, Srikanth R, Parsons A, et al. Effects of raloxifene on the endometrium in healthy postmenopausal women. *Ultrasound Obstet Gynecol* 1998; 12[Suppl 1]:36(abst).
145. Taylor KJW, Ramos I, Carter D, Morse SS, Snower D, Fortune K. Correlation of Doppler ultrasound tumor signals with neovascular morphologic features. *Radiology* 1988;166:57–62.
146. Folkman J, Watson J, Inger D, Hanahan D. Induction of angiogenesis during the transition from hyperplasia to neoplasia. *Nature* 1989;339:58–61.
147. Hillard TC, Bourne TH, Whitehead MI, Crayford TV, Wollins WP, Campbell S. Differential effects of transdermal estradiol and sequential progestogens on impedance to flow within the uterine arteries of postmenopausal women. *Fertil Steril* 1992;58:959–963.
148. De Ziegler D, Cedars M. Doppler: a refinement to standard transvaginal ultrasonography for the gynecologist. *Semin Reprod Endocrinol* 1992;10:34–44.
149. Scholtes MCW, Wladimiroff JW, van Rijenhjm, Hop WCJ. Uterine and ovarian glow velocity wave forms in the normal menstrual cycle: a transvaginal Doppler study. *Fertil Steril* 1989;52:981–985.
150. Kurjak A, Kupesic-Urek S, Schulman H, Salud I. Transvaginal color flow Doppler in the assessment of ovarian and uterine blood flow in infertile women. *Fertil Steril* 1991;56:870–873.
151. Bourne T, Hillard T, Whitehead MI, Crook D, Campbell S. Evidence for a rapid effect of estrogens on the arterial status of postmenopausal women. *Lancet* 1990; 1:1470–1471.
152. Jackson S, Vyas S. A double-blind, placebo controlled study of postmenopausal oestrogen replacement therapy and carotid artery pulsatility index. *Br J Obstet Gynaecol* 1998;105:408–412.
153. La Sala GB, Cantarelli M, Gaddi O, et al. Noninvasive evaluation of cardiovascular hemodynamics during multiple follicular stimulation, late luteal phase and early pregnancy. *Fertil Steril* 1989;51:796–802.
154. Vielle JC, Morton MJ, Burry K, Nameth M, Speroff L. Estradiol and hemodynamics during ovulation induction. *J Clin Endocrinol Metab* 1986;63: 721–724.
155. Bourne TH, Campbell S, Steer CV, Royston P, Whitehead MI, Collins WP. Detection of endometrial cancer by transvaginal ultrasonography with color flow imaging and blood flow analysis: a preliminary report. *Gynecol Oncol* 1991:40: 253–259.
156. Weiner Z, Beck D, Rottem S, Brandes JM, Thaler I. Uterine artery flow velocity waveforms and color flow imaging in women with perimenopausal bleeding. *Acta Obstet Gynecol Scand* 1993;72:162–166.
157. Sladkevicius P, Valentin L, Marsal K. Endometrial thickness and Doppler velocimetry of the uterine arteries as discriminators of endometrial status in women with postmenopausal bleeding: a comparative study. *Am J Obstet Gynecol* 1994;171:722–728.
158. Candiani GB, Belloni C, Maggi R, Colombo G, Frigoli A, Carinelli S. Evaluation of different surgical approaches in the treatment of endometrial cancer at FIGO stage I. *Gynecol Oncol* 1990;37:6–8.
159. Peters WA III, Andersen WA, Thornton WN Jr, Morley GW. The selective use of vaginal hysterectomy in the management of adenocarcinoma of the endometrium. *Am J Obstet Gynecol* 1983;146:285–291.
160. Hata K, Hata T, Kitao M. Intratumoral blood flow analysis in endometrial cancer: does it differ among individual tumor characteristics? *Gynecol Oncol* 1996; 61:341–344.
161. Schink JC, Rademaker AW, Miller DS, Lurain JR. Tumor size in endometrial cancer. *Cancer* 1991;67:2791–2794.
162. Lobermair A, Tempfer C, Wasicky R, Kaider A, Hefler L, Kainz C. Prognostic significance of tumor angiogenesis in endometrial cancer. *Obstet Gynecol* 1999; 93:367–371.
163. Cacciatore B, Lehtovirta P, Wahlstrom T, Ylostalo P. Preoperative sonographic evaluation of endometrial cancer. *Am J Obstet Gynecol* 1989;160:133–137.
164. Bidzinski M, Lemieszczuk B. The value of TS in the assessment of myometrial and cervical invasion in corpus uterine neoplams. *Eur J Gynecol Oncol* 1993; 14[Suppl]:86–91.
165. Sahakian V, Syrop C, Turner D. Endometrial carcinoma: transvaginal ultrasonography prediction of depth of myometrial invasion. *Gynecol Oncol* 1991;43:217–219.
166. Karisson B, Norstrom A, Granerg S, Wikland M. The use of endovaginal ultrasound to diagnose invasion of endometrial carcinoma. *Ultrasound Obstet Gynecol* 1992;2:35–39.
167. Gordon AN, Fleischer AC, Reed GW. Depth of myometrial invasion in endometrial cancer: preoperative assessment of TV ultrasonography. *Gynecol Oncol* 1990;39:321–327.
168. Shipley CF, Smith ST, Dennis EJ, Nelson GH. Evaluation of pretreatment transvaginal ultrasonography in the management of patients with endometrial carcinoma. *Am J Obstet Gynecol* 1992;167:406–412.
169. Artner A, Bosze P, Gonda G. The value of ultrasound in preoperative assessment of the myometrial and the cervical invasion in endometrial carcinoma. *Gynecol Oncol* 1994;54:147–151.
170. Weber G, Merz E, Bahlmann F, Mitze M, Weikel W, Knapstein PG. Assessment of myometrial infiltration and preoperative staging by transvaginal ultrasound in patients with endometrial carcinoma. *Ultrasound Obstet Gynecol* 1995;6: 362–367.
171. Gabrielli S, Marabini A, Bevini M, et al. Transvaginal sonography vs. hysteroscopy in the preoperative staging of endometrial carcinoma. *Ultrasound Obstet Gynecol* 1996;7:443–446.
172. Del Maschio A, Vanzulli A, Sironi S, et al. Estimating the depth of myometrial involvement by endometrial carcinoma: efficacy of transvaginal sonography vs. MR imaging. *AJR Am J Roentgenol* 1993;160:533–538.
173. Conte M, Guariglia L, Benedetti P, Scambia G, Cento R, Mancuso S. Transvaginal ultrasound evaluation of myometrial invasion in endometrial carcinoma. *Obstet Gynecol Invest* 1990;29:224–226.
174. Teefey SA, Stahl JA, Middleton WD, et al. Local staging of endometrial carcinoma: comparison of transvaginal and intraoperative sonography and gross visual inspection. *AJR Am J Roentgenol* 1996;166:547–552.
175. Hricak H, Rubinstein LV, Gherman GM, Karstaedt N. MR imaging evaluation of endometrial carcinoma: results of an NCI cooperative study. *Radiology* 1991; 179:829–832.
176. Murakami T, Kurachi H, Nakamura H, et al. Cervical invasion of endometrial carcinoma—evaluation by parasagittal MR imaging. *Acta Radiol* 1995;36: 248–253.
177. Gruboeck K, Jurkovic D, Lawton F, Savvas M, Tailor A, Campbell S. The diagnostic value of endometrial thickness and volume measurements by three-dimensional ultrasound in patients with postmenopausal bleeding. *Ultrasound Obstet Gynecol* 1996;8:272–276.
178. Bonilla-Musoles F, Raga F, Osborne NG, Blanes J, Coelho F. Three-dimensional hysterosonography for the study of endometrial tumors: comparison with conventional transvaginal sonography, HSG, hysteroscopy. *Gynecol Oncol* 1997;65: 245–252.
179. Feldman S, Berkowitz RS, Tosteson ANA. Cost-effectiveness of strategies to evaluate postmenopausal bleeding. *Obstet Gynecol* 1993;81:968–975.
180. Weber AM, Belinson JL, Bradley LD, Piedmonte MR. Vaginal ultrasonography versus endometrial biopsy in women with postmenopausal bleeding. *Am J Obstet Gynecol* 1997;177:924–929.

Treatment of the Postmenopausal Woman: Basic and Clinical Aspects, Second Edition, edited by Rogerio A. Lobo, Lippincott Williams & Wilkins, Philadelphia © 1999.

CHAPTER 48

Ovarian Screening by Ultrasound

Richard Jaffe

The ovaries are located posterior to the broad ligament and anterior to the iliac vessels. During the reproductive years, they are identified by multiple follicles or corpora lutea. The ovaries undergo significant changes during the menstrual cycle, but, on average, their volume measures 6 to 7 cm^3 during the reproductive years and is 2 to 3 cm^3 at the time of menopause.

Postmenopausal ovaries have been reported to be visualized by transvaginal ultrasonography in 64% to 81% of women (1–3). The postmenopausal ovary is small, shrunken, and inert and thus difficult to visualize or palpate. Although shrunken and inert, small cystic findings are often picked up on transvaginal ultrasound. Although authors differ on the management of these findings, most agree that single-appearing cysts less than 5 cm in diameter can be handled conservatively (4–6).

Transvaginal ultrasonography is the gold standard for evaluating normal and abnormal ovaries. The most common ultrasonographic finding is the cystic ovary, which represents a wide pathophysiologic spectrum. The most common cystic findings are follicular cysts, corpus luteum cysts, and polycystic ovaries. These cysts usually appear as thin-walled hypoechoic structures and are usually unilateral. Hemorrhage occasionally occurs with these cysts, and low-level echoes will appear on ultrasonography (Fig. 48.1). The most common benign tumors seen during the reproductive years are dermoid cysts and endometriomas (Fig. 48.2).

Most ovarian neoplasms occur at the end of reproductive age or during menopause. It is often difficult to distinguish ultrasonographically among the different tumors, as characteristics are shared by different types of tumors. The major diagnostic parameters are thickness and regularity of tumor wall, presence or abscess of septa, echogenesis of

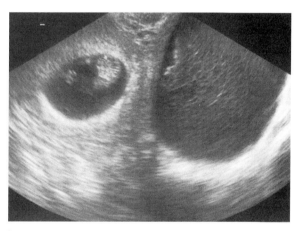

FIG. 48.1. Hemorrhagic corpus luteum in an 8-week pregnancy.

the content, and presence or absence of solid tissue or internal projections (Fig. 48.3).

Color Doppler velocimetry is now frequently used in the evaluation of adnexal masses. The rationale behind the use of Doppler velocimetry is that tumors are associated with increased angiogenesis and hypervascularity. Neovascularization in a tumor consists of pathologic and tortuous, dilated, at times saccular vessels that do not maintain the classical organization of arterioles, venules, and capillaries. These newly formed vessels lack the muscular layer. This muscular wall maintains a relatively high resistance index and pulsatility index in normal tissues. Because this regulatory function is lacking, these vessels may demonstrate a continuous high diastolic flow, a smaller difference between systolic and diastolic peaks, and a low pulsatility. Because the needs of a relatively fast-growing tumor tissue are increased, the velocity of the flow is higher. Because of the multiple arteriovenous communications, a highly vascularized area will appear on the screen. Several authors have reported on their experiences in differentiating malignant from benign tumors of the ovaries by using color

R. Jaffe: Division of Obstetric and Gynecological Ultrasound, Department of Obstetrics and Gynecology, Sloane Hospital for Women, Columbia Presbyterian Medical Center, New York, New York 10032.

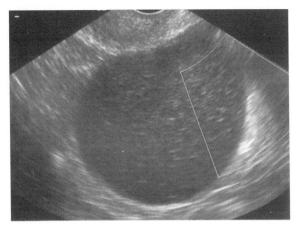

FIG. 48.2. Endometria with characteristic low-level echoes.

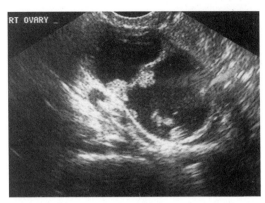

FIG. 48.4. Malignant ovarian mass demonstrating irregular walls, thick septa, and solid projections.

Doppler velocimetry and special scoring systems that can be used (2,7–10).

Malignant tumors show low resistance index (RI) and pulsatility index (PI) scores as a result of increased diastolic flow (Fig. 48.4). The flow can be detected in the center of the tumor, if tumor necrosis occurs, or adjacent to the necrotic area. Systolic velocities are somewhat higher, and there is usually absence of the diastolic notch (present in a normal arterial flow pattern between systolic and the diastolic components of the waves). Flow can also be appreciated in the septum, if such a structure exists.

Benign masses demonstrate higher impedances to flow (higher RI and PI), a more peripherally located vessel pattern, and lower maximal systolic velocities; the diastolic notch is usually present.

Data from the available literature suggest that the true-positive rate or, in other words, the percentage of malig-

nant masses with a low RI or PI is about 90% to 95% (9,11,12). The false-positive rate or the percentage of benign masses with a low RI or PI is about 2% to 5%. Negative predictive values are uniformly high, in the rage of 98%.

Ovarian cancer is the most deadly gynecologic malignancy. Poor prognosis is directly related to advanced disease at time of diagnosis. It has been proposed that screening early detection will be the only means by which survival can be improved. A review of prospective screening studies shows that ultrasound screening can detect ovarian cancer in asymptomatic women, but there was no evidence that this improves long-term survival. The major problem with ultrasound screening is that the number of cases is small, and false positives are high, with large numbers of women undergoing unnecessary surgery.

At present the use of ultrasound should be considered as promising but should be considered as one of several measures to aid in the preventative health care of women.

REFERENCES

1. Rodriguez MH, Platt LD, Medanis AL, et al. The use of transvaginal sonography for evaluation of postmenopausal ovarian size and morphology. *Am J Obstet Gynecol* 1988;159:810.
2. Sassone AM, Timor-Tritsch IE, Artuer A, et al. Transvaginal sonographic characterizated of ovarian disease and evaluation of a new scoring system to predict ovarian malignancy. *Obstet Gynecol* 1991;78:70.
3. Gollub E, Westhoff C, Timor-Tritsch IE. Transvaginal sonography in 230 healthy menopausal women. *Ultrasound Obstet Gynecol* 1993;3:422–425.
4. Goldstein SR, Subramanyan B, Snyder JR, et al. The postmenopausal cystic adnexal mass: The potential role of ultrasound in conservative management. *Obstet Gynecol* 1989;73:8–10.
5. Hall DA, McCarthy KA. The significance of the postmenopausal single adnexal cyst. *J Ultrasound Med* 1986;5:503–505.
6. Rubin MC, Preston AI. Adnexal masses in postmenopausal women. *Obstet Gynecol* 1987;70:578–581.
7. Fleischer AC, Rodgers WH, Kepple DM, et al. Color Doppler sonography of ovarian masses: A multiparameter analysis. *J Ultrasound Med* 1993;12:41.
8. Kurjak A, Predani M. New scoring system for predicting of ovarian malignancy based on transvaginal color Doppler sonography. *J Ultrasound Med* 1992;11:631.
9. Bourne T, Campbell S, Steer C, et al. Transvaginal color flow imaging: A possible new screening technique for ovarian carcinoma. *BMJ* 1989;229:1367.
10. Lerner JP, Timor-Tritsch IE, Federman A, Abramowich G. Transvaginal sonographic characterization of ovarian masses using an improved heightened system. *Am J Obstet Gynecol* 1994;170:81–85.
11. Kurjak A, Zalud I, Jurkovic D, et al. Transvaginal color Doppler for the assessment of pelvic circulation. *Acta Obstet Gynecol Scand* 1989;68:131–135.
12. Weiner Z, Thaler I, Beck D, et al. Differentiating malignant from benign ovarian tumors with transvaginal color flow imaging. *Obstet Gynecol* 1992;79:159–162.

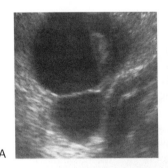 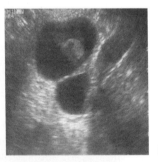

A B

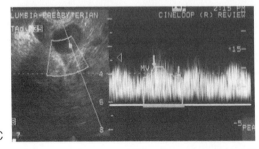

C

FIG. 48.3. Low resistance to flow demonstrated by Doppler velocimetry in a cystadenocarcinoma of ovary.

Treatment of the Postmenopausal Woman: Basic and Clinical Aspects, Second Edition, edited by Rogerio A. Lobo, Lippincott Williams & Wilkins, Philadelphia © 1999.

CHAPTER 49

Patients at High Risk for Ovarian Carcinoma

Thomas C. Randall and Stephen C. Rubin

A minority of cases of ovarian cancer occur in patients who are known to be at high risk for the disease because of a strong family history or because of a mutation in a cancer susceptibility gene. The identification and management of such patients remains highly controversial, yet the new availability of genetic testing, combined with the significant morbidity and mortality associated with ovarian cancer, have aroused great interest in these issues in the general public. Any clinician caring for women is therefore well advised to become familiar with the utility and clinical implications of this new technology.

Clinicians commonly encounter two major groups of patients who seek information about hereditary ovarian cancer. Women with ovarian cancer are often interested in determining whether they carry a mutation that would place their family members at increased risk. Women who do not have ovarian cancer often seek advice from their doctors about inherited cancer syndromes because they feel that they may be at increased risk. The current clinical value of genetic testing is still somewhat uncertain because the meaning of a positive or negative test is often unclear, and the effectiveness of subsequent interventions is unproven. Although much of the published material has focused on these uncertainties (1), genetic testing has tremendous potential to reduce the morbidity and mortality of cancer for women at risk for inherited malignancies. Here we provide a brief overview of the major causes of hereditary ovarian cancer, and we suggest a strategy for approaching patients who either perceive themselves to be at high risk for ovarian cancer or who have ovarian cancer and are interested in determining the likelihood that they carry a genetic mutation.

BACKGROUND

About 10% of cases of ovarian cancer occur in women with multiple cases of ovarian cancer, breast cancer, or

T.C. Randall, S.C. Rubin: Division of Gynecologic Oncology, Department of Obstetrics and Gynecology, University of Pennsylvania Medical Center, Philadelphia, Pennsylvania 19104.

other adenocarcinoma in their families (2). Epidemiologic studies confirmed this observation (3), and algorithms were created to estimate the risk that an unaffected individual from such a family might develop cancer. Many of these families appeared to have autosomal dominant transmission of cancer of the ovary and/or breast. It was in these families with unusually high rates of breast and ovarian cancer that linkage studies were performed that ultimately led to the identification of several genes that, when altered in the germline, confer an increased risk of ovarian cancer.

FAMILIAL OVARIAN CANCER SYNDROMES

Studies of families with multiple cases of ovarian cancer yielded the observation that such cohorts appear to belong to one of three major syndromes: the breast/ovarian cancer syndrome, the site-specific ovarian cancer syndrome, and ovarian cancer associated with the hereditary nonpolyposis colon cancer syndrome (HNPCC) or Lynch syndrome type II. Before the identification of the involved cancer susceptibility genes, estimates of cancer risk were based on epidemiologic studies. Patients with the breast/ovarian cancer syndrome or site-specific ovarian cancer were reported to have a risk of ovarian cancer related to the number of first-degree relatives with ovarian cancer; studies suggested that women with one or more first-degree relatives with breast cancer face a 50% increase in their risk of ovarian cancer, whereas women with first-degree relatives who have ovarian cancer face a 50% increased risk of developing breast cancer (4). Case-control and tumor registry-based studies have shown that having a first-degree relative with ovarian cancer confers relative risk of developing the disease of 3.6, yielding an absolute risk of about 5% (5). If two or more first-degree relatives have ovarian cancer, the estimated risk for an unaffected woman is between 7% and 50% (6).

Hereditary nonpolyposis colorectal carcinoma syndrome is a familial syndrome in which colon cancer susceptibility is inherited in an autosomal dominant pattern;

in some families this is also associated with endometrial cancers and less frequently with other adenocarcinomas, including ovarian cancer (7). The ovarian cancer risk is relatively low (about 5%) in this uncommon syndrome.

A relatively small number of women, therefore, might be identified as being at high risk for ovarian cancer based on a carefully obtained family history alone. Genetic screening for mutations in cancer susceptibility genes can improve on this risk assessment by determining which members of high-risk families are mutation carriers.

OVARIAN CANCER SUSCEPTIBILITY GENES

Genetic linkage studies were performed using microsatellite markers to track the gene loci that cosegregate with disease status within families highly affected by cancer, such as those that were used to describe the hereditary cancer syndromes. Microsatellites are repetitive oligonucleotide sequences (e.g., CACACA . . . etc.) that are found interspersed throughout the genome. These markers are often different lengths in different individuals, and a given individual's two copies of a microsatellite marker may be different, representing genetic material inherited from each parent. By amplifying microsatellite markers by PCR and separating them by gel electrophoresis, one can identify the segregation of these alleles within a family. By evaluating a large panel of such markers within a cancer-prone family, one can determine which markers sort with the disease state. Because of genetic recombination in meiosis, genetic markers will be less likely to sort with disease the further they are on a chromosome from the responsible gene; thus, statistical models have been developed to award a score that increases as the marker is increasingly associated with disease within a given pedigree. By performing extensive studies of this kind using large families with many members affected by breast and/or ovarian cancer, researchers were able to determine the location of the *BRCA1* gene on chromosome 17q21 (8), and the gene was subsequently cloned in 1994 (9). It was noted that not all families with familial breast cancer susceptibility were linked to *BRCA1*, and subsequently *BRCA2* was localized to chromosome 13q12-13 in 1994 (10) and cloned soon thereafter (11).

Genetic screening of families with hereditary breast/ovarian cancer syndrome and site-specific ovarian cancer syndrome has revealed that the majority of hereditary breast/ovarian cancer (12) and virtually all site-specific ovarian cancer (13) are linked to germline mutations in *BRCA1*. It thus appears that site-specific ovarian cancer syndrome may be a variant of hereditary breast/ovarian cancer in which breast cancer has been either not expressed or not detected. Similar linkage analyses of families with HNPCC identified the DNA mismatch repair gene *hMSH2* as responsible for a subset of families

with HNPCC (14). Because this gene was found to be a homolog of bacterial DNA mismatch repair genes, other human homologs of these genes, *hMLH1, hPMS1,* and *hPMS2,* were identified and subsequently found to be altered in affected members of some HNPCC families (15,16).

IDENTIFICATION OF PATIENTS WITH CANCER SUSCEPTIBILITY MUTATIONS

The identification and cloning of cancer susceptibility genes has generated considerable attention and interest from both the professional and lay public, even though only a small minority of cancer appears to be caused by inherited mutations in these genes. Although patients have been found to have germline mutations in one of these genes in the absence of a significant family history, no published study has convincingly shown a case of ovarian cancer caused by a somatic mutation in one of the above-mentioned genes. Thus, acquired mutations in *BRCA1, BRCA2,* or one of the mismatch repair genes do not appear to play a significant role in the development of sporadic ovarian cancers.

Because testing for a mutation is expensive and interpretation of the results is complex, it is helpful to estimate which patients have an increased chance of carrying a germline mutation. Couch and colleagues (17) screened blood samples from all patients with breast cancer who presented for evaluation at a breast cancer risk evaluation program and found that the chance of a woman with breast cancer carrying a germline mutation in *BRCA1* was increased if a patient had developed breast cancer before the age of 55, was from a family in which at least one member had ovarian cancer, was from a family in which any individual had developed both breast and ovarian cancer, or was of Ashkenazi Jewish ancestry. Although these investigators found that the proportion of women with breast cancer and a positive family history who were found to be carriers of *BRCA1* mutations was smaller (15%) than had been previously estimated (45%) (18), they also found that women with early-onset breast cancer who had family histories of both breast and ovarian cancer had very high rates of *BRCA1* germline mutations (17% to 97%), consistent with previous estimates based on families that included ovarian cancer. Neuhausen and colleagues evaluated blood samples from international investigators that were submitted to a proprietary diagnostic genetics laboratory for complementary direct sequencing of the entire coding sequences of *BRCA1* and *BRCA2* (19). They found an increased likelihood (at least 10% chance) of carrying a germline mutation in either of these genes in women who had breast cancer before age 45 and who had a family history of ovarian cancer, women who had bilateral breast cancer before age 50 and had a family history of breast or ovarian cancer, women who had ovarian cancer before age 50 regardless of family history, and Ashkenazi Jewish women who developed breast cancer before the age of 50 regardless of family history.

Neither of these two studies present population-based data, and the reader should remember that, although these data offer the potential to create algorithms to determine the potential value of genetic screening for women in various clinical situations, the ultimate decision as to whether screening is warranted is best left to the patient. Many patients who are thought to be at very high risk for carrying a genetic mutation may elect not to undergo genetic screening, and another patient who had been predicted to be quite unlikely to carry a mutation might find great satisfaction in the results of such a test. Such algorithms also appear to be flawed as applied to patients with ovarian cancer. Rubin and colleagues screened blood samples from 115 consecutive ovarian cancer patients for germline mutations in *BRCA1, BRCA2, hMSH2,* and *hMLH1* and found that a positive family history for breast and/or ovarian cancer was a poor predictor of carrying a germline mutation in one of these genes (20). Thus, family history is an imperfect indicator of a germline mutation in a cancer susceptibility gene in patients with ovarian cancer.

Only limited data exist regarding the likelihood that a women with a mutation in *BRCA1* or *BRCA2* will develop cancer of the ovary or breast. Ford and colleagues studied 33 families with breast and ovarian cancer linked to *BRCA1* and found that for women from these families who had a mutation, the risk of developing breast cancer by age 70 was 87%, and the risk of developing ovarian cancer was 44% (21). These data suggest that the penetrance of *BRCA1* is very high; that is, the presence of the genotype (a mutation) is very likely to be expressed as a phenotype (cancer). In contrast, Struewing and colleagues studied 5,087 Ashkenazi Jews from a single geographic area who volunteered to complete a questionnaire and give a blood sample for a study on cancer genetics (22). The blood specimens were screened for three specific mutations, 185delAG and 5382insC from *BRCA1,* and 6174delT from *BRCA2,* which exist at a frequency of approximately 1% in this ethnic group. Among this more population-based sample of participants, the risk that an individual with a mutation would develop breast cancer by age 70 was 56%, and the risk of ovarian cancer was 16%. Thus, it appears that the risk of developing cancer if one has a mutation may be higher for individuals from families in which there are many people affected by inherited cancers. Presumably, these patients have additional environmental or genetic exposures that make them more likely to develop cancer than women from families that do not have very high rates of breast or ovarian cancer. Cancer is a complex, multigenic phenomenon, and these data emphasize how difficult it is to determine who will develop cancer, even in the age of molecular diagnosis.

Patients seeking information about cancer susceptibility from their physicians often do so because of the occurrence of multiple cancers within a family. Often these histories are not suggestive of family cancer syndromes, and the patient can be reassured that her family history does not suggest a risk of ovarian or breast cancer that is greater than that of the general population (see Fig. 49.1). Patients with family histories that suggest an increased genetic susceptibility to cancer (Fig. 49.2) can take action based on the risk of breast or ovarian cancer that is conferred by family history alone, or they can have genetic testing. If genetic testing is chosen, two questions

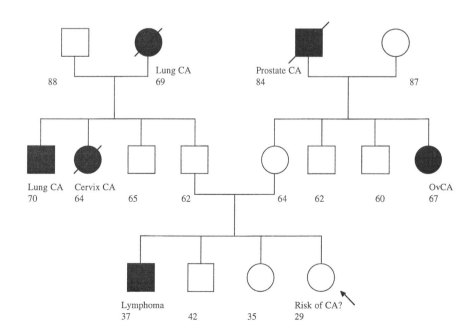

FIG. 49.1. This family cohort suggests the occurrence of multiple sporadic cancers. Because the family history does not suggest a familial cancer syndrome, the patient seeking advice regarding her need for genetic testing (arrow) can be advised that she does not appear to have a risk of developing breast or ovarian cancer greater than that of the general population.

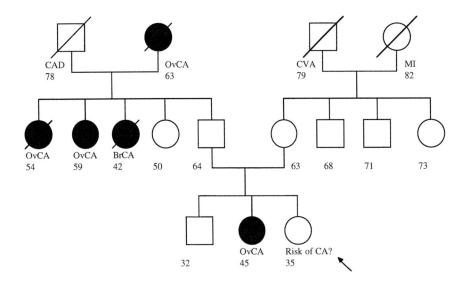

FIG. 49.2. Hereditary breast/ovarian cancer. In this family, ovarian cancer appears to be transmitted in an autosomal dominant fashion. Note that an unaffected parent, in this case the patient's father, can transmit cancer susceptibility to his offspring. Identification of *BRCA1* mutation in this family and testing of the patient seeking information (*arrow*) would help her make important decisions about cancer screening or prophylactic surgery.

must be answered: first, does the family harbor a germline mutation in a cancer susceptibility gene, and, second, does the individual in question carry the mutation? To answer these questions, a member of the family with breast or ovarian cancer must be tested. If a mutation is identified in the affected family member, then other family members who are at risk may be screened for that mutation. In high-risk populations, such as women of Ashkenazi Jewish ancestry, one should consider screening the entire sequence of *BRCA1* and *BRCA2* even if a particular mutation has been identified within a family (23).

Multiple technologies are available to screen the genes in question for mutations. These include single-strand conformational polymorphism (SSCP) analysis, the protein truncation test (PTT), conformation-sensitive gel electrophoresis (CSGE), and direct sequencing of the entire coding portions of the gene. Elaboration of the mechanics of each of these techniques is beyond the scope of this discussion, but all have imperfect sensitivity, and many geneticists estimate that even direct sequencing has a sensitivity of about 80%. Initial screening studies suggested a clustering effect in that one of the 20 most common *BRCA1* abnormalities accounted for about 70% of the mutation families evaluated worldwide, and in some ethnic groups such as Ashkenazi Jews, a small number of so-called founder mutations appear to account for the majority of mutations. As more population-based screening studies are performed, however, a greater variety of mutations are identified (24).

Given the complexity of cancer genetics and the rapid pace of clinical and molecular research, the practitioner may be well advised to refer patients interested in obtaining information regarding genetic susceptibility to cancer to an oncologist or genetic counselor with expertise in these issues. Once a patient has been to a genetic counseling and testing facility, however, she is likely to return

to her original caregiver to seek advice about any suggested treatments. Specifically, a patient with a positive test may seek advice from her gynecologist regarding risk modification interventions that might be undertaken. In general, the actions that a patient may undertake include cancer screening and prophylactic surgery.

SCREENING OF WOMEN WITH MUTATIONS

No screening modality has been identified to date that reliably detects early ovarian cancers in the general population. Large prospective trials of ultrasonography, CA125 measurements, or multimodal screening have failed to demonstrate that ovarian cancers can be detected before they have metastasized. In one study 5,500 women over age 40 had annual CA125 measurements (25). If the CA125 value was elevated, more intensive surveillance with pelvic exam, transabdominal ultrasound, and repeat CA125 measurements was undertaken. Among 165 women with elevated CA125 levels, six were found to have ovarian cancer (only two of whom had stage I disease), and three women with normal CA125 levels subsequently were found to have ovarian cancer. Similarly, a review of multiple trials of ovarian cancer screening revealed that among 36,208 women who had been screened, only 29 cases of ovarian cancer had been detected, 12 of whom had stage I disease (26). Thus, although one might expect a higher yield from screening patients with familial ovarian cancer, the data from trials studying unselected populations suggest that screening may not reliably detect ovarian cancer while it is in a curable stage.

PROPHYLACTIC OOPHORECTOMY

Prophylactic surgery to prevent cancer is warranted when patients are at high risk, and the reduction of risk is felt to justify the morbidity of the intervention. Prophylactic oophorectomy can frequently be performed as an outpatient procedure, and the intervention, unlike prophylactic mastectomy, is generally not disfiguring. For menopausal or postmenopausal patients there is minimal physiologic change. Thus, the procedure is often appropriate for patients with significant family histories of breast and/or ovarian cancer, especially those who have been shown to have germline mutations in cancer susceptibility genes.

Before deciding on prophylactic oophorectomy, the patient and her gynecologist should realize that the level of benefit of this intervention is unknown, for several reasons. As discussed earlier, the exact risk posed by having a family history, or even of having a germline mutation in BRCA1 or another cancer susceptibility gene, is still unknown. The risk of developing cancer appears to be increased in patients from families with multiple affected members, but it is difficult to anticipate what the risk will be for an individual. To complicate matters, it is unclear what risk of "ovarian-like" carcinoma persists after prophylactic oophorectomy has been performed for a germline mutation. For example, there has not been time to establish the risk of developing primary peritoneal cancer after prophylactic oophorectomy for a germline BRCA1 mutation. In a retrospective study by Tobacman and colleagues, 28 women, each of whom had two or more first-degree relatives with ovarian cancer, underwent prophylactic oophorectomy (27). After 1 to 20 years of follow-up, three of these women developed primary peritoneal cancers. In another study (28), 324 patients thought to be at high risk for ovarian cancer based on their family histories underwent prophylactic oophorectomy. After 1 to 27 years of follow-up, six of these women had developed primary peritoneal cancers. Thus, there appears to be a small but significant risk of developing primary peritoneal cancer in patients with family histories of ovarian cancer. The incidence of ovarian cancer itself in these women is expected to be elevated, but the exact magnitude of this increase is unknown, and thus, the reduction in cancer conferred by prophylactic oophorectomy is impossible to determine. Struewing and colleagues published the results of a multicenter trial in which 44 women who had undergone prophylactic oophorectomy were compared to 346 women who had not undergone prophylactic oophorectomy (29). All these women had first-degree relatives with either breast or ovarian cancer. After comparison to tumor registry data and adjustment for patient mix, there was an apparent trend toward a protective effect of prophylactic oophorectomy, but this trend was not significant. Whether this trend would become significant given more patients or longer follow-up, and what the effect would be of selecting only patients from such families who are shown to have germline mutations in BRCA1 or BRCA2, are issues that need to be addressed in further investigations.

SUMMARY

The patient who is at high risk for ovarian cancer because of a significant family history faces difficult decisions: there is no proven screening regimen that will reliably detect ovarian cancer in a curable stage, and the benefits of prophylactic oophorectomy have yet to be confirmed. These deficits notwithstanding, we recommend that women with significant family histories obtain genetic counseling and genetic screening if they feel that they would be interested in prophylactic surgery. If a mutation has been identified within a family, and the patient is found to be a carrier, then we encourage her to follow an intensified cancer screening regimen with CA125 and pelvic exams, with periodic endovaginal ultrasounds. We encourage mutation carriers to undergo prophylactic surgery at the completion of childbearing. Because many patients with germline mutations may develop ovarian cancer after the menopause, however, a considerable benefit can still be anticipated for middle-aged women who choose to undergo prophylactic surgery.

Patients who are from families with germline mutations who are shown not to carry the mutation may be reassured that they have a risk of ovarian cancer that is similar to that of the general population. Some patients are found not to have mutations but have been unable to have family members who are affected by cancer tested. Because not all familial ovarian cancer is explained by mutations in known genes, these women can not necessarily be reassured and might best be counseled according to their family history alone. Specifically, if such a patient is not shown to carry a mutation but has a strong family history for breast or ovarian cancer, we would still consider offering prophylactic oophorectomy based on the risk conferred by her family history alone. Information is limited on the meaning and utility of genetic testing for ovarian cancer and on the utility of any intervention we may take based on that information, so patients should be encouraged to undergo testing and surveillance and or prophylactic surgery under the auspices of a clinical trial.

Many women, especially those who are menopausal or postmenopausal, may only desire information or genetic screening and prophylactic surgery for the benefit of their daughters or other younger relatives. Given the current limitations in our understanding of the implications and value of genetic screening, it seems reasonable to encourage these women to defer evaluation until more information is available or to take part in a clinical trial that will help to clarify these issues.

REFERENCES

1. ASCO Subcommittee on Genetic Testing for Cancer Susceptibility. Statement of the American Society of Clinical Oncology: genetic testing for cancer susceptibility. J Clin Oncol 1996;14:1730–1736.

2. Lynch HT, Bewtra C, Wells JC, Schuelke GS, Lynch JF. Hereditary ovarian cancer: clinical and biomarker studies. In: Lynch HT, Kulander S, eds. *Cancer genetics in women*. Boca Raton: CRC Press, 1987:49–97.
3. Lynch HT, Harris RE, Guirgis HA, et al. Familial association breast/ovarian cancer. *Cancer* 1978;41:1543–1547.
4. Thompson WD, Schildkraut JM. Family history of gynecologic cancers: relationships to the development of breast cancer prior to the age of 55. *Int J Epidemiol* 1991;20:595–602.
5. Amos CI, Struewing JP. Genetic epidemiology of epithelial ovarian cancer. *Cancer* 1993;71:566–572.
6. Piver MS, Baker TR, Piedmonte M, Sandecki AM. Epidemiology and etiology of ovarian cancer. *Semin Oncol* 1991;18:177–185.
7. Watson P, Lynch HT. Extracolonic cancer in hereditary nonpolyposis colorectal cancer. *Cancer* 1993;71:677–685.
8. Hall JM, Lee MK, Newman B, et al. Linkage of early-onset familial breast cancer to chromosome 17q21. *Science* 1990;250:1684–1689.
9. Miki Y, Swensen J, Shattuck-Eidens D, et al. A strong candidate for the breast and ovarian cancer susceptibility gene *BRCA1*. *Science* 1994;266:66–71.
10. Wooster R, Neuhausen S, Mangion J, et al. Localization of a breast cancer susceptibility gene, *BRCA2,* to chromosome 13q12-13. *Science* 1994;265:2088–2090.
11. Wooster R, Bignell G, Lancaster J, et al. Identification of the breast cancer susceptibility gene *BRCA2*. *Nature* 1995;378:789–791.
12. Narod SA, Ford D, Devilee P, et al. Genetic heterogeneity in 145 breast-ovarian cancer families. *Am J Hum Genet* 1995;56:254–264.
13. Steichen-Gersdorf E, Gallion HH, Ford D, et al. Familial site-specific ovarian cancer is linked to *BRCA1* on 17q12-21. *Am J Hum Genet* 1994;55:870–875.
14. Leach FS, Nicolaides FS, Papadopoulos N, et al. Mutations of mutS homolog in hereditary nonpolyposis colon cancer. *Cell* 1994;75:1215–1225.
15. Nicolaides NC, Papadopoulos N, Liu B, et al. Mutations of two PMS homologues in hereditary non-polyposis colon cancer. *Nature* 1994;371:75–80.
16. Papadopoulos N, Nicolaides NC, Wei Y-F, et al. Mutation of a mutL homolog in hereditary colon cancer. *Science* 1994;263:1625–1629.
17. Couch FJ, DeShano ML, Blackwood MA, Calzone K, Stopfer J, Campeau L, et al. BRCA1 mutations in women attending clinics that evaluate the risk of breast cancer. *N Engl J Med* 1997;336:1409–1415.
18. Easton DF, Bishop DT, Ford D, Crockford GP. Genetic linkage analysis in familial breast and ovarian cancer: results from 214 families. *Am J Hum Genet* 1993;52:678–701.
19. Shattuck-Eidens D, Oliphant A, McClure M, et al. *BRCA1* sequence analysis in women at high risk for susceptibility mutations: risk factor analysis and implications for genetic testing. *JAMA* 1997;278:1242–1250.
20. Rubin SC, Blackwood MA, Bandera CB, et al. *BRCA1, BRCA2,* and *HNPCC* gene mutations in an unselected ovarian cancer population: relationship to family history and implications for genetic testing. *Am J Obstet Gynecol* 1998;178:670–677.
21. Ford D, Easton DF, Bishop DT, et al. Risks of cancers in *BRCA1* mutation carriers. *Lancet* 1994;343:692–695.
22. Struewing JP, Hartge P, Wacholder S, et al. The risk of cancer associated with specific mutations of *BRCA1* and *BRCA2* among Ashkenazi Jews. *N Engl J Med* 1997;336:1401–1408.
23. Randall TC, Bell KA, Chiu HC, Rebane B, Rubin SC, Boyd J. Germline mutations in *BRCA1* and *BRCA2* in a patient with breast and ovarian cancer: molecular genetic and clinical implications. *Gynecol Oncol* 1998;70:432–434.
24. Szabo CI, King MC. Population genetics of *BRCA1* and *BRCA2*. *Am J Hum Genet* 1997;60:1013–1020.
25. Einhorn N, Sjovall K, Knapp RC, et al. Prospective evaluation of serum CA125 levels for early detection of ovarian cancer. *Obstet Gynecol* 1992;80:14–18.
26. Westhoff C. Current status of screening for ovarian cancer. *Gynecol Oncol* 1994;55:S34–S39.
27. Tobacman JK, Tucker MA, Kase R, Greene MH, Costa J, Fraumeni JF. Intraabdominal carcinomatosis after prophylactic oophorectomy in ovarian-cancer-prone families. *Lancet* 1982;2:795–798.
28. Piver MS, Jishi MF, Tsukuda Y, Nava G. Primary peritoneal carcinoma afer prophylactic oohorectomy in women with a family history of ovarian cancer. *Cancer* 1993;71:2751–2755.
29. Struewing JP, Watson P, Easton DF, Ponder BAJ, Lynch HT, Tucker MA. Prophylactic oophorectomy in inherited breast/ovarian cancer families. *Monogr Natl Cancer Inst* 1995;17:33–35.

Risk-Benefit Assessment

In the final analysis, it is the woman's decision as to whether she will receive hormonal replacement in the postmenopausal years. This is particularly relevant if estrogen is being prescribed when there are no specific symptoms such as hot flashes or vulvovaginal irritation. While estrogen is clearly cost-effective as a prophylactic treatment of postmenopausal women and results in an increased longevity and quality of life, the fear of side effects may be sufficient for some women to choose not to use estrogen. Unless a woman is convinced of the need or benefits of such therapy, compliance on continuance will always be an issue. It has been found that most women only comply with hormonal therapy for the first 2 to 3 years. It is equally clear, nevertheless, that it is long-term treatment that results in the major benefits of increased longevity in postmenopausal women.

Nevertheless, when I council women on this difficult decision, I tell them that treatment should remain flexible. A decision to use hormones need not be a lifelong commitment. Alternatives and adjunctive therapies may be considered and each woman's need is different depending on her symptoms and risk factors. Using lower doses is also another option. These points and others will be found in this section on risk-benefit assessment.

In the first chapter, Annlia Paganini-Hill discusses the epidemiological evidence for the risks and benefits of hormonal therapy. We have clearly observed a reduction in all cause mortality with the use of hormones in several studies. The increase in longevity is about 1 to 3 years. Cost-benefit analysis is a difficult area of assessment. Anna Tosteson, Milton Weinstein, and Isaac Schiff beautifully handle this. They conclude that hormonal therapy is cost-effective whether looking at more favorable or less favorable scenarios. The figure of $15,000 to $25,000 per year of life saved, compares favorably with the accepted treatment of hypertension. The cost savings are probably greater in terms of quality years of life and if they factor in a reduction in cardiovascular morbidity and mortality. In the last chapter in this section, Donna Shoupe discusses contraindications to therapy. Donna's perspective is that these are extremely rare and hormonal therapy may be an option for women whom we have traditionally thought had a contraindication.

Treatment of the Postmenopausal Woman: Basic and Clinical Aspects, Second Edition, edited by Rogerio A. Lobo, Lippincott Williams & Wilkins, Philadelphia © 1999.

CHAPTER 50

Morbidity and Mortality Changes with Estrogen Replacement Therapy

Annlia Paganini-Hill

About one-third of a woman's life is now after the menopause. The lowered estrogen levels occurring during this period can produce effects on many organs of the body. To enhance their later years and to prevent or delay some chronic diseases of aging, some postmenopausal women choose to use estrogen replacement therapy (ERT). The ERT can alleviate hot flushes and night sweats, relieve vaginal atrophy, prevent bone loss and osteoporotic fractures, reduce the incidence of cardiovascular disease, and decrease mortality. However, ERT increases the risks of endometrial and breast cancers. Recent evidence suggests it may also lower risk of colorectal cancer and Alzheimer's disease.

OSTEOPOROSIS AND FRACTURES

Nearly half of the 40 million women in the United States over age 50 have osteoporosis, and 1.3 million per year endure fractures (1). Hip fractures, the most serious consequence of osteoporosis, occur in 240,000 women each year and kill 40,000. Each hip fracture costs about $21,000 for the first year of care (2).

Estrogen replacement therapy is the most effective method of retarding bone loss in postmenopausal women. The large number of controlled clinical trials that have assessed the effect of estrogen on bone density consistently showed that estrogen prevents or delays bone loss (3). In the latest findings from the Postmenopausal Estrogen/Progestin Interventions trial of 875 women, those on estrogen (with and without progestin) for 3 years averaged bone-density gains of 5.1% in their spines and 2.3% in their hips, while women on placebo lost bone density (4).

A. Paganini-Hill: Department of Preventive Medicine, University of Southern California School of Medicine, Los Angeles, California 90089.

Epidemiologic case-control and cohort studies have shown a reduction in hip and wrist fractures with ERT (3,5,6). A summary analysis of these studies found the pooled relative risk of hip fracture was 0.7 for estrogen users compared to nonusers, with risk decreasing with increasing duration of estrogen use (6). Starting estrogen within a few years of menopause appears to give more protection against fractures than starting later (7). However, hormone therapy given to women many years past menopause also beneficially affects bone (8). The limited data available suggest that combination therapy with estrogen plus progestin provides the same degree of protection against fractures as estrogen alone (7). After treatment is stopped, estrogen's effects on bone and fracture dissipate (9), suggesting the need for long-term therapy.

CARDIOVASCULAR DISEASE

Cardiovascular disease (CVD) is the leading cause of death in American women, with 365,000 deaths each year (10). Ischemic heart disease accounts for more than half of these deaths and is a leading cause of hospitalization.

Over three dozen observational studies have investigated the relationship between estrogen and CVD. Most indicate that ERT reduces CVD risk by 30% to 50% (11–14). More than 20 prospective cohort studies have found a protective effect of estrogen on myocardial infarction, ischemic heart disease, coronary heart disease (CHD), and all cardiovascular disease, both fatal and nonfatal events. A metanalysis for 16 prospective studies yielded a pooled summary relative risk for CHD of 0.70 (13). Evidence from many epidemiologic studies indicates that current estrogen users enjoy greater protection against CHD than past users; the summary relative risk for current estrogen use was 0.50 (13). The estrogen effect is observed for angiographically defined coronary artery disease as well as clinical disease (15,16). Furthermore, the lowered risk appears to be independent of other CVD risk factors.

Although many studies examined the relationship of hormone replacement therapy (HRT) and CVD risk, most looked at the effect of estrogen alone. The limited data suggest that adding progestin to the estrogen therapy will not eliminate, but may attenuate, the benefits of estrogen on CVD (13).

ENDOMETRIAL CANCER

Endometrial cancer is the fourth most common cancer in U.S. women, with an annual incidence of 34,900 cases and 6,000 deaths each year (17).

Over three dozen studies have confirmed the strong association between endometrial cancer and ERT (18). Women who have used unopposed estrogen are at greater risk of endometrial cancer than never-users. Risk increases with higher doses and longer durations of ERT and persists for several years after discontinuation of estrogen. Women using ERT for 10 years or more have nearly a tenfold increased risk. Five years or more after stopping estrogen, risk is still increased more than twofold. Thus, patients who have received ERT require careful posttreatment surveillance. Although risk of early-stage and noninvasive endometrial cancer is greater than that of late-stage invasive disease, the risks of disseminated endometrial cancer and endometrial cancer death are also increased.

The substantial increase in risk of endometrial cancer leads most physicians to add a progestin to the treatment regimen for women with an intact uterus. Although progestin can prevent the development of endometrial hyperplasia and successfully treat endometrial hyperplasia that develops in women on unopposed estrogen (19,20), the epidemiologic data on endometrial cancer and combination therapy are limited and contradictory (18).

BREAST CANCER

As the most common cancer in U.S. women, breast cancer will affect more than 10% of women in their lifetime. In 1997, 180,200 new cases developed, and 43,900 deaths from breast cancer occurred (17).

Numerous studies have reported on the association between ERT and breast cancer risk. The Collaborative Group on Hormonal Factors in Breast Cancer recently reanalyzed about 90% of the worldwide epidemiologic evidence on the association of breast cancer risk and HRT (21). Data from 51 studies conducted in 21 countries were analyzed centrally. The two main findings are based on over 53,000 postmenopausal women with a known age at menopause, of whom 33% had used HRT. First, while women are using HRT and in the 5 years after they cease use, breast cancer risk increases 2.3% with each year of use. Among women who use estrogen for 5 years or more, the relative risk is 1.35. Second, 5 years or more after ceasing use, no excess risk persists. Neither estrogen type nor dose markedly affected the results. The risk estimates also did not vary significantly between users of estrogen alone and those using estrogen with progestin. However, the cancers diagnosed in women who had used HRT were less advanced clinically than the cancers diagnosed in never-users.

Although estrogen slightly increases the risk of developing breast cancer, its effect on risk of dying from breast cancer is controversial. The American Cancer Society's Cancer Prevention Study showing a 16% decreased risk of fatal breast cancer among women who had ever used estrogen (22) supports several other investigations (23–25). However, the Nurses' Health Study reported increased mortality from breast cancer associated with estrogen use for 5 years or more (26).

MORTALITY

Prospective studies suggest that ERT users have a longer life expectancy than nonusers (25,27–31). The evidence strongly indicates that mortality is decreased 20% to 60% among ERT users. Fewer deaths from CHD and other cardiovascular disease account for most of the improved survival. The association of ERT with reduced mortality was related both to duration (25,29) and to recency of estrogen use (25,29,31).

Few studies have looked at the effect of combined estrogen-progestin therapy. Like unopposed estrogen therapy, combined therapy appears to reduce mortality as well (30,31).

COLORECTAL CANCER

Colorectal cancer is the third most common cancer in incidence among U.S. women. In 1997, 64,800 women were diagnosed with colorectal cancer, and 27,900 died of the disease (17).

Although more than two dozen epidemiologic studies have examined the relationship of ERT and colorectal cancer, results are inconsistent. A metanalysis of 14 studies found the overall relative risk from all studies to be 0.92 (95% confidence interval, CI 0.74–1.15) (32). Summary relative risks for colon cancer (based on 11 studies) and for rectal cancer (based on eight studies) separately were 1.04 (95% CI 0.80–1.53) and 0.89 (95% CI 0.46–1.74). Many of these studies were of modest size and included small numbers of women who had used ERT. More recent studies have found RRs ranging from 0.5 to 0.8, especially among current/recent users (28,33–38).

ALZHEIMER'S DISEASE

Today Alzheimer's disease (AD) affects 4.5 million Americans and claims more than 100,000 lives annually.

With no cure or means of prevention, the number of AD patients will increase to 14 million by the middle of the next century.

The year 1994 brought the first report of a significantly reduced AD risk among women who had used ERT (39). Risk was 30% lower in estrogen users compared to never users. In the next 3 years, nine studies analyzed the relationship of AD and estrogen use (40). All but one estimated the relative risk of AD to be at least 45% lower among ERT users. The strongest support for a protective effect of estrogen comes from four longitudinal studies in which information on ERT was collected prospectively before the presumptive onset of dementia symptoms (41–44). Three found a decreased AD risk among estrogen users (42–44).

Findings of a dose-response relationship would strengthen the argument for a causal relationship between ERT and reduced AD risk. Although dose-response data are sparse, one study found a significant trend of decreasing risk with increasing dose of the oral conjugated estrogen used for the longest time (42). And two (42,43) of three (42–44) found a significant trend of decreasing risk with increasing duration.

THE LEISURE WORLD COHORT STUDY

The Leisure World Cohort Study provides an opportunity to look at the effects of ERT on various disease outcomes simultaneously in a community setting.

Materials and Methods

The author and her colleagues are conducting a prospective cohort study of 13,979 residents of Leisure World Laguna Hills, a California retirement community (25,39,42,45–50). Most residents are white, moderately affluent, and well educated. In 1981 we mailed residents a health survey with detailed questions on use of estrogens during menopause (including routes of administration—oral, injectable, vaginal—and doses, duration of therapy, and years of use). For the most commonly used oral conjugated estrogen, Premarin, pill color was used to help identify the dosage(s) taken.

Questionnaires were returned by 8,877 women; 27 did not provide information on estrogen use. The remaining 8,850 women (median age 73 years) were analyzed for the effect of ERT on morbidity and mortality from several diseases.

The cohort is followed for all hospital admissions to three local hospitals and for cancer from five hospitals and from the Cancer Surveillance Programs of Los Angeles and Orange Counties. Death certificates are obtained for decedents identified from the records of the local county health department, the obituary columns of the local newspaper, annual mailings to the cohort, information provided by relatives and friends, and search of national and commercial death indices.

Duration was evaluated as the total number of years of all types of ERT, regardless of route of administration. Dose was available only for women taking oral conjugated estrogens. The reported dose is that taken for the longest time. Eighty-nine percent of estrogen users had used oral estrogen for at least part of the time, and 62% had used only this form of ERT.

Results

By December 31, 1995, 4,045 deaths had occurred among these 8,850 women, who had contributed 97,878 woman-years of follow-up. Of the 4,987 women who had used ERT, 1,984 had died, and 2,061 deaths occurred among the 3,863 nonusers. The tables show the age-adjusted relative risk (RR) estimates by estrogen use for morbidity of and mortality from several chronic diseases.

The ERT was associated with a significant reduction in mortality (Table 50.1). In this population, ever-users of ERT had nearly a 15% lower overall death rate (RR 0.87, 95% CI 0.82–0.93). Most of this reduced mortality reflected fewer deaths from cardiovascular disease (acute myocardial infarction, ischemic heart disease, and chronic forms of heart disease).

Recent use of ERT was associated with the lowest death rate. The reduction in the risk of death from all causes (RR 0.78, 95% CI 0.70–0.87) in this subgroup may be an underestimate of the actual protection afforded recent users because of changes in ERT use throughout the follow-up period. The data on estrogen use were gathered at the onset of the study—up to 14 years before death of some study participants. Individuals reporting estrogen use at the start of the study might have stopped use of ERT during the follow-up period. Similarly, women not using estrogens at enrollment may have begun taking them. This would attenuate any real association between ERT use and the diseases of interest.

Cancer deaths were less frequent in ERT users than in nonusers (RR 0.83, 95% CI 0.72–0.95). Deaths from colon cancer were particularly reduced (RR 0.72, 95% CI 0.49–1.06). In contrast, we observed no effect on mortalities from all other causes of death.

This population-based cohort study confirms that the risk of endometrial cancer increases sharply with increasing duration of ERT (p for trend < 0.0001) (Table 50.2). We found no clear effect of pill dose on risk, although 26% of Premarin users in our cohort reported using multiple pill doses. Although women who had used ERT within 1 year of completing the original questionnaire had a very high risk (RR 10, 95% CI 5.7–18), the risk remained elevated even in women who had ceased taking ERT 15 years or more earlier (RR 3.3, 95% CI 1.7–6.4).

We found no increased incidence of or mortality from breast cancer among ever-users, long-term users, or recent users of ERT in this cohort. The reduction in breast cancer mortality among current estrogen users (RR 0.60,

TABLE 50.1. *Age-adjusted relative risks and numbers of deaths for specific causes by ERT use: Leisure World Cohort, 1981–1995*

ERT use	Endometrial cancer (179,182)		Breast cancer (174)		Colon cancer (153)		All cancers (140–208)		All other causes	
	RR	No.	RR	No.	RR	No.	RR	No.	RR	No.
Estrogen use										
No	1.00	7	1.00	68	1.00	56	1.00	391	1.00	591
Yes	2.06	20	0.89	80	0.72	52	0.83[b]	421	0.95	612
Dose (mg)										
≤0.625	3.67[b]	11	0.67	18	0.62	13	0.77[a]	116	0.85	152
≥1.25	1.13	4	0.99	31	0.63	15	0.80[a]	138	1.00	195
Duration (years)										
≤3	3.12[a]	9	0.74	20	0.86	19	0.87	134	0.98	203
4–14	1.73	6	1.04	33	0.67	17	0.93	167	0.94	199
≥15	1.60	5	0.91	26	0.52[a]	12	0.68[c]	110	0.90	183
Years since last use										
≥15	3.01[a]	9	0.86	25	0.88	21	0.90	150	0.95	243
2–14	1.55	6	1.14	39	0.55[a]	15	0.82[a]	158	0.96	212
0–1	1.40	4	0.60	15	0.70	14	0.74[b]	105	0.88	131

[a]$p < 0.05$.
[b]$p < 0.01$.
[c]$p < 0.001$.

95% 0.34–1.06) is possibly a result of less extensive disease at diagnosis because of increased medical surveillance or better health awareness among women using these medications or a fundamental difference in the biologic behavior of ERT-associated cancer versus that occurring in non-ERT users.

Incidence of both colon and rectal cancer was lower in ERT users than nonusers. This reduction was even more pronounced among recent estrogen users (RR 0.70, 95% CI 0.45–1.09 for colon cancer and RR 0.52, 95% CI

0.21–1.31 for rectal cancer). Similarly, colon cancer mortality was lower in women who had used estrogen.

Estrogen replacement therapy was not consistently associated with low risk of hip fractures, even after therapy of long duration.

Using a nested-case-control study nested within our cohort, we found that estrogen users were at decreased risk of Alzheimer's disease and related dementias (42). The risk for women who had ever used estrogen was one-third below that of women who had never used estrogen

TABLE 50.2. *Age-adjusted relative risks and incidence numbers of specific cancers by ERT use: Leisure World Cohort, 1981–1995 (7.701 women with no history of cancer)*

ERT use	Endometrial cancer[a] (179,182)		Breast cancer (174)		Colon cancer (153)		Rectal cancer (154)	
	RR	No.	RR	No.	RR	No.	RR	No.
Estrogen use								
No	1.00	17	1.00	178	1.00	97	1.00	22
Yes	4.98[d]	89	0.84	204	0.82	103	0.77	25
Dose (mg)								
≤0.625	6.04[d]	36	0.76	57	0.59[b]	22	0.56	6
≥1.25	5.53[d]	29	0.86	74	0.81	34	0.64	8
Duration (years)								
≤3	2.95[c]	21	0.81	59	0.91	35	0.62	6
4–14	4.39[d]	32	0.91	78	0.71	31	0.96	12
≥15	11.4[d]	36	0.83	65	0.82	33	0.49	5
Years since last use								
≥15	3.31[c]	19	0.79	58	1.02	41	1.18	10
2–14	4.13[d]	32	0.84	77	0.72	34	0.60	8
0–1	10.2[d]	38	0.93	68	0.70	26	0.52	6

[a]Among 4,682 nonhysterectomized women with no history of cancer.
[b]$p < 0.05$.
[c]$p < 0.001$.
[d]$p < 0.0001$.

TABLE 50.3. *Age-adjusted relative risks and numbers of cases of Alzheimer's disease, senile dementia, dementia, and senility combined by ERT use: Leisure World Cohort, 1981–1995*

ERT use	No. cases	No. controls	Relative risk
Estrogen			
No	150	615	1.00
Yes	96	578	0.65[a]
Dose (mg)			
≤0.625	27	141	0.78[a]
≥1.25	21	156	0.54[a]
Duration (years)			
≤4	17	81	0.72
5–14	18	116	0.61[a]
15+	14	115	0.54[a]

[a]$p < 0.05$.
Adapted from ref. 42.

(RR 0.65, 95% CI 0.49–0.88) (Table 50.3). The risk decreased with both increasing dose (p for trend = 0.01) and increasing duration (p for trend = 0.01) of estrogen.

RISK–BENEFIT ANALYSES

Various risk–benefit analyses of ERT have been performed (51–57). These show ERT to be beneficial in terms of financial costs and overall mortality, especially for hysterectomized women and women at increased risk of heart disease. Grady et al. estimated a 1.1-year increase in life expectancy among hysterectomized women who take estrogen (54). In women with CHD, treatment with unopposed estrogen would extend life an average of 2.1 years. Col et al. found that HRT should increase the life expectancy of most women, with gains exceeding 3 years in women at greatest risk of CHD and lowest risk of breast cancer (57). Even a small reduction in risk of cardiovascular disease by ERT leads to substantial benefits in terms of morbidity, mortality, and costs because it is so common. The lifetime risk of a 50-year-old white woman dying of CHD is 31%, ten times greater than her risk of dying from either osteoporotic fracture or breast cancer (58). Henderson et al. (59) concluded that ERT would reduce mortality from cardiovascular disease in postmenopausal women by 5,350 per 100,000 per year and save 250,000 lives annually from heart attack and stroke. Hillner and his co-workers (51) estimated that if estrogens reduce fractures by 50% and cardiovascular death by 57%, then the use of ERT results in a gain of 2.61 "quality-adjusted" years. The benefits of a substantial reduction in osteoporotic fractures and cardiovascular disease are far greater than increased incidence of endometrial and breast cancers. Substantiation of the suggested decreased risks of colorectal cancer and Alzheimer's disease would tip the scale even further to the beneficial side.

WHAT'S NEXT?

All the information about these effects of ERT comes from observational epidemiologic studies. These findings do not provide conclusive evidence of efficacy because of the potential influence of selection bias, recall bias, and confounding variables. A major concern of past studies is the possible self-selection of ERT by women with other health-promoting habits and the differential interaction with the medical care system between users and nonusers (60). The possibility exists that women who use ERT are different from nonusers in some unquantified but confounding way. Women taking estrogen after the menopause are more likely to be white, educated, upper middle class, lean, and more compliant, to exercise more, have more interaction with the medical community, receive more screening tests and advice, and have lower blood pressure and fasting plasma glucose levels than nonusers, thereby being at lower risk of heart disease than women without ERT (60–62). Petitti et al. (27) observed a reduced risk of death from accidents, homicide, and suicide in ERT users, suggesting that behavioral traits and/or personality factors are associated with estrogen use. In most observational studies, no information is available on why a woman was or was not prescribed estrogen or chose to use or not to use or continue to use estrogens. It is not always possible to quantify and adjust for these factors when studying the risks and benefits of ERT. A clinical trial with random assignment of women to estrogen and placebo groups would ensure that the estrogen and not some characteristic of estrogen users accounts for the beneficial effects observed among estrogen users.

The addition of a progestin to the HRT regimen may also cause the risks and benefits to balance differently. Progestin does not impair the effect of estrogen on bone (63). No substantial epidemiologic data describe the effect of estrogen-progestin therapy on cardiovascular disease risk. However, if the estrogen-progestin combination reverses some favorable lipoprotein changes caused by ERT (64,65), this could reduce its cardiovascular protection. Combining estrogen with progestin protects against the risk of estrogen-induced endometrial hyperplasia and may reduce the risk of endometrial cancer, but conclusive evidence of an effect on endometrial cancer mortality is lacking. Whether the addition of progestin modifies the risk of breast cancer is also controversial.

It is important to continue efforts to measure the effects of various routes of administration, doses, and formulations of ERT on disease outcome, to ensure that the observed effects are not a consequence of the characteristics of estrogen users but of the estrogen itself, and to assess the effect of combined estrogen-progestin therapy on each risk and benefit.

RECOMMENDATIONS

It is difficult to determine with certainty whether the benefits of ERT (e.g., relief of menopausal symptoms, preservation of bone mass, improved lipoprotein profiles, reduced risk of CVD) outweigh its potential risks (e.g., endometrial and breast cancers) and inconvenience (e.g., vaginal bleeding, headache, weight gain, daily administration) in a specific postmenopausal woman. Individual women have different risks of various conditions depending on their risk factors for those diseases. For example, the risk of fracture for an individual correlates with her bone mass; the risk of breast cancer is associated with family history of the disease; the risk of CVD depends on lipoprotein levels and cigarette use.

It is important for women to receive counseling about the potential risks and benefits so they can make an informed decision about therapy. Decisions about the long-term use of ERT for individual patients should consider potential benefits, risks, uncertainties, and the patient's values. All women should receive information about alternatives for risk prevention (exercise, diet, smoking cessation, calcium intake, etc.). Comparing overall death rates assumes that a death from one cause is the same as a death from another cause. However, some women fear cancer more than heart disease. Some may dislike taking medications to prevent a disease that may never develop. Also, some women may be more concerned about the immediate consequences on quality of life rather than life expectancy. Ideally, the patient should make the decision after weighing the risks and benefits she finds important: "since an individual woman gains the benefits and suffers the consequences of treatment, her preferences should be respected" (66).

Whether a woman takes ERT or not should be her informed decision.

REFERENCES

1. Booher DL. Estrogen supplements in menopause. *Cleve Clin J Med* 1990;57:154–160.
2. Johnell O. The socioeconomic burden of fractures: Today and in the 21st century. *Am J Med* 1997;103(2A):20S–26S.
3. Genant HK, Baylink DJ, Gallagher JC. Estrogens in the prevention of osteoporosis in postmenopausal women. *Am J Obstet* 1989;161:1842–1846.
4. The Writing Group for the PEPI Trial. Effects of hormone therapy on bone mineral density. Results from the Postmenopausal Estrogen/Progestin Interventions (PEPI) Trial. *JAMA* 1996;276:1389–1396.
5. Lindsay R, Cosman F. Primary osteoporosis. In: Coe FL, Favus MJ, eds. *Disorders of bone and mineral metabolism*. New York: Raven Press, 1992:831–888.
6. World Health Organization. *Assessment of fracture risk and its application to screening for postmenopausal women. WHO Technical Report Series 843.* Geneva: WHO, 1994.
7. Cauley JA, Seeley DG, Ensrud K, et al. Estrogen replacement therapy and fractures in older women. Study of the Osteoporotic Fractures Research Group. *Ann Intern Med* 1995;122:9–16.
8. Lufkin EG, Wahner HW, O'Fallon WM, et al. Treatment of postmenopausal osteoporosis with transdermal estrogen. *Ann Intern Med* 1992;117:1–9.
9. Ettinger B, Grady D. The waning effect of postmenopausal estrogen therapy on osteoporosis. *N Engl J Med* 1993;329:1192–1193.
10. National Center for Health Statistics. *Vital statistics of the United States 1992. Vol II: Mortality, Part A.* Hyattsville, MD: US Department of Health and Human Services, 1996.
11. Stampfer MJ, Colditz GA. Estrogen replacement therapy and coronary artery disease: a quantitative assessment of the epidemiologic evidence. *Prev Med* 1991;20:47–63.
12. Barrett-Connor E, Bush TL. Estrogen and coronary heart disease in women. *JAMA* 1991;265:1861–1867.
13. Grodstein F, Stampfer M. The epidemiology of coronary heart disease and estrogen replacement in postmenopausal women. *Prog Cardiovasc Dis* 1995;38:199–210.
14. Bush TL. Evidence for primary and secondary prevention of coronary artery disease in women taking oestrogen replacement therapy. *Eur Heart J* 1996;17(Suppl D):9–14.
15. Sullivan JM. Coronary arteriography in estrogen-treated postmenopausal women. *Prog Cardiovasc Dis* 1995;38:211–222.
16. O'Keefe JH Jr, Kim SC, Hall RR, Cochran VC, Lawhorn SL, McCallister BD. Estrogen replacement therapy after coronary angioplasty in women. *J Am Coll Cardiol* 1997;29:1–5.
17. American Cancer Society. *Cancer facts and figures—1997.* Atlanta, GA: American Cancer Society, 1997.
18. Grady D, Gebretsadik T, Kerlikowske K, Ernster V, Petitti D. Hormone replacement therapy and endometrial cancer risk: a meta-analysis. *Obstet Gynecol* 1995;85:304–313.
19. Gelfand MM, Ferenczy A. A prospective 1-year study of estrogen and progestin in postmenopausal women: effects on the endometrium. *Obstet Gynecol* 1989;74:398–402.
20. Thom MH, White PJ, Williams RM, et al. Prevention and treatment of endometrial disease in climacteric women receiving oestrogen therapy. *Lancet* 1979;2:455–457.
21. Collaborative Group on Hormonal Factors in Breast Cancer. Breast cancer and hormone replacement therapy: Collaborative reanalysis of data from 51 epidemiological studies of 52,705 women with breast cancer and 108,411 women without breast cancer. *Lancet* 1997;350:1047–1059.
22. Willis DB, Calle EE, Miracle-McMahill HL, Heath CW Jr. Estrogen replacement therapy and risk of fatal breast cancer in a prospective cohort of postmenopausal women in the United States. *Cancer Causes Control* 1996;7:449–457.
23. Bergkvist L, Adami HO, Persson I, Hoover R, Schairer C. The risk of breast after estrogen and estrogen-progestin replacement. *N Engl J Med* 1989;321:293–297.
24. Hunt K, Vessey M, McPherson K. Mortality in a cohort of long-term users of hormone replacement therapy: an updated analysis. *Br J Obstet Gynaecol* 1990;97:1080–1086.
25. Henderson BE, Paganini-Hill A, Ross RK. Decreased mortality in users of estrogen replacement therapy. *Arch Intern Med* 1991;151:75–78.
26. Colditz GA, Hankinson SE, Hunter DJ, et al. The use of estrogens and progestins and the risk of breast cancer in postmenopausal women. *N Engl J Med* 1995;332:1589–1593.
27. Petitti DB, Perlman JA, Sidney S. Noncontraceptive estrogens and mortality: long-term follow-up of women in the Walnut Creek Study. *Obstet Gynecol* 1987;70:289–293.
28. Folsom AR, Mink PJ, Sellers TA, Hong C-P, Zheng W, Potter JD. Hormonal replacement therapy and morbidity and mortality in a prospective study of postmenopausal women. *Am J Public Health* 1995;85:1128–1132.
29. Ettinger B, Friedman GD, Bush T, Quesenberry CP Jr. Reduced mortality associated with long-term postmenopausal estrogen therapy. *Obstet Gynecol* 1996;87:6–12.
30. Schairer C, Adami H-O, Hoover R, Persson I. Cause-specific mortality in women receiving hormone replacement therapy. *Epidemiology* 1997;8:59–65.
31. Grodstein F, Stampfer MJ, Colditz GA, et al. Postmenopausal hormone therapy and mortality. *N Engl J Med* 1997;336:1769–1775.
32. MacLennan SC, MacLennan AH, Ryan P. Colorectal cancer and oestrogen replacement therapy. A meta-analysis of epidemiologic studies. *Med J Aust* 1995;162:491–493.
33. Calle EE, Miracle-McMahill HL, Thun MJ, Heath CW Jr. Estrogen replacement therapy and risk of fatal colon cancer in a prospective cohort of postmenopausal women. *J Natl Cancer Inst* 1995;87:517–523.
34. Newcomb PA, Storer BE. Postmenopausal hormone use and risk of large-bowel cancer. *J Natl Cancer Inst* 1995;87:1067–1071.
35. Persson I, Yuen J, Bergkvist L, Schairer C. Cancer incidence and mortality in women receiving estrogen and estrogen-progestin replacement therapy—long-term follow-up of a Swedish cohort. *Int J Cancer* 1996;67:327–332.
36. Grodstein F, Martinez ME, Giovannucci EL, et al. Postmenopausal hormone use and colorectal cancer in the Nurses' Health Study. *Am J Epidemiol* 1996;143(Suppl):S63.
37. Troisi R, Schairer C, Chow W-H, Schatzkin A, Brinton LA, Fraumeni JF Jr. A prospective study of menopausal hormones and risk of colorectal cancer (United States). *Cancer Causes Control* 1997;8:130–138.
38. Kampman E, Potter JD, Slattery ML, Caan BJ, Edwards S. Hormone replacement therapy, reproductive history, and colon cancer: a multicenter, case-control study in the United States. *Cancer Causes Control* 1997;8:146–158.
39. Paganini-Hill A, Henderson VW. Estrogen deficiency and risk of Alzheimer's disease in women. *Am J Epidemiol* 1994;140:256–261.
40. Paganini-Hill A. Alzheimer's disease in women. Can estrogen play a preventive role? *Female Patient* (in press).
41. Brenner DE, Kukull WA, Stergachis A, et al. Postmenopausal estrogen replacement therapy and the risk of Alzheimer's disease: A population-based case-control study. *Am J Epidemiol* 1994;140:262–267.

42. Paganini-Hill A, Henderson VW. Estrogen replacement therapy and risk of Alzheimer's disease. *Arch Intern Med* 1996;156:2213–2217.
43. Tang M-X, Jacobs D, Stern Y, et al. Effect of oestrogen during menopause on risk and age at onset of Alzheimer's disease. *Lancet* 1996;348:429–432.
44. Kawas C, Resnick S, Morrison A, et al. A prospective study of estrogen replacement therapy and the risk of developing Alzheimer's disease: The Baltimore Longitudinal Study of Aging. *Neurology* 1997;48:1517–1521.
45. Paganini-Hill A, Ross RK, Henderson BE. Prevalence of chronic disease and health practices in a retirement community. *J Chron Dis* 1986;39:699.
46. Paganini-Hill A, Ross RK, Henderson BE. Postmenopausal oestrogen treatment and stroke: a prospective study. *BMJ* 1988;297:519–522.
47. Henderson BE, Paganini-Hill A, Ross RK. Estrogen replacement therapy and protection from acute myocardial infarction. *Am J Obstet Gynecol* 1988;159:312–317.
48. Paganini-Hill A, Ross RK, Henderson BE. Endometrial cancer and patterns of use of oestrogen replacement therapy: a cohort study. *Br J Cancer* 1989;59:445–447.
49. Paganini-Hill A, Chao A, Ross RK, Henderson BE. Exercise and other factors in the prevention of hip fracture: the Leisure World Study. *Epidemiology* 1991;2:16–25.
50. Paganini-Hill A. The benefits of estrogen replacement therapy on oral health: the Leisure World Cohort. *Arch Intern Med* 1995;155:2325–2329.
51. Hillner BE, Hollenberg JP, Pauker SG. Postmenopausal estrogens in the prevention of osteoporosis. Benefit virtually without risk if cardiovascular effects are considered. *Am J Med* 1986;80:1115–1127.
52. Miller AB. Risk/benefit considerations of antiestrogen/estrogen therapy in healthy postmenopausal women. *Prev Med* 1991;20:79–85.
53. Cheung AP, Wren BG. A cost-effectiveness analysis of hormone replacement therapy in the menopause. *Med J Aust* 1992;156:312–316.
54. Grady D, Rubin SM, Petitti DB, et al. A cost-effectiveness analysis of hormone replacement therapy in the menopause. *Ann Intern Med* 1992;117:1016–1037.
55. Daly E, Vessey MP, Barlow D, Gray A, McPherson K, Roche M. Hormone replacement therapy in a risk–benefit perspective. *Maturitas* 1996;23:247–259.
56. Zubialde JP, Lawler F, Clemenson N. Estimated gains in life expectancy with use of postmenopausal estrogen therapy: a decision analysis. *J Fam Pract* 1993;36:271–280.
57. Col NF, Eckman MH, Karas RH, et al. Patient-specific decisions about hormone replacement therapy in postmenopausal women. *JAMA* 1997;277:1140–1147.
58. Cummings SR, Black DM, Rubin SM. Lifetime risks of hip, Colles', or vertebral fracture and coronary heart disease among white postmenopausal women. *Arch Intern Med* 1989;149:2445–2448.
59. Henderson BE, Ross RK, Paganini-Hill A, Mack TM. Estrogen use and cardiovascular disease. *Am J Obstet Gynecol* 1986;154:1181–1186.
60. Barrett-Connor E. Postmenopausal estrogen and prevention bias. *Ann Intern Med* 1991;115:455–456.
61. Barrett-Connor E, Wingard DL, Criqui MH. Postmenopausal estrogen use and heart disease risk factors in the 1980s. *JAMA* 1989;261:2095–2100.
62. Cauley JA, Cummings SR, Black DM, Mascioli SR, Seeley DG. Prevalence and determinants of estrogen replacement therapy in elderly women. *Am J Obstet Gynecol* 1990;163:1438–1444.
63. Gallagher JC, Kable WT, Goldgar D. Effect of progestin therapy on cortical and trabecular bone: comparison with estrogen. *Am J Med* 1991;90:171–178.
64. Tikkanen MJ, Kuusi T, Nikkilä EA, Sipinen S. Post-menopausal hormone replacement therapy: effects of progestogens on serum lipids and lipoproteins. A review. *Maturitas* 1986;8:7–17.
65. Sherwin BB, Gelfand MM. A prospective one-year study of estrogen and progestin in postmenopausal women: effects on clinical symptoms and lipoprotein lipids. *Obstet Gynecol* 1989;73:759–766.
66. Cummings SR. Evaluating the benefits and risks of postmenopausal hormone therapy. *Am J Med* 1991;91(Suppl 5B):14S–18S.

Treatment of the Postmenopausal Woman: Basic and Clinical Aspects, Second Edition, edited by Rogerio A. Lobo, Lippincott Williams & Wilkins, Philadelphia © 1999.

CHAPTER 51

Cost-Effectiveness Analysis of Hormone Replacement Therapy

Anna N. A. Tosteson, Milton C. Weinstein, and Isaac Schiff

In the United States alone, it is estimated that by the year 2005 there will be 25.3 million women between the ages of 50 and 64 who would be potentially eligible for hormone replacement therapy (1). The estimated cost of treating these women with hormone replacement therapy, considering only the cost of the drugs and monitoring, is $5 billion per year (2). In a society of limited resources, it is imperative that the net cost of hormone replacement therapy be weighed in relation to its net impact on health outcome. Cost-effectiveness analysis (3), which considers the costs, risks, and benefits of health interventions jointly, provides an ideal framework for the economic evaluation of hormone replacement therapy. By combining clinical, epidemiologic, and economic data, cost-effectiveness analysis attempts to answer the question: Is the additional benefit of alternate health interventions worth the additional cost? In this chapter, we address this question by reviewing the literature and updating existing estimates of the cost-effectiveness of hormone replacement therapy in the menopause.

ESTIMATED IMPACT OF HORMONE REPLACEMENT THERAPY ON HEALTH

The multifaceted effects of hormone replacement therapy include its impact on symptoms of the menopause, endometrial cancer, breast cancer, heart disease, and

osteoporosis. Accounting for the occurrence of these risks and benefits is a complex undertaking. To understand the impact of the relative risks of hip fracture, coronary heart disease, breast cancer, and endometrial cancer that are associated with hormone replacement therapy on overall health, one must consider the absolute risks of these events (4). Cummings et al. (5) estimated lifetime risks of mortality from hip fracture and coronary heart disease for 50-year-old white perimenopausal women as 2.8% and 31%, respectively. Lifetime risks of mortality from breast cancer and endometrial cancer have been estimated as 2.8% and 0.7%, respectively (6). These figures are useful to keep in mind when considering the cost-effectiveness evaluation.

Recent epidemiologic studies have reported a reduction in overall mortality for women using hormone replacement therapy relative to nonusers (7–9). Since 1980 there have been many published reports that have estimated the impact of hormone replacement therapy on overall health as measured by changes in event rates or changes in overall life expectancy using decision-analytic models (10). We review selected reports (Table 51.1) before describing the components of cost-effectiveness evaluation in detail and presenting revised estimates of cost-effectiveness.

Weinstein (11) first considered the impact of unopposed estrogen replacement therapy in a population of postmenopausal women by including the risks of endometrial hyperplasia and cancer, hip and wrist fractures, and gallbladder disease as well as effects on menopausal symptoms. A small net change in life expectancy was reported for women who were age 50 at initiation of unopposed estrogen, ranging from 0.04 to 0.06 years for 10- and 15-year treatment durations, respectively. Effects on quality of life were found to be potentially decisive, when measured in terms of quality-adjusted life years

A. N. A. Tosteson: Departments of Medicine and Community and Family Medicine, Dartmouth Medical School, Lebanon, New Hampshire 03756.
M. C. Weinstein: Department of Health Policy and Management, Harvard School of Public Health, Boston, Massachusetts 02115.
I. Schiff: Department of Obstetrics and Gynecology, Harvard Medical School, Boston, Massachusetts 02114.

TABLE 51.1. *Studies that have estimated the impact of hormone replacement therapy on overall health*

Authors	Year of publication	Unopposed estrogen	Combined therapy	Symptoms considered?	Patient ages	Duration (years)	Breast cancer	Fracture	Heart disease	Endo Ca	Other risks	Endpoints
Weinstein (11)	1980	Yes	No	Yes	50, 55	10, 15	No	Hip/wrist	No	Yes	Yes	Cost, LE, QALY
Weinstein and Schiff (12)	1982	Yes	Yes	Yes	50	5, 10, 15	Yes	Hip/wrist	No	Yes	No	Cost, LE, QALY
Henderson et al. (13)	1988	Yes	Yes	No	65–74	10	Yes	Hip	Yes	Yes	No	Mortality/100,000
Weinstein and Tosteson (2)	1990	Yes	Yes	Yes	50	5, 15	Yes	Hip	No	Yes	No	Cost, LE, QALY
Tosteson et al. (14)	1990	No	Yes	No	50	5, 10, 15, Life	Yes	Hip	Yes	No	No	Cost, LE, QALY
Tosteson and Weinstein (15)	1991	Yes	Yes	Yes	50	10, 15	Yes	Hip	Yes	No	No	Cost, LE, QALY
Cheung and Wren (16)	1992	Yes	Yes	Yes	50	5, 10, 15	Yes	Hip/wrist	Yes	Yes	No	Cost, LE, QALY
Grady et al. (17)	1992	Yes	Yes	No	50	Long-term	Yes	Hip	Yes	Yes	Yes	LE
Col et al. (18)	1997	Yes	Yes	No	50	Long-term	Yes	Hip	Yes	No	No	LE

(QALY). Later, this work was augmented and updated to consider treatment with estrogen combined with progestins (2,12). In regard to the impact of treatment on endometrial cancer and hyperplasia, fractures of the wrist and hip, and breast cancer, small net increases in life expectancy were reported only for women receiving long-term combined therapy.

Henderson et al. (13) considered 10-year durations of unopposed estrogen and combined estrogen-progestin therapy in 65- to 74-year old women and estimated the change in mortality per 100,000 for women receiving these treatments relative to women receiving no intervention. Effects of ischemic heart disease mortality were included. Under their assumptions, a reduction in mortality of 230/100,000 was estimated for women receiving unopposed estrogen who had not had a hysterectomy. For women who had a previous hysterectomy, a greater reduction in mortality (256/100,000) was predicted. For estrogen combined with progestin, a reduction in mortality of 163/100,000 was projected. The differences between projected outcomes with unopposed estrogen and with combined therapy resulted primarily from the greater reduction in ischemic heart disease mortality that was assumed for unopposed estrogen (48% vs. 31% for combined therapy).

Tosteson et al. (14) considered the use of combined therapy in postmenopausal asymptomatic women who had not had a previous hysterectomy. In addition to universal estrogen-progestin therapy at menopause, selective treatment strategies involving an initial bone density measurement were evaluated. This analysis, which considered hip fracture risk, also showed a modest increase in life expectancy. An update of this work (15) included assumptions regarding breast cancer and ischemic heart disease mortality and estimated net increases in life expectancy both for unopposed estrogen in women with a uterus and for combined therapy in women with a previous hysterectomy that ranged from 0.13 to 0.24 years for 10- and 15-year treatment durations, respectively.

Using Australian data combined with data from the epidemiologic literature, Cheung and Wren (16) evaluated both unopposed and combined therapies in symptomatic and asymptomatic women. Their risk–benefit analysis assumed relative risks for hip and wrist fractures, endometrial cancer, and breast cancer that were identical to those of Weinstein and Schiff and also included risk of mortality from myocardial infarction. Although undiscounted life expectancies were not reported, changes in life expectancy were consistent with previous reports.

Grady et al. assessed the impact of hormone replacement therapy on life expectancy (17) and provided estimates of the impact of therapies on average asymptomatic postmenopausal women and on postmenopausal women at risk for heart disease, breast cancer, and osteoporosis under a variety of assumptions. Meta-analytic techniques were used to estimate the relative risks and

benefits of hormone replacement therapy, but costs and quality of life were not considered. A gain in life expectancy of 0.9 year was estimated for women receiving unopposed estrogen, and a gain of 1.0 year for women receiving combined therapy under the assumption that the only difference between unopposed and combined therapies is to eliminate the increased risk of endometrial cancer. When progestin was assumed to also reduce the coronary heart disease benefit by 66% and to increase the risk of breast cancer by twofold, the overall difference in life expectancy relative to no intervention was reduced to 0.1 years. These gains in projected life expectancy are larger than those estimated in previous studies, because it was assumed that women taking long-term hormone replacement therapy would have a decreased risk of coronary heart disease death for the remainder of their lives. Relative to the estimates reported (above) for the average 50 year old women, women at risk for coronary heart disease were estimated to have larger gains in life expectancy and women at risk for breast cancer were estimated to have smaller gains in life expectancy.

More recently, Col et al. (18) evaluated the net impact of long-term hormone replacement therapy use on life expectancy for 50-year-old cohorts of women at various underlying risks of breast cancer, coronary heart disease, and hip fracture. Most women were projected to have longer life expectancy with hormone replacement therapy use; however, the minority of women without any risk factors for coronary heart disease or hip fracture who had two first-degree relatives with breast cancer would be harmed by hormone replacement therapy. This study did not address the potential benefits (i.e., relief of menopausal symptoms) or harms (i.e., treatment side effects) of hormone replacement therapy on quality of life.

In addition to the risk–benefit estimates, each of the cost-effectiveness analyses have estimated the net change in cost associated with hormone replacement therapy. Each highlighted circumstances in which hormone replacement therapy in the menopause is reasonably cost-effective in comparison to other accepted medical practices. In the sections that follow we define each component of the risk–benefit equation and make updated estimates of cost-effectiveness based on current evidence. First, however, we describe the clinical management strategies that we will evaluate.

CLINICAL STRATEGIES FOR EVALUATION

We consider the clinical management of two groups of patients who are assumed to be age 50 at the time of menopause. First, for women who have had a previous hysterectomy, we evaluate 10- and 15-year courses of unopposed estrogen beginning at menopause such as 0.625 mg conjugated equine estrogen taken daily. Second, for women with a uterus, we evaluate 10- and 15-year courses of estrogen combined with progestin, such as

0.625 mg of conjugated equine estrogen given daily through the month with 5 to 10 mg of medroxyprogesterone acetate given on days 1 through 13 of the month, or combined continuous regimens of 0.625 mg of conjugated equine estrogens and medroxyprogesterone acetate, 2.5 mg daily. Progestins are added to offset the increase in endometrial hyperplasia and endometrial cancer that has been associated with unopposed estrogen (19,20). Although the routine use of hormone replacement in the menopause has not been advocated (21), the clinical treatments evaluated here represent common clinical practice (22).

COST-EFFECTIVENESS ENDPOINTS

Net Effectiveness

For each strategy, net effectiveness is measured as the change in life expectancy (ΔLE) or in quality-adjusted life expectancy ($\Delta QALE$) for patients treated with hormone replacement therapy compared to patients who receive no treatment. The components of change in life expectancy are associated with breast cancer, coronary heart disease, and osteoporotic fractures of the hip and are denoted as $\pm\Delta LE_{BRCA}$, $\pm\Delta LE_{CHD}$, and $\pm\Delta LE_{HIP}$, respectively. For quality-adjusted life expectancy, components of quality are associated with morbidity from the hip fracture, symptom relief, and side effects associated with treatment, which are denoted as $\pm\Delta Q_{HIP}$, $\pm\Delta Q_{SYMPT}$, and $\pm\Delta Q_{SIDE}$, respectively.

Net Cost

For each strategy, net resource cost is measured as the change in average direct medical cost (ΔC) for patients treated with hormone replacement therapy compared to patients who receive no treatment. Components of change in net resource cost are associated with hormone replacement therapy, long-term nursing home care, breast cancer, hip fracture, and coronary heart disease and are denoted as $\pm\Delta C_{HRT}$, $\pm\Delta C_{NH}$, $\pm\Delta C_{BRCA}$, $\pm\Delta C_{HIP}$, $\pm\Delta C_{CHD}$, respectively. Estimates of direct medical cost are made from the societal perspective, and all costs are represented in 1992 U.S. dollars.

Cost-Effectiveness Ratio

Incremental cost-effectiveness ratios are used to compare the ratio of additional cost to additional health benefit when hormone replacement therapy is compared with the option of no intervention. For analyses that assess additional cost per additional year of life saved, the ratio is defined as:

$$\frac{\Delta C}{\Delta LE} = \frac{\pm \Delta C_{HRT} \pm \Delta C_{HIP} \pm \Delta C_{NH} \pm \Delta C_{BRCA} \pm \Delta C_{CHD}}{\pm \Delta LE_{HIP} \pm \Delta LE_{BRCA} \pm \Delta LE_{CHD}}$$

For analyses that include quality-of-life considerations, the cost-effectiveness ratio is defined as:

$$\frac{\Delta C}{\Delta QLE} = \frac{\pm \Delta C_{HRT} \pm \Delta C_{HIP} \pm \Delta C_{NH} \pm \Delta C_{BRCA} \pm \Delta C_{CHD}}{\pm \Delta LE_{HIP} \pm \Delta LE_{BRCA} \pm \Delta LE_{CHD} \pm \\ \Delta Q_{HIP} \pm \Delta Q_{SYMPT} \pm \Delta Q_{SIDE}}$$

When included in the cost-effectiveness ratio, all components of net change in life expectancy and cost are discounted at a rate of 5% per year. This accounts for the differential timing of events and has the effect of weighing near-term costs and health effects more heavily in the cost-effectiveness equation.

DECISION-ANALYTIC MODEL

To assess the lifetime impact of the hormone replacement therapy regimens described above on each component in the cost-effectiveness equation, we used a previously described Markov state-transition model (14) with modified assumptions about the relative risks associated with treatment. This model follows a cohort of women who are initially well at age 50 until death or age 99 and keeps track of the annual incidence of hip fracture and associated sequelae, placement in a nursing home, coronary heart disease death, and death from other causes. Breast cancer and coronary heart disease costs were not included as endpoints in the Markov state-transition model. Therefore, a separate analysis estimates the impact that hormone replacement therapy has on breast cancer incidence, and impact on the cost of heart disease is not evaluated.

DATA AND ASSUMPTIONS

In this section, we review the impact that clinical strategies of treating women at menopause with 10- or 15-year courses of hormone replacement therapy have on each component of the cost-effectiveness equation. To estimate the cost-effectiveness of hormone replacement therapy under optimal conditions, we assume 100% compliance with prescribed therapy, recognizing that this is an optimistic assumption (23). The annual cost of therapy, including the drug, physician visits, and monitoring, is estimated at $263 for unopposed estrogen and $340 for combined therapy. Two quality weights, which represented the proportion of a year of life in perfect health that a women would be willing to trade for a year in her current state of health, were used to estimate the impact that alleviation of symptoms of the menopause and side effects of treatment have on overall quality-adjusted life expectancy. A weight of 0.99 (−3 days per year) was given to women who were adversely affected by the symptoms of menopause, and a weight of 0.997 (−1 day per year) was given to women who were adversely affected by combined estrogen-progestin therapy.

Osteoporosis and Sequelae

Osteoporosis is common among postmenopausal women, and the complications of osteoporosis frequently include fractures of the wrist, vertebrae, and hip (24). Here, we focus on the impact that hormone replacement therapy has on the incidence of hip fracture. Hip fractures are the most dramatic of the common osteoporotic fractures and are associated with significant morbidity, mortality, and cost (25).

The Markov state-transition model keeps track of the bone mineral density distribution of women entering the model at age 50. The initial bone mineral density distribution used in the model is the average of the intertrochanteric and cervical regions of the femur for 45- to 54-year-old women in Rochester, Minnesota (26). As the cohort ages, bone mineral densities are updated based on age-related rates of loss reported for the same population (27). Thus, annual probabilities of hip fracture are estimated as a function of initial bone mineral density and age.

Epidemiologic data show that age-related bone loss is stopped or slowed (28,29) in women receiving hormone replacement therapy. We assumed that the age-related loss of bone mineral density stops with treatment and resumes and continues as it would have at menopause when treatment is terminated. These assumptions were shown by Tosteson et al. (14) to be consistent with the relative risks associated with long-term estrogen exposure as reported in epidemiologic studies (30,31).

An increase in mortality following hip fracture, which increases with age and with increasing comorbidity, has been reported by several investigators (32–38). The Markov state-transition model (14) assumed that 50% of the mortality observed in the Rochester, Minnesota cohort in the year following hip fracture was related to the hip fracture. Thus, the probability of death from hip fracture was 0.06 for women aged 50 to 59 and 70 to 79 years, 0.03 for women aged 60 to 69 years, and 0.11 for women age 80 years or more.

Persons who survive the hip fracture may require long-term placement in a nursing home. The rate of nursing home placement was estimated from the 1984 National Hospital Discharge Survey with adjustment for patients who were discharged from the nursing home within 1 year of admission. The probability of remaining in a nursing home at 1 year following hip fracture ranged from 0 for women aged 50 to 59 years to 0.30 for women age 85 years or older. In analyses that considered quality of life, it was assumed that women would become disabled at the same rate that they entered the nursing home for long-term care following hip fracture (39).

Quality weights for hip fracture and its sequelae were taken from a study by Hillner et al. (38,39). The quality weights in the year the fracture occurred, which reflected acute morbidity for an uncomplicated hip fracture, a disabling hip fracture, and a fracture requiring long-term nursing home placement, were 0.95, 0.76, and 0.36, respectively. The quality weights associated with long-term disability or nursing home placement were 0.8 and 0.4, respectively.

Costs for the acute care of the hip fracture ranged from $17,440 among 50- to 59-year-old women to $20,590 among women age 80 years and older. The details of these cost estimates, which have been updated to 1992 dollars, are given elsewhere (14).

Breast Cancer

The association between postmenopausal estrogen use and breast cancer has been addressed by many conflicting epidemiologic studies and was the subject of two recent meta-analyses (17,40). An analysis that combined dose-response slopes and reported relative risks of breast cancer by duration of treatment showed no increased relative risk of breast cancer after 5 years of use but a relative risk of 1.3 (CI 1.2–1.6) after 15 years of use (40). A more recent analysis, which included additional cohort studies, estimated a relative risk of breast cancer among women who used estrogens for 8 years or more compared with nonusers of 1.25 (CI 1.04–1.51) (17). Based on these data, we assumed a relative risk of 1.25 for women treated with unopposed estrogen for 10 years and assume that this increased risk applies from year 5 of treatment to 2 years past termination of therapy (41). For 15-year treatment durations, a relative risk of 1.25 is assumed for years 5 to 10 of treatment, and a relative risk of 1.3 is assumed for years 11 to 15, with the risk returning to 1.25 for 2 years following termination of therapy.

The literature on the risk of breast cancer and combined estrogen-progestin therapy is sparse and conflicting (17). Therefore, analyses are completed for combined therapy under two alternate assumption sets. Under the favorable scenario, combined estrogen-progestin therapy is assumed to have no impact on breast cancer risk. Under the unfavorable scenario, combined therapy is assumed to increase the risk of breast cancer by 50%, based on biologically plausible hypotheses that progestin may increase breast cancer risk (42).

The estimated cost of an incident case of breast cancer, which did not include the cost of terminal care, was based on Medicare data and reflected a charge of $10,850 for noninvasive breast cancers (43). Quality-of-life adjustments were not made for breast cancer. All other assumptions are described in detail elsewhere (12).

Coronary Heart Disease

Findings of epidemiologic studies have consistently shown that women receiving estrogen replacement therapy are at lower risk of coronary heart disease than nonusers. Two recent meta-analyses evaluated the association between unopposed estrogen and heart disease (17,44). One meta-analysis reported a relative risk of 0.50 (CI 0.43–0.56) for women who had ever used estrogen compared with nonusers when internally controlled cohort studies and cross-sectional angiography studies were summarized (44). Another study reported a summary relative risk of coronary heart disease mortality of 0.63 (95% CI 0.55–0.72) for ever users of estrogen compared with nonusers (17). Because our model addresses death from coronary heart disease rather than coronary heart disease incidence, we have used a relative risk of 0.63 for women receiving unopposed estrogen and assumed that this benefit applies for the duration of treatment. Annual probability of death from heart disease was derived from U.S. life tables (45).

The data on estrogen combined with progestin and coronary heart disease risk are limited. Preliminary data from a European study have shown that women receiving estrogen and norgestrel have a relative risk of coronary heart disease of 0.53 compared with nonusers (46). This, combined with studies that suggest that the mechanism of benefit provided by estrogen goes beyond estrogen's favorable impact on lipoproteins (47–49), which are dampened by progestins (50,51), indicate that combined regimens may also offer cardioprotective benefits. Here, we assume that under the favorable scenario, combined estrogen-progestin therapy reduces the incidence of coronary heart disease mortality by 37%. Under the unfavorable scenario, combined therapy is assumed to reduce the incidence of coronary heart disease mortality by only 20%.

No quality-of-life adjustments are made for coronary heart disease. An Australian study (16) estimated the average savings per patient treated that would result if hormone replacement therapy decreased risk of death from myocardial infarction by 50% in users as $67 and $110 (converted to 1992 U.S. dollars) for 10- and 15-year treatment durations, respectively. Because these figures reflect the Australian health care system, they are not readily translated into U.S. dollars. To adequately assess the impact of coronary heart disease on net cost, a model of incident coronary heart disease and associated costs is required. Thus, savings associated with decreases in coronary heart disease are not included.

Nursing Home Placement and Death from Other Causes

Annual probability of long-term placement in a nursing home for causes other than hip fracture was estimated from the literature (52). Average nursing home costs were updated to 1992 dollars and were based on the daily rate published for skilled nursing homes (53). The annual cost was estimated at approximately $37,000. U.S. lifetables were used to estimate annual probabilities of death from other causes (45).

IMPACT ON HEALTH

Life Expectancy

All strategies were found to extend life from 0.06 to 0.24 years (Table 51.2). The largest projected increase in life years was for women with a uterus who received estrogen combined with progestin for 15 years under the favorable assumption that combined therapy did not increase risk of breast cancer and decreased risk of coronary heart disease death by 37%.

Quality-Adjusted Life Expectancy

When quality of life was considered, all strategies resulted in a net increase in life expectancy. On average, side effects associated with combined therapy, which reduced overall quality of life by 1 day per year, were estimated to result in losses of 0.03 and 0.04 years of life for the 10- and 15-year treatment durations, respectively. In contrast, when symptoms of menopause were viewed as decreasing overall quality of life by 3 days per year,

TABLE 51.2. *Net change in undiscounted life expectancy, quality components, and cost for hormone replacement regimens*

| | Unoppposed estrogen in women without a uterus | | Estrogen combined with progestin in women with a uterus | | | |
| | | | Favorable scenario | | Unfavorable scenario | |
	10 years	15 years	10 years	15 years	10 years	15 years
Components of life expectancy (undiscounted)						
LE$_{HFX}$	0.0519	0.0732	0.0519	0.0732	0.0519	0.0732
LE$_{BRCA}$	-0.0325	-0.0417	—	—	-0.0429	-0.0647
LE$_{CHD}$	0.0843	0.1652	0.0843	0.1652	0.0465	0.0892
Net life expectancy	0.1037	0.1967	0.1362	0.2384	0.0555	0.0977
Components of cost (discounted)						
C$_{HRT}$	$2,086	$2,765	$2,709	$3,592	$2,709	$3,592
C$_{HFX}$	-429	-592	-429	-592	-429	-592
C$_{NH}$	-919	-1,229	-919	-1,229	-919	-1,229
C$_{BRCA}$	41	50	—	—	53	77
Net cost	$779	$994	$1,361	$1,770	$1,414	$1,848

TABLE 51.3. *Summary of assumptions concerning increased (↑), decreased (↓), or unchanged (→) risks of hormone replacement therapy*

Event	Unopposed estrogen in women with a previous hysterectomy	Combined estrogen-progestin therapy in women with a uterus	
		Favorable scenario	Unfavorable scenario
Hip fracture incidence	↓	↓	↓
Breast cancer incidence	↑ 25–30%	→	↑ 50%
Coronary heart disease death	↓ 37%	↓ 37%	↓ 20%

symptom relief associated with any form of treatment resulted in a gain of 0.11 years.

IMPACT ON COST

Although there were savings associated with several components of cost, the cost of the drug and monitoring, which ranged from an average of $2,086 to $3,592 per patient treated, far outweighed the estimated savings (Table 51.2). The largest savings were from decreased nursing home usage for persons treated with hormone replacement therapy compared to persons who were not treated. However, we did not estimate the costs that would be saved from decreases in the incidence of coronary heart disease. It is possible that this component of the cost equation could lead to greatly reduced costs and to potential savings in women at risk for coronary heart disease.

COST EFFECTIVENESS RELATIVE TO NO INTERVENTION

For each strategy and set of assumptions (Table 51.3), we estimated the cost per year of life saved relative to a strategy of no intervention. Our estimates of cost per year of life saved range from $15,300 for 15 years of unopposed estrogen to $81,800 under the unfavorable scenario for 15 years of combined therapy. Most costs per year of life saved were in the $15,000 to $25,000 range (Table 51.4). Such cost-effectiveness ratios compare favorably

with the ratios that have been estimated for other commonly accepted medical practices, such as the treatment of mild to moderate diastolic hypertension ($15,800 to $89,800 per year of life saved, inflated to 1992 dollars) (54). When costs per quality-adjusted year of life saved are computed, the ratios were even more favorable, with the exception of combined therapy in women who are asymptomatic and bothered by the side effects of the medication (Table 51.4).

LIMITATIONS

Several factors were not considered in our analysis. First, the only osteoporotic endpoint that we considered was hip fracture. Fractures of the wrist and vertebrae are commonly associated with osteoporosis and are prevalent among older postmenopausal women. Consideration of these painful fractures would further reduce the costs per quality-adjusted year of life saved that are associated with hormone replacement therapy.

Second, we evaluated the long-term (10- and 15-year duration) use of hormone replacement in perimenopausal women but did not evaluate lifetime use of hormone replacement therapy. We did not discuss surgical menopause in young women because the generally accepted standard of care is to use unopposed estrogen replacement therapy in these women. We also did not address the effectiveness or cost-effectiveness of treating older postmenopausal women with hormone replacement therapy (55).

TABLE 51.4. *Cost per year of life saved and per quality-adjusted year of life saved for each intervention[a]*

	Unopposed estrogen in women with a uterus		Estrogen combined with progestin in women with a uterus			
			Favorable scenario		Unfavorable scenario	
	10 years	15 years	10 years	15 years	10 years	15 years
Cost per year of life saved	$21,900	$15,300	$30,400	$23,900	$81,800	$56,000
Cost per quality-adjusted year of life saved						
No symptoms/no side effects	$14,500	$11,100	$21,600	$17,900	$39,700	$32,000
No symptoms/side effects	$14,500	$11,100	$36,200	$26,300	$139,000	$70,000
Symptomatic/no side effects	$5,600	$5,700	$9,200	$9,700	$11,800	$13,000
Symptomatic/side effects	$5,600	$5,700	$11,100	$11,600	$14,900	$16,600

[a]Both costs and life years are discounted in the cost-effectiveness ratio computation.

Third, we have not estimated the savings that would be associated with hormone replacement therapy from reduced incidence of coronary heart disease. Because coronary heart disease is common and can be costly, the savings from heart disease averted may outweigh the costs of hormone replacement therapy. This is most likely among women who are at risk for coronary heart disease.

Fourth, we have not addressed the issue of screening women using bone densitometry to assist in their decision of whether or not to take hormone replacement therapy. This option has been addressed for the asymptomatic perimenopausal women with a uterus (14). For women who have had a hysterectomy, the screening issue is moot because the cardioprotective benefits of hormone replacement therapy far outweigh its impact on the complications of osteoporosis. We also did not address the cost-effectiveness of new pharmaceutical agents that have been approved for prevention of osteoporosis. These agents include alendronate, a bisphosphonate (56), and raloxifene, a selective estrogen receptor modulator or SERM (57). SERMs have agonistic actions on bone and lipids that mimic the actions of estrogen but cause no stimulatory effect on the breast or uterine tissues. To the extent that women choose to take long-term hormone replacement therapy to prevent osteoporosis, the cost-effectiveness of hormone replacement therapy relative to these agents should be considered as data become available.

Finally, our analysis did not consider the use of unopposed estrogens in women with a uterus. A recent analysis highlighted the role of unopposed estrogen in increasing life expectancy (17). However, patients' perceptions of risks of cancer associated with hormone replacement therapy (endometrial cancer, breast cancer) often outweigh the perceived benefits (reduced incidence of heart disease and complications of osteoporosis). Thus, although unopposed estrogen may be more effective (and cost-effective) than combined therapy, it may be an unacceptable treatment option for many women and physicians. The choice of whether or not to take hormone replacement therapy remains a very personal decision to be undertaken by each individual in consultation with her physician. This decision can be assisted with an accurate understanding of the risks and benefits of alternate approaches.

SUMMARY

The expected costs and life years for women using long-term estrogen or estrogen combined with progestin compared with women receiving no intervention were estimated. For combined therapy, estimates were made under both a favorable and unfavorable scenario. For all other treatment regimens and assumptions, hormone replacement therapy was found to increase net life expectancy. The impact of hormone replacement therapy on quality of life was substantial, especially among

women suffering from the symptoms of menopause or among women adversely affected by the side effects of estrogen combined with progestin. When costs were considered, hormone replacement therapy was found to increase cost of care; however, savings associated with incident coronary heart disease cases were not estimated. Although costs were increased, the additional cost per year of life saved for most hormone replacement therapy regimens was in the range of $15,000 to $25,000. Thus, from society's standpoint, the cost-effectiveness of hormone replacement therapy compares favorably with other commonly accepted medical interventions. The cost-effectiveness of long-term hormone replacement therapy for women concerned about osteoporosis prevention will need to be reevaluated relative to new osteoporosis prevention agents such as alendronate and raloxifene as additional data become available.

REFERENCES

1. US Department of Commerce, Bureau of the Census. *Projections of the population of the United States, by age, sex, and race: 1983 to 2080. Current population reports. Population estimates and projections. Series P-25, number 952.* Washington, DC: US Government Printing Office, 1984.
2. Weinstein MC, Tosteson ANA. Cost-effectiveness of hormone replacement. *Ann NY Acad Sci* 1990;592:162–172.
3. Eisenberg JM. Clinical economics: A guide to the economic analysis of clinical practices. JAMA 1989;262:2879–2886.
4. Goldman L, Tosteson ANA. Uncertainty about postmenopausal estrogen: Time for action, not debate. *N Engl J Med* 1991;325:800–802.
5. Cummings SR, Black DM, Rubin SM. Lifetime risks of hip, Colles', or vertebral fracture and coronary heart disease among white postmenopausal women. *Arch Intern Med* 1989;149:2445–2448.
6. Seidman H, Mushinski MN, Gelb SK, Silverberg E. Probabilities of eventually developing or dying of cancer: United States, 1985. *CA* 1985;35:36–56.
7. Grodstein F, Stampfer MJ, Colditz GA, et al. Postmenopausal hormone therapy and mortality. *N Engl J Med* 1997;336:1769–1775.
8. Folsom A, Mink P, Sellers T, Hong C, Zheng W, Potter J. Hormonal replacement therapy and morbidity and mortality in a prospective study of postmenopausal women. *Public Health Briefs* 1995;85:1128–1132.
9. Ettinger B, Friedman GD, Bush T, Quesenberry CP. Reduced mortality associated with long-term postmenopausal estrogen therapy. *Obstet Gynecol* 1996;87:6–12.
10. Whittington R, Faulds D. Hormone replacement therapy: II. A pharmacoeconomic appraisal of its role in the prevention of postmenopausal osteoporosis and ischemic heart disease. *PharmacoEconomics* 1994;5:513–554.
11. Weinstein MC. Estrogen use in postmenopausal women: costs, risks and benefits. *N Engl J Med* 1980;303:308–316.
12. Weinstein MC, Schiff I. Cost-effectiveness of hormone replacement therapy in the menopause. *Obstet Gynecol Surv* 1982;38:445–455.
13. Henderson BE, Ross RK, Lobo RA, Pike MC, Mack TM. Reevaluating the role of progestogen therapy after the menopause. *Fertil Steril* 1988;49(Suppl):9S–15S.
14. Tosteson ANA, Rosenthal DI, Melton LJ III, Weinstein MC. Cost effectiveness of screening perimenopausal white women for osteoporosis: Bone densitometry and hormone replacement therapy. *Ann Intern Med* 1990;113:594–603.
15. Tosteson ANA, Weinstein MC. Cost-effectiveness of hormone replacement therapy after menopause. In: Christiansen C, ed. *Hormone replacement and its impact on osteoporosis.* Bailliere's Clin Obstet Gynaecol 1991;5:943–959.
16. Cheung AP, Wren BG. A cost-effectiveness analysis of hormone replacement therapy in the menopause. *Med J Aust* 1992;156:312–316.
17. Grady D, Rubin SM, Petitti D, et al. Hormone therapy to prevent disease and prolong life in postmenopausal women. *Ann Intern Med* 1992;117:1016–1037.
18. Col NF, Eckman MH, Karas RH, et al. Patient-specific decisions about hormone replacement therapy in postmenopausal women. *JAMA* 1997;277;1140–1147.
19. Persson I, Adami H, Bergkvist L, et al. Risk of endometrial cancer after treatment with oestrogens alone or in conjunction with progestogens: results of a prospective study. *BMJ* 1989;298:147–151.
20. Voigt LF, Weiss NS, Chu J, Daling JR, McKnight B, Van Belle G. Progestagen supplementation of exogenous oestrogens and risk of endometrial cancer. *Lancet* 1991;338:274–277.
21. US Preventive Services Task Force. Estrogen prophylaxis. *Am Fam Physician* 1990;42:1293–1296.
22. Utian WH. Consensus statement on progestin use in postmenopausal women. *Maturitas* 1988;11:175–177.
23. Ravnikar V. Compliance with hormone therapy. *Am J Obstet Gynecol* 1987;156:1332–1334.

24. Riggs BL, Melton LJ III. Involutional osteoporosis. *N Engl J Med* 1986;314: 1676–1686.
25. Cummings SR, Kelsey JL, Nevitt MC, O'Dowd KJ. Epidemiology of osteoporosis and osteoporotic fractures. *Epidemiol Rev* 1985;7:178–208.
26. Melton LJ III, Wahner HW, Richelson LS, O'Fallon WM, Riggs BL. Osteoporosis and the risk of hip fracture. *Am J Epidemiol* 1986;124:254–261.
27. Melton LJ III, Kan SH, Wahner HW, Riggs BL. Lifetime fracture risk: An approach to hip fracture risk assessment based on bone mineral density and age. *J Clin Epidemiol* 1988;41:985–994.
28. Ettinger B, Genant HK, Cann CE. Long-term estrogen replacement therapy prevents bone loss and fractures. *Ann Intern Med* 1985;102:319–324.
29. Quigley MET, Martin PL, Burnier AM, Brooks P. Estrogen therapy arrests bone loss in elderly women. *Am J Obstet Gynecol* 1987;156:1516–1523.
30. Weiss NS, Ure CL, Ballard JH, Williams AR, Daling JR. Decreased risk of fractures of the hip and lower forearm with postmenopausal use of estrogens. *N Engl J Med* 1980;303:1195–1198.
31. Kiel DP, Felson DT, Anderson JJ, Wilson PWF, Moskowitz MA. Hip fracture and the use of estrogens in postmenopausal women: The Framingham study. *N Engl J Med* 1987;317:1169–1174.
32. Pettiti DB, Sidney S. Hip fracture in women: Incidence, in-hospital mortality and five-year survival probabilities in members of a pre-paid health plan. *Clin Orthop Rel Res* 1989;246:150–155.
33. Weiss NS, Liff JM, Ure CL, Ballard JH, Abbott GH, Daling JR. Mortality in women following hip fracture. *J Chron Dis* 1983;36:879–882.
34. Mossey JM, Mutran E, Knott K, Craik R. Determinants of recovery 12 months after hip fracture: The importance of psychosocial factors. *Am J Public Health* 1989;79:279–286.
35. Kenzora JE, McCarthy RE, Lowell JD, Sledge CB. Hip fracture mortality: Relation to age, treatment, preoperative illness, time of surgery and complications. *Clin Orthop Rel Res* 1984;186:45–56.
36. Kreutzfeld J, Haim M, Bach E. Hip fracture among the elderly in a mixed urban and rural population. *Age Aging* 1984;13:111–119.
37. Dahl E. Mortality and life expectancy after hip fractures. *Acta Orthop Scand* 1980;51:163–170.
38. Miller CW. Survival and ambulation following hip fracture. *J Bone Joint Surg* 1978;7:930–934.
39. Hillner BE, Hollenberg JP, Pauker SG. Postmenopausal estrogens in prevention of osteoporosis: Benefit virtually without risk if cardiovascular effects are considered. *Am J Med* 1986;80:1115–1117.
40. Steinberg KK, Thacker SB, Smith SJ, et al. A meta-analysis of the effect of estrogen replacement therapy on the risk of breast cancer. *JAMA* 1991;265:1985–1990.
41. Colditz GA, Stampfer MJ, Willet WC, Hennekens CH, Rosner B, Speizer FE. Prospective study of estrogen replacement therapy and risk of breast cancer in postmenopausal women. *JAMA* 1990;264:2648–2653.
42. Key TJA, Pike MC. The role of oestrogens and progestagens in the epidemiology and prevention of breast cancer. *Eur J Cancer Clin Oncol* 1988;24:29–43.
43. Eddy DM. Screening for breast cancer. *Ann Intern Med* 1989;111:389–399.
44. Stampfer MJ, Colditz GA. Estrogen replacement therapy and coronary heart disease: A quantitative assessment of the epidemiologic evidence. *Prev Med* 1991; 20:47–63.
45. National Center for Health Statistics. *Vital Statistics of the United States, 1983, Vol II, part B.* Washington, DC: US Government Printing Office, 1986.
46. Persson I, Falkeborn M, Lithell H. The effect on myocardial infarction risk of estrogens and estrogen-progestin combinations (abstract). In: *Sixth International Congress on the Menopause.* Bangkok, Thailand: Parthenon Publishing, 1990: 223.
47. Pines A, Fisman EZ, Levo Y, et al. The effects of hormone replacement therapy in normal postmenopausal women: Measurements of Doppler-derived parameters of aortic flow. *Am J Obstet Gynecol* 1991;164:806–812.
48. Adams MR, Kaplan JR, Manuck SB, et al. Inhibition of coronary artery atherosclerosis in 17-beta estradiol in ovariectomized monkeys. Lack of an effect of added progesterone. *Arteriosclerosis* 1990;10:1051–1057.
49. Bush TL, Barrett-Connor E, Cowan LD, et al. Cardiovascular mortality and noncontraceptive use of estrogen in women: results from the Lipid Research Clinics Program Follow-up Study. *Circulation* 1987;75:1102–1109.
50. Ottosson UB, Johansson BG, von Schoultz B. Subfractions of high-density lipoprotein cholesterol during estrogen replacement therapy: A comparison between progestogens and natural progesterone. *Am J Obstet Gynecol* 1985;151: 745–750.
51. Wahl P, Walden C, Knopp R, et al. Effect of estrogen/progestin potency on lipid/lipoprotein cholesterol. *N Engl J Med* 1983;308:862–867.
52. Cohen MA, Tell EJ, Wallack SS. The lifetime risks and costs of nursing home use among the elderly. *Med Care* 1986;24:1161–1172.
53. National Center for Health Statistics. Use of nursing homes by the elderly: Preliminary data from the 1985 National Nursing Home Survey. *DHHS pub. no. (PHS)87-1250, Vital and Health Statistics, no. 135.* Hyattsville, MD: US Public Health Service, 1987.
54. Edelson JT, Weinstein MC, Tosteson ANA, Williams L, Lee TH, Goldman L. Long-term cost-effectiveness of various initial monotherapies for mild to moderate hypertension. *JAMA* 1990;263:408–413.
55. Resnick NM, Greenspan SL. "Senile" osteoporosis reconsidered. *JAMA* 1989; 261:1025–1029.
56. Hosking D, Chilvers CED, Christiansen C, et al, for the Early Postmenopausal Intervention Cohort Study Group. Prevention of bone loss with alendronate in postmenopausal women under 60 years of age. *N Engl J Med* 1998;338:485–492.
57. Delmas P, Bjarnason N, Mitlak B, et al. Effects of raloxifene on bone mineral density, serum cholesterol concentrations, and uterine endometrium in postmenopausal women. *N Engl J Med* 1997;337:1641–1647.

Treatment of the Postmenopausal Woman: Basic and Clinical Aspects, Second Edition, edited by Rogerio A. Lobo, Lippincott Williams & Wilkins, Philadelphia © 1999.

CHAPTER 52

Contraindications to Hormone Replacement Therapy

Donna Shoupe

As the list of known benefits of estrogen replacement therapy (ERT) continues to grow, it becomes increasingly more difficult to deny treatment to potential candidates. The lowered risk of cardiovascular disease, osteoporosis, and dementia added to the benefits of better skin quality, urogenital health, dental preservation, and greater sense of well-being weigh heavily when compared to the negative risks. In the past, the contraindications of hormone replacement therapy (HRT) were based either on theory or extra. Now, as more relevant information is obtained, and as more options become available, ERT can be safely utilized by almost all postmenopausal women, including those with a wide range of medical problems. The question of whether or not to use HRT is now often replaced with a question of which low-dose regimen to use or which nonoral route is most appropriate.

The growing interest in the menopause is reflected by the explosion of media coverage, a growing number of consumer books, and the large numbers of conferences focusing on health issues for women over 40. Until recently, most women saw breast cancer as their major health threat and often avoided ERT on the basis of this one issue. There is now better dispersal of information regarding all of the health threats to women and better coverage of the beneficial role of estrogens in decreasing death and disability from heart disease, dementia, and osteoporosis, thus allowing for more balanced decision making. Of course, the huge influx of alternative medicines, new antiresorptive agents, countless products offered by compounding pharmacies, and the availability of estrogen alternatives complicate the playing field as never before. But physicians now have better-educated patients, a growing list of excellent studies, better, lower

dosages, and many new tools (bone density studies, bone turnover tests, blood flow and vascular studies), which mean better health care in the long-run.

ABSOLUTE CONTRAINDICATIONS TO ESTROGEN REPLACEMENT THERAPY

Absolute contraindications to ERT and HRT include undiagnosed vaginal bleeding, acute liver disease, acute thrombosis or emboli, and current breast or endometrial cancer (Table 52.1). The first three conditions are short-term problems, and following their resolution, ERT/HRT may be safely prescribed. Following thromboembolic disease, a nonoral route of ERT may be preferable because of the absence of an effect of transdermally administered estrogen on hepatic protein synthesis, in particular, clotting factors (1). Other medical conditions and potential contraindications are discussed below.

Estrogen Replacement Therapy and Breast Cancer

Until recently, ERT was contraindicated in women with a past history of breast cancer. Recent studies now

TABLE 52.1. *Contraindications to ERT/HRT*

Severe active liver disease
Acute thrombophlebitis or thromboembolic event
Current breast cancer
Current endometrial cancer
Undiagnosed vaginal bleeding
Known or suspected pregnancy
Relative contraindications
History of breast cancer
History of endometrial cancer
Chronic liver disease
Pancreatic disease

D. Shoupe: Department of Obstetrics and Gynecology, University of Southern California Women's and Children's Hospital, Los Angeles, California 90033.

suggest that in selected patients, ERT does not promote an earlier recurrence or decrease survival time and additionally provides the known benefits of therapy (2–11). There are currently many diverse strategies for management of postmenopausal women with breast cancer, especially in regard to the use or nonuse of HRT. In a recent study of postmenopausal women with early-stage breast cancer, 7% of the women eligible for the study were already taking HRT (3).

Most of the women with a history of breast cancer are either naturally postmenopausal or have experienced an early menopause following chemotherapy or hormonal manipulations. In either case, these women suffer health consequences from an estrogen-deficient state and often complain of hot flushes, insomnia, vaginal atrophy and dryness, depressed mood, and cognitive changes. For those with successful treatment of the tumor, survival extends for many years, thus exposing them to many years of the consequences of estrogen deficiency.

The major arguments against the use of HRT in women with a personal history of breast cancer have been based on theoretical reasoning originating from observations linking estrogen with breast cancer (Table 52.2). The arguments criticizing the prohibition against the use of HRT in these patients are equally convincing (Table 52.3). Although there are still many unknowns, many clinical studies have addressed this problem.

In the growing number of clinical trials to date (3–11), none has shown an increased risk of tumor recurrence with HRT. In one study where 25 patients previously treated for breast cancer received HRT for relief of menopausal symptoms, the overall survival rate was 96% with no adverse effect on cancer outcome (10). DiSaia et al. followed 77 breast cancer survivors on HRT (11).

After 15 years, 71 of 77 (92%) had no evidence of disease. The authors concluded that renewed HRT does not cause recurrence. In the largest study to date, 90 women were treated with continuous estrogen/progestin therapy (MPA 50 mg/day) and matched with 180 nonuser controls. The risk of recurrence was significantly lower in the hormone users compared with the controls (4).

Although these studies are encouraging, caution is still necessary. The relationship of tumor receptor status and nodal status to HRT remains unknown. Additionally, women who have remained disease-free for 10 to 15 years still have a small risk of recurrence. However, as a woman ages, other risks such as osteoporosis and cardiovascular disease may play a more important role in her overall survival than her risk of dying from breast cancer. In order to make the best decision regarding whether or not to use HRT, the patient and physician should discuss the potential risks and benefits that are known and unknown (12). Factors to consider are the menopausal symptoms, potential for estrogen deficiency diseases to occur, and the type and stage of tumor.

In selected patients, HRT may improve the quality of life without shortening the length of life. The postmenopausal women who are most often considered for replacement therapy are those who are 5 to 10 years from diagnosis and remain disease-free. Although these patients have an excellent prognosis, recurrence rates of up to 5% per year have been reported in some series. There are current efforts to establish other prognostic factors such as the presence of axillary nodal disease, tumor size, and hormone receptor status that may aid in selecting appropriate candidates for ERT. The American College of Obstetrics and Gynecology recommends that clinicians base their decision on whether or not to use ERT

TABLE 52.2. *Arguments that link estrogen with breast cancer*

- Breast cancer is 100 times more common in women than in men.
- Breast cancer risk relates to reproductive markers such as age at menarche, first pregnancy, and menopause.
- Serum estrogen levels predict breast cancer risk.
- Incidence of breast cancer higher in men who have excessively high estrogen levels, such as transsexuals or those with metastatic prostatic cancer.
- Estrogen is implicated in the etiology of breast cancer.
- Long-term use of HRT increases the risk or breast cancer.
- Many breast cancers have a substantial proportion of cells with estrogen receptors, and estrogen may have a proliferative effect on those cells.
- Antiestrogenic drugs or ovarian ablation has been shown to be effective in women with advanced disease.
- Breast cancer is significantly decreased in women undergoing oophorectomy before age 50 or in women with premature menopause.
- Obesity, an independent risk factor for breast cancer, is also linked with high estrogen levels. Obese postmenopausal women have decreased sex-hormone-binding globulin and higher peripheral conversion rates of androstenedione to estrone, creating increased circulating estrogen levels.
- Decreasing endogenous estrogen levels by oophorectomy, adrenalectomy, or antiestrogen therapy (tamoxifen, raloxifen) may temporarily arrest tumor cell growth.
- Tamoxifen treatment significantly increases survival compared with nontreated controls and reduces the risk (38%) of contralateral primary breast cancer.
- Estrogen stimulates the proliferation of breast cancer cells *in vitro*.

TABLE 52.3. *Arguments criticizing the prohibition of the use of HRT in breast cancer patients*

- Estrogen is indirectly implicated in the etiology of breast cancer.
- Circulating levels of estrogen in peri- or postmenopausal women may have little influence on breast cancer risk.
- Data on HRT and breast cancer risk are conflicting, even regarding long-term use, and if anything, risk seems to be tied to at least 5 years of exposure.
- The exact mechanisms of the interaction between estrogen and the estrogen-receptor-positive cells are not known, and cell control rather than cell kill may be a key factor in controlling the disease.
- Tamoxifen is not simply an antiestrogen but also has estrogenic properties (i.e., on lipids and bone).
- The present experience, although limited, at least does not show a burst of metastases following HRT in breast cancer survivors.
- Pharmacologic doses of estrogen have been shown to induce breast cancer regression rather than promotion.
- Approximately 10% of patients with estrogen-receptor-negative tumors response to antiestrogens like tamoxifen, suggesting that estrogen is not the only "clue" to tumor growth.
- Pregnancy following previously treated breast cancer is no longer associated with an unfavorable prognosis. It is rather the young age of the pregnant woman and the advanced stage of the disease (rather than the pregnancy and its high hormone levels) that confer the poor outcome. Some studies have shown a survival advantage for patients who become pregnant after primary treatment.
- Breast cancer may remain occult for many years before its clinical presentation, and therefore, large numbers of women with breast cancer have had prolonged exposure to estrogens (i.e., OCs or ERT). Generally, no adverse effect on survival rates for either has been shown. In fact, a significantly higher survival rate is reported for breast cancer patients who previously used HRT or were using HRT at the time of diagnosis.
- Estrogen may be considered as a promoter rather than an initiator. This would be consistent with the earlier diagnosis and better prognosis associated with patients on ERT when the diagnosis is made. The nonestradiol estrogens are either weak promoters or function as antipromoters and protect against cancer growth and spread.

on the theoretical risk of recurrence as well as the potential health benefits. An informed consent should be documented and, when applicable, the treating oncologist contacted.

If the decision is made to use estrogen, the lowest effective dose is recommended. Some advocate that a medium-dose progestogen be added (4). In one study using an estrogen and progestin regimen, there was a lower rate of death and a 50% reduction in recurrent or new breast cancer (13,14). These favorable results, according to the authors, were a response to the suppressant activity of the progestogen on breast cell mitosis.

Other Options

In patients who suffer from vaginal dryness, urge or stress incontinence, or frequent urinary tract infections, use of vaginal estrogen cream (one-third to one-half tube twice weekly) or an estrogen-releasing vaginal ring (Estring) may be beneficial (15,16). Medroxyprogesterone acetate alone, 20 mg/day orally, is often effective for relief of hot flushes (17).

Tamoxifen, given at doses of 20 to 40 mg/day, is often used as adjunctive therapy for breast cancer. An overview of the large number of randomized trails of tamoxifen in the treatment of breast cancer showed a significant reduction in mortality in tamoxifen-treated women over the age of 50 compared with untreated controls (18). Improved survival with tamoxifen was noted in patients with both positive and negative nodes and also in those with both

positive and negative estrogen receptor status. A worldwide collaborative study of 75,000 patients showed a significant reduction in annual recurrence and death rates in women on tamoxifen and a 39% reduction in the risk of contralateral breast cancer (19).

Five studies report that tamoxifen decreases low-density lipoprotein (LDL)-cholesterol and total cholesterol and increases the high-density lipoprotein (HDL)-cholesterol ratio by a mean of 14% (20–24). These data suggest that tamoxifen may offer, at least in part, one of the major benefits of ERT, retarding the development of atherosclerosis. In addition, tamoxifen is effective in preventing bone loss in postmenopausal women (24,25). Although there is evidence that tamoxifen ameliorates urogenital atrophy (26,27), it does not relieve hot flushes and may not have the beneficial effect on brain function and dementia. Additionally, the estrogenic effects of tamoxifen therapy increase the risk of endometrial hyperplasia (18% to 27%) and endometrial cancer (0.3% to 1.4%) (21). Unlike the endometrial cancer associated with unopposed estrogen, which tends to be well differentiated and early stage, tamoxifen-associated endometrial cancer tends to be more aggressive and more often fatal.

The combination of continuous progestogen with tamoxifen therapy is reported to improve outcomes for women regarding both breast and uterine cancers without reducing the quality of life (14). Additionally, in a well-conducted study, no detrimental interaction between tamoxifen and HRT was noted in four areas including serum cholesterol, bone mineral density, fibrinogen, and antithrombin III.

Raloxifene, a new selective estrogen receptor modulator, is now approved for prevention and treatment of osteoporosis in postmenopausal women. Raloxifene also appears to decrease breast cancer risk and has a beneficial effect on lipids (29). Unfortunately, raloxifene may not have cardioprotective effects (30) or brain protection. Trials of raloxifene with ERT or HRT are pending and should produce interesting results.

Benign Breast Disease

There have been many studies documenting the safety of HRT use in women with a history of benign breast disease. In an analysis of 10,366 consecutive breast specimens in 3,303 women, Dupont et al. showed a protective effect of ERT in women with an original pathology specimen of atypical hyperplasia, proliferative disease without atypia or in those without proliferative disease (28). Most studies in postmenopausal women with benign breast disease show no significant increase in breast cancer after HRT, although a few of the studies show increased risk in certain subgroups such as epithelial hyperplasia or papillomatosis (30–32).

Ovarian Cancer

Estrogens have not been convincingly linked with development of ovarian cancer. Hoover et al. reported that the relative risk in users was 2.4 (CI 1.0–4.8) (33) while several case-control studies have shown no association (34–36) or a decreased risk 0.89 (37) and 0.6 (CI 0.4–0.8) (38). Theories regarding causative factors, suggest that the development of ovarian cancer is related to gonadotropin stimulation thus elevations in gonadotropins in early menopause many be associated with an increased risk. Oral contraceptive suppress gonadotropin release and have a protective effect. Generally, it is felt or any type of epithelial damage, either through irritants or *incessant ovulation,* plays a major role in the development of ovarian cancer. After examining ovaries, removed in women being operated on for endometrial cancer, Resta et al. (39) reported that the ovarian epithelium was more likely to be hyperplastic or metaplastic in women with endometrial cancer. These authors suggested that the hormonal milieu, including high estrogen levels, leading to endometrial cancer may also play a role in ovarian cancer.

Many studies demonstrate no detrimental effect of ERT or HRT given to women with a history of ovarian cancer. In one retrospective study of selected ovarian cancer patients receiving ERT, the relative risk of death was 0.63 (CI 0.3–1.34) when compared to women not receiving estrogen (40). With few exceptions, studies using high-dose progestogens (500 to 1,000 mg medroxyprog-esterone acetate daily) to treat ovarian cancer have had disappointing results, suggesting that the tumor is not influenced directly by sex steroids.

Endometrial Cancer

There are a number of reports suggesting that ERT can safely be prescribed for patients with stage I endometrial cancer following treatment (41,42). In 1990, a committee opinion of the American College of Obstetricians and Gynecologists stated that for women with a past history of endometrial cancer, "estrogens could be used for the same indications as for any other woman, except that the selection of appropriate candidates should be based upon prognostic indicators and the risk the patient is willing to assume. The sense of well-being afforded by amelioration of menopausal symptoms or the need to treat atrophic vaginitis or osteoporosis may outweigh the risk of stimulating tumor growth."

It is of interest to note that patients with hormone-dependent endometrial adenocarcinomas have a low risk of recurrence. However, grade 1 lesions, which are most likely to respond adversely to ERT, tend to recur late (43). Therefore, ERT in any patient treated for endometrial cancer always carries some risk with respect to cancer recurrence. However, the long-term protection from disability and death from cardiovascular disease, osteoporosis, and dementia seems to justify the risk for many patients with this disease. Additionally, there are a great deal of reassuring data. In a retrospective study of 47 women receiving ERT and 174 controls, the ERT-treated group experienced a longer disease-free survival (44). A similar study also confirmed these findings (42), and in two observational reports involving over 50 patients receiving ERT following endometrial cancer, none had recurrences (45,46).

There are various recommendations regarding the length of time that should be allowed to elapse from cancer treatment before ERT or HRT is begun (47). There are clinicians who advocate immediate treatment (48), especially in selected low-risk groups (Table 52.4), as retrospective studies report improved overall survival. For others, because 60% to 80% of recurrences occur within 2 years, waiting for this time period minimizes the risk of

TABLE 52.4. *Low-and high-risk groups for recurrence with use of ERT following endometrial cancer*

Low-risk group
1. Stage I disease, steroid-receptor negative
2. Steroid-receptor-positive tumors with all of the following: superficial or no myometrial penetration, negative nodes, and negative peritoneal cytology

High-risk group
1. Steroid-receptor-positive tumors with one of the following: deep myometrial penetration, positive nodes, positive peritoneal cytology, or stage II or higher

starting ERT in patients with possible residual cancer. In the meantime, treatment with oral or intramuscular medroxyprogesterone acetate is effective in alleviating hot flushes and affords some protection against bone loss.

Combination oral contraceptives have been shown to decrease the risk of endometrial cancer by about one-half. Obesity has been linked with endometrial cancer, probably through its effect on circulating estrogen levels.

Cardiovascular Disease

Heart disease is the leading cause of death of American women and men. Estrogen replacement therapy reduces the risk of developing coronary heart disease, especially in women at risk for heart disease, and should be prescribed accordingly. Although the use of ERT/HRT reduced the overall risk of death in nurses participating in the Nurses Health Study, the largest reduction in mortality (50% reduced risk of death) was in the current hormone users who had at least one coronary risk factor (69% of all participants) (RR 0.51, CI 0.46–0.57 compared to never users) (49). Coronary risk factors included current smoking, high cholesterol levels, high blood pressure, diabetes, parental history of premature myocardial infarction, and body-mass index ≥ 29.

Estrogen appears to prevent the increase in fibrinogen associated with menopause (50,51), promotes vasodilation of the coronary artery endothelium and vascular smooth muscle, counters the tendency toward vasospasm in athlersclerotic coronary artery (52), and increases blood flow (53). Long-term benefits of estrogen appear to be a direct protection from athlerosclerotic changes in the endothelium including decreased platelet aggregation and less plaque accumulation (54). Surgical menopause predisposes to increases in cardiovascular disease and myocardial infarction (54–56) as a result of loss of these protective effects of endogenous estrogen.

Coronary Heart Disease and Myocardial Infarction

There has been concern that ERT might cause increased risk of thrombosis in coronary arteries already stenotic from known atherosclerosis. On the contrary, the protection from progression of disease or death with ERT/HRT seen in women with or without risk factors without known cardiovascular disease is extended for those with documented disease. In women with angiographically proven coronary artery stenosis, ERT users have an increased survival rate (97%) at 10 years compared to nonusers (60%) (57). Combined estrogen-progestin therapy (HRT) appears to offer a similar protection.

In a prospective study, in almost 9,000 women with a history of angina or myocardial infarction (MI), after 7.5 years, continuous users had a relative risk of mortality of 1 versus 1.6 in never users ($p < 0.01$) (58). In a retro-

spective cohort study of 726 women (mean age 66.2 years) who had survived a first MI, the relative risk for reinfarction, adjusted for age, was 6.4 (CI 0.32–1.30) for current users and 0.9 (0.62–1.31) for past estrogen replacement. The all-cause mortality associated with current use was 0.5 (CI 0.25–1.00) (59). Estrogen replacement after first myocardial infarction is not associated with increased risk of reinfarction or mortality. Transdermal therapy may be the best option in those with advanced vascular disease.

Hypertension

In postmenopausal normotensive women, HRT does not increase blood pressure and often lowers it (60–64). Although there is little information available, all studies indicate that HRT is safe to use with concomitant hypertensive medicines (65). Despite these reports and the accepted benefits of HRT, some clinicians are unwilling to prescribe HRT to their hypertensive patients. In a postal survey, 61/191 clinicians (30%) reported that they were reluctant to prescribe HRT if blood pressure was difficult to control (66). This concern is likely related to confusion that has linked ERT to the side effects associated with oral contraceptives.

Climacteric women with hypertension are candidates for ERT (67). Because the transdermal route of ERT administration lowers levels of renin substrate (angiotensinogen) compared to oral administration (68), transdermal treatment may the best option in women with difficult-to-control hypertension. Declines in blood pressure with oral estrogen are also documented (69). In a nonrandomized, prospective, observational study of almost 9,000 women, the relative risk of mortality in hypertensive continual ERT users was 1.15 versus 1.54 for hypertensive women who had never used ERT ($p < 0.01$) (58).

Diabetes Mellitus

Postmenopausal women with diabetes have an especially high rate of vascular disease and complications and are a group that should be specifically targeted to receive HRT (70). In addition to a long-term lowered risk of cardiovascular disease in general, potential benefits of HRT include decreased insulin resistance (71–75), decreased thrombotic response, improved endothelial function, decreased hypertension, decreased microalbuminuria, decreased platelet adhesion, increased HDL-cholesterol levels, and decreased LDL (71–77).

Analysis of postchallenge glucose and insulin levels from the Rancho-Bernardo cohort suggest that oral ERT was associated with lower fasting insulin levels and that this difference was independent of age, obesity, or differential hormone use by women with known glucose intolerance (73). The PEPI trail, the first major randomized placebo-controlled trial of HRT, also showed that women on active treatment had lightly lower fasting insulin and glucose levels, although the 2-hour post-glucose-challenge levels were slightly higher than those of the placebo group (50). Women with glucose intolerance taking ERT had significantly lower fasting plasma glucose concentrations (5.8 vs. 6.8 mmol/L) compared to nonusers. Other groups suggest that this improved insulin sensitivity with ERT is lost with the addition of an androgenic progestogen such as norethisterone (53) and, to a lesser degree, by adding medroxyprogesterone acetate or micronized progesterone (50,71).

These results are consistent with findings in NIDDM patients on a euglycemic hyperinsulinemic clamp technique that showed a significant reduction in hepatic glucose production and improvements in HbA1c following oral ERT (75). In animal models, the development of diabetes as well as the significant declines in insulin release and number of β-cells that occurred as a result of oophorectomy were reversed by oral administration of ERT (78,79).

Transdermal estrogens either have a small effect (77,80,81) or do not affect insulin sensitivity (53). In a 3-month study, transdermal estradiol (0.05 mg) was associated with a small decrease in insulin levels and an increase in C-peptide levels (a measure of pancreatic responsivity to glucose), while oral conjugated estrogen (0.625) admistration was associated with slightly lower glucose levels and no change in insulin or C-peptide (77). In a larger study comparing oral conjugated estrogen (0.625 mg) and norgestrel (0.15 mg) to transdermal estradiol (0.05 mg) and norethindrone acetate (0.25 mg), there was a 15% decline in insulin sensitivity in both groups by the end of 18 months (81).

Use of Transdermal or Low-Dose ERT

There are many conditions in which consideration should be given to administering either transdermal or low-dose therapy (Table 52.5). Transdermal products are

TABLE 52.5. *Conditions in which transdermal or, in some cases, very-low-dose oral ERT should be considered*

Gallstones or gallbladder disease
Hypertriglyceridemia
History of venous thrombosis or thrombotic event (without an identifiable risk factor)
Poorly controlled hypertension
Vascular disease
Recent myocardial infarction
Poor mobility
Recent trauma
Postoperative
Migraine headaches
Malabsorption
Chronic hepatic dysfunction

especially useful in patients with known vascular disease, hypertriglyceridemia, immobility, extensive surgery, migraines, and history of thrombotic problems (82,83). The use of oral ERT or HRT slightly increases the risk of venous thrombosis (84,85). Study of coagulation profiles in healthy menopausal women show either small or no significant change in response to oral ERT (86). In a cross-sectional study of almost 5,000 women, oral ERT and HRT users had lower levels of fibrinogen, antithrombin III, and protein C, although protein C and factor VII were higher in users of ERT as opposed to users of HRT or nonusers (71). Use of transdermal estradiol avoids the first-pass effect on the liver and thus has no adverse effect on clotting parameters. Levels of antithrombin III are reported to be higher following transdermal ERT compared to oral ERT (68).

Estrogen replacement therapy is not contraindicated for women with a history of migraine headaches, although the headaches may get worse in about 3% of women who start ERT (87). Estrogens help to regulate cerebral vasomotor tone by altering neurotransmitter function (88,89). Because of the findings that acute estrogen withdrawal is implicated in the onset of migraines (90) and that percutaneous estrogens are used to treat menstrual migraines (91), it is suggested that transdermal ERT may be the route of choice in migraineurs. The gradual and infrequent addition of progestins is also recommended.

Conditions Under Which Low-Dose or Very-Low-Dose ERT/HRT Should Be Considered

There are numerous conditions where low-dose or very-low-dose ERT/HRT should be considered (Table 52.6). Obese postmenopausal women have increased circulating endogenous estrogen levels, and often the dose of ERT needs to be reduced so that circulating estrogen levels are similar to those in normal-weight patients receiving ERT. Obese women have an increased risk of cardiovascular disease and appear to have the greatest beneficial protection from cardiovascular events from taking ERT (49).

Minimizing side effects, especially bleeding problems and breast tenderness, may maximize compliance and promote continued long-term use of ERT. Low-dose (0.3

TABLE 52.6. *Conditions in which lower-dose ERT/HRT should be considered*

History of symptomatic endometriosis or leiomyomata
Bleeding problems on standard therapy
Side effects on standard therapy
Obesity
Patient reluctance to use ERT
Perimenopausal symptoms
Elderly or petite

mg conjugated estrogen or esterified estrogens) therapy protects against bone loss and appears to offer cardiovascular protection (92,93). Very-low-dose therapy is an option in the elderly or in patients who continue to have problems on low-dose therapy. In postmenopausal patients with bleeding or other problems occurring with standard treatment regimens of HRT, reduced dosages are preferable to having the patient stop therapy completely. Consideration of adequate calcium intake, increased exercise, reduced fat and carbohydrate diet, and lifestyle changes to reduce cardiovascular risk are important adjunctive measures. Consideration of addition of androgen therapy to low-dose estrogen therapy rather than increasing the estrogen dose is advised in selected patients, especially those who have had an oophorectomy. Androgen plus estrogen therapy is often beneficial in treating or preventing osteoporosis, resistant hot flushes, or libido problems.

Clinical Problems in Which ERT Is Not Contraindicated

A common clinical problem is how to treat a patient with known endometriosis. Continuous estrogen, estrogen plus progestogen, estrogen plus androgen, or progestogen alone are all options. Most patients do well on standard low-dose therapy.

REFERENCES

1. Chetkowshi RH, Meldrum DR, Steingold KA, et al. Biological effects of transdermal estradiol. N Engl J Med 1986;314:1615.
2. Wilie AG, Opfell RW, Margileth DA. Hormone replacement thearpy in breast cancer. Lancet 1993;342:1232.
3. Vassilopou-Sellin R, Theriault R. Randomized prospective trial of estrogen replacement therapy treatment for localized breast cancer patients' responses and opinions. Cancer 1996;78:1043–1049.
4. Eden JA, Bush T, Nand S, Wren BG. A case-controlled study of combined continuous estrogen-progestin replacement therapy among women with a personal history of breast cancer. J North Am Menopause Soc 1995;2:67–72.
5. Stoll BA, Parbhoo R. Treatment of menopausal symptoms in breast cancer patients. Br Med J 1988;312:1646–1647.
6. Di Saia PJ. Hormone replacement therapy in patients with breast cancer. Cancer 1993;71(Suppl):1490–1500.
7. Powles TJ, Hickish T, Casey S, O'Brian M. Hormone replacement therapy after breast cancer. Lancet 1993;341:60–61
8. Bluming AZ, Wile AG, Schain W, et al. Hormone replacement therapy in women with previous treated primary breast cancer. Proc Annu Meet Am Soc Clin Oncol 1996;15:134.
9. Eden J, Wren BG. Hormone replacement therapy after breast cancer: A review. Cancer Treat Rev 1996;22:335–343.
10. Wilie AG, Opfell RW, Margileth DA. Hormone replacement in previously treated breast cancer patients. Am J Surg 1993;165:372–375.
11. DiSaia PJ, Odicino F, Grosen EA, et al. Hormone replacement therapy in breast cancer. Lancet 1993;342:1232
12. Henrich JB. The postmenopausal estrogen/breast cancer controversy. JAMA 1992;268:1900–1902.
13. Wren B. Hormonal therapy and genital tract cancer. Curr Opin Obstet Gynecol 1996;8:38–41.
14. Eden JA, Bush T, Nand S, Wren BG. A case-control study of combined continuous estrogen-progestogen replacement therapy among women with a personal history of breast cancer. Menopause 1995;2:7–73.
15. Thorneycroft IH. Practical aspects of hormone replacement therapy. Prog Cardiovasc Dis 1995;38(3):243–254.
16. Henriksson L, Stjernquist M, Boquist L, et al. A comparative multicenter study of the effects of continuous low-dose estradiol released from a new vaginal ring versus estriol vaginal pessaries in postmenopausal women with symptoms and signs of urogenital atrophy. Am J Obstet Gynecol 1994;171(3):624–632.
17. Robustelli della Cuna G, Pavesi L, Preti P, Baroni M. High dose medroxyprogsterone acetate in breast cancer: controlled studies. Adv Clin Oncol 1988;1:45–58.
18. Early Breast Cancer Trialists' Collaborative Group. Effects of adjuvant tamoxifen and cytotoxic therapy on mortality in early breast cancer. N Engl J Med 1988;319:1681–1692.
19. Spicer D, Pike MC, Henderson BE. The question of estrogen replacement therapy in patients with a prior diagnosis of breast cancer. Oncology 1990;4:49.
20. Breunning PF, Bonfrer JMG, Hart AAM, et al. Tamoxifen serum lipoprotens and cardiovascular risk. Br J Cancer 1988;58:497–499.
21. Sismondi P, Biglia N, Giai M, et al. Metabolic effects of tamoxifen in postmenopause. Anticancer Res 1994;14:2237–2244.
22. Fisher B, Costantino J, Redmond C. A randomized trial evaluating tamoxifen in the treatment of patients with node-negative breast cancer who have estrogen-receptor positive tumors. N Engl J Med 1989;320:479.
23. Early Breast Cancer Trialists' Group. Systemic treatment of early breast cancer by hormonal, cytotoxic, or immune therapy. Lancet 1992;339(1):71.
24. Turken S, Siris E, Seldin D, Flaster E, Hyman G, Lindsay R. Effects of tamoxifen on spinal bone density in women with breast cancer. J Natl Cancer Inst 1989;81:1086–1088.
25. Love RR, Mazess RB, Torney DC, Barden HS, Newcomb PA, Jordan VC. Bone mineral density in women with breast cancer treated with adjuvant tamoxifen for at least two years. Breast Cancer Res Treat 1988;12:297–301.
26. Ferrazzi E, Cartei G, Mattarazzo R, Fiorentino M. Oestrogen-like effect of tamoxifen on vaginal epithelium. Br Med J 1977;1:1351–1352.
27. Boccardo F, Bruzzi P, Rubagotti A, Nicolo G, Russo R. Estrogen-like action of tamoxifen on vaginal epithelium in breast cancer patients. Oncology 1981;38:281–285.
28. Dupont WD, Page DL. Risk factors for breast cancer in women with proliferative breast disease. N Engl J Med 1985;312:146.
29. Draper MW, Flowers DE, Huster WJ, Neild JA, Harper KD, Arnaud C. A controlled trial of raloxifene: Impact on bone turnover and serum lipid profile in healthy postmenopausal women. J Bone Miner Res 1996;11:835–842.
30. Clarkson T, Anthony MS, Jerome CP. Lack of effect of raloxifene on coronary artery atherosclerosis of postmenopausal monkeys. J Clin Endocrinol Metab 1998;83:721–726.
31. Brinton LA, Hoover R, Fraumeni JF, et al. Menopausal oestrogens and breast cancer risk: An expanded case-control study. Br J Cancer 1986;54:825–832.
32. Ross RK, Paganini-Hill A, Gerkins VR, et al. A case control study of menopausal estrogen therapy and breast cancer. JAMA 1980;243:1635–1639.
33. Hoover R, Gray LA, Fraumeni JF. Stilbestrol and the risk of ovarian cancer. Lancet 1977;2:533.
34. Weiss NS, Lyon JL, Krishnamurthy S, et al. Noncontraceptive estrogen use and the occurrence of ovarian cancer. J Natl Cancer Inst 1982;68:95.
35. Kaufman DW, Kelly JP, Welch WR, et al. Noncontraceptive estrogen use and epithelial ovarian cancer. Am J Epidemiol 1989;130:1142.
36. Kaufman DW, Palmer JR, deMouzon J, et al. Estrogen replacement therapy therapy and the risk of breast cancer: Results from the case-control surveillance study. Am J Epidemiol 1991;134:137.
37. Wu ML, Whittemore AS, Paffenbarger RS, et al. Personal and environmental characteristics related to epithelial ovarian cancer, Part 1: Reproductive and menstrual events and oral contraceptive use. Am J Epidemiol 1988;128:1216.
38. Hartge P, Hoover R, McGowan L, et al. Menopause and ovarian cancer. Am J Epidemiol 1988;127:990.
39. Resta L, DeBenedictis G, Scordari MD, et al. Hyperplasia and metaplasia of ovarian surface epithelium in women with endometrial cancer: Suggestion for a hormonal influence in ovarian cancer. Am J Epidemiol 1983;117:128.
40. Eeles RA, Tan S, Wilshaw E, et al. Hormone replacement therapy and survival after surgery for ovarian cancer. BMJ 1991;302:259.
41. Creasman WT, Henderson D, Hinshaw W, et al. Estrogen replacement therapy in the patient treated for endometrial cancer. Obstet Gynecol 1986;67:326–330.
42. Lee RB, Burke TW, Park RC. Estrogen replacement therapy following treatment for stage I endometrial carcinoma. Gynecol Oncol 1990;36:189–191.
43. Morrow CP. Endometrial cancer. In: Morrow CP, Curtis JP, Townsend DS, eds. Synopsis of gynecologic oncology, 4th ed. New York: Churchill Livingstone, 1993:191–192.
44. Creasman WT. Estrogen replacement therapy: is previously treated cancer a contraindication? Obstet Gynecol 1991;77:308.
45. Baker DP. Estrogen replacement therapy in patients with previous endometrial carcinoma. Compr Ther 1990;16:28–35.
46. Bryant GW. Administration of estrogen to patients with a previous diagnosis of endometrial adenocarcinoma. South Med J 1990;83:725–726.
47. Barakat RR. The Creasman article reviewed. Oncology 1992;6:26.
48. Creasman WT. Recommendations regarding estrogen replacement therapy after treatment of endometrial cancer. Oncology 1992;6:23–26
49. Grodstein F, Stampfer MJ, Colditz GA, et al. Postmenopausal hormone therapy and mortality. N Engl J Med 1997;336:1769–1775.
50. The Writing Group for the PEPI Trial. Effects of estrogen or estrogen/progestin regimens on heart disease risk factors in postmenopausal women. JAMA 1995;273:199–208.
51. Meilahn EN, Kuller LH, Matthews KA, et al. Hemostatic factors according to menopausal status and use of hormone replacement therapy. Ann Epidemiol 1992:2;445–455.
52. Adams MR, Washburn SA, Wagner JD, et al. Arterial changes, estrogen defi-

ciency and effects of hormone replacement. In: Lobo RA, ed. *Treatment of the postmenopausal women: basic and clinical aspects.* New York: Raven Press, 1994.

53. Sarrel PM. Blood flow. In: Lobo RA, ed. *Treatment of the postmenopausal women: basic and clinical aspects.* New York: Raven Press, 1994.

54. Shoupe D, Brenner PF, Mishell DR. Menopause. In: Lobo RA, Mishell DR, Paulson RJ, Shoupe D, eds. *Mishell's textbook of infertility, contraception, and reproductive endocrinology.* Boston: Blackwell, 1997.

55. Rosenberg L, Hennekens CH, Rosner B, et al. Early menopause and the risk of myocardial infarction. *Am J Obstet Gynecol* 1981;139:47–51.

56. Falkeborn M, Pearsson I, Adami HO, et al. The risk of acute myocardial infarction after oestrogen and oestrogen-progestogen replacement. *Br J Obstet Gynaecol* 1992;99:821–828.

57. Sullivan JM, Vander-Zwagg R, Hughes JP, et al. Estrogen replacement and coronary artery disease: effect on survival in postmenopausal women. *Arch Intern Med* 1990;150:2557–2562.

58. Henderson BE, Paganini-Hill A, Ross RKL. Decreased mortality in users of esrogen replacement therapy. *Arch Intern Med* 1991;151:75–78.

59. Newton K, Newton M, Lacrois AZ, et al. Estrogen replacement therapy and prognosis after first myocardial infarction. *Am J Epidemiol* 1997;145:269–277.

60. Pfeffer RI, Kurosaki TT, Charlton SK. Estrogen use and blood pressure in later life. *Am J Epidemiol* 1979;110;469–478.

61. von Eiff AW, Piotz EJ, Beck KJ, Czernik A. The effects of estrogens and progestins on blood pressure regulation of normotensive women. *Am J Obstet Gynecol* 1971; 4:31–47.

62. Christiansen C, Christensen MS, Hagen C, et al. Effects of natural estrogen/gestagen and thiazide on coronary risk factors, in normal postmenopausal women. *Acta Obstet Gynecol Scand* 1981;60:407–412.

63. Lind T, Cameron EC, Hunter WM, et al. A prospective controlled trial of six forms of hormone replacment therapy given to postmenopausal women. *Br J Obstet Gynaecol* 1979;86(Suppl 3):1–29.

64. Perry I, Beever M, Beevers DG, Leusley D. Oestrogens and cardiovascular disease. *BMJ* 1988;297:1127.

65. Christiansen C, Christensen MS, Hagen C, et al. Effects of natural estrogen/gestagen and thiazide on coronary risk factors in normal postmenopausal women. *Acta Obstet Gynecol Scand* 1981;60:407–412.

66. Gyh Lip. Do clinicians prescribe HRT for hypertensive postmenopausal women? *Br J Clin Pract* 1995;49(2):61–64.

67. The fifth report of the Joint National Committee on Detection, Evaluation, and Treatment of High Blood Pressure. *Arch Intern Med* 1993;153:154–183.

68. de Lignieres B, Basdevant A, Thomas G, et al. Biological effects of estradiol-17β in postmenopausal women: Oral versus percutaneous administration. *J Clin Endocrinol Metab* 1986;62:536–541.

69. Wren BG, Troutledge AD. The effect of type and dose of oestrogen on the blood presssure of post-menopausal women. *Maturitas* 1983;5:135–142.

70. Miller VT, Muesing RA, LaRosa JC, Timmons MC. ERT. Weighing the risks and benefits. *Patient Care* 1990;24:30–48.

71. Nabulsi AA, Folsom AR, White A, et al. Association of hormone-replacement therapy with various cardiovascular risk factors in post-menopausal women. *N Engl J Med* 1993;328:1069–1075.

72. Luotola H, Pyorala T, Loikkanen M. Effects of natural oestrogen/progestogen substitution therapy on carbohydrate and lipid metabolism in post-menopausal women. *Maturitas* 1986;8:245–253.

73. Barrett-Connor E, Laasko M. Ischaemic Heart disease risk in postmenopausal women. Effects of estrogen use on glucose and insulin levels. *Arteriosclerosis* 1990;10:531–534.

74. Stevenson JC, Crook D, Godsland IF, Collins P, Whitehead MI. Hormone replacement therapy and the cardiovascular system. *Drugs* 1994;47(Suppl 2):35–41.

75. Brussard HE, Gevers, Leuven JA, Kluft C, Krans HMJ. Oestrogen replacement improves insulin response, lipoproteins and fibrinolysis in women with NIDDM. *Diabetologia* 1995;38:A25.

76. Cagnacci A, Soldani R, Carriero PL, et al. Effects of low doses of transdermal 17β-estradiol on carbohydrate metabolism in postmenopausal women. *J Clin Endocrinol Metab* 1992;74:1396–1400.

77. Bailey CJ, Ahmed-Sorour H. Role of ovarian hormone in the long-term control of glucose homeostasis: the effects on insulin secretion. *Diabetologia* 1980;19: 475–481.

78. Shi K, Mizuno A, Sano T, Ishida K, Shima K. Sexual differences in the incidence of diabetes mellitus in Otsuka-Long-Evans-Tokoshima fatty rats: effects of castration and sex-hormone replacement on its incidence. *Metabolism* 1994;43: 1214–1220.

79. Chetkowski RJ, Meldrum DR, Steingold KA, et al. Biologic effects of transdermal estradiol on carbohydrate metabolism in postmenopausal women. *J Clin Endocrinol Metab* 1992;74:1396–1400.

80. Stevenson JC, Crook D, Dodsland IF, et al. Oral versus transdermal hormone replacement therapy. *Int J Fertil* 1993;38S:30–35.

81. Crook D, Cust MP, Gangar KR, et al. Comparison of transdermal and oral estrogen-progestin replacemnt therapy: Effects on serum lipids and lipoproteins. *Am J Obstet Gynecol* 1993;166:950–955.

82. Walsh BW, Schiff I, Rosner B, et al. Effects of postmenopausal estrogen replacement on the concentrations and metabolism of plasma lipoproteins. *N Engl J Med* 1991;325:1196–1204.

83. Jick H, Derby LE, Myers MW, et al. Risk of hospital admission for idiopathic venous thromboembolism among users of postmenopausal oestrogens. *Lancet* 1996;348:981–983.

84. Grodstein F, Stampfer JM, Goldhaber SZ, et al. prospective study of exogenous hormones and risk of pumonary embolism in women. *Lancet* 1996;348:983–987.

85. Notelovitz M, Kitchens C, Ware M, et al. Combination estrogen and progestogen replacement therapy does not adversely affect coagulation. *Obstet Gynecol* 1983; 62:596–600.

86. Kaiser HJ, Meienberg O. Deterioration or onset of migraine under oestrogen replacement therapy in the menopause. *J Neurol* 1993;240:195–197.

87. Ferrari MD. Biochemistry of migraine. *Pathol Biol* 1992;40:287–292.

88. Welch KMA, Darnley D, Simkins RT. The role of estrogen in migraines: A review and hypothesis. *Cephalalgia* 1984;4:227–236.

89. Mattson RH, Rebar RW. Contraceptive methods for women with neruological disorders. *Am J Obstet Gynecol* 1993;168:2027–2032.

90. De Lignieres B, Vincens M, Mauvaia-Jarvis P, et al. Prevention of menstrual migraine by percutaneous oestradiol. *BMJ* 1986;293:1540.

91. Colditz DA, Hankinson SE, Hunter DJ, et al. The use of estrogens and progestins and the risk of breast cancer in postmenopausal women. *N Engl J Med* 1995;332: 1389.

92. Mohle-Beotani JC, Gorosser S, Whittemore AS, Malec M, Kampert JB, Paffenbarger RS Jr. Body, size, reproductive factors and breast cancer survival. *Prev Med* 1988;17:634–642.

93. Colditz G, Hankinson SE, Hunter DJ, et al. The use of estrogens and progestins and the risk of breast cancer in postmenopausal women. *N Engl J Med* 1995;332: 1589–1593.

Alternatives to Sex Steroid Therapy and Adjunctive Measures

In this section a number of "alternatives" will be considered for postmenopausal women. We designed this section to complement the section on lifestyle (Section VIII).

Expanding upon the data presented in Chapter 41 on "Complementary Medicine," Tom Clarkson and his colleagues provide a more in-depth look at considering phytoestrogens for therapy. They point out some of the areas (e.g., cognitive function) where we still have substantial gaps in our knowledge base. Next is a discussion about the possible uses of dehydroepiandrosterone (DHEA) by Peter Casson and John Buster. Apart from the consideration of using DHEA as an androgen, discussed earlier, they critically assess the use of DHEA for longevity and cardiovascular health, insulin resistance, and immune function. Bob Marcus and Andrew Hoffman next provide a summary of the potential uses of growth hormones (GH). Although GH therapy is attractive to consider for reversing some of the effects of old age, the data so far are not as promising. Changes in body habits do not appear to translate into improvements in muscle mass or strength. Next Ralf Zimmermann reviews the biology of melatonin—whether melatonin may be considered as an adjunct for sleep disorders and for mood alterations such as depression. The last chapter in this section is by Felicia Cosman and Bob Lindsay; they discuss the choice of selective estrogen receptor modulators (SERMs) as an alternative therapy. While SERMs do not provide relief from hot flushes and appear to have similar risks as oral estrogen in terms of venous thrombosis they provide an alternative for concerns such as osteoporosis. An attractive characteristic feature of SERMs is an inhibitory effect on breast tissue proliferation and therefore beneficial effect for breast cancer prevention. As pointed out, strong data are available for bone maintenance and osteoporosis but we need more data for cardiovascular effects as well as for cognitive function. Several newer SERMs will be available shortly. The most recent data on raloxifene was confirmatory of earlier reports. In the Multiple Outcomes of Raloxifene Evaluation (MORE) trial, venous thromboembolic disease was increased threefold, they did not increase uterine cancer risk and invasive breast cancers were decreased by 76% over the three years. This benefit, however, was confirmed to estrogen receptor positive tumors (1).

REFERENCE

1. Cummings SR, Eckert S, Krueger KA, et al. The effect of raloxifene on risk of breast cancer in postmenopausal women: results from the MORE randomized trial. Multiple Outcomes of Raloxifene Evaluation. *JAMA* 1999;281:2189–97.

Treatment of the Postmenopausal Woman: Basic and Clinical Aspects, Second Edition, edited by Rogerio A. Lobo, Lippincott Williams & Wilkins, Philadelphia © 1999.

CHAPTER 53

Clinical Efficacy of Phytoestrogens

Pharmacology and Biology

Thomas B. Clarkson, Mary S. Anthony, and J. Mark Cline

A large number of plants, primarily the legumes, contain compounds referred to as phytoestrogens (also called isoflavones) (1,2), which bind to the estrogen receptor and are generally weak agonists but may have both estrogen agonist and antagonist properties (3). Soybeans are a particularly rich source of phytoestrogens, containing 1 to 3 mg of phytoestrogens per gram of soy protein. The phytoestrogens of soybeans are genistein (4), daidzein (5), and glycitein (6,7). The molecular structures of soy phytoestrogens have some common features with 17β-estradiol (Fig. 53.1).

Coumestrol, another important phytoestrogen, is present in soybean sprouts (6) but in much higher amounts in alfalfa and clover sprouts (8). Among foods commonly consumed by human beings, mung bean sprouts contain particularly high concentrations of coumestrol (1 mg/100 g) (9). Coumestrol is a relatively rare component of human diets, is more estrogenic than genistein and daidzein, and its potential benefits for postmenopausal women have not been studied (9).

The classical estrogenic effects of the more potent phytoestrogens are well known from early reports of reproductive tract responses induced in domestic animals such as sheep (10) and subsequently in a variety of other species and laboratory rodents. An interesting aspect of early work with rodent models was the observation that phytoestrogens operated as both estrogen agonists and antagonists, depending on the presence of other estrogens (11). Previously, phytoestrogens were considered to be merely "weak estrogens" because their binding affinity for the estrogen receptor was considerably less than that of estradiol. Currently, with recent understanding of differences in estrogen

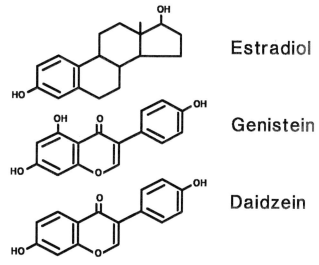

FIG. 53.1. Molecular structure of 17β-estradiol compared with genistein and daidzein.

receptors α and β, that view must be revised. Some phytoestrogens have relatively high affinity, relative to estradiol, for estrogen receptor β (12). The soy phytoestrogen genistein, for example, has a sixfold greater affinity for the ER-β relative to the ER-α. Given the different tissue distributions of the α and β forms of the receptor (12), there is the potential for tissue-selective effects of genistein.

Soy protein, isolated so as not to remove the phytoestrogens, usually contains about 1.2 mg/g protein as genistein, 0.5 mg/g protein as daidzein, and only small quantities of glycitein. These phytoestrogens occur in soybeans as conjugates, primarily β-glucosides, acetylglucosides, and malonylglucosides. Not all soy protein isolates contain phytoestrogens because some processes used to make the isolates use an alcohol extraction step, which removes the

T. B. Clarkson, M. S. Anthony, and J. M. Cline: Comparative Medicine Clinical Research Center, Wake Forest University School of Medicine, Winston-Salem, North Carolina 27157.

TABLE 53.1 *Genistein and daidzein concentrations of some foods (mg/100 g)*

Foods	Genistein	Daidzein
Soybean flour (Soyolk)	97	68
Kikkoman firm tofu	21	8
Nasoya soft tofu	19	7
Hatcho miso	15	14
Soy drink (Soy Alternative)	2	0.7
Soy-milk formula (Jevity Isotonic)	0.3	0.03
Sunflower seed	0.1	0.008
Chick peas	0.08	0.01
Mung bean sprouts	2	0.7
Chinese soy sauce	TR	0.02
Broccoli	0.007	0.005
Peanuts	0.08	0.05

Modified from ref. 9.

TABLE 53.2. *Characteristics of an ideal estrogen for postmenopausal replacement[a]*

	Ideal	CEE/ estradiol	Soy phytoestrogens
Bone	+	+	?
Lipoproteins	+	+	+
Coronary arteries	+	+	+
Brain	+	+	?
Breast	–	+	?
Endometrium	–	+	–
Genitourinary	+	+	?

[a]Estrogen action: +, agonist; –, antagonist; ?, unknown.

phytoestrogens (13). A summary of genistein and daidzein concentrations reported for some common foods is presented in Table 53.1. Most studies of soy phytoestrogen effects on postmenopausal women have used 50 to 90 mg of total isoflavones per day (14–19). Such doses are difficult to obtain in the usual daily diet of omnivores and so are generally provided in a soy protein isolate supplement.

BASIS FOR STUDIES OF THE POTENTIAL BENEFITS OF SOY PHYTOESTROGENS FOR POSTMENOPAUSAL HORMONE REPLACEMENT THERAPY

The major health benefits of current postmenopausal hormone replacement therapy (HRT) are widely recognized; however, despite the benefits, compliance is generally poor, about 20% (20). Lack of compliance with traditional HRT relates to the non-tissue-specific agonist properties of the currently used estrogens—conjugated equine estrogens (CEE) in the United States and 17β-estradiol (E2) in Europe. Although the estrogen agonist properties of CEE and E2 are beneficial for bones, brains (probably), lipoprotein metabolism, coronary arteries, and the genitourinary system, they have the disadvantage of also being estrogen agonists for breast and endometrium. The estrogen agonist properties of mammalian estrogens for breast appear to be associated with a relative risk for breast cancer of between 1.2 and 1.4 depending on the length of treatment (21,22). The estrogen agonist effects of the mammalian estrogens on the endometrium necessitate the use of a progestin to prevent endometrial cancer among women having a uterus. The progestin most commonly used in the United States is medroxyprogesterone acetate (MPA). Addition of MPA results in continued menstrual periods, depression, and mood swings (23,24). There is also growing evidence that MPA does not diminish, and may increase, the breast cancer risk associated with estrogen replacement therapy (25).

To be more acceptable to postmenopausal women, the HRT must have the benefits of traditional estrogens and

lack the potential for increasing risk for breast cancer or the necessity of administering a progestin to protect against endometrial cancer. In Table 53.2 are presented the characteristics of an ideal target-tissue-specific estrogen. The experimental evidence that soy phytoestrogens have some and lack some of these ideal characteristics are presented in this chapter.

METABOLISM OF SOY PHYTOESTROGENS

The origin, formation, and metabolism of phytoestrogens in animals (1,26) and man (27–29) have been the subject of review reports. There is a great deal of variability in the absorption and metabolism of the isoflavones in both human beings (30) and monkeys (unpublished data). In order for the isoflavones to be absorbed, the glycosylated forms of genistein and daidzein that are most common in soy foods must first be metabolized to aglycones during digestion (31). Gut bacteria can further metabolize these isoflavones to other estrogenic compounds that are also absorbed: daidzein to equol, dihydrodaidzein, and/or o-desmethylangolensin; genistein to 4-ethylphenol. However, there is evidence that only about two-thirds of human beings have the gut bacteria required to metabolize daidzein to equol (32). Although there is much *in vitro* evidence to suggest that genistein is the active isoflavone for chronic disease prevention (33–35), there are two studies that suggest that daidzein and/or its metabolites might be more effective (36,37). Hodgson and colleagues (37) found that equol and o-desmethylangolensin were more potent inhibitors of *in vitro* lipoprotein oxidation in serum than daidzein or genistein. We recently presented data suggesting an association between plasma concentrations of the metabolites of daidzein (equol, dihydrodaidzein, and o-desmethylangolensin) and plasma lipoprotein responses (Symposium on Phytoestrogen Research Methods, Tucson, AZ, September 21–24, 1997). There was no significant association between lipoprotein response and genistein concentrations. In order to establish an association between the isoflavone concentrations and beneficial health outcomes and to determine which of the isoflavones or its metabolites are most important, both the parent compounds (genistein, daidzein) and their metabolites (4-ethylphenol, equol, dihydrodaidzein, *o*-desmethyl-angolensin) must be measured in future research.

SOY PHYTOESTROGEN EFFECTS ON HOT FLUSHES

There are some epidemiologic data suggesting that diets rich in soybean estrogens (SBE) reduce the incidence of hot flushes. European women have about an 80% incidence of hot flushes, whereas women in China and Singapore (where consumption of SBE is high) have an incidence of about 20% (38). Murkies and colleagues (17) found that consumption of a dietary supplement containing soy flour reduced the incidence of hot flushes by about 40%. Burke et al. (15) have conducted a preliminary study in postmenopausal women comparing treatment with a soy isolate given either once a day or in a split dose twice a day. Once-daily treatment had no effect on hot flushes, but twice-daily treatment reduced the severity of hot flushes. Harding and collaborators (39) have reported a reduction in the number of hot flushes in postmenopausal women with severe vasomotor symptoms when they were treated with soy protein supplementation in a short-term, crossover design study. There are several longer-term clinical trials under way to further assess the effects of soy phytoestrogens on menopausal symptoms.

PHYTOESTROGEN EFFECTS ON POSTMENOPAUSAL BONE LOSS

The evidence concerning the effectiveness of soy protein and soy isoflavones on preservation of bone density is conflicting. Arjmandi et al. (40) evaluated the bone density of ovariectomized rats in which soy replaced casein in the diet (20% by weight) or that were treated with estradiol. The addition of soy inhibited bone loss, but not to the extent achieved with estradiol treatment (Fig. 53.2).

Blair et al. (41) reported on the effect of the soy phytoestrogen genistein in maintaining bone (measured as ash weights) of ovariectomized rats. In that study, bone ash weight for animals treated with the soy phytoestrogen genistein was found to be about 110% of that for ovariectomized controls. These same authors reported that genistein suppresses osteoclastic activity both *in vitro* and *in*

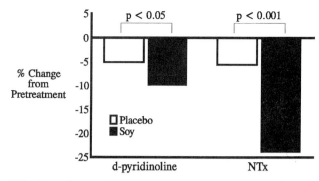

FIG. 53.3. Change from pretreatment in urinary concentrations of *d*-pyridinoline or cross-linked N-telopeptides (NTx) among women treated with casein (placebo) or with a phytoestrogen-containing soy isolate. (Modified from ref. 45.)

vivo. Soy phytoestrogens have been reported in an abstract to be equivalent to CEE in maintaining bone mass of ovariectomized rats (42).

Indirect evidence for bone protection by soy phytoestrogen comes from data reported on the use of ipriflavone (an isoflavonic derivative that is daidzein with an isopropyl group). Ipriflavone maintains bone density of premenopausal women being treated with GnRH agonists (43) and of postmenopausal women (44).

More direct evidence comes from a recent report by Bonaccorsi and his colleagues (45). They administered 60 g/day of a soy isolate containing 1.7 mg of phytoestrogens per gram to postmenopausal women and used 60 g/day of casein as the placebo. The effect on bone was evaluated using two biomarkers. A summary of their data is shown (Fig. 53.3).

In another short-term study (18), postmenopausal women were treated with 40 g of soy protein isolate with phytoestrogen doses of either 56 or 90 mg per woman per day for 6 months. A control group was treated with 40 g of casein protein with no phytoestrogens. Bone density was assessed by dual-energy x-ray absorptiometry. The higher-dose phytoestrogen group had significant increases in bone density compared to the casein group for the lumbar spine and similar trends at other skeletal sites.

We have found that soy phytoestrogens did not protect against bone loss among postmenopausal cynomolgus monkeys fed diets low in calcium (46). We shall seek a better understanding of the possible relationship between dose of soy phytoestrogens and measures of bone metabolism in the future.

CARDIOPROTECTIVE EFFECTS OF SOY PHYTOESTROGENS

Cardioprotective Components of Soy

Isoflavones (Phytoestrogens)

Recent studies have suggested that an alcohol-extractable component of soy protein lowers plasma cho-

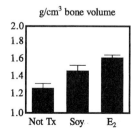

FIG. 53.2. Comparison of the effects of soy and estradiol on bone volume of ovariectomized rats. The data are means ± SE. (Modified from ref. 40.)

TABLE 53.3. *Effects of proteins and isoflavones on plasma lipoprotein concentrations in male and female cynomolgus monkeys[a]*

	Casein	Soy(−)	Soy(+)	Casein vs. Soy(−)	Casein vs. Soy(+)	Soy(−) vs. Soy(+)
					p Values	
LDL- and VLDL-cholesterol (mg/dL)						
Female	437 ± 24	403 ± 22	303 ± 23	0.31	0.0002	0.003
Male	417 ± 24	387 ± 22	250 ± 22	0.36	<0.0001	<0.0001
HDL-cholesterol (mg/dL)						
Female	42 ± 4	50 ± 3	62 ± 3	0.10	0.0001	0.008
Male	38 ± 3	46 ± 3	58 ± 3	0.03	<0.0001	0.002

[a]Means ± SEM; means are adjusted for baseline variable.
From ref. 51.

lesterol. Balmir et al. (47) fed one group of rats an alcohol extract of soy protein in a casein-based diet, and another group was fed the identical diet with casein as the source of protein but without the extract added. Low-density lipoprotein (LDL)-cholesterol concentrations were significantly lower in the group fed the diet with the alcohol-extractable soy components added. Sugano and Koba (48) found that a methanol-extracted soy fraction was not as effective as the unextracted fraction in maintaining low plasma cholesterol concentrations in rats.

Our own work further supports the hypothesis that soy isoflavones play a primary role in modulating plasma lipid and lipoprotein concentrations (49). In a crossover study in young rhesus monkeys, we fed diets containing soy protein isolate from which the isoflavones had been extracted with ethanol [Soy(−)] or with the isoflavones intact [Soy(+)] (isolates from Protein Technologies International, St. Louis, MO). We found that plasma LDL- plus very-low-density lipoprotein (VLDL)-cholesterol concentrations were significantly lower with the Soy(+) diet in both male and female subjects. Additionally, in the female monkeys, consumption of the Soy(+) diet resulted in significantly improved high-density lipoprotein (HDL)-cholesterol concentrations relative to when they were fed the Soy(−) diet.

This finding prompted us to examine the relative contributions of the soy protein amino acids and soy isoflavones and to extend the findings in the previous study to include atherosclerosis (50,51). We randomized 85 male and 75 female cynomolgus monkeys *(Macaca fascicularis)* into one of three treatment groups: (a) casein and lactalbumin as the source of protein (Casein), (b) the Soy(−) diet described above, and (c) the Soy(+) diet described above. All were fed the diets for 14 months, during which time cardiovascular disease risk factors, including plasma lipids, were measured.

The diets were identical in the percent of energy from protein (18.5%), fat (40.6%), and carbohydrate (40.9%) and had the same amount of cholesterol (0.31 mg/kcal). There were no isoflavones in the Casein diet, low levels (equivalent to 16 mg per person per day) in the Soy(−) diet,

and about tenfold higher amounts of isoflavones (equivalent to 143 mg per person per day) in the Soy(+) diet. These human equivalencies for isoflavone consumption are calculated assuming an average daily energy intake of 2,000 kcal based on averages for people in Western countries.

Plasma lipoprotein concentrations are shown in Table 53.3. Because monkeys have relatively low plasma triglyceride concentrations, the LDL- plus VLDL-cholesterol is nearly all in the LDL fraction. For both male and female monkeys, the group fed the Soy(−) diet had only slightly lower LDL- plus VLDL-cholesterol concentrations than the Casein group, but the group fed the Soy(+) diet had LDL- plus VLDL-cholesterol concentrations significantly lower than both the Soy(−) and Casein groups. There were also beneficial effects on HDL-cholesterol, as the Soy(−) group had higher HDL-cholesterol concentrations than the Casein group, and the Soy(+) group had the highest concentrations.

Peptides

Data from our monkey studies have provided evidence that soy protein or some peptide component of soy protein is necessary for the isoflavones to affect plasma lipoprotein concentrations.

Soy protein consists of discrete groups of peptides that can be separated on the basis of their molecular sizes by ultracentrifugation (52) or by gel filtration (53). Soy protein has four major peptide fractions that have been called 2S, 7S, 11S, and 15S on the basis of their sedimentation rates. The 2S fraction accounts for about 20% of the extractable protein. The 7S fraction accounts for about one-third of the extractable protein and is also called conglycinin. The 11S fraction, also called glycinin, accounts for about one-third of the protein. The 15S fraction accounts for about 10% of the protein. There are no data available to us about the isoflavone concentrations in the four peptide fractions (i.e., it is possible that the isoflavones are preferentially in one fraction or another). There is evidence from Sirtori's group that the 7S peptide is of particular importance in lipoprotein metabolic effects. Lovati et al. (54), using Hep-G2 cells in culture, found an upregulation of LDL receptor when the 7S globulin was added to the culture medium. In an earlier paper, Lovati and colleagues (55) provided evidence that the 11S globulin, compared to the 7S globulin, had a smaller effect on uptake and degradation of LDL by Hep-G2 cells, and the effect of 11S was not dose dependent. Sirtori et al. (56) extended these *in vitro* studies to *in vivo* studies with rats and reported that the 7S peptide reduced total plasma cholesterol concentrations by about 35%.

Another approach to the separation of soy peptides is by hydrolysis and separation into soluble and insoluble fractions. The soluble fraction markedly increases plasma cholesterol when fed to rats. The peptide fraction (the high-molecular-weight fraction, HMF) markedly lowers plasma cholesterol when fed to rats, and much of the effect seems to be through increasing the bile acid production and the binding of the bile salts to the HMF, thereby increasing bile acid excretion (57,58).

EFFECTS OF SOY PHYTOESTROGENS ON CARDIOVASCULAR RISK FACTORS AND THE CARDIOVASCULAR SYSTEM OF SURGICALLY POSTMENOPAUSAL MONKEYS

Plasma Lipoproteins

The effect of the SBE on plasma lipoprotein concentrations appears to be one of their most robust physiologic effects. We have reported on the effect of soy protein with its phytoestrogens removed and with soy protein containing its phytoestrogens on the plasma lipids and lipoproteins of premenopausal rhesus monkeys (49). The SBE decreased total plasma and LDL-C concentrations ($p = 0.009$ and 0.003, respectively) and increased HDL-C concentrations ($p = 0.05$). Plasma concentrations of Apo-A$_1$ were increased ($p = 0.04$) and Lp(a) decreased ($p = 0.03$). We also compared the effect of SBE and CEE for their effects on plasma lipoprotein concentrations of surgically postmenopausal cynomolgus monkeys (59). Table 53.4

summarizes the effects of the two estrogen replacement therapies after 12 months of treatment. Both CEE and SBE decreased plasma concentration of total cholesterol and low-density plus very-low-density cholesterol equivalently. The SBE increased high-density lipoprotein concentrations, but such an effect was not seen with CEE. Plasma triglyceride concentrations increased in response to CEE but not to SBE treatment. These effects are expressed as a percentage difference from the untreated control group.

Coronary Arteries

We have reported recently that soy isoflavones markedly reduce coronary artery atherosclerosis of male cynomolgus monkeys fed a moderately atherogenic diet (50). Data concerning CEE and soy isoflavone effects in postmenopausal monkeys are being collected currently. We have shown in previous studies that iliac arteries are good surrogates for coronary arteries. In our current CEE/soy isoflavone monkey study we determined the pretreatment atherosclerosis extent in one iliac artery and thus can now compare change in plaque size in the contralateral artery after treatment. Data are complete on only a portion of the cases, but a preliminary analysis of the data is shown in Fig. 53.4. The data suggest that SBE is equivalent to CEE in inhibiting atherosclerotic plaque progression.

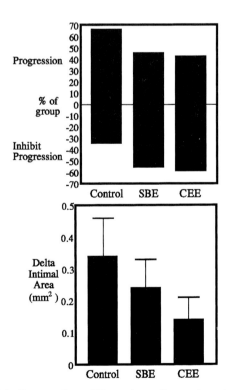

FIG. 53.4. Progression of iliac artery atherosclerosis in surgically postmenopausal female cynomolgus monkeys treated with alcohol-extracted soy protein [Soy(–)] ($n = 38$), intact soy protein (SBE, $n = 53$), or conjugated equine estrogens (CEE, $n = 38$). Modified from ref. 36.)

TABLE 53.4. *Effects of SBE and CEE on plasma lipids, lipoproteins, and apolipoproteins in postmenopausal cynomolgus monkeys*[a]

Variable	SBE	CEE	p Values: SBE vs. CEE
TPC	↓ 16%	↓ 17%	NS
Triglycerides	↓ 3%	↑ 73%	<0.0001
HDL-C	↑ 16%	↓ 11%	<0.0001
LDL + VLDL-C	↓ 22%	↓ 19%	NS
TPC:HDL-C	↓ 30%	↑ 2%	0.005
Lp(a)	↓ 8%	↓ 11%	NS
Apo-A1	↑ 14%	↓ 5%	0.0001

[a]Results are expressed as percent difference from the untreated control group.
Adapted from ref. 59.

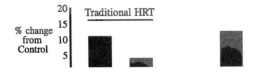

FIG. 53.5. Amount of coronary artery dilation measured during quantitative angiography of surgically postmenopausal cynomolgus monkeys treated with conjuncted equine estrogens (CEE), CEE plus medroxyprogesterone acetate (MPA), or premenopausal monkeys treated with soy phytoestrogens

Based on studies of coronary artery reactivity, soy isoflavones have estrogen-like effects on coronary arteries. We have studied the effects of SBE treatment, CEE treatment, and treatment with CEE plus MPA on the ability of female atherosclerotic cynomolgus monkeys to dilate their coronary arteries in response to perfusion with acetylcholine. We found that SBE treatment improved vascular reactivity relative to controls fed soy protein without phytoestrogens (60). The SBE treatment is equivalent to CEE treatment and is better than CEE plus MPA in modulating coronary artery dilation (Fig. 53.5) (61).

Results of these studies indicate that soy phytoestrogens have beneficial effects on coronary arteries and may be a useful therapeutic intervention for women at risk for CHD.

POTENTIAL OF SOY PHYTOESTROGENS FOR BREAST CANCER PROTECTION

There are several lines of evidence that support a causal relationship between soy phytoestrogens and cancer prevention. The first piece of evidence is derived from cross-cultural comparisons of cancer incidence (Fig. 53.6). The rates of breast cancer are lower in Japan, where soy is a staple of the diet, than in the United States, where very little soy is eaten (63). Migrant studies also support environmental factors, which likely includes diet, as

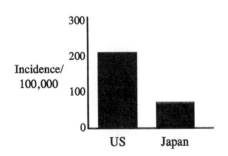

FIG. 53.6. Age-adjusted breast cancer incidence for women 35 to 74 years of age, expressed per 100,000 women, in the United States and Japan. (Modified from ref. 62.)

important in the pathogenesis of breast cancer because the rate of breast cancer increases among Japanese who emigrate to the United States (64,65). Although these comparisons do not directly implicate soy or its phytoestrogens, the data do support such an association.

A second line of evidence supporting a possible role for soy in breast cancer prevention is based on observational studies. From a review by Messina and colleagues (66) and five studies since then (65,67–70), there are seven studies that found significantly reduced risk of breast cancer with increasing soy consumption and two that found no significant association. The consistency of these findings supports a protective association. This association is stronger for premenopausal women than postmenopausal women; thus, a protective effect of soy phytoestrogens may be through a mechanism of antagonizing estrogenic effects (L. Kohlmeier, *personal communication*).

More convincing evidence for a phytoestrogen–cancer association is from animal studies. Barnes and colleagues (31) found a reduction in carcinogen-induced mammary tumor number and/or size among rats treated with soy protein isolate with the phytoestrogens intact compared to those fed the isolate from which the phytoestrogens had been extracted. Constantinou et al. (71) found that rats treated with purified genistein had reduced carcinogen-induced tumor multiplicity relative to vehicle-treated rats. Lamartiniere (72) found that rats treated neonatally with genistein were protected against carcinogen-induced mammary tumors later in life. A number of other studies in rodent models have recently been reviewed; the overwhelming weight of evidence is in favor of a breast-cancer protective effect (73,74).

In a recent study of hormone replacement therapy and its alternatives, adult, surgically postmenopausal female macaques *(Macaca fascicularis)* were treated continuously with either estradiol (E_2), isoflavone-containing soy isolate (SBE), or E_2 plus SBE (75). Doses were equivalent on a caloric basis to 1 mg/woman/day of micronized estradiol, and 129 mg/woman/day for soy isoflavones. After 6 months of replacement therapy, histopathologic, morphometric, and immunohistochemical measurements of mammary glands were done. A summary of the results of that study is presented in Fig. 53.7.

Estradiol treatment increased cell proliferation in both lobules and large ducts. The SBE treatment had no statistically significant effect on proliferation. Of particular importance was the finding that addition of SBE to the E_2 treatment markedly attenuated the E_2- induced proliferation.

The mechanisms by which phytoestrogens produce their breast cancer protective effects *in vivo* are still poorly understood. Despite the relatively large number of demographic, epidemiologic, and *in vivo* observations indicating a protective role of soy isoflavones against breast cancer, there is, in fact, some concern about the

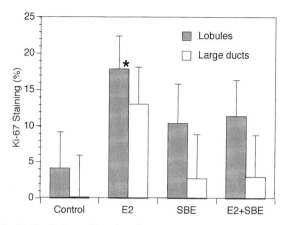

FIG. 53.7. Cell proliferation (as percentage of cells stained with the marker Ki-67) in mammary gland tissues of surgically postmenopausal cynomolgus monkeys given no treatment (control) or treated with estradiol (E₂), soybean phytoestrogens (SBE), or E₂ plus SBE. *$p < 0.05$ compared with untreated control monkeys. (From ref. 75.)

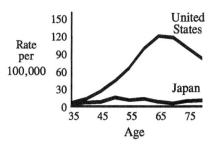

FIG. 53.8. Age-specific endometrial cancer incidence in women in the United States and Japan. (Modified from ref. 63.)

ENDOMETRIAL EFFECTS OF THE SOY PHYTOESTROGENS

Both cross-cultural and experimental data tend to support the conclusion that the soy phytoestrogens, at reasonable doses (less than 200 mg/day), do not have endometrial estrogen agonist effects and, to the contrary, are endometrial estrogen antagonists. The cross-cultural data relate to the low rates of endometrial cancer among Japanese women consuming their native diet (Fig. 53.8).

The experimental data come from a recent study of hormonal replacement therapy and its alternatives. Adult, surgically postmenopausal female macaques *(Macaca fascicularis)* were treated continuously with either estradiol (E₂), isoflavone-containing soy isolate (SBE), or E₂ plus SBE. Doses were equivalent on a caloric basis to 1 mg/woman/day for estradiol and 129 mg/woman/day for soy isoflavones. After 6 months of replacement therapy, histopathologic, morphometric, and immunohistochemical measurements of endometrium and mammary glands were done.

Increases in endometrial thickness, gland area, and epithelial proliferation were induced by E₂ and E 2-SBE.

potential for phytoestrogens to act as breast cancer promoters. This concern is based primarily on *in vitro* studies of breast cancer cells (76) as well as yet unpublished studies of tumor cells injected into nude mice (W. Helferich, *personal communications*). These studies have shown evidence that phytoestrogens can augment, rather than inhibit, estrogen-stimulated cell growth (77). By design, these studies circumvent the carcinogenic process (i.e., the cells are cancerous at the outset of the study) and do not account for the complex interplay of endocrine and paracrine effects operative in the normal breast. Of additional concern are the limited observations of Petrakis et al. (78) and McMichael-Phillips et al. (16), which indicate that breast cell proliferation may increase in women consuming soy isolates. However, phytoestrogens also have other actions that may play an important role in their cancer-preventive effect, such as inhibition of steroid-hormone-metabolizing enzymes (79) and tyrosine protein kinases (80). Isoflavones inhibit cell proliferation in estrogen receptor (ER)-negative as well as ER-positive breast cancer cell lines (81), suggesting that they have actions that are independent of their estrogenicity. Genistein inhibits the formation of free radicals thought to be important in mutagenesis and tumor promotion (35). Soy isoflavones also may have antiangiogenic effects, which may impede tumor progression (82). We believe that the preponderance of data indicates a lack of traditional estrogenicity of soy isoflavones in the breast and a well-documented anticarcinogenic effect. However, physicians should maintain some concern about potential risks, and future studies should include ascertaining the effects of isoflavones on the breast at a variety of doses, from levels attainable in the Western diet (30 mg/day) to levels approximately five times those seen in an Asian diet (i.e., 480 mg).

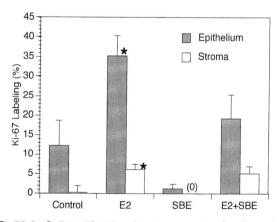

FIG. 53.9. Cell proliferation (as percentage of cells stained with the marker Ki-67) in endometrial tissues of surgically postmenopausal cynomolgus monkeys given no treatment (control) or treated with estradiol (E₂), soybean phytoestrogens (SBE), or E₂ plus SBE. *$p < 0.05$ compared with untreated control monkeys. (From ref. 75.)

Morphometric changes were accompanied by increased epithelial expression of the proliferation marker Ki-67. The effects of E₂ were antagonized by the addition of SBE, as indicated by decreased Ki-67 staining (Fig. 53.9). Progesterone receptor (PR) expression was induced by E₂ but not by SBE, indicating lack of a classical estrogenic effect; the induction of PR was also antagonized by SBE in the E₂ plus SBE group. Effects on induction of estrogen receptor were similar but did not achieve statistical significance.

Although a clinical study has not yet been done, the evidence suggest the possibility that soy phytoestrogens could be used as a progestin to protect the endometrium from low doses of mammalian estrogen. Such combined use of mammalian and soy estrogens might maximize cardiovascular benefit and bone protection and at the same time provide protection for both breast and uterus.

EFFECTS OF SOY PHYTOESTROGENS ON BRAIN AND COGNITIVE FUNCTION

Evidence is increasing that treatment of postmenopausal women with mammalian estrogens favorably influences both memory and cognitive function (83,84). Although the mechanisms remain uncertain, it likely has to do with the effect of estrogen treatment on synaptic plasticity (85), the regulation of dendritic spine densities (86), and the regulation of relative levels of choline acetyltransferase and neurotropic factors (87).

Data are sparse concerning whether soy isoflavones have either estrogen agonist or antagonist effects on brain. Two preliminary observational reports have prompted us to address the issue actively. In a report from the Honolulu-Asia Aging Study, an association was reported between consistently high levels of tofu consumption in midlife of men and low cognitive test scores ($p = 0.02$) (88). Rice and co-workers (89) studied Japanese-American women living in King County, Washington. The subjects were 65 years or older and were participants in a population-based study of aging and memory. Estrogen users consuming tofu less than three times per week were less likely to be cognitively impaired than were estrogen nonusers. On the other hand, estrogen users consuming tofu more than three times per week were not protected from cognitive impairment. Although both studies may be confounded in ways not yet clear, they do provide concerns that should be addressed in future human and animal studies.

Murphy and Segal (90) have reported on the effect of genistein alone and combinations of estradiol and genistein on the dendritic spine density of cultured rat hippocampal neurons. The addition of estrogen to the cultured hippocampal neurons markedly increased dendritic spine density. That the system could measure an estrogen antagonist effect is shown by the inhibition by tamoxifen of estrogen-induced dendritic spines. In their system genistein was neither an estrogen agonist nor did it antagonize the estrogen effect.

We have used surgically postmenopausal retired breeder rats to compare the effects of estradiol and purified soy phytoestrogens on molecular processes important in cognition. We have chosen to measure mRNA for choline acetyltransferase (ChAT) and brain-derived neurotropic factor (BDNF), two factors believed to play an important role in protection of cholinergic neurons that are essential for learning and memory (87,91,92). In this experiment we treated retired breeder rats with either oral estradiol, soy phytoestrogens, or no hormone replacement for 8 weeks. Both estradiol and the soy phytoestrogens upregulated the message for BDNF and ChAT. The soy phytoestrogen effects were as pronounced as those of estradiol.

SUMMARY

Although there are considerable cross-cultural and observational data that support the hypothesis that soy phytoestrogens might be a viable alternative to traditional hormone replacement therapy for some women, the more conclusive experimental data are just beginning to be available. However, before soy phytoestrogens are used widely for postmenopausal hormone replacement, there are a number of unanswered questions that require investigation. We have summarized what is currently known and some unanswered questions below.

Cardiovascular Effects

Both observational and experimental data are reassuring that soy with its phytoestrogens is likely to provide postmenopausal cardioprotection. There are data in both animals and human beings that show beneficial effects on plasma lipids and lipoproteins. In addition, data from animal studies have shown inhibition of atherosclerosis progression.

Endometrial Effects

Data from both cross-cultural and experimental studies support the conclusion that soy phytoestrogens, at doses less than about 200 mg/day, do not have adverse proliferative effects on the endometrium. There are some data from nonhuman primates that suggest it may serve as an estrogen antagonist at usual estrogen replacement doses. However, there are, as yet, no data in women supporting this latter effect.

Dose and Form of Soy Phytoestrogens

The optimum dose of soy phytoestrogens for any postmenopausal outcome has not been determined. Neither has the question of whether purified soy isoflavones are active in the absence of some amount of soy protein.

Putative Breast Cancer Protective Effect of Soy Phytoestrogens

Although observational studies and experimental data provide evidence of a breast cancer protective effect of soy phytoestrogens, a few studies are not consistent with that conclusion. Future studies must actively seek to clarify their putative protective effect.

Postmenopausal Bone Loss

Because surgically postmenopausal monkeys treated with the equivalent of a woman's dose of 120 mg of soy isoflavones do not have bone protection, it is uncertain whether the rodent studies can be generalized to women. There are two preliminary reports in postmenopausal women that suggest a beneficial effect of soy protein supplementation. However, both studies were relatively short term.

Hot Flushes

It remains unclear what the effect of soy phytoestrogens is on hot flushes and whether there is a safe dose that is also effective for this symptom.

Genitourinary Function

There are no data that would lead one to assume a beneficial effect of soy phytoestrogens on postmenopausal genitourinary function.

Brain and Cognitive Function

Of utmost importance is the need for a clear understanding of whether soy phytoestrogens have beneficial or deleterious effects for preserving cognitive function and preventing Alzheimer's disease.

REFERENCES

1. Price KR, Fenwick GR. Naturally occurring oestrogens in foods—a review. *Food Addict Contam* 1985;2:73–106.
2. Reinli K, Block G. Phytoestrogen content of foods—a compendium of literature values. *Nutr Cancer* 1996;26:123–148.
3. Markiewicz L, Garey J, Adlercreutz H, Gurpide E. *In vitro* bioassays of nonsteroidal phytoestrogens. *J Steroid Biochem Mol Biol* 1993;45:399–405.
4. Walter ED. Genistin (an isoflavone glucoside) and its aglucone, genistein, from soybeans. *J Am Chem Soc* 1941;63:3273–3276.
5. Eldridge A, Kwolek WF. Soybean isoflavones: effect of environment and variety on composition. *J Agr Food Chem* 1983;31:394–396.
6. Naim M, Gestetner B, Kirson I, Birk Y, Bondi A. A new isoflavone from soy beans. *Phytochemisty* 1973;22:237–239.
7. Kuduo S, Shimoyamada M, Imura T, Uchida T, Okubo K. A new isoflavone glycoside in soybean seeds (Glycine Max Merrill), glycetin 7-0-D-(6"-0-acetyl)-glucopyranoside. *Agr Biol Chem* 1991;55:859–860.
8. Franke AA, Custer LJ, Cerna CM, Narala KK. Quantitation of phytoestrogens in legumes by HPLC. *J Agr Food Chem* 1994;42:1905–1913.
9. Adlercreutz H, Mazur W. Phyto-oestrogens and western diseases. *Ann Med* 1997;29:95–120.
10. Lindner HR. Occurrence of anabolic agents in plants and their importance. *Environ Qual Safety Suppl* 1976;5:151–158.
11. Folman Y, Pope GS. The interaction in the immature mouse of potent oestrogens with coumestrol, genistein and other utero-vaginotrophic compounds of low potency. *J Endocrinol* 1966;34:215–225.
12. Kuiper GGJM, Carlson B, Grandien K, et al. Comparison of the ligand binding specificity and transcript tissue distribution of estrogen receptors α and β. *Endocrinology* 1997;138:863–870.
13. Anderson RL, Wolf WJ. Compositional changes in trypsin inhibitors, phytic acid, saponins and isoflavones related to soybean processing. *J Nutr [Suppl]* 1995;125:581S–588S.
14. Baird DD, Umbach DM, Lansdell L, et al. Dietary intervention study to assess estrogenicity of dietary soy among postmenopausal women. *J Clin Endocrinol Metab* 1995;80:1685–1690.
15. Burke GL, Hughes CL, Anthony MS. The potential use of a dietary soy supplement as a post-menopausal hormone replacement therapy. *Am J Clin Nutr* (in press).
16. McMichael-Phillips DF, Harding C, Morton M, et al. Effects of soy protein supplementation on epithelial proliferation in the normal human breast. *Am J Clin Nutr* 1998;68(Suppl 6):1431S–1435S.
17. Murkies AL, Lombard C, Strauss BJG, Wilcox G, Burger HG, Morton MS. Dietary flour supplementation decreases post-menopausal hot flushes: Effect of soy and wheat. *Maturitas* 1995;21:189–195.
18. Potter SM, Baum JA, Teng H, Stillman RJ, Erdman JW Jr. Soy protein and isoflavones: their effects on blood lipids and bone density in postmenopausal women. *Am J Clin Nutr* 1998;68(Suppl 6):1375S–1379S.
19. Wilcox G, Wahlqvist ML, Burger HG, Medley G. Oestrogenic effects of plant foods in postmenopausal women. *BMJ* 1990;301:905–906.
20. Brett KM, Madans JH. Use of postmenopausal hormone replacement therapy: estimates from a nationally representative cohort study. *Am J Epidemiol* 1997;145:536–545.
21. Colditz GA, Egan KM, Stampfer MJ. Hormone replacement therapy and risk of breast cancer: Results from epidemiologic trials. *Am J Obstet Gynecol* 1993;168:1473–1480.
22. Collaborative Group on Hormonal Factors in Breast Cancer. Breast cancer and hormone replacement therapy: collaborative reanalysis of data from 51 epidemiological studies of 52,705 women with breast cancer and 108,411 women without breast cancer. *Lancet* 1997;350:1047–1059.
23. Ravnikar VA. Compliance with hormone therapy. *Am J Obstet Gynecol* 1987;156:1332.
24. Ravnikar VA. Compliance with hormone replacement therapy: Are women receiving the full impact of hormone replacement therapy's preventive health benefits? *Women's Health Issues* 1992;2:75–82.
25. Colditz GA, Hankinson SE, Hunter DJ, et al. The use of estrogens and progestins and the risk of breast cancer in postmenopausal women. *N Engl J Med* 1995;332:1589–1593.
26. Müller H-M, Hofman J, Mayr U. Stoffwechsel und Wirkung von Phytoöstrogenen beim Tier. *Übers Tierernährg* 1989;17:47–84.
27. Adlercreutz H. Lignans and phytoestrogens. Possible preventive role in cancer. In: Horwitz C, Rozen P, eds. *Progress in diet and nutrition*. Basel: S. Karger, 1988:165–176.
28. Setchell KDR, Adlercreutz H. Mammalian lignans and phyto-oestrogens. Recent studies on their formation, metabolism and biological role in health and disease. In: Rowland I, ed. *Role of the gut flora in toxicity and cancer*. London: Academic Press, 1988:315–345.
29. Adlercreutz H, Mousavi Y, Loukovaara M, Hämäläinen E. Lignans, isoflavones, sex hormone metabolism and breast cancer. In: Hochberg R, Naftolin F, eds. *The new biology of steroid hormones. Serono Symposia publications from Raven Press, Vol 74*. New York: Raven Press, 1991.
30. Xu X, Harris KS, Wang H-J, Murphy PA, Hendrich S. Bioavailability of soybean isoflavones depends upon gut microflora in women. *J Nutr* 1995;125:2307–2315.
31. Barnes S, Kirk M, Coward L. Isoflavones and their conjugates in soy foods: Extraction conditions and analysis by HPLC-mass spectrometry. *J Agric Food Chem* 1994;42:2466–2474.
32. Cassidy A, Bingham S, Setchell KDR. Biological effects of a diet of soy protein rich in isoflavones on the menstrual cycle of permenopausal women. *Am J Clin Nutr* 1994;60:333–340.
33. Barnes S, Peterson TG, Coward L. Rationale for the use of genistein-containing soy matrices in chemoprevention trials for breast and prostate cancer. *J Cell Biochem* 1995;Suppl 22:181–187.
34. Shimokado K, Umezawa K, Ogata J. Tyronsine kinase inhibitors inhibit multiple steps of the cell cycle of vascular smooth muscle cells. *Exp Cell Res* 1995;220:266–273.
35. Wei H, Bowen T, Cai Q, Barnes S, Wang Y. Antioxidant and antipromotional effects of the soybean isoflavone genistein. *Proc Soc Exp Biol Med* 1995;208:124–130.
36. Anthony MS, Clarkson TB. Comparison of soy phytoestrogens and conjugated equine estrogens on atherosclerosis progression in postmenopausal monkeys. *Circulation* (in press).
37. Hodgson JM, Croft KD, Puddey IB, et al. Soybean isoflavonoids and their metabolic products inhibit *in vitro* lipoprotein oxidation in serum. *J Nutr Biochem* 1996;7:664–669.
38. Tang GWK. The climacteric of Chinese factory workers. *Maturitas* 1994;19:177–182.
39. Harding C, Morton M, Gould V, McMichael-Phillips D, Howell A, Bundred NJ. Dietary soy supplementation is oestrogenic in menopausal women. *Am J Clin Nutr* (in press).
40. Arjmandi BH, Alekel L, Hollis BW, et al. Dietary soybean protein prevents bone loss in an ovariectomized rat model of osteoporosis. *J Nutr* 1996;126:161–167.

41. Blair HC, Jordan SE, Peterson TG, Barnes S. Variable effects of tyrosine kinase inhibitors on avian osteoclastic activity and reduction of bone loss in ovariectomized rats. *J Cell Biochem* 1996;61:629–637.

42. Anderson JJ, Ambrose WW, Garner SC. Orally dosed genistein from soy and prevention of cancellous bone loss in two ovariectomized rat models. *J Nutr* 1995;125:799S.

43. Gambacciani M, Spinetti A, Piaggesi L, et al. Ipriflavone prevents the bone mass reduction in premenopausal women treated with gonadotropin hormone-releasing hormone agonists. *Bone Miner* 1994;26:19–26.

44. Valente M, Bufalino L, Castigloione GN, et al. Effects of 1-year treatment with ipriflavone on bone in postmenopausal women with low bone mass. *Calcif Tissue Int* 1994;54:377–380.

45. Bonaccorsi G, Albertazzi P, Costantino D, et al. Soy phytoestrogens and bone. *North Am Menopause Soc Meetings* 1997:44.

46. Jayo MJ, Anthony MS, Register TC, Rankin SE, Vest T, Clarkson TB. Dietary soy isoflavones and bone loss: A study in ovariectomized monkeys. *J Bone Miner Res* 1996;11(Suppl 1):S228.

47. Balmir F, Staack R, Jeffrey E, et al. An extract of soy flour influences serum cholesterol and thyroid hormones in rats and hamsters. *J Nutr* 1996;126:3046–3053.

48. Sugano M, Koba K. Dietary protein and lipid metabolism: a multifunctional effect. *Ann NY Acad Sci* 1993;676:215–222.

49. Anthony MS, Clarkson TB, Hughes CL Jr, Morgan TM, Burke GL. Soybean isoflavones improve cardiovascular risk factors without affecting the reproductive system of peripubertal rhesus monkeys. *J Nutr* 1996;126:43–50.

50. Anthony MS, Clarkson TB, Bullock BC, Wagner JD. Soy protein versus soy phytoestrogens in the prevention of diet-induced coronary artery atherosclerosis of male cynomolgus monkeys. *Arterioscler Thromb Vasc Biol* 1997;17:2524–2531.

51. Anthony MS, Clarkson TB, Williams JK. Effect of soy isoflavones on atherosclerosis potential mechanisms. *Am J Clin Nutr* 1998;68(Suppl 6):1390S–1393S.

52. Naismith WEF. Ultracentrifuge studies on soya bean protein. *Biochim Biophys Acta* 1955;16:203–210.

53. Hasegawa K, Kusano T, Mitsuda H. Fractomation of soybean protein by gel filtration. *Agric Biol Chem* 1963;27:878–890.

54. Lovati MR, Manzoni C, Corsini A, Granata A, Fumagalli R, Sirtori CR. 7S globulin from soybean is metabolized in human cell culures by a specific uptake and degradation system. *J Nutr* 1996;126:2831–2842.

55. Lovati MR, Manzoni C, Corsini A, et al. Low density lipoprotein receptor activity is modulated by soybean globulins in cell culture. *J Nutr* 1992;122:1971–1978.

56. Sirtori CR, Even R, Lovati MR. Soybean protein diet and plasma cholesterol: from therapy to molecular mechanisms. *Ann NY Acad Sci* 1993;676:188–201.

57. Sugano M, Yamada Y, Yoshida K, Hashimoto Y, Matsuo T, Kimoto M. The hypocholesterolemic action of the undigested fraction of soybean protein in rats. *Atherosclerosis* 1988;72:115–122.

58. Sugano M, Goto S, Yamada Y, et al. Cholesterol-lowering activity of various undigested fractions of soybean protein in rats. *J Nutr* 1990;120:977–985.

59. Anthony MS, Clarkson TB, Hughes CL. Plant and mammalian estrogen effects on plasma lipids of female monkeys. *Circulation* 1994;90:I-235.

60. Honoré EK, Williams JK, Anthony MS, Clarkson TB. Soy isoflavones enhance coronary vascular reactivity in atherosclerotic female macaques. *Fertil Steril* 1997;67:148–154.

61. Williams JK, Honoré EK, Washburn SA, Clarkson TB. Effects of hormone replacement therapy on reactivity of atherosclerotic coronary arteries in cynomolgus monkeys. *J Am Coll Cardiol* 1994;24:1757–1761.

62. Ursin G, Bernstein L, Pike MC. Breast cancer. In: Doll R, Fraumeni JF, Muir CS, eds. *Trends in cancer incidence and mortality, Vol 19/20.* Plainview, NY: Cold Spring Harbor Laboratory Press, 1994:241–264.

63. Parkin DM, Muir CS, Whelan SL, Gao YT, Ferlay J, Powell J. *IARC scientific publication no. 120: cancer incidence in five continents.* VI. Lyon: International Agency for Research on Cancer, 1992.

64. Shimizu H, Ross RK, Bernstein L, Yatani R, Henderson BE, Mack TM. Cancers of the prostate and breast among Japanese and white immigrants in Los Angeles County. *Br J Cancer* 1991;63:963–966.

65. Wu AH, Ziegler RG, Horn-Ross PL, et al. Tofu and risk of breast cancer in Asian-Americans. *Cancer Epidemiol Biomarkers Rev* 1996;5:901–906.

66. Messina MJ, Persky V, Setchell KDR, Barnes S. Soy intake and cancer risk: a review of the *in vitro* and *in vivo* data. *Nutr Cancer* 1994;21:113–131.

67. Hirose K, Tajima K, Hamajima N, et al. A large-scale, hospital-based case-control study of risk factors of breast cancers according to menopausal status. *Jpn J Cancer Res* 1995;86:146–154.

68. Yuan J-M, Wang Q-S, Ross RK, Henderson BE, Yu MC. Diet and breast cancer in Shanghai and Tianjin, China. *Br J Cancer* 1995;71:1353–1358.

69. Ingram D, Sanders K, Kolybaba M, Lopez D. Case-control study of phyto-oestrogens and breast cancer. *Lancet* 1997;350:990–994.

70. Greenstein J, Kushi L, Zheng W, et al. Risk of breast cancer associated with intake of specific foods and food groups. *Am J Epidemiol* 1996;144:S36.

71. Constantinou AI, Mehta RG, Vaughan A. Inhibition of N-methyl-N-nitrosourea-induced mammary tumors in rats by the soybean isoflavones. *Anticancer Res* 1996;16:3293–3298.

72. Lamartiniere CA, Moore J, Holland M, Barnes S. Neonatal genistein chemoprevents mammary cancer. *Proc Soc Exp Biol Med* 1995;208:120–123.

73. Barnes S. Effect of genistein on *in vitro* and *in vivo* models of cancer. *J Nutr* 1995;125:777S–783S.

74. Hawrylewicz EJ, Zapata JJ, Blair WH. Soy and experimental cancer: animal studies. *J Nutr* 1995;125:698S–708S.

75. Foth D, Cline JM. Effect of mammalian and plant estrogens, tamoxifen, and medroxyprogesterone acetate on epithelial proliferation in the mammary glands and uteri of macaques. *Am J Clin Nutr* 1998;68(Suppl 6):1413S–1417S.

76. Mäkelä S, Davis VL, Tally WC, et al. Dietary estrogens act through estrogen receptor-mediated processes and show no antiestrogenicity in cultured breast cancer cells. *Environ Health Perspect* 1994;102:572–578.

77. Mäkelä S, Poutanen M, Lehtimaki J, Kostian ML, Santti R, Vihko R. Estrogen-specific 17 β-hydroxysteroid oxidoreductase type 1 (E.C. 1.1.1.62) as a possible target for the action of phytoestrogens. *Proc Soc Exp Biol Med* 1995;208:51–59.

78. Petrakis NL, Barnes S, King EB, et al. Stimulatory influence of soy protein isolate on breast secretion in pre- and postmenopausal women. *Cancer Epidemiol Biomarkers Prev* 1996;5:785–794.

79. Baker ME. Origins of regulation of gene transcription by steroid, retinoid and thyroid hormones. In: Hochberg RB, Naftolin F, eds. *The new biology of steroid hormones.* New York: Raven Press, 1991:187–202.

80. Akiyama T, Ishida JSN, Ogawara H, et al. Genistein, a specific inhibitor of tyrosine-specific protein kinases. *J Biol Chem* 1987;262:5592–5595.

81. Peterson G, Barnes S. Genistein inhibition of the growth of human breast cancer cells: independence from estrogen receptors and the multi-drug resistance gene. *Biochem Biophys Res Commun* 1991;179:661–667.

82. Fotsis T, Pepper M, Adlercreutz H, Hase T, Montesano R, Schweigerer L. Genistein, a dietary ingested isoflavonoid, inhibits cell proliferation and *in vitro* angiogenesis. *J Nutr* 1995;125:790S–797S.

83. Sherwin BB. Estrogenic effects on memory in women. *Ann NY Acad Sci* 1994;743:213–231.

84. Sherwin BB. Hormones, mood and cognitive functioning in postmenopausal women. *Obstet Gynecol* 1996;87:20S–26S.

85. Naftolin F, Leranth C, Perez J, Garcia-Segura LM. Estrogen induces synaptic plasticity in adult primate neurons. *Neuroendocrinology* 1993;57:935–939.

86. Woolley CS, McEwen BS. Estradiol regulates hippocampal dendritic spine density via an N-methyl-D-aspartate receptor-dependent mechanism. *J Neurosci* 1994;14:7680–7687.

87. Gibbs RB, Wu D, Hersh LB, Pfaff DW. Effects of estrogen replacement on the relative levels of choline acetyltransferase, *trkA* and nerve growth factor messenger RNAs in the basal forebrain and hippocampal formation of adult rats. *Exp Neurol* 1994;129:70–80.

88. White L, Petrovitch H, Ross GW, Masaki K. Association of mid-life consumption of tofu with late life cognitive impairment and dementia: the Honolulu-Asia Aging Study. *Neurobiol Aging* 1996;S17:5121.

89. Rice MM, Graves AB, Larson EB. Estrogen replacement therapy and cognition: role of phytoestrogens. *Gerontologist* 1995;35:169.

90. Murphy DD, Segal M. Regulation of dendritic spine density in cultured rat hippocampal neurons by steroid hormones. *J Neurosci* 1996;16:4059–4068.

91. Lapchak PA. Nerve growth factor pharmacology: application to the treatment of cholinergic neurodegeneration in Alzheimer's disease. *Exp Neurol* 1993;124:16–20.

92. Singh M, Meyer EM, Millard WJ, Simpkins JW. Ovarian steroid deprivation results in a reversible learning impairment and compromised cholinergic function in female Sprague-Dawley rats. *Brain Res* 1994;644:305–312.

Treatment of the Postmenopausal Woman: Basic and Clinical Aspects, Second Edition, edited by Rogerio A. Lobo, Lippincott Williams & Wilkins, Philadelphia © 1999.

CHAPTER 54

Alternative Therapy

Dehydroepiandrosterone Replacement in the Menopause

Peter R. Casson and John E. Buster

In adults, dehydroepiandrosterone (DHEA) and dehydroepiandrosterone sulfate (DHEA-S) collectively circulate in levels far exceeding those of any other steroid (1). These hormones are secreted almost exclusively by the reticularis zone of the adrenal cortex (2). Dehydroepiandrosterone sulfate levels are high in fetal life, drop precipitously with birth, remain negligible in childhood, and then climb at 6 to 8 years, reaching peak levels in the third decade of life. This peripubertal increase in adrenal androgens, termed "adrenarche," occurs concurrent with growth of the adrenal zona reticularis (3). Subsequently, DHEA-S levels decline markedly with age (Fig. 54.1); in the elderly, they are about 10% to 20% of the reproductive age peak (4). This decline is sometimes called "adrenopause" and occurs concurrent with involution of the zona reticularis (Fig. 54.1) (5). This fluctuating pattern of adrenal androgen secretion is unique to humans and certain primates (6).

Is adrenopause simply an epiphenomenon of aging, or is it a true senescent endocrine deficiency state of aging similar to menopause? If the latter situation is true, restitution of the physiologic adrenal androgen milieu of the early reproductive years in elderly individuals may very well have salutary effects. These questions have only recently come to the fore in the scientific community but are now the subject of active investigation in numerous centers around the world. However, there is much lay speculation about DHEA, and it is now widely touted in the mass media as a panacea for aging. Although not present in foodstuffs, DHEA is considered a "food supplement"; it is thus exempt from FDA regulation. A large and well-organized nutritional supplement industry widely markets this compound for a multitude of presumed indi-

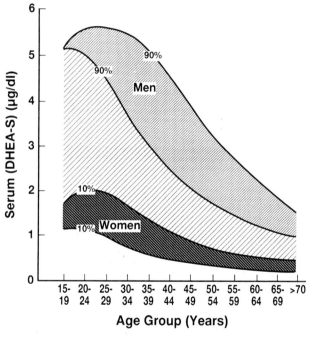

FIG. 54.1. The decline in serum DHEA-S with advancing age in men and women. (From ref. 4.)

cations. This has led to widespread and unregulated use of varying dosages and preparations of this potent oral steroid, a sure recipe for disaster.

Interest in DHEA replacement germinated with animal studies indicating it may have antioncogenic, cardioprotective, antiobesity, insulin sensitizing, antiosteoporotic, immune, and cognitive enhancing properties. Unfortunately, extrapolation of these results to humans is limited, as the animal models used have negligible endogenous adrenal androgen levels, and the DHEA doses used were extremely supraphysiologic. Thus, it

P. R. Casson, J. E. Buster: Department of Obstetrics and Gynecology, Baylor College of Medicine, Houston, Texas 77030.

remains in the realm of clinical research to determine whether the salutary effects of DHEA replacement exist. Unfortunately, the clinical literature is fraught with problems, which include the use of varying DHEA doses, preparations, and routes of administration. Study designs are sometimes suboptimal. Further, epidemiologic studies addressing the relationship between endogenous serum DHEA-S levels and various disease outcomes are of limited utility. Single serum DHEA-S values may not accurately reflect adrenal androgen reserve or the rate of adrenal androgen decline with age in a particular individual. Finally, DHEA-S values are also subject to multiple confounding factors, including smoking, alcohol use, obesity, gender, and race.

Nonetheless, about 30 trials addressing DHEA replacement exist in the literature, with several more under way at the present time. This chapter attempts to summarize the the clinical literature to date and provide an overview of the state of the art of DHEA replacement as it stands today.

DHEA AND CARDIOPROTECTION

Animal evidence implies a cardioprotective effect from exogenously administered DHEA. In a rabbit model of accelerated atherogenesis (heterotopic heart transplantation or aortic balloon injury), DHEA retarded disease progression in a lipoprotein-independent fashion (7,8). Despite these data, the epidemiologic literature on the cardioprotective effects of the adrenal androgens is more controversial. The initial evaluation of the Rancho Bernardo cohort indicated that an increase in serum DHEA-S of 100 µg/dL was associated with a 36% reduction in overall and a 48% reduction in cardiovascular mortality, even after adjustment for multiple risk factors (9). This effect, however, was seen only in men, although another study of this cohort did demonstrate a significant association between high DHEA-S levels and elevated high-density lipoprotein (HDL) in women (10). The most recent evaluation of this cohort, published in 1995, demonstrated a mild cardioprotective effect with elevated DHEA-S levels in both men and women (11).

Other epidemiologic data are similarly equivocal. Some reports imply an inverse relationship between DHEA-S levels and premature myocardial infarction (MI) in young men (12,13). DHEA-S is also lower in men with angiographically demonstrated coronary artery disease (14) and in heart transplant patients with accelerated posttransplant atherosclerosis (15). However, other studies have not demonstrated a reproducible cardioprotective effect of DHEA (16–18). Unrecognized confounding factors may impact DHEA levels and may explain these equivocal results. Factors that increase adrenal androgen levels include cigarette smoking (19), alcohol consumption (20), and obesity (21). Conversely, DHEA-S levels are attenuated by estrogen replacement (Fig. 54.2)

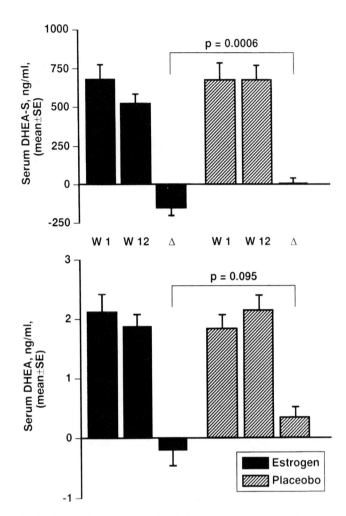

FIG. 54.2. The effect of physiologic postmenopausal estrogen replacement therapy on circulating DHEA-S and DHEA. In this randomized, prospective, blinded, placebo-controlled trial of 28 subjects, estrogen suppressed circulating DHEA-S and DHEA levels. (From ref. 20.)

(20,22), chronic illness (23), and hyperinsulinemia (24). There is also a strong heritable and racial component to individual DHEA-S levels (25).

Thus, it remains the task of clinical trials of DHEA replacement to determine whether any cardioprotective effect exists. In a prospective double-blind, randomized trial of ten healthy young men, Nestler and colleagues administered DHEA (1,600 mg/day) or placebo over 28 days (26) and observed a decline in low-density lipoprotein (LDL) in the DHEA group. However, subsequent clinical trials of DHEA replacement in various populations have demonstrated either no effect on lipids (27) or overall androgenization (28). As seen in Fig. 54.3, we have shown that 6 months of 25 mg of oral micronized DHEA given to postmenopausal women results in a 12% decline in HDL, with a concurrent decline in apolipoprotein A1 (Apo-A1), indicative of increased atherogenic risk (29). In perimenopausal women, Barnhardt and col-

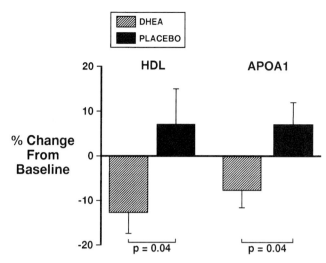

FIG. 54.3. Fasting serum high-density lipoprotein (HDL) and apolipoprotein A₁ (APOA1) after 6 months of treatment with 25 mg/day of oral micronized DHEA or placebo. Over the 6-month period, adverse changes in the HDL and Apo-A₁ levels are seen (29). (n = 6 and 7 in placebo and DHEA arms, respectively.)

leagues observed that oral DHEA (50 mg/day) given over 3 months also induced a progressive decline in total cholesterol and HDL (30). It may very well be, therefore, that oral administration of DHEA, even in low doses, may adversely affect the lipoprotein profile of women.

However, as with estrogen replacement, the cardioprotective effect of DHEA may not be entirely lipoprotein mediated. Other plausible cardioprotective mechanisms postulated on the basis of human trials include a fibroblast antiproliferative effect (31), glucose-6-phosphate dehydrogenase inhibition (32), decreased platelet aggregation (33), or increased fibrinolysis (34). DHEA may also have an indirect inotropic effect on the aged heart by augmenting serum insulin-like growth hormone (IGF-1) levels (27,29,35). It may also have secondary beneficial cardiac effects via its antiobesity and insulin-sensitizing actions.

DHEA AND OBESITY

In both rodents and dogs, DHEA supplementation appears to have antiobesity effects (36,37). Again, the clinical trials are more equivocal. Nestler and colleagues, giving 1,600 mg/day of DHEA in young men over a month, demonstrated a decline in body weight and an increase in lean body mass (26). However, two further investigations in the same population or in obese young men did not confirm these results (38,39). In elderly men and women, Yen and colleagues performed a double-blind, parallel, randomized controlled trial of 100 mg/day of oral DHEA administration, showing increased lean body mass in both sexes and decreased fat mass in men but not in

women (35). We have done a 1-month study of 25 mg/day of oral micronized DHEA administered to older men and also noted decreased weight with increased lean body mass (40), but we have not seen any reproducible effects on body morphology in postmenopausal women. Thus, if there is an effect of DHEA replacement on obesity in humans, the effect appears mild and may also be gender-limited.

DHEA AND INSULIN SENSITIVITY

In rats, DHEA administration reduces the onset and ameliorates the severity of genetic and drug-induced diabetes (42). A case report of DHEA treatment of severe type II diabetes with subsequent improvement has been described (43). Seventeen-hour infusions of intravenous DHEA in women with polycystic ovarian disease have been noted to increase postreceptor pyruvate dehydroge-

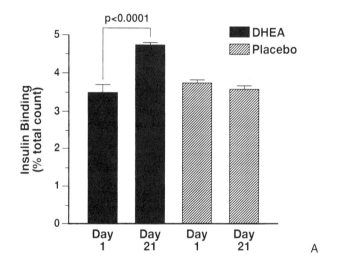

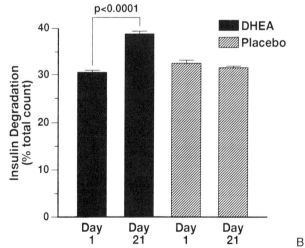

FIG. 54.4. Increases in T-lymphocyte insulin binding **(A)** and degradation **(B)** in 11 postmenopausal women after 3 weeks of 50 mg/day of oral micronized DHEA or placebo. The DHEA significantly enhanced binding and degradation, both considered markers of tissue insulin sensitivity. (From ref. 41.)

nase (PDH) activity, thought a postreceptor marker of insulin effect (44).

These studies prompted us to examine whether DHEA replacement may augment insulin sensitivity in older men and women. In a placebo-controlled, double-blind cross-over trial in postmenopausal women (with 3-week treatment periods and a 2-week washout), we found that 50 mg/day of oral micronized DHEA augmented T-lymphocyte insulin binding and degradation (41), a marker of clinical insulin sensitivity (Fig. 54.4). This enhanced insulin effect was associated with a trend toward decreased areas under the curve (AUC) for glucose and insulin after an oral glucose load. Subsequently, we performed a parallel, blinded, randomized, controlled trial giving 50 mg/day of oral micronized DHEA to postreproductive women (45). We measured insulin sensitivity with an intravenous glucose tolerance test, with data analysis by the minimal modeling technique, and found DHEA replacement has an ameliorating effect on observed study-induced declines in insulin sensitivity, as shown in Fig. 54.5.

Despite these data, other studies have not shown an insulin-sensitizing effect of DHEA (27). However, Diamond and colleagues recently demonstrated that application of 10% DHEA cream for 12 months in older women resulted in significant declines in basal glucose and insulin levels (46). In an early study of 1,600 mg/day of DHEA replacement in obese young men, HbA_{1c} did decline (38). In summary, it appears that if an insulin-sensitizing effect of DHEA exists, it may well not be dramatic and be gender limited (to women).

DHEA AND BONE TURNOVER

Although data on DHEA and bone metabolism are limited, the observation that the pattern of bone gain and

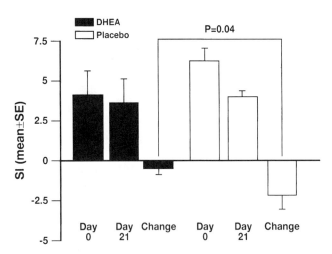

FIG. 54.5. Insulin sensitivity (SI) before and after treatment with oral, micronized DHEA, 50 mg/day, or placebo. A study in stress-induced drop in SI in the placebo group was ameliorated by DHEA, indicating an insulin-sensitizing effect. (From ref. 5.)

loss in human life closely parallels of adrenal androgen secretion provides tantalizing evidence of an association between the two phenomena. Some epidemiologic investigations have correlated bone loss with DHEA-S levels, particularly in the very elderly (47). Other rationales for a role of DHEA in bone turnover include the existence of frequent and disastrous bone loss with long-term corticosteroid administration, a situation in which adrenal androgen secretion is greatly reduced to negligible levels (48). Interleukin 6 (IL-6), a mediator of bone reabsorption in osteoporosis, decreases with DHEA supplementation (49).

In vitro studies in this area also show promise. In human osteoblast cell cultures, DHEA has a mitogenic effect, mediated through transforming growth factor-β (TGF-β) and the androgen receptor (50). This effect is not blocked by 5α-reductase or 3β-hydroxysteroid dehydrogenase (3β-HSD) inhibition, indicating a direct DHEA/androgen receptor effect or an effect mediated by Δ^5 metabolites of DHEA.

Despite these hints that DHEA may play a role in bone turnover, the clinical data remain limited. In our 3-week and 6-month studies in postmenopausal women, we have measured urinary hydroxyproline, hydroxylysine, and collagen cross-links and have not seen DHEA-induced effects (29,41). In similar populations, others have not seen bone mineral density (BMD) changes with dual-energy x-ray absorptiometry scans, albeit with short durations of treatment (35). However, a recent study by Labrie et al., using 12 months of DHEA 10% cream applied topically, demonstrated increases in BMD at the hip in conjunction with declines in plasma bone alkaline phosphatase and urinary hydroxyproline (51). Serum osteocalcin, a marker of bone formation, was increased twofold over control values. Whether or not DHEA replacement has bone-sparing effects remains an area for further investigation.

DHEA REPLACEMENT AND THE GROWTH HORMONE/INSULIN-LIKE GROWTH FACTOR AXIS

Growth hormone (GH) declines markedly with age and itself has been under scrutiny as a possible hormonal replacement therapy to prevent some of the sequelae of aging (52). Studies with recombinant GH (rGH) demonstrate some promise in increasing muscle mass, strength, and well-being in elderly individuals (53,54). However, this therapy is expensive and requires daily injection.

The effects of GH are in large part mediated by either hepatic or end-organ production of insulin-like growth factor (IGF-1), otherwise known as somatomedin (55). In several clinical trials of DHEA replacement in aged individuals, serum IGF-1 levels, both total and free, were increased in concert with decreasing IGF-1 binding protein-3 (IGFBP-3) values. This was first demonstrated by Morales and colleagues in a placebo-controlled study in men and women (27) and subsequently confirmed by Yen (35) and by ourselves (29) in 6-month and year-long trials. Diamond and colleagues have also demonstrated an augmentation of serum IGF-1 levels and action with 12 months of 10% DHEA cream in 15 postmenopausal women (46). Thus, it appears certain that in both men and women, physiologic DHEA replacement augments serum IGF-1 levels by about 50%, about the same magnitude of increase with rGH. This effect may be related to augmentation of the hepatic and end-organ IGF-1 secretory response to circulating GH. That this augmentation of IGF-1 secretion may have clinical benefits is demonstrated by Yen's and colleagues finding of increased muscle strength in men with DHEA replacement (35).

DHEA AND IMMUNE FUNCTION

In aging individuals, a decline in cell-mediated immune competence is thought to occur, a phenomenon termed "immunosenescence" (56). This decline in immune function may be mediated by decreased interleukin-2 (IL-2) or lymphocyte IL-2 receptor levels and is also associated with increased IL-6. The concept that the age-related decline in DHEA levels may be linked to immunosenescence was first given credence by Schwartz and colleagues, who demonstrated that DHEA supplementation prevents spontaneous or mutagen-induced carcinogenesis in rats (57). Although the DHEA doses used were extremely high, subsequent studies in mice have demonstrated that both *in vivo* and *in vitro* DHEA augments lymphocyte IL-2 production (58). In humans, an *in vitro* study indicates that DHEA augments lymphocyte IL-2 production (59).

There are now increasing clinical data demonstrating the immunoaugmentory effects of physiologic DHEA replacement in the elderly. Fifty milligrams of DHEA-S, given twice a day at the time of vaccination, increases influenza (but not tetanus) titer response over that seen with placebo (60). In another randomized, blinded trial, 7.5 mg of subcutaneous DHEA-S given at the time of influenza vaccination increases the hemagglutination inhibition (HI) antibody response, particularly in subjects with lower initial titers and lower serum endogenous DHEA-S levels (61). However, the effects seen in both studies are not large.

In 1993, we demonstrated that DHEA significantly augments natural killer cell (NK cell) cytotoxicity and number in postreproductive women and decreases stimulated lymphocyte IL-2 response (49). Yen's group subsequently confirmed these data in a 6-month study giving 100 mg of oral DHEA to elderly men and women (35) and also demonstrated increases in serum IL-2 levels and lymphocyte expression of surface IL-2 receptor.

It appears now that one of the more clearly delineated effects of DHEA replacement in humans is functional enhancement of the aging immune system. Whether this finding results in clinically significant beneficial effects is an issue that remains to be addressed.

COGNITIVE EFFECTS

DHEA has demonstrated neurotropic action at the GABA receptor. This steroid enhances the maze performance of mice and has a beneficial effect on memory in these animals (63,64). It also promotes the growth of mouse brain explants *in vitro* (65).

Human studies are more limited. In a single-dose, double-blind, randomized, controlled trial, DHEA significantly augmented rapid eye movement (REM) sleep over placebo (66). Given the benefits of REM sleep to overall sleep quality, this finding may contribute to the postulated enhancement in well-being seen in subjects given DHEA, as shown by Morales (27). She and her colleagues demonstrated a libido-independent increase in a sense of well-being (as measured by objective scales) with DHEA (50 mg/day).

BIOAVAILABILITY OF DHEA PREPARATIONS

The bioavailability of orally administered adrenal androgens was first reported in 1982 in the form of a case report describing administration of 25 mg/day of DHEA-S for 1 year to a 19-year-old with hypogonadal hypogonadism (67). Administration of this compound did not result in puberty, but serum DHEA-S rose to peripubertal levels (200 to 250 µg/dL), with development of high testosterone levels (150 ng/dL). Thus, even at this early stage, significant bioconversion of orally administered adrenal androgen to more potent androgens was demonstrated. Later, Nestler and colleagues gave 1,600 mg/day of DHEA to five healthy young men for 28 days (26). Surprisingly, at this dose they increased serum DHEA-S levels only 2.5- to 3.5-fold. Androstenedione increased twofold, and estrone, estradiol, SHBG, and total and free testosterone remained unaltered. However, Mortola and colleagues later used the same doses given to postmenopausal women and demonstrated significant elevations in all downstream androgens to supraphysiologic levels, with androgenization of both glucose tolerance and lipid profiles (28).

The use of physiologic replacement doses was then considered by investigators working in the area, on the basis of the fact that the combined production rates of DHEA and DHEA-S are in the range of 50 mg/day. We performed an initial dose-ranging study to ascertain what levels of our oral micronized DHEA preparation (*Belmar Pharmacy, Lakewood, CO*) were needed to reproduce the premenopausal adrenal androgen milieu without adverse androgenization. On the basis of these single-dose studies, we postulated that the optimal oral replacement dose of this preparation of DHEA was 50 mg/day. Concurrently, we addressed the issue of nonoral administration

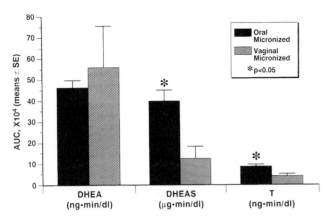

FIG. 54.6. Ratios of areas under the curve for DHEA-S, DHEA, and T after oral administration of 300 mg of micronized or unmicronized DHEA or placebo (*n* = 7). DHEA-S/T and DHEA-S/DHEA ratios are significantly increased with micronization. (From ref. 69.)

by performing a randomized, placebo-controlled, blinded, single-dose trial of oral compared to vaginal micronized DHEA administration (69). After DHEA administration, we sampled blood over a 12-hour period and generated AUCs for DHEA, DHEA-S, and testosterone (T). Comparison of these AUCs seen in Fig. 54.6 shows that the with oral administration there is significant bioconversion to DHEA-S and T; with vaginal administration, this bioconversion is dramatically attenuated, and most of the DHEA appears in the circulation as the native steroid.

In our 3-week trial of 50 mg/day of oral micronized DHEA in postmenopausal women, we demonstrated supraphysiologic elevations of 23-hour postdose DHEA-S and T, indicating that oral bioavailability of this preparation was more efficient than initially postulated and that 25 mg/day may be a more appropriate dose (41). However, in a subsequent study, 25 mg/day of oral micronized DHEA, administered to older women over 6 months, as seen in Fig. 54.6, was subject to significant dose attenuation (29). At the end of the trial, serum DHEA and DHEA-S levels (again 23-hour postdose levels) were not significantly different from placebo values (Fig. 54.7). Thus, we feel that any further trials of DHEA supplementation would require dose titration on the basis of serum DHEA-S and T values to overcome this dose-attenuation effect. Also, given the adverse lipid effects seen with oral administration, the possibility of nonoral (vaginal, sublingual, or transcutaneous) administration becomes germane to avoid a putative hepatic first-pass effect. Indeed, DHEA 10% cream has been effectively administered transcutaneously with physiologic elevations of downstream metabolites. Importantly, in these studies, there were also changes in the GH axis and in bone turnover, indicating that even with nonoral administration, beneficial salutary effects exist and, thus, may not be mediated by hepatic first-pass effect (46,51).

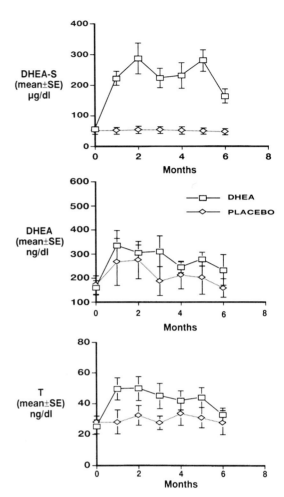

FIG. 54.7. Monthy serum dehydroepiandrosterone (DHEA), dehydroepiandrosterone sulfate (DHEA-S), and testosterone (T) levels after daily administration of 25 mg of oral micronized DHEA (*n* = 6 and 7 in placebo and DHEA arms, respectively). These values are 23-hour postdose nadir levels. DHEA-S, DHEA, and T all decrease toward placebo values by 6 months, indicating time-dependent reduction in bioavailability (dose attenuation) (*n* = 6 and 7 in placebo and DHEA arms, respectively).

Much more investigation needs to be done on doses of DHEA and routes of administration used in human trials. The future of DHEA replacement therapy may very well lie with nonoral administration.

SIDE EFFECTS

Although the possibility of adverse effects of this potent oral steroid exists, in the literature to date only one side effect has been noted (68). This occurred in one of our single-dose studies: a woman was given 150 mg and developed transient jaundice and hepatic dysfunction a week later. Her baseline blood serum, assayed retrospectively, demonstrated false-positive hepatitis C titers and positive antimitochondrial antibodies. Thus, whether or not her hepatic dysfunction was a direct result of DHEA administration is not known, but the previously documented effects of oral steroids, particularly androgens, give pause for concern (71).

Although no other side effects have been noted, the lipid changes seen in women, both in our 6-month study and in Barnhardt and colleagues' investigation, raise some concern about chronic oral administration of this compound (29,30). Additionally, the theoretical potential for side effects such as hirsutism are cogent because of the rapid biotransformation of this compound to the more potent androgens when administered orally. Finally, in animal models of oral DHEA administration, increases in liver size and induction of hepatic carcinoma have been seen (71,72). In men, the possible effects of chronic DHEA administration on subclinical prostate cancer or benign prostatic hyperplasia must also be considered carefully.

CONCLUSION

It appears that physiologic DHEA administration to aging humans may have multiple beneficial effects. In men, but possibly not in women, it may have an antiobesity effect. Conversely, in women, but possibly not in men, DHEA may have an insulin-sensitizing effect. DHEA may beneficially affect bone turnover and clearly augments the GH/IGF-1 axis. Additionally, DHEA is quite likely an immunoaugmentory hormone, reducing some of the declines in immune competence seen with aging.

It is still puzzling how DHEA achieves these effects. Several investigators have noted either a membrane-bound or cytosolic DHEA receptor (73,74), but despite intensive effort, this work remains to be replicated. Alternately, Labrie and colleagues postulate that DHEA may act by virtue of end-organ bioconversion to a mix of estrogenic and androgenic metabolites, which, in turn, would interact with androgen and estrogen receptors to create a set of tissue-unique physiologic effects (76). This potential mechanism of action of DHEA is termed "intracrinology" and remains the most plausible theory of DHEA action at present.

DHEA may also act in humans to exert multiple beneficial effects by augmenting end-organ and hepatic production of IGF-1 in response to GH. It has now been well demonstrated that IGF-1 is an immunoaugmentory substance in its own right (55). Insulin-like growth factor-1 receptors and effects are noted in bone, muscle, and fat (55). Such an augmentation of IGF-1 effect would also result in overall decline in serum GH levels by virtue of hypothalamic–pituitary negative feedback and thus result in a beneficial effect on insulin sensitivity. Indeed, IGF-1 therapy is in clinical trials as a treatment for diabetes (76).

Clearly, the issue of DHEA replacement as an antiaging therapy is rapidly evolving. Future studies of DHEA

replacement in humans are needed, with dose titration, possibly nonoral administration, and with and without concurrent estrogen replacement. Even more important is the development of basic science investigations into this area, looking at the mechanism of adrenarche and adrenopause and the secretory control of DHEA and DHEA-S. Finally, elucidating a mechanism of action could explain the multiple beneficial effects of these compounds and would lend credence to this field.

Unfortunately, at this point, popularization of this compound has far outpaced credible scientific investigation. At present, we do not recommend using DHEA clinically because of its possible side effects. However, the future of DHEA replacement has great potential for attenuating some aspects of aging, and the subject is certainly worthy of further concentrated investigation.

REFERENCES

1. Casson PR, Buster JE. DHEA administration to humans: panacea or palaver? *Semin Reprod Endocrinol* 1995;13:247–256.
2. Endoh A, Kristiansen SB, Casson PR, et al. The zona reticularis is the site of biosynthesis of dehydroepiandrosterone and dehydroepiandrosterone sulfate in the adult human adrenal cortex, resulting from its low expression of 3β-hydroxysteroid dehydrogenase. *J Clin Endocrinol Metab* 1996;81(10):3558–3565.
3. Dhom G. The prepuberal and puberal growth of the adrenal (adrenarche). *Beitr Pathol* 1973;150:357–377.
4. Orentreich N, Brind JL, Rizer RL, et al. Age changes and sex differences in serum dehydroepiandrosterone sulfate concentrations throughout adulthood. *J Clin Endocrinol Metab* 1984;59:551–555.
5. Kreiner E, Dohm G. Altersveranderungen de menschlichen Nebenniere. *Zbl Allg Pathol Anat* 1979;123:351–356.
6. Sapolsky RM, Vogelman JH, Orentreich N, et al. Senescent decline in serum dehydroepiandrosterone sulfate concentrations in a population of wild baboons. *J Gerontol* 1993;48:B196–B200.
7. Eich DM, Nestler JE, Johnson DE, et al. Inhibition of accelerated coronary atherosclerosis with dehydroepiandrosterone in heterotopic rabbit model of cardiac transplantation. *Circulation* 1993;87:261–269.
8. Gordon GB, Bush DE, Weisman HF. Reduction of atherosclerosis by administration of dehydroepiandrosterone. *Adv Enzyme Regul* 1987;26:355–382.
9. Barrett-Connor E, Goodman-Gruen D. Dehydroepiandrosterone sulfate does not predict cardiovascular death in postmenopausal women. *Circulation* 1995;91:1757–1760.
10. Barrett-Connor E, Khaw KT, Yen SSC. A prospective study of dehydroepiandrosterone sulfate, mortality, and cardiovascular disease. *N Eng J Med* 1986;315:1519–1524.
11. Barrett-Connor E, Goodman-Gruen D. The epidemiology of DHEA-S and cardiovascular disease. *Ann NY Acad Sci* 1995;774:259–270.
12. Mitchell LE, Sprecher DL, Borecki IB, et al. Evidence for an association between dehydroepiandrosterone sulfate and nonfatal premature myocardial infarction in males. *Circulation* 1995;89:89–93.
13. Slowinska-Srzednicka J, Zgliczynski S, Ciswicka-Sznajderman M, et al. Decreased plasma dehydroepiandrosterone sulfate and dihydrotestosterone concentrations in young men after myocardial infarction. *Atherosclerosis* 1989;79:197–203.
14. Herrington DM, Gordon GB, Achuff SC, et al. Plasma dehydroepiandrosterone and dehydroepiandrosterone sulfate in patients undergoing diagnostic coronary angiography. *J Am Coll Cardiol* 1990;16:862–870.
15. Herrington DM. DHEA and coronary atherosclerosis. *Ann NY Acad Sci* 1995;774:271–280.
16. Contoreggi CS, Blackman MR, Andres R, et al. Plasma levels of estradiol, testosterone, and DHEAS do not predict risk of coronary artery disease in men. *J Androl* 1990;11:460–470.
17. Rice T, Sprecher DL, Borecki IB, et al. The Cincinnati myocardial infarction and hormone family study: family resemblance for dehydroepiandrosterone sulfate in control and myocardial infarction families. *Metabolism* 1993;42:1284–1290.
18. Newcomer LM, Manson JE, Barbieri RL, et al. Dehydroepiandrosterone sulfate and the risk of myocardial infarction in US male physicians: a prospective study. *Am J Epidemiol* 1994;140:870–877.
19. Khaw KT, Tazuke S, Barrett-Connor E. Cigarette smoking and levels of adrenal androgens in post menopausal women. *N Engl J Med* 1987;318:1705–1709.
20. Tazuke S, Khaw KT, Barrett-Connor E. Exogenous estrogen and endogenous sex hormones. *Medicine* 1992;71:44–50.
21. Field AE, Colditz GA, Willett WC, et al. The relation of smoking, age, relative

weight, and dietary intake to serum adrenal steroids, sex hormones, and sex hormone-binding globulin in middle-aged men. *J Clin Endocrinol Metab* 1994;79: 1310–1316.

22. Casson PR, Elkind-Hirsch KE, Carson SA, et al. Effect of postmenopausal estrogen replacement on circulating androgens. *Obstet Gynecol* 1997;90(6):995–998.

23. Casson PR, Hornsby PJ, Buster JE. DHEA—adrenal androgens, insulin resistance and cardiovascular disease. *Semin Reprod Endocrinol* 1996;14(1):29–34.

24. Nestler JE, Clore JN, Strauss JR III, Blackard WG. The effects of hyperinsulinemia on serum testosterone, progesterone, dehydroepiandrosterone sulfate and cortisol levels in normal women and in a woman with hyperandrogenism, insulin resistance and acanthosis nigricans. *J Clin Endocrinol Metab* 1987;64:180–184.

25. Rotter JI, Wong L, Lifrak ET, et al. A genetic component to the variation of dehydroepiandrosterone sulfate. *Metabolism* 1985;34:731–736.

26. Nestler JE, Barlascini CO, Clore JN, et al. Dehydroepiandrosterone reduces serum low density lipoprotein levels and body fat but does not alter insulin sensitivity in normal men. *J Clin Endocrinol Metab* 1987;64:180–184.

27. Morales AJ, Nolan JJ, Nelson JC, et al. Effects of replacement dose of dehydroepiandrosterone in men and women of advancing age. *J Clin Endocrinol Metab* 1994;78:1360–1367.

28. Mortola J, Yen SSC. The effects of dehydroepiandrosterone on endocrine-metabolic parameters in postmenopausal women. *J Clin Endocrinol Metab* 1990;71: 696–704.

29. Casson PR, Santoro N, Elkind-Hirsch KE, et al. Postmenopausal dehydroepiandrosterone (DHEA) administration increases insulin-like growth factor-I (IGF-I) and decreases high density lipoprotein (HDL): a six month trial. *Fertil Steril* 1998;70:107–110.

30. Barnhart KT, Rader D, Freeman E, et al. The effect of DHEA replacement on the endocrine and lipid profiles of perimenopausal women. *Fertil Steril* 1997;abstract O-081.

31. Saenger P, New M. Inhibitory action of dehydroepiandrosterone (DHEA) on fibroblast growth. *Experientia* 1976;33:966–967.

32. Lopez SA, Krehl WA. *In vivo* effect of dehydroepiandrosterone on red blood cells glucose-phosphate dehydrogenase. *Proc Soc Exp Biol Med* 1967;126:776–778.

33. Lesse RL. *The effects of DHEA on atherogenesis and platelet function.* Paper presented at the Dehydroepiandrosterone and Aging Conference, New York Academy of Sciences, Washington, DC, June, 1995.

34. Beer NA, Jakubowicz DJ, Matt DE, et al. *Oral dehydroepiandrosterone (DHEA) administration produces plasma levels of plasminogen activator (t-PA) in men.* Paper presented at the Dehydroepiandrosterone and Aging Conference, New York Academy of Sciences, Washington, DC, June, 1995.

35. Yen SCC, Morales AJ, Khorram O. Replacement of DHEA in aging men and women: potential remedial effects. *Ann NY Acad Sci* 1995;775:128–142.

36. Yen TT, Allan JV, Pearson DV. Prevention of obesity in Avy/A mice by dehydroepiandrosterone. *Lipids* 1997;12:409–413.

37. MacEwen EG, Kurzman ID. Obesity in the dog: role of the adrenal steroid dehydroepiandrosterone (DHEA). *J Nutr* 1991;121:S51–S55.

38. Usiskin KS, Butterworth S, Clore JN, et al. Lack of effect of dehydroepiandrosterone in obese men. *Int J Obesity* 1990;14:457–463.

39. Welle NB, Jozefowics R, Statt M. Failure of DHEA to influence energy and protein metabolism in humans. *J Clin Endocrinol Metab* 1990;71:1259–1264.

40. Ghusn HF, Taffet G, Jaweed MM, et al. DHEA improves lean body mass of older men. 1998.

41. Casson PR, Faquin LC, Stentz FB, et al. Replacement of dehydroepiandrosterone (DHEA) enhances T-lymphocyte insulin binding in postmenopausal women. *Fertil Steril* 1995;3(5):1027–1031.

42. Coleman DL, Leiter EH, Schwizer RW. Therapeutic effects of dehydroepiandrosterone (DHEA) in diabetic mice. *Diabetes* 1982;31:830–833.

43. Buffington CK, Pourmotabbed G, Kitabchi AE. Case report: amelioration of insulin resistance in diabetes with dehydroepiandrosterone. *Am J Med Sci* 1993; 306:320–324.

44. Schriock ED, Buffington CK, Givens JR, et al. Enhanced post-receptor insulin effects on women following dehydroepiandrosterone infusion. *J Soc Gynecol Invest* 1994;1:74–78.

45. Bates GW, Egerman RS, Umstot ES, et al. Dehydroepiandrosterone attenuates study-induced declines in insulin sensitivity in postmenopausal women. *Ann NY Acad Sci* 1995;774:291–293.

46. Diamond P, Cusan L, Gomez JL, et al. Metabolic effects of 12-month percutaneous dehydroepiandrosterone replacement therapy in postmenopausal women. *J Endocrinol* 1996;150:S43–S50.

47. Wild RA, Buchanan JR, Myers C, et al. Declining adrenal androgens: an association with bone loss in aging women. *Proc Soc Exp Biol Med* 1987;186:355–360.

48. Abraham GE. Ovarian and adrenal contribution to peripheral androgens during the menstrual cycle. *J Clin Endocrinol Metab* 1974;39:340.

49. Casson PR, Anderson RN, Herrod HG, et al. Oral dehydroepiandrosterone in physiologic doses modulates immune function in postmenopausal women. *Am J Obstet Gynecol* 1993;169:1536–1539.

50. Kasperk CH, Wakley GK, Hierl T, et al. Gonadal and adrenal androgens are potent regulators of human bone cell metabolism in vitro. *J Bone Miner Res* 1997;12(3): 464–471.

51. Labrie F, Diamond P, Cusan L, et al. Effect of 12-month dehydroepiandrosterone replacement therapy on bone, vagina, and endometrium in postmenopausal women. *J Clin Endocrinol Metab* 1997;82(10):3498–3505.

52. Lamberts SWJ, Vandenbeld AW, Vanderly AJ. The endocrinology of aging. *Science* 1997;278:419–424.

53. Cuttica CM, Castoldi L, Ggorrini GP, et al. Effects of six-month administration of recombinant human growth hormone to healthy elderly subjects. *Aging* 1997;9(3): 193–197.

54. Sassolas G. Potential therapeutic applications of growth hormone in adults. *Horm Res* 1994;42:72–78.

55. Clark R. The somatogenic hormones and insulin-like growth factor-1: stimulators of lymphopoiesis and immune function. *Endocrine Rev* 1197;18(2):157–179.

56. Thoman ML, Weigle WO. The cellular and subcellular bases of immunosenescence. *Adv Immunol* 1989;46:331–361.

57. Schwartz AG, Pashko LL. Cancer chemoprevention with the adrenocortical steroid dehydroepiandrosterone and structural analogs. *J Cell Biochem* 1993:17G: 73–79.

58. Daynes RA, Dudley DJ, Araneo BA. Regulation of murine lymphokine production *in vivo: dehydroepiandrosterone is a natural enhancer of interleukin 2 synthesis by helper T cells.* Eur J Immunol 1990;20:793–802.

59. Suzuki T, Suzuki N, Daynes RA, et al. Dehydroepiandrosterone enhances IL-2 production and cytotoxic effector function of human T cells. *Clin Immunol Immunopathol* 1991;61:202–211.

60. Araneo BA, Dowell T, Woods MA, et al. DHEAS as an effective vaccine adjuvant in elderly humans. *Ann NY Acad Sci* 1995;774:232–248.

61. Degelau J, Guay D, Hallgren H. The effect of DHEAS on influenza vaccination in aging adults. *J Am Geriatr Soc* 1997;45:747–751.

62. Robel P, Baulieu EE. Neurosteroids: biosynthesis and function. *Trends Endocrinol Metab* 1994;5:1–8.

63. Flood JF, Roberts E. Dehydroepiandrosterone sulfate improves memory in aging mice. *Brain Res* 1988;448:178–181.

64. Melchior CL, Ritzmann RF. Dehydroepiandrosterone enhances the hypnotic and hypothermic effects of ethanol and pentobarbital. *Pharmacol Biochem Behav* 1992;43:223–227.

65. Roberts E. Dehydroepiandrosterone (DHEA) and its sulfate (DHEAS) as neural facilitators: effects on brain tissue in culture and on memory in young and old mice. A cyclic GMP hypothesis of action of DHEA and DHEAS in nervous system and other tissues. In: Kalimi M, Regelson W, eds. *The biologic role of dehydroepiandrosterone (DHEA).* Berlin: Walter de Gruyter, 1990:43–64.

66. Friess E, Trachsel L, Guldner J, et al. DHEA administration increases rapid eye movement sleep and EEG power in the sigma frequency range. *Am J Physiol* 1995;268:E107–E113.

67. Cohen HN, Hay ID, Beastall GH, et al. Failure of adrenal androgen to induce puberty in familial cytomegalic adrenocortical hypoplasia. *Lancet* 1982;12: 1471–1472.

68. Buster JE, Casson PR, Straughn AB, et al. Postmenopausal steroid replacement with micronized dehydroepiandrosterone: preliminary oral bioavailability and dose proportionality studies. *Am J Obstet Gynecol* 1992;166:1163–1170.

69. Casson PR, Straughn AB, Milem CA, et al. Delivery of dehydroepiandrosterone (DHEA) in premenopausal women: Effects of micronization and non-oral administration. *Am J Obstet Gynecol* 1996;174:649–653.

70. Casson PR, Carson SA. Androgen replacement therapy in the menopause: myth and reality. *Int J Fertil* 1996;41(4):412–422.

71. Milewich L, Catalina F, Bennett M. Pleotropic effects of dietary DHEA. *Ann NY Acad Sci* 1995;774:149–170.

72. Rao MS, Subbarao V, Yelandi AV, et al. Hepatocarcinogenicity of dehydroepiandrosterone in the rat. *Cancer Res* 1992;52:2977–2979.

73. Imai A, Ohno T, Tamaya T. Dehydroepiandrosterone sulfate-binding sites in plasma membrane from human uterine cervical fibroblasts. *Experientia* 1992;48: 999–1002.

74. Miekle AW, Dorchuck RW, Araneo BA, et al. The presence of dehydroepiandrosterone-specific receptor binding complex in murine T cells. *J Steroid Biochem Mol Biol* 1992;42:293–304.

75. Labrie F, Belanger A, Simard J, et al. DHEA and peripheral androgen and estrogen formation: Intracrinology. *Ann NY Acad Sci* 1996;774:16–28.

76. Kolaczynski JW, Caro JF. Insulin-like growth factor-1 therapy in diabetes: physiologic basis, clinical benefits, and risks. *Ann Intern Med* 1994;120(1):47–55.

Treatment of the Postmenopausal Woman: Basic and Clinical Aspects, Second Edition, edited by Rogerio A. Lobo, Lippincott Williams & Wilkins, Philadelphia © 1999.

CHAPTER 55

Growth Hormone as Therapy for Postmenopausal Women

Robert Marcus and Andrew R. Hoffman

Few publications in recent memory have generated as much public interest as did the 1990 report by Rudman et al. (1), describing the results of treating a small group of elderly men with recombinant human growth hormone (GH) for 6 months. In that study, GH increased lean body and bone mass, decreased adiposity, and apparently restored skin thickness to that of a 50-year old man. Study participants gave enthusiastic testimony on national television, claiming improved mood, libido, and muscle strength, all ascribing improvement to GH. Although GH prescriptions available at "over-the-border" Mexican spas and from nonorthodox practitioners have long been a subtext in "antiaging" therapy (2), its "legitimization" by the Rudman et al. study precipitated enormous interest on the part of the public, the media, and the medical community, which continues today.

The rationale underlying the potential use of growth hormone as a therapy for older people includes the following factors: (a) aging is associated with declines in the secretory capacity of GH and its intermediary, insulin-like growth factor-1 (IGF-1); (b) aging is associated with changes in body composition resembling those in younger patients with "true" GH deficiency caused by pituitary disorders; and (c) the somatic changes of aging may improve by exogenous GH replacement.

Testing this rationale was not possible when growth hormone available for human use was derived only from human pituitary glands. However, with the availability of recombinant human GH, daily treatment has become a plausible, albeit expensive notion. Several reports have now been published of the effects of GH administration

R. Marcus, A. R. Hoffman: Geriatrics Research, Education, and Clinical Center and the Medical Service, Department of Veterans Affairs Palo Alto Health Care System, and the Division of Endocrinology, Gerontology and Metabolism, Department of Medicine, Stanford University, Palo Alto, California 94304.

on healthy older women and men. This chapter summarizes that experience. Although its primary focus is on studies in postmenopausal women, valuable insights from result of studies in men will also be discussed, where appropriate. The US Food and Drug Administration (FDA) has recently approved the use of GH for adults with adult-onset growth hormone deficiency resulting from specific pituitary disorders. Consideration of that syndrome lies beyond the scope of this chapter, but some of the body composition and metabolic changes induced by GH seen in those patients, which are highly relevant to this discussion, are briefly summarized.

EFFE|CTS OF AGE ON THE GROWTH HORMONE–INSULIN-LIKE GROWTH FACTOR-1 AXIS

The growth hormone–insulin-like growth factor-1 (GH–IGF-1), or somatotropic, axis is composed of several distinct elements: the hypothalamus, which regulates GH secretion via its overall balance between an inhibitory peptide (somatostatin) and a smaller GH-releasing hormone (GHRH); the somatotropic cells of the anterior pituitary gland, which synthesize and secrete GH in a pulsatile fashion; the liver, which is stimulated by GH to secrete IGF-1 and its major binding protein, IGF binding protein 3 (IGFBP-3) into the systemic circulation; and peripheral tissues, such as bone or fat, which respond directly to GH by producing IGF-1, which acts locally in an auto or paracrine fashion, but does not materially affect circulating IGF-1 concentrations. Progressive deficits in all components of the somatotropic axis accompany normal aging (Table 55.1).

No central unifying basis has been proven to underlie these changes, although some evidence suggests that depression of central cholinergic tone in the aging brain

TABLE 55.1. *Age-related changes (deficits) in the GHRH-GH-IGF axis*

1. ⇓ Central cholinergic tone leading to increased hypothalamic somatostatin
2. ⇓ Hypothalamic GHRH mRNA and expression of pituitary GHRH receptors
3. ⇓ Pituitary GH mRNA
4. ⇓ GHRH-induced GH secretion *in vivo* and *in vitro*
5. ⇓ GH secretory pulse frequency
6. ⇓ Circulating GH
7. ⇓ Serum GH-BP and GH half-life
8. ⇓ IGF-1 response to GH and to GHRH
9. ⇓ Serum IGF-1 and IGFBP-3 levels

GHRH, growth hormone releasing hormone; IGF, insulin-like growth factor; BP, binding protein.

leads to enhanced somatostatinergic activity which, in turn, depresses the somatotropic axis (3,4).

EFFECTS OF AGE ON BODY COMPOSITION

The decrease in bone and lean body mass and the increase in adiposity that occur with age have become axioms of gerontology and geriatric medicine. Several mechanisms have been proposed to explain these changes. With age, total daily energy expenditure generally decreases, representing a reduction in physical activity. As this reduction is not generally accompanied by lowered energy intake, both body weight and adiposity increase. By lowering the daily mechanical stimulus to bone, reduced physical activity would also aggravate age-related bone loss. Similarly, age-related deficits in reproductive, adrenal, or somatotropic hormones might lead, alone or in combination, to these somatic alterations. Rudman et al. (1) first proposed that the decreased action of the GH–IGF-1 axis underlies some of the features of normal aging, including osteopenia, muscle atrophy, frailty, and disordered sleep. The causes of these changes are undoubtedly complex, with no single theory likely to prove decisive. Nonetheless, the notion that an age-related decline in somatotropic function contributes to a catabolic diathesis eventuating in frailty, falls, and fractures in elderly people led some authors to define a syndrome complex, named "the somatopause" (5).

GROWTH HORMONE EFFECTS IN PATIENTS WITH ADULT-ONSET GROWTH HORMONE DEFICIENCY

Several European centers first called attention to a clinical syndrome in adults with chronic, organically based growth hormone deficiency (6). Despite sufficient adrenal, thyroid, and reproductive hormone replacement, these patients (a) were easily fatigued; (b) had little drive; (c) did poorly in work and in relationships; (d) had

excess adiposity and low muscle and bone mass; and (e) had a relatively high incidence of premature cardiovascular mortality.

Several clinical trials have examined the effects of growth hormone replacement in such patients, leading to its FDA approval in 1997 (7–12). These studies uniformly report GH to increase lean mass by several kilograms and to decrease fat, primarily visceral fat, by at least several kilograms as well. Skeletal results showed greater variability, probably related to treatment duration. However, when patients are treated with GH beyond 1 year, gains in bone mass have been observed (13–15).

Growth hormone-deficient adults have a high prevalence of visceral obesity (7,10), hypertriglyceridemia, and low circulating concentrations of high density lipoprotein (HDL) cholesterol (16). In one study (17), they also had increased activity of other cardiovascular risk factors, plasminogen activator inhibitor-1 (PAI-1), and fibrinogen. Circulating insulin concentrations appear to be elevated in GH-deficient patients, suggesting insulin resistance as an underlying feature for many of these abnormalities. A solid metabolic foundation, therefore, exists for the observed increase in atherosclerotic cardiovascular morbidity and mortality in these patients.

Growth hormone promotes insulin resistance in children and adults, which also appears to be the case in GH-deficient adults (18). This effect is transient, however, and resolves within several weeks. Growth hormone decreases total serum cholesterol concentrations, and it is associated with decreases in low-density (LDL) cholesterol and increased HDL cholesterol. Triglyceride concentrations do not change significantly with GH. Thus, GH appears to ameliorate, or at least not to aggravate, the major lipoprotein cardiovascular risk factors. A worrisome finding, however, is that GH has increased the concentration of another cardiovascular risk factor, Lp(a) in some reports (19).

Reduced lean mass in growth hormone-deficient adults is associated with deficits in muscle strength (20,21). Several trials examined the effect of GH replacement on muscle strength. Results have been inconsistent; one report showed an increase in limb-girdle force (22), but others showed no significant changes in isometric quadriceps force (21,22) despite clear increases in muscle cross-sectional area. In one 3-year study, quadriceps strength improved substantially (11). Thus, as with changes in bone mass, treatment duration may be a critical predictor of response. It should be remembered that peak muscle strength is not the only component of muscle performance and that changes in muscle endurance and fatigue properties could occur without any change in maximal power. In this regard, Cuneo et al. (23) showed that GH improved exercise endurance in GH-deficient patients.

SHORT-TERM EFFECTS OF GROWTH HORMONE IN OLDER MEN AND WOMEN

Growth hormone administration to older men and women for 1 to 4 weeks consistently results in restoration of circulating IGF-1 concentrations to within the normal range for young adults, promotes conservation of urinary nitrogen and sodium retention, and increases bone remodeling activity (24,25). Measurements of body composition show GH treatment to be associated with increased lean mass and loss of adipose tissue. Such treatment is not without important side effects. In these studies, fluid retention, an almost universal consequence of sodium conservation, was of sufficient magnitude to produce peripheral edema, breast tenderness, and carpal tunnel suppression. Insulin sensitivity is also acutely impaired by GH administration, but this phenomenon appears to be transient.

Sophisticated assessment of protein turnover in one study showed that GH treatment of older women increased muscle protein synthesis, but the long-term impact of that effect on body composition was not understood for two reasons. First, it seems unlikely that net positive protein synthesis can persist long-term in a person who is beyond the growth years. That is, a new equilibrium state, where protein synthesis and breakdown are equal, must eventually be established, and it is not clear from a single 4-week study when that equilibrium point is reached. Second, and more importantly, the measurement of muscle mass by available noninvasive methods is highly confounded by the accumulation of water that attends GH administration. For example, radiologic methods based on differential tissue density (e.g., dual-energy x-ray absorptiometry [DEXA]) cannot distinguish between an increase in tissue protein and an increase in tissue water. At least one study has clearly shown GH treatment to be associated with significant gains in intracellular water, beyond that which is obligatorily tied to protein accumulation. Thus, literature claims about improvements in muscle protein must be viewed with caution in the absence of measurements of body fluid compartments.

SUSTAINED GROWTH HORMONE TREATMENT OF OLDER MEN AND WOMEN

Three clinical trials have reported the effects of growth hormone in healthy older men (1,26) and women (27). In the studies in men, participants were selected on the basis of low circulating IGF-1 and treatment duration was 6 months. The study in women had no IGF-1 selection criterion, and treatment duration was 12 months.

1. Rudman et al. (1) reported the most widely publicized GH trial to date. In a randomized fashion, 21 elderly men received placebo or GH (0.03 mg/kg three times per week) for 6 months. The most dramatic treatment response was a significant increase in lean mass, as determined by ^{40}K analysis. Bone density was assessed at nine different sites by dual photon absorptiometry, and a 1.6% increase in lumbar spine mineral density was reported. No significant change in skinfold estimates of adiposity was observed. Measurements of skin thickness indicated gains to values generally observed in 50-year old men.

The results of this experiment were provocative and interesting, but several interpretive concerns require discussion. The ^{40}K data provide convincing evidence of a true increase in lean mass. It must be noted, however, that total body lean mass includes both somatic (muscle) and visceral protein. Although it may be tempting to conclude that GH had expanded the muscle compartment, careful analysis of lean tissue distribution following a 12-week GH treatment schedule in younger men indicated much of this effect to be on visceral protein (28).

As discussed, a second issue confounding interpretation of this and other GH studies is the substantial increase in body water that rapidly follows GH administration accompanied by the failure of noninvasive methods used to assess body composition (e.g., DEXA) to distinguish water from tissue. In the Rudman et al. study (1), it seems highly likely that at least some of the increase in "lean mass" and much of the change in skin thickness was confounded by increased body water.

It would not be accurate to leave an impression that the only effects of growth hormone in this study were potentially beneficial. Inadequate scrutiny was given to lipoprotein or other metabolic risk factors. It should also be noted that an attempt to prolong this 6-month study into a year-long intervention led to discontinuation of treatment by a substantial number of participants who developed manifestations of carpal tunnel compression or gynecomastia (29).

2. Papadakis et al. (26) recently presented the results of a trial that addressed the effects of growth hormone on functional status of 52 elderly men, mean age 75 years. Participants were given GH (0.03 mg/kg) or placebo, three times each week, for 6 months. This dose of GH was sufficient to restore circulating IGF-1 concentrations to within the normal range for young men. At study completion, the GH group had shown a 4.3% increase in lean mass and a 13% decrease in fat mass, whereas body composition remained stable in the placebo group. No statistically or clinically significant differences were observed in grip strength or in endurance. One scale of cognitive function, the Trail B test, showed significant improvement with GH, whereas the placebo group showed deterioration. Other cognitive tests, however, did not show a consistent response. Mini-Mental Examination scores deteriorated by 0.4 units with GH, improving slightly with placebo, whereas performance on a Digit Symbol Substitution test was identical between groups. The authors concluded that, although GH improved body composition in this group of healthy older men, such

improvement was not associated with corresponding changes in functional ability. Finally, this study confirmed the experience that GH produces a high prevalence of side effects. In particular, edema was observed in 65% of participants who received GH.

Although the report of Papadakis et al. (26) establishes the important point that changes in body composition do not necessarily translate into functional benefit, it does have limitations. GH was administered for only 6 months to a cohort of healthy men in robust health. Particularly in regard to cognitive function, baseline test scores may have been so high that the possibility of measurable improvement was remote. Considerably longer treatment duration would be required if GH protected against loss of functional capacity, rather than actually increasing it. The same issues of fluid balance that were discussed above also confound this study. Nonetheless, as opposed to the 6-month study of Rudman et al. (1) that addressed symptoms and function in a nonquantitative manner, the results Papadakis et al. (26) found provide no support for a conclusion that GH improves functioning of elderly men.

3. Holloway et al. (27) conducted a year-long trial of recombinant GH in healthy elderly women. Nineteen women were assigned to receive GH at an initial daily dose of 0.043 mg/kg, but after several weeks, a 50% dose reduction was necessitated by side-effects, primarily fluid retention and edema. Thirteen women assigned to GH and 14 women assigned to placebo completed 6 months of drug treatment. Six women in the GH group had taken a stable dose of replacement estrogen, permitting the effects of recombinant GH to be assessed separately by estrogen status. GH increased IGF-1 in all subjects, with greater rises observed in estrogen-deficient women (308 ng/mL) than in those who received estrogen replacement (230 ng/mL), and no changes in IGF-1 occurred with placebo. Skinfold thickness measurements showed an 11% decrease in fat mass and a 9% decrease in adiposity after 6 months of GH treatment. No significant difference in nitrogen balance was seen in either group at 6 months, but GH increased creatinine clearance significantly by 9.2%. GH dramatically increased markers of bone turnover, with more pronounced effects in women who were not taking estrogen. The traditional bone resorption marker, urinary hydroxyproline, increased by 20% in those taking estrogen and by 80% in those who did not, and the more contemporary resorption marker, total urinary pyridinolines, increased by 44% and 75% in these subgroups. The bone formation marker, osteocalcin, increased in concentration by more than 60% in women not receiving estrogen replacement, but did not change in women on estrogen replacement. No changes in any turnover marker was seen in the placebo group. GH did not alter blood pressure or circulating L-thyroxine, but a transient increase in serum triiodothyronine was observed at 3 months. GH decreased LDL cholesterol in those not on estrogen, but otherwise no significant changes in circulating lipoproteins or fibrinogen were observed.

Eight women assigned to GH and 14 placebo-treated women remained on blinded treatment for a full year. Analysis of this cohort showed persistence of the 6 month changes in IGF-1 and bone turnover. GH did not increase bone mineral density (BMD) at the lumbar spine or hip, but the placebo group experienced 1.7% and 3.0% decreases of BMD at the trochanter and Ward's triangle. The results of this trial indicate that GH can be administered to healthy elderly women without obvious adverse effects on major cardiovascular risk factors, and that effects of such treatment are modulated by concurrent estrogen replacement therapy. Although GH was a powerful initiator of bone remodeling, it seemed unlikely as monotherapy to achieve major improvement in bone mass. The results also justify a conclusion that the clinical utility of GH in older women is constrained by a high prevalence of side-effects, particularly fluid retention and carpal tunnel syndrome.

In this study it was shown that nitrogen balance at 6 months did not differ from baseline values. Although nitrogen conservation clearly occurs early in the course of GH therapy, one cannot expect sustained positive nitrogen balance to occur after linear growth has stopped. Thus, a return to an equilibrium state, where protein synthesis and breakdown are the same, is predictable. What is not indicated by these data, however, is whether GH has produced this new equilibrium condition in the face of more rapid protein turnover. In addition, the rise in endogenous creatinine clearance lends support to the notion discussed above that GH can improve visceral (in this case renal) protein status.

EFFECTS OF GROWTH IN COMBINATION WITH OTHER MODALITIES IN OLDER MEN AND WOMEN

Growth Hormone, Exercise, and Muscle Strength

Along with characteristic changes of normal aging in body composition, muscle strength also decreases, and these reductions in muscle strength contribute to frailty and risk for fracture. Older adults can increase muscle strength with exercise training (30,31), but strength gains quickly level off, with only modest increases thereafter, despite continued training. To determine whether age-related deficits in the somatotropic axis limit the degree to which muscle strength improves with resistance training, Taaffe et al. (32) conducted a double-blind, placebo-controlled exercise trial. Eighteen healthy men, aged more than 65 years, underwent progressive weight training for 14 weeks to invoke a trained state. Participants were then randomly assigned to receive either recombinant human GH (0.02 mg/kg body weight/day) or placebo, while undertaking a further 10 weeks of strength training. Sequential measurements were made of muscle strength, and body composition was assessed by DEXA. For each major muscle group, maximal strength increased impressively for both groups over 14 weeks of training, with little improvement thereafter. Highly significant increases in muscle strength ranged from 24% to 62%, depending on muscle group. Baseline plasma IGF-1 concentrations were similarly low in both groups (106 ng/mL)—approximately half that observed in healthy young adults. In the GH group, IGF-1 levels increased to 255 ng/mL at week 15 and 218 ng/mL at week 24. In the placebo group, IGF-1 increased slightly to 119 ng/mL at 24 weeks. GH had no effect on muscle strength for any muscle group at any time, and no systematic intergroup differences in muscle strength were observed at any time during the study (Fig. 55.1). Body weight did not change in either group, but lean body mass increased and fat mass decreased in men receiving GH. Vastus lateralis muscle biopsies showed similar increases in cross-sectional fiber areas in both the GH and placebo groups, and GH treatment led to no change in muscle GH or IGF-1 receptor content, or IGF receptor messenger RNA, either following the initial exercise period or in response to GH treatment (33). These data indicate clearly that replacement therapy with GH does not augment the strength or hypertrophy response to strength training in elderly men. They suggest that deficits in GH secretion do not underlie the time-dependent level-ing off of muscle strength gains seen with training in the elderly, and provide no support for the popular view of growth hormone as an ergogenic aid.

Growth Hormone, Calcitonin, and Bone Mass

The possibility that growth hormone might provide an anabolic stimulus to achieve increased bone mass in adults has been attractive because it directly stimulates IGF production, and stimulates IGF-1 type collagen synthesis in osteoblastic cells (34–36). In a classic experiment (37), administration of GH to adult dogs increased bone mass; recombinant human GH also has been shown to maintain trabecular bone mass in primates rendered hypogonadal by a gonadotropin-releasing hormone analog (38). Thus, a combination of *in vitro* and *in vivo* evidence suggests the conclusion that GH or IGF-1 might represent an effective strategy to improve bone mass.

As described, we found no skeletally anabolic effect of 6 to 12 months of growth hormone monotherapy in women (27). This was surprising, considering that earlier work with pituitary-derived hormone, showed that GH increased bone density when given in combination with the anti-resorptive hormone, calcitonin (39,40). Several features of those studies may have actually restricted the magnitude of a GH treatment effect. Non-availability of recombinant GH necessitated the use of hormone of uncertain potency. Hormone supply was sufficiently low to restrict the size of treatment groups, thereby jeopardizing statistical power. Holloway et al. (41), therefore, undertook to evaluate the utility of combined GH-antiresorptive therapy by using recombinant GH in a large study cohort. This placebo-controlled, randomized clinical trial involved 2-month cycles of 7 days of GH (0.02 mg/kg/day) followed by 5 days of CT (100 U/day) (or their respective placebos), carried out recurrently for 2 years, with follow-up bone density assessment at 3 years. Each 12-day treatment cycle was followed by 44 days of supplemental calcium only. Eighty-four healthy women with lumbar spine BMD more than 1 SD below the average value for a healthy 25-year-old white woman volunteered for this study. Treatment endpoints included BMD at the lumbar spine and proximal femur by DEXA, biochemical markers of bone turnover, and circulating IGF-1.

Seventy-two women completed the 2-year protocol. Growth hormone treatment increased IGF-1 concentrations from low baseline values (112 ng/mL) to the young normal range ~(430 ng/mL). Groups receiving GH (with or without calcitonin) increased lumbar spine BMD at 2 years by 2.70 ± 0.81% and 1.72 ± 0.74%, whereas no change occurred in women in the placebo groups (Fig. 55.2). Significant increases in total hip BMD of 1% to 2% were observed for the growth hormone plus placebo group, with a nonsignificant trend in the GH plus calcitonin group. For the femoral trochanter, significant

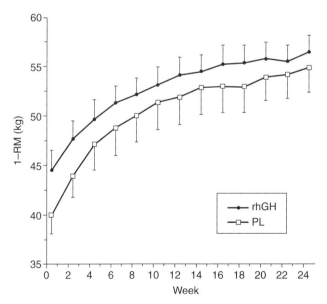

FIG. 55.1. Effect of growth hormone (GH) on muscle strength response to resistance training in elderly men. Subjects underwent strength training for 24 weeks. After 14 weeks, they were randomly assigned to receive daily placebo or GH (0.02 mg/kg/day) injections for the next 10 weeks. No strength difference exists at any time point between groups. (From Taaffe DR, Pruitt L, Reim J, et al. Effect of recombinant human growth hormone on the muscle strength response to resistance exercise in elderly men. *J Clin Endocrinol Metab* 1994;79:1361–1366; with permission.)

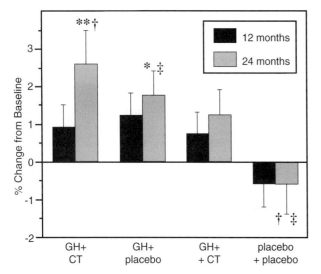

FIG. 55.2. Effect of cyclic growth hormone (GH) and calcitonin on lumbar spine body mass index. Results are given as percent changes from baseline (mean ± SEM). *$p < 0.05$; **$p < 0.01$ (versus baseline). † and ‡, Groups sharing these symbols differed significantly. (From Holloway L, Kohlmeier L, Kent K, Marcus R. Skeletal effects of cyclic recombinant human growth hormone and salmon calcitonin in osteopenic postmenopausal women. *J Clin Endocrinol Metab* 1997;82: 1111–1117; with permission.)

increases were observed for the GH plus calcitonin and placebo plus calcitonin groups only. No significant change in femoral neck BMD was observed in any group. Women taking replacement estrogen had the same BMD response as those who were estrogen-deficient. No significant increase in BMD was observed between 24 and 36 months in 62 women who returned for a 3-year measurement. In response to GH, short-term increases in resorption and formation markers were observed, but these had decreased before the next treatment cycle. No long-term changes in resorption markers were observed, but women in the GH groups showed a sustained rise in circulating osteocalcin over the entire 2-year protocol. Thus, although GH given cyclically with or without calcitonin for 2 years achieved statistically significant increases in BMD of the lumbar spine and selected areas of the hip in postmenopausal women, these gains were less marked than those that are routinely achieved with estrogen or bisphosphonates, and they were associated with a relatively high incidence of adverse experiences. Therefore, it is unlikely that cyclic GH, with or without calcitonin, will prove clinically useful in the treatment of postmenopausal women with osteoporosis.

CONCLUSIONS

Although changes in GH–IGF-1 axis function can contribute to acquired biochemical, body composition, and functional changes of normal human aging, they certainly do not provide a sole or even major explanation for these changes. The concept that GH "replacement" would materially benefit the daily function of older men and women finds little support in the controlled clinical trials reported to date (42). Further, GH, either as monotherapy or in combination with antiresorptive medication, seems not to offer a clinically useful strategy for the treatment of osteoporosis. GH may yet prove to have clinical utility for older men and women in the management of other clinical syndromes, such as visceral obesity, but insufficient data currently exist to justify any conclusions in this regard.

REFERENCES

1. Rudman D, Feller AG, Nagraj HS, et al. Effects of human growth hormone in men over 60 years old. *N Engl J Med* 1990;323:1.
2. Klatz R. *Grow young with HGH.* New York: Harper Collins, 1997:1–368.
3. Pepeu G, Casamenti F, Pepeu IM, Scali C. The brain cholinergic system in ageing mammals. *J Reprod Fertil* 1993;46(Suppl):155.
4. Müller EE, Cella SG, De Gennaro Colonna V, Parenti M, Cocchi D, Locatelli V. Aspects of the neuroendocrine control of growth hormone secretion in ageing mammals. *J Reprod Fertil* 1993;46(Suppl):99.
5. Hoffman AR, Pyka G, Lieberman SA, Ceda GP, Marcus R. The Somatopause. In: Muller EE, Cocchi D, Locatelli V, eds. *Growth hormone and somatomedins during lifespan.* Berline: Springer-Verlag, 1993:265.24.
6. De Boer H, Blok GJ, van der Veen VA. Clinical aspects of growth hormone deficiency in adults. *Endocr Rev* 1995;16:63–86.
7. Salomon F, Cuneo RD, Hesp R, Sönksen PH. The effects of treatment with recombinant human growth hormone on body composition and metabolism in adults with growth hormone deficiency. *N Engl J Med* 1989;321:1797–1803.
8. Whitehead HM, Boreham C, McIlrath EM, et al. Growth hormone treatment of adults with growth hormone deficiency: results of a 13-month placebo controlled cross-over study. *Clin Endocrinol* 1992;36:45–52.
9. Binnerts A, Swart GR, Wilson JHP, et al. The effect of growth hormone administration in growth hormone deficient adults on bone, protein, carbohydrate and lipid homeostasis, as well as body composition. *Clin Endocrinol* 1992;37:79–87.
10. Bengtsson B-Å, Eden S, Lonn L, et al. Treatment of adults with growth hormone deficiency with recombinant human GH. *J Clin Endocrinol Metab* 1993;76: 309–317.
11. Jorgensen JOL, Thuesen L, Muller J. Three years of growth hormone treatment in growth hormone-deficient adults: near normalization of body composition and physical performance. *Eur J Endocrinol* 1994;130:224–228.
12. Johansson G, Rosen T, Lindstedt G, Bosaeus I, Bengtsson B-Å. Effect of 2 years of growth hormone treatment on body composition and cardiovascular risk factors in adults with growth hormone deficiency. *Endocrinol Metab* 1996;4(Suppl A): 3–12.
13. Degerblad M, Bengtsson B-Å, Bramnert M, et al. Reduced bone mineral density in adults with growth hormone deficiency: increased bone turnover during 12 months of GH substitution. *Eur J Endocrinol* 1995;133:180–188.
14. Vandeweghe M, Taelman P, Kaufman JM. Short and long-term effects of growth hormone treatment on bone turnover and bone mineral content in adult growth hormone-deficient males. *Clin Endocrinol* 1993;39:409–415.
15. Kann P, Piepkorn B, Schehler B, et al. Replacement therapy with recombinant human growth hormone in GH-deficient adults. Effects on bone metabolism and bone mineral density in a 2-year prospective study. *Endocrinol Metab* 1995; 2(Suppl B):103–110.
16. Rosen T, Eden S, Larson G, Wilhelmsen L, Bengtsson B-Å. Cardiovascular risk factors in adult patients with growth hormone deficiency. *Acta Endocrinol* 1993; 129:195–200.
17. Johansson JO, Landin K, Tengborn L, Rosen T, Bengtsson B-Å. High fibrinogen and plasminogen activator inhibitor activity in growth hormone-deficient adults. *Arterioscler Thromb Vasc Biol* 1994;14:434–437.
18. O'Neal DN, Kalfas A, Dunning PL. The effect of 3 months of recombinant human growth hormone (GH) therapy on insulin and glucose-mediated glucose disposal and insulin secretion in GH-deficient adults: a minimal model analysis. *J Clin Endocrinol Metab* 1994;79:975–983.
19. Johansson JO, Oscarsson J, Rosen T, et al. Effects of 1 year of growth hormone therapy on serum lipoprotein levels in growth hormone-deficient adults. Influence of gender and Apo(a) and Apo(E) phenotypes. *Arterioscler Thromb Vasc Biol* 1995;15:2142–2150.
20. Cuneo RC, Salomon F, Wiles CM. Skeletal muscle performance in adults with growth hormone deficiency. *Horm Res* 1990;33(Suppl 4):55–60.
21. Rutherford OM, Beshyah SA, Johnston DG. Quadriceps strength before and after growth hormone replacement in hypopituitary adults: relationship to changes in lean body mass and IGF-I. *Endocrinol Metab* 1994;1:41–47.
22. Cuneo RC, Salomon F, Wiles CM, Hesp R, Sonksen PH. Growth hormone treat-

ment in growth hormone-deficient adults. I. Effects on muscle mass and strength. *J Appl Physiol* 1991;70:688–694.

23. Cuneo RC, Salomon F, Wiles CM, Hesp R, Sonksen PH. Growth hormone treatment in growth hormone-deficient adults. II. Effects on exercise performance. *J Appl Physiol* 1991;70:695–700.

24. Marcus R, Butterfield G, Holloway L, et al. Effects of short-term administration of recombinant human growth hormone to elderly people. *J Clin Endocrinol Metab* 1990;70:519–527.

25. Thompson JL, Butterfield, GE, Marcus R, Hintz RL, Van Loan M, Ghiron L, Hoffman AR. The effects of recombinant human insulin-like growth factor-I and growth hormone on body composition in elderly women. *J Clin Endocrinol Metab* 1995;80:1845–1852.

26. Papadakis MA, Grady D, Black D, et al. Growth hormone replacement in healthy older men improves body composition but not functional ability. *Ann Intern Med* 1996;124:708–716.

27. Holloway L, Butterfield G, Hintz RL, Gesundheit N, Marcus R. Effect of recombinant human growth hormone on metabolic indices, body composition, and bone turnover in healthy elderly women. *J Clin Endocrinol Metab* 1994;79:470–479.

28. Yarasheski KE, Campbell JA, Smith K, et al. Effect of growth hormone and resistance exercise on muscle growth in young men. *Am J Physiol* 1992;262: E261–E267.

29. Cohn L, Feller AG, Draper MW, Rudman IW, Rudman D. Carpal tunnel syndrome and gynaecomastia during growth hormone treatment of elderly men with low circulating IGF-I concentrations. *Clin Endocrinol* 1993;39:417–25.

30. Charette S, McEvoy L, Pyka G, Snow-Harter C, Guido D, Wiswell RA, Marcus R. Muscle hypertrophy response to resistance training in older women. *J Appl Physiol* 1991;70:1912–1916.

31. Pyka G, Lindenberger E, Charette S, Marcus R. Muscle strength and fiber adaptations to a year-long resistance training program in elderly men and women. *J Gerontol* 1994;49:22–27.

32. Taaffe DR, Pruitt L, Reim J, et al. Effect of recombinant human growth hormone on the muscle strength response to resistance exercise in elderly men. *J Clin Endocrinol Metab* 1994;79:1361–1366.

33. Taaffe DR, Jin IH, Vu Hoffman AR, Marcus R. Lack of effect of recombinant human growth hormone on muscle morphology and growth hormone-insulin-like-growth factor expression in resistance-trained elderly men. *J Clin Endocrinol Metab* 1996;81:421–425.

34. Stracke H, Schultz A, Moeller D, Rossol S, Schatz H. Effect of growth hormone on osteoblasts and demonstration of somatomedin C/IGF-1 in bone organ culture. *Acta Endocrinol* (Copenh) 1984;107:16–24.

35. Chenu C, Valentin-Opran A, Chavassieux P, Saez S, Meunier PJ, Delmas PD. Insulin like growth factor I hormonal regulation by growth hormone and by 1,25(OH)$_2$D$_3$ and activity on human osteoblast-like cells in short-term cultures. *Bone* 1990;11:81–86.

36. Barnard R, Ng KW, Martin TJ, Waters MJ. Growth hormone (GH) receptors in clonal osteoblast-like cells mediate a mitogenic response to GH. *Endocrinology* 1991;128:20.

37. Harris WH, Heaney RP. Effect of growth hormone on skeletal mass in adult dogs. *Nature* 1969;273:403–404.

38. Mann DR, Rudman CG, Akinbami MA, Gould KG. Preservation of bone mass in hypogonadal female monkeys with recombinant human growth hormone administration. *J Clin Endocrinol Metab* 1992;74:1263–1269.

39. Aloia JF, Vaswani A, Kapoor A, Yeh JK, Cohn SH. Treatment of osteoporosis with calcitonin, with and without growth hormone. *Metabolism* 1985;34:124–129.

40. Aloia JF, Vaswani A, Meunier PJ, et al. Coherence treatment of postmenopausal osteoporosis with growth hormone and calcitonin. *Calcif Tissue Int* 1987;40: 253–259.

41. Holloway L, Kohlmeier L, Kent K, Marcus R. Skeletal effects of cyclic recombinant human growth hormone and salmon calcitonin in osteopenic postmenopausal women. *J Clin Endocrinol Metab* 1997;82:1111–1117.

42. Marcus R, Reaven G. Growth hormone—ready for prime time? *J Clin Endocrinol Metab* 1997;82:725–726.

Treatment of the Postmenopausal Woman: Basic and Clinical Aspects, Second Edition, edited by Rogerio A. Lobo, Lippincott Williams & Wilkins, Philadelphia © 1999.

CHAPTER 56

Melatonin

Ralf C. Zimmermann

CHEMISTRY, SYNTHESIS, AND METABOLISM

The indole derivative *N*-acetyl-5-methoxytryptamine, which is better known as melatonin, was discovered by Lerner et al. (1) in 1958. This hormone is mainly synthesized by pinealocytes located in the pineal gland (2,3). The pineal gland is a small cone-shaped structure attached to the roof of the third ventricle between the superior colliculi immediately adjacent to the habenular commissure (4). Melatonin is produced from the essential amino acid tryptophan, which is taken up by the gland passively from the blood stream. Blood tryptophan shows a circadian rhythm (5) which very likely does not influence melatonin production as the concentration of the melatonin precursor 5-hydroxytryptamine in the pineal gland is high (6). Tryptophan is converted to 5-hydroxytryptophan in a reaction catalyzed by the enzyme tryptophan hydroxylase. The next step in melatonin production is the decarboxylation of 5-hydroxytryptophan by an L-amino-decarboxylase, which converts it to 5-hydroxytryptamine better known under the name serotonin. Serotonin is then converted to L-acetyl-5-hydroxytryptamine by an arylalkylamine *N*-acetyltransferase (AANAT), the rate limiting step. This enzyme, which was cloned recently, plays a key role in the regulation of melatonin production (7). The human AANAT gene is located on chromosome 17q25. O-methylation of *N*-acetyl-5-hydroxytryptamine produces the hormone melatonin. Melatonin, which is lipophilic and hydrophilic, can leave and enter cells by simple diffusion. It is transported in the blood in an albumin-bound form and cleared quickly (half-life less than 40 minutes). Melatonin is metabolized in the liver to 6-hydroxymelatonin, which undergoes conjugation to either sulfate or glucuronide and is excreted mainly into urine (Fig. 56.1) (6).

R. C. Zimmermann: Departments of Obstetrics & Gynecology and Psychiatry, Columbia University College of Physicians & Surgeons, New York, New York 10032.

The enzyme arylalkylamine *N*-acetyltransferase controls the daily rhythm in pineal melatonin production and blood melatonin concentration. The activity of this enzyme increases substantially at night in the absence of light, but is inhibited in the presence of light (6). Regulation of the expression of this gene occurs through (β_1-receptors, which are located in the membrane of pinealocytes. Binding of norepinephrine or a compound with (β-agonist activity will stimulate a $G_{stimulatory}$ protein complex, which via adenylyl cyclase will produce c-AMP, which will activate a c-AMP–dependent protein kinase to phosphorylate a c-AMP response element binding protein (CREB) to form phosphorylated CREB. It is possible that this process might be enhanced by norepinephrine's action on the β_1-adrenergic receptor located in the membrane of pinealocytes. The night:day ratios of pineal AANAT mRNA varies from more than 150 in the rat to 1.5 in sheep. Tissue-specific AANAT mRNA expression in the human is high in the pineal gland and the retina, low in other areas of brain, and nondetectable in peripheral tissues (8). It is of note that repeated stimulation of the pinealolcyte with norepinephrine does not tonically elevate AANAT activity or AANAT mRNA. Therefore, stimulation of β_1-receptors seems to induce a second mechanism which counteracts AANAT activity. Fos-related antigen 2 and inducible c-AMP early response protein (ICER) are two candidates that might function as such inhibitory factors (7).

REGULATION OF MAMMALIAN PINEAL MELATONIN RHYTHM AND DETECTION IN BLOOD

The rhythm of pineal melatonin secretion is regulated by a well-characterized neural circuit that drives the activity of pinealocytes to produce and secrete melatonin (9). Circadian stimulatory signals originate in the suprachiasmatic nucleus (SCN), the principal circadian

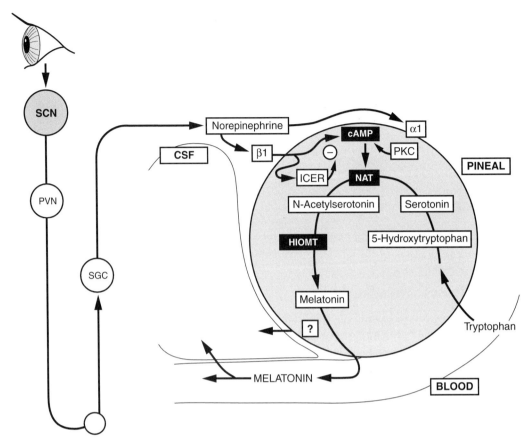

FIG. 56.1. Schematic representation of the synthesis and secretion of melatonin by the pineal gland, and of its regulation by circadian and photoperiod signals. SCN, hypothalamic suprachiasmatic nuclei; PVN, hypothalamic paraventricular nuclei; SCG, superior cervical ganglia; CSF, cerebrospinal fluid; NAT, N-acetyltransferase; HIOMT, hydroxyindole-O-methyltransferase; ICER, cAMP-induced gene transcription regressor.

pacemaker in the mammalian brain; they are transmitted to the pineal gland through the hypothalamic paraventricular nucleus via the medial forebrain bundle to the intermediolateral cell column of the upper spinal cord which, in turn, innervates superior cervical ganglia (9). These ganglia innervate the pineal gland with norepinephrine-containing fibers. Release of this neurotransmitter increases AANAT mRNA as described (10). The SCN is the circadian pacemaker that is not dependent on the dark–light cycle, but functions autonomously. Input or entrainment pathways establish the precise period and phase of the pacemaker (i.e., it assures appropriate adjustment to the 24-hour light–dark cycle). Light, an *entrainment* signal or *Zeitgeber*, acts through the retinohypothalamic pathway to reset the clock (SCN), and via the SCN it makes subtle adjustments in the duration and intensity of stimulation of the pineal gland and its output signal melatonin. Blind individuals with abnormal retinal processing or a defective retinohypothalamic tract can have free-running rhythms (11). How powerful the input signal light is in altering SCN activity and its impact on the pineal gland and melatonin secretion is exemplified

by the following example: Light exposure at a high melatonin state such as nighttime blocks the SCN/pineal gland transmission, thereby terminating norepinephrine release into the pineal extracellular space, which promptly lowers melatonin production and release (12, 13). Extraretinal circadian phototransduction is also possible, and it might have implications for the development of new treatments for sleep and circadian rhythm disorders in the near future (13a).

Blood melatonin concentration is low during the daytime (20 to 25 pmol/L), and increases at night with peak levels between 2 AM and 4 AM to levels between 150 and 200 pmol/L (1 pg/mL = 4.31 pmol/L) (14). A similar pattern is seen when metabolites of melatonin are measured in urine; for example 24-hour measurements of 6-hydroxymelatonin sulfate reflect 24-hour plasma melatonin secretion adequately (15). Melatonin production or secretion is not influenced by gender. Wide interindividual variation in melatonin secretion is seen, but the intraindividual secretion pattern is relatively stable (16,17).

As mentioned, blind people whose retina is no longer competent to inform the SCN about light and darkness through the retinohypothalamic tract still secrete melatonin in a circadian fashion, but this secretion might no longer be entrained to light (i.e., the rhythm is free running). This is one of the reasons why these individuals might suffer from sleep-related problems (11). The importance of extraretinal circadian phototransduction in blind people is not known.

MELATONIN RECEPTORS AND EFFECTS OF MELATONIN ON THE SUPRACHIASMATIC NUCLEUS

Following the introduction of 2-(^{125}I)iodomelatonin analogues, specific melatonin receptors were identified in the SCN but not in the pars tuberalis of the pituitary gland in the human (18,19). Melatonin receptors, which have also been identified in other areas of the brain including the preoptic area, cerebral cortex, and thalamus of some mammals, could mediate the hypnotic effects of this hormone (20). Melatonin receptors in nonneuronal tissue are found in cerebral arteries, ovarian granulosa cells, Leydig cells of the testis, prostate epithelial cells, and renal tubular cells (6). The physiologic significance of these receptors in nonneuronal tissue is currently not clear. The dissociation constant (Kd) of this receptor is less than 100 pM (i.e., it is physiologically meaningful). The human melatonin receptor has been cloned recently by molecular biologic techniques (20,21). At least two receptor subtypes, Mel 1a and Mel 1b, are coupled to $G_{inhibitory}$ proteins. The chromosomal locations are 4q35.1 and 11q21–22 (20), respectively. It has been shown recently that the Mel 1a receptor involves both inhibition of adenylyl cyclase and potentiation of phospholipase activation (22). Melatonin binding leads to a functional change in the SCN. Cultured SCN *in vitro*, SCN continues 24-hour oscillations with neuronal firing being maximal corresponding to the light phase and the firing being minimal corresponding to the dark phase of the animals before killing (23). Administration of melatonin during the peak firing rate of the SCN *in vitro* causes acute inhibition of neuronal firing in these animals (23). This acute inhibitory activity of melatonin on neuronal firing seems to be mediated by Mel 1a receptors through activation of potassium channels activated by the βγ subunits of pertussis toxin-sensitive G proteins, which is consistent with Mel 1a signalling through $G_{inhibitory}$ proteins (23). This acute suppressive effect of melatonin on SCN multiunit firing is abolished in Mel 1a receptor-deficient mice (23).

Application of physiologic melatonin concentrations to the SCN *in vitro* experiments at specific time points can reset the neuronal circadian rhythms (24). Phase shifting activity by melatonin to reset the SCN is greatest prior to the onset of darkness, with robust advances of 2 to 4 hours occurring in subsequent neuronal rhythms (24). The phase shifting effect of melatonin, which is distinct from the acute inhibitory effect of melatonin on neuronal

firing, might involve protein kinase C (25) and nitric oxide (26). This effect may be mediated by the Mel 1a receptor as Mel 1a receptor knockout mice (23) continue to show the phase shift phenomenon in response to melatonin despite the lack of Mel 1a receptors. Therefore, multiple signalling pathways might be used by the Mel 1a and Mel 1b receptors for different physiologic effects on the SCN. Detection of melatonin receptor-mediated alterations in gene expression, which might mediate these distinct effects of melatonin on the SCN, has just begun to be analyzed (6).

The expression of melatonin receptors is a dynamic process, which might show a circadian variation in their binding capacity as is exemplified in the SCN. Maximal binding of ^{125}I-iodomelatonin to rat SCN melatonin receptors occurs late in the day and minimal binding in the early morning around 4 a.m. (27). Gauer et al. (27) speculated that daily variations in plasma melatonin concentrations could be implicated in the regulation of the density of melatonin binding sites in the SCN and pars tuberalis, possibly by a mechanism of desensitization of the melatonin binding sites by melatonin itself. If this is correct, administration of high doses of melatonin might not be innocuous as it could downregulate its own melatonin receptors. Also based on the observations discussed above, timing of exogenously administered melatonin might be crucial to cause a shift in circadian rhythms.

PHYSIOLOGIC AND PATHOPHYSIOLOGIC ASPECTS OF MELATONIN SECRETION

Physiology

In a natural setting, entrainment by melatonin may be most important during early development when retina-mediated light information cannot be processed (28). Maternal melatonin secretion rhythms are maintained during pregnancy (29,30). During fetal life, at a time when the retina-SCN pathway has not yet formed, melatonin produced by the mother provides the developing SCN with entraining information. This fetal maternal information keeps the fetal clock entrained and in tune with the outside world until retina-mediated entrainment becomes functional during postnatal life (28). Babies up to the age of 3 months do not have a well-developed circadian rhythm (31). Nighttime melatonin secretion peaks during early childhood and then drops sharply until early adulthood (32). It had been speculated that the sharp decline in melatonin secretion that occurs in late childhood might be involved in the initiation of puberty, but no strong data are available to support this assumption. Melatonin continues to decrease significantly with age; similarly, the time during which melatonin remains elevated at night also decreases with age (33). Studies in women during the perimenopause period reveal that the decline in melatonin precedes follicle-stimulating hormone increase during menopause with a decline of 41% in the age group 40 to 44 years, and a further decline of 35% between the age groups 50 to 54 years and 55 to 59 years (34). Whether this decline in melatonin secretion contributes to the development of menopause or to menopausal symptoms and signs is questionable. An association between the quality of sleep and the amount of melatonin secreted has been noted, especially in the elderly (35). Animal studies, which included mice whose ovaries no longer functioned, (similar to menopause) seemed to show that the aging process could be slowed down by pineal grafting of young pineal glands from young animals on to aging animals. It was speculated that this inhibitory effect on aging might possibly be mediated by melatonin (36). Obviously, if these findings could be replicated, this would have important consequences in the management of menopause and aging (see below).

Body temperature fluctuates during the 24-hour time period, with temperature being higher during the daytime when compared with nighttime. The drop in nighttime temperature can be reversed by exposure to bright light. Because this effect is mediated by melatonin, melatonin, therefore, decreases core body temperature (37,38). The temperature-lowering effect of melatonin might be of therapeutic interest, as hot flushes are associated with an increase temperature. No studies are available to answer this question.

Melatonin secretion changes with alterations in the length of daytime encountered in the different seasons of the year. This has powerful effects on reproductive function in seasonal breeding animals, but, if present, its effect on human reproduction seems to be minimal (39,40). Melatonin secretion does not change in different phases of the menstrual cycle or by the administration of oral contraceptives (14,16). Melatonin receptors have been identified in human granulosa cells (41), and this hormone stimulates progesterone production by human granulosa cells (42). Also melatonin seems to concentrate in follicular fluid (43). The physiologic significance of these observations is not clear. A possible association of the 24-hour melatonin secretion pattern and the initiation of the luteinizing hormone (LH) has been observed (44,45).

Pathophysiology

Nocturnal melatonin secretion is amplified in women with functional hypothalamic amenorrhea (46,47). It is not clear whether increased melatonin concentration is a contributing factor in causing amenorrhea by influencing LH-releasing hormone secretion or an epiphenomenon. Short-term administration of supraphysiologic doses of melatonin (60 to 300 mg), which creates supraphysiologic levels, in the periovulatory period did not prevent ovulation (45,48). Long-term use of high-dose melatonin (4 months, 300 mg/day) seems to decrease the midcycle

LH surge. It has been suggested that a combination of high-dose melatonin with a progestin derivative (norethindrone) could be used as an estrogen-free oral contraceptive pill (48). Acute elevations of melatonin occur during fasting (49) and sustained exercise (50). The importance of these observations regarding possible impacts on reproduction currently are not clear. Travelling across several time zones creates a situation in which the body's circadian rhythms, including melatonin secretion, are temporarily not properly synchronized to the prevailing light–dark cycle, which might cause jet lag (51). While readjusting their circadian rhythm to local time, individuals experience difficulty sleeping, among other signs and symptoms. Chronic circadian disturbance encountered in shift work might cause many of the health and social problems reported by shift workers, including chronic sleep problems.

COMPOUNDS THAT ALTER MELATONIN SECRETION

As alterations in melatonin secretion might have an impact on the circadian rhythm and possibly sleep, it is important to be aware of substances which influence melatonin secretion. Nonsteroidal antiinflammatory drugs (e.g., aspirin or ibuprofen) can lower melatonin secretion. These medications interfere with the production of prostaglandins, which can influence melatonin production in the pinealocyte (52). As would be expected from the regulation of melatonin secretion, β-blockers (e.g., atenolol) abolish the nocturnal rise of melatonin secretion (15). Similarly, presynaptic blockage of norepinephrine production with α-methyl-para-tyrosine attenuates the nocturnal melatonin peak (53). It is of note that subjects taking this compound complain of sleep disturbances for several days after stopping this medication, which could be related to the disruption of the circadian rhythm of melatonin secretion. Some of the calcium channel blockers and the α2 receptor agonist clonidine decrease melatonin secretion (54,55). Decreased intracellular Ca^{2+} levels seem to interfere with melatonin production, and presynaptic α2 receptors decrease norepinephrine release. The sedative-hypnotics of the benzodiazepine type (e.g., diazepam and alprazolam), which act on the γ-aminobutyric acid complex type A receptor complex, lower melatonin secretion (56,57). Antidepressants such as the norepinephrine reuptake inhibitor, desipramine, and monoamine oxidase (MAO) inhibitors seem to increase plasma melatonin secretion (58,59). Serotonin reuptake inhibitors can increase or decrease melatonin secretion (60,61). Therefore, different types of antidepressant medications might interfere with the circadian rhythm or magnitude of melatonin secretion. Caffeine and alcohol might decrease melatonin secretion, especially when consumed at nighttime (62,63). Dexamethasone decreases melatonin secretion

(64). Alterations in plasma tryptophan concentration can increase or decrease melatonin secretion (65,66).

THERAPEUTIC INTERVENTIONS USING MELATONIN

Circadian Rhythms

Jet lag is caused by travelling across several time zones within several hours. The internal clock (i.e., the SCN) is not synchronized with the daytime–nighttime rhythm at the place of arrival. Jet lag can cause insomnia, fatigue, irritability, and poor concentration. It is easier to adapt when flying west, when the day is stretched, than flying east when the day is compressed. A possible explanation is that the body clock operates on a 25-hour rhythm when no clues are given to the SCN (67). To alleviate jet lag symptoms, it is recommended to take low doses of melatonin 1 to 2 hours prior to going to be bed in the place of destination for several days (68,69). In addition to other environmental clues, such as light, melatonin helps to reset the clock faster. Taking melatonin at a time corresponding to the beginning of the sleep period at the point of destination starting a few days prior to departure can inconvenience people significantly because of side effects, such as drowsiness. Most of the data available seem to demonstrate that starting treatment after arrival seems to produce similar positive results when compared with starting to take melatonin several days prior to departure (70). Therefore, it is recommended to take a dose of 5 mg of melatonin 1 to 2 hours before bedtime after arrival at your destination (67,68,70). Exposure to sunlight after arrival also might help to reset the SCN (71). When travelling more than six times zones, avoiding bright light exposure at certain times might become important in facilitating readaptation and a nomogram has been developed, which helps to avoid exposure to light at these critical periods (72).

Shift Work

Switching from working during the daytime to working at night is very taxing as the sleep–wake cycle is opposite to the light–dark cycle of the environment. To improve adjustment to these conditions, workers can expose themselves to artificial bright light at night, which resets the SCN and lowers melatonin levels (73–76). In addition, avoiding exposure to bright light during the daytime and taking melatonin (0.5 to 5 mg) prior to sleep seems to improve daytime sleep and alertness (67,74,77). It is not clear how beneficial an attempt to shift the sleep–wake cycle is, if the change in the work schedule is short term ($\leq$4 weeks).

It is of note that air travelers do adjust their circadian rhythm faster than shift workers. Melatonin production that prevents the desired phase shift is suppressed by sunlight exposure, which is generally much brighter then than the indoor light exposure for shift workers. Sunlight is also available to help shift the endogenous circadian pacemaker (71).

Sleep Disturbances

Sleep disturbances increase with age. Possible reasons for the high frequency of sleep complaints in elderly people are primary endogenous age-related sleep disorders, increased likelihood of disease that interferes with sleep, and drug use, which can cause secondary sleep disorders (78). Therefore, review type of nonprescription and prescription drugs used before beginning treatment with melatonin in patients with insomnia physical disorders, mental health problems including depression and anxiety disorders, improper sleep environment, inadequate sleep habits, circadian cycle abnormalities, and substance abuse (79). It might also be prudent to collect nocturnal urine, preferably in 3-hour intervals, to detect a decrease in melatonin secretion or a shift in its peak secretion (78). To document improvement, a subjective sleep diary should be kept and, if possible, an actigraph be used to estimate sleep variables (78) for a limited period of time of melatonin use on sleep quality and quantity. Because of the metabolism of orally administered melatonin, slow release capsules such as the one used by Garfinkel et al. (78) might be preferable (2 mg, Circadin, *Neurim Pharmaceutical, Tel Aviv, Israel*). Wurtman and Zhdanova (80) had similar positive results in sustaining sleep in elderly insomniacs using an oral dose of melatonin (0.3 mg). Therefore, in a carefully screened group of patients suffering from insomnia, a trial of melatonin might be indicated before switching the patient to more powerful medication such as benzodiazepines, which have more side effects. Patients suffering from delayed sleep phase syndrome might possibly benefit from melatonin treatment (81).

Unproven Benefits From Melatonin

Melatonin secretion can be decreased in patients with psychiatric disorders, especially depression (82). Some forms of depression seem to involve disregulation in the central nervous system of norepinephrine and serotonin containing neurons and postsynaptic receptors (83,84). Therefore, at least from a theoretical standpoint, an attractive hypothesis is that alterations in melatonin secretion reflect disease states as both systems also play an important role in the regulation of melatonin secretion (53,66). Unfortunately, no consistent changes in melatonin secretion have been found reflecting depression (32,85). Therefore, melatonin measurements cannot be used to diagnose depression, and treatment of depression with melatonin is not appropriate. Seasonal affective disorder, which is characterized by recurrent episodes in autumn and winter of depression, hypersomnia, and augmented appetite, fulfills the criteria of a rhythm disorder (86). These patients show a change in core temperature rhythms, but melatonin rhythm and amplitude seem to be unchanged (86). The preferred therapy is timed exposure to bright light, and it is not clear whether melatonin administration might be beneficial to this group of patients (86). Melatonin secretion does not seem to be altered in premenstrual syndrome (87). Patients suffering from anorexia nervosa might have elevated melatonin blood levels, but this has no therapeutic implications (88).

In very high pharmacologic doses, melatonin works as an antioxidant, possibly through non–receptor-mediated mechanisms. It has been claimed that this property of melatonin might have a preventive effect on illnesses affected by free radicals (67). As stated by Reppert and Weaver (28) this antioxidant effect requires melatonin concentrations approximately 100 times greater than the physiologic melatonin secretion (< 1 nm). Therefore, an antioxidant effect of melatonin may have some therapeutic application, but definitely not to the extent claimed in self-help books (67).

It has been claimed that melatonin can reverse aging (89). Some have studied strains of mice with a well-described genetic defect in pineal melatonin biosynthesis which therefore could not make melatonin (28,36). In some of these melatonin-deficient mice strains, lifespan increased by 20%, but not in female C57BL/6 mice. The lifespan was actually shortened in the mouse strain C3H/He secondary to reproductive tract tumors (28,36). Thus, no evidence indicates that melatonin administered to melatonin-producing mice can increase longevity. The suggestion that melatonin may increase longevity in humans is based on pure speculation (28).

SUMMARY

Molecular biology has been able to disperse some of the myth surrounding melatonin: melatonin production sites can be clearly identified by detecting message and protein from AANAT in specific tissues; specific melatonin receptors can be identified by detecting message and protein in specific tissues; activation of specific signalling pathways used by the different melatonin receptors can be detected. Also, knockout models will help to clarify the physiologic action of this hormone as well as it pathophysiologic states. This grounding in molecular biology will help to develop sound therapeutic applications for melatonin. It would be regrettable if melatonin did not find its proper place in the therapeutic armamentarium because unfounded claims might discredit well-defined positive actions of this fascinating hormone.

ACKNOWLEDGMENT

I would like to thank James Olcese, PhD from the Institute of Hormone and Fertility Research, University of Hamburg for reading the manuscript and his valuable suggestions.

REFERENCES

1. Lerner AB, Case JD, Takashi Y, et al. Isolation of melatonin, pineal factor that lightens melanocytes. *Journal of the American Chemical Society* 1958;80:2587.
2. Cardinali DP. Melatonin. A mammalian pineal hormone. *Endocr Rev* 1981;2:327–346.
3. Reiter RJ. The pineal and its hormones in the control of reproduction in mammals. *Endocr Rev* 1980;1:109–131.
4. Preslock JP. The pineal gland: basic implications and clinical correlations. *Endocr Rev* 1984;5:282–308..
5. Krahn LE, Lu PY, Klee G, Delgado PR, Lin S-C, Zimmermann RC. Examining tryptophan function: a modified technique for rapid tryptophan depletion. *Neuropsychopharmacology* 1996;15:325–328.
6. Olcese J. Cellular and molecular mechanisms mediating melatonin action. *The Aging Male* 1988;1:1–17.
7. Klein DC, Roseboom PH, Coon SL. New light is shining on the melatonin rhythm enzyme. The first postcloning view. *TEM* 1996;7:106–112.
8. Coon SL, Mazuruk K, Bernard M, et al. The human serotonin N-acetyltransferase (EC 2.3.187) gene: structure, chromosomal location and tissue expressions. *Genomics* 1996;34:76–84.
9. Moore RY. Neural control of the pineal gland. *Behav Brain Res* 1996;73:125–130.
10. Roseboom PH, Coon SL, Baler R, et al. Melatonin synthesis: analysis of the > 150-fold nocturnal increase in serotonin N-acetyltransferase mRNA in the rat pineal gland. *Endocrinology* 1996;137:3033–3044.
11. Lockley SW, Skene DJ, Arendt J, Tabandeh H, Bird AC, Defrance R. Relationship between melatonin rhythms and visual loss in the blind. *J Clin Endocrinol Metab* 1997;82:3763–3770.
12. Lewy AJ, Wehr TA, Goodwin FK, Newsome DA, Markey SP. Light suppresses melatonin secretion in humans. *Science* 1980;210:1267–1269.
13. Bispink G, Zimmermann RC, Weise HC, Leidenberger F. Influence of melatonin on the sleep independent component of prolactin secretion. *J Pineal Res* 1990;8:97–106.
13a.Campbell SS, Murphy PJ. Extraocular circadian phototransduction in humans. *Science* 1998;279:396–399.
14. Berga SL, Yen SSC. Circadian pattern of plasma melatonin concentrations during four phases of the menstrual cycle. *Neuroendocrinology* 1990;51:606–612.
15. Arendt J, Bojkowski C, Franey C, Wright J, Marks V. Immunoassay of 6-hydroxymelatonin sulfate in human plasma and urine. Abolition of the 24-hour rhythm with atenolol. *J Clin Endocrinol Metab* 1985;60:1166–1173.
16. Delfs TM, Baars S, Fock F, Schumacher M, Olcese J, Zimmermann RC. Sex steroids do not alter melatonin secretion in the human. *Hum Reprod* 1994;9:49–54.
17. Arendt J. Radioimmunoassayable melatonin: circulating patterns in man and sheep. *Progr Brain Res* 1979;52:249–258.
18. Reppert SM, Weaver DR, Rivkees SA, Stopa EG. Putative melatonin receptors in a human biological clock. *Science* 1988;242:78–81.
19. Weaver DR, Stehle JH, Stopa EG, Reppert SM. Melatonin receptors in human hypothalamus and pituitary: implications for circadian and reproductive responses to melatonin. *J Clin Endocrinol Metab* 1993;76:295–301.
20. Reppert SM, Weaver DR, Godson C. Melatonin receptors step into the light: cloning and classification of subtypes. *Trends Pharmacol Sci* 1996;17:100–102.
21. Reppert SM, Weaver DR, Ebisawa T. Cloning and characterization of mammalian melatonin receptor that mediates reproductive and circadian responses. *Neuron* 1994;13:1177–1185.
22. Godson C, Reppert SM. The Mel 1a melatonin receptor is coupled to parallel signal transduction pathways. *Endocrinology* 1997;138:397–404.
23. Liu C, Weaver DR, Jin X, Shearman LP, Pieschl RL, Gribkoff VK, Reppert SM. Molecular dissection of two distinct actions of melatonin on the suprachiasmatic circadian clock. *Neuron* 1997;19:91–102.
24. Gillette MU, McArthur AJ. Circadian actions of melatonin at the suprachiasmatic nucleus. *Behav Brain Res* 1996;73:135–139.
25. McArthur AJ, Hunt AE, Gillette MU. Melatonin action and signal tansduction in the rat suprachiasmatic circadian clock; activation of protein kinase C at dusk and dawn. *Endocrinology* 1997;138:627–634.
26. Starkey SJ. Melatonin and 5-hydroxytryptamine phase advance the rat circadian clock by activation of nitric oxide synthesis. *Neurosci Lett* 1996;211:199–202.
27. Gauer F, Masson-Pevet M, Skene DJ, Vivien-Roels B, Pevet P. Daily rhythms of melatonin binding sites in the pars tuberalis and suprachiasmatic nuclei; evidence for a regulation of melatonin receptors by melatonin itself. *Neuroendocrinology* 1993;57:120–126.
28. Reppert SM, Weaver DR. Melatonin madness. *Cell* 1995;83:1059–1062.
29. Zimmermann RC, Schröder S, Baars S, Schumacher M, Weise HC. Melatonin and prolactin secretion during pregnancy. *Acta Endocrinol* 1989;120 (Suppl 1):224–225.
30. Kivelä A. Serum melatonin during pregnancy. *Acta Endocrinol* 1991;124:233–237.
31. Jaldo-Alba F, Munoz-Hoyos M, Molina-Carballo A, Molina-Font J, Acuna-Cas-

troviejo D. Light deprivation increases plasma levels of melatonin during the first 72 h of life in human infants. *Acta Endocrinol* 1993;129:442–445.

32. Waldhauser F, Ehrhart B, Forster E. Clinical aspects of the melatonin action: impact of development, aging, and puberty involvement of melatonin in psychiatric disease and importance of neuroimmunoendocrine interactions. *Experientia* 1993;49:671–681.

33. Nair NPV, Hariharasubramanian N, Pilapil C, Isaac I, Thavundayil JX. Plasma melatonin—an index of brain aging in humans. *Biol Psychiatry* 1986;21:141–150.

34. Vakkuri O, Kivela A, Leppäluoto J, Valtonen M, Kauppila A. Decrease in melatonin precedes follicle-stimulating hormone increase during menopause. *Eur J Endocrinol* 1996;135:188–192.

35. Haimov I, Laudon M, Zisapel N, et al. Sleep disorders and melatonin rhythms in elderly people. *BMJ* 1994;300:167.

36. Pierpaoli W, Regelson W. Pineal control of aging: effect of melatonin and pineal grafting on aging mice. *Proc Natl Acad Sci U S A* 1994;91:787–791.

37. Strassman RJ, Qualls CR, Lisansky EJ, Peake GT. Elevated rectal temperature produced by bright light is reversed by melatonin infusion in men. *J Appl Physiol* 1991;71:2178–2182.

38. Cagnacci A, Elliott JA, Yen SSC. Melatonin: a major regulator of the circadian rhythm of core temperature in humans. *J Clin Endocrinol Metab* 1992;74:447–452.

39. Cagnacci A, Volpe A. Influence of melatonin and photoperiod on animal and human reproduction. *J Endocrinol Invest* 1996;19:382–411.

40. Kauppila A, Kivela A, Pakarinen A, Vakkuri O. Inverse seasonal relationship between melatonin and ovarian activity in humans in a region with a strong seasonal contrast in luminosity. *J Clin Endocrinol Metab* 1987;65:823–828.

41. Yie SM, Niles LP, Younglai EV. Melatonin receptors on human granulosa cell membranes. *J Clin Endocrinol Metab* 1995;80:1747–1749.

42. Webley G, Luck M. Melatonin directly stimulates the secretion of progesterone by human and bovine granulosa cells in vitro. *J Reprod Fertil* 1986;78:711–717.

43. Brzezinski A, Seibel MM, Lynch HJ, Deng M-H, Wurtman RJ. Melatonin in human preovulatory follicular fluid. *J Clin Endocrinol Metab* 1987;64:865–867.

44. Brzezinski A, Lynch HJ, Wurtman RJ, Seibel MM. Possible contribution of melatonin to the timing of the luteinizing hormone surge. *N Engl J Med* 1987;316:550–551.

45. Zimmermann RC, Schröder S, Baars S, Schumacher M, Weise HC. Melatonin and the luteinizing hormone surge. *Fertil Steril* 1990;54:612–618.

46. Berga SL, Mortola JF, Yen SSC. Amplification of nocturnal melatonin secretion in women with functional hypothalamic amenorrhea. *J Clin Endocrinol Metab* 1988;66:242–244.

47. Brzezinsky A, Lynch HJ, Seibel MM, Nader, Wurtman RJ. The circadian rhythm of plasma melatonin during the normal menstrual cycle and in amenorrheic women. *J Clin Endocrinol Metab* 1988;66:891–895.

48. Voordouw BCG, Euser R, Verdonk RER, et al. Melatonin and melatonin-progestin combinations alter pituitary-ovarian function in women and can inhibit ovulation. *J Clin Endocrinol Metab* 1992;74:108–117.

49. Beitins IZ, Barkan A, Klibanski A, et al. Hormonal responses to short term fasting in postmenopausal women. *J Clin Endocrinol Metab* 1985;60:1120–1126.

50. Carr DB, Reppert SM, Bullen B, et al. Plasma melatonin increases during exercise in women. *J Clin Endocrinol Metab* 1981;53:224–225.

51. Bellamy N. The jet lag phenomenon: etiology, pathogenesis, clinical features, and management. *Modern Med Can* 1986;41:717–732.

52. Cardinali D, Ritta MN, Pereya E. Role of prostaglandins in rat pineal neuroeffector junction. Changes in melatonin and norepinephrine release in vitro. *Endocrinology* 1982;111:530–534.

53. Zimmermann RC, Krahn L, Klee G, Delgado P, Ory S, Lin S-C. Inhibition of presynaptic catecholamine synthesis with α-methyl-para-tyrosine attenuates nocturnal melatonin secretion in humans. *J Clin Endocrinol Metab* 1994;79:1110–1114.

54. Meyer AC, Nieuwenhuis JJ, Meyer BJ. Dihydropyridine calcium antagonists depress the amplitude of the plasma melatonin cycle in baboons. *Life Sci* 1986;39:1563–1569.

55. Lewy A, Siever LJ, Markey SP. Clonidine reduces plasma melatonin levels. *J Pharm Pharmacol* 1986;38:555–556.

56. Monteleone P, Forziati D, Maj M. Preliminary observations on the suppression of nocturnal plasma melatonin levels by short-term administration of diazepam in humans. *J Pineal Res* 1989;6:253–258.

57. McIntyre I, Burrows GD, Norman TR. Suppression of nocturnal plasma melatonin by a single dose of the benzodiazepine alprazolam in humans. *Biol Psych* 1988;24:105–108.

58. Skene D, Bojkowski C, Arendt J. Comparison of the effects of acute fluvoxamine (Luvox) and desipramine administration on melatonin and cortisol production in humans. *Br J Clin Pharmacol* 1994;37:181–186.

59. Oxenkrug G, McIntyre I, McCauley R, Yuwiler A. Effect of selective monoamine oxidase inhibitors on rat pineal melatonin synthesis in vitro. *J Pineal Res* 1988;5:99–109.

60. Demisch K, Demisch L, Bochnik HJ, Nickelson T, Althoff PH, Schöffling K, Rieth R. Melatonin and cortisol increase after fluvoxamine. *Br J Clin Pharmacol* 1986;22:620–622.

61. Childs PA, Rodin I, Martin NJ, Allen NHP, Plaskett L, Smythe PJ, Thompson C. Effect of fluoxetine (prozac) on melatonin secretion in patients with seasonal affective disorder and matched controls. *Br J Psychiatry* 1995;166:196–198.

62. Wright KP. Badia P, Myers BL. Hakel M. Effects of caffeine, bright light, and their combination on nighttime melatonin and temperature during 2 nights of sleep deprivation. *J Sleep Res* 1995;24:458.

63. Ekman AC, Leppaluoto J. Vakkuri O. Ethanol inhibits melatonin secretion in healthy volunteers in a dose-dependent randomized double blind cross-over study. *J Clin Endocrinol Metab* 1993;77:780–783.

64. Demisch L, Demisch K, Nickelson T. Influence of dexamethasone on nocturnal melatonin production in healthy adult subjects. *J Pineal Res* 1988;5:317–322.

65. Hajak G, Huether G, Blanke J, et al. The influence of intravenous L-tryptophan on plasma melatonin and sleep in men. *Pharmacopsychiatry* 1991;24:17–20.

66. Zimmermann RC, McDougle C, Schumacher M, Olcese J, Mason JW, Heninger GR, Price LH. Effects of acute tryptophan depletion on nocturnal melatonin secretion in humans. *J Clin Endocrinol Metab* 1993;76:1160–1164.

67. Reiter RJ, Robinson J. *Melatonin. Breakthrough discoveries that can help you.* New York: Bantam Books, 1995.

68. Petri K, Dawson AG, Thompson L, Brook R. A double-blind trial of melatonin as a treatment for jet lag in an international cabin crew. *Biol Psychiatr* 1993;33:526–530.

69. Claustrat B, Brun J, David M, Sassolas G, Chazot G. Melatonin and jet lag: confirmatory results using a simplified protocol. *Biol Psych* 1992;32:705–711.

70. Lino A, Silvy S, Condorelli L, Rusconi AC. Melatonin and jet lag: treatment schedule. *Biol Psych* 1993;34:587.

71. Lewy AJ, Saeeduddin A, Sack L. Phase shifting the human circadian clock using melatonin. *Behav Brain Res* 1996;73:131–134.

72. Daan S, Lewy AJ. Scheduled esposure to daylight: a potential strategy to reduce jet lag following transmeridian flight. *Psychopharmacol Bull* 1984;20:566–568.

73. Bojkowski CJ, Aldhous ME, English J, Franey C, Poulton AL, Skene DJ, Arendt J. Suppression of nocturnal plasma melatonin and 6-sulfatoxymelatonin by bright and dim light in man. *Horm Metab Res* 1987;19:437–440.

74. Eastman C, Stewart K, Mahoney M, Liu L, Fogg L. Dark goggles and bright light improve circadian rhythm adaptation to nightshift work. *Sleep* 1994;17:535–543.

75. Dawson D, Encel N, Sushington K. Improving adaptation to simulated night shift: timed exposure to bright light versus daytime melatonin administration. *Sleep* 1995;18:11–21.

76. Dawson D, Encel N, Lushington K. Improving adaptation to simulated night shift: timed exposure to bright light versus daytime melatonin administration. *Sleep* 1995;18:1139–1142.

77. Folkard S, Arendt J, Clark M. Can melatonin improve shift workers tolerance of the night shift. Some preliminary findings. *Chronobiol Int* 1993;10:315–320.

78. Garfinkel D, Laudon M, Zisapel N. Improvement of sleep quality in elderly people by controlled-release melatonin. *Lancet* 1995;346:541–544.

79. Sahelian R. *Melatonin. Nature's sleeping pill.* Garden City Park, NY, Avery Publishing Group, 1995:42–43.

80. Wurtman RJ, Zhdanova I. Improvement of sleep quality by melatonin. *Lancet* 1995;346:1491.

81. Stankov B, Fraschini F, Oldani F. Melatonin and delayed sleep phase syndrome: ambulatory polygraph evaluation. *Neuroreport* 1994;5:132–134.

82. Wetterberg L, Beck Frijs J, Kjellman BF, Ljunggren JG. Circadian rhythms in melatonin and cortisol secretion in depression. *Adv Biochem Psychopharmacol* 1984;39:197–205.

83. Schatzberg AF, Schildkraut JJ. Recent studies on norepinephrine systems in mood disorders. In: Bloom FE, Kupfer DJ, eds. *Psychopharmacology. The fourth generation of progress.* New York: Raven Press, 1995:911–920.

84. Maes M, Meltzer HY. The serotonin hypothesis of major depression. In: Bloom FE, Kupfer DJ, eds. *Psychopharmacology. The fourth generation of progress.* New York: Raven Press, 1995:933–944.

85. Rubin RT, Heist EK, McGeoy SS, Hanada K, Lesser IM. Neuroendocrine aspects of primary endogenous depression. XI. Serum melatonin measures in patients and matched control subjects. *Arch Gen Psychiatry* 1992;49:558–567.

86. Wirt-Justice A. Biological rhythms in mood disorder. Recent studies on norepinephrine systems in mood disorders. In: Bloom FE, Kupfer DJ, eds. *Psychopharmacology. The fourth generation of progress.* New York: Raven Press, 1995:999–1018.

87. Mortola JF. The premenstrual syndrome. In: Adashi E, Rock J, eds. *Reproductive medicine.* New York: Raven Press, 1996:1635–1647.

88. Kennedy SH, Brown GM, McVey G, Garfinkel PE. Pineal and adrenal function before and after refeeding in anorexia nervosa. *Biol Psychiatr* 1991;30:216–224.

89. Pierpaoli W, Regelson W. *The melatonin miracle.* New York: Simon and Schuster, 1995.

Treatment of the Postmenopausal Woman: Basic and Clinical Aspects, Second Edition, edited by Rogerio A. Lobo, Lippincott Williams & Wilkins, Philadelphia © 1999.

CHAPTER 57

Selective Estrogen Receptor Modulators

Felicia Cosman and Robert Lindsay

Estrogen is the most frequently prescribed medication in the United States. In postmenopausal women, estrogens are the most effective treatment for menopausal symptoms such as hot flushes (also called flashes) and urogenital atrophy (1–2). Estrogen, which is also the leading pharmacologic regimen for the prevention and therapy of osteoporosis, is approved by the US Food and Drug Administration (FDA) for this purpose (3–5). Estrogens exert multisystem effects, including a probable decrease in the risk of heart disease and possibly stroke, only in part through beneficial effects on blood lipids (6). Furthermore, evidence is accumulating to suggest that estrogens exert positive effects on the central nervous system, possibly reducing the incidence and severity of Alzheimer's type dementia and maintaining normal cognitive function in healthy postmenopausal women (7–8).

However, because many women are concerned that breast cancer risk can be modestly increased after long-term estrogen treatment (9,10), the use of estrogens is often restricted to a duration of insufficient length to provide significant effects on disease outcomes. Long-term compliance is often estimated to be 15% to 40% (11). The fear of breast cancer is so profound that many women mistakenly view it as the most common cause of death, and reductions in risk of heart attack and osteoporotic fracture are often not sufficient to counteract this fear. In addition, the stimulatory action of estrogen on the uterine endometrium, although easily controlled with progestin, also remains an issue, because for many regimens, regular vaginal bleeding is necessary to protect the endometrium. Furthermore, the risk of uterine cancer can be increased with some hormone replacement regimens even when progestins are given (12,13). The increased risk of deep venous thrombosis, breast tenderness and engorgement, as well as the perception that hormone

replacement is associated with weight gain are other reasons that limit long-term use of this therapy.

It is likely that an agent that maintains the benefits of estrogens but avoids the risks would be used by many postmenopausal women for overall health maintenance. Drugs in the class now called "selective estrogen receptor modulators" (SERMS), previously called "antiestrogens" (Fig. 57.1), hold this promise. Some of these agents act as antagonists in human reproductive tissues, but act as partial agonists on the skeletal system and on serum lipoproteins. They might, therefore, be alternatives for prevention of osteoporosis, particularly in women with an increased risk of breast or uterine cancer, or in those women who are not willing to take estrogen because of the fear of breast or uterine cancer.

SELECTIVE ESTROGEN RECEPTOR MODULATORS

Definition and Mode of Action

The term "antiestrogens" has been largely replaced because it is a misleading term for many of the agents, including those to which it was originally applied, for example, clomiphene and tamoxifen. Most agents in clinical use or in clinical trials are those which retain some estrogen agonist activity in addition to maintaining some antagonist activity. The drugs are, therefore, better named mixed estrogen agonist/antagonists or partial agonist antiestrogens. The term "SERM" has come into vogue because it implies that these drugs have agonist properties on some estrogen receptive tissues and antagonist properties on others. This term can also be used to encompass the concept of partial estrogen agonist activity on some estrogen receptors. Currently under development are several drugs that are pure estrogen antagonists and, therefore, true antiestrogens, which do not seem to exert any estrogen agonist effects on any of the estrogen receptors throughout the body (14). These medications (ICI 164,384

F. Cosman, R. Lindsay: Department of Clinical Medicine, Columbia University College of Physicians & Surgeons, New York, New York 10032.

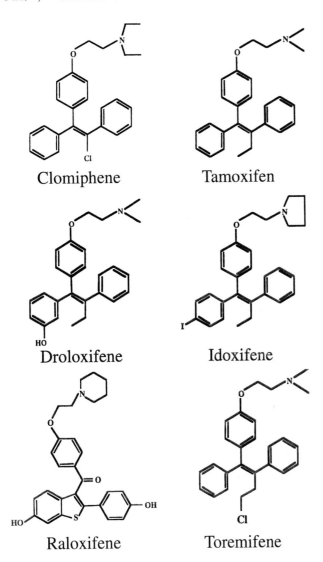

FIG. 57.1. Structure of selective estrogen receptor modulators (SERMS) in clinical use or clinical development.

cellular estrogen receptor subtypes (ER-α and ER-β) have been identified (18). The distribution of these receptors is complex with both types being expressed in reproductive versus nonreproductive tissues, although in general, with an apparent predominance of ER-α expression in reproductive tissues and ER-β expression in nonreproductive tissues (19). To some extent, differences in activity of a SERM on reproductive tissues versus other tissues could be explained by the difference in agonist versus antagonist activity at these two different receptor subtypes. That is, a drug such as raloxifene, could exert antagonist activity on breast and uterus (through the α receptor) and agonist activity on the skeleton and lipoproteins (through the β receptor). The issue is clearly more complicated, however, in that some SERMS can have differential effects even in organs with the same predominant type of estrogen receptor (e.g., tamoxifen has largely antagonistic effects on the breast but partial agonist effects on the uterus). Moreover, many organs such as the brain contain both α and β receptors, making it difficult to know which effect will predominate if divergent effects occur on the two receptors.

Another level of complexity regarding the mechanism of SERM actions is that different drugs that bind the same estrogen receptor can exert different effects (20). Pure antiestrogen action might be caused by the inability of the receptor–drug complex to achieve an appropriate functional conformation or a reduction in estrogen receptor density from increased turnover of the receptor (21,22). Partial agonist SERMS induce different conformations of the drug–receptor complex. The variable conformations induced bind, with different affinities, auxiliary proteins (co-repressors or coactivators), which either inhibit or potentiate subsequent gnomic actions (23). Finally, certain SERMS, such as raloxifene, can promote transcription of genetic material outside of the usual estrogen response element (24,25). Thus, we might expect that each SERM could produce a somewhat different spectrum of activity.

When comparing the SERMS with each other and with estrogens for clinical purposes, we need to consider the following issues for the target clinical dose of the medication: (a) In what tissues does the agent have an estrogen agonist effect and in what tissues does it have an estrogen antagonist or neutral effect? (b) In those tissues in which an estrogen-agonist effect exists, how does the potency compare with estrogen? (c) In those tissues in which an estrogen antagonist effect is found, how does the potency compare with that of the pure antiestrogens (ICI compounds 164,384 and ICI 182,780)?

Drugs in Clinical Use or Clinical Development

Clomiphene

Clomiphene was one of the first SERMs studied, and is a nonsteroidal triphenylethylene SERM. Some of its

and ICI 182,780) might be particularly useful for the treatment of breast cancer or benign proliferative diseases such as endometriosis or uterine fibroids. Pure estrogen antagonists have antiestrogenic effects on the uterus in the ovariectomized rat (no increase in uterine weight), whereas, tamoxifen produces changes more modest than those attributed to estrogens (15–17). Furthermore, when estrogen is given in combination with a SERM such as tamoxifen, only partial inhibition of the expected increase in uterine weight occurs, whereas the pure antagonists completely inhibit the expected estrogen-stimulated increment in uterine weight. Moreover, different target organ tissues might have differential sensitivities to these agonist/antagonist agents. For example, it is theoretically possible to find a dose of a pure antiestrogen that can result in uterine atrophy but not reduce bone density (14).

The major actions of the SERMS are thought to occur through interaction with the estrogen receptor. Two intra-

opposing biologic activities relate to its mixture of geometric isomers, with the *trans* isomer possessing antiestrogenic activity and the *cis* isomer possessing estrogenic activity. Although this agent was effective at reducing fertility in rodents, it actually increased fertility in humans and is currently used most frequently as an ovulation inducer in women trying to conceive. This fertility-enhancing effect appears to be mediated by estrogen antagonist effects on the neuroendocrine axis with a subsequent stimulation of gonadotropin secretion (20). Clomiphene also has some activity against advanced breast cancer (26,27), but studies of its efficacy were stopped because of the emergence of tamoxifen for this indication, the higher toxicity associated with chronic clomiphene use, and the less robust effect seen with this compound versus tamoxifen (28). Clomiphene probably has some estrogen agonist skeletal activity in ovariectomized rats (29–31), but human studies have been conducted. Several cohort investigations suggest that cyclical use of clomiphene for infertility might increase the risk of ovarian cancer (32–35).

Tamoxifen

Tamoxifen, also a nonsteroidal triphenylethylene compound, was first studied in rodent models as a possible postcoital contraceptive, such as clomiphene; however, in women, it was later found to induce ovulation. Similarly to clomiphene, this agent exerts estrogen antagonist effects on the neuroendocrine axis, boosting gonadotropin production, and increasing menopausal symptoms. The major development of this compound, however, has been as adjuvant chemotherapy for breast cancer. Tamoxifen has been shown conclusively in an abundance of clinical trials to decrease the risk of contralateral breast cancer and increase disease-free survival in patients with breast cancer at multiple stages of the disease (36). Furthermore, tamoxifen appears to prevent some breast cancer in high risk women without previous cancer (37,38). Because of an overall breast cancer incidence reduction of approximately 45%, the Breast Cancer Prevention Trial was terminated early, at 4.5 years (39).

Tamoxifen was initially expected to show negative effects on the skeleton because it was assumed that "antiestrogen" action would dominate there just as it did in the breast. Early cross-sectional, retrospective and, finally, prospective studies in patients with breast cancer given tamoxifen, however, did not demonstrate these negative effects and, in fact, showed neutral or even positive effects on the skeleton (40–49). Love et al. (50) subsequently studied 140 breast cancer patients randomized to receive tamoxifen versus placebo for 2 years. Lumbar spine mass in the tamoxifen-treated group increased significantly compared with placebo losses; radius losses were steeper in placebo-treated versus tamoxifen-treated patients.

Two prospective studies have also been performed in normal postmenopausal women without history of breast cancer. In late postmenopausal women (average time from menopause 11 years, $n = 57$), spine mass increased in tamoxifen-treated patients over two years (1.4% vs. loss of 0.7% in placebo group) but only a minimal effect was seen in total body bone mineral (group difference 0.5% at 2 years) and no effect on hip bone mass (51). In the other study (52), bone loss occurred in premenopausal patients ($n = 125$) treated with tamoxifen, but small bone gains occurred in the postmenopausal group ($n = 54$) in both spine and hip (Fig. 57.2). These investigations demonstrated that tamoxifen could exert a net antiestrogenic effect in the presence of normal premenopausal estrogen levels but a net estrogenic effect when estrogen levels are low as seen in postmenopausal women. Histomorphometric studies and bone turnover assessments corroborate the estrogenlike actions in estrogen-deficient women (48–51, 53–55). Moreover, the National Cancer Institute (NCI)-sponsored Breast Cancer Prevention Trial, documented that fracture incidence was reduced by about 30%, although this was apparently not statistically significant (39). These fracture data do not include vertebral deformity incidence because routine spine radiographs were not performed in this study.

Tamoxifen also appears to possess some of the beneficial effects of estrogen against heart disease. Two breast cancer studies using adjuvant tamoxifen reported occurrence of coronary heart disease. In the Scottish Breast Cancer Study, fatal myocardial infarction was 63% less common in those patients who received tamoxifen than in those who did not (56). In the Stockholm Breast Cancer Study, incidence of cardiac disease requiring hospital admission was 32% less common in those allocated to receive tamoxifen after breast cancer surgery (57). The reduction in coronary heart disease risk may be related in part to a reduction in total plasma cholesterol (12%), reduction in low-density lipoprotein (LDL) cholesterol (20%), or reduction in lipoprotein a (34%). Little if any effect has been seen on high-density lipoprotein (HDL) and triglyceride levels increase slightly. It is unknown whether tamoxifen exhibits lipoprotein-independent mechanisms of reducing coronary atherosclerosis such as reducing LDL oxidation or affecting vasodilation through nitric oxide and prostacyclin or endothelin-1 production (6,58). Not all data are consistent, however; in the Breast Cancer Prevention Trial, apparently no reduction was seen in the risk of myocardial infarction (39).

In summary, tamoxifen could potentially be useful as a breast cancer preventive agent or as an overall health maintenance agent in postmenopausal women on the basis of breast cancer, heart disease, and osteoporosis risk reduction because of the respective estrogen antagonist properties on the breast and estrogen agonist properties on the liver and skeleton. Its use in normal women

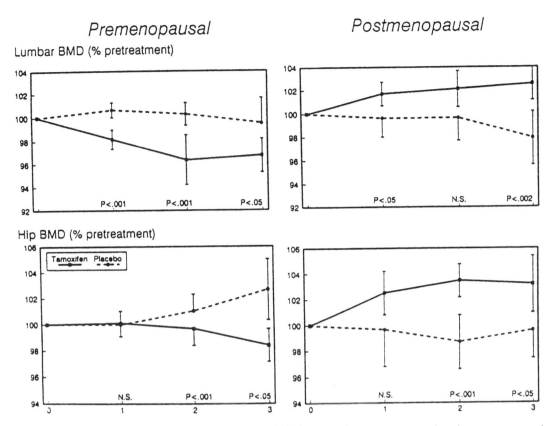

FIG. 57.2. Changes in bone mass of the spine and hip in normal postmenopausal and premenopausal women given tamoxifen over a 2-year period. (From Powles TJ, Kanis JA, Tidy A, Ashley S. Effect of tamoxifen on bone mineral density measured by dual-energy x-ray absorptiometry in healthy premenopausal and postmenopausal women. *J Clin Oncol* 1996;14:78–84; with permission.)

is limited by several specific problems, however. It is a sufficiently powerful estrogen agonist in the endometrium such that it causes an increase in malignant uterine tumors in humans as well as nonmalignant pathologic uterine conditions, including endometrial and endocervical polyps, fibroid tumors, adenomyosis, and endometrial hyperplasia (59–70). It also increases the frequency of ovarian cysts (65,66), but no evidence indicates that ovarian cancer incidence is increased with tamoxifen use (70–73). Tamoxifen increases the risk of hepatic tumors and DNA adducts in rodents given tamoxifen, suggesting a possible increase in the risk of hepatocellular carcinoma (74,75). This has not been demonstrated in humans, however, where only two cases of hepatocellular carcinoma have been reported during adjuvant chemotherapy with tamoxifen (76,77). Furthermore, studies indicate that hot flushes occur with increased frequency in postmenopausal (10% to 20%) as well as premenopausal women (60%) given tamoxifen (78–80). Whether this will translate into any effects on the central nervous system long-term is unknown. Ocular toxicity (81–90), thrombocytopenia (91), and deep venous thrombosis (70,91–93) are other potential adverse effects.

Raloxifene

Raloxifene, a nonsteroidal benzothiophene derivative, originally developed to treat breast cancer, is now approved by the FDA for prevention of osteoporosis in women after menopause. Raloxifene, appears to have an advantage over tamoxifen by retaining the beneficial effects of tamoxifen, but resulting in less estrogenic uterine stimulation. It is also at least as potent, if not more so, as an estrogen antagonist on the breast, although as yet no direct head-to-head comparisons have been made (39,94,95). (One is currently being planned by the NCI).

In a short-term, 8-week preliminary trial of raloxifene in 251 healthy, postmenopausal women, two doses of raloxifene were tested against estrogen and placebo (96). Bone turnover variables were reduced below placebo; these reductions were similar to those seen with estrogen for all markers except osteocalcin in the lower dose raloxifene group. Likewise, urinary calcium was similarly reduced to that seen with estrogen. Histomorphometric study showed that bone quality appeared to be totally normal under the influence of raloxifene (97), and calcium metabolism studies indicated changes similar to those seen with estrogen (98). Data from rodent models indicate that the protective effect of raloxifene on bone mass is associated with an increase in bone strength (99).

The clinical bone program for raloxifene is now extensive with 3-year follow-up in the phase III early postmenopausal prevention studies (approximately 1,200 women) now complete, and a 2-year extension underway. A 6-month study comparing raloxifene with unopposed conjugated equine estrogen has also been completed (98). The treatment program, Multiple Outcomes of Raloxifene Efficacy (MORE), evaluating older women for multiple end organ effects is also well underway and involves more than 7,000 women.

Data from the ongoing phase III trials of raloxifene have now been published (100). Healthy postmenopausal women (*n* = 601) aged between 45 and 60 years, within 2 to 8 years of menopause, with lumbar spine mass in the normal or low bone mass range were recruited into the trial. After baseline evaluation, patients were randomized to receive one of three raloxifene doses or placebo. Bone density, bone turnover, and lipid biochemistry were evaluated serially over 2 years. A total of 149 subjects (25%) dropped out of the study. Bone turnover decreased between 20% and 40% over the course of the study. Bone mass increased at all measured sites, including the lumbar spine, total hip, and total body, with all raloxifene doses resulting in increments between 1% and 2%, compared with losses in the placebo group of about 1% at each site (Fig. 57.3). Therefore, at 2 years, differences between raloxifene and placebo treated patients averaged 2.5% at all skeletal sites. Notably, bone mass changes were nearly identical at all skeletal sites, which is distinct from what is usually seen with antiresorptive therapy,

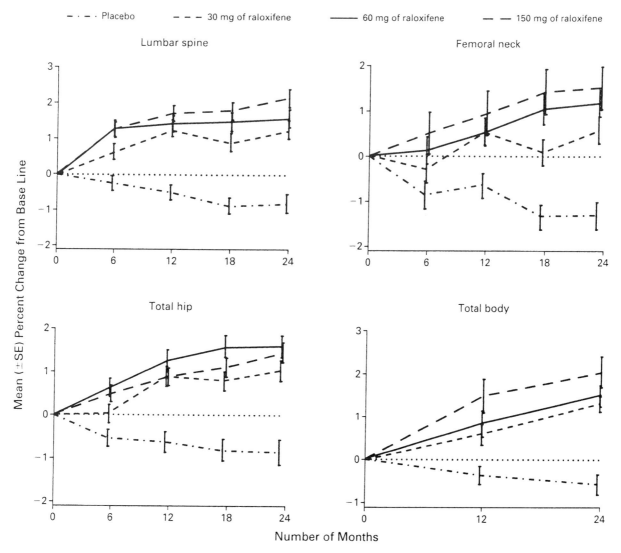

FIG. 57.3. Data from the ongoing phase III trials of raloxifene. (From Delmas PD, Bjarnason NH, Mitlak BH, et al. Effects of raloxifene on bone mineral density, serum cholesterol concentrations, and uterine endometrium in postmenopausal women. *N Engl J Med* 1997;337:1641–1647; with permission.)

such as estrogens and alendronate, where a much larger spine increment occurs in contrast to the hip or total body increment. Furthermore, the bone mass increment in the spine was lower than that attributable to estrogen in the estrogen comparator study (97). Finally, bone mass changes were very similar to those seen in a comparable group of normal postmenopausal women given tamoxifen in a European study (52). Preliminary data from the MORE osteoporosis treatment study, suggest that vertebral fracture occurrence is reduced by 40% to 60%, without a significant effect on peripheral fracture occurrence yet at 2 years (101).

As with tamoxifen, raloxifene has an estrogen agonist effect on several serum lipoproteins, but the potency of the effect differs from estrogen. In a study comparing raloxifene (60 and 120 mg) to hormone replacement therapy (HRT; conjugated equine estrogen 0.625 mg plus medroxyprogesterone acetate 2.5 mg), LDL was lowered to a similar extent by raloxifene and HRT (12% to 14%) but lipoprotein a was lowered only 7% to 8% by raloxifene in contrast to 19% by HRT (102). Furthermore, HRT increased total HDL cholesterol by 11%, whereas raloxifene produced no total HDL increment. Consistently, the HDL-2 subclass was increased 33% by HRT compared with 15% to 17% increases with raloxifene. All of these differences would suggest that HRT would be a better protector against atherogenesis that raloxifene. However, two other independent variables indicate raloxifene appears superior. Raloxifene did not increase triglyceride levels significantly, whereas HRT resulted in a 20% increase. Moreover, raloxifene lowered fibrinogen by 12% to 14%, compared with no effect for HRT. Both of these effects would suggest a superior effect of raloxifene against atherogenesis. Therefore, based on biochemical changes alone, it is difficult to compare the theoretical potency of protective effect by raloxifene versus HRT against vascular disease. Changes in serum lipoproteins are only one mechanism by which estrogens protect against heart disease, however. In monkeys, treatment with conjugated equine estrogen resulted in a 70% reduction in coronary artery plaque size, whereas raloxifene had no effect at either low or high dose (103). In contrast, in ovariectomized rabbits, raloxifene reduced aortic cholesterol accumulation (104). Clinical trial data with heart disease outcomes in humans are lacking for both raloxifene and estrogens but are soon to be forthcoming.

Unlike both tamoxifen and estrogen, raloxifene does not appear to stimulate uterine tissue (97,100). Approximately 400 women had serial transvaginal ultrasonography over the 2 years in the multicenter European study (99). No significant difference was found in endometrial thickness at any time during the study between raloxifene and placebo treated patients.

Unlike estrogen, but similarly to tamoxifen, raloxifene increases the incidence of hot flushes slightly (97,100). Furthermore, as with both estrogen and tamoxifen, raloxifene increases the risk of venous thromboembolism (70,91–93,97,105–107). Effects on the brain and urogenital tissues are unknown.

Drugs Currently Under Development

Toremifene (a chlorinated derivative of tamoxifen), which has similar effects on uterine tissue as tamoxifen, but perhaps more potent effects on breast cancer, has recently been approved for treatment of breast cancer. Droloxifene (3-hydroxytamoxifen) and idoxifene (an iodinated tamoxifen derivative) are both being tested for anticancer and antiosteoporotic properties. Neither toremifene nor droloxifene has been shown to induce hepatic tumors in rodents (unlike tamoxifen). Both pure antiestrogenic ICI agents, 164,384 and 182,780, which are analogues of 7-β estradiol with a long alkylamine side chain, are also being tested for antibreast cancer treatment potential. Levomeloxifene is an additional SERM in clinical development for prevention and treatment of osteoporosis.

CONCLUSION

We are still in the infancy of the study of drugs in the SERM class. Some of the benefits of a drug such as raloxifene are known; however, ultimate target organ outcomes such as incidence of heart attack and fracture are still to be determined. Long-term effects on other systems also, such as perineal tissues and central nervous system, also need to be ascertained. The fact that certain SERMS can actually reduce the risk of breast cancer occurrence is incredibly exciting and it is virtually the first time that a medication has been shown to reduce cancer risk substantially. These drugs, therefore, have tremendous potential for reducing the risk of a multitude of chronic diseases in some groups of postmenopausal women. A more complete understanding of the pharmacology and mechanisms of actions of these agents will ultimately help us design the truly perfect estrogen or estrogen/SERM combination regimen to achieve all of the desired effects.

REFERENCES

1. Ettinger B. Overview of estrogen replacement therapy: a historical perspective. *Proc Soc Exp Biol Med* 1998;217:2–5.
2. Ulmsten U. Some reflections and hypotheses on the pathophysiology of female urinary incontinence. *Acta Obstet Gynecol Scand* 1997;76:3–8.
3. Cauley JA, Seeley DG, Ensrud K, et al. Estrogen replacement therapy and fractures in older women. Study of osteoporotic fractures research group. *Ann Intern Med* 1995;122:9–16.
4. Lindsay R, et al. Prevention of spinal osteoporosis in oophorectomised women. *Lancet* 1980;2:1151–1154.
5. Lufkin EG, et al. Treatment of postmenopausal osteoporosis with transdermal estrogen. *Ann Intern Med* 1992;117:1–9.
6. Nasr A, Breckwoldt M. Review. Estrogen replacement therapy and cardiovascular protection: lipid mechanisms are the tip of an iceberg. *Gynecol Endocrinol* 1998;12:43–59.
7. Henderson VW. The epidemiology of estrogen replacement therapy and Alzheimer's disease. *Neurology* 1997;48:S27–S35.
8. Yaffe K, Sawaya G, Lieberburg I, Grady D. Estrogen therapy in postmenopausal women: effects on cognitive function and dementia. *JAMA* 1998;9:688–695.

9. Zumoff B. Does postmenopausal estrogen administration increase the risk of breast cancer? Contributions of animal, biochemical, and clinical investigative studies to a resolution of the controversy. *Proc Soc Exp Biol Med* 1998;217: 30–37.
10. Collaborative Group on Hormonal Factors in Breast Cancer. Breast cancer and hormone replacement therapy: collaborative reanalysis of data from 51 epidemiological studies of 52,705 women with breast cancer and 108,411 women without breast cancer. *Lancet* 1997;350:10-47–1059.
11. Ravnikar VA. Compliance with hormone replacement therapy: are women receiving the full impact of hormone replacement therapy preventative health benefits? *Women's Health Issues* 1992;2:75.
12. Beresford SA, Weiss NS, Voigt LF, McKnight B. Risk of endometrial cancer in relation to use of oestrogen combined with cyclic progestogen therapy in postmenopausal women. *Lancet* 1997;349:458.
13. Udoff L, Langenberg P, Adashi EY. Combined continuous hormone replacement therapy: a critical review [see Comments]. *Obstet Gynecol* 1995;86:306–316.
14. Wakeling AE. Clinical implications of target organ-specific actions of selective antiestrogens. In: Lindsay R, Dempster DW, Jordan VC, eds. *Estrogens and antiestrogens, basic and clinical aspects*. Philadelphia: Lippincott-Raven, 1997: 165–173.
15. Wakeling AE, Bowler J. Steroidal pure antiestrogens. *J Endocrinol* 1987;112: R7–R10.
16. Wakeling AE, Dukes M, Bowler J. A potent specific pure antiestrogen with clinical potential. *Cancer Res* 1991;51:3867–3873.
17. Dukes M, Miller D, Wakeling AE, Waterton JC. Antiuterotrophic effects of a pure antiestrogen ICI 182,780: magnetic resonance imaging in ovariectomized monkeys. *J Endocrinol* 1992;135:239–247.
18. Kulper GGJM, Enmark E, Pelto-Huikko M, Nilsson S, Gustafsson J-A. Cloning of a novel estrogen receptor expressed in rat prostate and ovary. *Proc Natl Acad Sci U S A* 1996;93:5925–5930.
19. Enmark E, Pilto-Huikko M, Grandien K, et al. Human estrogen receptor β-gene structure, chromosomal localization, and expression pattern. *J Clin Endocrinol* 1997;82:4258–4265.
20. Baker VL, Jaffe RB. Clinical uses of antiestrogens. *Obstet Gynecol Surv* 1995; 51:45–59.
21. Fawell SE, White R, Hoare S, Sydenham M, Page M, Parker MG. Inhibition of estrogen receptor-DNA binding by the pure antiestrogenic ICI 164,384 appears to be mediated by impaired receptor dimerization. *Proc Natl Acad Sci U S A* 1990;87:6883–6887.
22. Dauvois S, Danilian PS, White R, Parker MG. Antiestrogen ICI 164,384 reduces cellular estrogen receptor content by increasing its turnover. *Proc Natl Acad Sci U S A* 1992;89:4037–4041.
23. Brzozowski AM, Pike ACW, Dauter Z, et al. Molecular basis of agonism and antagonism in the oestrogen receptor. *Nature* 1997;389:753–758.
24. Yang NN, Venugopalan M, Hardikar S, Glasebrook A. Identification of an estrogen response element activated by metabolites of 17-β-estradiol and raloxifene. *Science* 1996;273:1222–1225.
25. Yang NN, Venugopalan M, Hardikar S, Glasebrook A. Correction: raloxifene response needs more than an element. *Science* 1997;275:1249.
26. Herbst AL, Griffiths CT, Kistner RW. Clomiphene citrate in disseminated mammary carcinoma. *Cancer Chemother Rep* 1964;43:39–41.
27. Hecker E, Vegh I, Levy CM, et al. Clinical trial of clomiphene in advanced breast cancer. *Eur J Cancer* 1974;10:747–749.
28. Clark JH, Markaverich BM. The agonistic-antagonistic properties of clomiphene: a review. *Pharmacol Ther* 1982;15:467–519.
29. Wilson TM, Henke BR, Momtahen TM, et al. 30[4-(1,2,-Diphenylbut-1-enyl)phenyl] acrylic acid: a nonsteroidal estrogen with functional selectivity for bone over uterus in rats. *J Med Chem* 1994;37:1550–1552.
30. Beall PT, Misra LK, Young RL, et al. Clomiphene protects against osteoporosis in the mature ovariectomized rat. *Calcif Tissue Int* 1984;36:123–125.
31. Ke HZ, Simmons HA, Pirie CM, Crawford DT, Thompson DD. Droloxifene, a new estrogen antagonist/agonist, prevents bone loss in ovariectomized rats. *Endocrinology* 1995;136:2435–2441.
32. Rossing MA, Daling JR, Weiss NS, Moore DE, Self SG. Ovarian tumors in a cohort of infertile women. *N Engl J Med* 1994;331:771–776.
33. Whittemore AS, Harris R, Itnyre J, Collaborative Ovarian Cancer Group. Characteristics relating to ovarian cancer risk: collaborative analysis of 12 US case control studies. II: Invasive epithelial ovarian cancers in white women. *Am J Epidemiol* 1992;136:1184–1203.
34. Spirtas R, Kaufman SC, Alexander NJ. Fertility drugs and ovarian cancer: red alert or red herring? *Fertil Steril* 1993;59:291–294.
35. Harris R, Whittemore AS, Intyre J, Collaborative Ovarian Cancer Group. Characteristics relating to ovarian cancer risk: collaborative analysis of 12 US case control studies. III: Epithelial tumors of low malignant potential in white women. *Am J Epidemiol* 1992;136:1204–1211.
36. Pritchard K. Effects on breast cancer: clinical aspects. In: Lindsay R, Dempster DW, Jordan VC, eds. *Estrogens and antiestrogens*. Philadelphia: Lippincott-Raven, 1997:175.
37. Redmond CK, Wickerham DL, Cronin WM, Fisher B, Costantino J. The NSABP Breast Cancer Prevention Trial (BCPT): a progress report. *Proc Am Soc Clin Oncol* 1993;112:69.
38. Powles TJ, Tillyer CR, Jones AL, et al. Prevention of breast cancer with tamoxifen—an update on the Royal Marsden Hospital pilot programme. *Eur J Cancer* 1990;26:680–684.
39. Breast Cancer Prevention Trial. NCI Press Release 4/6/98.
40. Love RR, Mazess RB, Tormey DC, Barden HS, Newcomb PA, Jordan VC. Bone mineral density in women with breast cancer treated with adjuvant tamoxifen for at least two years. *Breast Cancer Res Treat* 1988;12:297–301.
41. Fornander T, Rutqvist LE, Sjoberg HE, Blomqvist L, Mattsson A, Glas U. Long-term adjuvant tamoxifen in early breast cancer: effect on bone mineral density in postmenopausal women. *J Clin Oncol* 1990;8:1019–1024.
42. Cuzick J, Allen D, Baum M, et al. Long term effects of tamoxifen. *Eur J Cancer* 1993;29A:15–21.
43. Gotfredsen A, Christiansen C, Palshof T. The effect of tamoxifen on bone mineral content in premenopausal women with breast cancer. *Cancer* 1984;53: 853–857.
44. Fentiman IS, Caleffi M, Rodin A, Murby B, Fogelkman I. Bone mineral content of women receiving tamoxifen for mastalgia. *Br J Cancer* 1989;60:262–264.
45. Turken S, Siris E, Seldin D, Flaster E, Hyman G, Lindsay R. Effects of tamoxifen on spinal bone density in women with breast cancer. *J Natl Cancer Inst* 1989;71:1086–1088.
46. Ryan WG, Wolter J, Bagdade JD. Apparent beneficial effects of tamoxifen on bone mineral content in patients with breast cancer: preliminary study. *Osteoporosis Int* 1991;2:39–41.
47. Fentiman IS, Saad Z, Caleffi M, Chaudary MA, Fogelman I. Tamoxifen protects against steroid induced bone loss. *Eur J Cancer* 1992;28:684–685.
48. Kristensen B, Ejlertsen B, Dalgaard P, et al. Tamoxifen and bone metabolism in postmenopausal low risk breast cancer patients: a randomized study. *J Clin Oncol* 1994;12:992–997.
49. Ward RL, Morgan G, Dalley D, Kelly PJ. Tamoxifen reduces bone turnover and prevents lumbar spine and proximal femoral bone loss in early postmenopausal women. *J Bone Miner Res* 1993;22:87–94.
50. Love RR, Mazess RB, Barden HS, et al. Effects of tamoxifen on bone mineral density in postmenopausal women with breast cancer. *N Engl J Med* 1992;326: 852–856.
51. Grey AB, Stapleton JP, Evans MC, Tatnell MA, Ames RW, Reid IR. The effect of the antiestrogen tamoxifen on bone mineral density in normal late postmenopausal women. *Am J Med* 1995;99:636–641.
52. Powles TJ, Hickish T, Kanis JA, Tidy A, Ashley S. Effect of tamoxifen on bone mineral density measured by dual energy x-ray absorptiometry in healthy premenopausal and postmenopausal women. *J Clin Oncol* 1996;14:78–84.
53. Wright CDP, Mansell RE, Gazet JC, Compston JE. Effect of long term tamoxifen treatment on bone turnover in women with breast cancer. *BMJ* 1993;306: 429–430.
54. Wright CDP, Garrahan NJ, Stanton M, Gazet JC, Mansell RE, Compston JE. Effect of long term tamoxifen therapy on cancellous bone remodeling and structure in women with breast cancer. *J Bone Miner Res* 1994;9:153–159.
55. Kenny AM, Prestwood KM, Pilbeam CC, Raisz LG. The short term effects of tamoxifen on bone turnover in older women. *J Clin Endocrinol Metab* 1995; 80: 3287–3291.
56. McDonald CC, Stewart HJ. Fatal myocardial infarction in the Scottish adjuvant tamoxifen trial. The Scottish Breast Cancer Committee. *Br Med J* 1991;303: 435–437.
57. Rutqvist LE, Mattsson A, for the Stockholm Breast Cancer Study Group. Cardiac and thromboembolic morbidity among postmenopausal women with early stage breast cancer in a randomized trial of adjuvant tamoxifen. *J Natl Cancer Inst* 1993;85:1398–1406.
58. Clarkson TB, Anthony MS. Effects on the cardiovascular system: basic aspects. In: Lindsay R, Dempster DW, Jordan CV, eds. *Estrogens and antiestrogens: basic and clinical aspects*. Philadelphia: Lippincott-Raven Publishers, 1997:89–118.
59. Neven P, DeMuylder X, van Belle Y, Campo R, Vanderick G. Tamoxifen and the uterus. *BMJ* 1994;309:1313–1314.
60. Lahti E, Blanco G, Kauppila A, et al. Endometrial changes in postmenopausal breast cancer patients receiving tamoxifen. *Obstet Gynecol* 1993;81:660–664.
61. Thylan S. Tamoxifen treatment and its consequences. *Hum Reprod* 1995;10: 2174–2178.
62. Cohen I, Rosen DJD, Shapira J, et al. Endometrial changes in postmenopausal women treated with tamoxifen for breast cancer. *Br J Obstet Gynaecol* 1993; 100:567–570.
63. Jaiyesimi IA, Buzdar AU, Decker DA, Hortobagyi GN. Use of tamoxifen for breast cancer: twenty-eight years later. *J Clin Oncol* 1995;113:513–529.
64. Kedar RP, Bourne TH, Powles TJ, et al. Effects of tamoxifen on uterus and ovaries of postmenopausal women in a randomized breast cancer prevention trial. *Lancet* 1994;343:1318–1321.
65. Shushan A, Peretz T, Uziely B, Lewin A, Mor-Yosef S. Ovarian cysts in premenopausal tamoxifen-treated women with breast cancer. *Am J Obstet Gynecol* 1996;174:141–144.
66. Cohen I, Rosen DJD, Altaras M, et al. Tamoxifen treatment in premenopausal breast cancer patients may be associated with ovarian overstimulation, cystic formations and fibroid overgrowth. *Br J Obstet Gynaecol* 1993;100:567–570.
67. Wolf DM, Jordan VC. Gynecologic complications associated with long-term adjuvant tamoxifen therapy for breast cancer. *Gynecol Oncol* 1992;45: 118–128.
68. Morgan MA, Gincherman Y, Mikuta JJ. Endometriosis and tamoxifen therapy. *Int J Gynaecol Obstet* 1994;45:55–57.
69. Uziely B, Lewin A, Brufman G, Dorembus D, Mor-Yosef S. The effect of tamoxifen on the endometrium. *Breast Cancer Res Treat* 1993;26:101–105.

70. Fisher B, Costantino JP, Redmond CK, et al. Endometrial cancer in tamoxifen-treated breast cancer patients: findings from the National surgical Adjuvant Breast and Bowel Project (NSABP) B-14.*J Natl Cancer Inst* 1994;86:527–537.

71. Cook LS, Weiss NS, Swartz SM, et al. Population based study of tamoxifen therapy and subsequent ovarian, endometrial and breast cancer. *J Natl Cancer Inst* 1995;87:1359–1364.

72. Rutqvist LE, Johansson H, Signomklao T, et al. Adjuvant tamoxifen therapy for early stage breast cancer and second primary malignancies. *J Natl Cancer Inst* 1995;87:645–651.

73. Stewart HJ, Knight GM. Tamoxifen and the uterus and endometrium. *Lancet* 1989;8643:375.

74. Williams GM, Iatropoulos MJ, Djordjevic MV, Kaltenberg OP. The triphenylethylene drug tamoxifen is a strong liver carcinogen in the rat. *Carcinogenesis* 1993;14:315–317.

75. Hard GC, Iatropoulos MJ, Jordan K, et al. Major differences in the hepatocarcinogenicity and DNA adduct forming ability between toremifene and tamoxifen in female Crl: CD(BR) rats. *Cancer Res* 1993;53:3919–3924.

76. Fornander T, Turqvist LE, Cedermark BV, et al. Adjuvant tamoxifen in early breast cancer: occurrence of new primary cancers. *Lancet* 1989;1:117–120.

77. Martin EA, Rich KJ, White INH, et al. ^{32}P—Post labeled DNA adducts in liver obtained from women treated with tamoxifen. *Carcinogenesis* 1995;16:1651–1654.

78. Heel RC, Brogden RN, Speight TM. Tamoxifen: a review of its pharmacological properties and therapeutic use in the treatment of breast cancer. *Drugs* 1978;16:1–24.

79. Mouridsen HT, Palshof T, Patterson J, et al. Tamoxifen in advanced breast cancer. *Cancer Treat Rev* 1978;5:131–141.

80. Sawka CA, Pritchard KI, Paterson AHG, et al. Role and mechanism of action of tamoxifen in premenopausal women with metastatic breast carcinoma. *Cancer Res* 1986;46:3152–3156.

81. Ashford AR, Donev I, Tiwari RP, et al. Reversible ocular toxicity related to tamoxifen therapy. *Cancer* 1988;61:33–35.

82. Kaiser-Kupfer MI, Lippman ME. Tamoxifen retinopathy. *Cancer Treat Rep* 1978;62:315–320.

83. Heier JS, Dragoo RA, Enzenauer RW, Waterhouse WJ. Screening for ocular toxicity in asymptomatic patients treated with tamoxifen. *Am J Ophthalmol* 1994;117:772–775.

84. Mendonca Costa R, Dhooge MRP, Van Wing F, DeRouck AF. Tamoxifen retinopathy: a case report. *Bull Soc Belge Ophtalmol* 1990;238:161–168.

85. Gerner EW. Ocular toxicity of tamoxifen. *Ann Ophthalmol* 1989;21:420–423.

86. Mihm LM, Barton TL. Tamoxifen-induced ocular toxicity. *Ann Pharmacol* 1994;28:740–741.

87. Bently CR, Davies G, Aclimandos WA. Tamoxifen retinopathy: a rare but serious complication. *BMJ* 1992;304:495–496.

88. Longstaff S, Sigurdsson H, O Keeffe M, Osgton S, Preece P. A controlled study of the ocular effects of tamoxifen in conventional dosage in the treatment of breast carcinoma. *Eur J Cancer Clin Oncol* 1989;25:1805–1808.

89. Pavlidis N, Petris C, Briassoulis E, et al. Clear evidence that long-term, low dose tamoxifen treatment can induce ocular toxicity. *Cancer* 1992;69:2961–2964.

90. Chang T, Gonder JR, Ventresca MR. A case report. Low dose tamoxifen retinopathy. *Can J Ophthalmol* 1992;27:148–149.

91. Fisher B, Costantino J, Redmond C, et al. A randomized clinical trial evaluating tamoxifen in the treatment of patients with node-negative breast cancer who have estrogen-receptor-positive tumors. *N Engl J Med* 1989;320:479–484.

92. Enck RE, Rios CN. Tamoxifen treatment of metastatic breast cancer and antithrombin III levels. *Cancer* 1984;53:2607–2609.

93. Pemberton KD, Melissari E, Kakkar VV. The influence of tamoxifen in vivo on the main natural anticoagulants and fibrinolysis. *Blood Coagul Fibrinolysis* 1993;4:935–942.

94. Cummings SR, Eckert S, Krueger KA, et al. The effect of raloxifene on risk of breast cancer in post-menopausal women: results from the MORE randomized trial. *JAMA* 1999;2189–2197.

95. Jordan et al. American Society Clinical Oncology. Presentation 5/98.

96. Draper MW, Flowers DE, Huster WJ, Neild JA, Harper KD, Arnaud C. A controlled trial of raloxifene (LY139481) HC1: impact on bone turnover and serum lipid profile in healthy postmenopausal women. *J Bone Miner Res* 1996;11:835–842.

97. Evista (Raloxifene hydrocholoride). Product circular. Eli Lilly and Company, 1997, Indianapolis, IN.

98. Heaney RP, Draper MW. Raloxifene and estrogen: comparative bone remodeling kinetics. *J Clin Endrocrinol* 1997;82:3425–3429.

99. Turner CH, Sato M, Bryant HU. Raloxifene preserves bone strength and bone mass in ovariectomized rats. *Endocrinology* 194;135:2001–2005.

100. Delmas PD, Bjarnason NH, Mitlak BH, et al. Effects of raloxifene on bone mineral density, serum cholesterol concentrations, and uterine endometrium in postmenopausal women. *N Engl J Med* 1997;337:1641–1647.

101. Ettinger B, Black D, Cummings S, et al. Raloxifene reduces the risk of incident vertebral fractures: 24 month interim analysis (abstract). *Osteoporos Int* 1998;8(Suppl. 3):11.

102. Walsh BW, Kuller LH, Wild RA, et al. Effects of raloxifene on serum lipids and coagulation factors in healthy postmenopausal women. *JAMA* 1998;279:1445–1455.

103. Clarkson TB, Anthony MS, Jerome CP. Lack of effect of raloxifene on coronary artery atherosclerosis of postmenopausal monkeys. *J Clin Endocrinol* 1998;83:721–726.

104. Bjarnason NH, Haarbo J, Byrjalsen I, Christiansen C. Raloxifene inhibits aortic accumulation of cholesterol in ovariectomized, cholesterol-fed rabbits. *Circulation* 1997;96:1964–1969.

105. Daly E, Vessey MP, Hawkins MM, et al. Risk of venous thromboembolism in users of hormone replacement therapy. *Lancet* 1996;348:977–980.

106. Grodstein F, Stampfer MJ, Goldhaber SZ, et al. Prospective study of exogenous hormones and risk of pulmonary embolism. *Lancet* 1996;348:983–987.

107. Jick H, Derby LE, Myers MW, et al. Risk of hospital admission for idiopathic venous thromboembolism among users of postmenopausal oestrogens. *Lancet* 1996;348:981–983.

SECTION XII

Management of
the Postmenopausal Woman

In this section, important aspects pertinent to the care of the postmenopausal woman will be discussed. The first discussion will argue for the need of a specialized center for the care of postmenopausal women. The second chapter discusses the design of clinical trials and what requirements need to be met for FDA approval. The third gives the reader a flavor of the prospective clinical trials recently published and still underway which will help guide decision making in the treatment of postmenopausal women.

Morris Notelovitz has had vast experience in setting up medical centers or "clinics." In Chapter 58, he describes how he has set up several successful centers. An integrated, multidisciplinary center for comprehensive health care, created specifically for women, is the key to success. Next Chris Holinka and Jim Pickar describe the conduct of clinical trials and what is required to achieve FDA-approval. It is a long and expensive road! There are different requirements depending on the indication. This chapter should be useful for those readers who are involved in clinical trials as well as for practitioners who are waiting for products to be marketed. In the final chapter in this section, Jenny Kelsey and Bob Marcus review for us the status of various clinical trials. In the final analysis it will be prospective randomized clinical trials which will guide our decisions and recommendations that should be evidence-based. As pointed out, however, this guidance is confined only to the results of the trials using specific regimens. As was the case in HERS, we will be left primarily with data on a fixed continuous combined estrogen-progestogen regimen for women with a uterus.

Treatment of the Postmenopausal Woman: Basic and Clinical Aspects, Second Edition, edited by Rogerio A. Lobo, Lippincott Williams & Wilkins, Philadelphia © 1999.

CHAPTER 58

Integrated Adult Women's Medicine: A Model for Women's Healthcare Centers

Morris Notelovitz

In welcoming remarks to participants at the 4th International Congress on the Menopause (October, 1984), I noted:

> "The needs of women vary during the climacteric. Latent changes in the early phase have the potential for significant morbidity in the later years; by early recognition and prevention, conditions such as osteoporosis and atherogenic cardiovascular disease may be ameliorated or even prevented. It is for this reason that the theme for the Congress of Climacteric Medicine and Science—A Societal Need—has been chosen. By recognizing the needs of the total woman, the expertise of the primary care physician (gynecologist or family practitioner) is complemented by the skills and talents of nutritionists, exercise physiologists, psychologists and social counselors. Traditional health care specialists, in turn, need to work with the basic and social scientist" (1).

These comments were based on my research and clinical experience at the Menopause Clinic, Addington Hospital, Durban, RSA (1968) and at the Center for Climacteric Studies, University of Florida, Gainesville (1980).

Climacteric medicine is still not recognized as a medical entity, but increasing awareness of recognizing the needs of the total woman has led to the initiative to establish women's healthcare centers. No agreed-on formula exists and, indeed, no meaningful literature relates to the subject (2). The model described in this article is derived from an appreciation of the various biologic events that have an impact on women during their premenopausal and postmenopausal life cycle, and on the experience from 10 years of private practice experience at the Women's Medical & Diagnostic Center, Gainesville, Florida (1986–1996). This experience led to the concept of climacteric medicine being expanded to include the care of younger premenopausal women and conditions

not associated with climacteric per se, hence, the revised descriptor, "Integrated Adult Women's Medicine."

THE PRINCIPLES

The menopause is a natural life event that all women experience. With advances in healthcare, the life expectancy of women in Western and Asian societies has increased to the point where most women can expect to live 30 years beyond their last menstrual period. The key to achieving longevity is to reach age 65 years. After this milestone women can anticipate living between 19.5 and 23.1 more years (3). With this increased longevity, however, conditions associated with aging have also increased, including cardiovascular disease (and related risk factors), osteoporosis, urinary incontinence, Alzheimer's disease, cancer (breast and colon), arthritis, and failure of the sensory organs of hearing and vision. It is the management of these and related conditions that forms the scientific basis for the concept of integrated adult women's medicine.

Three basic issues have an impact on the design of healthcare centers for women:

1. The healthcare needs of women involve organ systems remote from the pelvis—the domain of the traditional primary care physician for women (gynecologist).
2. The pathogenesis of diseases, such as cardiovascular disease (4) and osteoporosis (5) precede the menopause by at least three decades. Thus, for preventive measures to succeed, patient advice and care should commence in early adolescence (Fig. 58.1)
3. Alterable factors such as exercise, lifestyle, diet, and social habits can have an impact on the future health and well-being of women, as much as does a physio-

M. Notelovitz: Women's Medical & Diagnostic Center, Gainesville, Florida 32605.

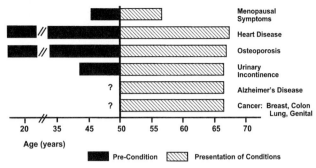

FIG. 58.1. Defining the medical practice: climacteric medicine. For preventive measures to succeed, patient advice and care should commence in early adolescence.

logic hormone deficiency associated with the menopause. For example, in the recent Finnish Twin Study (6), level of physical activity and not familial factors influenced premature mortality. Compared with their sedentary cohorts, conditioned female twins reduced their risk of death by 76% (odds ratio 0.24).

From this understanding, I developed the concept of climacteric and adult women's medicine to incorporate the following principles.

1. Recognition of the woman as a total person.
2. Meeting her healthcare needs across the spectrum of her climacteric and beyond (age 30 onward).
3. Inclusion of preventive as well as curative programs. Thus, services such as exercise prescription and nutritional advice should be available as an adjunct (or an alternative) to hormone therapy and other disease-specific medications.
4. Provision of diagnostic technologies for the early diagnosis of latent disease, for individualization of healthcare and monitoring of response to therapy.

For this comprehensive and integrated approach to succeed, a center that provides for the patient's total healthcare has to be cost-effective and provide long-term benefits to both the individual and to society. The center also has to be economically viable. Experience at the Women's Medical & Diagnostic Center (WMDC) has found the following to be essential:

1. Consumer education. Only an educated consumer can make informed decisions regarding her own healthcare needs.
2. Centralized technology. To make treatment decisions, certain diagnostic modalities should be available to individualize treatment regimens and monitor progress and treatment. This assists with treatment compliance (7,8).
3. Multidisciplinary staffing. This needs to include primary and gynecologic care and medical subspecialists (radiologists, cardiologists, rheumatologists, and so forth); paramedical professionals (physical thera-

pists; exercise physiologists; counselor), and appropriately trained nursing and clinical staff.
4. By housing all of the above in one facility, the various professionals can function as a team supervising the health of one individual. Important cost savings are seen in terms of overhead expenses and, of course, convenience to the patient.

Healthcare centers for women should avoid medicalization of the menopause. Nonmedical alternatives should be made available. However, the prevalence of various age and menopause-related diseases are a reality. The earlier they are detected and treated, the better. Only a comprehensive approach involving a multidisciplinary healthcare team and the selective use of appropriate diagnostic technology can optimize the healthcare of women.

THE PRACTICE

Primary Target Population

Climacteric medicine (as previously defined) involves the ambulatory care of women aged between 35 to 65 years and incorporates both preventive and curative healthcare. Adult women's medicine incorporates the management of young adult women (i.e., the care of women aged from 16 to 35 (Fig. 58.2). This provides the potential for optimal preventive medicine by emphasizing diet and exercise and lifestyle modification from an early age. Many chronic conditions may be prevented by simple and inexpensive measures. For instance, where osteoporosis is concerned, it is now established that exercise and calcium supplementation in teenagers leads to greater bone mineral accrual and the potential for an enhanced peak bone mass (9,10). The greater this peak bone mass, the lower is the risk for osteoporosis (5). In addition, osteoporosis risk factors, such as eating disorders and menstrual irregularities, can be readily detected and appropriately treated.

Also, childhood obesity increases the risk of obesity in adulthood (11) and, therefore, the risk of diseases such as

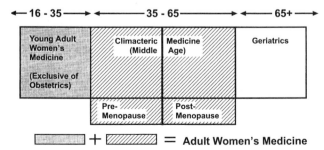

FIG. 58.2. Defining the medical practice: integrated adult women's medicine. This model allows the potential for optimal preventive medicine by emphasizing diet and exercise and lifestyle modification from an early age.

diabetes and coronary artery disease. A recent study confirmed that the children of parents with coronary artery disease were overweight in childhood (12). The implication for early lifestyle and exercise intervention is self-evident.

Instruction in safe sexual habits and effective contraception is yet another benefit younger women derive, both for their future reproductive potential and for their later postmenopausal health. For example, long-term use of oral contraceptives significantly reduces the risk of ovarian and endometrial cancer, and does not increase the risk of breast cancer (13). It has been the experience at the WMDC that obstetric care should not be included in an adult women's center.

Geriatrics is a recognized speciality with specific patient and clinic requirements; however this practice was not incorporated into the WMDC model. However, many elderly women need to be evaluated (dual-energy x-ray absorbtiometry [DEXA] testing) and treated (with specific medications and physical therapy) for conditions such as osteoporosis. In addition, elderly women require annual physical examination with cancer surveillance (Pap smears and mammograms), screening for colon disease (using guaiac tests, sigmoidoscopies and selective colonoscopies), and other common health problems. These include the evaluation and management of recurrent urinary tract infections and, particularly, urinary incontinence, which requires urodynamic testing. Urinary incontinence, which is probably the most common condition in older women, consistently and significantly reduces quality of life. A recent study confirmed that a simple questionnaire regarding voiding and leaking patterns serves as a valuable tool to detect this problem (14). Additional age-related problems that frequently occur are uterovaginal prolapse, arthritis, and visual and hearing impairment. Thus, in reality, senior citizen healthcare *is* an important extension of adult women's medicine. Therefore, in practice, mainly the frail elderly are referred for geriatric care .

Staffing

Type of Practice

In the traditional practice of women's curative medicine, patients are treated according to their presenting problem and the physician's area of interest. In contrast, climacteric and adult women's medicine targets the whole woman with a multidisciplinary, integrated approach, emphasizing (but not limited to) preventive care.

Apart from routine gynecologic evaluations and management, women obviously need treatment for nonreproductive complaints such as influenza and bronchitis. Women are also subject to potential life-threatening diseases such as cardiovascular disease, hypertension, osteoporosis, and metabolic and endocrine disorders, as well as common non–life-threatening conditions such as

arthritis, urinary incontinence, and visual and hearing impairment. Screening for breast, colon, lung, and genital tract cancers forms an essential core of clinical services that should be offered. Essential, too, are the emotional, psychological, and career needs of women.

Medical Staff: Adult Women's Generalist

A team approach is needed to optimize adult women's care. In practice, the medical services are best coordinated by a primary care adult women's generalist who functions as a gate keeper. As illustrated in Fig. 58.3, management of each case is determined by the adult women's generalist (AWG) after the screening and diagnostic procedure identifies either no problem or a primary (or latent) problem requiring medical attention. This process ensures cohesive integrated and cost-effective care. The AWG has to be well-rounded in primary care and internal medicine, and appropriately trained to perform gynecologic procedures such as colposcopy, endometrial biopsies, and pelvic ultrasound. The AWG could also be a board certified gynecologist, provided the physician is experienced in general internal medicine. Supervised physician assistants or nurse practitioners function very successfully and as cost-effectively as do AWGs.

Specialists and Consultants

Summarized in Fig. 58.4 is the staffing structure of the WMDC from 1986 to 1995. The four ambulatory care providers were full-time employees. The consultants were contracted for their services, all of which were provided at WMDC. This approach, which was test marketed, was enthusiastically endorsed by patients, who appreciated receiving individualized and total healthcare at a single facility. A panel of additional consultants was formed that included specialists in rheumatology, endocrinology, neurology, psychiatry, general and cosmetic surgery, and physiatry. These services were provided in the consultants private office.

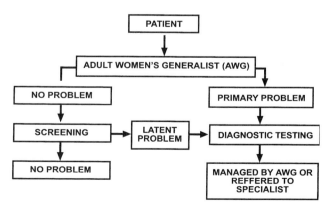

FIG. 58.3. A model for a team approach to adult women's medicine.

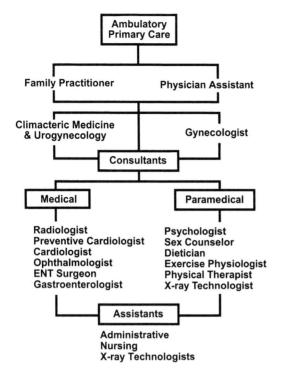

FIG. 58.4. Implementing the practice: a model for integrated women's medicine at the Women's Medical & Diagnostic Center, Gainesville, Florida.

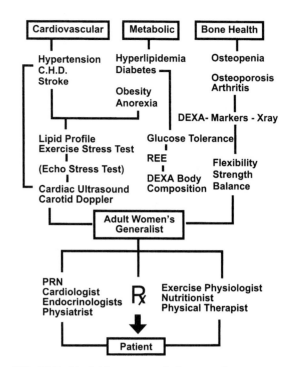

FIG. 58.5. Model for a prescriptive exercise program.

Paramedical Staff

The paramedical personnel comprise an essential component of the adult women's health team. Professionals included psychologists (in general and sex counseling) who offered traditional therapies, including treatment with biofeedback for stress management and certain aspects of sexual dysfunction; a dietitian provided evidence-based advice regarding weight loss using (selectively) resting energy expenditure testing (using indirect calorimetry), DEXA body composition analysis and computer-assisted dietary analysis. The physical therapy department concentrated on the management of problems related to arthritis, osteoporosis, and urinary incontinence (caused by pelvic floor muscle dysfunction). Finally, individualized prescriptive exercise regimens were developed by an exercise physiologist (under medical supervision) for the treatment of special medical entities (e.g., hypertension, diabetes, osteoporosis). All patients had an on-site exercise stress test (under the supervision of a cardiologist) and additional selective tests according to their medical condition (e.g., DEXA testing if they had osteoporosis) (Fig. 58.5). Both aerobic and resistive exercises were prescribed. The exercise program was conducted off-site under the guidance of a trained physical therapist or exercise physiologist.

The administrative staff, nurses, and x-ray technicians were critical to the success of the program at the WMDC. All were thoroughly schooled in both the philosophy and the practice of adult women's medicine. Their input was invaluable in reassuring patients that their care was in the hands of trained professionals. Much of the education and counseling of patients, and their reassurance *vis-á-vis* treatment protocols (and the anticipated response or potential side-effects) was undertaken by the nurses. X-ray technologists were trained to recognize abnormalities (e.g., in mammograms, x-rays films, or DEXA tests) and were encouraged to consult with the on-site physicians so that additional views or tests could be ordered prior to the patient leaving the center. Patients were often scheduled for physician consultations immediately after testing.

Patient Reporting and Compliance

All patients received individualized written reports summarizing the outcome of their visit. Full reports were sent to referring physicians. Compliance was high, which was probably due to having the patient appropriately educated to the point where she participated in her treatment decision. Ready telephonic access to trained and knowledgeable nurses was frequently favorably commented upon as well as the appointment reminders sent via mail and telephone.

CLINIC DESIGN

Clinic design focused on respect for the individual and an understanding of her medical needs. The ambience and decor of a center sets the tone for the practice. Regional tastes vary. Thus, the colors, finishings, and background, music for example, need to be tailored to the clientele. Research and clinical experience at the WMDC, however, has identified the type of customized patient examination furnishing and gowns, for example, that are universally acceptable and complementary to the overall relaxed nonmedical environment of the facility.

Central to the design is a floor plan that is convenient for the patient and labor saving for the staff. To facilitate this goal, services relevant to a given condition should be clustered according to the diagnostic and therapeutic requirements of that condition. An example is illustrated in Fig. 58.6. Osteoporotic-related fractures are associated with reduced bone mass, microarchitectural deterioration, and falls. Thus, the technology needed to evaluate bone health and strength (DEXA, bone ultrasound, and x-ray studies) is contiguous with the physical therapy department where balance, posture, and muscle strength and flexibility are evaluated. The x-ray technologists are also trained in specimen collection, techniques for the evaluation of bone remodeling, and other relevant biochemical tests, which are required either before or after the DEXA evaluation. Where relevant, impairment with hearing and inner ear dysfunction is evaluated by ear nose and throat (ENT) technicians; problems with visual acuity are evaluated by trained ophthalmic nurses. Both paramedicals are supervised by an ENT specialist and an ophthalmologist, who also consult with patients for hearing and visual problems unrelated to their risk for falling. Placement together of these seemingly unrelated diagnostic modalities also leads to patient-initiated cross-referral: a patient scheduled for an eye test realizes that she needs a bone density test and vice versa.

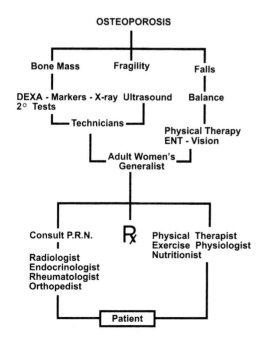

FIG. 58.6. Clinic design: cluster system.

Similar paradigms cluster technology and personnel for cardiovascular health evaluation, obesity management, cancer screening, urinary incontinence, and certain specialized team clinical services such as the premenstrual syndrome and an eating disorder clinic.

TECHNOLOGY: CLINICAL RESEARCH AND CONSUMER EDUCATION

It is important to recognize, that integrated adult women's medicine does not exist as an approved medical discipline. However, the development of various technologies allows physicians to evaluate patients selectively and to acquire objective information, thus facilitating the practice of evidence-based medicine. As such, specific and lower dose regimens can be prescribed for a given condition and the therapeutic response monitored with dosage adjustment made accordingly. Simply, prevention of disease for many conditions—such as osteoporosis—has now become a reality. Hormone therapy (15) and some of the new antiresorptive drugs (16) have been shown to reduce vertebral fracture risk by 50% to 90%. Newer tissue-specific drugs are being developed and evaluated for total menopausal healthcare (17). The use of natural products, such as phytoestrogens, holds great promise. In certain societies (e.g., Japan), phytoestrogens have been linked with a much lower prevalence of cardiovascular disease and breast and endometrial cancer (18) when taken as part and parcel of their daily diet.

The key is convenient and cost-effective technology for use in clinical medicine that identifies biologic markers that are closely linked to the pathogenesis of a given disease. Evaluation of evolving technology and participation in clinical drug trials are important activities that provide two advantages: early familiarity with cutting-edge technology and therapies, and research revenues that complement clinical income.

Most women are unaware of the existence or the advantage of comprehensive healthcare. Even when available, services that are regarded as preventive in nature may not be reimbursable. This was certainly the situation when the WMDC was first established. Yet, as the programs offered at the WMDC became known, women recognized the personal benefit they would derive, and they became paying patients.

The message is clear: educated women can (and do) make informed decisions. The difficulty is what is the best way to educate them about their health. Educational materials should be available and well-displayed in the office. The WMDC had a special lounge set aside for group discussions and a small library is situated within the room. It is advisable to review the reading materials available on the subject of menopause. Much is written, but relatively few texts are authored by individuals qualified or experienced in climacteric care. At WMDC we provide additional educational services that include a 1-

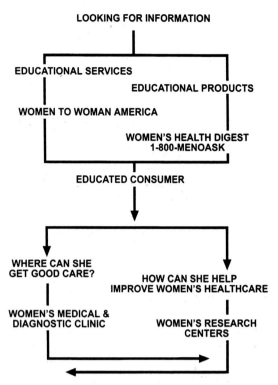

FIG. 58.7. Model for integrating consumer education with clinical services and research.

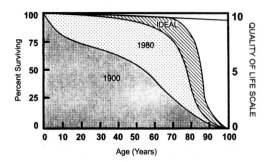

FIG. 58.8. Ideal survival and quality of life curve. (Modified from Fries HF, Green LW, Levine S. Health preservation and the compression of mortality. *Lancet* 1989;1:481; with permission.)

800 call-in service with recorded messages on different aspects of the menopause, and a quarterly medical journal written for lay consumption (Fig. 58.7). The importance of consumer education should not be underestimated. Approximately 95% of patients attending the WMDC were self-referrals—by friends who experienced the facility and through articles on the menopause in magazines that included information about the WMDC. In fact, women from 42 states have sought consultation or ongoing care after learning about the WMDC through the national media.

CONCLUSION

A biologic limit exist to the lifespan. Fries et al. (19) conceptualized the "rectangularization" of life, with the goal of maintaining physical and mental function as long as possible, until the inevitable and, it is hoped, acute point of decline and eventual death (Fig. 58.8). The practice of climacteric and adult women's medicine attempts to maximize the active life expectancy of women and to allow them a full vigorous and independent life. A vital issue in this quest may be preventive measures in young adulthood which, if extended into later life, would raise the level of wellness to an even higher plane by eliminating the risk of two of the most prevalent chronic disabilities associated with the older woman—osteoporosis and cardiovascular disease.

Climacteric medicine is a discipline waiting to be born. In short, it can be defined as preventive medicine for women (and men) in their middle years, and it has as its basic premise consideration of the whole individual, with the objective of achieving a healthy mind in a healthy body in a healthy environment. As such, it may be regarded as a national insurance policy. A healthy middle-age population will be a productive population; by preventing or ameliorating chronic illnesses much of the need for and cost of long-term geriatric care can be avoided. We have noted the benefit of preventive medicine in obstetrics and dentistry. Why should the climacteric be any different? It is in this context that climacteric medicine has emerged as a science and has become a societal need (1).

Preventive medicine, in fact, is practiced by a wide variety of healthcare professionals, both on an individual basis (e.g., doing Pap smears and ordering mammograms) and at a societal level (e.g., immunization). However, preventive medicine has not been the major thrust of healthcare in the United States and in most other countries. This stems in part from prioritization of the healthcare dollar and because of inadequate education of medical students and residents in training. With the current demand for cost-containment in healthcare and the obvious monetary savings associated with the prevention of disease and disability, preventive and primary care are now being recognized as essential components of a reformed health system (20). Women's healthcare centers provide the ideal environment for the practice of preventive medicine.

REFERENCES

1. Notelovitz M. Climacteric medicine and science: a societal need. In: Notelovitz M, Van Keep P, eds. *The climacteric in perspective.* Boston, MTP Press, 1986:19–21.
2. Notelovitz M. Is there a need for menopause clinics: In: Mulutidisciplinary Perspectives on Menopause. *Ann NY Acad Sci* 1990;592:239–241.
3. Hammond C. Menopause and hormone replacement therapy: an overview. *Obstet Gynecol* 1996;87:2S–15S.
4. Van Horn L, Greenland P. Prevention of coronary artery disease is a pediatric problem. *JAMA* 1997;278:1779–1780.
5. Notelovitz M. Post-menopausal osteoporosis. A practical approach to its prevention. *Acta Obstet Gynecol Scand Suppl* 1986;134:67–80.

6. Kujala UM, Kaprio J, Sarna S, Koskenvuo M. Relationship of leisure-time physical activity and mortality. The Finnish Twin Cohort. *JAMA* 1998;279:440–444.

7. Cook B, Notelovitz M, Rector C, Krischer J. An osteoporosis education and screening program: results and implications. *Patient Education and Counseling* 1991;17:135–145.

8. Silverman SS, Greenwald M, Klein RA, Drinkwater BL. Effect of bone density information on decisions about hormone replacement therapy: a randomized trial. *Obstet Gynecol* 1997;89:321–325.

9. Lloyd T, Martel J, Rollings N, et al. The effect of calcium supplementation and Tanner stage on bone density, content and area in teenage women. *Osteoporosis Int* 1996;6:276–283.

10. Boot AM, de Ridar MAJ, Pols H, et al. Bone mineral density in children and adolescents: relation to puberty, calcium intake and physical activity.¨20*J Clin Endocrinol Metab* 1997;82:57–62.

11. Whitaker RC, Wright JA, Pepe MS, et al. Predicting obesity in young adulthood from childhood and parental obesity. *N Engl J Med* 1997;337:869–873.

12. Rao W, Srinivasan SR, Valdez R, et al. Longitudinal changes in cardiovascular risk from childhood to young adulthood in offspring of parents with cardiovascular disease. The Bogalusa Heart Study. *JAMA* 1997;278:1749–1754.

13. Kaunitz AM, Benrubi GI. The good news about hormonal contraception and gynecological cancer. *The Female Patient* 1998;23:43–51.

14. Robinson D, Pearce KF, Preisser JS, et al. Relationship between patient reports of urinary incontinence symptoms and quality of life measures. *Obstet Gynecol* 1998;91:224–228.

15. Notelovitz M. Estrogen therapy and osteoporosis: principles and practice. *Am J Med Sci* 1997;313:2–12.

16. Black DM, Cummings SR, Karpf DB, et al. Randomized trial of effect of alendronate on risk of fractures in women with existing vertebral fractures. *Lancet* 1996;348:1535–1541.

17. Delmas P, Bjarnason N, Mitlak B, et al. Effects of raloxifene on bone mineral density, serum cholesterol concentrations and uterine endometrium in post-menopausal women. *N Engl J Med* 1997;337:1641–1647.

18. Aldercreutz H, Mazur W. Phyto-oestrogens and western diseases. *Ann Med* 1997;29:95–120.

19. Fries HF, Green LW, Levine S. Health preservation and the compression of mortality. *Lancet* 1989;1:481.

20. Eggert RW, Parkinson MD. Preventive medicine and health system reform. Improving physician education, training and practice. *JAMA* 1994;272:688–693.

Treatment of the Postmenopausal Woman: Basic and Clinical Aspects, Second Edition, edited by Rogerio A. Lobo, Lippincott Williams & Wilkins, Philadelphia © 1999.

CHAPTER 59

Clinical Studies in Hormone Replacement Therapy

Christian F. Holinka and James H. Pickar

Remarkable progress has been made since the early days of this century when hormonal steroids were initially isolated and synthesized, and synthetic derivatives were developed. In this scientific journey from laboratory to life, profertility drugs have been developed, contraceptive agents produced, and postmenopausal hormone replacement has become standard practice. Yet, frequently, little is known about the complex process of clinical development required for the approval of drugs for human use. This chapter provides an introduction to the design and conduct of clinical studies required in support of drug approval for the treatment of the postmenopausal woman. Emphasis is on the clinical development of products for hormone replacement therapy (HRT).

For marketing approval of a new drug in the United States, adequate and well-controlled studies testing solid scientific hypotheses should be conducted consistent with regulatory requirements set forth by the Food and Drug Administration (FDA). Additionally, the International Conference on Harmonization (ICH) Technical Requirements for Registrations of Pharmaceuticals for Human Use guidelines emphasize the need for global development programs. This harmonization can have an impact on the design and implementation of a significant number of studies. The FDA has acknowledged the importance of working with regulatory authorities outside the United States in a number of ways, such as its recent (Federal Register, October 1997) effort to develop guidelines for safety reporting that take into account ICH safety update report guidelines. In this final rule amending its expedited safety reporting regulations for human drugs and biological products, the FDA has modified its agreements concerning reporting periods, standards, and formats established with the ICH and the World Health Organization Council for Organizations of Medical Sciences.

Although globalization is beginning to affect the conduct of studies, implementation of changes worldwide will proceed in a manner consistent with country-specific regulatory requirements. These effects are not yet entirely clear, nor have they been fully implemented. This chapter will use the existing United States regulatory requirements as a framework for discussion of the conduct of clinical studies in hormone replacement therapy.

The present-day regulatory environment of preclinical and clinical drug development is the result of a long legislative evolution. Up to 1906 no comprehensive federal statutes for drug development and approval existed. As a result of increasing public concern about the lack of oversight and standards and sometimes haphazard handling of drug substances, the *Pure Food and Drug Act* was passed in 1906. The Act prohibited the interstate transportation of adulterated and misbranded drugs and foods, but otherwise provided no regulatory requirements regarding drug safety and efficacy. This Act remained the principal statute until 1937, when more than 100 individuals died from a marketed product, Elixir of Sulfanilamide, which contained the antifreeze diethylene glycol as a solubilizer. This tragedy provided pressure for stricter legislation of drug safety and led to the passage of the *Food, Drug and Cosmetics Act of 1938*, which required premarketing approval of a drug based on its safety profile. However, the Act fell short in several important aspects. Drugs marketed prior to 1938 were exempt from review; proof of the benefits claimed in the drug's labeling was not required; and active approval of marketing applications by the FDA was not necessary. Unless the FDA objected to the new drug application within 60 days, the drug was automatically approved.

C.F. Holinka: President, PharmConsult, New York, New York 10014.

J.H. Pickar: Women's Health Research, Wyeth-Ayerst, Radnor, Pennsylvania 19087.

It required yet another tragedy to advance the regulation for drug approval to modern standards. A sedative and antinausea drug, thalidomide, approved and sold in some countries in Europe, but not approved in the United States, was prescribed to an estimated 20,000 people. Epidemiologic evidence soon emerged that linked thalidomide use by pregnant women to birth defects, such as severely shortened limbs. In 1962, the drug was banned worldwide. That same year an amendment to the Food, Drug and Cosmetics Act was passed (the *Kefauver-Harris Amendment*) that provides the core regulatory basis for modern clinical development. It requires that all new drugs be proved effective as well as safe, and that clinical investigations be well controlled. Most importantly, the *Amendment* requires an affirmative act by the FDA for marketing approval of a new drug rather than automatic approval within a certain period after submission of the *New Drug Application* (NDA) unless the FDA objects.

CLINICAL STUDIES

General Requirements

The current requirement of submission to the FDA of an *Investigational New Drug Application* (IND) before clinical studies are begun is an outgrowth of that agency's concern for public safety expressed in the *Kefauver-Harris Amendment* as well as a means of protecting the participants in clinical studies. In addition to the IND, adverse effect reporting was established, the concept of "good manufacturing practices" was initiated as a regulatory tool, and informed consent by study subjects was instituted.

The *IND Rewrite of 1987* added to the importance of the *Investigator's Brochure*, which is a significant part of the application. The FDA requires that this document provide the following information to those conducting clinical studies:

A brief description of the drug substance and formulation, including the structural formula, if known.

A summary of the pharmacologic and toxicologic effects of the drug in animals and, to the extent known, in humans.

A summary of the pharmacokinetics and biologic disposition of the drug in animals and, if known, in humans.

A summary of information relating to safety and effectiveness in humans obtained from prior clinical studies, including foreign studies, with appended reprints of published articles on such studies when useful.

A description of possible risks and side effects to be anticipated on the basis of prior experience with the drug under investigation or with related drugs, and of precautions or special monitoring to be done as part of the investigational use of the drug.

The *IND Rewrite of 1987* also required that there be protocols which included the following:

- A statement of the objectives and purpose of the study;
- Investigators qualifications;
- Information on the facility where the study was to be conducted;
- Criteria for subjects selection and exclusion and an estimate of the number of subjects to be studied;
- A description of the design of the study, including the kind of control group to be used, if any, and a description of the methods to be used to minimize bias on the part of subjects, investigators, and analysis;
- The method for determining the dose(s) to be administered, the planned maximal dosage, and the duration of individual patient exposure to the drug;
- A description of the observations and measurements to be made to fulfill the objectives of the study;
- A description of clinical procedures, laboratory tests, or other measures to be taken to monitor the effects of the drug in human subjects and to minimize risk.

Standardization of Institutional Review Board (IRB) and informed consent requirements was established in a federal regulation in 1991 for all federal agencies that regulate clinical research. IRBs are responsible for the initial and continuing review and approval of all studies and for ensuring that the rights and welfare of the subjects are protected. Before entering a study, an individual must sign an informed consent form which states that the subject's participation in the trial is voluntary and that the subject may refuse to participate, or withdraw from the trial at any time without penalty. The consent form must also explain the study in language the subject can understand and must include a statement on reasonably expected benefits and reasonably foreseeable risks or inconveniences to the subject.

Clinical studies are conducted with new compounds only after an appropriate preclinical program has been undertaken in which the drug has been thoroughly tested in animals. Clinical trials are generally divided into three phases that are usually conducted sequentially, although there may be some overlapping.

Phase 1 studies first introduce the drug to humans under rigorously monitored conditions. The studies are designed to determine the side effects of a drug at increasing dose levels and to evaluate its metabolism and pharmacologic action. Phase 1 studies are expected to yield sufficient information about the drug to permit the design of well-controlled, scientifically sound phase 2 studies. Depending on the drug, phase 1 studies can require between 20 and 80 normal volunteers, or patients in the disease category for which the drug is intended. New progestins for the treatment of postmenopausal women, for example, are subject to extensive phase 1 trials.

Phase 2 studies evaluate the effectiveness and side effects of a drug at different dose levels. In addition to safety data, these studies are expected to yield information on the lowest effective dose and to identify a suboptimal dose level. Phase 2 studies are usually conducted in a study population of several hundred subjects.

Phase 3 studies are long-term safety and efficacy studies designed on the basis of results from phase 2 studies. They are generally large and can include up to several thousand subjects. Phase 3 studies are conducted in support of an indication for the investigational drug.

The entire body of data from phase 1 to phase 3 studies, together with data from preclinical studies and all other available data about the drug, such as those from scientific publications, is then submitted in a NDA for approval of the indication. Data on the clinical safety and efficacy, their analysis and the discussion of their clinical relevance, make up a major part of the NDA. Also included is detailed information on the manufacturing of the drug as well as the proposed labeling.

Specific Requirements for Hormone Replacement Therapy Studies

Hormone replacement therapy studies usually require volunteers who are at least 1 year past their last menstrual period. Because the true onset of menopause (i.e., the occurrence of the last menstrual period) is frequently obscured in individuals taking HRT, the levels of follicle-stimulating hormone (FSH) and 17β-estradiol (E2) may be evaluated to ensure postmenopausal status. FSH levels of 50 IU/L or above and E2 levels 20 pg/mL or below are frequently considered to indicate postmenopausal status. However, the methodology for FSH analysis has greatly advanced since the initial requirement of $\geq$ 50 IU/L FSH. Therefore, when analyzed by contemporary state-of-the-art methods, postmenopausal FSH levels may well be lower than 50 IU/L (1). Similarly, postmenopausal estradiol levels may be assay-dependent.

Apart from the requirements to ascertain postmenopausal status, studies have specific inclusion criteria. Vasomotor studies, for example, require a highly symptomatic study population, whereas studies designed to evaluate the efficacy of a drug for the treatment of established osteoporosis will recruit ambulatory outpatients with one or more osteoporosis-related vertebral fractures or bone mineral density (BMD) values $\geq$ 2 standard deviations below the mean peak BMD for premenopausal women (2). Studies for the prevention of osteoporosis would have a separate set of criteria. In addition to inclusion criteria, specific exclusion criteria and washout periods from previous HRT are stipulated in clinical protocols.

VASOMOTOR STUDIES

Postmenopausal estrogen depletion or changes in estrogen levels are accompanied by vasomotor disturbances and atrophic vaginal changes in a large number of women. It has been estimated that 25% of postmenopausal women seek medical care for these problems (3). Data from an early study, presented in Fig. 59.1, illustrate the effectiveness of estrogen in the treatment of hot flushes, also referred to as flashes, (4). A striking feature shown in this figure is the substantial placebo effect on the reduction of hot flushes. Vasomotor studies must, therefore, include a placebo group or active comparator to determine true treatment effects. Usually, vasomotor studies also include the evaluation of vaginal cytology to collect efficacy data for the treatment of vulvovaginal atrophy.

Clinical studies to collect data in support of the vasomotor indication are randomized, double-blind multicenter trials usually conducted over a treatment period of 3 months, preceded by 2 weeks of baseline observations. Based on the expected treatment effect, statistical calculations are used to estimate the number of patients required in each study arm. Two double-blind, randomized studies are usually required for approval, one of which must be placebo-controlled; the other can use an approved estrogen as an active control group. The primary data analysis must show a clinically and statistically significant reduction in the frequency and severity of hot flushes compared with the placebo group, or efficacy equal to or greater than that observed in the active control group (5).

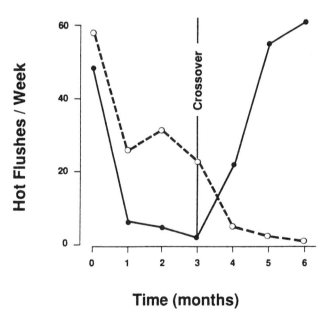

Time (months)

FIG. 59.1. Effects of estrogen (solid line) and placebo (broken line) on vasomotor symptoms during 3 months of treatment and after double-blind crossover of treatment. Vasomotor studies are generally conducted for 3 months, preceded by a 2-week baseline period. Maximal therapeutic effects are usually apparent after 1 month of treatment. (From Coope J, Thomson JM, Poller L. Effects of 'natural oestrogen' replacement therapy on menopausal symptoms and blood clotting. *Br Med J* 1975;4:139–143; with permission.)

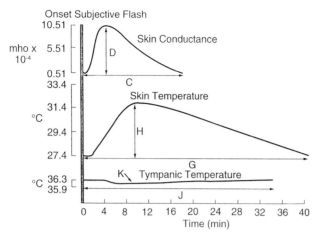

FIG. 59.2. Objective parameters and their time course for the assessment of the hot flush. (From Meldrum DR. The pathophysiology of postmenopausal symptoms. *Semin Reprod Endocrinol* 1983;1:11–17; with permission.)

The study population consists of women after natural or surgical menopause who experience seven to eight moderate to severe hot flushes per day or 60 per week during a 2-week baseline period. Moderate hot flushes are characterized by a sensation of heat with perspiration

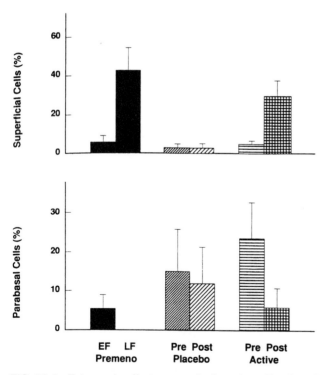

FIG. 59.3. Estrogenic effects on vaginal cytology. Parabasal (immature) and superficial (mature) cells are expressed as percentages of the total vaginal epithelial cell population. Changes during the early (EF) and late (LF) follicular phases of the normal menstrual cycle are presented for comparison. (From Laufer LR, DeFazio JL, Lu JKH, et al. Estrogen replacement therapy by transdermal estradiol administration. *Am J Obstet Gynecol* 1983;146:533–540; with permission.)

but without impairment of daily activities, whereas severe hot flushes result in the disruption of daily activities (5). Frequency and severity of hot flushes are evaluated subjectively by every study subject, who keeps daily records that also include information on the incidence of waking episodes and night sweats. The incidence of hot flushes can also be assessed by objective endpoints such as temperature increases and changes in conductance of the skin (6), as illustrated in Fig. 59.2.

Approval for the treatment of vulvar and vaginal atrophy requires the demonstration of therapeutic estrogen effects on vaginal epithelium, as shown by a shift from a predominantly immature squamous epithelial cell population (parabasal cells) to predominantly mature cells (superficial cells) (7). Typical effects of estrogen replacement are illustrated in Fig. 59.3. In clinical studies, the *Maturation Index*, expressed as percentages of parabasal, intermediate, and superficial cells, is evaluated from cell samples of the lateral vaginal wall. Alternatively, hormonal responsiveness can be estimated by the maturation value, which assigns a numerical value to each cell population (parabasal = 0; intermediate = 0.5, mature = 1.0). By that measure, 0 indicates an exclusively immature population whereas increasing values toward 1 denote increasing maturation.

HYPERPLASIA STUDIES

The association between unopposed estrogen and endometrial hyperplasia, and the possible progression from hyperplasia to cancer were first recognized over half a century ago (8). This association has now been well documented with regard to estrogen replacement therapy (9). Compelling evidence indicates that adjunctive progestin confers effective protection against estrogen-induced endometrial hyperplasia (10–13).

The rationale for the addition of progestin to estrogen is the protection against endometrial cancer. In clinical studies, the incidence of hyperplasia is the only acceptable surrogate endpoint for endometrial cancer (5) because hyperplasia has been shown to predict the development of adenocarcinoma, although a progression from hyperplasia to cancer is observed only in a minority of individuals, and predominantly in cases of atypical hyperplasia (14). In this context, note should be taken of the existence of estrogen-independent endometrial cancers that are unlikely to be prevented by progestins (15).

Hyperplasia studies are large and may require as many as 100 trial sites. Reported studies consist of five or more treatment groups with at least one hundred, but usually several hundred subjects per group (12,13). For drug approval, a 12-month dose-ranging, double-blind, randomized pivotal trial is required to identify the lowest adjunctive progestin dose to protect the endometrium against hyperplasia or cancer. In addition, bleeding patterns are carefully monitored and recorded on daily diary cards (16). An estrogen-only treatment group is required to estimate the hyperplasia rate in the absence of progestin when that rate has not previously been defined for the specific estrogen and estrogen dose. Women who develop hyperplasia are discontinued from the study and receive appropriate medical care.

Endometrial biopsies are scheduled at study entry and at 6 or 12-month intervals thereafter (12,13). Unscheduled biopsies are performed at any time, if medically indicated. Two independent pathologists, who are blinded to study treatment and to each other's readings, evaluate the biopsies by standard criteria for diagnosis of endometrial hyperplasia. In cases of diagnostic differences regarding hyperplasia between the two readers (i.e., when one reader records hyperplasia and the other non-hyperplasia), a third pathologist, also blinded, will read the slides. The majority diagnosis of the three readings is then used for analysis. Quantitative analysis of the variability between the readers is required as a validation of the diagnostic classification scheme (5).

OSTEOPOROSIS STUDIES

Osteoporosis affects an estimated 75 million people in the United States, Europe, and Japan (17). Prevention and treatment of this disease have major beneficial consequences for public health and healthcare costs. It has been known for several decades that HRT prevents postmenopausal bone loss when started shortly after menopause, and that it is effective even after bone loss has occurred (18). The bone-sparing effects of estrogen are illustrated in Fig. 59.4.

For phase 3 clinical trials, regulatory guidelines anticipate that studies for treatment of established osteoporosis will be initiated before the start of trials for prevention of osteoporosis. From the FDA's point of view, it is desirable to have interim data from treatment studies as well as appropriate data from preclinical studies in two animal species before prevention trials are initiated. Ordinarily, bone mineral density (BMD) as an endpoint is sufficient for approval of the prevention indication only if efficacy has already been demonstrated in a treatment study with a fracture endpoint.

However, in the guidelines, primary efficacy endpoints are defined differently, depending on the class of drugs: estrogens or nonestrogens (2). The incidence of new vertebral fractures is a necessary efficacy endpoint in treatment studies with a nonestrogenic new drug, whereas BMD is adequate for prevention studies. For estrogens, the primary endpoint is the same for prevention and treatment, namely, BMD, because the relationship between fracture risk and BMD has already been validated for patients receiving estrogen.

Osteoporosis prevention studies should be randomized, double-blind, placebo-controlled, and with multiple dosage arms sufficient to enable assessment of the minimal effec-

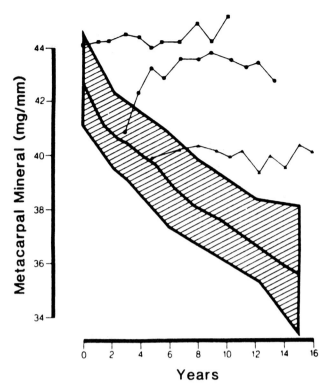

FIG. 59.4. Prevention of bone loss by estrogen replacement therapy started shortly after oophorectomy, or 3 and 6 years after oophorectomy.

tive dose. The minimal study duration is 2 years; the minimal sample size is that calculated to demonstrate adequately the safety and efficacy of the investigational drug.

Studies of treatment of osteoporosis in patients with fractures should be double-blind and randomized, with either placebo or active drug in the control group. In studies using an active control group, sample size calculations must be such that sufficient subjects are enrolled to detect a meaningful difference between the test drug and the active control if such a difference exists. The number of subjects can be higher in trials designed to study the efficacy of HRT regimens in the treatment of osteoporosis than in the prevention of osteoporosis.

CARDIOPROTECTION

The greatest overall benefit of HRT as a measure of preventive medicine may well be its cardioprotective effect (19,20). In fact, postmenopausal estrogen deprivation has been viewed as a major cardiovascular risk factor that rivals other established risk factors (21). Observational studies have suggested that estrogen replacement therapy reduces the risk of coronary heart disease (CHD) in postmenopausal women by approximately 50% (22, 23).

The mechanisms underlying the cardioprotective action of estrogen are incompletely understood and their elucidation is currently being pursued along a broad front of multidisciplinary research. Favorable effects of HRT on lipid profiles have been demonstrated in several large, randomized, double-blind studies (23,24), but favorable lipid patterns account for only a part of the cardioprotection.

Prospective primary and secondary prevention studies with sufficient power to detect meaningful differences are large, long, costly, and complex to manage. The ongoing Women's Health Initiative (WHI) primary prevention trial is designed to study a variety of outcomes including cardiovascular endpoints in approximately 63,000 women over an average of approximately 9 years. The Women's International Study of Long Duration Oestrogen After Menopause (WISDOM) primary prevention study to be conducted in the United Kingdom and 11 other countries is expected to enroll 34,000 women for a 10-year study period. The Heart and Estrogen Progestin Replacement Study (HERS) secondary prevention trial will complete shortly; it includes nearly 2,800 participants being studied for an average of 4.75 years. Prospective trials to investigate the beneficial effects of HRT on the central nervous system (i.e., the prevention or delay of Alzheimer's disease) are likely to be equally complex.

SAFETY ASSESSMENTS

Clinical trials in support of marketing approval for a new drug, or of approval for an additional indication for a marketed drug, must document thoroughly the safety of a drug, in addition to its efficacy. Standard safety assessments in HRT studies include physical and gynecologic examinations, mammography, Papanicolaou (Pap) smear, and laboratory tests (hematology, chemistry and urinalysis). Women with a uterus are closely monitored for endometrial hyperplasia. Prolonged vaginal bleeding in women receiving unopposed estrogen may suggest an increased risk of endometrial hyperplasia (26). In cases of severe or prolonged bleeding, a biopsy may be indicated. Additional special metabolic parameters (e.g., lipid profiles, coagulation factors, and carbohydrate metabolism) are usually evaluated in HRT studies (24,25) because of favorable or potentially unfavorable hormonal effects on those parameters.

All treatment-emergent adverse events, whether related to the investigational drug, are recorded throughout the study. An adverse event is considered serious if it is fatal or immediately life-threatening, requires or prolongs inpatient hospitalization, causes permanent or significant disability, is the result of an overdose, is a congenital abnormality or cancer, or requires medical or surgical intervention to prevent permanent sequelae.

THE CHALLENGE FOR THE FUTURE

Nearly 10 years ago it was proposed that HRT, because of its substantial benefits, should be considered for all women, and the benefits be weighed against the risks (27). A large body of additional evidence in support of this statement has since accumulated. The overall major benefits of HRT, compared with its risks, together with the sizable numbers of women eligible for this measure of preventive medicine, present a special challenge to the development of new drugs and to further studies of approved products.

To increase continuance with HRT remains a major challenge. Extended continuance with any voluntary measure in preventive medicine depends to a large extent on subject motivation and physician support. Hormone replacement therapy is a long-term elective therapy. Extensive public programs of education with respect to HRT and menopause, as well as a range of therapies and modes of administration, are likely to enhance continuance. Continuing research into new compounds, new methods of administering HRT, and lower doses of existing therapies all offer the possibility of improved outcomes and better continuance because therapies can be better tailored to individual needs. Accordingly, a number of novel products, such as percutaneous (28) or vaginal (29) delivery systems, and new regimens are now under development or being considered for development.

Reduction of hormonal doses without compromising efficacy is another challenge. For example, the development of short phases of adjunctive progestin treatment together with constant estrogen (i.e., a regimen of 3 days estrogen-only alternating with 3 days estrogen-progestin combined) has been proposed with the aim of achieving the effects of a continuous combined regimen at lower progestin doses (30). However, additional clinical evaluation is needed to properly evaluate both this regimen and long-cycle therapies.

Safety concerns, and especially the fear of breast cancer, remain a deterrent to HRT use. Data from large prospective clinical trials are needed to put these concerns in perspective. The development of compounds with maximal benefits with respect to vasomotor symptoms, osteoporosis, and cardioprotection, and without effects on breast and endometrium, represents a major challenge. In the past few years, encouraging results have been seen with the emergence of selective estrogen receptor modulators (31), with each new generation offering improvements over the preceding one for the prevention of osteoporosis. However, these compounds do not prevent or treat vasomotor symptoms and their role in cardiovascular protection remains to be defined. The recent discovery of a novel human estrogen receptor (32) opens up promising possibilities for other selective receptor modulators in the service of the overall goal of producing estrogenic compounds that are effective in the treatment of the postmenopausal woman with the potential of fewer side effects.

REFERENCES

1. Pandian MR, Odell WD, Carlton E, Fisher DA. Development of third-generation immunochemiluminometric assays of follitropin and lutropin and clinical application in determining pediatric reference ranges. *Clin Chem* 1993;39:1815–1819.
2. Division of Metabolism and Endocrine Drug Products, US Food and Drug Administration. *Clin 04/01/94 Draft Guidelines for Preclinical and Clinical Evaluation of Agents Used in the Prevention and Treatment of Postmenopausal Osteoporosis.*
3. Notelovitz M. Estrogen replacement therapy: indications, contraindications, and agent selection. *Am J Obstet Gynecol* 1989;161: 1832–1841.
4. Coope J, Thomson JM, Poller L. Effects of 'natural oestrogen' replacement therapy on menopausal symptoms and blood clotting. *Br Med J* 1975;4:139–143.
5. FDA HRT Working Group. *Guidance for Clinical Evaluation of Combination Estrogen/Progestin-Containing Drug Products Used For Hormone Replacement Therapy of Postmenopausal Women.* March 20, 1995.
6. Meldrum DR. The pathophysiology of postmenopausal symptoms. *Seminars in Reproductive Endocrinology* 1983;1:11–17.
7. Laufer LR, DeFazio JL, Lu JKH, et al. Estrogen replacement therapy by transdermal estradiol administration. *Am J Obstet Gynecol* 1983;146:533–540.
8. Gusberg SB. Precursors of corpus carcinoma: estrogens and adenomatous hyperplasia. *Am J Obstet Gynecol* 1947;54:905–927.
9. Grady D, Gebretsadik T, Kerlikowske K, Ernster V, Petitti D. Hormone replacement therapy and endometrial cancer risk: a meta-analysis. *Obstet Gynecol* 1995;85: 304–313.
10. Voigt LF, Weiss NS, Chu J, Daling JR, McKnight B, van Belle G. Progestagen supplementation of exogenous oestrogens and risk of endometrial cancer. *Lancet* 1991;338:274–277.
11. Persson I, Adami H-O, Bergkvist L, Lindgren A, Pettersson B, Hoover R, Schairer C. Risk of endometrial cancer after treatment with oestrogens alone or in conjunction with progestogens: results of a prospective study. *BMJ* 1989;298:147–151.
12. Woodruff JD, Pickar JF, for The Menopause Study Group. Incidence of endometrial hyperplasia in postmenopausal women taking conjugated estrogens (Premarin) with medroxyprogesterone acetate or conjugated estrogens alone. *Am J Obstet Gynecol* 1994;170:1213–1223.
13. The Writing Group for the PEPI Trial. Effects of hormone replacement therapy on endometrial histology in postmenopausal women. *JAMA* 1996;275:370–375.
14. Kurman RJ, Kaminski PF, Norris HJ. The behavior of endometrial hyperplasia. A long-term study of 'untreated' hyperplasia in 170 cases. *Cancer* 1985;56:403–412.
15. Holinka CF. Aspects of hormone replacement therapy. *Ann NY Acad Sci* 1994;734: 271–284.
16. Archer DF, Pickar JH, Bottiglioni F, for The Menopause Study Group. Bleeding patterns in postmenopausal women taking continuous combined or sequential regimens of conjugated estrogens with medroxyprogesterone acetate. *Obstet Gynecol* 1994;83:686–692.
17. Anonymous. Consensus development conference: prophylaxis and treatment of osteoporosis. *Am J Med* 1991;90:107–110.
18. Lindsay R. Sex steroids in the pathogenesis and prevention of osteoporosis. In: Riggs BL, Melton LJ, eds. *Osteoporosis.* New York: Raven Press, 1988:333–358.
19. Lobo RA, Speroff L. International consensus conference on postmenopausal hormone therapy and the cardiovascular system. *Fertil Steril* 1994;61:592–595.
20. Barrett-Connor E. The menopause, hormone replacement, and cardiovascular disease: the epidemiologic evidence. *Maturitas* 1996;23: 227–234.
21. Herrington DM. Estrogen and heart disease: trials to prevent tribulations. *Maturitas* 1997;27:199–202.
22. Stampfer M, Colditz G. Estrogen replacement therapy and CHID: a quantitative assessment of the epidemiologic evidence. *Prev Med* 1991;20:47–63.
23. Bush T. The epidemiology of cardiovascular disease in postmenopausal women. *Ann NY Acad Sci* 1990;592:263–271.
24. Lobo RA, Pickar JH, Wild RA, Walsh B, Hirvonen E, for The Menopause Study Group. Metabolic impact of adding medroxyprogesterone acetate to conjugated estrogen therapy in postmenopausal women. *Obstet Gynecol* 1994;84:987–995.
25. The Writing Group for the PEPI Trial. Effects of estrogen/progestin regimens on heart disease risk factors in postmenopausal women. *JAMA* 1995;273:199–208.
26. Pickar JH, Archer DF, for The Menopause Study Group. Is bleeding a predictor of endometrial hyperplasia in postmenopausal women receiving hormone replacement therapy? *Am J Obstet Gynecol* 1997;177:1178–1183.
27. Mishell, DR. Estrogen replacement therapy: an overview. *Am J Obstet Gynecol* 1989;161:1825–1827.
28. Moyer DL, de Lignieres B, Driguez P, Pez JP. Prevention of endometrial hyperplasia by progesterone during long-term estradiol replacement: influence of bleeding pattern and secretory changes. *Fertil Steril* 1993;59:992–997.
29. Ross D, Cooper AJ, Pryse-Davies J, Bergeron C, Collins WP, Whitehead MI. Randomized, double-blind, dose-ranging study of the endometrial effects of a vaginal progesterone gel in estrogen-treated postmenopausal women. *Am J Obstet Gynecol* 1997;177:937–941.
30. Casper RF, MacLusky NJ, Vanin C, Brown TJ. Rationale for estrogen with interrupted progestin as a new low-dose hormonal replacement therapy. *J Soc Gynecol Invest* 1996;3:225–234.
31. Hol T, Cox MB, Bryant HU, Draper M. Selective estrogen receptor modulators and postmenopausal women's health. *Journal of Women's Health* 1997;6:523–531.
32. Mosselman S, Polman J, Dijkema R. ERb: identification and characterization of a novel human estrogen receptor. *FEBS Lett* 1996;392:49–53.

Treatment of the Postmenopausal Woman: Basic and Clinical Aspects, Second Edition, edited by Rogerio A. Lobo, Lippincott Williams & Wilkins, Philadelphia © 1999.

CHAPTER 60

Clinical Trials Addressing Critical Aspects of Postmenopausal Women's Health

Jennifer Kelsey and Robert Marcus

Several large intervention trials have been undertaken in recent years to evaluate ways of reducing disease occurrence among postmenopausal women. These trials are testing hormone replacement regimens, dietary modification, various dietary supplements, and aspirin. Recent trials are also evaluating pharmacologic agents for the prevention of osteoporosis and other conditions. This chapter describes several of the major randomized prevention trials that are currently in progress or were recently completed in the United States. Some of the material is adapted from a previous review of intervention trials in women (1).

THE POSTMENOPAUSAL ESTROGEN–PROGESTIN (PEPI) TRIAL

Observational epidemiologic studies have indicated that estrogen replacement therapy has a substantial protective effect against coronary heart disease morbidity and mortality (2). Replacement estrogen appears both to produce beneficial changes in circulating lipoproteins known to affect coronary heart disease (3–5) and to decrease fibrinogen levels (6,7). Some evidence suggests that progestins suppress the beneficial effect of estrogen alone on high-density lipoprotein (HDL)-cholesterol (4,8,9). Therefore, when it became part of clinical practice in the 1980s to add progestin to the estrogen for protection of the uterus, concern was expressed that this modification might negate the beneficial effects of estrogen alone. In addition, some researchers and clinicians were not convinced by results from observational studies that estrogen did indeed protect against coronary heart

disease, because some data suggested that healthier women who would be at lower risk for coronary heart disease anyway were more likely to use estrogen replacement therapy than less healthy women (10). These concerns were important considerations in the development of the Postmenopausal Estrogen/Progestin Interventions (PEPI) Trial.

The PEPI Trial, funded by the National Institutes of Health, was designed to examine the effects of unopposed estrogen and three estrogen–progestin regimens on various heart disease risk factors in women aged 45–64 years. The estrogen used was conjugated equine estrogen (Premarin, *Wyeth-Ayerst, Philadelphia, PA*). The heart disease risk factors included HDL-cholesterol, fibrinogen, insulin, and blood pressure (11). When the idea of such a trial was first proposed in the mid-1980s, a trial with coronary events or mortality as endpoints was considered too expensive. Therefore, it was decided to use predictors of coronary heart disease, rather than coronary heart disease itself, as endpoints. The selected endpoints were generally accepted as being independent predictors of coronary heart disease, and the relationships between their levels and risk of coronary heart disease were well established.

From December 1989 to February 1991, 875 women who were 1–9 years beyond last menses were randomized to one of the following five groups: (a) placebo, (b) conjugated equine estrogen (0.625 mg/day), (c) estrogen plus cyclic medroxyprogesterone acetate (10 mg/day) for the first 12 days of the 28-day cycle, (d) estrogen plus continuous medroxyprogesterone acetate (2.5 mg/day), and (e) estrogen plus micronized progesterone (200 mg/day) for the first 12 days of each 28-day cycle. Women were seen at frequent intervals during the 3 years of follow-up; once a year, physical examination, mammography, and endometrial biopsy were performed.

J. Kelsey: Division of Epidemiology, Department of Health Research and Policy, Stanford University, Stanford, California 94305.

R. Marcus: Department of Medicine, Stanford University, and the Geriatrics Research Education & Clinical Center, Veterans Affairs Medical Center, Palo Alto, California 94304.

During the 3 years of the trial, HDL-cholesterol decreased slightly in the placebo group (decrease of 1.2 mg/dL), increased in the two groups assigned to take estrogen plus medroxyprogesterone acetate (increases of 1.2 to 1.6 mg/dL), and increased more in the groups assigned to take conjugated estrogen plus cyclic micronized progesterone (increase of 4.1 mg/dL) and conjugated estrogen alone (increase of 5.6 mg/dL). Compared with placebo, all active treatment groups showed decreases in mean low-density lipoprotein (LDL)-cholesterol and increases in triglycerides. Fibrinogen levels increased to a greater extent in the placebo group than in any of the active treatment groups; the magnitude of the changes did not differ significantly among the active treatment groups. Systolic blood pressure increased and postchallenge insulin levels decreased during the 3 years approximately to the same extent in all groups. Compared with all other groups, unopposed estrogen was associated with a greatly increased incidence of adenomatous or atypical hyperplasia (34% vs. 1%) and of hysterectomy (6% vs. 1%). In fact, 40% of participants originally assigned to unopposed estrogen were taken off of it because of endometrial hyperplasia.

Results regarding HDL-cholesterol are of particular interest because some evidence suggests that HDL-cholesterol is an especially important predictor of coronary heart disease in women. Because women randomized to estrogen alone or to estrogen in combination with micronized progesterone had the greatest increases in HDL-cholesterol, these compounds would be expected to have the most favorable effect on incidence of coronary heart disease. However, the high proportion of women developing endometrial hyperplasia among those using estrogen alone dampens enthusiasm for this regimen. Thus, in this trial conjugated estrogen with cyclic micronized progestin had the most favorable effect on HDL-cholesterol among the regimens that were not associated with an increased risk for endometrial hyperplasia. However, the long-term effects of micronized progesterone have not been well studied. It should be pointed out that the preparation of micronized progesterone used in PEPI was specially formulated for the trial by the Schering-Plough Corporation (*Kenilworth, NJ*). That highly standardized formulation is not the same as micronized progesterones that can be obtained from a number of pharmacies around the United States. The license to market the PEPI formulation has been acquired by Solvay Pharmaceuticals (*Marietta, GA*), and the drug should be available by prescription in 1998.

The PEPI Trial is also providing information on other endpoints. For instance, the trial clearly showed that, compared with placebo, all the active treatment regimens had a favorable effect on bone mineral density in the lumbar spine and hip over the 3 years of the trial (12). Women in all treatment groups gained weight, but weight gain was greatest in women assigned to placebo and least in those taking unopposed estrogen. However, the magnitude of the difference between groups in weight gain was only approximately 1 kg over the 3-year period (13). Future reports from PEPI will focus on physical, cognitive, and affective symptoms, mammographic parenchymal density, carbohydrate metabolism, and other outcomes of interest.

Much useful information was gained from the PEPI Trial. Because women were randomized to the various treatment groups, this study adds substantially to the body of evidence from observational studies indicating that hormone replacement therapy (HRT) reduces the risk of coronary heart disease and that the association does not occur solely because healthier people tend to use HRT. The magnitude of the changes in HDL-cholesterol levels associated with use of estrogen alone or estrogen with micronized progestin suggest that the risk for coronary heart disease would be reduced by 20% to 25% among women using these compounds. The favorable effect on fibrinogen levels with or without the addition of progestin to estrogen has been confirmed in a more recent study (14), and would be expected to be associated with a further substantial decrease in risk for coronary heart disease. The increase in HDL-cholesterol and decrease in fibrinogen levels compared with placebo suggest that estrogen has both a long-term beneficial effect and an immediate effect, in turn indicating that the great degree of protection will be achieved in long-term current users. On the other hand, the finding of a 10% per year incidence of adenomatous or atypical endometrial hyperplasia among women in the estrogen alone group provides strong evidence that women taking this regimen should be under annual endometrial surveillance.

Limitations of the PEPI Trial include its use of predictors of coronary heart disease as endpoints rather than coronary heart disease itself, and its relatively short period of follow-up. Premarin was the only type of estrogen used in this trial; the effects of other types of estrogens or of estrogens administered transdermally cannot be evaluated from this study. In addition, this study had small numbers of racial and ethnic minorities, so that the results cannot necessarily be generalized to them. Thus, although the PEPI Trial was considerably less expensive than the large trials described below and provided much useful information, it leaves unanswered some key questions that can be properly addressed only in larger trials of longer duration.

THE WOMEN'S HEALTH INITIATIVE

The overall goals of the Women's Health Initiative (WHI) are to test methods of reducing the risk for cardiovascular disease, breast cancer, colorectal cancer, and osteoporotic fractures in women. It is the largest and most expensive research study ever funded by the National Institutes of Health (NIH). The WHI was originally proposed in 1991 by the then Director-designate of the NIH, Bernadette Healey. The concept of such a trial received a great deal of support from the Congressional Caucus on Women's Issues, and the study is funded by the US Congress as a separate line item in the NIH budget. It includes a randomized trial, an observational study, and a community prevention study. Only the randomized trial component of the Women's Health Initiative is considered here.

The randomized trial includes approximately 64,500 women aged between 50 and 79 years, of diverse racial or ethnic groups and socioeconomic status. Its three branches are designed to test hypotheses concerning the effects of (a) a low-fat dietary pattern, (b) hormone replacement, and (c) calcium and vitamin D supplementation. The coordinating center is at the University of Washington. Recruitment began in 16 Vanguard Clinical Centers in the fall of 1993. Twenty-four additional clinical centers were added in early 1995 (15,16). Recruitment was completed in early 1998.

Dietary Modification Branch

The dietary modification branch of the WHI has the primary aim of testing the hypothesis that a low-fat dietary pattern reduces the risks of breast cancer and colon cancer. A secondary hypothesis is that a low-fat dietary pattern reduces the risk of coronary heart disease.

Evidence that a diet high in fat increases the risk for breast cancer is derived mostly from comparisons of breast cancer incidence rates in countries with various levels of per capita fat consumption, studies of migrants from one country to another, and animal studies. Epidemiologic case-control studies suggest, at most, a weak association between fat consumption and risk of breast cancer. In a recent metaanalysis of cohort studies of the relationship between dietary fat intake during adulthood and breast cancer found no association (17). Also, it has been hypothesized that if a high-fat diet is involved in the cause of breast cancer, it may be fat intake early in life rather than in adulthood that is important (18).

On the other hand, evidence is strong that people who have diets high in meat, protein, and fat have an elevated risk of colon cancer, and that persons with diets high in vegetables and fibers are at reduced risk (19). It is uncertain which of these foods are actually of etiologic importance, because people who eat large amounts of meat, protein, and fat tend to eat relatively small quantities of vegetables and fibers. Nonetheless, most epidemiologists agree that this general dietary pattern is related to colon cancer risk.

It is generally accepted that a diet low in fat, saturated fat, and cholesterol lowers total cholesterol and LDL-cholesterol, both of which are risk factors for coronary heart disease. A diet low in fat may also reduce HDL cholesterol (20). Because, as mentioned above, a high HDL-

cholesterol level protects against coronary heart disease, especially in women (21,22), the net effect of the low-fat dietary pattern on coronary heart disease risk in women is not entirely clear.

Some 48,000 women are enrolled in the dietary modification branch of the trial. It is intended that women in the intervention group attain a diet with (a) total fat intake of no more than 20% of daily calories, (b) saturated fat intake less than 7% of daily calories, (c) at least five daily servings of fruits and vegetables, and (d) at least six daily servings of grain products. In addition, women in both the intervention and control groups are being provided with a standard packet of health promotion materials, including information on a healthy diet. Group meetings with a nutritionist and self-monitoring tools are also being used in an attempt to persuade the women in the intervention group to reach and maintain the low-fat dietary pattern. The average intervention period is expected to be 9 years.

Hormone Replacement Branch

When the WHI began, the primary aim of the hormone replacement branch was to test the hypotheses that estrogen replacement therapy with progestin and estrogen replacement therapy alone reduce the risk of coronary heart disease. Secondary hypotheses were that these same regimens reduce the risk of osteoporotic fractures and increase the risk of breast cancer.

As mentioned, almost all observational epidemiologic studies find that estrogen replacement therapy is associated with a reduced risk of coronary heart disease, but concern exists that a tendency for healthier women to use estrogen replacement therapy may make it appear that the beneficial effect is greater than it really is. Another concern is that the beneficial effects of a combined progestin and estrogen regimen on coronary heart disease may be less than those of estrogen alone (8,9). It has been known from randomized trials reported in the 1980s (23,24) that estrogen replacement therapy reduces loss of bone mass in women who have recently undergone either natural menopause or oophorectomy, and available evidence suggests that progestin and estrogen therapy together decrease loss of bone mass at least to the same extent as estrogen alone (12,25). Most observational studies suggest protection against hip and other fractures, especially among current long-term users (25). Results of studies concerned with the effect of HRT on breast cancer risk have been somewhat inconsistent, but a recent meta-analysis reported a relative risk of about 1.35 for women who had used estrogen alone for 5 or more years (26). The risk in women who had used estrogen and progestin was similar or slightly greater; numbers were too small to be certain.

Approximately 27,500 women are enrolled in the hormone replacement branch. Women without a uterus are randomized to either (a) conjugated equine estrogen alone (0.625 mg/day) or (b) placebo. At the beginning of enrollment, women with a uterus were randomized to one of three groups: (a) conjugated equine estrogen alone (0.625 mg/day), (b) conjugated equine estrogen (0.625 mg/day) plus continuous low-dose progestin (2.5 mg/day), and (c) placebo. However, when results of the PEPI Trial were published showing that a relatively high proportion of the women taking estrogen alone had to be taken off it because of endometrial hyperplasia, the women in this group were switched to the estrogen plus progestin group. WHI investigators have been working closely with the external Data and Safety Monitoring Board to develop algorithms that take into account risks and benefits and to consider early stopping criteria and trial reporting procedures (16).

Obtaining information on long-term risks and benefits of estrogen plus continuous low-dose progestin among women of various ages and racial or ethnic groups will be important for women considering using this regimen. Valuable data on adverse side effects such as uterine bleeding in women of various ages and on possible beneficial effects such as on memory will also be important. Nevertheless, several questions about the design of this trial have arisen. One major question is why it began before the results from the PEPI Trial were available, because the findings from the PEPI Trial brought about a major change in the hormone replacement branch shortly after it began. Second, it is unfortunate that only one regimen, conjugated estrogen with continuous low-dose progestin, is being tested in the women with an intact uterus, and that another single regimen, conjugated estrogens alone, is being tested in the women without a uterus. Even at the time the trial began many questions arose about the optimal dose of progestin and about other forms of estrogen. Now, just a few years after the WHI began, many more options are available to women regarding doses, modes of administration, and forms of estrogen and progestin. In addition, a selective estrogen-receptor modulator (SERM), raloxifene (to be discussed below), has now been approved by the FDA for postmenopausal therapy, and more SERMs are expected to be approved over the next few years. The hormone replacement branch, thus, will provide little information to assist women in deciding which of many possible regimens are likely to be optimal for them. A third problem is that if the primary aim is indeed to determine whether HRT affects the incidence of coronary heart disease, it would seem much more cost-effective if women at low risk for coronary heart disease had not been included in this branch. Finally, concern exists that as new information about risks and benefits of replacement therapy is reported from other on-going studies, women who have been randomized may wish to switch from their assigned treatment. To date, this has not proved to be a major problem, but as time goes on and women become aware of the large number of options available to them, this could become an important issue.

Calcium–Vitamin D Supplementation Branch

The primary aim of the calcium–vitamin D supplementation branch is to test the hypothesis that supplemental calcium and vitamin D reduce the risk of hip fracture. Secondary aims are that this supplementation reduces the risk of other fractures and of colorectal cancer.

Most randomized trials indicate that use of calcium supplementation somewhat retards loss of bone mass (27). Bone mass is a moderately strong predictor of hip fracture. Results from observational studies are inconsistent to whether supplemental or dietary calcium intake affects hip fracture risk. However, a randomized trial in frail older women in France (28) showed a substantial reduction in hip and other nonvertebral fracture incidence among elderly women taking supplemental calcium with vitamin D. In addition, an American study (29) showed that calcium supplementation reduced vertebral fracture incidence in older women who had already sustained at least one such fracture at baseline. Available evidence does not permit a firm conclusion to be drawn to whether the addition of vitamin D to supplemental calcium increases the protective effect against bone loss of calcium alone. Evidence is inconsistent to whether supplemental calcium and vitamin D protect against colorectal cancer (19).

Participants in the dietary modification and hormone replacement branches are invited at their 1-year anniversary to enroll in the calcium–vitamin D branch as well. It is expected that about 45,000 women will participate. Half of the participants are randomized to a regimen of calcium carbonate plus vitamin D and half are randomized to placebo.

This branch of the trial is the least costly and probably the least controversial. It is unlikely that these supplements will have adverse effects, and this component of the trial may increase knowledge about the long-term effects of this supplementation on fracture risk in women of different ages. Also, it may address the question of whether simultaneous HRT enhances any effect of calcium and vitamin D. It is unfortunate, however, that this trial was not designed to compare the effect of calcium supplementation alone compared with calcium supplementation plus vitamin D. This is likely to remain an important unanswered question.

THE HEART AND ESTROGEN/PROGESTIN STUDY

The primary objective of the Heart and Estrogen/Progestin Study (HERS) is to determine whether hormone replacement therapy is associated with a reduced risk of fatal coronary heart disease and nonfatal and fatal myocardial infarction among women with an intact uterus who have already been diagnosed with coronary heart disease (30). Secondary objectives are to examine the effects of HRT on other outcomes among women with diagnosed coronary heart disease. Among the other outcomes of interest are other cardiovascular changes such as venous thromboembolic events, cancer, osteoporotic fractures, uterine bleeding, and symptomatic side effects. The study is funded by Wyeth-Ayerst Laboratories (*Philadelphia, PA*).

From February 1993 to September 1994, 2,763 women aged younger than 80 years with coronary heart disease were enrolled in this double-blind randomized trial. The women were randomized either to a daily pill containing 0.625 mg conjugated estrogen plus 2.5 mg medroxyprogesterone acetate (Prempro, *Wyeth-Ayerst, Philadelphia, PA*) or to placebo. Annual follow-up of these women includes cardiovascular and gynecologic examinations, electrocardiogram, mammography, and a questionnaire concerned with various symptoms. The trial is scheduled to continue until mid-1998 (31).

This study should be able to address the question of whether this particular hormone replacement regimen protects against recurrence of coronary heart disease, not just uncovering predictors of it. Because coronary heart disease occurs in virtually all adult women to some extent, even if it is not clinically apparent, one could assume that the results from this study might apply to the general population of women as well. Nevertheless, one cannot be certain of this. The results will be available in a much shorter period of time and at a much lower cost than other studies based on much greater numbers of women not at particularly high risk for coronary heart disease. Unfortunately, only one type of hormone replacement regimen is being tested, so this study will be unable to provide much help to women trying to decide among the variety of replacement regimens now available. (Note: HERS was published in 1998; see the introduction to Section VII on page 329.)

THE WOMEN'S HEALTH STUDY

The Women's Health Study (WHS) was designed to be a randomized trial of the benefits and risks of low-dose aspirin, β-carotene, and vitamin E on cardiovascular disease and cancer (32,33). It is funded by the National Institutes of Health.

Considerable evidence suggests that low-dose aspirin reduces the risk of coronary heart disease (33). Low-dose aspirin reduces the tendency of platelets to aggregate, thus decreasing the likelihood that clots or thrombi will form. Randomized trials in both men and women have shown that aspirin reduces the risk for myocardial infarction, stroke, and vascular death among patients with cardiovascular disease. In 1982 the Physicians' Health

Study, a large randomized double-blind placebo-controlled trial of the primary prevention of cardiovascular disease in apparently health male physicians, was initiated to test the effects of aspirin and β-carotene on risk for cancer and cardiovascular disease. In 1988 the aspirin component of this trial was stopped prematurely because a substantially reduced risk of a first myocardial infarction had been noted among those assigned to take aspirin (34). However, the mortality rate from all cardiovascular causes was similar among those assigned aspirin and those not assigned aspirin, and the rate of moderate to severe or fatal hemorrhagic stroke was higher among the aspirin users, although this latter finding was based on small numbers. Thus, the balance of risks and benefits of aspirin use even among men is not entirely clear.

Several reasons are found for initiating a study of aspirin among women (33). Because the Physicians' Health Study included only men, any recommendations regarding aspirin use in women had to be extrapolated from men. Results from observational epidemiologic studies of the risk for cardiovascular disease among female aspirin users have been inconsistent. In addition, although women have lower rates of myocardial infarction than men, the rates of stroke are similar. Thus, the net balance of risks and benefits could be different in women and men.

Various epidemiologic and laboratory studies have suggested that antioxidants such as β-carotene and vitamin E can reduce the incidence of cardiovascular disease and cancer (35,36). Foods such as fruits and vegetables that are high in β-carotene and vitamin E also have relatively high levels of other substances that might inhibit cancer. Thus, whether supplementation with β-carotene and vitamin E (as opposed to other constituents of fruits and vegetables, either singly or in combination) will reduce the risk for cancer and cardiovascular disease is not known. Because any reduction in risk associated with antioxidants is expected to be on the order of only 20% to 30% (37), and because people with diets high in antioxidants are likely to have healthier than average lifestyles in other respects (38), a large randomized trial is needed to provide conclusive evidence of their beneficial effects.

With these considerations in mind, the WHS was started in 1991 (33). Female health professionals aged 45 years and older were recruited from among nurses, physicians, dentists, and other health professionals. A total of 39,876 women were randomized to one of eight combinations of placebo, aspirin, β-carotene, and vitamin E. A major reason for using health professionals was that it had been found in other studies that health professionals can provide accurate and complete information over long periods of time. Studies of health professionals can also be conducted entirely by mail at a considerable savings of money compared with trials in which participants must be seen at a central clinic.

In January, 1996, the β-carotene arm of the trial was stopped because results from the Physicians' Health

Study in men showed no overall evidence of benefit or risk for coronary heart disease or cancer after more than 10 years of use. In addition, two other trials suggested an increased risk for lung cancer and cardiovascular disease mortality among heavy smokers (mostly men) taking supplemental β-carotene (39,40). The aspirin and vitamin E components of the trial continue.

The WHS is a cost-effective way of testing hypotheses regarding the effects of use of aspirin and certain nutritional supplements in women. Although some might question the representativeness of the study population on which it is based, it is hard to see why findings from women health professionals, who come from a wide range of social classes and backgrounds, would not apply to other women as well.

THE BREAST CANCER PREVENTION TRIAL

The Breast Cancer Prevention Trial (BCPT), initiated by the NIH and with a coordinating center at the University of Pittsburgh, was a randomized double-blind placebo-controlled trial to test the efficacy of tamoxifen (Nolvadex, *Zeneca, Wilmington, DE*) in the prevention of breast cancer. It included women who were aged at least 35 years and whose risk of breast cancer was at least as high as that of an average 60-year-old woman in the United States. This trial will be described only briefly because it did not specifically focus on postmenopausal or perimenopausal women.

Tamoxifen, when used as a chemotherapeutic agent in women with breast cancer, has been shown to reduce the incidence of contralateral breast cancer and to delay breast cancer recurrence (41). Compared with other chemotherapeutic agents, serious side effects and adverse reactions have been reported to be rare (42–44). In view of these desirable properties, the BCPT was started to determine if tamoxifen can reduce the incidence of breast cancer in healthy women. A secondary aim was to determine whether tamoxifen reduces the incidence of cardiovascular diseases, as suggested by some previous trials. Osteoporotic fractures were also monitored, because a few studies had indicated some protection against loss of bone mass among postmenopausal women.

The trial was begun in 1992; it included 13,388 women assigned in equal numbers to tamoxifen or placebo. The trial was halted early in 1998, 14 months earlier than planned, because it showed a 45% reduction in breast cancer incidence among the women who took tamoxifen compared with the placebo group (45). No difference was found in the number of heart attacks in the two groups. Women in the tamoxifen group had 34% fewer fractures of the hip, wrist, and spine than those in the placebo group. Given the relatively young age distribution of the women in the trial, most of these fractures were probably of the spine and wrist, so the effect of tamoxifen on hip fracture remains unknown. Tamoxifen was associated with an increased incidence of three uncommon but serious conditions, including endometrial cancer, pulmonary embolism, and deep vein thrombosis.

The encouraging early results of the BCPT need to be interpreted with caution. First, in addition to the potentially life-threatening side effects mentioned, women taking tamoxifen often experience vasomotor symptoms such as hot flushes (46). These are sufficiently troublesome that compliance is sometimes a problem in breast cancer patients. Healthy women may be even less likely to take a medication that makes them feel uncomfortable. Among women in the trial for 3 years, noncompliance (defined as discontinuation of protocol therapy for other than a protocol-specific reason) was approximately 33% (Ford L, *personal communication*). Second, one study (47) reported an increased risk of hip fracture among breast cancer patients randomized to tamoxifen. This finding needs to be evaluated in other studies. Third, concern exists that tamoxifen may stimulate breast tumor growth in some patients (48). In both premenopausal and postmenopausal breast cancer patients who initially responded to tamoxifen but who later developed resistance, the breast tumors in some instances appear dependent on tamoxifen for growth. Finally, reports have been made of new primary breast cancers years after tamoxifen had been discontinued. In particular, a higher-than-expected incidence of estrogen-receptor negative contralateral tumors following tamoxifen treatment has been noted (48,49). In addition, in late 1995, the National Surgical Adjuvant Breast and Bowel Project stopped its study of long-term use of tamoxifen as adjuvant therapy for early stage breast cancer when routine review of data found no additional benefit for women taking tamoxifen for more than 5 years (50). Thus, many questions remain about the use of tamoxifen to reduce the incidence of breast cancer. Long-term follow-up is needed.

RECENT TRIALS OF AGENTS TO REDUCE BONE LOSS AND FRACTURE OCCURRENCE

Although estrogen has been administered for skeletal protection for several decades, trials conducted with adequate statistical power to assess the effect of osteoporosis regimens on bone fracture is a recent phenomenon. To a large degree, this situation reflects the fact that the FDA has only recently required that new osteoporosis drugs, other than estrogens and their analogs, be shown to decrease the incidence of fracture. This provision recognizes the experience from two clinical trials of sodium fluoride showing that increased bone mineral density is not necessarily synonymous with improvement in skeletal integrity (51,52).

Since 1994, the pharmaceutical industry has operated according to a comprehensive FDA Guidance (53) that prescribes the nature of preclinical (animal) studies that need to be carried out and the type of bone quality testing that needs to support evidence of changes in bone mass or bone mineral density. Consequently, during the 1990s several large, well-designed industry-sponsored multicenter clinical trials have been undertaken to test the skeletal benefits of new osteoporosis drugs in postmenopausal women. In this section we discuss published trials involving the potent bisphosphonate, alendronate, and the selective estrogen receptor modulator (SERM), raloxifene, both of which have received FDA approval for osteoporosis prevention.

Alendronate

Bisphosphonates is a term given to a group of drugs related to the naturally occurring molecule, pyrophosphate, in which the oxygen bridge is replaced by carbon, thus rendering the compound completely inaccessible to cleavage by alkaline phosphatases. The first generation bisphosphonate, etidronate (Didronel, *Procter and Gamble Pharmaceuticals, Cincinnati, OH*) has been used in the treatment of Paget's disease of bone since the 1960s. In the early 1990s, a strategy for applying this antiresorptive agent to conservation of bone mass and treatment of osteoporosis was reported in two independent studies (54,55). In both studies, the drug was administered cyclically, 2 weeks every 3 months, for several years. Cyclic administration was required because, unique among drugs of this class, etidronate at effective antiresorptive doses also inhibits the deposition of mineral on bone matrix, thereby increasing the risk for osteomalacia if use is continuous. Both studies clearly showed a beneficial effect of cyclic etidronate on bone mineral density. However, although several hundred women were enrolled, neither study actually achieved adequate statistical power to establish antifracture efficacy; consequently, the FDA did not approve this drug for an osteoporosis indication.

Fracture Intervention Trial

Subsequent generations of bisphosphonates show considerable improvement in the ratios of antiresorptive effects to mineralization inhibition, permitting their continuous use. One potent bisphosphonate, alendronate (Fosamax) was used in the largest osteoporosis clinical trial to date. Sponsored by the manufacturer (*Merck & Company, West Point, PA*), the Fracture Intervention Trial (FIT) enrolled approximately 6,000 women at multiple centers across the United States. FIT was actually a composite of two related but distinct studies. The first was an evaluation of antifracture efficacy of alendronate among approximately 2,000 women with evidence of vertebral compression fracture on entry to the trial (Vertebral Fracture Arm). The second arm enrolled approximately 4,000 women who fulfilled bone mineral density criteria for osteoporosis but who had not yet sustained a compression

deformity (Clinical Fracture Arm). Participants were randomized to receive placebo or alendronate (5 mg/day) with an intent to stay on the assigned regimen for 3 years. Unfortunately for the integrity of the study design, results of smaller phase 2 studies came to light during the course of the FIT trial, from which it was recognized that a 10 mg dose offered greater skeletal response without adding significantly to the incidence of adverse experiences. Therefore, the treatment dose was increased to 10 mg for the last year of the trial. Moreover, during year 3, the FIT Data Safety Monitoring Board determined that drug efficacy was established for the Vertebral Fracture Arm, and that it was not ethically justified to continue half of the women on placebo. Accordingly, the Vertebral Fracture Arm was brought to an early conclusion. Thus, although the FDA approved alendronate at a 10 mg daily dose for treatment of osteoporosis, much of the benefit documented by FIT represents the effect of the 5 mg dose. Despite the deviations from the original study protocol described above, the results from the FIT Vertebral Fracture Arm were dramatic (56). Women assigned to alendronate experienced a 50% reduction in new vertebral fracture, a 90% reduction in the incidence of multiple vertebral fractures, and a 50% reduction in all nonvertebral fractures. In addition, 22 hip fractures were observed for women assigned to placebo, and only 11 in the alendronate group. Women assigned to alendronate sustained less height loss than those on placebo. All of these results were statistically significant.

The substantial decrease in fracture incidence associated with alendronate exceeds that which could have been predicted from the observed elevations in bone mineral density and published relationships between bone mineral density deficit and fracture incidence. This result confirms the FDA's wisdom in requiring fracture incidence to be the primary endpoint of osteoporosis trials. The explanation for this discrepancy is not immediately clear, but it seems likely that a high rate of bone remodeling is itself conducive to fracture, and that effective suppression of remodeling by alendronate had a salutary effect independent of bone mineral density.

It was also found in FIT that approximately one of three vertebral fractures is actually symptomatic to the point that patients seek medical attention for fracture-related symptoms. Although it had been widely understood that many compression fractures were asymptomatic, FIT represents the first prospective confirmation and quantification of this view.

The FIT Clinical Fracture Arm has now been completed. Although the results have been presented at national meetings, a formal paper has not yet been published. From the presented results, it appears that alendronate did offer significant antifracture protection to women without a previous fracture. Even within this highly jeopardized group of women who met bone mineral density criteria for osteoporosis, those in the lowest tertile of bone mineral density experienced greater fracture protection than women in the higher tertiles. At present, FIT participants are being offered an opportunity to remain under observation for several additional years.

In FIT, as in all formal trials, alendronate has proved to be extremely well-tolerated. Concern had been seen about the propensity for this drug (as for most drugs of this class) to cause esophageal irritation and symptoms of heartburn. In FIT, the overall incidence of adverse experiences was very low, and the incidence of esophageal symptoms associated with alendronate did not differ from that observed with placebo. Although esophagitis occurs at low incidence (<10%) in clinical practice, it does remain the major adverse experience with alendronate, particularly among patients who neglect to take the medication exactly as prescribed (with a full glass of water and remaining in upright position for at least 30 minutes after taking the pill).

Early Postmenopausal Intervention Cohort

In 1997, the FDA extended approval of alendronate for the *prevention* of bone loss in recently menopausal women who choose not to take hormone replacement therapy. Evidence to support this indication included interim results from another large clinical trial (57). In the Early Postmenopausal Intervention Cohort (EPIC), 6,000 healthy women who were about 5 years postmenopausal were randomly assigned to receive placebo, alendronate at either 2.5 or 5 mg/day, or HRT. The HRT regimen differed by study center. Participants in the United States received 0.625 mg of conjugated estrogens and continuous medroxyprogesterone acetate (5 mg) on a daily basis. Women in European centers received estradiol plus norethindrone, an androgenic progestin. At the 2-year interim analysis, women in all active treatment groups had conserved and actually gained bone mineral density compared with the placebo group. However, women receiving HRT showed significantly greater gains in bone mineral density than women assigned to alendronate, and women in the European centers showed the greatest increases, presumably reflecting the additive skeletal effects of norethindrone. Thus, alendronate (5 mg/day) does constitute an effective alternative to HRT for skeletal protection of early menopausal women. However, the interim EPIC results show that alendronate is by no means superior to HRT for this purpose, and that presently no basis is found for recommending that women who are doing well on HRT be switched to alendronate.

Selective Estrogen Receptor Modulators

Selective estrogen receptor modulators (SERMS) are agents that produce estrogenlike effects on some tissues and antagonize estrogen in others. SERMs under development are those with actions mimicking the beneficial effects of estrogen on bone and lipid metabolism while antagonizing estrogen in reproductive tissue (58). The precise mechanisms by which SERMs produce these tissue-selective actions are not fully understood, but they appear to reflect characteristic changes in the three-dimensional structure of the estrogen receptor that are induced by binding of the drugs. Different SERMs may have different tissue-specific effects. Tamoxifen is one example of a SERM. Tamoxifen is a triphenyl-ethylene, which behaves as a partial agonist in the uterus, whereas raloxifene (Evista, *Eli Lilly & Co., Princeton, NJ*), a benzothiophene, behaves as a complete antagonist in the uterus. Thus, raloxifene was developed to have beneficial effects on bone and on lipid metabolism, while antagonizing estrogen in both the uterus and breast. In fact, preliminary data presented to the FDA suggested that raloxifene might reduce the risk of breast cancer. Accordingly, SERMs such as raloxifene have been proposed as an alternative to HRT in postmenopausal women for the prevention and treatment of osteoporosis and cardiovascular disease, and possibly the prevention of breast cancer, while not adversely affecting the uterus. Raloxifene is the first SERM to be approved by the FDA for postmenopausal therapy.

Raloxifene received FDA approval for osteoporosis prevention in early 1998. At its approved dose of 60 mg/day, raloxifene increases bone mineral density at the spine and hip. Raloxifene's skeletal protective effect has been shown by several relatively small placebo-controlled clinical trials carried out in North America and Europe, and by one somewhat larger study, in which raloxifene treatment for 2 years increased bone mineral density at the spine and hip by approximately 2% compared with placebo (59). This increase was slightly less than that which had been observed in various studies with HRT or alendronate therapy. Raloxifene was shown to be well-tolerated, although its antiestrogenic actions on the hypothalamus resulted in an increase in hot flushes in some women. Large multicenter phase 3 clinical trials of the antifracture efficacy of raloxifene are in progress.

CONCLUSION

Many options are now available to women around and after menopause to reduce both the extent of their menopausal symptoms and their risk for certain major diseases (although possibly to increase their risk for other diseases). Still more choices will be available in the near future. However, the *long-term* risks and benefits of many of these agents are largely unknown. The ongoing intervention trials should provide some information to help women make choices, but large gaps remain in our knowledge.

If compliance and retention are adequate, the Women's Health Initiative can provide some information about the long-term effects of what is currently considered to be a healthy diet and it should also quantify the long-term effects of supplementation with calcium and vitamin D. The Women's Health Study will be useful in determining whether aspirin and vitamin E supplementation reduce the frequency of occurrence of cardiovascular disease and cancer. These results may be particularly useful to healthy women who are averse to taking potent medications.

However, the major trials of hormone replacement therapy, such as the Women's Health Initiative and the Heart Estrogen/Progestin Study, are testing only single hormone replacement regimens compared with placebo. Now that a variety of doses and modes of administration of hormone replacement and new agents such as SERMs are available, these trials provide information for only a small degree of what needs to be known. Trials of the newer agents, such as alendronate, raloxifene, and tamoxifen, have not been sufficiently long to evaluate many potential important risks and benefits. Thus, continued monitoring through various types of studies, both observational and randomized, are extremely important. The appearance of SERMs makes even more complex a woman's decision about hormone replacement therapies. In individual cases, reliance on the results of large randomized trials may provide assistance but not necessarily determine the ultimate correct choice. It remains important for each woman and her physician to have a reasonable sense of individual risks in the skeletal, cardiovascular, breast, and other areas to reach a decision with potentially far ranging consequences.

REFERENCES

1. Kelsey JL, Marcus R. Intervention trials concerned with disease prevention in women. In: Casper RC, ed. *Women's health: hormones, emotions and behavior.* Cambridge: Cambridge University Press, 1998:219–242.
2. Grady D, Rubin SM, Petitti DB, et al. Hormone replacement to prevent disease and prolong life in postmenopausal women. *Ann Intern Med* 1992;117:1016–1037.
3. Walsh BW, Schiff I, Rosner B, Greenberg L, Ravnikar V, Sacks FM. Effects of postmenopausal estrogen replacement on the concentrations and metabolism of plasma lipoproteins. *N Engl J Med* 1991;325:1196–1204.
4. Lobo RA. Effects of hormonal replacement on lipids and lipoproteins in postmenopausal women. *J Clin Endocrinol Metab* 1991;73:925–930.
5. Bush TL, Barrett-Connor E, Cowan LD, et al. Cardiovascular mortality and noncontraceptive use of estrogen in women: results from the Lipid Research Clinics Follow-up Study. *Circulation* 1987;75:1102–1109.
6. Meilahn EN, Kuller LH, Matthews KA, Kiss JE. Hemostatic factors according to menopausal status and use of hormone replacement therapy. *Ann Epidemiol* 1992;2:445–455.
7. Nabulsi AA, Folsom AR, White A, et al. Association of hormone-replacement therapy with various cardiovascular risk factors in postmenopausal women. *N Engl J Med* 1993;328:1069–1075.
8. Tikkanen MJ, Kuusi T, Nikkila EA, Sipinen S. Post-menopausal hormone replacement therapy: effects of progestogens on serum lipids and lipoproteins: a review. *Maturitas* 1986;8:7–17.
9. Lobo RA, Pickar JH, Wild RA, Walsh B, Hirvonen E. Metabolic impact of adding medroxyprogesterone acetate to conjugated estrogen therapy in postmenopausal women. *Obstet Gynecol* 1994;84:987–995.
10. Rosenberg L. Hormone replacement therapy: the need for reconsideration. *Am J Pub Health* 1993;83:1670–1673.
11. The Writing Group for the PEPI Trial. Effects of estrogen or estrogen/progestin regimens on heart disease risk factors in postmenopausal women. The Postmenopausal Estrogen/Progestin Interventions (PEPI) Trial. *JAMA* 1995;237:199–208.
12. The Writing Group for the PEPI Trial. Effects of hormone therapy on bone mineral density. Results from the Postmenopausal Estrogen/Progestin Interventions (PEPI) Trial. *JAMA* 1996;276:1389–1396.
13. Espeland MA, Stefanick ML, Kritz-Silverstein D, Fineberg SE, Waclawiw MA, James MK, Greendale GA. Effect of postmenopausal hormone therapy on body weight and waist and hip girths. *J Clin Endocrinol Metab* 1997;82:1549–1556.
14. Koh KK, Mincemoyer R, Bui MN, et al. Effects of hormone-replacement therapy on fibrinolysis in postmenopausal women. *N Engl J Med* 1997;336:683–690.
15. Rossouw JE, Finnegan LP, Harlan WR, Pinn VW, Clifford C, McGowan JA. The evolution of the Women's Health Initiative: Perspectives from the NIH. *J Am Med Wom Assoc* 1995;50:50–55.
16. Prentice RL, Rossouw JE, Johnson SR, Freedman LS, McTiernan A. The role of randomized controlled trials in assessing the benefits and risks of long-term hormone replacement therapy: example of the Women's Health Initiative. *Menopause* 1996;3:71–76.
17. Hunter DJ, Spiegelman D, Adami H-O, et al. Cohort studies of fat intake and the risk of breast cancer—a pooled analysis. *N Engl J Med* 1996;334:356–361.
18. Colditz GA, Frazier AL. Models of breast cancer show that risk is set by events of early life; preventive efforts must shift focus. *Cancer Epidemiol Biomarkers Prev* 1995;4:567–571.
19. Potter JD, Slattery ML, Bostick RM, Gastur SM. Colon cancer: a review of the epidemiology. *Epidemiol Rev* 1993;15:499–545.
20. Institute of Medicine Committee to Review the NIH Women's Health Initiative. In: Thaul S, Hotra D, eds. *An assessment of the NIH Women's Health Initiative.* Washington, DC: National Academy Press, 1993.
21. Castelli WP. Cardiovascular disease in women. *Am J Obstet Gynec* 1988;158:1553–1560.
22. Bass KM, Newschaffer CJ, Klag MJ, Bush TL. Plasma lipoprotein levels as predictors of cardiovascular death in women. *Arch Intern Med* 1993;153:2209–2216.
23. Genant HK, Christopher CE, Ettinger B, Gordan GS. Quantitative computed tomography of vertebral spongiosa: a sensitive method for detecting early bone loss after oophorectomy. *Ann Intern Med* 1982;97:699–705.
24. Lindsay R, Hart DM, Clark DM. The minimum effective dose of estrogen for prevention of postmenopausal bone loss. *Obstet Gynecol* 1984;63:759–763.
25. Cauley JA, Salamone LM, Lucas FL. Postmenopausal endogenous and exogenous hormones, degree of obesity, thiazide diuretics, and risk of osteoporosis. In: Marcus R, Feldman D, Kelsey J, eds. *Osteoporosis.* San Diego: Academic Press, 1996:551–576.
26. Collaborative Group on Hormonal Factors in Breast Cancer. Breast cancer and hormone replacement therapy: collaborative reanalysis of data from 51 epidemiological studies of 52,705 women with breast cancer and 108,411 women without breast cancer. *Lancet* 1997;350:1047–1059.
27. Cumming RG. Calcium intake and bone mass: a quantitative review of the evidence. *Calcif Tissue Int* 1990;47:194–201.
28. Chapuy MC, Arlot ME, Duboef F, et al. Vitamin D3 and calcium to prevent hip fractures in elderly women. *N Engl J Med* 1992;327:1637–1642.
29. Recker RR, Hinders S, Davies KM, Heaney RP, Stegman MR, Lappe JM, Kimmel DB. Correcting calcium nutritional deficiency prevents spine fractures in elderly women. *J Bone Miner Res* 1996;11:1961–1966.
30. Schrott HG, Bittner V, Vittinghoff E, et al. Adherence to National Cholesterol Education Program treatment goals in postmenopausal women with heart disease. The Heart and Estrogen/Progestin Replacement Study (HERS). The Hers Research Group. *JAMA* 1997;277:1281–1286.
31. Grady D, Hulley SB, Furberg C. Venous thromboembolic events associated with hormone replacement therapy [Letter]. *JAMA* 1997;278:477.
32. Buring JE, Hennekens CH. The Women's Health Study: summary of the study design. *J Myocard Ischemia* 1992;4:27–29.
33. Buring JE, Hennekens CH. Randomized trials of primary prevention of cardiovascular disease in women. An investigator's view. *Ann Epidemiol* 1994;4:111–114.
34. Steering Committee of the Physicians' Health Study Research Group. Final report on the aspirin component of the ongoing Physicians' Health Study. *N Engl J Med* 1989;321:129–135.
35. Greenwald P, Kelloff G, Burch-Whitman C, Kramer BS. Chemoprevention. *CA Cancer J Clin* 1995;45:31–49.
36. Rich-Edwards JW, Manson JE, Hennekens CH, Buring JE. The primary prevention of coronary heart disease in women. *N Engl J Med* 1995;332:1758–1766.
37. Hennekens CH, Buring JE, Peto R. Antioxidant vitamins—benefits not yet proved. *N Engl J Med* 1994;330:1080–1081.
38. Serdula MK, Byers T, Mokdad AH, Simoes E, Mendlein JM, Coates RJ. The association between fruit and vegetable intake and chronic disease risk factors. *Epidemiology* 1996;7:161–165.
39. The Alpha-Tocopheral, Beta Carotene Cancer Prevention Study Group. The effect of vitamin E and beta carotene on the incidence of lung cancer and other cancers in male smokers. *N Engl J Med* 1994;330:1029–1035.
40. Omenn GS, Goodman GE, Thornquist MD, et al. Effects of a combination of beta carotene and vitamin A on lung cancer and cardiovascular disease. *N Engl J Med* 1996;334:1150–1155.
41. Early Breast Cancer Trialists' Collaborative Group. Systemic treatment of early breast cancer by hormonal, cytotoxic, or immune therapy. *Lancet* 1992;339:1–15, 71–85.
42. Nayfield SG, Karp JE, Ford LG, Dorr FA, Kramer BS. Potential role of tamoxifen in prevention of breast cancer. *J Natl Cancer Inst* 1991;83:1450–1459.
43. Powles TJ. The case for clinical trials of tamoxifen for prevention of breast cancer. *Lancet* 1992;340:1145–1147.

44. National Surgical Adjuvant Breast and Bowel Project (NSABP). NSABP Protocol P-1: a clinical trial to determine the worth of tamoxifen for preventing breast cancer. Pittsburgh: National Surgical Adjuvant Breast and Bowel Project, January 24, 1992 (Chairman: Dr. Bernard Fisher, University of Pittsburgh).

45. National Cancer Institute, Office of Cancer Communications. Breast cancer prevention trial shows major benefit, some risk. Press Release, April 6, 1998.

46. Bush TL, Helzlsouer KJ. Tamoxifen for the primary prevention of breast cancer: a review and critique of the concept and trial. *Epidemiol Rev* 1993;15:233–243.

47. Kristensen B, Ejlertsen B, Mouridsen HT, Andersen KW, Lauritzen JB. Femoral fractures in postmenopausal breast cancer patients treated with adjuvant tamoxifen. *Breast Cancer Res Treat* 1996;39:321–326.

48. DeGregorio MW, Maenpaa JU, Wiebe VJ. Tamoxifen for the prevention of breast cancer: No. 12 *Important Adv Oncol* 1995:175–185.

49. Rutqvist LE, Cerdermark B, Glas U, et al. Contralateral primary tumors in breast cancer patients in a randomized trial of adjuvant tamoxifen therapy. *J Natl Cancer Inst* 1991;83:1299–1306.

50. Anonymous. NSABP halts B-14 trial: no benefit seen beyond 5 years of tamoxifen use. *J Natl Cancer Ins* 1995;87:1829.

51. Riggs BL, Hodgson S, O'Fallon WM, et al. Effect of fluoride treatment on the fracture rate in postmenopausal women with osteoporosis. *N Engl J Med* 1990; 322:802–809.

52. Kleerekoper M, Peterson EL, Nelson DA, Phillips E, Schork MA, Tilley BC, Parfitt AM. A randomized trial of sodium fluoride as a treatment for postmenopausal osteoporosis. *Osteoporos Int* 1991;1:155–161.

53. Food and Drug Administration. *Guidelines for preclinical and clinical evaluation of agents used in the prevention and treatment of postmenopausal osteoporosis.* April 1994.

54. Storm T, Thamsborg G, Steiniche T, Genant HK, Sorenson OH. Effect of cyclical etidronate therapy on bone mass and fracture rate in women with postmenopausal osteoporosis. *N Engl J Med* 1990;322:1265–1271.

55. Watts NB, Harris ST, Genant HK, et al. Intermittent cyclical etidronate treatment of postmenopausal osteoporosis. *N Engl J Med* 1990;323:73–79.

56. Black D, Cummings SR, Karpf DB, et al. For the Fracture Intervention Trial Research Group. Alendronate reduces the risk of fractures in women with existing vertebral fractures: results of the Fracture Intervention Trial. *Lancet* 1996;348: 1535–1541.

57. Hosking D, Chilvers CED, Christiansen C, et al. Prevention of bone loss with alendronate in postmenopausal women under 60 years of age. *N Engl J Med* 1998; 338:485–492.

58. Bryant HU, Dere WH. Selective estrogen receptor modulators: an alternative to hormone replacement therapy. *Proc Soc Exp Biol Med* 1998;217:45–52.

59. Delmas PD, Bjarnason NH, Mitlak BH, et al. Effects of raloxifene on bone mineral density, serum cholesterol concentrations, and uterine endometrium in postmenopausal women. *N Engl J Med* 1997;337:1641–1647.

SECTION XIII

Hormonal Regimens

In this final section, hormonal regimens will be stressed with a forward-looking view. Strategies for regimens of the future have been presented by Göran N. Samsioe, Lars-Åke Mattsson, and M. Dören. In the closing chapter of the book my task is to put into perspective the issue of treatment and specifically that of hormonal treatment of postmenopausal women. Clearly, there is the option of no treatment and nonhormonal therapies as well. Choice is the operative word in contemplating therapy. A woman needs to be provided with a variety of options depending on her particular situation and possible risk factor. There also needs to be flexibility in prescribing with the full realization that a change or adjustment will likely be needed in the future. Philosophies on treatment vary considerably among the "experts" in the field and there is certainly room for controversy and further discussion. More clinical studies are sorely needed in this new field of medicine, which is only now coming into its own. Therefore I can only provide one view, that of my own, in terms of what I view to be appropriate treatment for today.

Treatment of the Postmenopausal Woman: Basic and Clinical Aspects, Second Edition, edited by Rogerio A. Lobo, Lippincott Williams & Wilkins, Philadelphia © 1999.

CHAPTER 61

Regimens for Today and the Future

Göran N. Samsioe, Lars-Åke Mattson, and M. Dören

Although treatment of sweats and hot flushes, also called flashes, remains an undisputed major indication for hormone replacement therapy (HRT), other potential benefits and problems can also come into play. A major issue in the postmenopausal period is quality of life. Osteoporotic fractures, cardiovascular disease, and possibly Alzheimer's disease are other major health hazards that could be positively influenced by HRT. National as well as multinational population surveys confirm that urogenital problems, especially impaired control of micturition, concern about one-third of women aged more than 55 years (1).

Although estrogen's mechanism of action is still not fully understood, major breakthroughs have been occurring during the last decade in understanding their receptor-mediated effects. These have included discovery of a second estrogen receptor, an interaction between estrogen receptors and other steroid receptors, and the role of cytokines in modifying receptor responses. This research has led to an increased understanding to why some substances (e.g., tamoxifen) could act as estrogen antagonists in some tissues and estrogen agonists in others. With this knowledge, it was possible to target the original molecular structure to create novel compounds with higher selectivity. These groups of substances, commonly referred to as "selective estrogen receptor modulators," display estrogen antagonism on breast and endometrial tissues and estrogen agonism on bone mass and markers of the cardiovascular system.

The potential drawbacks of long-term estrogen replacement therapy, especially risk of breast cancer, have generated interest in developing alternatives to the traditional estrogen treatment. Such alternatives include the use of naturally occurring compounds with estrogenic properties often referred to as "phytoestrogens."

It has become increasingly clear that the compulsory addition of progestogens to protect the endometrium from malignant transformation by estrogen stimulation is not without problems. Women may accept monthly bleeds around the menopause and during the following years, but with advancing age bleed-free regimens are clearly preferred (2).

This can be achieved in many women by using continuous combined regimens, but some women may bleed from an atrophic endometrium. Monitoring, surveillance, and treatment of bleeds from an atrophic endometrium remain a challenge as the cause of these atrophic bleeds is not fully understood, although much knowledge has been gained during the past few years (3). Transvaginal ultrasound and endometrial biopsy are meaningful techniques used to investigate unscheduled bleeding in the woman on HRT (4). Whether endometrial ablation by hysteroscopy will alleviate or even abolish the problem of uterine bleeding remains to be proved in well-designed studies with appropriate long-term follow-up. Progestogen influence needs to be fairly high to induce endometrial atrophy. This means that other progestogenic side effects are not uncommon in women using continuous combined HRT regimens.

Hence, we need to have more selective progestogens that are primarily designed as estrogen co-medications, also for use by elderly postmenopausal woman. Unfortunately, almost all data on pharmocokinetics and pharmacodynamics on estrogens, progestogens, and various estrogen–progestogen combinations inclusive of the continuous combined regimens are obtained in women aged less than 65 years, whereas the major target group for HRT may well be women older than this age group. For these reasons, we have insufficient data to guide us in the selection of the progestogen type, dose, or mode of administration.

Given its great potential, estrogen administration is a focus of preventive medicine. Cost-benefit analyses seem

G. Samsioe: Department of Obstetrics and Gynecology, Lund University Hospital, SE-221 85 Lund, Sweden.

L. Å. Mattson: Department of Obstetrics and Gynecology, Sahlgrens University Hospital, Göteborg, Sweden.

M. Dören: Wesstfalische Wilhems-Universitat, Munster, Germany.

649

to suggest that estrogens are cost-effective in women with symptoms and possibly also in women without a uterus. In the hysterectomized woman, estrogens can be given without progestogen co-medication. This implies that the only proved positive effect of progestogen use is its reduction of endometrial hyperplasia and endometrial cancer.

DEVELOPMENT OF ESTROGEN COMPONENTS

The predominant human natural estrogen present during the fertile period is 17β-estradiol. Hence, several hormone replacement therapies focus on its use. As with natural progesterone, similar problems arise with natural estradiol. We need to know what molecular substituents are responsible for the positive effects on symptoms and prevention and what molecular substituents can contribute to weight gain and influence breast tissues (i.e., the proliferation of glandular cells). The estradiol molecule could be particularly "tailored" to diminish or even abolish interaction with breast tissues.

Another feature is to look at the various components of conjugated equine estrogens (CEE). Although the major components are estrone and estrone sulfate, CEE contain a variety of compounds which display different estrogenic activities. In particular, the so-called α estrogens contained in CEE are of interest as they possess qualities different from the β compounds. The further characterization of the various components of conjugated estrogens and their biologic effects should stimulate future research into estrogen pharmacology and pharmacodynamics. It is also of extreme importance to try to identify the type of molecular infrastructure responsible for the various cardiovascular effects, such as antioxidative properties, vasodilation, and bone sparing factors.

Apart from these considerations, various new estradiol delivery systems have been introduced to improve the convenience of treatment and the potential for long-term use. A vaginal silicone ring that releases approximately 7.5 µg/day estradiol constantly over a period of 3 months seems to be valuable in the treatment of urogenital symptoms in estrogen-deprived women. A vaginal tablet containing 25 µg estradiol to be applied twice weekly is another alternative to vaginal creams containing estriol or conjugated estrogens. The ring system, originally designed for local treatment without the necessity of adding a progestogen in nonhysterectomized women for endometrial safety, can also be supplemented with a slow-release progesterone system or any progestogen capable of passing the vaginal epithelium for systemic treatment. Other forms of local treatment include estradiol eye drops designed for the treatment of postmenopausal keratoconjunctivitis sicca, although systemic absorption seems to be possible with its use (5).

Advances in transdermal patch technology has resulted in various forms of so-called matrix skin patches where the estradiol is incorporated into a nonethanol adhesive matrix. Skin reactions are apparently diminished compared with the original reservoir patches where the steroid is dissolved in an alcohol-based gel enclosed in a permeable membrane. The rate of drug delivery is controlled by diffusion rather than by use of a rate-limiting membrane as is the case with the reservoir patch. However, skin absorption might differ between women: in particular, little is known about this in the elderly and very old. The 7-day patch is another modification of the transdermal route that apparently yields more steady serum levels of estradiol compared with the twice weekly patches, particularly after patch application. Whether this is an advantage will be demonstrated after various systems have been in clinical use over some time. The acceptability for patients might be improved as the time intervals for patch change lengthen. Transdermal systems for even longer periods could be useful. Transdermal delivery is also possible using skin gels.

Long-acting delivery systems (e.g., estradiol implants) have been used for many years in various European countries. However, supraphysiologic blood levels are commonly seen associated with the phenomenon of symptom recurrence and tachyphylaxis. Non-biodegradable silicone-based implants could improve this type of replacement, because they would avoid peak levels after insertion and maintain lower, more constant estradiol levels in the range of the early to mid-follicular phase.

Newer regimens such as "long-cycle" therapy address the major adherence problem—uterine bleeding. Although it is an intriguing idea to space out the sequential administration of a progestogen to induce endometrial shedding, it should be noted that the long-term endometrial safety of the few combinations tested remains to be demonstrated (6,7). Sequential estrogen and progestogen treatment with monthly induced withdrawal bleeding cannot be replaced by "long-cycle" treatment as yet.

DEVELOPMENT OF PROGESTOGENS AND PROGESTERONE

An important task in future research is to delineate which constituents of the progesterone molecule yield different metabolic profiles. In other words, what molecular structures influence the endometrium and what molecular configurations lead to other potential negative effects (e.g., premenstrual syndrome symptoms [PMS] and lowering of high-density lipoprotein [HDL] cholesterol). Progestogens have been developed mostly for contraceptive use, but they are also used to treat various bleeding disorders in fertile life. More recently, progestogens for use in postmenopausal women have become an important factor also for the development of newer agents. The development of newer progestogens with fewer side effects and a more selective influence on the endometrium are obvious goals in this respect. One example of this is trimegestone. Trimegestone is well absorbed also by the percutaneous route. Clinical data, so far, apply only to the oral route using different doses of trimegestone (8). *In vitro* data further suggest that trimegestone potentiates the effects of 17β-estradiol on the proliferation and differentiation of human osteoblasts. Other examples include the antiandrogenic cyproterone acetate (CPA), a derivative of progesterone, and dienogest, a nortestosterone derivative. Dienogest has antiandrogenic properties on the sebaceous glands, although less pronounced than CPA. Norgestimate, which is partly metabolized to levonorgestrel, also has fewer androgenic side effects compared with levonorgestrel. CPA, dienogest, and norgestimate are already available in oral contraceptive formulations. Dydrogesterone, a compound closely related to natural progesterone, is another new alternative approved for the treatment of postmenopausal women in a sequential preparation with estradiol. It remains to be established in clinical practice whether these newer progestogens will provide both more individualized treatment choices for postmenopausal women and improve the overall tolerability of the frequency of PMS-like symptoms.

Estrogen patch administration has been favorably received; however, progestogens may have less of an impact via the transdermal route as some of them have very little or no first pass hepatic metabolism as exemplified by levonorgestrel. Other progestogens including progesterone may show a first pass metabolism. Natural progesterone displays a low oral bioavailability. Using newer microcrystallization techniques, it has been possible to achieve acceptable bioavailability by the oral route. However, this needs to be substantially improved as only a small fraction of orally administered progesterone is bioavailable. This means that progesterone has to be given in doses of 200 mg/day to ensure endometrial protection (9). Work is underway to modify the molecule so that it can penetrate into the body either via the skin or the oral route and then rapidly be degraded to natural progesterone.

A vaginal progesterone gel to be administered twice weekly for a period of 1 month at a dose of 45 mg has been shown to induce a secretory endometrium in the presence of mean serum progesterone levels as low as some 2 mg/mL, which is suggestive of a so-called first uterine pass effect in women with premature ovarian failure and ovarian dysgenesis (10). Endometrial safety remains to be demonstrated in clinical trials of postmenopausal women subjected to several months treatment. Other developments to improve acceptance by women without compromising endometrial safety are administration or use of various progestogens in either implant form or as an intrauterine device (IUD). One approved IUD releases levonorgestrel 20 μg daily for 5 years.

Intrauterine devices releasing levonorgestrel in combinations with estradiol administered orally or transder-

mally have been tested in perimenopausal women (11,12). Because the concentration of levonorgestrel in the uterine mucosa is several times greater than in serum, it might be ideal for endometrial protection. However, this type of device, which releases 20 μg/24 hours of levonorgestrel, was originally introduced for contraceptive purpose.

Recently, IUDs with lower concentrations of progestogens have been tested. Two different IUDs with a release rate of 5 and 10 μg/24 hours were reported to induce acceptable bleeding patterns, and they showed beneficial effects on lipid and lipoprotein metabolism when combined with oral estradiol valerate (2 mg) (12). A disadvantage with this type of device was that the progestogen reservoir covered by the rate-limiting membrane could be too thick for insertion into the uterus of a postmenopausal woman. A device with a thinner vertical arm should be developed for the use to be extended to postmenopausal women. A release rate of 5 to 10 μg/24 hours is sufficient for endometrial protection.

Another feature is to introduce newer regimens to reduce the progestogen dosage. An example of this is the so-called "on-and-off" therapy in which estrogens are given continuously but progestogens are given 3 days on and 3 days off. In such clinical trials bleeding patterns were acceptable.

Another area of controversy involves which type of progestogen would be more preferable—one that has similar pharmacokinetics to the administered estrogens (e.g., medroxyprogesterone acetate [MPA], norethisterone, or dydrogesterone) or a more long-acting progestogen such as desogestrel, levonorgestrel, or norgestimate).

THE ARTIFICIAL OVARY

Given major advancements in computer technology, it is intriguing to suggest the development of an artificial ovary. The idea is fairly simple; estrogen and progestogen implants already exist. The new feature would be to control the release rate from the outside using a remote control by which the woman could adjust the estrogen and progestogen dose to exactly match her needs at a given period of time. One possibility to mimic an artificial ovary is to use so-called "matrix patches." Such patches release a constant amount of estradiol or estradiol plus progestogen, commonly norethisterone or levonorgestrel. By using an estrogen patch and a combined patch and a pair of scissors a woman could find the dose that could fit her specific needs. The same concept holds true for hormone administration via various creams and gels applied to the skin; pessaries used intravaginally; and estradiol nasal spray, the latter under investigation in clinical trials. Potential future developments include oral slow release systems aimed at pulsatile release of sex steroids, which is another new intriguing way to apply physiologic hormone doses (Table 61.1)

TABLE 61.1. *Potential future developments*

Modified molecules of natural estrogens and progesterone
  Specific organ targeting
Selective estrogen receptor modulators
  Nonoral routes of administration
Selective progesterone receptor blocker
Improved systemic delivery of steroids via
  Slow-release-pulsatile-oral systems
  Transdermal systems including progesterone
  Vaginal administration
  Intrauterine devices designed for postmenopausal
    women
  With ultra-slow release
  Slow-release subcutaneous depot systems
New progestogens without non-beneficial psychotropic side
  effects
New concepts
  Long-acting systems with remote control
  Long-cycle therapies
  Interrupted administration of steroids
Nonhormonal alternatives to improve postmenopausal
  quality of life

DEVELOPMENT OF SELECTIVE ESTROGEN RECEPTOR MODULATORS

The modification of the so-called antiestrogens has led to the development of an array of substances known as "selective estrogen receptor modulators" (SERM). A recent review (13) highlighted their possibilities. Most of the published data refer to the use of raloxifene, a compound derived from the family of nonsteroidal benzothiophene, but modifications of this molecule inclusive of other so-called SERMs may well show improvements over the recently approved first SERM, raloxifene, to be used for the prevention of postmenopausal osteoporosis (14). Apart from decreasing bone turnover, raloxifene also shows beneficial effects on cardiovascular risk markers such as LDL cholesterol. Contrary to tamoxifen, raloxifene and other SERMs under clinical investigation do not display detrimental effects on the endometrium. In addition, preliminary data indicate that the incidence of breast cancer may be lower in raloxifene-treated women compared with controls. However, studies specifically designed to address the issue of breast cancer are needed until firm conclusions can be drawn.

PHYTOESTROGENS

A new way of addressing menopausal problems is based on the observations made in relation to the use of various diets and plant extracts. Not only the perception of menopausal symptomatology, but the pattern of many diseases including estrogen-dependent tumors are different between Eastern and Western societies. Indirect, epidemiologic evidence suggests that Asian phytoestrogen-rich diets, (in particular, those rich in soy products) may be associated with a decreased risk of endometrial cancer (15), premenopausal and postmenopausal breast cancer (16), and arterial diseases linked to cholesterol metabolism (17). A growing general interest is seen, not only from the medical community, in investigating the feasibility of using phytoestrogen-rich foods and plant extracts as adjuncts or even an alternative strategy to alleviate climacteric symptoms in postmenopausal women apart from estrogen replacement as a medication prescribed by doctors.

Some 100 plants, some of which are edible, with a variety of 30 specific compounds, are known to exhibit estrogenic activity in both humans and animals.

Phytoestrogens consist of a number of classes: isoflavones, lignans, coumestans, and fungal estrogens. Various legumes contain the isoflavones daidzein, genistein, formononetin, biochanin A, and the coumestan coumestrol.

Lignans are mainly found in cereals, vegetables, and oilseeds. The average Asian diet contains some 25 to 45 mg/day isoflavones compared with less than 5 mg in European diets. A variable bacterial metabolism in an important additional source of indirect supplementation with phytoestrogens. The isoflavones daidzein and genistein are known to exist either as aglycones, which are directly absorbable from dietary sources, or as one of three glucoside conjugates to be metabolized by intestinal bacteria into aglycones. The main lignan metabolites, enterolactone and enterodiol, are produced by colonic bacteria.

An *in vitro* model using the estrogen-specific enhancement of alkaline phosphatase activity in human endometrial adenocarcinoma cells suggests that phytoestrogens exert minimal estrogenic effects, at least in this system.

The clinical use of phytoestrogens has been shown to prevent postmenopausal bone loss. A *de novo* phytoestrogenic compound, 7-iso-propoxy-isoflavone or ipriflavone, is known to maintain bone density in early and late postmenopausal women with normal bone mass, osteopenia, and established osteoporosis (18), and it is registered in 20 countries for the prevention of postmenopausal osteoporosis. Other extracts of nonedible plants such as black kohosh are registered for oral treatment of climacteric, in particular vasomotor, symptoms in many European countries.

Evidence for the efficacy of phytoestrogen-rich diets and of various medications derived from natural source, some of which are combined with homeopathic substances, is far from being conclusive as appropriate long-term studies with meaningful sample sizes of postmenopausal women are missing. In particular, claimed benefits with regard to psychological symptoms have not been demonstrated (Table 61.2). (19–24).

Plant extracts from black kohosh, *Cimicifuga racemosa,* are not able to increase the uterine weight of immature mice or to cause proliferation of superficial cells in the vaginal epithelium in rats. Both effects are to be expected for substances with estrogenlike activity (25).

TABLE 61.2. *Clinical trials to assess the impact of phytoestrogens on climacteric symptoms and clinical endpoints*

Intervention	Patients	Outcome	Author
Dietary modifications			
Phytoestrogen-rich diet for 6 weeks	Postmenopausal women/Australia	Increased amount of vaginal superficial cells (soy and linseed episodes)	Wilcox et al 1990
2 weeks each with soy/red clover/linseed; open study, no controls	$n = 25$		
Isoflavone-rich diet (soy) for 4 weeks	Postmenopausal women/ North Carolina	Vaginal cytology + FSH/LH/SHBG; no change	Baird et al 1995
Control group: continuation of existing diet; randomized	$n = 66$ $n = 25$ (controls)		
Phytoestrogen-rich diet for 12 weeks	Postmenopausal women/ Australia	Reduction of hot flushes:	Murkies et al 1995
45 g soy flour/day Control group: wheat flour; double-blind, randomized	$n = 28$ $n = 30$ (controls)	−40% soy flour group −25% wheat flour group nonsignificant within-group differences	
Phytoestrogen-rich diet for 12 weeks— soy products	pre- and postmenopausal women/Israel	Reduction of hot flushes + vaginal dryness in the soy group	Brzezinski et al 1997
Controls: continuation of present, omnivorous diet; randomized	$n = 95$ $n = 50$ (controls)		
Phytoestrogen-rich diet for 12 weeks	Postmenopausal or ovariectomized women/Italy	Reduction of hot flushes:	Albertazzi et al 1998
60 g isolated soy protein/day Control group: casein; double-blind, randomized	$n = 51$ $n = 52$ (controls)	−45% soy group −33% controls $p < 0.01$	
Nonedible plant extract			
8 mg Cimicifuga racemosa/day or 0.625 mg CEE/day or placebo for 12 weeks double-blind, randomized	Pre- and postmenopausal women/Germany	Reduction of climacteric symptoms (Kupperman-index) within all groups; most pronounced in the Cimicifuga group (significant difference to placebo + estrogens)	Stoll 1987
	$n = 30/n = 10$ $n = 20$ (controls)		

CEE, conjugated equine estrogens; FSH, follicle-stimulating hormone; LH, luteinizing hormone; SHBG, sex hormone-binding globulin.

Whether phytoestrogens might play an active role in preventing arterial diseases and breast cancer, as already advocated, remains to be demonstrated in carefully designed studies.

Alternative methods for the relief of vasomotor symptoms are widely used among middle-aged women. In a questionnaire study, 45% of Swedish women reported current or past use of herbal compounds for the treatment of climacteric symptoms. A few randomized, placebo-controlled studies have been conducted to evaluate the efficacy of such compounds. Recently, a study compared ginseng extract with placebo on impact on quality of life in postmenopausal women. A total of 382 women were randomly allocated to receive either a ginseng extract or placebo. The ginseng extract had no effect on vasomotor symptoms but was superior to placebo by enhancing well-being and relieving somatic symptoms. No estrogenic effect exerted by the ginseng extract could be found as measured by maturity index, plasma follicle-stimulating hormone (FSH), and estradiol levels (26).

TIBOLONE

Tibolone is an interesting steroid that possesses weak estrogenic, progestogenic, and androgenic properties in one molecule. It is used in tablets of 2.5 mg and ingested daily on a continuous basis. Vaginal bleeds occur only rarely. It has similar effects to estrogens on vasomotor symptoms, and as it possesses some androgenic properties, it has psychotrophic effects, which are somewhat different from pure estrogens (27). Effects on bone seem to be similar to those of estrogens. Cardiovascular effects are largely unknown. Long-term lipid metabolic effects are small but include a transient decrease in HDL cholesterol (28).

ANDROGENS

In general, a paucity of well-controlled studies of androgens is striking despite the fact that testosterone has been in clinical use as an implant for many years in various countries. In particular, the advocated positive impact of androgens on psychological symptoms with special emphasis on sex drive (29) has not been as extensively studied as estrogen and progestogen replacement (30). Clearly, a need is seen for more knowledge about the applicability of androgen replacement as the ovary itself produces testosterone throughout life, which marks a distinctive difference to ovarian estradiol synthesis and might be of particular significance for the oophorectomized woman deprived of endogenous ovarian function.

Beyond the issue of testosterone, interest has been paid recently to the replacement of dehydroepiandrosterone (DHEA) (31), which is the adrenal precursor for testosterone. Whether the potential replacement of this steroid might have any additional advantage so far as well-being and various metabolic systems are concerned that is distinctly different from estrogen replacement throughout a specific period of postmenopausal life is currently unknown. The "adrenopause" can be defined as an age-related slow decline of adrenal function. The relationship between menopause and adrenopause needs more attention as the implications for the quality of life of an ever-growing elderly female population are formidable.

CONCLUSIONS

In conclusion, great health potentials exist by replacing the age-dependent loss of gonadal hormones in women. It is a challenge for clinical medicine to define those women who have the most to gain from such replacement to make it truly cost-effective.

REFERENCES

1. Barlow DH, Samsioe G, van Geelen JM. A study of European women's experience of the problems of urogenital ageing and its management. *Maturitas* 1997;27:239–248.
2. Stadberg E, Mattsson LÅ, Milsom I. Women's attitudes and knowledge about the climacteric period and its treatment. A Swedish population-based study. *Maturitas* 1997;27:109–116.
3. Smith S. Endometrial changes during the primenopausal years. In: Berg G, Hammar M, eds. *The modern management of the menopause*. London: Parthenon Publishing, 1994:201–206.
4. Parsons AK, Londono JL. Detection and surveillance of endometrial hyperplasia and carcinoma. In: Lobo RA, ed. *Treatment of the postmenopausal woman*. Philadelphia: Lippincott Williams & Wilkins, 1999:513–538.
5. Sator MO, Joura BA, Golaszewski T, et al. Treatment of menopausal keratoconjunctivitis sicca with topical estradiol. *Br J Obstet Gynaecol* 1998;105:100–102.
6. Ettinger B, Selby J, Citron JT, et al. Cyclic hormone replacement therapy using quarterly progestin. *Obstet Gynecol* 1994;83:693–700.
7. Cerin A, Heldaas K, Moeller B, for the Scandinavian Long Cycle Study Group. Adverse endometrial effects of long-cycle estrogen and progestogen replacement therapy. *N Engl J Med* 1996;334:668–669.
8. Ross D, Godfree V, Cooper A, et al. Endometrial effects of three doses of trimegestone, a new orally active progestogen, on the postmenopausal endometrium. *Maturitas* 1997;28:83–88.
9. The Writing Group for PEPI trial. Effects of estrogen or estrogen/progestin regimens on heart disease risk factors in postmenopausal women. The postmenopausal estrogen/progestin interventions (PEPI) trial. *JAMA* 1995;273:199–208.
10. Fanchin R, de Ziegler D, Bergeron C, et al. Transvaginal administration of progesterone. *Obstet Gynecol* 1997;90:396–401.
11. Suhonen SP, Allonen HO, Lähteenmäki P. Sustained-release estradiol implants and a levonorgestrel-releasing intrauterine device in hormone replacement therapy. *Am J Obstet Gynecol* 1995;172:562–567.
12. Wollter-Svensson L-O, Stadberg E, Andersson, K, et al. Intrauterine administration of levonorgestrel 5 and 10 μg/24h in perimenopausal hormone replacement therapy. A randomized clinical trial during one year. *Acta Obstet Gynecol Scand* 1997;76:449–454.
13. Tissue-specific estrogens—the promise for the future [Editorial]. *N Engl J Med* 1997;337:1686–1687.
14. Delmas P, Bjarnason N, Bruce H, et al. Effects of raloxifene on bone mineral density, serum cholesterol concentrations, and uterine endometrium in postmenopausal women. *N Engl J Med* 1997;337:1641–1647.
15. Goodman MT, Wilkens LR, Hankin JH, et al. Association of soy and fiber consumption with the risk of endometrial cancer. *Am J Epidemiol* 1997;146:294–306.
16. Ingram D, Sanders K, Kolybaba M, Lopez D. Case-control study of phyto-estrogens and breast cancer. *Lancet* 1997;350:990–994.
17. Anderson JW, Johnstone BM, Cook-Newell ME. Meta-analysis of the effects of soy protein intake on serum lipids. *N Engl J Med* 1995;333:276–282.
18. Gennari C, Adami S, Agnusdei D, et al. Effect of chronic treatment with ipriflavone in postmenopausal women with low bone mass. *Calcif Tissue Int* 1997;61:S19–S22.
19. Albertazzi P, Pansini F, Bonaccorsi G, et al. The effect of dietary soy supplementation on hot flushes. *Obstet Gynecol* 1998;91:6–11.
20. Baird DD, Umbach DM, Landsell L, et al. Dietary intervention study to assess estrogenicity of dietary soy among postmenopausal women. *J Clin Endocrinol Metab* 1995;80:1685–1690.
21. Brzezinski A, Adlercreutz H, Shaoul R, et al. Short-term effects of phytoestrogen-rich diet on postmenopausal women. *Menopause* 1997;4:89–94.
22. Murkies AL, Lombard C, Strauss BJG, et al. Dietary flour supplementation decreases post-menopausal hot flushes: effect of soy and wheat. *Maturitas* 1995;21:189–195.
23. Stoll W. Phytotherapeutikum beeinflusst atrophisches Vaginalepitel. Doppelblindversuch Cimicifuga vs Östrogenpräparat. (Translation from German: The impact of a phytotherapeutical drug on the vaginal epithelium. A double blind study to compare *Cimicifuga* and estrogen. *Therapeutikon* 1987;1:1–15.
24. Wilcox G, Wahlquist ML, Burger HG, Medley G. Oestrogenic effects of plant foods in postmenopausal women. *BMJ* 1990;301:905–906.
25. Einer-Jensen N, Zhao J, Andersen KP, Kristoffersen K. *Cimicifuga* and Melbrosia lack oestrogenic effects in mice and rats. *Maturitas* 1996;25:149–153.
26. Lindgren R, Mattsson L-Å, Meier W, Wiklund I. Has Ginsana G115 estrogenic effects when measured by maturity index, plasma FSH and estradiol. *Menopause* 1997;4:248.
27. Tax L, Goorissen EM, Kicovec PM. Clinical profile of Org OD 14. *Maturitas* 1987;1(Suppl):3–13.
28. Hänggi W, Lippuner K, Riesen W, et al. Long term influence of different postmenopausal hormone replacement regimens on serum lipids and lipoprotein(a): a randomised study. *Br J Obstet Gynaecol* 1997;104:707–717.
29. Sherwin B, Gelfand M. The role of androgen in the maintenance of sexual functioning in oophorectomized women. *Psychosom Med* 1987;49:397–409.
30. Nathorst-Böös J, Hammar M. Effects on sexual life—a comparison between tibolone and a continuous estradiol-norethisterone regimen. *Maturitas* 1997;26:15–20.
31. Casson P, Hornsby P, Ghusn H, Buster J. Dehydroepiandrosterone (DHEA) replacement in postmenopausal women: present status and future promise. *Menopause* 1997;4:225–231.

Treatment of the Postmenopausal Woman: Basic and Clinical Aspects, Second Edition, edited by Rogerio A. Lobo, Lippincott Williams & Wilkins, Philadelphia © 1999.

CHAPTER 62

Treatment of the Postmenopausal Woman: Where We Are Today

Rogerio A. Lobo

More than 5 years ago, the first edition of this book ended with my assessment of where we are in treating postmenopausal women. Now that an update is due, it is my perspective that the focus of this chapter should shift from a "how-to" format to one that outlines general principles in line with developments in the field. Although many of the treatment concepts and general principles are the same, more choices are now available, including many more alternatives. Also, the last few years have seen a much greater realization of the importance of women's health; this national and international focus has also been spirited by new developments and research in the field.

It is the approach to treatment that is important. This includes assessment of symptoms, if present, the needs of the woman, and her specific risk factors and family history. It is only in this context that the various choices and options can be considered. The ultimate question at the end of the decision tree should be: Will any of the available options improve the overall quality of life for the woman?

PROVIDING THE BEST CARE

Many cities around the world have centers or clinics for women's health. These vary from being comprehensive multidisciplinary centers that emphasize primary care for women to more specialized centers. These, in turn, may emphasize hormonal problems or may be devoted to cancer or cardiovascular screening. Some incorporate research and clinical trials, whereas others do not. A discussion of the organization of these centers is found in Chapter 58.

With the penetration of managed care in the United States it is increasingly difficult for a provider to spend sufficient time to assess the individual needs of each woman. Often paramedical personnel have been asked to carry out this task, which includes use of printed material and videotapes. Although many of these tools are useful and have been used to assess risks and benefits, prescribing patterns have tended to be fixed and inflexible. Unfortunately, this shotgun approach often has been inadequate in that the specific needs and characteristics of the patient have not been taken into account.

THE WOMAN'S PERCEPTION

So much of what women know about healthcare is derived from the media. In general, the more sensational the item is, the more noteworthy. Although breast cancer risk is a real and serious concern for all women, this fear drives all of decision-making, particularly regarding hormonal options. The decision analysis with hormonal therapies largely contrasts the risks and mortality of cardiovascular disease (CVD) with that of breast cancer.

TABLE 62.1. *Women's top health risks and causes of death**

Perception	%	Reality	%
Breast cancer	46	Heart disease	34
Unspecified cancer	16	Other cancers	12
Heart disease	4	Lung cancer	5
Acquired immune deficiency syndrome (AIDS)	4	Stroke	8
		Breast cancer	4
Uterine or ovarian cancer	3		

*Gallup poll for Walnut Marketing Board, National Center for Health Statistics 1995.

R. A. Lobo: Department of Obstetrics and Gynecology, Columbia University College of Physicians & Surgeons, New York, New York 10032.

TABLE 62.2. *Women who will develop breast cancer: Risk through years*

Decade of life	Incidence
Third	1 of 250
Fourth	1 of 77
Fifth	1 of 42
Sixth	1 of 36
Seventh	1 of 34
Eighth	1 of 45

Of the risk factors for breast cancer age is the most significant, with the risk being greatest for women in their seventies.
Source: Cancer Care Ontario

American women believe that the leading cause of death in women is from breast cancer (Table 62.1). They also perceive that only a small percentage of death is attributable to CVD. In reality, these perceptions are reversed. A statistic provides that one in three women after age 65 have some evidence of CVD. What is the comparable figure for breast cancer? Although it has been widely asserted that the incidence of breast cancer in women is approximately one in eight women, this is the lifetime risk. Age-specific data are quite different: 1 of 77 in the fourth decade and 1 of 42 in the fifth decade, rising to 1 of 45 when a woman is in her eighth decade (Table 62.2). In terms of mortality, because the case fatality rate of CVD is several times greater than that of breast cancer, even if the incidence of these two diseases were similar, many more women would die of CVD. Figure 62.1 shows the death rate according to different ages. Soon after menopause, at age 50 to 54 years, the death rate from breast cancer decreases and rises steadily for CVD. As noted in Fig. 62.1, the leading cause of cancer death in women is lung cancer. Overall 30% to 40% of women die of CVD and by age 55, 20% of all deaths are caused by CVD.

PREVENTATIVE STRATEGIES

How can we prevent the increased mortality rates? For lung cancer, it is clear that smoking cessation should be the message of all health providers. For breast cancer, risks include family history and reproductive variables such as the history of infertility, menarche, age of menopause, and age of first pregnancy. Preventative measures necessitate frequent self and provider examinations, and mammography annually for women after age 40. For CVD, assessment of family history and modifiable risk factors such as blood pressure, cholesterol level, exercise, diabetes, diet, smoking, and so forth are important. We also need to assess women in totality and not ignore surveillance for other cancers such as colon, ovary, and uterus. These cancers have been addressed in earlier chapters.

It is also important not to forget about bone mass. Particularly in the woman who is undecided about treatment options, obtaining bone mass screening has proved to be useful for decision-making and follow-up, particularly when we now have nonhormonal as well as many hormonal treatment options. At present, bone mass measurements are clearly superior to urinary biochemical assays for screening.

THE DECISION TO TREAT OR NOT TO TREAT

The first question to address is what is the reason to treat. Are there symptoms like hot flushes or is there a sig-

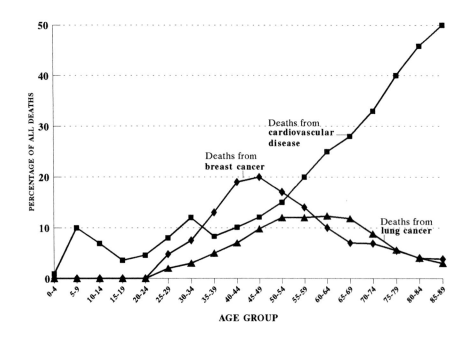

FIG. 62.1. Risks of breast cancer and lung cancer versus cardiovascular disease in various age categories. (Adapted from Phillips KA, Glendon G, Knight JA. Putting the risk of breast cancer in perspective. *New Engl J Med* 1999;340:141–144; with permission.)

nificant concern for osteoporosis? Good evidence indicates that short-term therapy with estrogen, particularly with lower doses, is not associated with significant risks. Therefore, in a woman suffering with hot flushes, no need is seen to commit for long-term therapy, and a short-term approach may be embarked upon. However, a more difficult question always arises in the woman who may be older and has no major complaints. Her family history, risk profile, and perhaps bone mass assessment are valuable adjuncts to help in decision-making. Depending on these variables, the choice may be for natural supplements, nonhormonal treatments such as a bisphosphonate, a selective estrogen receptor modulator, or estrogen. The wide array of options now available is extremely valuable in helping a woman feel comfortable with her decision.

Overall, in my view sufficient data exist to suggest that all cause mortality is reduced in women who receive estrogen, principally because of a reduction in CVD (1–3). This large effect also counterbalances any potential increase in breast cancer mortality, even if this risk is as high as a relative risk (RR) of 1.6 or greater (Fig. 62.2). Yet, the woman who has seen her mother suffer from breast cancer will probably choose not to use estrogen. The existing data we have would suggest that in women with a family history of breast cancer, the risk is not increased further with estrogen, and all cause mortality is decreased in these women to a similar degree as reported in the several observational cohorts (4).

The decision to use estrogen need not be a long-term commitment. Estrogen can be used for short-term treatment of symptoms, and with the lowest dose, which can control hot flushes; or by the vaginal route for symptoms of dryness or dyspareunia. Ultimately we will have more data from prospective trials to allow even more data-driven decision-making. I refer here to the anticipated results of the Women's Health Initiative, which will be

available in the next 5–10 years. Although it is my speculation that these results will not alter current recommendation, findings will provide new and important data for us to reflect on to help our patients.

WHAT ARE THE TREATMENT OPTIONS?

Natural supplements are extremely popular. However, few have been proven to provide benefit for symptoms. Among those that have received the scrutiny of controlled trials, only black kohosh, genistein, and soy-based products have been shown to be effective for hot flushes. Dose is important and large doses are needed to achieve benefit on a statistical basis. Although some data are available for soy-based products, no convincing data exist about efficacy for vaginal health, bone mass, or improvements in CVD or brain function. Because it is known that plant-based estrogens (e.g., genistein) bind to estrogen receptors (ERβ > ER), on a theoretical basis, large doses may pose some risk for estrogen responsive cancers such as breast cancer, although conventional thinking is that these products are protective for the breast.

Adequate calcium and vitamin D are important adjuncts. Antioxidants, particularly vitamin E and C have been shown to be beneficial. Use of steroids such as dehydroepiandrosterone (DHEA) (in lower doses) can be useful in some women and this has been reviewed earlier.

In the women with osteoporosis, who cannot or chooses not to use estrogen, bisphosphonates are available. Doses of alendronate for prevention (5 mg) or treatment (10 mg) have been shown to be beneficial. However, gastrointestinal side effects are common; newer generation products promise to be better tolerated. Here also are new data that suggest a synergism between the action of bisphosphonates and estrogen (5).

Selective estrogen receptor modulators (SERMs) are a newer class of compounds, which add to our armamentarium. With raloxifene use, we now know that bone mass improves and vertebral fracture risk is reduced with 60 mg daily. However, apart from a reduction in total and low-density lipoprotein (LDL)-cholesterol, the data for any true benefit for CVD remains unclear and is still under investigation. A benefit of no endometrial proliferation is attractive for women with a uterus. However, it is not beneficial for hot flushes (and may induce these symptoms), nor is it beneficial for vaginal atrophy. We also do not know if there are any beneficial or detrimental effects on the brain; we believe there are cognitive benefits associated with estrogen use. A small increase in venous thrombosis occurs with raloxifene use. Nevertheless, in that women have different needs, raloxifene remains an option for some women, particularly those who are at high risk for, or who have had breast cancer in the past, and are not bothered by hot flushes.

In terms of estrogen treatment, many products and routes of administration are available, and these have

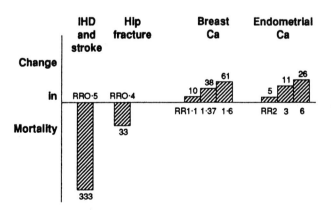

FIG. 62.2. Annual change in mortality per 100,000 estrogen users at ages 65 to 74 years. Mortality changes are based on the case fatality rate and the relative risk (RR) for ischemic heart disease (IHD) and stroke, hip fractures, brease cancer (Ca), and endometrial Ca. (Adapted from Henderson et al. *Fertil Steril* 1988;49(Suppl 5):9S–15S; and Ross et al. *Lancet* 1989;1–505; with permission.)

been reviewed in many of the preceding chapters. All things considered, efficacy of estrogen has been demonstrated for symptoms, CV benefit, osteoporosis, reduction in Alzheimer's risk, and improved cognition and quality of life. As noted, all cause mortality is reduced by 40% among estrogen users. The strong association of breast cancer risk with estrogen has not been proved, and if it occurs it is likely to be in the range of a 20% to 30% increased risk (RR:1.2–1.3) and to occur with long-term use. It is also likely to be related to dose. Therefore, one strategy may be to provide the minimal effective dose for a given indication. It is known that for some women a lower dose of estrogen is protective for osteoporosis (particularly with 1,500 mg of calcium) and some women may also have protection for CVD (6). It is important for these reasons not to be dogmatic about requiring full doses such as the equivalent of 0.625 mg of conjugated equine estrogens (CEE) in all women. Some women have symptoms such as breast tenderness, which are only decreased by using a lower dose. At the same time some women require larger doses for symptomatic relief and it is known that doses larger than the equivalent of 0.625 mg of CEE are needed by some women to maintain bone mass. The strategy for these adjustments is beyond the scope of this chapter. My personal philosophy of estrogen use is to attempt to use lower doses eventually when contemplating prolonged treatment. Particularly in older women, dose requirements are likely not to be as high. This is also important for control of uterine bleeding and to avoid any potential side effects. With lower dose therapy, adjuncts (calcium, antioxidants, and so forth) become more important.

In the last few years, it has become clear that a small risk of venous thrombosis exists with standard doses of oral estrogen (about 20 to 25 cases/100,000 women). This is approximately double the normal or baseline rate, but is still one third of the rate of normal pregnancy (60/100,000). Lower doses and nonoral preparations may reduce this risk further. Hypertension, on the other hand, is not a major risk factor; it occurs as an idiosyncratic reaction with oral estrogen. Alterations in type of estrogen, dose, and route of administration are also useful strategies for this unusual occurrence.

As mentioned, the new area of excitement, therapeutically, is the influence of estrogen on brain function. Reductions in Alzheimer's disease risk has been discussed. Improvements in mood, quality of life, cognition, and memory are important attributes for long-term therapy. These parameters have not been factored in as yet in decision analysis models. Clearly, these reasons are likely to substantially influence the decision to use estrogen for some women. What we do not know as yet are many of the specifics such as dose requirements for these effects. This is such an important issue for some women that even some with contraindications to estro-

gen (e.g., breast cancer) are willing to use estrogen with complete informal consent. This complicated issue, because it is so individually determined, and because of the paucity of good data has not been reviewed.

As an adjunct to adequate estrogen therapy, some women appear to need some androgen. Women who have been oophorectomized and some normal postmenopausal women are androgen deficient. Indeed, all women taking oral estrogen will be testosterone deficient in that sex hormone-binding globulin (SHBG) is raised (almost twofold) and, as a result, free or unbound testosterone plummets. With this knowledge, the addition of androgen in low dose is reasonable. The only preparation available in the United States employs low doses of methyl testosterone, although a low dose patch is in development and in some centers the testosterone pellet and transdermal gels are also used. Nevertheless, efficacy for the improvement in psychosexual function with many of these preparations, as yet, has not been established. Another option is lower doses of DHEA (e.g., 25 mg), as has been mentioned earlier.

THE PROGESTOGEN QUESTION

One of the final frontiers in this field is how to adequately protect the uterus with a progestin, yet avoid potentially harmful effects. For some women, progestin treatment interferes substantially with the enthusiasm for estrogen use. It induces bleeding, premenstrual syndrome (PMS)-like symptoms and is known to attenuate some of the CV benefits of estrogen. The attenuating effects are primarily reductions in high-density lipoprotein (HDL)-cholesterol (cholesterol and LDL-cholesterol are not affected), blood flow, and vasomotion; carbohydrate metabolism can also be affected, as is an interference with the improvement in stress reactivity with estrogen. Although unproven, it is plausible that the lack of secondary CV protection in the Heart and Estrogen–Progestin Study (HERS) (7) was because of the initial use of a fixed combination of estrogen and progestin in older women with compromised CV function. It has been my personal preference not to use a fixed combination or higher doses of progestins in women with CVD.

To avoid some of these concerns, newer progestin preparations have been studied. It was suggested in the Postmenopausal Estrogen–Progestin (PEPI) Trial (8), which only used surrogate endpoints of CV function, that oral micronized progesterone (200 mg) was advantageous. Also vaginal therapies allow an enhancement of uterine delivery while minimizing systemic effects. Specifically, targeting the uterus with a progesterone interuterine device (IUD) has been studied, and newer progestin IUDs for postmenopausal women will be introduced in the next few years. Many of these thoughts were discussed at the first international progestogen consensus

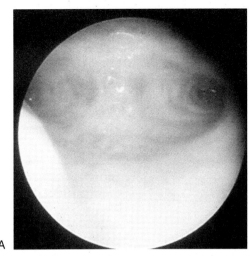

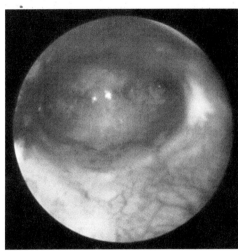

FIG. 62.3. A: Atrophic endometrium in a postmenopausal woman not on hormone therapy. **B:** Dilated vessels in endometrium of a woman on continuous combined hormone replacement therapy. (Adapted from Bruno de Lignières et al. *Contemporary OB/GYN* 1998;43:10–17; with permission.)

meeting in 1989 and were updated at the second symposium, which was held recently (9).

To minimize bleeding, fixed continuous combinations have been used and a newer intermittent progestin regimen (cyclophasic) is being introduced. Although all these regimens are beneficial for many women, some do not respond and tend to bleed unpredictably. It is now known that some women are particularly sensitive to continuous progestin therapy. Although the endometrium is atrophic, a vascularity pattern develops, probably induced by vascular endothelial growth factor (VEGF) (Fig. 62.3). This leads to continuous bleeding and is only ameliorated by a change in the regimen.

CONCLUSION

As stated, the aim of treatment is efficacy for specific symptoms and risk profiles. It is imperative, also, that any treatment helps to improve the quality of life. We have seen several developments since the last edition of this volume and many more are on the horizon. These innovations are important and necessary to provide choice and flexibility in prescribing for the postmenopausal women. Highlighting this need is the fact that continuance (compliance) remains a major problem in this field, with all types of therapy. Although part of this problem is one of education and the establishment of an adequate dialogue between the woman and her provider, more options will also be helpful. We look forward to the next few years as more therapies emerge and new clinical data become available.

REFERENCES

1. Henderson BE, Paganini-Hill A, Ross RK. Decreased mortality in users of estrogen replacement therapy. *Arch Intern Med* 1991;75–78.
2. Ettinger B, Friedman GD, Bush T, Quesenberry CP Jr. Reduced mortality associated with long-term postmenopausal estrogen therapy. *Obstet Gynecol* 1996;87:6–12.
3. Grodstein F, Stampfer MJ, Colditz GA, et al. Postmenopausal hormone therapy and mortality. *N Engl J Med* 1997;336:1769–1775.
4. Sellers TA, Mink PJ, Cerhan JR, et al. The role of hormone replacement therapy in the risk for breast cancer and total mortality in women with a family history of breast cancer. *Ann Intern Med* 1997;127:973–980.
5. Lindsay R, Cosman F, Lobo RA, et al. Addition of alendronate to ongoing hormone replacement therapy in the treatment of osteoporosis: A randomized, controlled clinical trial. *J Clin Endocrinol Metab* 1999 (in press).
6. Lobo RA. Current clinical uses of low-dose estrogen therapy. *Contemp OB/GYN* 1998;43(Suppl):4–26.
7. Hulley S, Grady D, Bush T, et al. Randomized trial of estrogen plus progestin for secondary prevention of coronary heart disease in postmenopausal women. *JAMA* 1998;280:605–613.
8. Writing Group for the PEPI Trial. Effects of estrogen or estrogen/progestin regimens on heart disease risk factors in postmenopausal women. *JAMA* 1996;273:1389–1396.
9. Lobo RA, Fraser IS. Update on progestogen therapy. *J Reprod Med* 1999;44(Suppl 2):139–227.

Subject Index

Note: Page numbers followed by an f refer to figures, those followed by t refer to tables.

relationship to menopausal
status, 344f
oral contraceptives-related, 83, 85
pathogenesis of, 335–338
phytoestrogens and, 455,
579–582, 584
postmenopausal risk of, 58
risk factors for, 79, 84t, 338–349
estrogen deficiency, 332
gender-related, 332
glucose intolerance, 79, 350t
insulin resistance, 391–392,
392t
obesity, 423–425
sexual function effects, 440
β-Carotene, 641–642
Carotid arteries, atherosclerosis of,
hormone replacement
therapy and, 210–211, 210f
Carpal tunnel syndrome, 598
Caruncles, urethral, 4
Catecholamines, estrogen-induced
potentiation of, 345
Catechol estrogens, 97
Catheterization, urinary, 223, 224
Cell death
amyloid-induced, 239, 239f
estrogen-mediated, 237–241
Central nervous system
effect of estrogen on, 189–190
effect of sex steroids on, 231–246
action mechanisms of, 233–237
in neurologic disorders, 231
in neuronal growth and
development, 237–241
structural and functional
effects, 232–233
as sex steroid source, 231–232
Cerebrovascular disease. See Stroke
Cervical cancer, 441, 521
Chemotherapy
as premature ovarian failure
cause, 14
as secondary amenorrhea cause, 17
Childbearing. See also Pregnancy
during perimenopause, 29–30
Chlamydial infections, 224, 225
Cholesterol. See also
Hypercholesterolemia
age-related increase in, 349
antihypertensive drug-related
increase of, 420–421
dietary intake of, 417–418
lowering of, 8
Choline acetyltransferase, 180, 236,
256

Cholinergic system, effect of
estrogen on, 236
Cholinesterase inhibitors, 242
Chromosomal abnormalities
of aborted fetuses, 24
maternal age relationship of, 26
in premature ovarian failure, 14,
16, 16t, 19–20
Chromosomal evaluation, of
hypergonadotropic
amenorrhea patients, 19–20
Chronic illness, 335f
androgen production in, 148,
151–152
Chylomicrons, 369
Cigarette smoking. See Smoking
Cimicifugae racemosa (black
cohosh), 172–173, 455, 652,
653t, 657
Circadian rhythm
of bone turnover markers,
297–298, 298f
of growth hormone secretion,
77
of melatonin secretion, 603–605,
606, 607
Cirrhosis, obesity as risk factor for,
423
Clauberg test, 110–111, 110t
Climacteric, See also Menopause,
natural
definition of, 43, 69
Climacteric medicine, 621–627
Clinical studies/trials
of Alzheimer's disease treatment,
266–267
of hormone replacement therapy,
629–635
cardioprotective effects,
633–634
hyperplasia studies, 632–633,
632f
osteoporosis prevention and
treatment, 631, 633, 633f
regulatory requirements for,
629–631
safety assessment in, 634
vasomotor studies, 631–632,
631f, 632f
of women's health interventions,
637–646
Clomiphene, 612–613, 612f
estrogen receptor affinity of, 96
Clomiphene citrate, 15
Clomiphene citrate challenge test,
65

Clonidine
cognitive function effects of,
180
as hot flash therapy, 167–168,
171–172, 172f
Coagulation
atherosclerosis and, 402
coronary artery heart disease and,
343, 345, 349, 402
estrogen and, 129, 397, 403
hormone replacement therapy
and, 572
thrombosis and, 399–400
Cognitive function
estrogen in, 183, 183f, 185, 236,
255–257, 257f
neuroendocrine basis of,
255–257, 256f, 257f
in estrogen deficiency, 269–270
gender differences in, 270
effect of ginko on, 456–457
glucose in, 239–240
growth hormone in, 597
hormone replacement therapy
effects, 266–267
in Alzheimer's disease, 259
phytoestrogens in, 584, 585
sex hormones in, 231, 235–236
Cold medications, as urinary
incontinence cause, 216
Collagen, 203–212
age-related changes in, 204
of bone, 204–210
as connective tissue component,
203–204
as osteoporosis risk marker, 207
of skin, 208, 209–210
types of, 203
Colon cancer
age-related incidence of, 463,
463f, 474f
dietary factors in, 639
hereditary, 541–542
hormone replacement therapy
and, 102
prevalence of, 513
Colposuspension, 223
Complementary medicine, 453–459
Connective tissue, 203–204
Contraception. See also Oral
contraceptives
during perimenopause, 79
Copper, dietary, 430
Coronary arteries
atherosclerosis of. See
Atherosclerosis